Cardiorespiratory
Physiotherapy

To Barbara, Jennifer and Ammani

Cardiorespiratory Physiotherapy

ADULTS AND PAEDIATRICS

Fifth Edition

EDITED BY

ELEANOR MAIN BSc BA MSc PhD FCSP

Professor of Physiotherapy and Director of UCL Postgraduate Physiotherapy Programme, UCL School of Life and Medical Sciences, University College London, London, UK

LINDA DENEHY BAppSc(Phty) GradDipPhysio(Cardiothoracic Phty) PhD

Professor and Head, Department of Physiotherapy, Melbourne School of Health Sciences, Faculty of Medicine, Dentistry and Health Sciences, University of Melbourne, Melbourne, Australia

FOREWORD BY
BARBARA A WEBBER FCSP DSc(Hons)
Formerly Head of Physiotherapy, Royal Brompton Hospital, London, UK

JENNIFER A PRYOR PhD MBA MSc FNZSP MCSP
Formerly Senior Research Fellow in Physiotherapy, Royal Brompton & Harefield NHS Trust; Honorary Lecturer, University College London and Imperial College London, London, UK

S AMMANI PRASAD GradDipPhys FCSP
Cystic Fibrosis Manager, Respiratory Unit, Great Ormond Street Hospital for Children NHS Trust, London, UK

ELSEVIER   Edinburgh   London   New York   Oxford   Philadelphia   St Louis   Sydney   Toronto   2016

ELSEVIER

ISBN 978-0-7020-4731-2

Notices

Knowledge and best practice in this field are constantly changing. As new research and experience broaden our understanding, changes in research methods, professional practices, or medical treatment may become necessary.

Practitioners and researchers must always rely on their own experience and knowledge in evaluating and using any information, methods, compounds, or experiments described herein. In using such information or methods they should be mindful of their own safety and the safety of others, including parties for whom they have a professional responsibility.

With respect to any drug or pharmaceutical products identified, readers are advised to check the most current information provided (i) on procedures featured or (ii) by the manufacturer of each product to be administered, to verify the recommended dose or formula, the method and duration of administration, and contraindications. It is the responsibility of practitioners, relying on their own experience and knowledge of their patients, to make diagnoses, to determine dosages and the best treatment for each individual patient, and to take all appropriate safety precautions.

To the fullest extent of the law, neither the Publisher nor the authors, contributors, or editors, assume any liability for any injury and/or damage to persons or property as a matter of products liability, negligence or otherwise, or from any use or operation of any methods, products, instructions, or ideas contained in the material herein.

For Elsevier
Senior Content Strategist: Rita Demetriou-Swanwick
Content Development Specialist: Sally Davies, Nicola Lally
Project Manager: Julie Taylor
Designer/Design Direction: Miles Hitchen
Illustration Manager: Brett MacNaughton
Illustrator: TNQ and V. Heim

your source for books,
journals and multimedia
in the health sciences

www.elsevierhealth.com

 Working together to grow libraries in developing countries

www.elsevier.com • www.bookaid.org

The publisher's policy is to use paper manufactured from sustainable forests

Printed in Italy

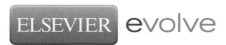

Register today

To access your Evolve Resources visit:

evolve.elsevier.com/Main/cardiorespiratory

Register today and gain access to:

- Bank of 350 images

CONTENTS

Foreword ix

About the Editors... xi

Preface.. xiii

Acknowledgements xv

Contributors... xvii

1 ANATOMY AND PHYSIOLOGY OF THE RESPIRATORY AND CARDIAC SYSTEMS 1
MANDY JONES ■ ALEX HARVEY ■ ELEANOR MAIN

2 CLINICAL ASSESSMENT 47
Adults.. 48
AMANDA THOMAS ■ LYNDAL J MAXWELL

Infant and Child 74
ELEANOR MAIN

The Acutely Ill or Deteriorating Patient 77
SARAH KEILTY

3 THORACIC IMAGING.............................83
Adults.. 84
CONOR D COLLINS ■ SUSAN J COPLEY

Paediatrics 108
JOY L BARBER ■ CHRISTOPHER D GEORGE

4 CARDIAC AND CARDIOVASCULAR DISEASES 125
ANDREW D HIRSCHHORN ■ SEAN F MUNGOVAN ■ DAVID A B RICHARDS

5 RESPIRATORY DISEASES 163
ANNE E HOLLAND ■ JENNIFER A ALISON
WITH A CONTRIBUTION FROM ALEX HARVEY AND MANDY JONES

6 OUTCOME MEASUREMENT IN CARDIORESPIRATORY PHYSIOTHERAPY PRACTICE.................195
SELINA M PARRY ■ LINDA DENEHY
WITH CONTRIBUTIONS FROM CLAIRE E BALDWIN, BRONWEN CONNOLLY, ELIZABETH H SKINNER, SALLY J SINGH, SARAH RAND, CRAIG A WILLIAMS

7 PHYSIOTHERAPY INTERVENTIONS 248
ELEANOR MAIN
WITH CONTRIBUTIONS FROM SUE BERNEY, LINDA DENEHY, MICHELLE CHATWIN, MARK R ELKINS, DANIEL FLUNT, AMANDA J PIPER, ANNEMARIE L LEE, BREDGE MCCARREN, HARRIET SHANNON, SARAH RAND, ROSEMARY MOORE, BARBARA A WEBBER, MARIE T WILLIAMS

8 OPTIMIZING ENGAGEMENT AND ADHERENCE WITH THERAPEUTIC INTERVENTIONS 402
MANDY BRYON

9 ADULT INTENSIVE CARE......................415
JENNIFER PARATZ ■ GEORGE NTOUMENOPOULOS ■ ALICE Y M JONES ■ CLAIRE FITZGERALD

10 PAEDIATRIC INTENSIVE CARE 455
Paediatric Mechanical Support......................... 456
STEWART REID ■ MARK J PETERS

Physiotherapy Management of Ventilated Infants and Children 473
ELEANOR MAIN ■ ALICIA J SPITTLE

11 UPPER ABDOMINAL AND CARDIOTHORACIC SURGERY FOR ADULTS.......................................513
DOA EL-ANSARY ■ JULIE C REEVE ■ LINDA DENEHY
WITH CONTRIBUTIONS FROM SULAKSHANA BALACHANDRAN, MICHELLE MULLIGAN

**12 PHYSICAL ACTIVITY AND
    REHABILITATION** 579

Physical Activity and Physical Fitness
in Health and Disease 580
CHRIS BURTIN ▪ VASILEIOS ANDRIANOPOULOS ▪
MARTIJN A SPRUIT

Pulmonary Rehabilitation 586
KATY MITCHELL ▪ FABIO PITTA ▪ ANNE E
HOLLAND ▪ ANNEMARIE L LEE ▪ LINDA DENEHY

Cardiac Rehabilitation 597
JULIE REDFERN ▪ JENNIFER JONES

**13 CARDIORESPIRATORY MANAGEMENT
    OF SPECIAL POPULATIONS** 639
LINDA DENEHY ▪ ELEANOR MAIN
*WITH CONTRIBUTIONS FROM SARAH SMAILES, ANITA PLAZA,
JENNIFER PARATZ, LEANNE WILLIAMS, CLAIRE BRADLEY,
JACQUELINE L LUKE, JACQUELINE ROSS, BROOKE WADSWORTH,
KATE J HAYES, PRUE E MUNRO, PAUL AURORA, HELENA VAN
ASWEGEN, CRAIG A WILLIAMS, SARAH RAND, CATHERINE L
GRANGER, SUE BERNEY, AMY NORDON-CRAFT, LINDA DENEHY*

APPENDIX – NORMAL VALUES, CONVERSION
    TABLE AND ABBREVIATIONS 757

Index 767

EVOLVE RESOURCES
(evolve.elsevier.com/Main/cardiorespiratory):
▪ bank of 350 images

FOREWORD

As previous editors of this textbook we feel very fortunate to have two remarkably busy professors of physiotherapy who have carried forward the editorship of this book. They are both actively involved in leading cardiorespiratory physiotherapy research and in teaching under- and postgraduate physiotherapists – Eleanor Main in London and Linda Denehy in Melbourne.

The editors have brought together a wealth of knowledge and evidence-based practice in respiratory and cardiac medicine, physiotherapy and assessment techniques. Expert clinicians have contributed important new material in cardiorespiratory care. This international collaboration will facilitate further progress for the benefit of both physiotherapists and patients.

Despite improvements in the design, quality and rigour of allied healthcare research, there remains a paucity of evidence and a lack of clarity for best practice in some clinical areas. In physiotherapy research the 'gold-standard' randomized controlled trial is often fraught with difficulty because of the inability to conceal treatment allocation from participants. This can create uncontrollable bias resulting from patient preference, particularly in studies which involve a long-term burdensome intervention. Therefore clinical expertise currently remains an important element of evidence-based practice.

There have been many changes in healthcare provision and we have come a long way since the early days of 'chest physiotherapy' and 'postural drainage' prescribed by medical practitioners. This edition recognizes physiotherapists as highly skilled independent practitioners who are integral members of the multidisciplinary team. Their considerable depth of knowledge and ability to interpret the many and ever-increasing investigative tests enable them to identify appropriate treatments, exercise or education programmes which meet the needs of individual patients.

This comprehensive new edition will be a great asset to both undergraduate and postgraduate physiotherapists and other health professionals interested in respiratory and cardiac problems. The increase in research and improvements in clinical practice, undertaken during the 23-year lifetime of this textbook, are in part due to imaginative methods, advances in technology and education by enthusiastic clinicians and academics such as our two new editors. We believe that this edition will inspire another generation of physiotherapists to advance our profession.

BARBARA A WEBBER
JENNIFER A PRYOR
S AMMANI PRASAD
2016

ABOUT THE EDITORS

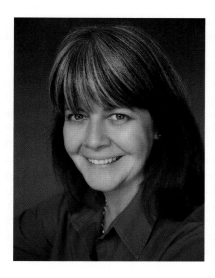

ELEANOR MAIN

Eleanor Main has been involved with clinical physiotherapy, teaching and research at Great Ormond Street Hospital for Children and the Institute of Child Health at University College London for almost 24 years. She qualified as a physiotherapist at the University of the Witwatersrand, South Africa (1988) and worked as a paediatric physiotherapist at both the Red Cross Children's Hospital in Cape Town and then Great Ormond Street Hospital in London. She completed a BA (English and Psychology) at UNISA in South Africa (1991), an MSc in research methods from King's College, London (1995) and a PhD in paediatric respiratory physiology from University College London (2001).

She was appointed as Lecturer in Children's Physiotherapy Research at UCL in 2001, promoted to Senior Lecturer in 2007 and to Professor of Physiotherapy in 2015. She has been programme director for the UCL postgraduate Certificate, Diploma and MSc in physiotherapy at UCL since 2005 and has supervised five PhD students and 79 MSc project dissertations to date. In 2011 she was awarded a Fellowship of the Chartered Society of Physiotherapy in London for her 'significant contribution to education, teaching and learning in the field of cardiorespiratory and paediatric physiotherapy'. Eleanor's primary research interests relate to outcome measurement and clinical efficacy studies in physiotherapy. This research, resulting in more than 80 peer-reviewed publications, and attracting over £2.8 million in project grant funding so far, has resulted in substantive advances in the understanding of assessment and treatment of children who require physiotherapy.

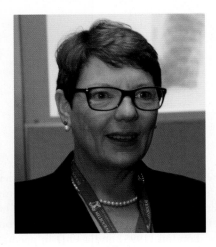

LINDA DENEHY

Linda Denehy is a PhD-qualified physiotherapist who is Head of the Department of Physiotherapy at the University of Melbourne, Australia. Linda graduated in physiotherapy in Melbourne and spent 20 years as a clinician managing respiratory medicine, thoracic surgery and ICU patients both in Melbourne and at the Brompton Hospital in London. She has been a teaching and research academic for nearly 20 years and obtained her PhD in 2002 in the management of patients having upper abdominal surgery. Linda developed curricula in cardiorespiratory physiotherapy both for undergraduate and for postgraduate students and led the implementation of the new three-year doctor of physiotherapy entry to practice course at the University of Melbourne. She has supervised 30 higher degree research students to completion and has extensive research expertise in the area of cardiorespiratory physiotherapy, particularly in patient populations who are acutely unwell, including patients after major surgery and critically ill patients. She has published more than 100 research publications in peer-reviewed journals and 15 invited editorials or book chapters and has been invited to more than 25 national and international meetings as a keynote speaker. These include the European Respiratory Society in 2014 and the American Thoracic Society in 2014 and 2016. She is currently involved in developing international guidelines for ICU mobility and outcome measures in ICU. Linda has been successful in obtaining funding from more than 30 applications of over $6 million Australian dollars for research into physiotherapy and rehabilitation, including as a chief investigator on five nationally competitive grants in rehabilitation after critical illness, lung cancer and breathlessness in COPD. She reviews for national and international competitive granting bodies and for several international scientific journals including *Lung Cancer*, *Intensive Care Medicine*, *Critical Care Medicine* and *Thorax*. Her research has contributed to evidence-led practice, clinical guidelines and improved patient-centred outcomes.

PREFACE

It has been a real privilege to be invited to co-edit the fifth edition of this core international cardiorespiratory textbook. It has always been an important text for undergraduate students around the world but is also an enduringly valuable reference text for both experienced and novice practitioners involved with cardiorespiratory care.

There have been some interesting and important advances in cardiorespiratory physiotherapy in the nine years since the first printing of the fourth edition, and we have tried hard to include as many of the new ideas and new pieces of evidence as possible. Having said that, we acknowledge without reserve that we 'stand on the shoulders of giants', and many of the essential timeless features of the earlier editions remain intact.

Before we started, we asked clinical and university staff and students what they most wanted to see in this new edition and, as a result, we have made changes that we think will enhance the book. Some of the changes involved updating information or reorganizing where it is found in the text, and some are entirely new chapters. For example, the new first chapter is an overview of cardiorespiratory anatomy and physiology essentials, with wonderful new illustrations, which we hope will be an outstanding clinical reference. Similarly, the assessment chapter, now doubled in length, provides an expanded and structured systematic approach to clinical cardiorespiratory assessment. Other new chapters include two dedicated to cardiac and respiratory problems or pathology, an outcome measures chapter,

a chapter on the principles of exercise and physical activity in cardiorespiratory populations and a chapter on cardiorespiratory rehabilitation of special populations, for example, children or those with obesity, cancer, liver disease or burns. Also new is the structure of the Physiotherapy Interventions chapter (previously Techniques), which is now problem-based rather than alphabetical, and which hopefully will facilitate a clearer clinical reasoning pathway for students or novice practitioners.

In general, topics related to the care of children with cardiorespiratory problems have now been incorporated into appropriate sections of text throughout the book, either because there is significant overlap in approach or care between adults and children, or because understanding children with cardiorespiratory problems facilitates better care of individuals through the lifespan: problems in childhood frequently continue into adulthood. An exception is the division between the adult and paediatric ICU chapters, because differences in the reasons for hospital admission and clinical and physiotherapy management of these populations remain substantial.

We are excited about and proud of the new edition and hope that it continues to serve physiotherapy professionals in cardiorespiratory care around the world for many years to come.

EM
LD
London and Melbourne 2016

ACKNOWLEDGEMENTS

We are indebted to all the expert contributors to this edition for the many tireless hours of work they have surrendered to the cause. Many of the contributors were new and, on the whole, represent a truly international perspective on cardiorespiratory physiotherapy. A few chapters involve collaborative writing partnerships between countries, and this enriches the text and assures that physiotherapy practice can ultimately aim to reach consensus about best practice internationally.

We are also so very grateful to Barbara Webber, Jennifer Pryor and Ammani Prasad (the 'giants' referred to in the Preface – although not in actual size!), for their extraordinary dedication over several decades to the clinical and academic advancement of cardiorespiratory physiotherapy care. The continued and growing appeal of this textbook over the past 23 years is testament to their work, the high quality of the book's content and its ongoing usefulness in clinical practice.

It has been a pleasure working with Elsevier on this text and all the members of the editorial and production team: Rita Demetriou-Swanwick, Sally Davies, Julie Taylor, Nicola Lally, Brett MacNaughton, Miles Hitchen, Jo Collett, Kirsty Guest, Tharangini Sakthivel and Rupa Rai. Thank you also to the Elsevier illustrators for doing such a lovely job.

Finally we are eternally thankful to our colleagues, families and friends who helped us choose the front cover design and have tolerated neglect during this production, largely, but not exclusively without complaint! Colin, Daniel, Callum, the Shire folk, Gabrielle, Andrew and Lara, when you read your signed copies carefully, you'll know it was worth it!

EM
LD
2016

CONTRIBUTORS

JENNIFER A ALISON MSc PhD DipPhty
Professor of Respiratory Physiotherapy, University
of Sydney; Clinical Specialist, Pulmonary
Rehabilitation, Royal Prince Alfred Hospital,
Sydney, Australia

VASILEIOS ANDRIANOPOULOS MSc
Clinical Exercise Physiologist, CIRO+ Research and
Development, Horn, Netherlands

PAUL AURORA MRCP PhD
Consultant in Paediatric Respiratory Medicine and
Paediatric Lung Transplantation, Great Ormond
Street Hospital for Children NHS Foundation
Trust; Honorary Senior Lecturer, UCL Institute of
Child Health, London, UK

SULAKSHANA BALACHANDRAN PhD
BPhysio(Hons)
Senior Physiotherapist, Epworth HealthCare,
Melbourne, Australia

CLAIRE E BALDWIN PhD BPhysio(Hons)
Lecturer in Physiotherapy, Acute Care, University of
South Australia, Adelaide; Physiotherapist, Flinders
Medical Centre, South Australia, Australia

JOY L BARBER MBBS MA FRCR
Radiology Registrar, St George's University Hospitals
NHS Foundation Trust, London, UK

SUE BERNEY BPhysio PhD
Associate Professor, Manager of Physiotherapy
Department, Austin Health, Melbourne, Australia

CLAIRE BRADLEY BSc MSc
Senior Physiotherapist, King's College Hospital NHS
Foundation Trust, London, UK

MANDY BRYON PhD
Consultant Clinical Psychologist, Great Ormond
Street Hospital for Children NHS Foundation
Trust, London, UK

CHRIS BURTIN MSc PhD
Clinical Researcher in Respiratory Physiotherapy,
Faculty of Medicine and Life Sciences, Hasselt
University, Diepenbeek, Belgium

MICHELLE CHATWIN PhD BSc(Hons)
PHYSIOTHERAPY
Consultant Physiotherapist in Respiratory Support,
Royal Brompton Hospital, London, UK

CONOR D COLLINS FRCPI FRCR
Consultant Radiologist, St Vincent's University
Hospital, Dublin, Ireland; Associate Clinical
Professor, University College, Dublin, Ireland

BRONWEN CONNOLLY BSc(Hons) MSc PhD
Consultant Clinical Research Physiotherapist, Critical
Care, Guy's & St Thomas' NHS Foundation Trust,
London, UK

SUSAN J COPLEY MB BS MD FRCR FRCP
Consultant Radiologist and Reader in Thoracic
Imaging, Imperial College Healthcare NHS Trust,
London, UK

LINDA DENEHY BAPPSC(PHTY) GRADDIPPHYSIO(CARDIOTHORACIC PHTY) PHD
Professor and Head, Department of Physiotherapy, Melbourne School of Health Sciences, Faculty of Medicine, Dentistry and Health Sciences, University of Melbourne, Melbourne, Australia

DOA EL-ANSARY BAPPSC(PHTY) INTCERT OMT PHD APAM
Senior Lecturer, Lead: Engagement, Faculty of Medicine, Dentistry and Health Sciences, Physiotherapy Department, University of Melbourne, Melbourne, Australia; Research Fellow, HeartWeb, Melbourne; Research Fellow, Clinical Research Institute, Westmead, Sydney, Australia

MARK R ELKINS BA BPHTY MHSC PHD
Clinical Associate Professor, Sydney Medical School, University of Sydney; Research Education Consultant, Centre for Education and Workforce Development, Sydney Local Health District, Sydney, Australia

CLAIRE FITZGERALD BSC(HONS) MSC MCSP
Clinical Specialist Respiratory Physiotherapist, London North West Healthcare NHS Trust; Senior Teaching Fellow, MSc Advanced Physiotherapy, University College London, London, UK

DANIEL FLUNT BAPPSC(PHTY, HONS)
Senior Physiotherapist, Department of Respiratory and Sleep Medicine, Royal Prince Alfred Hospital, Sydney, Australia

CHRISTOPHER D GEORGE FACADMED FRCS FRCR
Consultant Radiologist, Epsom and St Helier University Hospitals NHS Trust; Examiner, Royal College of Radiologists; Honorary Senior Lecturer, St George's University of London, London, UK

CATHERINE L GRANGER BPHYSIO(HONS) PHD
Lecturer, Department of Physiotherapy, Melbourne School of Health Sciences, Faculty of Medicine, Dentistry and Health Sciences, University of Melbourne, Melbourne, Australia; Research Lead, Department of Physiotherapy, Royal Melbourne Hospital, Melbourne, Australia

ALEX HARVEY BSC(HONS) MSC MCSP SRP
Physiotherapy Lecturer, Brunel University, Middlesex; Senior Teaching Fellow, University College London, London, UK

KATE J HAYES BPHYSIO MPHYSIO(CARDIO)
Senior Clinician Physiotherapist, Cardiothoracic Unit, Alfred Health, Melbourne, Australia

ANDREW D HIRSCHHORN BAPPSC(PHTY) PHD
Senior Associate Physiotherapist, Westmead Private Physiotherapy Services; Research Fellow, Clinical Research Institute, Westmead; Honorary Research Fellow, Department of Physiotherapy, University of Melbourne, Melbourne, Australia

ANNE E HOLLAND BAPPSC(PHYSIO) PHD
Professor of Physiotherapy, Alfred Health and La Trobe University, Melbourne, Australia

ALICE Y M JONES PHD FACP
Honorary Professor, Faculty of Health Sciences, University of Sydney, Sydney; Adjunct Professor, School of Allied Health, Griffith University, South East Queensland, Australia

JENNIFER JONES PHD MSC BSC(HONS) PGCERTED
Director of Croí Prevention Programmes, Training and Education, Croi Cardiac Foundation, Galway, Ireland; Adjunct Senior Lecturer, Discipline of Health Promotion, National University of Ireland, Galway, Ireland; Reader in Physiotherapy, Brunel University; Honorary Research and Teaching Associate, Imperial College London, London, UK

MANDY JONES PHD MSC MCSP SRP
Course Director MSc (pre-registration) Physiotherapy, Brunel University, Middlesex, UK

SARAH KEILTY MSc MCSP
Consultant Physiotherapist, Respiratory and Critical
Care, Guy's and St Thomas' NHS Foundation
Trust, London, UK

ANNEMARIE L LEE BPHYSIO MPHYSIO PHD
Senior Lecturer, Physiotherapy, University of
Melbourne, Melbourne, Australia

JACQUELINE L LUKE BSc(PHYSIO, HONS)
Senior Clinician, Victoria Liver Transplant Unit,
Austin Health, Melbourne, Australia

ELEANOR MAIN BSc BA MSc PHD FCSP
Professor of Physiotherapy and Director of UCL
Postgraduate Physiotherapy Programme, UCL
School of Life and Medical Sciences, University
College London, London, UK

LYNDAL J MAXWELL BAPPSc(PHTY)
GRADDIP(CARDIOTHORACIC PHTY)
MAPPSC(CARDIOPULMONARY PHTY) PHD
Senior Lecturer in Physiotherapy, School of
Physiotherapy, Faculty of Health Sciences,
Australian Catholic University, North Sydney,
Australia

BREDGE MCCARREN BSc MAPPSc(PHTY)
GRADDIPPHYSIO(CARDIOTHORACIC) PHD
Senior Lecturer, Western Sydney University, Penrith,
Australia

KATY MITCHELL MSCP PHD
Research Associate, University Hospitals of Leicester
NHS Trust, Leicester, UK

ROSEMARY MOORE BAPPSc(PHTY)
GRADDIPPHYSIO(CARDIOTHORACIC)
MPHYSIO(RESEARCH) PHD
Physiotherapist/Research Fellow, Institute for
Breathing and Sleep, Austin Health, Heidelberg,
Australia

MICHELLE MULLIGAN BMED MBA AFRACMA
FAICD FANZCA
Specialist Anaesthetist, Sydney, Australia

SEAN F MUNGOVAN BAPPSc(PHTY) MPHIL
Principal Physiotherapist, Westmead Private
Physiotherapy Services, Westmead Private
Hospital, Sydney, Australia; Director, The Clinical
Research Institute, Sydney, Australia; Honorary
Fellow, Department of Physiotherapy, Faculty of
Medicine, Dentistry and Health Sciences,
University of Melbourne, Melbourne, Australia

PRUE E MUNRO BPHYSIO GRADDIPHLTHMGT
Senior Clinician Physiotherapist, Alfred Health,
Melbourne, Australia

AMY NORDON-CRAFT PT DSC
Assistant Professor, Physical Therapy Program,
University of Colorado, Anschutz Medical
Campus, Denver, USA

GEORGE NTOUMENOPOULOS BAPPSc BSc
GRADDIPCLINEPID PHD
Associate Professor of Physiotherapy, Australian
Catholic University, North Sydney; Consultant
Physiotherapist, Physiotherapy Department, St
Vincent's Hospital, Darlinghurst, Australia;
Honorary Consultant Physiotherapist,
Physiotherapy Department, Guy's and St Thomas'
NHS Foundation Trust, London, UK

JENNIFER PARATZ MPHTY PHD FACP
Principal Research Fellow, Griffith University; Senior
Research Fellow, School of Medicine, University of
Queensland, Brisbane, Australia

SELINA M PARRY BPHYSIO(HONS) GRAD CERT
UNI TEACHING PHD
Lecturer, Department of Physiotherapy, Melbourne
School of Health Sciences, Faculty of Medicine,
Dentistry and Health Sciences, University of
Melbourne, Melbourne, Australia

MARK J PETERS PHD MBCHB MRCP FRCPCH
Professor of Paediatric Intensive Care, Institute of
Child Health, University College London;
Consultant Paediatric and Neonatal Intensivist,
Great Ormond Street Hospital NHS Foundation
Trust, London, UK

AMANDA J PIPER BAPPSC(PHTY) MED PHD

Senior Physiotherapist, Department of Respiratory and Sleep Medicine, Royal Prince Alfred Hospital; Clinical Senior Lecturer, Faculty of Medicine, University of Sydney, Sydney, Australia

FABIO PITTA PT PHD

Professor of Physiotherapy, Universidade Estadual de Londrina, Londrina, Brazil

ANITA PLAZA BPHTY(HONS)

Consultant Physiotherapist, Professor Stuart Pegg Adult Burn Centre, Royal Brisbane and Women's Hospital, Brisbane, Australia

SARAH RAND BA BSC MSC

Senior Teaching Fellow, University College London Institute of Child Health, London, UK

JULIE REDFERN BAPPSC(PHTY, HONS) BSC PHD

Associate Professor, Sydney Medical School, University of Sydney; Head of Cardiovascular Health Services and Public Health Program, The George Institute for Global Health, Sydney, Australia

JULIE C REEVE GRADDIPPHYS MSC PHD

Senior Lecturer in Physiotherapy, Faculty of Health and Environmental Studies, Auckland University of Technology, Auckland, New Zealand

STEWART REID MA(OXON) MB BCH FRCA

Consultant, Paediatric Anaesthesia and Paediatric Intensive Care Medicine, Royal Belfast Hospital for Sick Children, Belfast, UK

DAVID A B RICHARDS OAM BSC(MED) MBBS MD FRACP FCSANZ FACC

Cardiologist, Westmead Private Hospital, Sydney, Australia; Cardiologist, Liverpool Hospital, Liverpool, UK; Honorary Associate Professor, Department of Medicine, University of Sydney, Australia; Conjoint Associate Professor, Department of Medicine, University of New South Wales, Sydney, Australia

JACQUELINE ROSS BAPPSC(PHTY) GRADDIPNEUROSCIENCE

Senior Clinician Physiotherapist, Victorian Spinal Cord Service, Austin Health, Melbourne, Australia

HARRIET SHANNON BSC(HONS) MA PHD MCSP

Senior Teaching Fellow, University College London, Institute of Child Health, UK

SALLY J SINGH PHD FCSP

Professor of Pulmonary and Cardiac Rehabilitation, Centre of Exercise and Rehabilitation Science, University Hospitals of Leicester NHS Trust and Leicester University, Leicester, UK

ELIZABETH H SKINNER BPHYSIO(HONS) PHD

Director, Physiotherapy Research, Western Health; Senior Intensive Care Unit Physiotherapist, Western Health; Honorary Research Fellow, University of Melbourne; Honorary Research Fellow, Monash University, Melbourne, Australia

SARAH SMAILES BSC(HONS) MCSP PHD

Physiotherapy Consultant, St Andrew's Centre for Plastic Surgery and Burns, Broomfield Hospital; Visiting Clinical Fellow, Postgraduate Medical Institute, Anglia Ruskin University, Chelmsford, UK

ALICIA J SPITTLE PHD MPHYSIO, BPHYSIO

Associate Professor, University of Melbourne; Principal Research Fellow, Murdoch Childrens Research Institute; Senior Physiotherapist, Royal Women's Hospital, Parkville, Australia

MARTIJN A SPRUIT PT PHD

Scientific Advisor, Department of Research and Education, CIRO+ Center of Expertise for Chronic Organ Failure, Horn, Netherlands; Associate Professor in Cardiopulmonary Rehabilitation at REVAL – Rehabilitation Research Center, BIOMED – Biomedical Research Institute, Faculty of Medicine and Life Sciences, Hasselt University, Diepenbeek, Belgium

AMANDA THOMAS MAPPSC(EX & SPSC) BAPPSC(PHYS) MCSP
Clinical Specialist Physiotherapist, Critical Care Outreach, The Royal London Hospital, Barts Health NHS Trust, London, UK; Vice President, International Confederation of Cardiorespiratory Physical Therapy, Clinical Advisor, United Kingdom Confidential Enquiry into Patient Outcome and Death, London, UK

HELENA VAN ASWEGEN BSC(HONS) MSC PHD
Associate Professor, Department of Physiotherapy, Faculty of Health Sciences, University of the Witwatersrand, Johannesburg, South Africa

BROOKE WADSWORTH BSC PHTY(HONS) MPHIL
Advanced Physiotherapist, Princess Alexandra Hospital, Brisbane, Australia

BARBARA A WEBBER FCSP DSC(HONS)
Former Head of Physiotherapy, Royal Brompton Hospital, London, UK

CRAIG A WILLIAMS BED(HONS) MSC PHD FACSM FBASES
Professor of Paediatric Physiology and Health, University of Exeter, Exeter, UK

LEANNE WILLIAMS BSC MCSP
Clinical Specialist Physiotherapist, London, UK

MARIE T WILLIAMS PHD GRADCERT(CARDIORESPIRATORY PHYTY) BAPPSC(PHYTY)
Associate Professor and Associate Head of School: Research, School of Health Sciences, University of South Australia, Adelaide, Australia

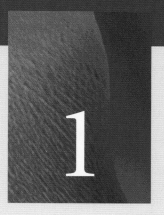

1

ANATOMY AND PHYSIOLOGY OF THE RESPIRATORY AND CARDIAC SYSTEMS

MANDY JONES ■ ALEX HARVEY ■ ELEANOR MAIN

CHAPTER OUTLINE

INTRODUCTION TO RESPIRATION 2

UPPER RESPIRATORY TRACT 3

THE BRONCHIAL TREE 4

THE LUNGS AND PLEURAE 5

SURFACE MARKINGS OF THE LUNGS 8
The Right Lung 8
The Left Lung 8
The Pleura 9

THE THORACIC CAGE 9
Movements of the Ribs 9

MUSCLES OF RESPIRATION 11
Diaphragm 11
Intercostals 13
Accessory Muscles of Inspiration 13
Muscles of Forced Expiration 13

RESPIRATORY MECHANICS 13
Respiratory Pressures 13
Ventilation 14

MUCOCILIARY TRANSPORT SYSTEM 15
Cilia 15
Aqueous (Sol) Layer 15
Viscous (Gel) Layer 15

COLLATERAL VENTILATION 15

AIRWAYS RESISTANCE 16
Airway Innervation 16
Site of Highest Resistance 16
Poiseuille's Law 16
Clinical Relevance of Poiseuille's Law 16
Consequences of Increased Airway Resistance 17
Clinical Signs of Airflow Limitation 17
Problems Associated with Airflow Limitation 17
Reversal of Airflow Limitation 17

RESPIRATORY COMPLIANCE 18
Factors Affecting Lung Compliance 18

Altered Lung Compliance 18
Closing Volume 18
Pulmonary Surfactant 18
Altered Chest Wall Compliance 19
Consequences of Reduced Total Lung Compliance 19

CONTROL OF BREATHING 19
Origin of Breathing 19
Respiratory Control Centres (RCCs) 19
The Medullary Control Centres 19
The Pontine Control Centres 20
Higher Brain Centres 20
Clinical Failure of the Respiratory Control Centres 20
Ondine's Curse 20
Respiratory Control Feedback Mechanism 20
Clinical Failure of the Effectors 20
Respiratory System Sensors 21
Mechanoreceptors 21
Irritant Receptors 21
Juxta-Capillary Receptors 21
Proprioceptors 21
Spinal Cord Reflexes 21
Nasopulminary Reflexes 21
Chemoreceptors 21
Peripheral Chemoreceptors 22
Central Chemoreceptors 22
Stimulation of the Central Chemoreceptors 22
Central Chemoreceptors and COPD 22
Clinical Relevance of Hypercapnic COPD 23
Loss of Hypoxic Drive 23
Increased $\dot{V}/\dot{Q}$ Mismatch 23
Haldane Effect 23

LUNG VOLUMES & VENTILATION 23
Lung Volumes 23
Lung Capacities 23

Factors Affecting Lung Volumes 23
Clinical Relevance of Lung Volumes and
Capacities 24
Measuring Lung Volumes and Capacities 25
Why Assess Spirometry? 25
Ventilation Terminology 25
Anatomical Dead Space 25
Alveolar Dead Space 25
Physiological Dead Space 25
Alveolar Ventilation 25
Clinical Relevance of Alveolar Ventilation 26
Alteration of Alveolar Ventilation 26

GAS EXCHANGE 26
Fick's Law and Gas Exchange 27
Concentration Gradient and Gas Solubility 27
Transit Time of Red Blood Cell (RBC) 28
Thickness of the Alveolar Membrane 28
Surface Area of Alveolar Membrane 28
Ventilation and Perfusion Matching ($\dot{V}/\dot{Q}$) 28
Distribution of Ventilation in Healthy Lung 28
Distribution of Perfusion in Healthy Lung 29
$\dot{V}/\dot{Q}$ Matching in the Self-Ventilating Adult 29
Maintaining $\dot{V}/\dot{Q}$ Matching 30
Hypoxic Pulmonary Vasoconstriction (HPV) 30
Pulmonary Capillary Recruitment 30
Diagnosis of $\dot{V}/\dot{Q}$ Mismatch 30
Bronchiole Response 30
Transport of Oxygen and Carbon Dioxide 31
Oxygen Transport 31
Oxygen and Haemoglobin 31
Haemoglobin's Affinity for Oxygen 32
The Oxygen Dissociation Curve 32
Why Does O_2 Need to Dissociate? 32
Factors Affecting Hb Affinity for O_2 32
Diphosphoglycerate (DPG) 32

Carbon Dioxide Transport 33
Carbon Dioxide and Haemoglobin 33
Carbon Dioxide as Bicarbonate 33
Carriage From Tissue to Lungs 33
THE EFFECT OF GROWTH AND AGEING ON
RESPIRATION 34
Embryonic Period (Weeks 3–5) 34
Pseudoglandular Period (Weeks 6–16) 34
Canalicular Period (Weeks 17–24) 34
Terminal Sac Period (Week 24–Term) 34
RESPIRATORY SYSTEM: ANATOMICAL AND
PHYSIOLOGICAL DIFFERENCES BETWEEN
CHILDREN AND ADULTS 35
Anatomical Differences in the Respiratory System
between Children and Adults 35
Physiological Differences in the Respiratory System
between Children and Adults 38
INTRODUCTION TO CARDIAC ANATOMY AND
PHYSIOLOGY 40
Layers of the Heart Wall 41
Heart Valves 41
Coronary Circulation 41
Cardiac Cycle 41
Heart Sounds 42
Electrical Conductivity of the Heart 42
Electrical Conductivity and Electrocardiogram
(ECG) 43
Autonomic Regulation of Heart Rate 44
Blood Pressure 44
Stroke Volume 44
Total Peripheral Resistance 45
Renal System 45
Auto Regulation of Blood Pressure 45
REFERENCES AND FURTHER READING 46

INTRODUCTION TO RESPIRATION

The supply of oxygen to body tissues is essential to life. As well as nutrients, cells require oxygen in order to release energy as part of tissue metabolism. As the cells use oxygen, they produce carbon dioxide, which is a metabolic waste product and is toxic if allowed to accumulate.

The primary function of the respiratory system is to supply the body with oxygen taken from atmospheric air, and to dispose of carbon dioxide. This complex process is known as respiration and is com-

prised of four stages: ventilation, external respiration, gas transport and internal respiration (Marieb and Hoehn 2013).

The respiratory system is responsible for two of these stages: ventilation and external respiration. Ventilation is the movement of air in and out of the lungs, and external respiration (pulmonary gas exchange) is the diffusion of oxygen from the lungs to the blood, and carbon dioxide from the blood to the lungs. To achieve this, air is drawn by conductive flow into the alveoli and presented to the gas-exchanging surface where the process of exchange occurs by diffusion. The carriage of air through the airways depends on the size and patency of the tubes as well as on the compliance of the lung and power of the respiratory muscles.

Gas transport is the transportation of oxygen and carbon dioxide to/from the lungs in the blood, and this is dependent on the cardiovascular system. The final stage is internal respiration, and this is the movement of oxygen from the blood to the cells and carbon dioxide from the cells to the blood.

In health, the human cardiorespiratory system has a substantial reserve capacity to cope with the demands of exercise or illness. Breathlessness or fatigue is not normally a feature of resting activity. In patients with heart or lung disease, the erosion of physiological reserve eventually imposes limitations upon the activities of daily life.

UPPER RESPIRATORY TRACT

The 'upper respiratory tract' (Fig. 1-1) is the term for the extra-thoracic components of the respiratory system. It broadly consists of the nose, the pharynx, the larynx and the trachea.

The nose has a number of important functions, including warming, humidifying (moistening) and filtering the air. As a result, respiratory physiotherapists encourage patients who are not breathless to inhale through the nose rather than the mouth. The nose also provides a resonance chamber for speech and contains olfactory (smell) receptors.

Respiratory mucosa lines the nasal cavity. This is ciliated epithelium that contains goblet cells. Goblet cells secrete mucus and this serves to trap inhaled particles. Cilia are microscopic hair-like projections that move rhythmically to sweep the mucus and any trapped particles towards the pharynx.

Just proximal to the nostrils is the nasal vestibule. This contains short, thick hairs called 'nasal vibrissae'. These hairs filter large particles, e.g. dust, from the inspired air. Proximal to the nasal vestibule is the nasal cavity and this contains three mucosa-covered projections that protrude medially from the lateral walls. These projections are the superior, middle and inferior nasal conchae (otherwise known as 'nasal turbinates'). The nasal conchae increase the mucosal surface area and increase turbulence through the nasal cavity,

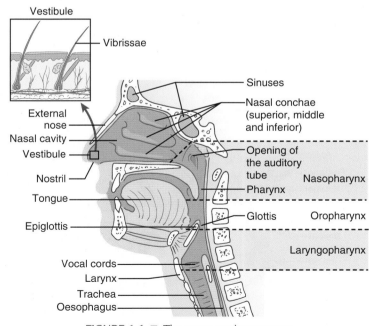

FIGURE 1-1 ■ The upper respiratory tract.

which serves to slow airflow. This allows time for the air to be warmed, filtered and humidified. The nasal mucosa is also supplied with a large number of sensory nerve endings. When irritated by inhaled particles, these sensory nerve endings will trigger a sneeze reflex.

The pharynx is commonly termed the 'throat' and is divided (from superior to inferior) into the nasopharynx, the oropharynx and the laryngopharynx. Only air moves through the nasopharynx, whereas both food and air pass through the oropharynx and laryngopharynx. The laryngopharynx is the point of bifurcation which leads to the larynx anteriorly and the oesophagus posteriorly.

The lungs are protected from food substances by the flap-like epiglottis that closes over the larynx during swallowing. The larynx contains the vocal cords and so is essential for voice production. Vocal cord (glottic) function is also essential for an effective cough mechanism.

The trachea, or windpipe, descends from the larynx into the thorax and is situated anterior to the oesophagus. It contains numerous cartilaginous C-shaped rings that support the anterior and lateral aspects of the trachea. These rings help to prevent tracheal collapse during the pressure changes associated with breathing. They are open posteriorly to allow the oesophagus to expand anteriorly as food is swallowed.

THE BRONCHIAL TREE

The branching pattern of airways is often referred to as the 'bronchial tree'. The airways divide and subdivide again. In all, there are approximately 23 generations (divisions) of airway in the human lung (Fig. 1-2).

The trachea bifurcates into the right and left main bronchi, which then supply their respective lungs. This point of bifurcation is termed the 'carina'. The right main bronchus branches off from the trachea at an angle of 20–30 degrees, while the left main bronchus branches off at an angle of 45–55 degrees. As the right main bronchus is more vertical than the left, aspirated food and drink are more likely to end up in the right lung if the person is in an upright position.

Each main bronchus then divides into lobar bronchi: three on the right and two on the left. Each lobar bronchus supplies the lobe of a lung and subdivides into segmental bronchi and then bronchi and bronchioles of ever decreasing size. Finally, terminal bronchioles divide into respiratory bronchioles. Respiratory bronchioles are hybrid structures and are part bronchiole, part alveoli. The respiratory bronchioles then give rise to the 300 million alveoli that are present in a healthy adult.

The structure of the airways changes towards the lung peripheries. The bronchioles lack cartilage but

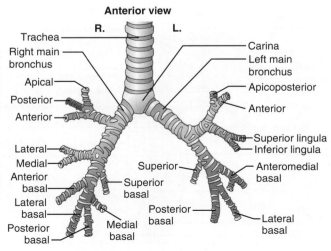

FIGURE 1-2 ■ The bronchial tree.

still have a relative abundance of smooth muscle. Hence the cartilage that maintains airway patency is absent, and constriction of the smooth muscle significantly reduces airway calibre in these small airways.

The calibre of the airways reduces through their generations and the major resistance to gas flow is normally in the upper airway. The larger airways are supported by cartilage, while the smaller airways are held patent by the radial traction of the surrounding lung so that their calibre increases with the volume of the lung. The diameter of these airways is also controlled by neural tone, which is predominantly parasympathetic.

The conducting zone of the lung includes the upper respiratory tract and the airway divisions up to and including the terminal bronchioles. The function of the conducting zone is to transport gas in and out of the lungs. The respiratory zone is where gas exchange takes place and includes the respiratory bronchioles and alveoli (Fig. 1-3).

Disruption of airway function can occur through obstruction to a large airway by, for example, a tracheal tumour. It may also occur because of more widespread disease in asthma, when the calibre of large numbers of smaller airways is affected by episodic alteration of smooth muscle contraction, mucosal oedema and intraluminal secretions. In chronic bronchitis, obstruction occurs by mucosal thickening and mucus secretion, but in emphysema the mechanism is different. Though seldom occurring in isolation from other forms of airway obstruction, the result of parenchymal emphysema is to weaken the elastic structure which maintains radial traction on the airways and allows them to close too early in expiration.

THE LUNGS AND PLEURAE

The cone-shaped lungs are located in the thoracic cage and are positioned vertically around the heart. The two lungs contain millions of alveoli within a fibro-elastic matrix. They do not have a very rigid structure and are held in contact with the rib cage by negative pressure between the pleural surfaces. The resting volume of the lung is determined by the outward spring of the rib cage and the inward elastic recoil of the lung matrix. Expansion and contraction of the lung involves the controlled stretching or relaxation of the lung by the respiratory muscles. The position of lung resting volume can be influenced if the lung is stiffer than usual (as in interstitial disease) or if it is more compliant (as when damaged by emphysema).

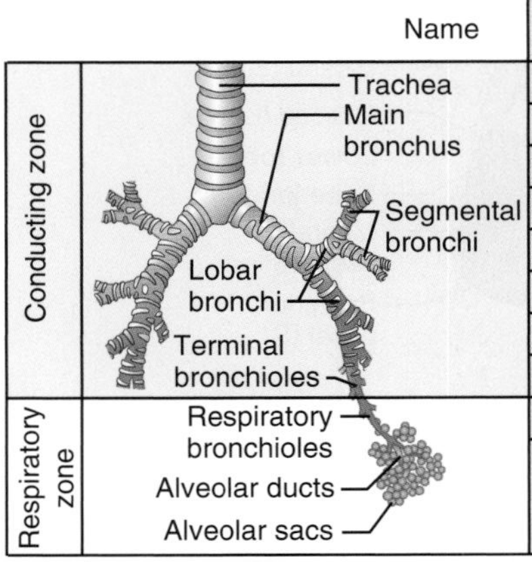

	Name	Division	Diameter (mm)	How many?	Cross-sectional area (cm²)	Epithelium	Goblet cells	Ciliated cells	Glands	Hyaline cartilage	Smooth muscle	Elastic fibers
Conducting zone	Trachea	0	15-22	1	2.5							
	Main bronchus	1		2								
		2		4								
	Segmental bronchi	3										
		4	1-10									
	Lobar bronchi	5										
		6-11		10 000								
	Terminal bronchioles	12-15	0.5-1	20 000	100							
Respiratory zone	Respiratory bronchioles	16-23		80 000 000	5000							
	Alveolar ducts Alveolar sacs	24	0.3	300 000 000-600 000 000	>1 000 000							

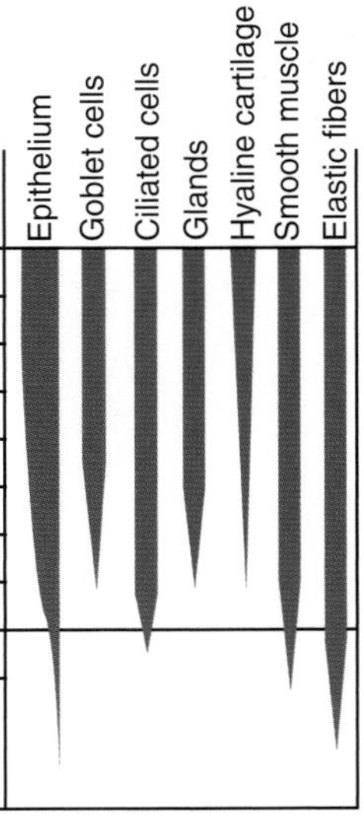

FIGURE 1-3 ■ Conducting and respiratory zones.

The lungs are divided into **lobes** (Fig. 1-4). The right lung is larger and has three lobes: upper, middle and lower. The left lung has just two lobes: upper and lower. The left lung is smaller because the heart is situated to the left of midline and therefore some of the space of the left lung is taken up by the heart (cardiac notch).

The lobes of the lungs are separated by **fissures**. The right lung is divided by the horizontal fissure (separates the upper and middle lobe) and the oblique fissure (separates the lower lobe from the upper and middle lobe). The left lung only has two lobes and therefore just has an oblique fissure (between the upper and lower lobe).

Each lobe of lung is divided into **bronchopulmonary segments**. There are 10 bronchopulmonary segments in the right lung, and eight in the left lung. A bronchopulmonary segment is a functionally and

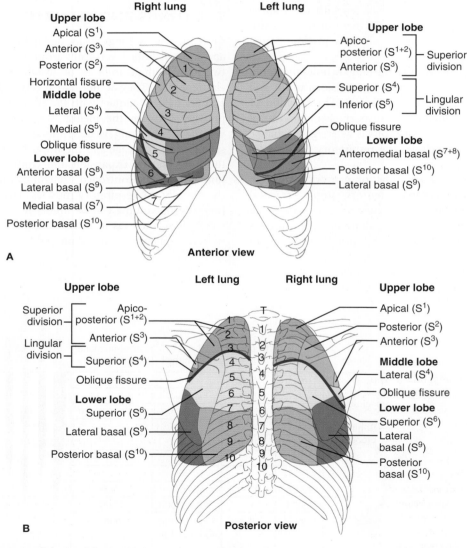

FIGURE 1-4 ■ Lung lobes and fissures. **(A)** Anterior view. (Superior basal segments not visible in anterior view.) **(B)** Posterior view.

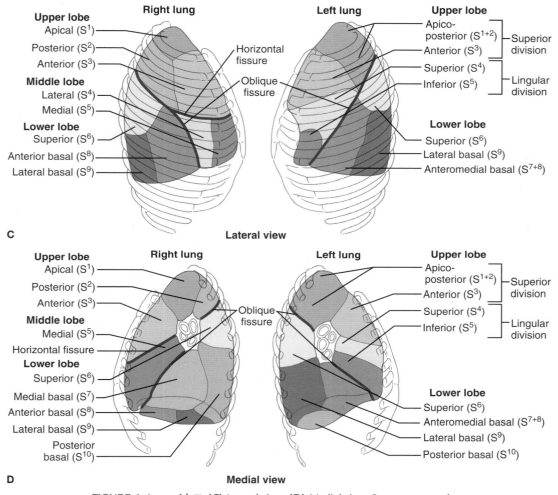

FIGURE 1-4, cont'd ■ **(C)** Lateral view. **(D)** Medial view. S, segment number.

anatomically independent unit of lung which has its own segmental bronchus, artery and vein. Segments are separated from one another by connective tissue septa. This means that if an isolated tumour or disease is present in one bronchopulmonary segment, it can be surgically removed (segmentectomy), causing minimal disruption to adjacent segments of lung. Respiratory physiotherapists should be familiar with the names of the bronchopulmonary segments and the anatomical position of each segmental bronchus. This anatomical knowledge is required in order to perform gravity-assisted positioning (GAP), which is used to promote drainage of excess bronchopulmonary

secretions. Specific segmental bronchi are positioned perpendicular to gravity in order to drain the affected bronchopulmonary segment (see Fig. 1-2).

The lungs are covered with a thin double-layered serous sac called the **'pleural membrane'**. The outer layer of the membrane is the **parietal pleura** and the inner layer is the **visceral pleura** (Fig. 1-5). The parietal pleura lines the inner surface of the thoracic wall and the superior surface of the diaphragm. The visceral pleura covers the outer surface of the lungs and also lines the fissures. The potential space between the parietal and visceral pleurae is the pleural cavity, and this contains a small amount of pleural fluid which is

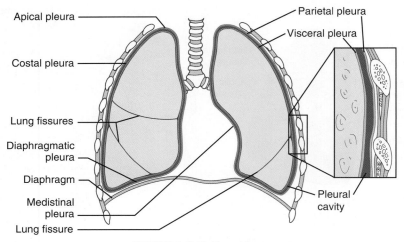

Apical pleura

Costal pleura

Lung fissures

Diaphragmatic pleura

Diaphragm

Medistinal pleura

Lung fissure

Parietal pleura

Visceral pleura

Pleural cavity

FIGURE 1-5 ■ Pleural layers.

secreted by the pleurae. **Pleural fluid** acts as a lubricant, allowing the two pleural layers to glide over each other during inspiration and expiration. The pleural fluid also acts to increase surface tension and therefore 'locks' the two pleural layers together. This can be compared to a wet plastic bag – when wet, the two sides of the plastic bag are difficult to separate. This means that the lungs will cling to the chest wall throughout inspiration and expiration. The visceral pleura is innervated by the autonomic nervous system (ANS) and so is not sensitive to pain. However, the parietal pleura is highly sensitive to pain due to innervation from the phrenic and intercostal nerves. As a result, pleural disease such as pleuritis (inflammation of the pleurae) can cause a severe, sharp stabbing pain.

SURFACE MARKINGS OF THE LUNGS

Respiratory physiotherapists should be able to surface mark the outline of the lungs, pleurae and fissures. In particular, surface marking the lungs may be the best way to visually learn that the lower lobes are positioned posteriorly. This knowledge may enable more accurate auscultation of the lungs.

The Right Lung

Anteriorly, the apex of the right lung is situated 2–3 cm superior to the medial third of the clavicle. The medial border of the lung descends through the sternoclavicular joint and close to midline to the level of the sixth rib. The inferior border goes from the sixth rib in the mid-clavicular line, to the eighth rib in the mid-axillary line, to the 10th rib posteriorly. Posteriorly, the apex of the lung is level with T1 and the medial border of the lung is approximately 2 cm from midline and descends from the level of T1 to T10. The **horizontal fissure** (separating the upper lobe from the middle lobe) follows the line of the fourth rib anteriorly and ends where it meets the oblique fissure in the mid-axillary line. The **oblique fissure** (separating the lower lobe from the upper and middle lobes) runs posteriorly from T3 and descends diagonally. It roughly follows the line of the medial border of the scapula with the arm abducted to 90 degrees. It forms a junction with the end of the horizontal fissure in the mid-axillary line and ends anteriorly at the level of the sixth rib in the mid-clavicular line.

The Left Lung

The outline of the left lung is the same as the right lung, except that there is a cardiac notch on the left. Anteriorly, the medial border of the left lung deviates laterally by 3–4 cm at the level of the fourth rib. It then descends vertically to the level of the sixth rib in the mid-clavicular line. The remaining outline of the left lung is exactly the same as the right. There is no horizontal fissure on the left lung, only an oblique.

The Pleura

The pleura follows the outline of the lung except that the inferior border of the pleura is situated two ribs below the inferior border of the lung. Anteriorly, the inferior border of the pleura runs from the level of the eighth rib in the mid-clavicular line, to the 10th rib in the mid-axillary line and the 12th rib posteriorly. This two-rib difference between the outline of the lung and the pleura is not representative of the pleural space; it simply represents full inspiration.

THE THORACIC CAGE

To maintain their shape, the lungs depend on the support of the rib cage, negative pressure between the pleural surfaces and the patency of the airways and alveoli. The expansion of the rib cage by the respiratory muscles is responsible for the tidal flow of gas into and out of the lungs. Over the past few years there has been increasing awareness of the importance of dysfunction of the respiratory muscles and the bony rib cage in contributing to respiratory failure. Such conditions include myopathies and polio, as well as skeletal malformations such as scoliosis, which decrease rib cage compliance and reduce the effectiveness of the musculature.

The respiratory muscles include the diaphragm as the major muscle of inspiration and the intercostal muscles and scalenes. The latter, together with the sternocleidomastoids, are known as the 'accessory muscles', of respiration because they assist, but do not play a primary role, in breathing. Weakness of the respiratory muscles will eventually lead to ventilatory failure, which may first become apparent during the night as an exaggeration of normal nocturnal hypoventilation (Shneerson 1988).

The thoracic cage is cone shaped with its wider end inferiorly. It is made up of the thoracic vertebrae dorsally, the ribs laterally and the sternum and costal cartilages anteriorly.

One function of the thoracic cage is to protect the heart, lungs and great vessels. It also provides support for the pectoral girdle and upper limbs, and provides a point of attachment for neck, trunk and upper limb muscles. Finally, the rib cage allows the movement necessary for breathing.

There are 12 pairs of ribs and they slope inferiorly as they curve anteriorly. All the ribs attach posteriorly to the thoracic vertebrae. Ribs are termed 'true', 'false' or 'floating' according to their anterior attachment. The **true ribs** (1–7) attach directly to the sternum by individual costal cartilages. The **false ribs** (8–10) attach to the sternum indirectly, each joining the costal cartilage immediately above it. The **floating ribs** (11–12) have no anterior attachment (Fig. 1-6).

The **head** of the rib attaches to the thoracic vertebrae posteriorly. It is wedge shaped and has two articular facets which articulate with the upper border of the body of its own vertebra and the lower border of the body of the vertebra above. So the head of rib 8 will articulate with the upper part of the body of T8 and the lower part of the body of T7. These articulations are the **costovertebral joints**. The **neck** of the rib is the narrowed area just lateral to the head. The **tubercle** is lateral to the neck and has a small oval articular facet. This facet articulates with the transverse process of the same-numbered thoracic vertebra (rib 8 with transverse process of T8). This articulation is the **costotransverse joint**. The **shaft** makes up the majority of the rib. The **rib angle** is approximately 3 cm lateral to the tubercle and is where the shaft angles sharply forwards (see Fig. 1-6).

Movements of the Ribs

The dimensions of the thorax must change in order for respiration to occur. The vertical, transverse and antero-posterior (AP) diameters of the thorax increase during inspiration and decrease during expiration. This rib movement is brought about by the inspiratory muscles (external intercostals and diaphragm).

Rib 1 is capable of very little movement because it is so short and firmly attached to the manubrium by the first costal cartilage. The anterior ends of ribs 2–5 are raised during inspiration, along with the body of the sternum. This increases the AP diameter of the thorax and is known as **'pump handle movement'**.

Inspiration causes the anterior ends of ribs 8–10 to move in an upwards and outwards direction. This increases the transverse diameter of the thorax. The resultant upward and outward movement of the shaft of the ribs has been compared to lifting the handle from the side of a bucket and is termed **'bucket handle movement'** (Palastanga & Soames, 2012) (Fig. 1-7).

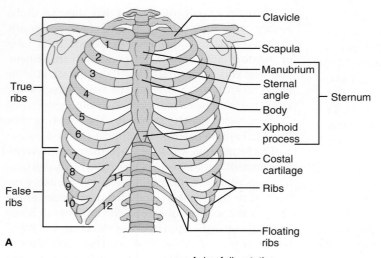

A

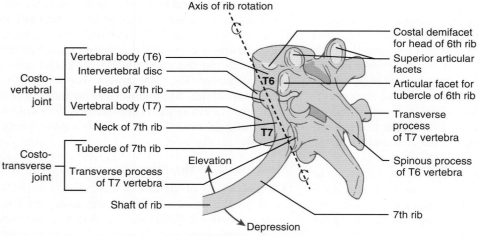

B   **Left posterolateral view**

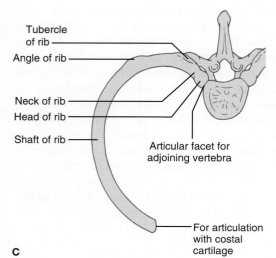

C

FIGURE 1-6 ■ **(A)** Rib cage. **(B)** and **(C)** Costovertebral and costotransverse joints. The head of rib articulates with two adjacent vertebral bodies and the disc between them, and the tubercle of rib articulates with the transverse process of a vertebra. The rib moves up and down around an axis that traverses the head and neck of rib.

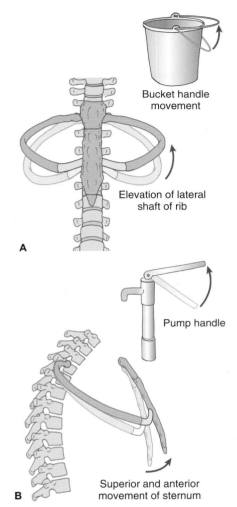

FIGURE 1-7 ■ Bucket and pump handle rib movement is caused by the anterior ends of ribs 8-10 moving upwards and outwards during inspiration. **(A)** Increasing transverse dimension. **(B)** Increasing antero-posterior (AP) dimension.

Ribs 6 and 7 are capable of both pump and bucket handle movement. Ribs 11–12 do not contribute to increasing the diameter of the thorax as they have no anterior attachment.

MUSCLES OF RESPIRATION

Diaphragm

The diaphragm is the main muscle of inspiration. It is a musculotendinous sheet which separates the thorax from the abdomen. It is a large, dome-shaped muscle and is lower posteriorly than anteriorly. The right hemidiaphragm sits 1–2 cm higher than the left hemidiaphragm due to the presence of the liver on the right. The superior surface of the diaphragm is covered with the parietal pleura. The pericardium which encloses the heart is attached to the central tendon of the diaphragm. The diaphragm has three openings to allow structures to pass between the thorax and the abdomen (**oesophageal opening**, **aortic opening** and **vena caval opening**) (Palastanga & Soames, 2012) (Fig. 1-8).

The diaphragm is innervated by the phrenic nerve (remember that 'C3, 4, 5 keep the diaphragm alive!').

The diaphragm has three sets of fibres: **sternal**, **costal** and **lumbar**. These fibres are all named according to their origin. All fibres converge into a central trefoil shaped (clover leaf) tendon. The **sternal** fibres of the diaphragm arise from the posterior surface of the xiphoid process. The fibres run upwards and medially to insert into the anterior border of the central tendon. The **costal** fibres make up the majority of muscle fibres of the diaphragm and arise from the inner surface of the lower six ribs and their costal cartilages. The fibres run upwards and medially to insert into the anterolateral part of the central tendon. The **lumbar** fibres arise in part from two crura. The right crus is larger and originates from the anterolateral aspects of the bodies and intervertebral discs of L1–L3. The left crus arises from the bodies and discs of L1 and L2. The two sets of crural fibres are united opposite the disc between T12 and L1 to form an arch which is the aortic opening (median arcuate ligament). Both sets of crural fibres insert into the central tendon. The remainder of the lumbar fibres arise from the medial and lateral arcuate ligaments which are lateral to the crura (see Fig. 1-8).

When contracting, the diaphragm descends and increases the vertical diameter of the thorax. During quiet breathing, the diaphragm descends just 1–2 cm (from the level of T8 to T9). However, in deep inspiration it can descend as much as 10 cm. Further descent of the diaphragm is prevented by compression of the abdominal organs. In this situation the central tendon now becomes the fixed point (reversed origin and insertion) and further contraction of the diaphragm causes upward and outward movement of the ribs and forwards movement of the sternum.

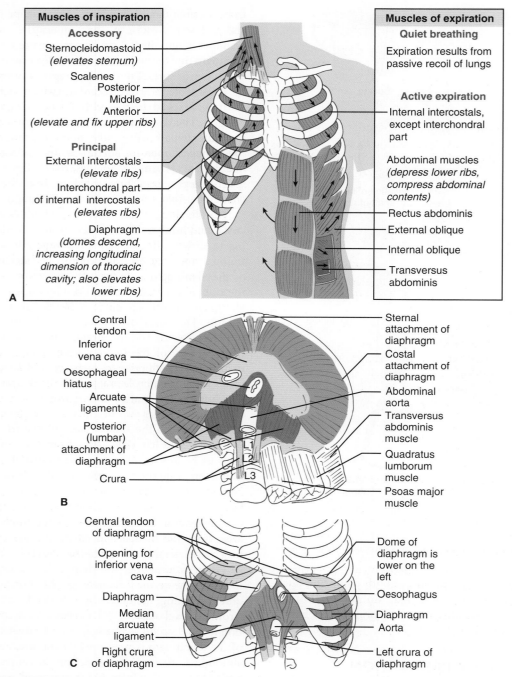

FIGURE 1-8 ■ Muscles of respiration. **(A)** Intercostal and accessory muscles. **(B)** and **(C)** The diaphragm.

Intercostals

The intercostal muscles pass between adjacent ribs. They span the intercostal space and there are 11 pairs between ribs 1 to 12. There are three layers of intercostals: external, internal and innermost (see Fig. 1-8). The intercostals are innervated by the intercostal nerves (T1–11).

The **external intercostals** are muscles of inspiration and form the outermost intercostal layer. They pass from the inferior border of the rib above to the superior border of the rib below. The fibres run diagonally in a downwards and forwards direction. Contraction of the external intercostals results in the rib below being pulled up towards the rib above, causing elevation of the rib cage (pump and bucket handle movement).

The interosseous part of the **internal intercostals** are muscles of expiration (the interchondral part of the internal intercostals are inspiratory muscles), and they form the middle intercostal layer. They pass from the inferior border of the rib above to the superior border of the rib below. The fibres run diagonally in a downwards and backwards direction, which is the opposite direction to the external intercostals. Contraction of the internal intercostals assists with forced expiration by drawing the ribs together and depressing the rib cage.

The **innermost intercostals** form the deepest intercostal layer and run in the same direction as the internal intercostals. Their function is probably to stabilize the chest wall, preventing the intercostal spaces from 'being sucked in' on inspiration and from 'bulging out' during expiration.

Accessory Muscles of Inspiration

There are a number of muscles that can assist with deep inspiration or during episodes of respiratory distress. These include the scalenes and sternocleidomastoid. The **scalenes** (anterior, middle and posterior) attach to ribs 1 and 2 and can therefore elevate the rib cage. **Sternocleidomastoid** can also bring about elevation of the rib cage due to the action of the sternal head which attaches to the manubrium, and the clavicular head which attaches to the clavicle. Other possible accessory muscles of inspiration include pectoralis minor and pectoralis major. Use of the accessory muscles of inspiration can be a sign of respiratory distress.

Muscles of Forced Expiration

Expiration is normally a passive process brought about by relaxation of the diaphragm and external intercostals which then allows elastic recoil of the lungs. Forced expiration such as when coughing or sneezing is brought about by the internal intercostals and the abdominal muscles. Contraction of the abdominal muscles causes the abdominal contents to push up against the diaphragm, which then reduces the vertical diameter of the thorax. During strenuous physical activity, expiration becomes forced or active in order to increase respiratory rate to the level required to meet metabolic demand. In the absence of strenuous activity, use of the abdominal muscles during expiration can be another sign of respiratory distress.

RESPIRATORY MECHANICS

Respiratory Pressures

Before describing the different respiratory pressures, it is important to understand the term '**atmospheric pressure**'. Atmospheric pressure is the pressure exerted by the gases in the air. It is the sum of all the partial pressures of gases in the air (including nitrogen, oxygen and carbon dioxide) and is 760 mmHg at sea level. The partial pressure of nitrogen in inspired air is 593 mmHg (78% of 760 mmHg), while the partial pressure of oxygen is 159 mmHg (21% of 760 mmHg). Respiratory pressures are always described in relation to atmospheric pressure. Hence a negative respiratory pressure is less than atmospheric pressure, a positive respiratory pressure is greater than atmospheric pressure and a respiratory pressure of zero is equal to atmospheric pressure.

Intrapulmonary pressure (P_{pul}) or intra-alveolar pressure is the pressure within the alveoli. It falls with inspiration and rises with expiration. It is important to note that intrapulmonary pressure always eventually equalizes with atmospheric pressure; i.e. returns to 0 mmHg at the end of inspiration and at the end of expiration (Fig. 1-9).

Intrapleural pressure (P_{ip}) is the pressure within the pleural cavity and also decreases on inspiration and increases on expiration. However, intrapleural

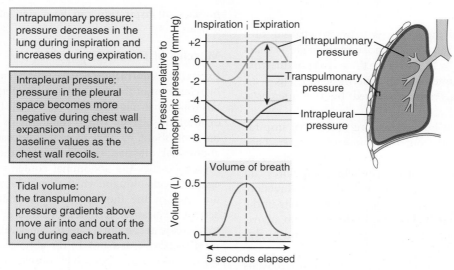

Intrapulmonary pressure: pressure decreases in the lung during inspiration and increases during expiration.

Intrapleural pressure: pressure in the pleural space becomes more negative during chest wall expansion and returns to baseline values as the chest wall recoils.

Tidal volume: the transpulmonary pressure gradients above move air into and out of the lung during each breath.

FIGURE 1-9 ■ Volume and pressure changes during inspiration and expiration.

pressure is always negative in relation to intrapulmonary pressure. This negative intrapleural pressure is created by two opposing forces: the tendency of the chest wall to expand outwards versus the tendency of the lungs to recoil inwards. The pleural fluid keeps the pleurae locked together.

Transpulmonary pressure ($P_{pul} - P_{ip}$) is the difference between the intrapulmonary and intrapleural pressures. The greater the transpulmonary pressure, the greater the size of the lungs (transpulmonary pressure is greatest at the end of inspiration).

A pneumothorax is the presence of air in the pleural space due to an abnormal communication between either the lung and the pleural space, or the atmosphere and the pleural space. This air in the pleural space will result in the loss of negative intrapleural pressure and the transpulmonary pressure will then become zero. As a result, the underlying lung will collapse. An intercostal drain restores the negative intrapleural pressure and the lung should then reinflate.

Ventilation

Ventilation is a mechanical process that depends on volume changes within the thorax. Volume changes leads to pressure changes, which then result in gas flow.

Gas flows into the lungs during inspiration and out of the lungs during expiration.

How do volume changes lead to pressure changes? If the volume of a container increases, then the gas molecules inside it are spaced further apart and therefore exert less pressure. If the volume of a container decreases then the gas will exert more pressure.

How do pressure changes result in gas flow? Gases always flow down pressure gradients, meaning they flow from high pressure to low pressure until the pressure has been equalized.

During quiet inspiration, the inspiratory muscles contract to increase thoracic cage diameter and lung volume. This increased volume causes a fall in intrapulmonary pressure and gas flows into the lungs down the pressure gradient. Air flow ceases when intrapulmonary pressure becomes equal to atmospheric pressure.

During quiet expiration, the inspiratory muscles relax and the lungs recoil passively. This reduces thoracic cage diameter and lung volume, which then leads to an increased intrapulmonary pressure. Gas now flows down the pressure gradient, from the lungs towards the mouth. Once again, gas flow will cease once intrapulmonary pressure reaches zero (equal to atmospheric pressure).

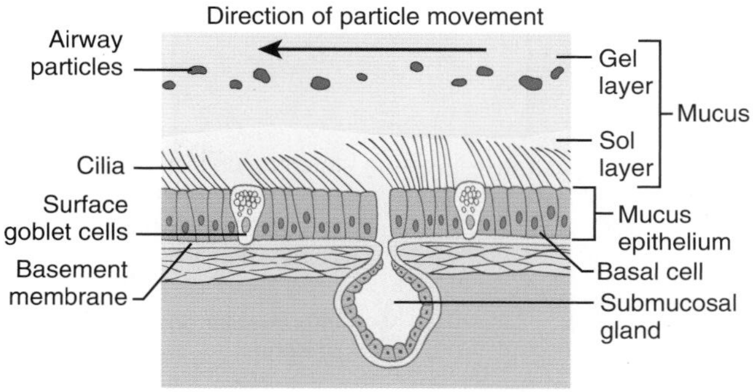

FIGURE 1-10 ■ Mucociliary transport (MCT) system.

MUCOCILIARY TRANSPORT SYSTEM

Ciliated epithelium is present in the upper respiratory tract and lines the airways down to the terminal bronchioles. Cilia are microscopic hair-like processes that are capable of rhythmic motion and are one of the three components of the mucociliary transport (MCT) system (Fig. 1-10). The MCT system sweeps mucus containing foreign particles towards the laryngopharynx, where the mucus is either swallowed or expectorated by coughing. It is therefore an important defence mechanism of the lung, reducing the incidence of respiratory infection.

The three components of the MCT system are

- Cilia
- Aqueous (sol) layer
- Viscous (gel) layer.

Cilia

The tips of the cilia hook into the gel layer to sweep it towards the laryngopharynx. The cilia situated below the larynx beat in an upwards direction, while the cilia above the larynx beat in a downwards direction. Cilia beat in a co-ordinated fashion at a frequency of approximately 20 cycles per second, which can propel mucus at a rate of 2 cm/min. Cilia demonstrate bi-directional movement. The power (effective) stroke moves mucus towards the mouth, while the recovery stroke enables the cilia to sweeps backwards and to the side (see Fig. 1-10).

Ciliary beat frequency can be reduced by a number of factors, including smoking, general anaesthesia and the inhalation of cold air.

The ultrastructure of cilia is extremely complex. Primary ciliary dyskinesia is an inherited condition where the cilia are structurally abnormal. As a result, cilia move in an uncontrolled way (dyskinesia) and the MCT system becomes ineffective.

Aqueous (Sol) Layer

For efficient ciliary motion, the cilia need to be bathed in the serous fluid that makes up the aqueous (sol) layer. It can also be referred to as 'periciliary fluid'. This thin, watery fluid extends most of the way up the shaft of the cilia. The fluid offers very little resistance to ciliary motion and actually seems to facilitate it. Ciliary movement will be impaired by both increased levels of periciliary fluid (e.g. pulmonary oedema), or by reduced levels (e.g. in dehydration).

Viscous (Gel) Layer

For most of the bronchial tree, goblet cells accompany the ciliated epithelium. Goblet cells secrete mucus, and mucus secretion volume is 10–100 mL per day in healthy adults. This viscous mucus forms the gel layer of the MCT system. It acts like flypaper, and foreign particles, cellular debris and microbes become trapped in it. Ciliary movement will become impaired in hypersecretory conditions such as cystic fibrosis and bronchiectasis due to the increased volume of the mucus layer or a depleted sol layer (cystic fibrosis).

COLLATERAL VENTILATION

Collateral channels of ventilation (Fig. 1-11) provide an alternative route for gas flow when peripheral airways are obstructed. These collateral channels may

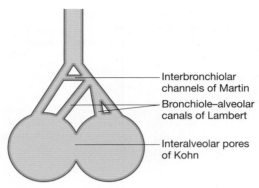

Interbronchiolar channels of Martin

Bronchiole–alveolar canals of Lambert

Interalveolar pores of Kohn

FIGURE 1-11 ■ Collateral ventilation pathways.

be 1–2 μm interalveolar (pores of Kohn), 25–30 μm bronchiole-alveolar (canals of Lambert) and 80–150 μm interbronchial (channels of Martin).

The average adult alveolus has somewhere between 5 and 20 pores of Kohn. These are not present in infants under the age of 1 year. Due to this lack of 'alveolar escape route', infants are at particular risk of barotrauma when positive pressure ventilation is applied to their lungs.

The resistance to airflow through collateral channels is extremely high because they are microscopically small. Therefore they are probably of little importance in the normal, healthy lung. However, collateral channels increase in number and have more of a role in obstructive lung disease, so that gas can find alternative routes to bypass obstructed airways.

If an airway is occluded by a sputum plug then the distal alveoli will collapse. A number of treatment techniques used by respiratory physiotherapists aim to recruit the channels of collateral ventilation in order to get air behind sputum plugs. The principle behind any of these treatment techniques is that by increasing lung volume, there will be increased airflow through the collateral channels. It is thought that this airflow will move the sputum plug more proximally, and will also recruit the atelectatic lung.

AIRWAYS RESISTANCE

'Airways resistance' refers to the resistance of the respiratory tract to airflow during inspiration and expiration. The amount of airways resistance is dependent on the calibre of the airway, therefore, *in general terms* the smaller the airway the greater the resistance.

Airway Innervation

The airways are innervated by the autonomic nervous system (ANS). The parasympathetic nervous system (PNS) directly innervates bronchial smooth muscle causing bronchoconstriction, which decreases airway calibre and increases airways resistance.

Sympathetic nervous system (SNS) receptors (β_2) are sited in airway walls and are stimulated by catecholamines, which relax bronchial smooth muscle, increase airway calibre and decrease airway resistance.

In health, airways resistance is low due to the balance between both branches of the ANS.

Site of Highest Resistance

The trachea and main airways are large calibre and therefore have low airways resistance. Although resistance to air flow is greatest in individual small airways, the total resistance to air flow contributed by the small airways taken together is very low because they represent a huge number of parallel pathways. Therefore under normal circumstances the greatest total airways resistance resides in the upper airways: oro and nasopharynx, larynx (approximately 40%) and medium-sized bronchi. These contain a high proportion of bronchial smooth muscle, and a high level of ANS innervation (alters calibre).

In health, airways resistance decreases as lung volume increases because the airways distend as the lungs inflate; wider airways have increased calibre and, therefore, lower airways resistance

Poiseuille's Law

Airways resistance is governed by Poiseuille's law, which states that the flow of gas through an airway is:

- directly proportional to the fourth power of its internal radius
- inversely proportional to its length
- inversely proportional to the viscosity of gas.

Clinical Relevance of Poiseuille's Law

As the length of airways does not change except during growth, and at sea level the viscosity of gas remains constant, a change in radius (airway calibre) is the most important factor affecting airway resistance. Resistance is in turn inversely proportional to airflow (and the fourth power of the internal radius), so a small change in radius leads to a big change in airway resistance. Halving the internal diameter of the radius, for example, will increase airway resistance by 16 and reduce airflow to $\frac{1}{16}$th of normal.

Respiratory diseases characterised by increased airways resistance and airflow limitation are called 'obstructive diseases', e.g. asthma, chronic obstructive pulmonary disease (COPD).

Any pathology which reduces the calibre of airways will lead to increased airways resistance, decrease airflow and cause airflow limitation. Airway calibre may be reduced by pathology inside the lumen of the airway or pathology outside the airway causing external compression.

Intra luminal pathology may include:

- bronchoconstriction
- bronchial secretions
- mucosal oedema
- airway remodelling
- tumour/mass
- inhaled foreign body.

Extra-luminal pathology may include:

- tumour/mass.

Loss of radial traction, bronchomalacia, trauma and stenosis may also affect airway calibre and airways resistance.

Consequences of Increased Airway Resistance

Decreased airway calibre
▼
Increased airways resistance
▼
Decreased airflow (airflow limitation)
▼
Increased work of breathing
▼
Breathlessness

Clinical Signs of Airflow Limitation

Clinically, a patient with airflow limitation secondary to obstructive respiratory disease may present with one or more of the following symptoms:

- increased work of breathing
  - accessory muscle recruitment
  - active expiration
  - pursed lip breathing

- fixed upper limbs
- soft-tissue recession
- prolonged expiration
- speaking in half sentences
- breathlessness
- wheeze
- fatigue
- reduced alveolar ventilation (V_A)
  - reduced partial pressure of oxygen (PaO_2)
  - increased partial pressure of carbon dioxide ($PaCO_2$).

Signs of obstruction and airflow limitation are always more apparent in expiration first. This is because expiration occurs secondary to passive recoil of the lung and is therefore already associated with shortening and narrowing of the airways. Any pathology which further decreases airway calibre will be most apparent in expiration. Airflow limitation can be assessed and measured using spirometry or a peak expiratory flow metre.

Problems Associated with Airflow Limitation

As airflow limitation is increased on expiration, patients with obstructive respiratory disease have difficulty fully breathing out. Consequently, some of their expiratory volume is not expelled and remains in the lungs increasing residual volume (RV). This is called 'air trapping' and causes the patient to become hyperinflated, giving rise to the characteristic barrel shaped chest associated with obstructive respiratory disease. Hyperinflation alters normal respiratory mechanics, as the diaphragm becomes flattened and unable to effectively contract, holding the thorax in an inspiratory position. This leads to reduced inspiratory flow, poor tidal volumes (V_Ts) and ultimately ventilation–perfusion ($\dot{V}/\dot{Q}$) mismatch. Prolonged inadequate V_A culminates in respiratory failure.

Reversal of Airflow Limitation

Intraluminal pathology leading to airflow limitation may be reversed by:

- pharmacology
  - bronchodilator therapy
    - inhibition of PNS
    - excitation of SNS
    - xanthine (directly affects bronchial smooth muscle)

- anti-inflammatory agents
  - □ corticosteroids
  - □ cytokine inhibitors
- diuretic therapy
- antibiotic therapy
- physiotherapy (airway clearance techniques)
- bronchoscopy
- surgery.

RESPIRATORY COMPLIANCE

Compliance refers to the distensibility (stretchiness) of an elastic structure. Physiologically, it refers to the change in pulmonary volume per unit of pressure change. Compliance is represented by the pressure–volume curve. In health, the respiratory system is highly compliant and needs very little pressure to change volume on inspiration; a 2 mmHg change in pleural pressure generates inspiratory flow. The lungs are most compliant above functional residual capacity (FRC).

The distensibility of the lungs is called 'lung compliance' and the distensibility of the chest wall is called 'chest wall compliance'. For effective inspiration to occur, *both* the lungs and chest wall must be compliant. Collectively, lung compliance plus chest wall compliance is called 'total lung compliance' or 'respiratory system compliance'.

Reduced Compliance

To maintain efficient inspiration, total lung compliance must be optimal. Therefore any pathology which reduces the compliance of *either* the chest wall *or* the lung will reduce total lung compliance and make inspiration more difficult. Respiratory disease characterized by reduced total lung compliance is classified as restrictive respiratory disease. Patients with restrictive respiratory disease have difficulty breathing in. This can be assessed and measured using spirometry.

Factors Affecting Lung Compliance

Lung compliance can change (reduced or increased) in various disease states.

Altered Lung Compliance

A change in compliance at either end of the pressure volume curve makes inspiration very difficult. Reduced

lung compliance makes the generation of a large pressure necessary to change volume.

- low lung volumes (FRC)
  - atelectasis
  - post surgery
  - prolonged recumbency in supine
- high lung volumes
  - hyperinflation
  - ageing
- reduced pulmonary surfactant
- pulmonary oedema
- consolidation
- interstitial fibrosis
  - idiopathic pulmonary fibrosis
- pleural effusion.

Closing Volume

FRC is the amount of air left in the lungs after tidal expiration (FRC = expiratory reserve volume (ERV) + RV). Within FRC is a critical level called 'closing volume', which is the point at which there is insufficient air left in the lungs to maintain lung inflation; subsequently, dynamic compression (collapse) of small airways and alveoli will occur. When closing volume is reached, inspiration falls below the lower inflexion point (LIP) on the pressure/volume curve, meaning a very large pressure is required to open airways and alveoli, increasing the work of breathing.

Closing volume increases with age, smoking, lung disease and position (supine > upright). Closing volume plus RV is called 'closing capacity (CC)'.

Pulmonary Surfactant

Pulmonary surfactant is a surface-active lipoprotein complex, secreted by type II alveolar cells. The main lipid component of surfactant (dipalmitoylphosphatidylcholine) reduces surface tension and increases pulmonary compliance. This prevents the lung collapsing at the end of expiration.

In humans, surfactant production begins in type II alveolar cells during the terminal sac stage of lung development. Lamellar bodies appear in the cytoplasm at about 20 weeks' gestation. Babies born prematurely before 28–32 weeks' gestation may develop infant respiratory distress syndrome (IRDS), characterized by poor lung compliance and increased work of breathing.

Reduced surfactant production

▼

Increased surface tension

▼

Decreased lung compliance

▼

Atelectasis

▼

Increased work of breathing/O_2 consumption

Altered Chest Wall Compliance

In this situation, the lungs are normal but inflation and inspiration is reduced secondary to reduced chest wall compliance. If the thorax is less compliant, it will prevent inflation of the underlying lung by providing an external limitation. Imagine trying to blow up a balloon inside a small box. The walls of the box limit the amount of inflation and distension of the balloon.

Reduced chest wall compliance may occur in the presence of:

- thoracic deformity
  - kyphosis
  - scoliosis
  - sternal deformity
- circumferential thoracic burn
- raised intra-abdominal pressure
  - abdominal distension
  - post-surgery
  - pregnancy
- obesity
- supine position
- ageing.

Consequences of Reduced Total Lung Compliance

Reduced total lung compliance produces an increased respiratory load, which leads to an increased work of breathing for the patient. In response, they may recruit the accessory muscles of respiration, which in turn increases O_2 demand and consumption. Over time, the respiratory muscles fatigue and V_A becomes inadequate, ultimately resulting in respiratory failure.

CONTROL OF BREATHING

'Control of ventilation' refers to the physiological mechanisms involved in the control of physiological ventilation, whereas gas exchange requirements primarily controls the rate of respiration (respiratory frequency).

Origin of Breathing

The respiratory system has no intrinsic driving system like the heart; therefore it is totally dependent on an external neural drive. The origin of breathing occurs in respiratory control centres (RCCs) in the brainstem and occurs automatically without any conscious effort.

The purpose of breathing is to provide adequate V_A, i.e. oxygen (O_2) delivery and carbon dioxide (CO_2) excretion. V_A alters in response to changing environmental or metabolic demands, e.g. exercise. Adequate V_A is essential to maintain a neutral acid–base balance (7.35–7.45 kPa), which provides an optimal environment for cellular function.

Respiratory Control Centres (RCCs)

There are four main centres in the brainstem which regulate respiration:

- Inspiratory centre (medulla)
- Expiratory centre (medulla)
- Pneumotaxic centre (pons)
- Apneustic centre (pons).

In general, the medullary respiratory centres provide output to the respiratory muscles (diaphragm, external and internal intercostals) and the pontine centres influence output from the medullary respiratory centres. Interaction of activity from these two centres establishes and modifies breathing (shortens inspiratory or expiratory phase or alters frequency) to meet metabolic demand or allow other activities such as speech, eating or singing.

The Medullary Control Centres

The medullary control centres contain two groups of respiratory neurones:

- Ventral respiratory group (VRG) controls
  - voluntary forced exhalation
  - increases force of inspiration
  - regulates rhythm of inhalation and exhalation.

- Dorsal respiratory group (DRG) controls
  - inspiratory movements and timing.

The Pontine Control Centres

- Pneumotaxic centre
  - coordinates speed of inhalation and exhalation
  - sends inhibitory impulses to inspiratory centre
  - provides fine tuning of respiration frequency.
- Apneustic centre
  - coordinates speed of inhalation and exhalation
  - sends stimulatory impulses to inspiratory centre
  - activates and prolongs long deep breaths.

Higher Brain Centres

Cortical inputs can temporarily override the intrinsic rhythm of the central control centres and lead to a voluntary increase or decrease of respiratory frequency, or alter breathing pattern to allow control of speech, singing or the ability to voluntarily hyperventilate, hypoventilate or breath hold.

- Cerebral cortex
  - cortical input can override intrinsic breathing pattern from RCC
  - voluntary pathways synapse with anterior horn cells (AHCs) in spinal cord
  - directly stimulate respiratory muscles
  - necessary for speech, eating, coughing.
- Hypothalamus and limbic systems
  - pain and emotional state can modulate RCC to produce apnoea or a gasp.

Clinical Failure of the Respiratory Control Centres

- Hypoventilation or absent ventilation can occur in the presence of
  - brainstem cerebral vascular accident (CVA) or tumour
  - raised intracranial pressure (ICP)
  - central sleep apnoea
  - Primary alveolar hypoventilation e.g. Ondine curse
  - decreased level of consciousness secondary to
    □ alcohol
    □ drugs
    □ pharmacology
    □ neurological event

- Hyperventilation can occur in the presence of
  - breathing dysregulation syndrome
  - anxiety
  - metabolic disease.

Ondine's Curse

Primary alveolar hypoventilation, known as Ondine's curse is a congenital central hypoventilation syndrome, but can also develop secondary to severe neurological brainstem trauma. It is a very rare and serious form of central nervous system failure due to an inborn failure of the autonomic control of breathing, leading to episodes of apnoea or breathing cessation during sleep. In a few patients with severe disease, apnoea may also occur while awake. The incidence is 1 in 200,000 live born children with 200 known cases worldwide.

Respiratory Control Feedback Mechanism

The RCCs are responsible for the generation and control of breathing. Medullary centres control basic inspiration and expiration; the frequency, timing and duration of each respiratory phase are fine-tuned by the pontine centres.

In addition, direct input from higher centres at both brain and spinal cord level can override basic rate as required. Output from the RCCs leads to depolarization and contraction of the effectors, i.e. respiratory muscles. Several different types of sensors monitor effector activity and provide constant feedback, which allows the RCCs to modify their output (respiratory frequency and depth) to meet metabolic demand (Fig. 1-12).

Clinical Failure of the Effectors

The effectors may fail in the presence of neuromuscular diseases of:

- nerves (for example injury to phrenic nerve leading to diaphragmatic weakness)
- the neuromuscular junction (for example myasthenia gravis)
- muscles (for example muscular dystrophy).

Alteration to respiratory mechanics or chest wall dysfunction may lead to failure of the effectors, for example:

- kyphoscoliosis
- obesity
- hyperinflation.

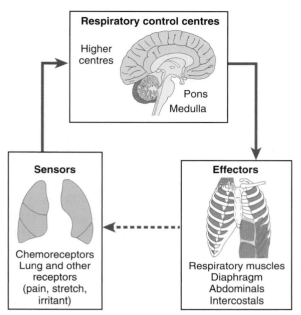

FIGURE 1-12 ■ Respiratory control centres (RCCs) and sensors.

Respiratory System Sensors

Several different types of sensors monitor respiration, providing direct feedback to the RCCs:

- chemoreceptors
  - central
  - peripheral
- mechanoreceptors
- irritant receptors
- juxta-capillary receptors
- proprioceptors.

Mechanoreceptors

High-threshold mechanoreceptors are sited in bronchial smooth muscle, trachea and visceral pleurae. They are stimulated by tension in airways and lung parenchyma during inflation, providing feedback to the RCCs to ensure an optimal level of inflation to meet activity and metabolic demand. A very large inflation can lead to a critical stretch of the lung parenchyma, eliciting the Hering-Breuer reflex to instruct the RCC to stop inspiration.

Irritant Receptors

Located in the epithelial surface of the nasal cavity, upper airways, larynx, trachea, and large bronchi, irritant receptors are stimulated by irritants such as noxious gases, cigarette smoke, dust, allergens, cold air or secretions. Feedback from irritant receptors can elicit a change in respiratory frequency or depth, induce a cough, sneeze or bronchospasm.

Juxta-Capillary Receptors

The alveolar capillaries located in the interstitium are richly supplied with sensory nerve endings called 'juxtacapillary receptors' or 'j-receptors'. These sensors are stimulated by the accumulation of fluid in alveoli or capillary walls secondary to inflammation or pulmonary oedema, leading to an increase in ventilation or an abnormal ventilatory pattern, e.g. Cheyne–Stokes respiration.

Proprioceptors

During early stages of exercise, impulses from proprioceptors and mechanoreceptors in muscle, ligaments and joint capsules stimulate respiratory neurones to increase the frequency and depth of respiration.

Spinal Cord Reflexes

Reflexes at spinal cord level lead to the activation and recruitment of respiratory accessory muscles to increase respiratory frequency and volume as a compensation mechanism secondary to hypoventilation, gasping and respiratory distress.

Nasopulminary Reflexes

Located in the nasal mucosa, triggered by a change in flow or air pressure in the nose, these reflexes provide feedback (via trigeminal nerve) to the RCCs to regulate deep breathing (increasing or decreasing) by altering excitation to the effectors.

Chemoreceptors

The most important of all the respiratory sensors are the chemoreceptors, which constantly sample arterial blood, providing feedback to the RCCs to maintain respiratory gases and pH within their normal range regardless of activity.

Peripheral Chemoreceptors

Peripheral chemoreceptors are located in the aortic arch between the ascending aorta and pulmonary artery (afferents in vagus nerve) and the carotid body at the bifurcation of the common carotid (afferents in glossopharyngeal nerve). Both sets of peripheral chemoreceptors sample surrounding arterial blood and are sensitive to arterial hypoxaemia, i.e. peripheral chemoreceptors are *only* stimulated when there is >40% reduction in PaO_2 (PaO_2 8 kPa or less). They both also have sensitivity to increased free hydrogen ion (H^+) concentration and are weakly sensitive to $PaCO_2$. Additionally, only the peripheral chemoreceptors in the carotid bodies are sensitive to a change in pH. Feedback from the peripheral chemoreceptors informs the RCCs to alter the frequency and depth of respiration to meet demand.

Central Chemoreceptors

Located bilaterally on the ventral surface of medulla, the central chemoreceptors are bathed in cerebrospinal fluid (CSF). At the blood–brain barrier (BBB), the concentration of CO_2 in CSF is equal to the concentration of CO_2 in arterial blood ($PaCO_2$). Central chemoreceptors are sensitive to free hydrogen ion (H^+) concentration, derived from CO_2 and demonstrate heightened sensitivity with mild hypoxia and acidosis. Central chemoreceptors are unaffected by oxygen concentration. Feedback from the central chemoreceptors to the RCCs is responsible for 70% of the drive to breathe. Once stimulated, the central chemoreceptors initiate a change in breathing pattern within 5 breaths (10–20 seconds).

Stimulation of the Central Chemoreceptors

CO_2 diffuses across the BBB and combines with water (H_2O) in CSF to form carbonic acid. Carbonic acid dissociates to form bicarbonate and free hydrogen ions.

$$CO_2 + H_2O \leftrightarrow H_2CO_3^- \leftrightarrow CO_3^- + H^+$$

The presence of free hydrogen ions increases acidity and reduces the pH of CSF, which directly stimulates the central chemoreceptors. The central chemoreceptors feedback to RCCs, which stimulate the effectors to increase the frequency and depth of ventilation until pH (CO_2/H^+) levels are back in normal range.

Conversely, when pH rises ($CO_2/H+$ low) the central chemoreceptors feedback to RCCs, which stimulate the effectors to decrease the frequency and depth of ventilation until pH ($CO_2/H+$) levels are back in normal range.

Additionally, the central chemoreceptors can provide central feedback to the RCCs, leading to an alteration in sympathetic and parasympathetic activity to alter blood pressure.

Central Chemoreceptors and COPD

In the presence of respiratory disease such as COPD, CO_2 may become chronically raised where the effectors are unable to alter respiratory frequency or depth. For example:

- hyperinflation
- alveolar destruction
- $\dot{V}/\dot{Q}$ mismatch
- altered respiratory mechanics
- effector failure.

In this situation, arterial blood and consequently CSF remain acidotic. The brain cannot function adequately with a deranged acid–base balance, so a compensatory mechanism is instigated.

$$CO_2 + H_2O \leftrightarrow H_2CO_3^- \leftrightarrow HCO_3^- + H^+$$

Normally, hydrogen carbonate (HCO_3^-) ions liberated from the dissociation of carbonic acid are excreted via the kidneys. In the presence of hypercapnia, HCO_3^- ions are transported across the BBB to combine with and 'buffer' free H^+ ions in the CSF, essentially 'neutralizing' their stimulation of the central chemoreceptors. This may take up to 3 days before being fully effective and is called 'metabolic compensation'. Effective buffering returns CSF pH to normal to facilitate effective cellular function; sensitivity of central chemoreceptors is reduced, but arterial blood CO_2 ($PaCO_2$) remains raised, producing a persistent acidosis (low pH).

When the central chemoreceptors are no longer sensitive to free H^+/CO_2 the COPD patient's drive to breathe falls to the peripheral chemoreceptors, which are sensitive to hypoxaemia; this is called 'hypoxic drive'.

Clinical Relevance of Hypercapnic COPD

Patients with COPD have large areas of low ventilation resulting in $\dot{V}/\dot{Q}$ mismatch, and are unable to alter ventilation to increase excretion of CO_2, leading to chronic hypercapnia. These patients with COPD will also be hypoxaemic and require supplemental oxygen therapy. However, if O_2 is given at high levels of concentration (above 28%) there is a risk of inducing further hypercapnia secondary to three mechanisms:

- loss of hypoxic drive
- increased $\dot{V}/\dot{Q}$ mismatch due to reversal of hypoxic pulmonary vasoconstriction (HPV)
- Haldane effect (oxygenated blood has a reduced capacity for carbon dioxide).

Loss of Hypoxic Drive

COPD patients with chronic hypercapnia have reduced sensitivity of central chemoreceptors and therefore rely on peripheral chemoreceptors to sense arterial hypoxaemia and provide a drive to breathe. As such, if the patient is given high dose therapeutic O_2; arterial hypoxaemia will be reversed, removing the remaining drive to breathe.

Increased $\dot{V}/\dot{Q}$ Mismatch

In the presence of respiratory disease such as COPD, areas of poor ventilation lead to reduced gas exchange and hypoxaemia. When PaO_2 falls to about 6 kPa (oxy-haemoglobin saturation (SaO_2) in low 80s), hypoxaemia is sensed by receptors in arterioles passing through the area of poor ventilation. This causes them to constrict to minimize $\dot{V}/\dot{Q}$ mismatch and provide increased blood flow to areas with better ventilation to facilitate gas exchange. This is called 'hypoxic pulmonary vasoconstriction (HPV)'. If the COPD patient is given high-dose therapeutic O_2, hypoxia in some areas of lung may be reduced due to an increased concentration gradient. Improved PaO_2 is sensed by arterioles leading to the reversal of HPV, once again causing perfusion of poorly ventilated lung and producing increased $\dot{V}/\dot{Q}$ mismatch (shunt).

Haldane Effect

Haemoglobin (Hb) has a strong affinity for O_2, but in the presence of hypoxaemia, CO_2 binds to Hb to be transported back to the lung. This is called the 'Haldane effect'. Conversely, if the COPD patient is given high dose therapeutic O_2, Hb dissociates from CO_2 in preference to bind with O_2. The dissociated CO_2 dissolves in plasma raising $PaCO_2$.

LUNG VOLUMES & VENTILATION

Although inflation and deflation of the lungs is continuous, the volume of air in the lungs varies at different points in the respiratory cycle and in health, is dependent on activity level. As a respiratory physiotherapist, it is important to understand the clinical relevance of lung volumes and how they may alter in the presence of dysfunction or disease. Lung volumes are measured directly; lung capacities are measured in multiples of two or more lung volumes (Fig. 1-13).

Lung Volumes

- V_T is the volume of air inspired during quiet respiration.
- Inspiratory reserve volume (IRV) is the volume air inspired from V_T to maximal inspiration.
- ERV is the volume of air expelled with forced expiration.
- RV is the volume of air left in lungs which cannot be expelled.

(Table 1-1)

Lung Capacities

- FRC is the volume of air left in the lungs at end of normal quiet expiration (ERV + RV).
- Vital capacity (VC) is the total volume of air from maximal inspiration to maximal expiration (IRV + V_T + ERV).
- Total lung capacity (TLC) is the volume from maximal inspiration to RV (IRV + V_T + ERV + RV).

(Figure 1-13, Table 1-2)

Factors Affecting Lung Volumes

- Body size: Taller people tend to have larger lung volumes. Obese people have smaller lung volumes as their chest wall is less compliant.
- Age: As a person gets older lung tissue loses elasticity and lung volumes increase. However, simultaneously, ageing leads to reduced compliance

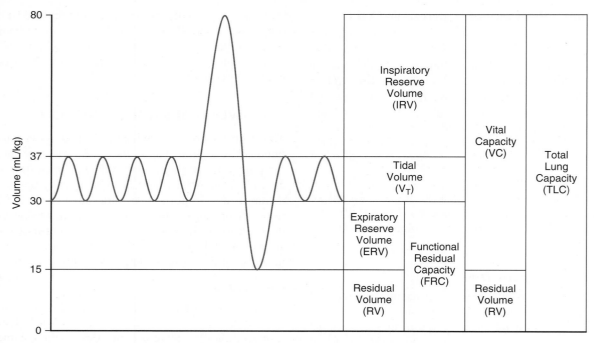

FIGURE 1-13 ■ Lung volumes and capacities.

TABLE 1-1		
Average Lung Volumes in Healthy Adults		
	VALUE (L)	
Volume	**Men**	**Women**
Inspiratory reserve volume	3.0	1.9
Tidal volume	0.5	0.5
Expiratory reserve volume	1.1	0.7
Residual volume	1.2	1.1

TABLE 1-2			
Average Lung Capacities in Healthy Adults			
	VALUE (L)		
Capacity	**Men**	**Women**	**Components**
Vital capacity	4.6	3.1	IRV & V_T & ERV
Functional residual capacity	2.3	1.8	ERV & RV
Total lung capacity	5.8	4.2	IRV & V_T & ERV & RV

ERV, Expiratory reserve volume; *IRV,* inspiratory reserve volume; *RV,* residual volume; V_T, tidal volume.

of the thoracic cage which is more pronounced than changes to lung elasticity. Therefore overall there is a reduction in lung volumes.

■ Gender: Men tend to be physically bigger than women and therefore have larger lung volumes.

■ Muscle training: Inspiratory muscle training increases lung volumes.

■ Respiratory disease: Respiratory disease may lead to an increase or decrease in lung volumes.

■ Altitude: People living at altitude have larger lung volumes in order to increase gas exchange where the partial pressure of oxygen is reduced.

Clinical Relevance of Lung Volumes and Capacities

■ V_T: an adequate V_T is necessary to maintain oxygenation and CO_2 clearance.

■ IRV: required to produce an effective cough and necessary to sustain increased level of activity or exercise.

■ FRC: essential to maintain distal lung patency on expiration. Within FRC, there is a critical value called closing volume. When FRC falls below closing volume, distal lung patency can no longer be maintained leading to atelectasis. Atelectasis is associated with reduced oxygenation, poor CO_2 clearance, an increased work of breathing, breathlessness and a reduced exercise tolerance.

■ RV: an increase in RV occurs in obstructive lung disease due to air trapping. This leads to altered respiratory mechanics, an increased work of breathing, reduced V_T, poor gas exchange and a reduced exercise tolerance.

■ VC: a VC of 1 L is the critical value used to identify if a patient is able to maintain spontaneous ventilation.

Measuring Lung Volumes and Capacities

V_T, VC, inspiratory capacity and IRV can be measured directly with a spirometer. These simple measurements form the basis of pulmonary function testing. As it is not possible to completely breathe out, measuring RV (and FRC) is more complex. Specialized testing is required using radiographic planimetry, body plethysmography, closed circuit dilution (the helium dilution technique) or nitrogen washout techniques.

Why Assess Spirometry?

As a physiotherapist, understanding spirometry will aid the clinical diagnosis and management of a patient with respiratory disease. In gross terms, respiratory disease is either categorized as obstructive (difficulty breathing out) or restrictive (difficulty breathing in), but in some cases both problems can co-exist. Spirometry is also often used as an objective measure to assess or monitor disease progression and deterioration during acute exacerbation, the efficiency of an inhaled drug or its delivery system.

Ventilation Terminology

An average adult has a V_T of 500 mL and has a respiratory frequency of 12 breaths per minute (approximately). Therefore the minute ventilation, the amount of air entering the lungs, is $12 \times 500 = 6.0$ L/min.

However, not all V_T which enters the lungs is used in gas exchange. 'Dead space' is the term for that part of the V_T that is *not* involved in gas exchange. There are 2 types of dead space:

■ anatomical dead space
■ alveolar dead space.

Together they are called 'physiological dead space'.

Anatomical Dead Space

The bronchial tree is divided into two zones (see Fig. 1-3):

■ conducting zone
■ respiratory zone.

The conducting zone consists of the trachea to the terminal bronchi. Air moves through the conducting zone by convection towards the alveolar membrane where gas exchange takes place. Within each tidal breath, 150 mL remains in the conducting zone and is therefore not used in gas exchange. This is called 'anatomical dead space'.

The respiratory zone extends from the respiratory bronchiole to the alveolus. Air moves through the respiratory zone by diffusion, culminating in gas exchange.

Alveolar Dead Space

'Alveolar dead space' is the term used to describe inspiratory gas reaching alveoli which is unable to participate in gas exchange due to an insufficient blood supply. In health, alveolar dead space is almost zero, but in disease, alveolar dead space may occur in the presence of a pulmonary embolus or ventilation of non-vascular air spaces, e.g. emphysematous bullae or cardiac shunt.

Physiological Dead Space

Physiological dead space is the sum of all parts of V_T which does *not* participate in gaseous exchange, i.e. anatomical dead space plus alveolar dead space. Therefore anything that affects anatomical or alveolar dead space will affect physiological dead space, e.g. age, gender, body size and posture and the instigation of mechanical ventilation and pulmonary disease.

Alveolar Ventilation

V_A is the amount of minute ventilation reaching the respiratory zone that can be used in gas exchange.

Tidal volume – anatomical dead space
= Alveolar ventilation

In an average adult

- 500 mL − 150 mL = 350 mL/breath
- 350 mL × 12 breaths per minute = 4.2 L/min.

Clinical Relevance of Alveolar Ventilation

Maintenance of V_A is of paramount importance because it determines the quantity of O_2 and CO_2 levels in alveolar gas (PAO_2, $PACO_2$) and subsequently arterial blood (PaO_2, $PaCO_2$). In particular, there is an inverse linear relationship between V_A and CO_2 levels, with $PACO_2$ decreasing as V_A increases. An alteration in V_A will lead to disruption of normal acid–base balance; both hypoxaemia and hypercapnia may occur with respiratory disease.

Other factors which affect the concentration of O_2 and CO_2 in arterial blood are

- the rate of O_2 consumption (VO_2)
- the rate of CO_2 production (VCO_2)
- Hb content of blood
- Hb affinity for O_2
- atmospheric pressure of O_2
- specific characteristics of the alveolar membrane.

Alteration of Alveolar Ventilation

Alveolar hypoventilation is defined as insufficient ventilation leading to raised levels of carbon dioxide (hypercapnia).

Hypoventilation may present
- localized to a particular lung, lobe or segment, e.g. secondary to infection, consolidation or atelectasis
- scattered through both lung fields, e.g. secondary to COPD or asthma
- generalized, e.g. secondary to pain, a reduced respiratory drive or reduced level of consciousness.

Hypoventilation leads to poor CO_2 excretion
- ↑ $PACO_2$ (alveolar concentration)
- ↑ $PaCO_2$ (plasma concentration)
- ↑ $CO_2 + H_2O \rightleftharpoons H_2CO_3 \rightleftharpoons HCO_3 + ↑ H^+$
- ↓ pH
- respiratory acidosis.

Alveolar hyperventilation is defined as excessive ventilation leading to reduced levels of carbon dioxide (hypocapnia).

Hyperventilation may occur secondary to
- anxiety/fear
- metabolic disease (hyperthyroidism)
- airway obstruction (asthma)
- parenchymal lung disease (pneumonia)
- neurological disorders (tumour)
- altitude.

Hyperventilation leads to excess CO_2 excretion:
- ↓ $PACO_2$ (alveolar concentration)
- ↓ $PaCO_2$ (plasma concentration)
- ↓ $CO_2 + H_2O \rightleftharpoons H_2CO_3 \rightleftharpoons HCO_3 + ↓ H^+$
- ↑pH
- respiratory alkalosis.

GAS EXCHANGE

The requirements of the average cell for oxygen are quite modest and a mitochondrion may need a partial pressure of oxygen (PO_2) of as little as 1 kPa (7.5 mmHg) to function effectively. At sea level, the atmospheric PO_2 is 20 kPa (150 mmHg) (fraction of inspired oxygen (FiO_2) = 0.21) and in the process of delivering oxygen to the cell, there is a loss along this gradient.

The mechanics of breathing produce inspiration and airflow into the lungs secondary to a change in volume and subsequently pressure. During inspiration air initially moves into the lungs via convection and passes through the conducting zone to the respiratory zone of the bronchial tree. In the most general terms, convection refers to the movement of currents within fluids (i.e. liquids, gases).

The first step is the dilution of inspired air with expired air within the alveolus. Each tidal breath (V_T) contains a portion of gas which will remain within the airways and not come into contact with the alveoli. This is known as the 'dead space ventilation' (V_D) and must be achieved before any effective V_A can take place:

$$V_T = V_D + V_A$$

Alveolar gas therefore contains a mixture of fresh gas and some expired CO_2 and the alveolar PO_2 is reduced to about 13.8 kPa (104 mmHg) before gas exchange begins.

Air moves along the smallest airways into the alveoli sacs by diffusion. The actual exchange of gases occurs across the capillaries in the alveoli sacs (alveolar membrane). 'Diffusion' refers to the process by which molecules intermingle as a result of kinetic energy of random motion. Diffusion is an extremely rapid process but can only occur over very small distances.

Fick's Law and Gas Exchange

Gas exchange takes place in the alveoli sac across the alveolar membrane, which is the boundary between the external environment and interior of the body (Fig. 1-14). Respiratory gases cross the respiratory membrane by diffusion, in accordance with Fick's law.

Fick's Law

- The rate of transfer of a gas through a sheet of tissue is proportional to
  - tissue area
  - difference in gas partial pressure between the two sides
  - diffusion constant
- inversely proportional to tissue thickness.

In the context of respiration and gas exchange, in accordance with Fick's law, diffusion is dependent on

- surface area of alveolar membrane
- concentration/pressure gradient
- gas solubility
- thickness of alveolar membrane
- ventilation/perfusion coupling.

Concentration Gradient and Gas Solubility

In the context of the respiratory gases, concentration is described using the term 'partial pressure'. Partial pressure describes the amount of gas dissolved in the plasma. For example, PaO_2 is the amount of O_2 dissolved in the plasma of arterial blood or $PvCO_2$ is the amount of CO_2 dissolved in the plasma of venous blood.

Partial pressures are equivalent to concentration gradients. The steeper the difference in partial pressure between gas in alveoli and capillary blood, the steeper the diffusion gradient producing faster and more efficient diffusion. Thus the partial pressure difference of 64 mmHg between deoxygenated venous blood in the pulmonary capillaries ($PvO_2 = 40$ mmHg) and the oxygen rich alveolus ($PAO_2 = 104$ mmHg), leads to rapid diffusion of O_2 from the alveolus

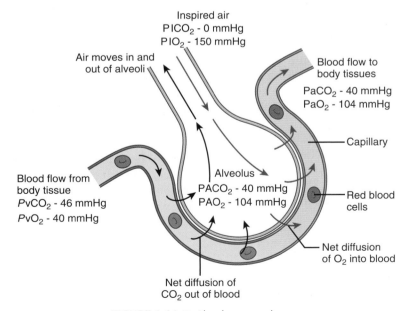

Inspired air
$PICO_2$ - 0 mmHg
PIO_2 - 150 mmHg

Air moves in and out of alveoli

Blood flow to body tissues
$PaCO_2$ - 40 mmHg
PaO_2 - 104 mmHg

Capillary

Blood flow from body tissue
$PvCO_2$ - 46 mmHg
PvO_2 - 40 mmHg

Alveolus
$PACO_2$ - 40 mmHg
PAO_2 - 104 mmHg

Red blood cells

Net diffusion of O_2 into blood

Net diffusion of CO_2 out of blood

FIGURE 1-14 ■ Alveolar gas exchange.

across the respiratory membrane into the pulmonary capillary.

The difference in partial pressure of CO_2 between the venous capillary ($PvCO_2 = 46$ mmHg) and the alveolus ($PACO_2 = 40$ mmHg) is much smaller at only 6 mmHg. However, as CO_2 is 20 times more soluble than O_2, only a small difference in partial pressure is necessary. Diffusion of CO_2 from venous capillary blood into the alveoli occurs extremely rapidly. Indeed, in the time available equal amounts of CO_2 and O_2 are exchanged across the respiratory membrane. Clinically, in respiratory disease where diffusion is impaired, O_2 will be primarily affected, as it is less soluble. A significant impairment is required to lead to poor CO_2 transfer.

Transit Time of Red Blood Cell (RBC)

During gas exchange, the total transit time of a RBC within the pulmonary capillaries is about 0.75 sec. However, in health, it normally only takes about 0.25 sec for O_2 equilibration to occur (i.e. gas exchange). This means that with normal partial pressures of O_2, there is a large time reserve; this provides a significant safety margin, which means the velocity of blood flow can significantly increase (i.e. during exercise) and still allow enough transit time for full RBC saturation with O_2 to be achieved.

Thickness of the Alveolar Membrane

The alveolar membrane is 0.5 to 1 μm thick (2000 times thinner than skin). Diffusion efficiency is highly dependent on distances involved; therefore an ultra-thin membrane facilitates rapid and efficient gas exchange.

Clinically, if the alveolar membrane becomes thickened, there is a greater distance between alveoli and capillary, leading to slower and or impaired diffusion, which may lead to hypoxaemia. Thickening of the alveolar membrane may occur due to inflammation, infection or fibrosis.

Surface Area of Alveolar Membrane

The adult lung contains around 300 million alveoli, which gives a gas exchange surface area in the region of 70–80 m^2 (40 times greater than the surface area of skin). Full lung surface area is not required for normal

activity, but additional recruitment of the gas exchange surface can be utilized to maintain acid–base balance during increased activity, e.g. during exercise.

In some respiratory diseases there is a marked loss of surface area available for gas exchange. Therefore even though diffusion may not be impaired, adequate oxygenation and carbon dioxide clearance cannot be maintained, leading to hypoxaemia and hypercapnia.

- temporary loss of surface area
  - bronchial obstruction (tumour, mucus plug)
  - atelectasis
  - consolidation
- permanent loss of surface area
  - emphysematous bullae.

Ventilation and Perfusion Matching ($\dot{V}/\dot{Q}$)

In respiratory physiology, the $\dot{V}/\dot{Q}$ ratio is the measurement used to describe efficiency and adequacy of matching between ventilation ($\dot{V}$) and perfusion ($\dot{Q}$) which are necessary for gas exchange.

- $\dot{V}$ ventilation
  - the air which reaches the lungs
- $\dot{Q}$ perfusion
  - the blood which reaches the lungs.

Inadequacy of either $\dot{V}$ or $\dot{Q}$ will have a significant impact on the oxygenation of blood and the removal of carbon dioxide. This is termed a '$\dot{V}/\dot{Q}$ mismatch'.

Distribution of Ventilation in Healthy Lung

The distribution of ventilation is affected by the pleural pressure gradient down the upright lung. Pleural pressure gradient is generated as a net result of the ribs trying to spring upward and outward and the lungs trying to recoil inward and downward (Fig. 1-15).

Pleural pressure becomes less negative down the upright lung. Therefore in the self-ventilating adult, lung parenchyma in the apices (non-dependent region) has the greatest initial volume (i.e. already expanded) with little additional capacity for volume change. The lung parenchyma in the bases (dependent region) is minimally expanded and can exhibit the greatest volume change as the dependent regions of lung are more compliant than the non-dependent regions. However, optimal ventilation occurs in the lower third

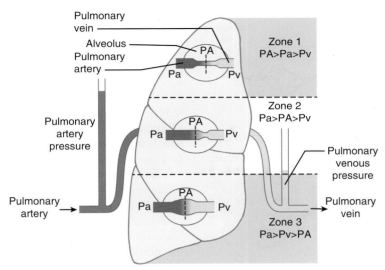

FIGURE 1-15 ■ Lung ventilation distribution. *PA*, alveolar pressure; *Pa*, pulmonary artery pressure; *Pv*, pulmonary venous pressure. *(Reproduced with permission from West, J.B., 2000. Respiratory Physiology: The Essentials, Lippincott. Williams & Wilkins, Philadelphia, p. 37.)*

of the lung, as the lung parenchyma in this region is partially expanded but still has increased capacity for further expansion and volume change. The distribution of ventilation is also influenced by differences in regional mechanics and airflow resistance.

Distribution of Perfusion in Healthy Lung

The distribution of perfusion increases down the healthy upright lung. The non-dependent–to–dependent increase in regional perfusion is influenced and affected by the interaction of alveolar, arterial and tissue pressure and the fractional geometry (branching) of the pulmonary artery. Gravity only has a limited affect (7%, 5%, and 25% of perfusion heterogeneity is due to gravity in the supine, prone and upright postures, respectively).

To aid the explanation of the distribution of perfusion, the lung can be divided into four zones. Zone 1 is not observed in the normal healthy human lung and refers to positive pressure ventilated non-perfused alveoli. In normal health, pulmonary arterial pressure exceeds alveolar pressure in all parts of the lung. Zone 2 refers to the region just above the level of the heart where blood flow may be intermittent, depending on *PA* or *Pa*, which may be influenced by high levels of positive end-expiratory pressure (PEEP), or

pulmonary hypotension. Zone 3 largely reflects the lungs in health. There is no external resistance to blood flow and blood flow is continuous throughout the cardiac cycle. Zone 4 is an additional theoretical region not shown in Figure 1-15. This zone is characterized by increased pulmonary vascular resistance caused by an increase in pulmonary interstitial pressure (*Pi*), in which $Pa > Pi > Pv > PA$, such as when lung volumes are low or in pulmonary oedema. This decrease in regional blood flow may be seen in the lung bases with conditions like acute respiratory distress syndrome (ARDS) (see Fig. 1-15).

$\dot{V}/\dot{Q}$ Matching in the Self-Ventilating Adult

In the self-ventilating adult, optimal $\dot{V}/\dot{Q}$ matching occurs in the dependent region of the lungs; the lower third, where perfusion is plentiful and the alveoli are maximally compliant and have the potential for expansion. The principles of $\dot{V}/\dot{Q}$ matching are utilized by respiratory physiotherapists when positioning patients who are hypoxic.

In health, ventilation in the lungs is met by ample blood supply from the pulmonary capillaries ($\dot{V}/\dot{Q}$ matching), facilitating effective gas exchange.

When $\dot{V}/\dot{Q}$ mismatch occurs due to **reduced ventilation** (e.g. secondary to a sputum plug disrupting

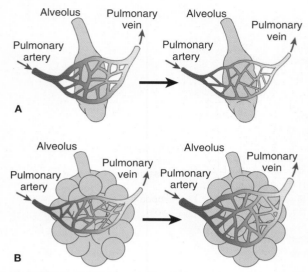

FIGURE 1-16 ■ Lung mechanisms for maintaining ventilation–perfusion ($\dot{V}/\dot{Q}$) matching. **(A)** In the event of good perfusion but poor alveolar ventilation (V_A) (collapse), reduced PO_2 and increased PCO_2 in the alveolus result in constriction of the pulmonary arterioles that supply it. Hence both alveolar ventilation and perfusion are reduced. **(B)** In the event of good alveolar ventilation but poor perfusion, increased PO_2 and reduced PCO_2 in the alveolus result in dilatation of the pulmonary arterioles that supply it. Hence both alveolar ventilation and perfusion are increased.

air flow), perfusion remains viable. An area of lung with no ventilation but good perfusion (and thus a $\dot{V}/\dot{Q}$ of 0) is termed a 'shunt' (Fig. 1-16).

When $\dot{V}/\dot{Q}$ mismatch occurs due to **reduced perfusion** (e.g. secondary to a pulmonary embolus disrupting blood flow), ventilation remains viable. An area with reduced perfusion but good ventilation (and thus a $\dot{V}/\dot{Q}$ of infinity) is termed 'alveolar dead space' (see Fig. 1-16).

Maintaining $\dot{V}/\dot{Q}$ Matching

It is vital to maintain $\dot{V}/\dot{Q}$ matching to achieve adequate gas exchange. In the presence of respiratory disease, a $\dot{V}/\dot{Q}$ mismatch triggers autoregulatory homoeostatic mechanisms to minimize the gas exchange deficit:

- HPV or dilatation
- bronchiole response (constriction or dilatation).

Hypoxic Pulmonary Vasoconstriction (HPV)

In respiratory disease, lung areas with reduced ventilation lead to poor gas exchange, and subsequent hypoxaemia and hypercapnia. When PaO_2 falls to about 6 kPa or SaO_2 is in the low 80s, hypoxia is sensed by receptors in arterioles. These arterioles constrict to reduce 'wasted perfusion' to areas of low ventilation in an attempt to minimize $\dot{V}/\dot{Q}$ mismatch. Blood flow is redirected to areas of lung with good ventilation to facilitate effective gas exchange.

Clinically, persistent HPV occurs in COPD. In this instance, pulmonary arterioles have a reduced diameter due to vasoconstriction and therefore an increased resistance to blood flow through them. Therefore to maintain blood flow to the lungs the right ventricle of the heart must work harder to push blood through these narrowed vessels. As a result, the right ventricle initially hypertrophies and then fails ultimately leading to right ventricular heart failure and cor pulmonale.

Pulmonary Capillary Recruitment

Conversely, in areas where ventilation is high, additional vessels in the pulmonary arteriole bed are recruited to optimize $\dot{V}/\dot{Q}$ matching and maximize gas exchange.

Diagnosis of $\dot{V}/\dot{Q}$ Mismatch

In respiratory disease where a $\dot{V}/\dot{Q}$ mismatch is suspected, patients undergo a $\dot{V}/\dot{Q}$ scan. This involves imaging of the distribution of air and blood in the lungs following the administration of radio-opaque markers.

Patient X's $\dot{V}/\dot{Q}$ scan reveals both a perfusion and ventilation deficit (Fig. 1-17). Therefore the underlying problem is a primary ventilatory defect with secondary compensatory HPV.

If the primary problem was reduced perfusion, a normal distribution of ventilation would still be seen.

Bronchiole Response

Bronchioles are highly sensitive to $PACO_2$. A high $PACO_2$ leads to bronchodilatation to increase CO_2 excretion (wider airways means reduced airway resistance and greater CO_2 clearance), in an attempt to normalize $PACO_2$ and $PaCO_2$. Conversely, a low $PACO_2$ leads to bronchoconstriction to reduce CO_2 excretion

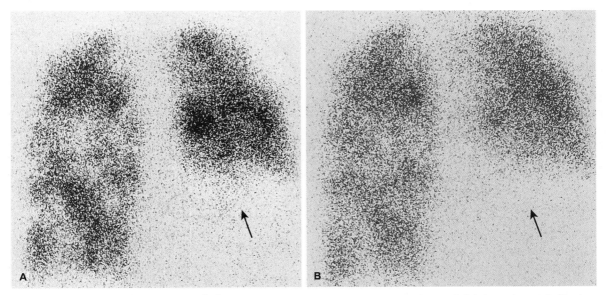

FIGURE 1-17 ■ Ventilation–perfusion ($\dot{V}/\dot{Q}$) scan reveals both a perfusion and ventilation deficit in patient X, indicating a primary ventilation defect with compensatory hypoxic pulmonary vasoconstriction. **(A)** Perfusion defect. **(B)** Ventilation defect. *(Reproduced with permission from Hansell, D.M., Lynch, D.A., McAdams, H.P., Bankier, A.A., 2009. Imaging of Diseases of the Chest, fifth ed. Mosby Elsevier, Philadelphia.)*

(narrower airways means increased airway resistance and less CO_2 clearance) in an attempt to normalize $PACO_2$ and $PaCO_2$

Transport of Oxygen and Carbon Dioxide

Oxygen and carbon dioxide are transported to and from the lungs in blood via several different methods. Oxygen is immediately bound to haemoglobin and released in the tissues under conditions of low oxygen tension or acidosis. Very little oxygen is carried in solution in the blood under conditions of normal pressure, although this can be increased in a hyperbaric chamber. By contrast, carbon dioxide is carried in the blood entirely in solution, mostly as bicarbonate. The difference between the two forms of carriage of the metabolic gases is fundamental to the interpretation of the measurement of arterial blood gases.

Oxygen Transport

Following diffusion at the alveolar membrane, 98.5% of O_2 is carried by the RBCs, called 'erythrocytes', combined with haemoglobin (SaO_2) and 1.5% of O_2 dissolves directly into the plasma (PaO_2).

Oxygen and Haemoglobin

Haemoglobin (Hb) is a complex molecule composed of four iron-containing haem groups, each attached to a polypeptide protein chain. The haem molecules are the O_2 binding sites where each of these four iron atoms can reversibly bind one O_2 molecule (oxyhaemoglobin). When all four binding sites are bound to O_2, it is called fully saturated. The process of O_2 binding is both rapid and reversible. After the first O_2 molecule binds to Hb, the shape of the haem molecule changes, which facilitates the faster binding of subsequent O_2 molecules. It takes <0.01 second to bind the first O_2 molecule but even less time to bind the second, third and fourth. This principle remains in the reverse situation of O_2 unloading at the tissues (deoxyhaemoglobin). In combination with Hb, blood can routinely transport 20 mL O_2 per 100 mL blood.

98% O_2 binds to Hb to produce oxyhaemoglobin (HbO_2).

$$HHb + O_2 \underset{\text{Tissues}}{\overset{\text{Lungs}}{\rightleftharpoons}} HbO_2 + H+$$

Haemoglobin's Affinity for Oxygen

At different points of the RBC's journey from the lung to the tissue, Hb changes its affinity for O_2, in a non-linear relationship which is represented by the sigmoid shaped oxygen dissociation curve. This alteration in Hb's affinity for O_2 serves to maximize and facilitate the process of O_2 loading at the lung and O_2 unloading at the tissue, increasing the efficiency of the O_2 transport mechanism.

The Oxygen Dissociation Curve

The oxygen dissociation curve (Fig. 1-18) describes the relationship between the partial pressure of O_2 either at the alveoli (PAO_2) or tissue level (PaO_2) and the degree to which Hb is saturated with O_2, i.e. how much O_2 is loaded (combined with Hb; SaO_2) and how much is given up (dissociated).

At the lung where PAO_2 is high, Hb has a high affinity for O_2 to facilitate maximum binding and loading in the RBC. As blood flows away from the lungs, initially very small amounts of O_2 are released from Hb as the surrounding PaO_2 remains high (between 10

and 14 kPa), producing the characteristic plateau phase of the curve. As PaO_2 falls to approximately 9 kPa, large amounts of O_2 are rapidly dissociated from Hb into the plasma, producing the steep portion of the curve. Finally, at the tissue, Hb has a decreased affinity for O_2, leading to dissociation and off-loading as the surrounding plasma level (PaO_2) has fallen below a critical value. This ensures the adequate delivery of O_2 to the tissues where it is required for metabolism and function. In health at rest, Hb only releases 25% of its O_2 cargo, as that is all the body requires. Therefore at rest, Hb remains 75% saturated; this safety margin allows increased amounts of O_2 to be available during exertion, e.g. exercise.

Why Does O_2 Need to Dissociate?

To fully understand the oxygen dissociation curve, the principles of gas exchange must be reviewed. Gas exchange (at both the lung and tissue) occurs via diffusion, which requires a concentration gradient. The necessary gradient is provided by PaO_2, i.e. the amount of O_2 dissolved in plasma, which must be maintained to drive gas exchange. Therefore before O_2 can move via diffusion to the tissue for utilization, the O_2 molecule must dissociate from Hb and dissolve into the plasma before passing through the capillary membrane into a cell. Hb can be thought of as a 'holding store' for O_2 until it is required to maintain the concentration gradient.

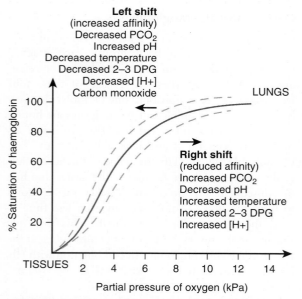

FIGURE 1-18 ■ Oxygen dissociation curve. When there is a high concentration of CO_2 (in the tissues), the curve moves down and towards the right. Carbon monoxide; DPG, diphosphoglycerate; H+, hydrogen ion; PCO_2, pressure of carbon dioxide.

Factors Affecting Hb Affinity for O_2

The rate at which Hb reversibly binds or releases O_2 is primarily regulated by PaO_2; however, other factors also affect Hb's affinity for O_2 such as temperature, pH, $PaCO_2$ and blood concentration of an organic chemical called 'diphosphoglycerate (DPG)'.

These factors interact to ensure there is adequate uptake of O_2 at the lung and adequate delivery of O_2 to the tissues.

Diphosphoglycerate (DPG)

RBCs do not possess mitochondria, so can only metabolize anaerobically. DPG is a by-product of RBC anaerobic metabolism or glycolysis. DPG rises with raised body temperature, altitude, exercise and in patients with chronic hypoxic lung conditions, e.g. COPD

Hb has a reduced affinity for O_2 where:

- PCO_2 is high (tissues)
- H^+ concentration is high ($\downarrow$pH)
- body temperature is increased
- DPG production is high.

In this situation, the O_2 dissociation curve 'shifts' down and towards the right, meaning that O_2 unloading to supply the tissues and CO_2 loading and removal from the tissues occurs more rapidly, e.g. exercise. This is called the 'Bohr effect'.

Conversely, Hb has an increased affinity for O_2 where:

- PCO_2 is low (lungs)
- H^+ concentration is low ($\uparrow$pH)
- body temperature is decreased
- DPG production is low.

In this situation, the O_2 dissociation curve 'shifts' up and towards the left, meaning that O_2 unloading at the tissues and CO_2 loading and removal from the tissues occurs *less* rapidly.

Carbon Dioxide Transport

Following diffusion across the capillary membrane, 20–30% of CO_2 is carried by the RBCs; combined with haemoglobin, 7–10% of CO_2 dissolves directly into the plasma ($PaCO_2$) and 60–70% is carried as bicarbonate.

Carbon Dioxide and Haemoglobin

Approximately 20–30% of CO_2 binds to the globin portion of the Hb molecule, forming a carbamino compound called 'carbaminohaemoglobin ($HbCO_2$)'. O_2 binds with the haem portion of the Hb molecule so there is no competition between O_2 and CO_2 for binding sites).

$$CO_2 + Hb \underset{\text{Tissues}}{\overset{\text{Lungs}}{\rightleftharpoons}} HbCO_2$$

Carbon Dioxide as Bicarbonate

Sixty to 70% of CO_2 is carried in the blood as bicarbonate and transported in this form from the tissues to the lungs. CO_2 combines with water to produce carbonic acid, which is an unstable compound that readily dissociates into bicarbonate and a free hydrogen ion. At the lung, the process is reversed to reproduce CO_2 gas and water ready for exhalation.

This conversion involves a series of chemical reactions which take place either in the plasma or in the RBC. In the plasma, the conversion rate is very slow; therefore the majority of CO_2 passes directly into the RBC which contains the enzyme carbonic anhydrase, which catalyses the reaction by 1000 times.

Carriage from Tissue to Lungs

$$CO_2 + H_2O \leftrightarrow H_2CO_3 \leftrightarrow HCO_3 + H^+$$

When there is a high concentration of CO_2 (in the tissues), the equation moves towards the right. When there is a low concentration of CO_2 (in the lungs), the equation moves towards the left and CO_2 and H_2O are excreted in the expired air.

The efficiency with which oxygen is transported from the atmosphere along the steps of the oxygen transport pathway to the tissues determines the efficiency of oxygen transport overall. The steps in the oxygen transport pathway include ventilation of the alveoli, diffusion of oxygen across the alveolar capillary membrane, perfusion of the lungs, biochemical reaction of oxygen with the blood, affinity of oxygen with haemoglobin, cardiac output (CO), integrity of the peripheral circulation and oxygen extraction at the tissue level (Wasserman et al 2011). At rest, the demand for oxygen reflects basal metabolic requirements. Metabolic demand changes normally in response to gravitational (positional), exercise and psychological stressors. When one or more steps in the oxygen transport pathway are impaired secondary to cardiopulmonary dysfunction, oxygen demand at rest and in response to stressors can be increased significantly. Impairment of one step in the pathway may be compensated by other steps, thereby maintaining normal gas exchange and arterial oxygenation. With severe impairment involving several steps, arterial oxygenation may be reduced, the work of the heart and lungs increased, tissue oxygenation impaired and, in the most extreme situation, multiorgan system failure may ensue.

While the oxygen transport pathway ensures that an adequate supply of oxygen meets the demands of the working tissues, the carbon dioxide pathway ensures that carbon dioxide, a primary by-product of metabolism, is eliminated. This pathway is basically the reverse of the oxygen transport pathway in that carbon dioxide is transported from the tissues, via the circulation, to the lungs for elimination. Carbon dioxide is a highly diffusible gas and is readily eliminated from the body. However, carbon dioxide retention is a hallmark of diseases in which the ventilatory muscle pump is operating inefficiently or the normal elastic recoil of the lung parenchyma is lost.

THE EFFECT OF GROWTH AND AGEING ON RESPIRATION

The embryological development of the lung can be divided into four stages (Inselman & Mellins 1981):

- embryonic period (gestational weeks 3–5)
- pseudoglandular period (gestational weeks 6–16)
- canalicular period (gestational weeks 17–24)
- alveolar sac period (gestational week 24–term).

Embryonic Period (Weeks 3–5)

The lung bud starts as an endodermal outgrowth of fetal foregut. The single tube thus formed soon branches into two, forming the major bronchi. By cell division, the process of growth continues until, at the end of this period, the major lung branches are formed.

Pseudoglandular Period (Weeks 6–16)

During this period the airways grow by dichotomous branching so that by week 16 all generations of the airway from trachea to terminal bronchioles (i.e. the preacinus) are formed. During this period the pulmonary circulation also develops, cartilage and lymphatic formation occur and cilia appear (week 10 onwards) (Langman 1977).

Canalicular Period (Weeks 17–24)

The respiratory bronchioles, alveolar ducts and alveoli (i.e. the acinus) start to develop during this time, simultaneously with the lung capillaries, thus preparing the lungs for their future role in gas exchange (Hislop & Reid 1974). The air–blood barrier first appears at week 19 and towards the end of this period, surfactant synthesis begins.

Terminal Sac Period (Week 24–Term)

Development of the pulmonary circulation continues and the respiratory bronchioles subdivide to form air spaces. Two different cell types (types I and II pneumocytes) line the air spaces. Type I pneumocytes flatten and elongate to cover the majority of the surface area of the saccular air spaces. Type II cells only occupy approximately 2% of the surface and are responsible for surfactant synthesis and storage (Greenough 1996). Surfactant is a phospholipid, which stabilizes surface tension in the alveolus and prevents alveolar collapse on expiration. Small quantities of surfactant are present at weeks 23–24 of gestation and the amount present gradually increases until a surge at about week 30. Birth itself and the onset of respiration stimulate further surfactant production.

Towards the end of the terminal sac period, the air spaces have developed into primitive multilocular alveoli. After birth, alveoli increase in size and number. The average number of alveoli in the newborn is 150 million. By the age of 3–4 years, the adult number of 300–400 million alveoli has been reached, but alveolar growth continues for the first 7 years (Hislop et al 1986). More recent estimations of mean alveolar number in adulthood have been 480 million (range 274–790 million), with alveolar number closely related to lung volume (Ochs et al 2004).

The most obvious differences between children and adults lie in the development of airway function. The airways develop faster than the alveoli, which may not reach maturity until about the seventh year. As the lung matrix develops, the airway walls remain strong and relatively patent. As a result, expiratory flow rates, although lower than in adulthood, are relatively high. In addition to airway patency, there are also developments in the behaviour of the chest wall with growth. In childhood, the musculoskeletal structures are immature and flexible. Rib cage distortion is often seen in childhood during illness, but disappears with growth and muscularization. The combination of airway patency and plasticity of the chest wall allows an interesting experiment. In childhood the RV is not determined by airway closure but by the strength of the expiratory muscles. Thus if children or young adults are hugged at the end of a forced expiration, more air can be expelled. After the age of 25 years, RV is determined by premature airway closure and the lungs cannot be emptied further.

The respiratory system reaches its peak in the third decade of life. Development of the lung continues from birth until the end of adolescence and starts to deteriorate after the age of 25 years. In the absence of disease there is sufficient reserve capacity to accommodate the requirements of old age.

After 25 years, the tissues become less elastic and the lung elastic recoil diminishes. Exercise capacity, as judged by oxygen consumption, shows a decline with age but it can be retarded by regular activity and accelerated by smoking or disease.

RESPIRATORY SYSTEM: ANATOMICAL AND PHYSIOLOGICAL DIFFERENCES BETWEEN CHILDREN AND ADULTS

The respiratory system in children differs significantly from adults, both anatomically and physiologically. These differences have important consequences for the physiotherapy care of children in terms of respiratory assessment, treatment and choice of techniques. Whereas the main reason for adult hospital emergency admissions is cardiac failure, the principal reason for hospital admissions in children aged 0–4 years is respiratory illness. The principles of adult cardiorespiratory physiotherapy management cannot be transposed directly to an infant with pulmonary pathology.

Anatomical Differences in the Respiratory System between Children and Adults

Rib Cage and Chest Shape

The cross-sectional shape of the infant thorax is cylindrical and not elliptical as in adolescents or adults. The ribs of the newborn infant are relatively soft and cartilaginous compared with the more rigid chest wall of older children and adults. They are also placed horizontally in relation to the sternum and vertebral column compared with the more oblique rib angle of adults. The bucket handle rib movement seen in older children and adults is therefore not possible. As the infant grows, and begins to develop an upright posture, the ribs develop a more oblique angle and the transverse diameter of the rib cage increases. The adult chest shape is achieved by 3 years of age (Openshaw et al 1984).

The intercostal muscles are poorly developed in infancy and contraction of the intercostal muscles is inefficient at improving thoracic volumes either by increasing the anteroposterior or transverse diameters

of the chest. Increased ventilatory requirements have to be met by increasing the respiratory rate rather than depth (Konno & Mead 1967).

Diaphragm

The angle of insertion of the infant diaphragm is horizontal compared with older children or adults, placing it at a mechanical disadvantage. The infant diaphragm has a lower relative muscle mass and a lower content of high-endurance muscle fibres, and thus is much more vulnerable to fatigue.

Maximal diaphragmatic activity during severe respiratory distress or respiratory obstruction leads to an inward movement of the lower rib cage instead of a downward movement of the diaphragm, as well as intercostal and sternal recession (Muller & Bryan 1979). Despite these disadvantages, the diaphragm is the main muscle of inspiration in the infant, since the intercostals are poorly developed. Ventilation in the infant is also more affected by impaired diaphragmatic function, for example by abdominal distension, hepatomegaly or phrenic nerve damage.

Preferential Nasal Breathing

The shape and orientation of head and neck in babies (large head, prominent occiput, short neck, large tongue, smaller retracted lower jaw, high larynx) mean that the airway is prone to obstruction in young infants. Young infants up to about 6 months of age are preferential nasal breathers and studies suggest that up to half of all neonates are unable to breathe through their mouths, except when crying, for the first few weeks of life (King & Booker 2004). The small nasal passages account for between 30% and 50% of the total airway resistance in neonates. The narrowest portion of the nasal airway has a cross-sectional area of about 20 mm^2. Therefore even a small amount of swelling or obstruction of the nasal passages of infants compromises breathing considerably and causes a disproportionate and detrimental effect on the work of breathing. Some young infants with upper respiratory tract infections and partial obstruction of their nasal passages can develop respiratory distress.

Position of Larynx

In the newborn infant, the larynx and hyoid cartilage are higher in the neck and closer to the base of the epiglottis, being at the level of C3 in a premature infant and C4 in a child compared with C5–C6 in the adult. The larynx descends with age, but its high position enables the infant to feed and breathe simultaneously for approximately the first 4 months of age.

This high position also provides some protection of the airway in infants younger than 4–6 months because it acts as a valve, which helps keep food in the mouth until the pharyngeal swallow is initiated. The airway has less anatomical protection, as the larynx assumes its lower position in the neck and is not as directly protected by the epiglottis. Then, poor closure of the airway or partial paralysis of the vocal folds may become more evident and coughing, choking or aspiration may occur.

Airway Diameter

The neonatal trachea is short (4–9 cm) and directed downward and posteriorly. The diameter of the trachea in the newborn is 4–5 mm and the diameter of an infant trachea is only about one-third that of an adult. This makes respiratory resistance higher and the work of breathing greater. Since the resistance to airflow through a tube is directly related to the tube length and inversely related to the fourth power of the radius of the tube, halving the radius of the trachea will increase its resistance (reduce flow) 16 times. Tracheal swelling as a result of endotracheal intubation or suction can therefore dramatically increase resistance to breathing. These factors give the lungs less reserve, so that a well-oxygenated infant with upper airway obstruction can become cyanotic in a matter of seconds.

In contrast to adolescents and adults, the narrowest part of the infant's airway is not the vocal cords, but the cricoid ring. Thus an uncuffed endotracheal tube provides a larger internal diameter compared with a cuffed tube and in children will successfully seal against in the circular subglottic ring. However, the inflexible cricoid ring also leaves children more vulnerable to mucosal oedema and post-extubation stridor. The right main bronchus is less angled than the left, making right mainstem intubation more likely.

At birth there is no further increase in the number of airways formed, but there is growth and development in their size. In the first few years of life, there is a significant increase in the diameter of the larger, more proximal airways (Hislop & Reid 1974). The smaller, more distal airways do not increase in diameter until nearer 5 years of age. This higher peripheral airways resistance is exacerbated by respiratory infections, which cause inflammation of the airways, for example in bronchiolitis, or in the presence of secretions.

Bronchial Walls

The bronchial walls are supported by cartilage, which begins to develop from 12 weeks' gestation and continues throughout childhood. The cartilaginous support of an infant's airways is much thinner than that of an adult, and predisposes the airways to collapse. However the bronchial walls contain proportionally more cartilage, connective tissue and mucous glands than do those of adults, but less smooth muscle; this makes the lung tissue less compliant. The lack of bronchial smooth muscle, particularly in the smaller bronchioles, may be one reason for the lack of response to bronchodilators under the age of 12 months. The β-receptors in infants are also immature, which further reduces any response to β-adrenergic bronchodilator therapy (Reid 1984). The high proportion of mucous glands in the major bronchi of infants makes the airways more susceptible to mucus obstruction.

Cilia

At birth the cilia are poorly developed, which increases the risk of secretion retention, especially in the premature infant. The airway obstruction caused by secretions in a neonate is much greater than in an adult whose airways are relatively large.

Alveoli and Surfactant

The respiratory system is not fully developed at birth, even in the term neonate, and postnatal maturation continues for a significant time. Although by 20–27 weeks' gestation lung acinar have formed, several types of epithelial cells can be differentiated, and the air–blood barrier is thin enough to support gas exchange; true alveoli develop only after about 36 weeks' gestation. A term newborn has an average of 150 million alveoli. The remainder of the eventual average of 400 million alveoli develop after birth, the vast majority within the first 2 years of life. Both the number and size of alveoli continue to increase postnatally until the chest wall stops growing. By 4 years of age, the adult number of 300 million may exist, although growth can continue until 7 years of age. The smaller alveolar size of an infant makes the infant more susceptible to alveolar collapse, and the smaller number of alveoli reduces the area available for gaseous exchange (Reid 1984).

Pulmonary surfactant is a mixture of phospholipids (90%) and apoproteins (10%), which act to reduce surface tension at the air–liquid interface in the alveolus, thereby preventing collapse of lung parenchyma at the end of expiration. Type II alveolar cells synthesize and secrete surfactant from 23 to 24 weeks' gestation. In preterm newborns, a deficiency of surfactant is a major factor in the development of neonatal respiratory distress syndrome (RDS). Male gender is a risk factor for neonatal RDS, bronchopulmonary dysplasia (BPD) and mortality. Boys with neonatal RDS seem to have more health problems than girls during the neonatal period.

Collateral Ventilation

Collateral ventilation is the means by which a distal lung unit can be ventilated, despite blockage of its main airway. Collateral ventilatory pathways are achieved by a network of interconnecting pathways linking different structures. Respiratory bronchioles are linked by channels of Martin. Canals of Lambert connect respiratory and terminal bronchioles with alveoli and their ducts; and adjacent alveoli are joined by openings in the alveolar wall, called 'pores of Kohn' (Menkes & Traystman 1977). However, none of these pathways exists at birth. The pores of Kohn develop between years 1 and 2, and the canals of Lambert do not appear until about 6 years of age. The collateral ventilatory channels between alveoli, respiratory bronchioles and terminal bronchioles are poorly developed until 2–3 years of age, predisposing towards alveolar collapse.

Internal Organs and Lymphatic Tissue

The lymphatic tissue (adenoids and tonsils) may be enlarged in the infant and the tongue is also relatively large. These factors may contribute to upper airway obstruction. The heart and other organs are also relatively large in infants, leaving less space for lung expansion. The heart can occupy up to half the transverse diameter of the chest in chest radiographs (Fig. 1-19).

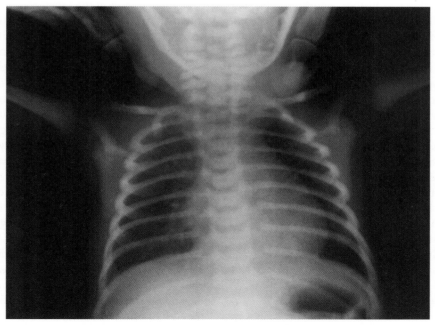

FIGURE 1-19 ■ Normal chest radiograph in a newborn.

Height and Exposure to Air Pollution

Because children breathe more rapidly compared with adults and because they spend more time outdoors being physically active, they tend to be more exposed to outdoor air pollution and allergens than do adults and have greater deposition of particulate matter. Their reduced height means they are also more exposed to vehicle exhausts and heavier pollutants that concentrate at lower levels in the air. There is substantial evidence linking air pollution with respiratory health problems and children are more vulnerable (Brauer et al 2007, Pénard-Morand et al 2005).

Physiological Differences in the Respiratory System between Children and Adults

Respiratory Compliance

Respiratory compliance is a measure of the pressure required to increase the volume of air in the lungs and reflects a combination of lung and chest wall compliance. The lung compliance of a child is comparable to that of an adult, being directly proportional to the child's size. However, compliance is reduced in the infant because of the high proportion of cartilage in the airways. The premature infant, who lacks surfactant, demonstrates a further significant decrease in compliance. The chest wall of an infant is cartilaginous and therefore very soft and compliant in comparison with the more calcified and rigid adult structure. The intercostal muscles are also less well equipped to stabilize the rib cage during diaphragmatic contraction. Neonates therefore have an imbalance between a relatively low outward recoil of their chest wall and normal inward elastic recoil, which means that they are prone to airway collapse. An awake, spontaneously breathing neonate will maintain its FRC by active measures including laryngeal braking, the initiation of inspiration before the end of passive expiration (intrinsic PEEP) and persistent inspiratory muscle activity throughout the respiratory cycle. These active mechanisms are lost during anaesthesia and result in a fall in FRC, airway closure, atelectasis and $\dot{V}/\dot{Q}$ mismatch.

Closing Volume

The closing volume is the lung volume at which closure of the small airways occurs. This volume plus the RV (the volume of gas left in the lungs following maximum expiration) is known as the CC. In the adult, CC usually occurs within FRC, i.e. the volume of gas left in the lungs following tidal expiration, whereas in the infant it is greater than FRC and can occur during tidal breathing. The higher closing volumes apparent in infants are due to greater chest wall compliance and reduced elastic recoil of the lungs than in the adult. Therefore airway closure may occur before the end of expiration, e.g. during expiratory chest vibrations, putting the infant at a much greater risk of developing widespread atelectasis, especially in the presence of lung disease, where lung volume is further reduced. In the event of respiratory distress, the infant grunts on expiration, adducting the vocal cords in an attempt to reduce the amount of gas expired, thus maintaining a higher FRC and minimizing alveolar collapse (Pang & Mellins 1975). Re-inflation of alveoli, once collapsed, is more difficult in the infant, who has to work considerably harder to overcome the effects of the compliant chest wall.

Ventilation and Perfusion

In the adult, both ventilation and perfusion are preferentially distributed to the dependent lung. The best gas exchange and $\dot{V}/\dot{Q}$ match will therefore be in the dependent region of the lung (Zack et al 1974). In the infant, however, ventilation is preferentially distributed to the uppermost lung (Davies et al 1985), whereas the perfusion remains best in the dependent regions. This leads to greater gas exchange in the uppermost lung (Heaf et al 1983), but an imbalance between ventilation and perfusion (Bhuyan et al 1989). In acutely ill children with unilateral lung disease, oxygenation may be optimized by placing the 'good' lung uppermost. However, this is contrary to the goal of improving ventilation to the diseased lung and facilitating secretion clearance, in which positioning and postural drainage would require the diseased lung to be uppermost. The therapist would have to balance their decision based on the stability, tolerance and current therapeutic priorities.

The difference in ventilation distribution between infants and adults is most likely due to the more compliant rib cage of the infant, which compresses the dependent areas of lung. In addition, while in the adult the weight of the abdominal contents provides a preferential load on the dependent diaphragm and therefore improves its contractility, in the infant this does not happen. The effect on both hemidiaphragms is similar, due to the abdomen being so much smaller and narrower (Davies et al 1985). It has been shown in adults that, when the diaphragm is inactivated, e.g. when ventilated under anaesthetic, the ventilation distribution changes to that of an infant (Rehder et al 1972). It is not yet known exactly when the ventilation distribution in the infant changes to that of an adult, but it is likely to be variable and dependent on lung health and musculoskeletal maturity.

Oxygen Consumption, Cardiac Output and Response to Hypoxia

Infants have a higher resting metabolic rate than adults and consequently have a higher oxygen requirement. Children have a higher SV and oxygen consumption per kilogram than adults; in infants this may exceed 6 mL/kg min^{-1}, twice that of adults. They support this higher output with a higher baseline heart rate (HR) but lower blood pressure than adults.

Neonatal myocardium has a large supply of mitochondria, nuclei and endoplasmic reticulum to support cell growth and protein synthesis, but these are non-contractile tissues, which render the myocardium stiff and non-compliant. This may impair filling of the left ventricle and limit the ability to increase the SV by increasing stroke volume (SV) (Frank Starling mechanism). SV in infants is therefore relatively fixed and the only way of increasing SV is by increasing HR.

The SNS is not well developed, predisposing the neonatal heart to bradycardia. An infant responds to hypoxia with bradycardia and pulmonary vasoconstriction, whereas the adult becomes tachycardic with systemic vasodilatation. The bradycardic response in infants is probably due to myocardial hypoxia and acidosis, but leads to an immediate reduction in SV and the development of further hypoxia.

Although anatomical closure of the foramen ovale can occur as early as 3 months of age, the channel remains 'probe patent' in 50% of children up to 5 years of age, and persists in about 30% of adults. Similarly, anatomical closure of the ductus arteriosus usually occurs between 4 and 8 weeks of age. Any stimulus, such as hypoxia or acidosis, that causes an increase in pulmonary vascular resistance during the neonatal period may allow these two potential channels to reopen, resulting in right-to-left shunting and increasing hypoxia (King & Booker 2004).

Muscle Fatigue

The respiratory muscles of infants tire more quickly than those of adults due to a much smaller proportion of fatigue-resistant muscle fibre (Keens & Ianuzzo 1979). There are two main muscle fibre types, type I and type II. Type I muscle fibres are slow twitch, high oxidative and slow to fatigue. Type II fibres are fast twitch, slow oxidative and tire quickly. Of the muscle fibres in the adult diaphragm, 55% are type I compared with only 30% in the infant. Premature infants tire even more easily as, at 24 weeks' gestation, only 10% of their muscle fibres are fatigue resistant (Muller & Bryan 1979). Excessive muscle fatigue results in apnoea. By 12 months of age the number of type I fibres equals that of an adult.

Breathing Pattern and Rapid Eye Movement Sleep

Irregular breathing patterns and episodes of apnoea are relatively common in neonates, especially if premature, and are related to immature cardiorespiratory control. Short spells of apnoea can be considered normal in these circumstances, but need careful monitoring as they may reflect hypoxic conditions.

During rapid eye movement (REM) sleep there is a reduction in postural tone and tonic inhibition of the infant's intercostal muscles such that the rib cage is even less well equipped to counteract the contraction of the diaphragm during inspiration (Muller & Bryan 1979). This reduces the efficiency of respiration, causes a drop in FRC and increases the work of breathing, predisposing the infant to apnoeic episodes (Muller & Bryan 1979). The premature infant is most at risk, spending up to 20 hours a day asleep, 80% of which may be in active REM sleep compared with 20% in adult sleep.

Response to Cold

Paediatric patients have an increased surface area per kilogram of body weight and lose heat to the environment more readily than adults. This is compounded by cold intravenous fluids, dry anaesthetic gases and exposure. Non-shivering thermogenesis in brown adipose tissue is the major mechanism of heat production during the first few months of life. Brown fat is specialized tissue located in the posterior of the neck, along the interscapular and vertebral areas, and surrounding the kidneys and adrenal glands. Metabolic heat production can increase up to two and a half times during cold stress. Shivering is a less economical form of heat production but does occur in severely hypothermic neonates. Hypothermia is a serious problem that can result in increased oxygen consumption, cardiac irritability and respiratory depression (King & Booker 2004).

INTRODUCTION TO CARDIAC ANATOMY AND PHYSIOLOGY

The heart is a roughly cone-shaped organ which is about the size of a fist. It lies diagonally between the lungs in the mediastinum, so that the wider upper portion (base) of the heart points towards the right shoulder and the lower tip of the heart (apex) points towards the left hip and rests on the diaphragm. The major blood vessels of the body emerge from the base.

The heart pumps blood around the body in order to provide cells with the oxygen and nutrients that are required for metabolism. The right side of the heart receives deoxygenated blood from the body and pumps it through the lungs in order for gas exchange to take place. The left side of the heart receives oxygenated blood from the lungs and pumps it around the body. Blood vessels that take blood away from the heart are called 'arteries' and blood vessels that bring blood back to the heart are called 'veins' (Fig. 1-20).

The heart has four chambers: the right and left atria superiorly and the right and left ventricles inferiorly. The atria are the receiving chambers of the heart and the larger ventricles are the pumping chambers.

In healthy individuals, blood cannot mix between the right and left sides of the heart. This is due to the presence of a dividing wall between the two atria (interatrial septum) and the two ventricles (interventricular septum).

The right atrium receives deoxygenated blood from the body via the superior and inferior vena cava. The blood then passes through the right tricuspid (or atrioventricular (AV)) valve into the right ventricle. It then passes through the pulmonary valve into the pulmonary artery and lungs (pulmonary circulation).

The left atrium receives oxygenated blood from the lungs via the pulmonary veins. Blood then passes through the left AV (or mitral) valve into the left ventricle. It then goes through the aortic valve into the aorta to be circulated around the body (systemic circulation).

The atria are much smaller and thinner walled then the ventricles. This is because the atria only have to squeeze blood into the adjoining ventricle, whereas the ventricles have to pump blood through the lungs (right ventricle) or around the body (left ventricle). The left ventricle is thicker walled than the right ventricle as it has to be more powerful in order to pump blood around the systemic circulation.

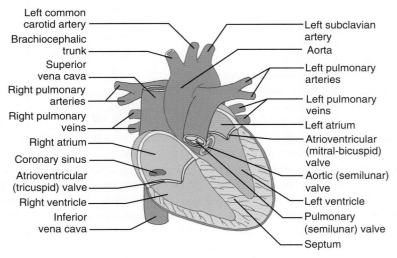

FIGURE 1-20 ■ Internal view of the heart.

Layers of the Heart Wall

The heart is surrounded by a double walled sac called the pericardium. The outer layer of the pericardium is made up of tough fibrous connective tissue and is called the fibrous pericardium. This protects the heart, prevents overfilling and anchors it to surrounding structures including the central tendon of the diaphragm. This attachment to the diaphragm explains why hyperinflated lungs and a flattened diaphragm will result in a thin, elongated heart on chest radiograph. The inner layer of the pericardium is the serous pericardium, which consists of two layers: the parietal pericardium and the visceral pericardium. The parietal pericardium lines the internal surface of the fibrous pericardium. The visceral pericardium is fused to the external layer of the heart wall, and is also known as the epicardium. There is a potential space between the parietal and visceral layers of the serous pericardium and this is called the 'pericardial cavity'. This cavity contains serous pericardial fluid which lubricates and creates a frictionless environment. It allows the parietal and visceral pericardial membranes to glide over one another as the heart beats. An increase in pericardial fluid will compress the heart and impair its ability to pump (cardiac tamponade).

The heart wall is made up of three layers: the epicardium, the myocardium and the endocardium. The epicardium is the outer layer and is the visceral pericardium. The bulkier myocardium is the middle layer and is mostly composed of cardiac muscle. The endocardium makes up the inner lining of the heart.

Heart Valves

Heart valves ensure that blood flows in one direction (from atria to ventricles to arteries). The heart valves open and close as a result of pressure differences on either side of the valve. When pressure is greater behind the valve, the leaflets open and blood flows through the valve. When pressure is greater in front of the valve, the leaflets shut.

The right AV valve has three leaflets or cusps and is called the tricuspid valve (remember that the tRIcuspid valve is on the RIght). The left AV valve has two cusps and is a bicuspid valve. It is also known as the mitral valve because it resembles the shape of a bishop's mitre. When the ventricles contract the valves shut preventing backflow (regurgitation) into the atria.

The pulmonary and aortic valves sit at the bases of the pulmonary artery and aorta, respectively. They are called 'semilunar valves (half moon)', as they each have three crescent shaped cusps. They prevent backflow from the great arteries into the ventricles.

Coronary Circulation

The blood supply to the heart is provided by the coronary arteries. The right and left coronary arteries arise from the base of the aorta. The left coronary has two main branches, which are the left anterior descending artery and the circumflex artery. The right coronary artery's main branches are the right marginal artery and the posterior descending artery (Fig. 1-21).

The coronary arteries are superficial as they are located in the epicardium, before sending branches deeper into the myocardium. This means they are relatively easily isolated for coronary artery bypass graft surgery. Blood flow to the myocardium occurs when the heart is relaxed as the blood vessels within the myocardium become compressed when the heart is contracting.

The coronary veins empty deoxygenated blood into the coronary sinus, which is located in the right atrium.

Cardiac Cycle

When the heart contracts it is termed 'systole' and when it relaxes it is termed 'diastole'. Both atria fill and contract together and both ventricles fill and contract together in sequence. The cardiac cycle refers to the mechanical events that occur with the flow of blood through the heart in one heartbeat. These mechanical events are preceded by electrical activity discussed below.

Early diastole: The whole heart is relaxed and the pulmonary and aortic valves are shut. The AV valves (tricuspid and mitral) are open and blood is flowing passively from the great veins (superior and inferior vena cavae and the pulmonary vein) through the atria into the ventricles.

Atrial systole: Following atrial depolarization (P wave), the atria contract forcing blood into the ventricles. This maximizes the volume of blood in the ventricles (end-diastolic volume). The atria now relax.

Isovolumetric contraction: Following ventricular depolarization (QRS complex) the ventricles contract causing ventricular pressure to rise and the AV valves

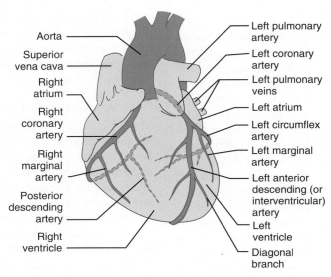

Aorta

Superior vena cava

Right atrium

Right coronary artery

Right marginal artery

Posterior descending artery

Right ventricle

Left pulmonary artery

Left coronary artery

Left pulmonary veins

Left atrium

Left circumflex artery

Left marginal artery

Left anterior descending (or interventricular) artery

Left ventricle

Diagonal branch

FIGURE 1-21 ■ Arterial blood supply to cardiac muscle.

to shut. The aortic and pulmonary valves are still shut at this point, so this contraction does not bring about any change in volume.

Ventricular ejection: As the pressure in the ventricles continues to rise, the aortic and pulmonary valves are forced open and blood is rapidly ejected into the great arteries (pulmonary artery and aorta). While the ventricles are in systole, the atria are in diastole and filling with blood.

Isovolumetric relaxation: Following ventricular repolarization (T wave), the ventricles relax and ventricular pressure drops. Blood in the aorta and pulmonary artery starts to flow back towards the heart causing the aortic and pulmonary valves to shut.

As the atria continue to fill, pressure on the atrial side of the AV valves will become greater than on the ventricular side and so the AV valves will open allowing ventricular filling to begin once more.

Heart Sounds

The heart sounds heard on auscultation are commonly termed 'lub dup'. This relates to the sound of the heart valves closing. The first sound (lub) is the sound of the AV valves closing. The second sound (dup) is created by the closing of the semilunar valves (pulmonary and aortic valves).

Electrical Conductivity of the Heart

The heart's muscle is made of specialized tissue and its ability to pump is controlled by an electrical conduction system that synchronizes the contraction of the heart chambers (Fig. 1-22). This ensures coordinated blood flow through the cardiac cycle to provide sufficient SV to maintain blood pressure and oxygen delivery to the body (Levick 2010).

An electrical stimulus is generated by the sino-atrial (SA) node or 'cardiac pacemaker'. This is a collection of specialized tissue located in the right atrium that spontaneously generates an electrical stimulus 60–100 times per minute. The wave of electrical activity generated by the SA node spreads through the right and left atria at a rate of 0.5 m/sec, initiating depolarization and contraction of both atria, which pushes blood through the open valves in to the corresponding ventricles

■ right atrium via tricuspid valve to right ventricle
■ left atrium via bicuspid (mitral) valve to left ventricle.

The electrical impulse travels to the AV node, where it is slowed down to 0.05 m/sec (AV delay) to allow sufficient time for atrial contraction and ventricular

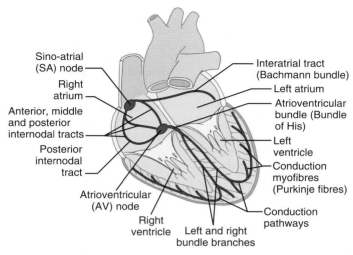

FIGURE 1-22 ■ Electrical conductivity of the heart.

filling. The electrical impulse then continues via the right and left bundle of His and Purkinje fibres, which cause ventricular depolarization and contraction.

■ Contraction of the right ventricle pushes blood through the pulmonary valve through the lungs for gas exchange.
■ Contraction of the left ventricle pushes blood through the aortic valve into the systemic circulation.

Each contraction of the ventricles represents one heartbeat. The atria contract a fraction of a second before the ventricles so their blood empties into the ventricles before the ventricles contract.

Electrical Conductivity and Electrocardiogram (ECG)

The electrical conduction system of the heart can be graphically represented on an ECG trace. The characteristic 'P-QRS-T' complex represents depolarization, contraction and repolarization of the atria and ventricles (Fig. 1-23).

The P wave indicates that the atria are electrically stimulated (depolarized) to pump blood into the ventricles. The first part of the P wave is flat and represents electrical impulse generation by the SA node. As both atria depolarize and subsequently contract, a peak is visible in the P-wave complex. The duration of the

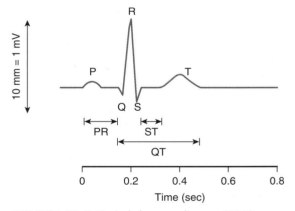

FIGURE 1-23 ■ Typical electrocardiogram (ECG) trace.

P wave should not exceed 0.08 sec. An abnormally wide P wave may be indicative of left atrial hypertrophy, as it would take a longer period of time for the impulse to travel through the larger atrial wall. The last part of the P wave is also flat, as the electrical impulse is held at the AV node. Following AV delay, the spread of electrical activity through both ventricles produces depolarization and contraction of the ventricles represented by the QRS complex.

'PR interval' refers to the time taken for atrial depolarization and AV delay. A normal duration of PR interval is 0.12–0.20 seconds. In situations where AV delay is increased, such as heart block, the PR interval may be lengthened. Conversely, PR interval may be shortened in situations where an impulse may arise from the AV node itself, such as Wolff-Parkinson-White syndrome.

The QRS complex indicates that the ventricles are electrically stimulated (depolarized) to pump blood out. Note the increased size of the peak in the QRS complex, indicating a greater muscle mass and therefore, an increased force of contraction from the ventricular myocardium compared to the relatively smaller atria. The QRS complex should not exceed 0.12 seconds; a longer duration is indicative of abnormal conductivity in the ventricles.

The ST segment indicates the amount of time from the end of the contraction of the ventricles to the beginning of the T wave. The ST segment is displaced or depressed in the presence of ischaemia and can become elevated following a myocardial infarction (MI). ECG changes may vary slightly depending on the exact location of the MI.

T wave: As the ventricles relax and repolarization takes place the T-wave can be seen. The T wave may become inverted in the presence of ischaemia.

An electrical impulse initiated at the SA node, which passes sequentially through the cardiac conducting system is described as 'sinus rhythm'.

Autonomic Regulation of Heart Rate

The ANS regulates the electrical conductivity of the heart, adjusting HR in response to various stimuli. The two branches of the ANS, the SNS (adrenergic system) and the PNS (cholinergic system) work reciprocally, meaning that as discharge from one branch increases, discharge from the other decreases.

Increased SNS activity will:

- increase HR via direct stimulation to the SA node (chronotropy) or the AV node (dromotropy or conduction velocity) and the myocardium
- release catecholamines, adrenaline and noradrenaline, and will increase HR.

Increased PNS activity will:

- decrease HR via direct stimulation (vagus nerve) to the SA and AV nodes and the myocardium.
- release of acetylcholine will decrease HR.

Physical factors such as level of physical activity and core body temperature will lead to a change in HR, secondary to ANS activation.

Blood Pressure

Blood pressure (BP) is defined as the pressure exerted by blood against the tunica interna (inner wall) of an artery. This pressure ensures that blood flows through the body between heart beats and provides adequate perfusion to maintain oxygen delivery.

Blood pressure is maintained via several physiological variables.

- HR: beats per minute
- SV: the volume of blood ejected from a ventricle per contraction
  - CO: the amount of blood ejected from a ventricle per minute (SV × HR)
- Total peripheral resistance (TPR): friction encountered by blood as it passes through a peripheral artery.

Blood pressure can be represented by the following equation:

$$BP = SV \times HR(CO) \times TPR$$

Therefore a change in any of the contributing physiological variables will lead to a change in BP.

Stroke Volume

In an average human heart, SV is approximately 70 mL/beat. When greater SV is required (e.g. during exercise, stress or with increased core body temperature), SV can be increased by three methods:

- Increased venous return (VR) (Frank Starling's law)
  - Frank Starling's law states that SV increases in response to an increase in the volume of blood filling the heart.
  - Increased blood filling produces a stretch to the cardiac muscle fibres producing an enhanced force of contraction.
  - Increased blood filling occurs with increased VR.
  - During exercise, increased activity of the skeletal muscle squeezes blood vessels and increases VR (pre-load).

- Negative pressure generated by the respiratory muscles aids VR by 'drawing' blood towards the heart from the lower limbs.
- VR is also increased via SNS stimulation, causing a small degree of vasoconstriction.
- Increased VR = increased volume of blood filling the heart and increased SV.
- Reduced after-load
  - After load is the pressure the ventricle must overcome to eject blood.
  - After-load for the right ventricle is the pressure in the pulmonary circulation (pulmonary artery pressure) and for the left ventricle is pressure in the aorta (systemic BP).
  - Additionally, if after-load is reduced (i.e. vasodilatation), for any given volume of blood in a ventricle, more SV can be ejected.
- Increased contractility of the ventricle (inotropy)
  - Cardiac muscle has the ability to increase the force of its contraction irrespective of the volume of blood filling; this is called' inotropy'.
  - Inotropy occurs secondary to SNS activation and SNS-induced release of catecholamines (from adrenal medulla), directly affecting the muscle fibres of the myocardium.
  - SNS activation also leads to an increased release of calcium ions (Ca^+), in a process called 'calcium-induced calcium release (CICR)'. CICR leads to increased cross-bridge formation and therefore, an enhanced force of contraction and increased SV.

Total Peripheral Resistance

In health, TPR is held in a mild state of vasoconstriction; from this baseline, TPR can be increased secondary to vasoconstriction or decreased secondary to vasodilatation of blood vessels to ensure BP is adequate to maintain homoeostasis. TPR alteration *predominantly* occurs via SNS activation, controlled by the vasomotor centre in the medulla oblongata in the brainstem.

Renal System

The renal system has an important role in the regulation of TPR and BP as a whole (see Auto Regulation of Blood Pressure). When BP is low, the kidneys release an enzyme called 'renin' into the blood. The presence of renin leads to a cascade of chemical reactions which convert the inert 'angiotensin I' to 'angiotensin II'. Angiotensin II is a potent vasoconstrictor, which when activated leads to an increase in TPR and subsequently, an increase in BP. Additionally, angiotensin I also stimulates the adrenal cortex to release a substance called 'aldosterone'. Aldosterone is a steroid hormone released from the adrenal cortex, which increases sodium ion (Na^+) reabsorption and potassium (K^+) excretion by the kidneys; the presence of increased blood Na^+ concentration leads to increased movement of water (via osmosis), increasing blood volume and therefore, VR and pre-load. Increased blood volume improves contractility via Frank Starling's law of the heart.

Other factors which influence TPR are:

- temperature
  - When the body's core temperature is reduced peripheral vasoconstriction may occur. Conversely, an increased core temperature leads to vasodilatation.
- chemicals
  - Substances such as nicotine (vasoconstriction, increased BP) and alcohol (vasodilatation, decreased BP) have an effect on the calibre of blood vessels and therefore BP.
- diet
  - In general, a diet high in salt, saturated fat and cholesterol adversely affects blood vessel calibre (narrows) and blood volume (increases), leading to increased BP.

Auto Regulation of Blood Pressure

BP is monitored and regulated by pressure receptors called 'baroreceptors', which are located in pressure receptor zones.

- high-pressure zones, e.g. carotid sinuses (bilaterally) and the aortic arch
- low-pressure areas, e.g. the venae cavae, pulmonary veins and both atria.

Baroreceptors send signals to the medulla of the brain stem, where ANS stimulation leads to the adjustment of mean arterial pressure by altering both the force and speed of the heart's contractions, as well as the TPR to maintain homoeostasis.

The renal system aids the long-term regulation of BP by altering TPR and blood volume. If blood volume is low, specialized cells in the hypothalamus are stimulated and trigger the release of antidiuretic hormone (ADH) from the pituitary gland. Release of ADH affects the renal collecting ducts and causes increased reabsorption of water (i.e. less urine is produced) to increase blood volume, VR and pre-load. Conversely, if blood volume is high, the kidneys will excrete more water, producing dilute urine to reduce blood volume, VR and pre-load.

REFERENCES AND FURTHER READING

Bhuyan, U., Peters, A.M., Gordon, I., Helms, P., 1989. Effect of posture on the distribution of pulmonary ventilation and perfusion in children and adults. Thorax 44, 480–484.

Brauer, M., Hoek, G., Smit, H.A., et al., 2007. Air pollution and development of asthma, allergy and infections in a birth cohort. Comment in Eur. Respir. J. 29 (5), 825–826.

Davies, H., Kitchman, R., Gordon, G., Helms, P., 1985. Regional ventilation in infancy: reversal of the adult pattern. NEJM 313, 1627–1628.

Greenough, A., 1996. Lung maturation. In: Greenough, A., Roberton, N.R.C., Milner, A. (Eds.), Neonatal Respiratory Disorders. Arnold, London, pp. 13–26.

Hansell, D.M., Lynch, D.A., Page McAdams, H., Bankier, A.A., 2009. Imaging of Diseases of the Chest, fifth ed. Mosby Elsevier, Philadelphia.

Heaf, D.P., Helms, P., Gordon, I., Turner, H.M., 1983. Postural effects on gas exchange in infants. NEJM 308 (25), 1505–1508.

Hislop, A., Reid, L., 1974. Development of the acinus in the human lung. Thorax 29, 90–94.

Hislop, A., Wigglesworth, J.S., Desai, R., 1986. Alveolar development in the human fetus and infant. Early Hum. Dev. 13, 1–11.

Inselman, L.S., Mellins, R.B., 1981. Growth and development of the lung. J. Pediatr. 98, 1–15.

Keens, T.G., Ianuzzo, C.D., 1979. Development of fatigue-resistant muscle fibers in human ventilatory muscles. Am. Rev. Respir. Dis. 119 (2), 139–141.

King, H., Booker, P.D., 2004. General principles of neonatal anaesthesia. Curr. Anaesth. Crit. Care 15, 302–308.

Konno, K., Mead, J., 1967. Measurement of the separate volume changes of rib cage and abdomen during breathing. J. Appl. Physiol. 22, 407–422.

Langman, J., 1977. Medical Embryology. Williams and Wilkins, Baltimore.

Levick, J.R., 2010. An Introduction to Cardiovascular Physiology, fifth ed. Hodder Arnold, London.

Marieb, Elaine N., Hoehn, Katja, 2013. Human Anatomy and Physiology, ninth ed. Pearson, Harlow, England.

Menkes, H.A., Traystman, R.J., 1977. Collateral ventilation. Am. Rev. Respir. Dis. 116, 287–309.

Muller, N.L., Bryan, A.C., 1979. Chest wall mechanics and respiratory muscles in infants. Pediatr. Clin. North Am. 26 (3), 503–516.

Ochs, M., Nyengaard, J., Jung, A., et al., 2004. Number of alveoli in the human lung. Am. J. Respir. Crit. Care Med. 169, 120–124.

Openshaw, P., Edwards, S., Helms, P., 1984. Changes in rib cage geometry during childhood. Thorax 39, 624–627.

Palastanga, N., Soames, R.W., 2012. Anatomy and Human Movement: Structure and Function: Structure and Function, sixth ed. Churchill Livingstone, London, UK.

Pang, L.M., Mellins, R.B., 1975. Neonatal cardiorespiratory physiology. Anesthesiology 43 (2), 171–196.

Pénard-Morand, C., Charpin, D., Raherison, C., et al., 2005. Long-term exposure to background air pollution related to respiratory and allergic health in schoolchildren. Clin. Exp. Allergy 35 (10), 1279–1287.

Rehder, K., Hatch, D.J., Sessler, A.D., Fowler, W.S., 1972. The function of each lung of anesthetized and paralyzed man during mechanical ventilation. Anesthesiology 37 (1), 16–26.

Reid, L., 1984. Lung growth in health and disease. Br. J. Dis. Chest 78, 113–132.

Shneerson, J., 1988. Disorders of Ventilation. Blackwell Science, Oxford, pp. 78–85.

Wasserman, K., Hansen, J., Sietsema, K., et al., 2011. Principles of exercise testing and interpretation: including pathophysiology and clinical applications. Lippincott Williams and Wilkins, Baltimore.

West, J.B., 2000. Respiratory Physiology: The Essentials, Lippincott. Williams & Wilkins, Philadelphia, p. 37.

Zack, M.B., Pontoppidan, H., Kazemi, H., 1974. The effect of lateral positions on gas exchange in pulmonary disease: a prospective evaluation. Am. Rev. Respir. Dis. 110, 49–55.

2

CLINICAL ASSESSMENT

Adults

AMANDA THOMAS ■ LYNDAL J MAXWELL

Infant and Child

ELEANOR MAIN

The Acutely Ill or Deteriorating Patient

SARAH KEILTY

CHAPTER OUTLINE

ADULTS 48
Introduction 48
Information Gathering 48
Subjective Assessment 48
  Breathlessness 49
  Cough 49
  Sputum 50
  Wheeze 50
  Chest Pain 51
  Incontinence 51
  Other Symptoms 51
  Disease Awareness 51
  Functional Ability 51
Objective Assessment 51
  A = Airway 54
  B = Breathing 55
  C = Circulation 64
  D = Disability 67
  E = Exposure 69
Using the Information from Clinical
Assessment 71
Documentation 71
Evaluating Outcome 73
Conclusion 73

INFANT AND CHILD 74
Introduction 74
Medical Notes 74
  Observation Charts and Investigations 74
Communication 74
  Discussion with the Relevant Carers 75
Physical Examination 75
Clinical Signs 75
Other Relevant Observations 77

THE ACUTELY ILL OR DETERIORATING
PATIENT 77
Introduction 77
Background 77
Assessment Technique 77
  A – Airway 78
  B – Breathing 78
  C – Circulation 79
  D – Disability 79
  E – Exposure 80
Actions and Communication 80
Conclusion 80
References 80

Adults

INTRODUCTION

Clinical assessment is part of the clinical reasoning process and involves identifying problems through the accurate recognition and interpretation of normal and abnormal signs and symptoms within a patient's presentation. Assessment is a process of gathering information about the patient by reviewing medical records, interviewing the patient and completing an objective assessment. Thorough assessment will allow the therapist to prioritize patient problems and establish a measurable baseline for evaluating response to physiotherapy interventions. It is important to recognize that assessment is a continuous process which occurs before, during and after each intervention.

Reliable clinical assessment and measurement should follow a systematic logical sequence to establish a process which is standardized, efficient and therefore repeatable. The components included within the assessment process may vary with the environment in which the patient is being assessed and their clinical need. For example, in the community the assessment process may concentrate on the patient's needs and goals, including functional measurement of exercise ability and quality of life (QOL) scales (see Chapter 6); whereas in the critical care environment the assessment process may concentrate on physiological systems and objective clinical findings alone (see Chapter 9).

The first part of this chapter largely refers to assessment of the adult patient, although much of the information is also relevant to the paediatric population. Specific considerations for the assessment of infants and children and normal values for these populations can be found towards the end of this chapter.

INFORMATION GATHERING

The first component of the clinical assessment relates to gathering relevant information from existing patient documentation. For example, existing documentation may be medical notes, a referral letter or test results such as a chest X-ray report. The following section is based on the patient having a hospital medical record. If there is limited or no existing documentation, the information is acquired during the subjective and objective assessments.

The format of records may differ from hospital to hospital, but will contain the same information. The first part contains the patient's personal details including name, date of birth, address, hospital number and referring doctor. It may also contain the medical diagnosis and reason for referral. Next is usually a medical summary which may include:

- *History of presenting condition (HPC):* A summary of the patient's current problems from the medical subjective assessment.
- *Previous medical history (PMH):* A summary of medical and surgical problems that the patient has had in the past. It may be written in disease-specific groupings or as a chronological account.
- *Drug history (DH):* A list of the patient's current medications (including dosage) and drug allergies.
- *Family history (FH):* A list of major diseases suffered by members of the immediate family.
- *Social history (SH):* A picture of the patient's social situation. Occupation and hobbies, both past and present, give information about the patient's lifestyle. Finally, history of smoking and alcohol is usually noted.
- *Patient examination* includes all information collected from the medical objective assessment.
- *Medical diagnosis and plan.*

Sections for test results contain any significant findings as they become available. These may include arterial blood gases (ABG), spirometry, blood tests, sputum analysis and radiological examinations. Notes from other healthcare professionals may also be found in the medical record and often follow the format shown, but with emphasis on the areas they manage.

SUBJECTIVE ASSESSMENT

The purpose of the physiotherapy subjective assessment is to confirm and clarify previously obtained information, and to seek any missing and physiotherapy-specific information. It should generally start with open-ended questions such as *'What is your main problem?'* or *'What troubles you most?',* allowing the patient to discuss the problems that are most important to them at that time. By asking open-ended questions, previously unmentioned problems may surface. As the interview progresses, questioning may become more focused on those important features that need clarification.

There are five main symptoms of cardiorespiratory disease:

- breathlessness (dyspnoea)
- cough
- sputum and haemoptysis
- wheeze
- chest pain.

Questions should be asked, as appropriate, to obtain a description, determine the behaviour and, in some situations, quantify these symptoms. The approach suggested by Maitland (Hengeveld & Banks 2013) for musculoskeletal pain can be adapted for patients with cardiorespiratory disorders. See also Table 2-2. Information should also be sought about activity/exercise limitation.

Breathlessness

Breathlessness is the subjective awareness of shortness of breath. In someone without cardiorespiratory disease this would be a normal sensation; for example, following exercise. When the awareness of breathing is unpleasant or uncomfortable, the term *dyspnoea* is used. It is the predominant symptom of both cardiac and respiratory disease. It also occurs in anaemia where the oxygen-carrying capacity of the blood is reduced, in neuromuscular disorders where the respiratory muscles are affected, and in metabolic disorders where there is a change in the acid–base equilibrium. Breathlessness is also a symptom in hyperventilation syndrome or dysfunctional breathing where psychological issues (e.g. anxiety) may also play a role.

Dyspnoea is a complex symptom which is the result of sensory feedback and cognitive and contextual factors. The duration and severity of breathlessness is most easily assessed through enquiries about the level of functioning in the recent and distant past. For example, a patient may say that 3 years ago he could walk up five flights of stairs without stopping, but now cannot manage even one flight. Some patients may deny breathlessness, as they have (unconsciously) decreased their activity levels so that they do not get breathless. They may only acknowledge breathlessness when it interferes with important activities, for example, bathing. The physiotherapist should always quantify breathlessness in terms of the level of function that the patient can achieve (see Chapters 6 and 7).

The description of the sensation (quality) of dyspnoea may vary depending on the cause and, more recently, research has documented an affective dimension of unpleasantness. Although this information is not sought clinically during the subjective assessment, this may change as our understanding of dyspnoea increases.

Breathlessness is usually worse during exercise and better with rest. An exception is hyperventilation syndrome where breathlessness may improve with exercise. Two patterns of breathlessness have been given specific names.

- *Orthopnoea* is breathlessness when lying flat
- *Paroxysmal nocturnal dyspnoea (PND)* is breathlessness that wakes the patient at night.

In the cardiac patient, lying flat increases venous return from the legs so that blood pools in the lungs, causing breathlessness. A similar pattern may be described in patients with severe asthma, but here the breathlessness is caused by nocturnal bronchoconstriction.

Further insight into a patient's breathlessness may be gained by enquiring about aggravating and relieving factors. Breathlessness associated with exposure to allergens and relieved by bronchodilators is typically found in asthma.

Cough

Coughing is a protective reflex that rids the airways of secretions (see Sputum), particulate matter or foreign bodies. Any stimulation of receptors located in the pharynx, larynx, trachea or bronchi may induce cough. Cough may be an occasional disturbance or repetitive and persistent, which is both troublesome and distressing. Important information about cough is its effectiveness, and whether it is productive or dry. Information about cough from the subjective assessment may be confirmed during the objective assessment.

Smokers may discount their early morning cough as being 'normal'. A chronic productive cough every day is a fundamental feature of chronic bronchitis and bronchiectasis. Recurrent coughing after eating or drinking is an important symptom of aspiration. Interstitial lung disease is characterized by a persistent, dry cough. Nocturnal cough is an important symptom of asthma in children and young adults, but in older patients it is more commonly due to cardiac failure. A loud, barking cough, which is often termed 'bovine', may signify laryngeal or tracheal disease. Drugs, especially β-blockers and some other antihypertensive agents, can cause a chronic cough. Chronic cough may cause fractured ribs (cough fractures) and hernias. Stress incontinence is a common complication of chronic cough, especially in women. As this subject is often embarrassing to the patient, specific questioning may be required (see Incontinence).

Sputum

In a normal adult, up to 100 mL of tracheobronchial secretions are produced daily and cleared subconsciously by swallowing. Sputum refers to excess tracheobronchial secretions that are cleared from the airways by coughing or huffing. Sputum may contain mucus, cellular debris, microorganisms, blood and foreign particles. Questioning should determine the colour and consistency of sputum, which may clarify the diagnosis and severity of disease (Table 2-1). An estimation of the volume should also be sought (1 teaspoon, 1 egg cup, half a cup, 1 cup).

Odour emanating from sputum signifies infection. In general, particularly offensive odours suggest infection with anaerobic organisms (e.g. aspiration pneumonia, lung abscess). Again findings from the subjective assessment may be confirmed during the objective assessment.

In patients with allergic bronchopulmonary aspergillosis (ABPA), asthma and occasionally bronchiectasis, sputum 'casts' may be expectorated. Classically these take the shape of the bronchial tree.

Haemoptysis is the presence of blood in the sputum. Frank haemoptysis can be life-threatening, requiring bronchial artery embolization or surgery. Isolated haemoptysis may be the first sign of bronchogenic carcinoma, even when the chest radiograph is normal. Patients with chronic infective lung disease often suffer from recurrent haemoptyses.

Wheeze

Wheeze is a whistling or musical sound produced by turbulent airflow through narrowed airways. These sounds are generally noted by patients when audible at the mouth. Stridor, the sound of an upper airway obstruction, is often mistakenly called 'wheeze' by patients. Heart failure may also cause wheezing in those

TABLE 2-1
Sputum Analysis

	Description	Causes
Saliva	Clear watery fluid	
Mucoid	Opalescent or white	Chronic bronchitis without infection, asthma
Mucopurulent	Slightly discoloured, but not frank pus	Bronchiectasis, cystic fibrosis, pneumonia
Purulent	Thick, viscous: ■ Yellow ■ Dark green/brown ■ Rusty ■ Redcurrant jelly	 *Haemophilus* *Pseudomonas* *Pneumococcus, Mycoplasma* *Klebsiella*
Frothy	Pink or white	Pulmonary oedema
Haemoptysis	Ranging from blood specks to frank blood, old blood (dark brown)	Infection (tuberculosis, bronchiectasis), infarction, carcinoma, vasculitis, trauma; also coagulation disorders, cardiac disease
Black	Black specks in mucoid secretions	Smoke inhalation (fires, tobacco, heroin), coal dust

patients with significant mucosal oedema. Wheezing is discussed in more detail later in this chapter.

Chest Pain

Chest pain in cardiorespiratory patients usually originates from musculoskeletal, cardiac, pleural or tracheal inflammation, as the lung parenchyma and small airways do not contain pain fibre innervation. Differential diagnosis of chest pain is important as pain of cardiac origin may require immediate medical intervention. Some of the features of chest pain of different origins are shown in Table 2-2.

Incontinence

Incontinence is a problem that is often aggravated by chronic cough (Orr et al 2001, Scottish Intercollegiate Guidelines Network 2004, Thakar & Stanton 2000). Coughing and huffing increase intra-abdominal pressure, which may precipitate urine leakage. Fear of this may influence compliance with physiotherapy. Thus identification and treatment of incontinence is important. Questions may need to be specific to elicit this symptom: When you cough, do you find that you leak some urine? Does this interfere with your physiotherapy?

Other Symptoms

Of the other symptoms a patient may report, a number have particular importance.

- *Fever (pyrexia)* is a common feature of infection, but low-grade fevers can also occur with malignancy and connective tissue disorders. Equally, infection may occur without fever, especially in immunosuppressed (e.g. chemotherapy) patients or those on corticosteroids. High fevers occurring at night, with associated sweating (night sweats), may be the first indicator of pulmonary tuberculosis. Fever as a symptom of cardiorespiratory disorders is non-specific and needs to be considered in the light of other findings.
- *Headache* is an uncommon feature of respiratory disease. Morning headaches in patients with severe respiratory failure may signify nocturnal carbon dioxide (CO_2) retention. Early morning ABG or nocturnal transcutaneous CO_2 monitoring are required for confirmation.

Disease Awareness

During the interview it is important to ascertain the patient's knowledge of his disease and treatment. The level of compliance with treatment, often difficult to assess initially, may become evident as rapport develops. These issues will influence the goals of treatment.

Functional Ability

It is important to assess the patient as a whole, enquiring about his daily activities. If the patient is employed, what does the job *actually* entail? For example, a surveyor may sit behind a desk all day, or may be climbing 25-storey buildings. The home circumstances should also be documented, in particular the number of stairs to the front door and within the house. With whom does the patient live? What roles does the patient perform in the home (shopping, housework, cooking)? Finally, questions concerning activities and recreation often reveal areas where significant improvements in QOL can be made. Functional ability may also be objectively assessed (see Objective Assessment).

OBJECTIVE ASSESSMENT

This component of clinical assessment refers to the physical examination of the patient and includes information which can be gathered from clinical investigations and tests. The objective assessment method described is used by multi-professional first responder training programs and those programs associated with rapid recognition of abnormal cardiorespiratory physiology (Nolan 2011, Robertson & Al-Haddad 2013, Thim et al 2012). The method uses a logical, systematic approach in a strict chronological order starting with examination of the airway, 'A', and progressing through breathing, 'B'; circulation, 'C'; disability, 'D' and exposure, 'E'. The systematic approach allows findings to be quickly assimilated and enables urgent priorities to be managed before moving on to the next component. The method is applicable across the spectrum of clinical presentations in cardiorespiratory health; however, the assessor should determine which component of assessment should be emphasized in each clinical setting. Documentation of the assessment findings within this systematic order permits standardization between professional groups, thus enabling clear communication of salient assessment features.

TABLE 2-2
Differential Diagnosis of Chest Pain

Structure	Causes	Location	Onset/Quality/Intensity	Aggravating/Relieving Factors and Associated Findings
Pulmonary				
Pleura (pleurisy)	Pleural infection or inflammation of the pleura Trauma (haemothorax) Malignancy	Unilateral, often localized	Rapid onset Sharp, stabbing Often 'catches' at a certain lung volume	Aggravated by deep breaths and coughing Relieved by anti-inflammatory medication Limits inspiration Not tender on palpation Associated findings may include: fever dyspnoea cough crackles pleural rub
Pulmonary embolus	DVT (secondary to immobilization, long distance travel)	Often lateral, on the side of the embolism but may be central	Sudden onset Sharp	Associated findings may include: dyspnoea tachypnoea tachycardia hypotension hypoxaemia (not significantly improved with oxygen therapy) haemoptysis if pulmonary infarction occurs unilateral swollen lower leg that is red and painful suggests DVT
Pneumothorax	Trauma Spontaneous Lung diseases (e.g. cystic fibrosis, AIDS) Iatrogenic (e.g. post central line insertion)	Lateral to side of pneumothorax	Sudden onset Sharp Severity depends on extent of mediastinal shift	Associated findings may include: dyspnoea decreased/absent breath sounds on side of pneumothorax increased percussion note tracheal deviation away from the side of the pneumothorax hypoxaemia
Tracheitis	Bacterial infection (e.g. *Staphylococcus* infection)	Central	Burning Constant	Aggravated by breathing
Tumours	Primary or secondary carcinoma Mesothelioma	May mimic any form of chest pain, depending on site and structures involved		Relieved by opiate and anti-inflammatory analgesia
Neuro-Musculoskeletal				
Rib fracture	Trauma Tumour Cough fractures (e.g. in chronic lung diseases, osteoporosis) Iatrogenic (e.g. surgery)	Localized point tenderness	Often sudden onset	Increases with inspiration

TABLE 2-2
Differential Diagnosis of Chest Pain (Continued)

Structure	Causes	Location	Onset/Quality/ Intensity	Aggravating/Relieving Factors and Associated Findings
Muscular	Trauma Unaccustomed exercise (excessive coughing during exacerbations of lung disease), accessory muscles may be affected	Superficial		Increases on inspiration and some body movements Relieved by rest, anti-inflammatory medication, ice/heat
Costochondritis and Tietze syndrome	Trauma Viral infection	Localized to one or more costochondral joints	With or without generalized, non-specific chest pain	Aggravated by sneezing, coughing, deep inspiration, twisting of the chest Reproducible pain, especially at the costochondral junctions Relieved by anti-inflammatory medication, ice/heat
Neuralgia	Thoracic spine dysfunction Tumour Trauma Herpes zoster (shingles)	Dermatomal distribution	Sharp or burning or paraesthesia	Anti-viral medications (if caused by herpes zoster)
Cardiac				
Acute coronary syndrome Angina Myocardial infarction	Ischaemic heart disease	Central, retrosternal with or without radiation to the jaw or upper extremities frequently on left	Pressure, tightness, squeezing, heaviness, burning Onset at rest is more suggestive of infarction	*Angina* Aggravated by exertion, exposure to cold, psychological stress Usually lasts less than 10 minutes Relieved by nitro-glycerine *Myocardial infarction* Duration variable; often more than 30 min Not relieved by nitro-glycerine Associated findings may include: nausea vomiting dyspnoea dizziness hypotension arrhythmias depending on severity of ischaemia
Pericardium (pericarditis)	Infection Inflammation Trauma Tumour	Retrosternal or towards cardiac apex; may radiate to left shoulder	Sharp May mimic cardiac ischaemia or pleurisy	May be relieved by sitting up and leaning forwards Associated findings may include: tachycardia pericardial friction rub
Mediastinal				
Dissecting aortic aneurysm	Trauma Atherosclerosis Marfan syndrome	Anterior chest, often radiating to back, between shoulder blades Poorly localized central chest pain	Sudden onset of unrelenting pain Tearing or ripping sensation; knifelike	Associated findings may include: dyspnoea unequal pulses or BP in both arms hypotension ischaemic leg pain reduced lower limb pulses

Continued on following page

	TABLE 2-2			
	Differential Diagnosis of Chest Pain *(Continued)*			
Structure	**Causes**	**Location**	**Onset/Quality/ Intensity**	**Aggravating/Relieving Factors and Associated Findings**
Oesophageal	Oesophageal reflux Trauma Tumour Vomiting (Boerhaave syndrome)	Retrosternal but can also be posterior in the lower back	Burning	Reflux: aggravated by lying flat or bending forwards after eating, relieved by antacids Oesophageal tears: mediastinal or subcutaneous air or pleural effusion may be seen on CXR
Mediastinal shift	Pneumothorax Rapid drainage of a large pleural effusion	Poorly localized central discomfort	Sudden onset Severe	

(BMJ Best Practice 2014; Lee 2004; Lee 2012)
CXR, Chest radiograph; *DVT,* deep vein thrombosis.

Each section of the structured objective examination described in the following paragraphs is divided into three or four component actions for ease of description. These actions are: observation, feel, listen and measure. The expert clinician may be able to complete these actions simultaneously and in a short time, whilst the novice may find it useful to deliberately organize their assessment actions separately.

A = Airway

This component of the objective assessment is concerned with collecting information regarding upper airway patency. Establishing patency of the upper airway is the most important component of performing a respiratory examination. Obstruction of the airway will ultimately lead to hypoxia and death. The most common cause of airway obstruction is an altered level of consciousness and pharyngeal obstruction by the tongue. Other causes of airway obstruction include inhalation of foreign bodies, vomitus or teeth; excessive pulmonary secretions; swelling or oedema and invasive tumours. Patency of the airway should be assessed using a structured process which will include the following actions.

Airway – Observation

Is the patient self-ventilating or requiring the assistance of an artificial airway to ensure airway patency? Forms of artificial airways include: a nasopharyngeal airway; an oropharyngeal airway; an endotracheal tube or a tracheostomy tube. Artificial airway security should be verified with inspection of tapes, ties and other holding devices. All artificial airways should be assessed for position and patency; for example, the inner lumen of a tracheostomy tube should be inspected to ensure it is not blocked by secretions and an endotracheal tube can be suctioned to determine if a catheter can pass unobstructed. Self-ventilating patients should be asked to open their mouth so a visual inspection can be made. Visual inspection will determine whether there is swelling or abnormality of the mouth, teeth, tongue or soft palate. The colour of the oral mucosa, lips and facial skin should be noted. Central cyanosis, seen on examination of the tongue and mouth, is caused by hypoxia where there is an increase in the amount of haemoglobin not bound to oxygen. The blueness is related to the quantity of unbound haemoglobin. Cyanosis is a late sign of airway obstruction.

Airway – Feel

Air movement into and out of a natural or artificial airway can be assessed by placing your hand to feel the flow of warm air against your skin during expiration. Simultaneous observation of chest rise and fall with air flow through an airway will assist in the determination of airway patency.

Airway – Listen

Is the airway clear? Can you hear any airway sounds? Normal quiet unobstructed breathing is almost inaudible at the mouth. Abnormal sounds heard at the mouth include: gurgling, when there is fluid in the upper airway; wheezing, with obstruction of the lower airways; stridor, with obstruction of the upper airway; crowing, caused by laryngeal spasm; grunting, caused by a flail chest; and snoring, caused when there is pharyngeal obstruction by the tongue. If the patient is conscious they should be asked a question so the sound quality of their response can be evaluated.

If the upper airway is not patent and the patient cannot protect the natural airway, an artificial airway should be immediately inserted (nasopharyngeal or oropharyngeal airway), oxygen applied and expert help requested. The lateral recovery position can be used to prevent aspiration of gastric secretions and airway opening interventions such as head tilt, chin lift or jaw thrust should be attempted. It would be negligent to continue the physical assessment until airway patency is established.

B = Breathing

The breathing component of the objective assessment relates to examination of the anatomical and physiological features which contribute to the process of breathing. The extent to which each item of this section is included in the physiotherapy assessment will depend on the clinical setting and presentation. To be able to examine breathing it is important to know the surface landmarks of the lungs (Fig. 2-1). Some important points are:

- The oblique fissure, dividing the upper and middle lobes from the lower lobes, runs from the spinous process of T2/3 posteriorly around the chest to the sixth costochondral junction anteriorly.
- The horizontal fissure on the right, dividing the right upper lobe from the right middle lobe, runs from the fourth intercostal space at the right sternal edge horizontally to the mid-axillary line, where it joins the oblique fissure.
- The diaphragm sits at approximately the sixth rib anteriorly, the eighth rib in the mid-axillary line and the 10th rib posteriorly.
- The trachea bifurcates just below the level of the manubriosternal junction.
- The apical segment of both upper lobes extends 2.5 cm above the clavicles.

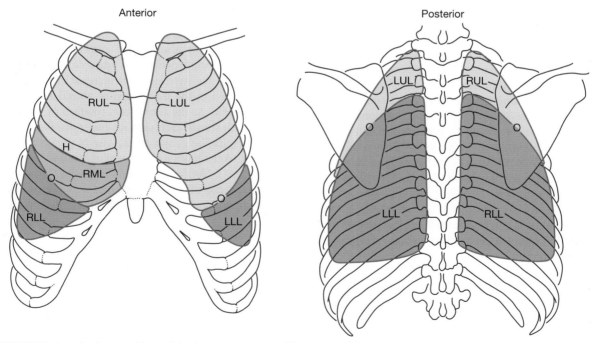

FIGURE 2-1 ■ Surface markings of the lungs: *H*, horizontal fissure; *O*, oblique fissure; *RUL*, right upper lobe; *LUL*, left upper lobe; *RML*, right middle lobe; *LLL*, left lower lobe; *RLL*, right lower lobe.

Breathing – Observation

Observation of the breathing component of objective assessment begins from initial patient contact. Does the patient appear short of breath, sitting on the edge of the bed or distressed? Is he able to speak; if so how long are his sentences? When he moves around or undresses, does he become distressed? Is the patient producing sputum; what is the colour, consistency and quantity of sputum?

Depending on the environment in which the assessment is occurring there are number of other features that can be assessed through observation. In the critically ill patient the level of ventilatory support should be determined, including the mode of ventilation, oxygen requirement, presence and patency of drains, thoracic epidurals and wounds. *Intercostal drains* are placed between two ribs into the pleural space to remove air, fluid or pus. The drain is attached to a bottle partially filled with sterile water, called an 'underwater seal drain' (see Chapter 9). The bottle should always be kept below chest level. Bubbling in the intercostal drain indicates air entering the tube from the pleural space. Fluid within the tube should oscillate or 'swing' with every breath. If no swing is apparent, the tube is not patent and requires medical attention. In certain situations the bottle may be connected to continuous suction. With practice, these observations will become automatic and can be subtly undertaken whilst introducing yourself to the patient.

Specific breathing components evaluated through observation are explored in the next sections and are best conducted by asking the patient to sit erect on the side of the bed or well positioned in bed with the thorax exposed. Observation of breathing cannot be undertaken when a patient is poorly positioned or slumped in the bed.

Chest Shape. The chest should appear symmetrical with the adult rib descending at approximately 45 degrees from the thoracic spine. The transverse diameter of the chest should be greater than the anteroposterior (AP) diameter. The thoracic spine should have a slight kyphosis. Common abnormalities of chest wall shape include:

- *Kyphosis:* An increase in thoracic spine flexion.
- *Scoliosis:* An excessive lateral curvature of the spine with vertebral rotation.

- *Kyphoscoliosis:* Scoliosis and an element of kyphosis. Kyphoscoliosis can cause a restrictive lung defect which may lead to respiratory failure.
- *Pectus excavatum* or 'funnel' chest: Is where part of the sternum is depressed inwards. This rarely effects lung function but may be corrected surgically for cosmetic reasons.
- *Pectus carinatum* or 'pigeon' or 'chicken' chest: Is where the sternum protrudes anteriorly. This may be present in children with severe asthma and rarely effects lung function.
- *Hyperinflation* or 'barrel chest': Is where the ribs lose their normal 45-degree angle with the thoracic spine and become almost horizontal. The AP diameter of the chest increases to almost equal the transverse diameter. This is commonly seen in severe emphysema.

Chest and Abdominal Movement. Normal quiet inspiration is characterized by small coordinated symmetrical increases in the *AP*, *transverse* and *vertical* diameters of the thorax. The increase in vertical diameter is achieved by diaphragm descent into the abdomen, resulting in anterior abdominal wall motion. Diaphragm contraction also elicits a small increase in the lower thoracic transverse diameter. The increase in AP diameter is the result of the anterior ends of the upper ribs moving forwards and upwards with anterior movement of the sternum. This increase in AP diameter is likened to the movement of an old-fashioned 'pump handle'. At the same time, rotation of the ribs around their sternal cartilaginous and spinal insertions during inspiration causes an increase in the transverse diameter, likened to the movement of a 'bucket handle' (see Fig. 1-7). Normal expiration is passive, caused by the elastic recoil of the lung and chest wall. Abnormalities of chest and abdominal wall motion may include:

- *Asymmetry:* When one side of the chest has reduced (or excessive) movement compared to the other. This can occur in acute lung collapse, haemothorax and simple and tension pneumothorax.
- *Abdominal distension:* Will impede descent of the diaphragm during inspiration and limit increases in the vertical diameter of the thorax. Abdominal distension may result from obesity, ascites, pregnancy, abdominal surgery and constipation.

- *Intercostal indrawing:* Occurs where the skin between the ribs is drawn inwards during inspiration. It may be seen in patients with severe inspiratory airflow resistance. Large negative pressures during inspiration suck the soft tissues inwards. Intercostal indrawing can be an important sign of respiratory distress in children.
- *Supraclavicular indrawing:* Occurs when the skin above the clavicle is drawn inwards during inspiration. It is also seen in patients with severe airflow resistance who generate high negative pressures during inspiration; for example, acute asthma.
- *Flail chest:* Occurs with multiple rib fractures when two or more breaks in each rib result in loss of integrity of the thoracic cage. During inspiration the loose segment is drawn inwards as the rest of the chest wall moves out. In expiration the reverse occurs.
- *Paradoxical breathing:* Is where the entire chest wall moves inwards on inspiration and outwards on expiration. Chest wall paradox occurs in bilateral diaphragm weakness or paralysis as observed in the patient with high cervical spinal cord injury. It is most apparent when the patient is supine.
- *Hoover sign:* Is paradoxical movement of the lower chest wall and occurs in patients with severe chronic airflow limitation who are extremely hyperinflated. As the dome of the flattened diaphragm cannot descend further, diaphragm contraction during inspiration pulls the lower ribs inwards.

Effort. Normal quiet breathing should occur with a regular rhythm and rate. The ratio of inspiratory to expiratory time (I : E ratio) is 1 : 2. Active inspiration should be approximately half the time of passive expiration. Maintenance of this rhythm should be achieved without discernable contraction of the primary muscles of respiration, accessory inspiratory muscles or abdominal wall muscles. Accessory inspiratory muscles are progressively recruited during exercise; however, contraction of these muscles at rest or alterations in the normal I : E ratio represent signs of dysfunction. The observable effort associated with breathing is often referred to as the 'work' of breathing. In pulmonary mechanics work is done when pressure causes a change in lung volume. The oxygen consumption (VO_2) associated with normal breathing is 3 mL/min and represents less than 5% of the total VO_2 at rest (Donahoe et al 1989). This energy is required to match elastic lung recoil and airway resistance, which are the two characteristics determining the work of breathing. An increased effort to breathe is characterized by the following observations.

- *Tachypnoea:* An increase in respiratory rate (RR) above 20 breaths per minute is considered abnormal and will contribute to an increased breathing effort.
- *Accessory inspiratory muscle use:* Accessory inspiratory muscle contraction during inspiration can increases the AP and transverse thoracic diameters of the thorax. Muscles which may be recruited to facilitate chest movements include the sternocleidomastoid, scalenes, trapezii and pectoral muscles (see Fig. 1-8).
- *Active expiration:* Expiration may be active with contraction of the abdominal and internal intercostal muscles.
- *Nasal flaring:* In adults and children is a sign of marked increases in respiratory effort and distress.
- *Prolonged expiration:* May be seen in patients with obstructive lung disease where expiratory airflow is severely limited by dynamic closure of the smaller airways. In severe obstruction the I : E ratio may increase to 1 : 3 or 1 : 4.
- *Pursed-lip breathing:* Is often seen in patients with severe airway disease. By opposing the lips during expiration, the airway pressure inside the chest is maintained, preventing the floppy airways from collapsing.

Pattern. In addition to the effort required to breathe and the observations described, it is important to be able to recognize commonly observed breathing patterns. Certain breathing patterns have been classified and are listed in Table 2-3.

Breathing – Feel

This action requires the examiner to palpate the structures and movement of the thorax. Using the surfaces of the fingers and hands the examiner can feel for areas of tenderness, skin temperature changes, swelling or masses. Specific assessment features that can be assessed through palpation are described.

TABLE 2-3
Breathing Patterns

Breathing Pattern	Description	Cause
	Eupnoea, normal breathing rate and pattern	
	Bradypnoea, abnormally slow RR of ≤10 breaths/min	Sleep, opiate analgesia, metabolic disorders, stroke, increased intracranial pressure
	Tachypnoea, an increase in breathing rate <20 breaths/min	Exercise, anxiety, metabolic acidosis, hypoxia, raised serum lactate
	Apnoea, total cessation in breathing for ≥10 seconds.	Traumatic head injury or stroke
	Hypoventilation, reduced RR and volume resulting in inadequate total ventilation	Sedation, opiate analgesia, morbid obesity, disorders causing increased arterial carbon dioxide
	Hyperventilation, increased rate and tidal volume (increased minute ventilation) which lowers arterial carbon dioxide concentration.	Stress, anxiety, hyperventilation syndrome (see Chapter 5).
	Hyperpnoea, normal RR but increased volume	Emotional stress and metabolic acidosis
	Biot breathing, rapid deep respiration (cluster gasps) with short pauses between sets	Spinal meningitis, medulla oblongata damage from stroke/trauma, prolonged opioid abuse Poor prognosis
	Kussmaul breathing, laboured, rapid, deep breathing (high minute ventilation).	Late stage severe metabolic acidosis, diabetic ketoacidosis or renal failure.
	Cheyne–Stokes breathing, gradual increases and decrease in respiration with periods of apnoea	Impending death, heart failure, morphine, stroke, traumatic brain injury, carbon monoxide poisoning, metabolic encephalopathy

TABLE 2-3		
Breathing Patterns *(Continued)*		
Breathing Pattern	**Description**	**Cause**
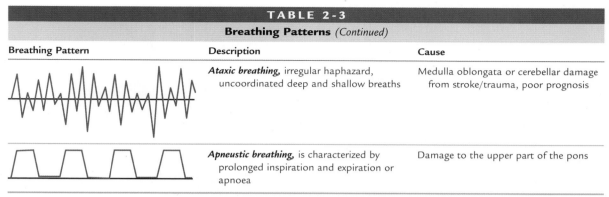	***Ataxic breathing***, irregular haphazard, uncoordinated deep and shallow breaths	Medulla oblongata or cerebellar damage from stroke/trauma, poor prognosis
	Apneustic breathing, is characterized by prolonged inspiration and expiration or apnoea	Damage to the upper part of the pons

RR, Respiratory rate.

Tracheal Position. The trachea is palpated to assess its position in relation to the sternal notch. Tracheal deviation indicates underlying mediastinal shift. The trachea may be pulled towards a collapsed or fibrosed upper lobe, or pushed away from a pneumothorax or large pleural effusion.

Chest Expansion. The examiner's hands are placed spanning the anterior segments of the lung bases, with the thumbs touching in the midline anteriorly. The patient is instructed to inspire slowly several times whilst the displacement of the thumbs is observed. Both sides should move equally, with a 3–5 cm displacement. A similar technique may be used posteriorlyas shown in Figure 2-2. Apical chest movement can be palpated by placing one hand over the upper chest anteriorly and one hand over the posterior upper chest. A comparison of AP apical movement of the left and right side of the chest should be made. In all cases, diminished or asymmetrical movement is abnormal and palpation of chest expansion may confirm observed asymmetry.

Subcutaneous Air. Air in the subcutaneous tissues of the chest, neck or face will result in a characteristic crackling in the skin or subcutaneous crepitation on palpation. *Subcutaneous air* occurs most commonly with pneumothorax but can be associated with pneumomediastinum (air in the mediastinum) and pneumoperitoneum (peritoneal air) where air can travel to the chest cavity through the fascial planes.

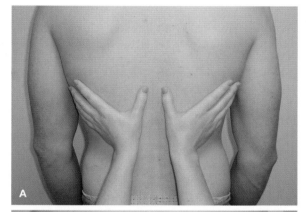
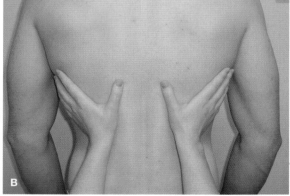

FIGURE 2-2 ■ Palpation of thoracic expansion. **(A)** Start of inspiration. **(B)** End of inspiration.

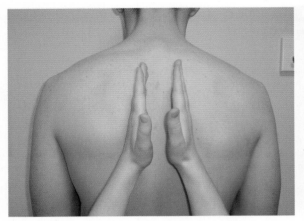

FIGURE 2-3 ■ Palpation of tactile fremitus using the ulnar border of the hands.

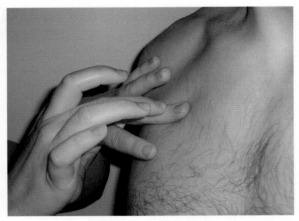

FIGURE 2-4 ■ Percussion note hand position.

Fremitus. Fremitus is a vibration felt on the body during palpation. Vocal or tactile fremitus is the palpation of speech vibrations transmitted through the chest wall to the examiner's hands. It is measured by asking the patient to repeatedly say 'ninety-nine' or 'blue moon' whilst the ulnar border of the examiner's hands are placed on both sides of the chest (Fig. 2-3). The hands are moved from apices to bases, anteriorly and posteriorly, comparing the vibration felt. Vocal fremitus is increased when the lung underneath is consolidated, as solid tissue transmits sound better. Vocal fremitus is decreased with a pneumothorax or a pleural effusion since the physical interface between the lung and examiners hands is increased. *Pleural fremitus* is the palpable vibration of the chest caused by friction between the visceral and parietal pleura. *Tussive fremitus* is vibration felt on the chest wall when a patient coughs. *Rhonchal* or bronchial fremitus is vibration felt on the chest wall caused by air moving through a large airway which is partially obstructed by secretions.

Breathing – Listen

This action requires the examiner to focus on the sounds associated with breathing. The examiner may have already noted breathing sounds when assessing the airway. Specific assessment features that can be assessed through listening are described.

Speech. What is the speech pattern – long fluent paragraphs without discernable pauses for breath, quick sentences, just a few words or is the patient too breathless to speak?

Quality of Cough. Instruct the patient to cough to assess the quality of their performance. Can the patient cough? Is the patient afraid to cough? Is the cough inhibited? Is the cough painful? Is the cough strong, tight, wheezy, productive or dry? A weak ineffective cough places the patient at risk of retained secretions, hypoxia and respiratory failure.

Percussion Note. Percussion is a method of tapping over the surface of the chest to determine the nature of the underlying structures. It is performed by placing the left hand firmly on the chest wall over an intercostal space. The distal interphalangeal joint of the middle finger on the left hand is tapped with the middle finger of the right hand using a wrist action (Fig. 2-4). A systematic percussion sequence should be adopted that allows the percussion of each lobe, comparing one side to the other, from lung apex to base, anteriorly and posteriorly (Fig. 2-5). Aerated lung will sound resonant, whilst consolidated lung sounds dull, and a pleural effusion sounds 'stony dull'. Increased resonance is heard when the chest wall is free to vibrate over an air-filled space, such as a pneumothorax.

Chest Auscultation. Auscultation is the process of listening and interpreting the sounds produced by air movement within airways and lungs with a stethoscope. The novice is instructed to follow

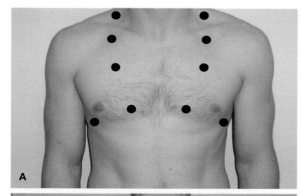

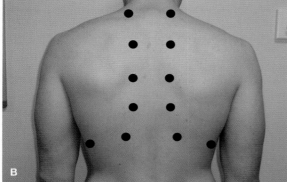

FIGURE 2-5 ■ Chest auscultation and percussion sites. **(A)** Anterior. **(B)** Posterior.

manufacturer's instructions for correct use of the stethoscope. The diaphragm of the stethoscope is used for listening to high-pitched breath sounds, and the earpieces should point slightly forwards to maximize sound transmission. Chest auscultation should be performed in a quiet environment, with the chest exposed and the stethoscope diaphragm placed directly on the skin. The patient is instructed to breathe deeply through an open mouth, since nasal turbulence can interfere with detection of breath sounds. A deep breath will increase turbulent flow in large airways and make the breath sounds louder. A systematic auscultation sequence should be adopted that allows the auscultation of each lobe, comparing one side to the other, from lung apex to base, anteriorly and posteriorly. A systematic auscultation sequence may incorporate up to 38 discreet chest wall positions (see Fig. 2-5).

Normal breath sounds (previously named 'vesicular') are generated by airflow-related turbulence in the trachea and large airways and are heard loudest directly over the trachea. Breath sounds heard over the lung periphery are softer and lower pitched than over the large airways since sounds generated in the large airways are filtered by lung tissue. Normal breath sounds can be heard all over the chest wall throughout inspiration and for a short period during expiration. There is a wide variation in the intensity of breath sounds depending on chest wall thickness. For example, breath sounds are diminished in obese patients since adipose tissue over the chest wall attenuates sound transmission. Normal and abnormal breath sounds are described in a variety of ways that include the characteristics of sound frequency, duration, timing, intensity and quality. Common descriptions and their meanings are provided in Table 2-4. The novice practitioner is encouraged to access interactive media websites (e.g. http://www.easyauscultation.com/lung -sounds.aspx, http://www.practicalclinicalskills.com/ breath-sounds-reference-guide.aspx) that provide audio recordings of normal and abnormal breath sounds for a true appreciation of the art of auscultation.

Vocal Resonance. Vocal resonance is the transmission of voice through the airways and lung tissue to the chest wall where it is heard through a stethoscope. It is tested by instructing the patient to say 'ninety-nine' repeatedly whilst the stethoscope is placed systematically to auscultate each lobe, comparing one side to the other, from lung apex to base, anteriorly and posteriorly (see Fig. 2-5). Over normal lung tissue, speech is low pitched and muffled. Consolidated lung transmits all sounds better, so speech is heard loud and clear and is described as 'bronchophony'. Whispered speech is not normally transmitted to the chest wall; however, over areas of consolidation a whispered '1, 2, 3' is clear and intelligible and is described as 'whispered pectoriloquy'. An increased resonance of vocal sounds transmitted through the chest wall can also be evaluated by asking the patient to say the letter 'e' whilst auscultating the chest. Over areas of consolidation the 'e' will sound like an 'a' and is described as 'aegophony'. Vocal resonance is decreased when the transmission of sound through the lung or from the lung to chest wall is impeded. This occurs with emphysema, pneumothorax, pleural thickening or pleural effusion.

TABLE 2-4	
Breath Sounds Descriptions	
Breath Sounds	**Description**
Normal breath sounds	Represent sound generated by turbulent airflow in the trachea and large airways which is attenuated (or filtered) by lung tissue in the periphery. Normal breath sounds vary according to stethoscope location. Sounds heard over the trachea and large bronchi have a loud, harsh, high pitched tubular quality that can be heard throughout inspiration and expiration and are called *'tracheal'* or *'bronchial'* sounds. Sounds heard over the hilar lung regions are softer bronchial sounds which may be louder during inspiration than expiration and are known as *'bronchovesicular'* sounds. Sounds heard over the periphery have a low pitched, soft blowing or rustling quality heard through inspiration but almost inaudible during expiration and are known as *'vesicular'* sounds.
Reduced breath sounds	Decreased intensity of breath sounds occurs for a number of reasons. Since breath sounds are generated by flow turbulence, a reduction in flow causes less sound. Patients who cannot breathe deeply will have globally diminished breath sounds. Similarly, reduced breath sounds may be heard when there is an increased sound attenuation in the periphery due to destruction of lung tissue or hyperinflation or an increase in the distance of the lung to the chest surface such as in obesity, pneumothorax or pleural effusion.
Absent breath sounds	Breath sounds may be absent when localized accumulation of air or fluid in the pleural space blocks sound transmission from the large airways. Similarly if the bronchus supplying an area of lung is obstructed (e.g. carcinoma, large sputum plug) sound transmission to the periphery will be blocked.
Bronchial breath sounds	Normal tracheal or bronchial sounds that are heard at the lung periphery. Any increase in airway fluid or lung tissue density will allow better sound transmission from the large airways. Consequently the sounds heard over an area of consolidated lung are similar to those heard over the trachea.
Wheeze	Continuous high-pitched musical tones produced by air vibrating in a narrowed airway heard during late inspiration and expiration. Airway diameter decreases during expiration but any cause of additional narrowing (bronchospasm, mucosal oedema, sputum, foreign bodies), will elicit wheeze. The pitch of the wheeze is related to the degree of narrowing. High-pitched wheezes indicate near total obstruction. A fixed, *monophonic* (single pitch) wheeze is caused by a single obstructed airway. *Polyphonic* (multiple pitch) wheeze is due to widespread airway narrowing. Localized wheeze may be caused by sputum retention and can change or clear after coughing.
Crackles	Discontinuous explosive popping or clicking sounds more commonly heard during inspiration than expiration, caused by the opening of previously closed small airways during inspiration causing transient airway vibration. Airway closure may occur due to fluid or exudate accumulation, low lung volumes or abnormalities of lung tissue. The cause of airway closure affects the acoustic properties ('fine' or 'coarse'); location ('localized' or 'widespread'); and timing of crackles throughout the respiratory cycle ('early' or 'late'). For example, localized crackles may occur in dependent alveoli, which are gradually closed by compression from the lung above. These crackles may resolve when the patient breathes deeply or coughs.
Pleural rub	Creaking, squeaking, grating or rubbing sounds that occur during inspiration and expiration caused by friction between the pleural surfaces. The pleura may be roughened by inflammation, infection or neoplasm.

Breathing – Measure

The breathing component of the objective examination incorporates a number of significant clinical investigations and measurements.

Respiratory Rate. Respiratory rate (RR) should be counted as the number of respiratory cycles in a minute with the patient resting comfortably. It is preferable that the patient is ignorant of the measurement since RR tends to increase when the patient is aware they are being observed. The normal adult respiratory rate is approximately 12–16 breaths/min. Respiratory rate is the most useful sign that a patient's breathing is compromised.

Oxygen Saturation. Oxygen saturation (SaO_2 and SpO_2) is defined as the ratio of oxyhaemoglobin to the total concentration of haemoglobin present in the blood. When arterial oxyhaemoglobin concentration is measured by an arterial blood gas it is called 'SaO_2'. When oxyhaemoglobin concentration is measured non-invasively by a pulse oximeter it is called 'SpO_2'. Normal values of oxygen saturation at sea level range from 96–99%. Saturation is determined by the characteristics of the non-linear oxyhaemoglobin dissociation curve, which relates oxyhaemoglobin saturation with the partial pressure of oxygen (PaO_2) in the blood. Rapid dissociation of oxygen and haemoglobin occurs below 90% saturation. Oxygen saturation does not reflect tissue oxygenation or the patient's ability to ventilate.

Fraction of Inspired Oxygen. Fraction of inspired oxygen (FiO_2) is defined as the percentage of inspired oxygen delivered to the patient. A patient breathing room air will inspire 21% oxygen, whilst oxygen delivery devices can provide an FiO_2 up to and including 100%.

Arterial Blood Gases. Arterial blood gases (ABG) can be sampled directly from the radial or femoral artery or withdrawn from an arterial catheter. Arterialized capillary samples may also be taken from the earlobe. The sampled blood is inserted into a gas analyser, which determines the pH, PaO_2, and partial pressure of CO_2 ($PaCO_2$), bicarbonate concentration (HCO_3^-) and base excess (BE). Some blood gas analysers can also report lactate, haemoglobin concentration and important electrolytes such as potassium (K). Normal values for ABG are given in Table 2-5.

TABLE 2-5		
Normal Arterial Blood Gas Values (kPa and mmHg)		
pH	7.35–7.45	
PaO_2	10.7–13.3 kPa	(80–100 mmHg)
$PaCO_2$	4.7–6.0 kPa	(35–45 mmHg)
HCO_3	22–26 mmol/L	
Base excess	−2 to +2	
Lactate	0.5–1 mmol/L	

FiO_2/PaO_2 Ratio. The PaO_2 is directly influenced by the FiO_2. The ratio is calculated by dividing the PaO_2 (mmHg) by the FiO_2 in decimal form. For example, a PaO_2 of 80 mmHg derived by breathing 40% FiO_2 (0.4) would generate a PaO_2/FiO_2 ratio of 200 mmHg. A PaO_2/FiO_2 ratio of 201–300 mmHg is one of the four defining criteria of acute lung injury, whilst a ratio of less than 200 represents one of the defining parameters of acute respiratory distress syndrome (Bernard et al 1994). The ratio is a useful indication of the degree to which the lungs are able to absorb delivered oxygen and a guide to the appreciation of effective gas exchange.

Lung Function Tests. The forced vital capacity (FVC), forced expiratory volume in 1 second (FEV_1) and the FEV_1/FVC% are effort-dependent, dynamic lung function parameters that can be measured using a spirometer which records volume of air expelled *over time*. The peak expiratory flow (PEF) is a measure of the highest expiratory flow that can be generated following maximal inspiration and can be measured with a hand-held peak flow metre. PEF is influenced by airway diameter and is a useful indication of the degree of bronchoconstriction in asthma. Some electronic spirometers are capable of recording both inspiratory and expiratory flow rates as a function of *volume* as well as *time*. The resulting flow–volume loops provide information regarding flow generation throughout the entire inspiratory and expiratory cycle, and the shape of the resultant curves indicate the anatomical location of airflow obstruction. The predicted values for these indices depend on age, height, sex and ethnicity.

Peak Cough Flow (PCF). Cough effectiveness can be quantified by measuring the maximum expiratory airflow generated during a cough with a peak flow metre. Normal values in adults range from 400 to 1200 L/min (Bianchi & Baiardi 2008). PCFs of greater than 60 L/min predict extubation outcome in patients without neuromuscular disease (Smina et al 2003), whilst patients with neuromuscular disorders have considerably poorer outcomes following decannulation from tracheostomy when the manually assisted PCF is less than 160 L/min following decannulation (Bach et al 2010, Bach & Saporito 1996). Cough augmentation should be considered when PCF falls below 260 L/min.

Respiratory Muscle Strength. *Maximum inspiratory pressure (P$_i$max)* is measured by making a maximal inspiratory effort against the closed valve of a pressure manometer after breathing out to residual volume. The value recorded is a negative inspiratory pressure and reflects the strength of the inspiratory muscles. *P$_i$*max is often measured to determine a patient's readiness for extubation. *Maximum expiratory pressure (P$_e$max)* is measured by making a maximal expiratory effort against the closed valve of a manometer after breathing in to total lung capacity. The value recorded is a positive expiratory pressure and reflects cough effectiveness particularly in neuromuscular disease.

Breathlessness. There are several scales that can be used to rate the sensation of breathlessness at rest and during exercise (e.g. the Modified Borg Scale (Borg 1982, Mahler et al 1987), the Medical Research Council (MRC) dyspnoea scale (Bestall et al 1999) and Dyspnoea-12 (Yorke et al 2010 & 2011). Use of these and other validated breathlessness scales (Johnson et al 2010) provide useful methods to evaluate physiotherapy interventions designed to reduce the perception of breathlessness.

Thoracic Imaging. Chest radiographs, thoracic imaging and ultrasonic techniques (see Chapter 3) illustrate the extent and severity of disease at a particular time point, although the chest radiograph changes may lag 1–2 days behind the clinical findings. Comparison with previous images provides a useful index of improvement or deterioration over time.

C = Circulation

This component of the objective assessment is concerned with collecting information regarding cardiovascular function, systemic hydration and fluid balance. This component includes the aspects of cardiovascular examination following the established 'look, feel, listen and measure' pattern. The experienced clinician will be capable of completing many components of this examination simultaneously. The extent to which each item of cardiovascular examination is included will depend on the clinical setting and presentation.

Circulation – Observation

Observation of the circulation begins with initial patient contact. Does the patient look pale or blue?

Changes in complexion may be due to anaemia or peripheral cyanosis, which may occur when peripheral circulation is poor due to low cardiac output. Is the patient diaphoretic? Excessive sweating is a nonspecific clinical sign with multiple causes but can be associated with myocardial infarction, febrile illnesses and septic shock. Are the lips and tongue moist or dry? Dry mucous membranes can be a sign of dehydration. Are there any obvious sources of insensible fluid loss or obvious external bleeding?

The environment will determine some features assessed through observation. For example, after cardiac surgery cardiac pacing wires that exit through the skin overlying the heart may be observed. In medical patients, pacemaker wires are introduced through one of the central veins and rest in the apex of the right ventricle. Care must be taken with all pacing wires as dislodgement may be life-threatening. The presence and level of cardiovascular support, including drugs to control blood pressure (inotropes) and cardiac output, and other mechanical devices used to support the circulation (e.g. left ventricular assist device), pulmonary artery catheters and central and peripheral venous lines should be noted. Single lines placed in small peripheral veins provide constant direct access to the bloodstream for the administration of intravenous (IV) fluids and drugs. Multi-lumen lines placed in the subclavian, internal jugular vein or femoral vein end in the venae cavae close to the right atrium. Central lines can be potentially dangerous, as disconnection of the line can quickly suck air into the central veins, causing an air embolus. Some patients may have an arterial line for continuous recording of blood pressure and repeated sampling of arterial blood. These lines are usually inserted in the radial or brachial artery. If accidentally disconnected, rapid blood loss will occur. Specific observational features which can reflect the circulation are described in the following sections.

Skin Turgor. Skin turgor is the ability of skin to deform and return to its normal elastic state. It is assessed by pinching the skin on the back of the hand or forearm and observing how quickly the skin returns to normal. Well-hydrated patients will not exhibit prolonged skin tenting. Decreased skin turgor is a late sign of dehydration.

Capillary Refill Time (CRT). Capillary refill time is the time taken for blood flow to return to capillaries after brief compression. It is measured by applying cutaneous pressure for 5 seconds on a fingertip held at heart level and counting the length of time it takes for blanching to recede once the pressure is removed. A normal CRT is less than 2 seconds. Delayed CRT is a common sign of dehydration and decreased peripheral perfusion and therefore reflects function of cardiac output and peripheral vascular resistance (Pickard et al 2011).

Peripheral Oedema. Peripheral oedema can be a sign of chronic cardiac failure but may also be found in patients with a low serum albumin, impaired lymphatic function or on high-dose steroids. Oedema may affect only the ankles, but with increasing severity it may progress up the legs to the sacrum.

Jugular Venous Pressure (JVP). On the side of the neck the JVP is seen as a pulsation in the jugular vein in the suprasternal notch between the attachments of the sternocleidomastoid muscle. It can be observed when the patient is lying at 45° with the neck rotated. A normal JVP at the base of the neck corresponds to a vertical height approximately 3–4 cm above the sternal angle, but above this height is considered elevated. The JVP provides a quick indication of the volume of blood in the great vessels entering the heart. JVP is elevated in right heart failure and may occur in patients with chronic lung disease complicated by *cor pulmonale*. In contrast, dehydrated patients may only have a visible JVP when lying flat.

Urine Colour and Quality. If the patient has a urinary catheter, brief inspection will identify if the urine is concentrated or cloudy. Dehydration can lead to decreased renal perfusion and oliguria. Cloudy urine can be a sign of urinary tract infection, which is a common cause of septic shock in the elderly.

Circulation – Feel

This action requires the examiner to palpate the patient to determine signs of cardiovascular compromise. Specific features of circulatory competence assessed through palpation include the following components.

Temperature. Cool pale limbs or digits are a sign of poor peripheral perfusion and cardiovascular compromise, including advanced shock. In contrast, the febrile septic patient may be peripherally vasodilated and extremely warm to touch.

Peripheral Pulses. Peripheral pulses can be felt at various sites around the body where the underlying artery is close to the surface. The radial pulse is commonly felt to assess heart rate and rhythm but the carotid, brachial and femoral pulses can also be palpated for this purpose. Dorsalis pedis on the superior surface of the foot lateral to the tendon of the great toe is often palpated to determine the integrity of distal blood flow in peripheral vascular disease. Determining equality between pulses (e.g. left and right radial or radial to femoral) can determine the presence of obstructive arterial disease or coarctation of the aorta. Reduced, thready or absent pulses are a sign of impaired blood flow or poor cardiac output. A bounding pulse may suggest sepsis.

Pulse Rate. If a strong pulse can be felt it should be counted for 60 seconds to manually estimate pulse rate. Tachycardia in adults is defined as a pulse rate greater than 100 beats/min at rest. Bradycardia is defined as a pulse rate less than 60 beats/min. Bradycardia may be a normal finding in athletes and may be caused by some cardiac drugs (especially β-blockers).

Pulse Rhythm and Quality. The pulse should be assessed for rhythm and quality. The peripheral pulse should occur regularly over the 60-second palpation period. Any extraneous additional beats should be noted and may represent ectopy. An irregular pulse may either be a recurring irregular pattern such as bigeminy or completely irregular such as atrial fibrillation. Experienced clinicians will also be able to detect subtle alterations in the quality of the palpated pulse. Since systolic blood pressure (SBP) decreases slightly (<10 mmHg) during inspiration, a subtle decrease in pulse amplitude during inspiration can be a normal clinical finding. A significant decrease in pulse amplitude during inspiration, known as *pulsus paradoxus*, suggests that SBP decreases in excess of 10 mmHg have occurred, such as with cardiac tamponade or pericarditis. A large volume pulse followed by a small volume pulse in repeating fashion is known as *pulsus alternans* and is a sign of severe cardiac failure. A collapsing pulse with an early peak is a sign of aortic regurgitation.

Circulation – Listen

This action requires the examiner to listen to the heart with a stethoscope. There are four discreet positions to listen to the heart sounds: the first position (aortic) is between the second and third intercostal space at the right sternal border; the second (pulmonic) is the same position at the left sternal border. Mitral sounds are heard best at the fifth left intercostal space mid-clavicular line. Tricuspid sounds are heard at the fourth left intercostal space lateral to the sternum. Each position should be auscultated with the patient reclined to 45 degrees. The normal heart sounds represent closure of the four heart valves. The first heart sound is caused by closure of the mitral and tricuspid valves, whilst the second sound is due to closure of the aortic and pulmonary valves. A third heart sound indicates cardiac failure in adults, but may be normal in children. A third sound is attributed to vibration of the ventricular walls caused by rapid filling in early diastole. The fourth heart sound is caused by vibration of the ventricular walls in late diastole as the atria contract and may be heard in heart failure, hypertension and aortic valve disease. A murmur is the sound generated by turbulent flow through a valve. The murmur of valve incompetence is caused by back flow across the valve, whilst stenotic valves generate murmurs by turbulent forwards flow.

Circulation – Measure

This action requires the examiner to gather objective data related to cardiovascular function and may include the following.

Body Temperature. Body temperature can be measured in a number of ways. Aural temperatures are the most convenient method in adults, although oral, axillary and rectal temperature may also be measured. Body temperature is maintained within the range 36.5–37.5°C. *Pyrexia* is elevation of the body temperature above 37.5°C, and is associated with an increased metabolic rate. For every 1°C rise in body temperature, there is a 10% increase in VO_2 and CO_2 production (Manthous et al 1995), resulting in a compensatory increase in heart rate and RR.

Electrocardiogram (ECG). Electrocardiogram is a transthoracic recording of the electrical activity of the heart measured from up to 12 electrodes placed in standardized positions around the chest wall. An ECG monitor allows the electrical signals recorded on the chest wall to be transduced to a digital display that provides a real-time representation of the cardiac cycle. The waveforms seen on the ECG reflect the underlying mechanical events of cardiac contraction. Analysis of the ECG is used for diagnosis of common cardiac dysfunction including myocardial infarction and atrial fibrillation. Detailed information about ECG measurement and interpretation is covered in Chapter 4.

Blood Pressure (BP). Contraction of the heart during systole increases peak arterial or 'systolic' pressure. During cardiac relaxation the arterial pressure drops to a minimum or 'diastolic' pressure. Blood pressure is measured by placing a sphygmomanometer cuff around the upper arm, and listening over the brachial artery with a stethoscope. Cuff inflation above systolic pressure compresses the artery inhibiting flow so that no brachial pulse is audible. Slowly releasing the cuff pressure until the pressure within the artery is greater than the pressure outside the artery allows blood flow to recommence, and an audible pulse can be heard through the stethoscope. This pressure is recorded as the systolic pressure. As the cuff pressure drops further the pressure within the artery is greater than that of the cuff throughout the cardiac cycle, turbulent flow abates and the pulse disappears again. This point defines the diastolic pressure. Normal adult blood pressure is between 95/60 and 140/90 mmHg. *Hypertension* is defined as a blood pressure greater than 145/95 mmHg. *Hypotension* is defined as a blood pressure less than 90/60 mmHg. *Postural hypotension* is a drop in blood pressure of more than 5 mmHg between lying and sitting or standing, and may be due to decreased circulating blood volume, or loss of vascular tone.

Central Venous Pressure (CVP). CVP is the pressure at the tip of an indwelling central venous catheter in the vena cava close to the right atrium of the heart. CVP represents the pressure associated with blood returning to the heart and closely reflects pressure within the right atrium. Normal values are 2–6 mmHg. CVP is elevated in right heart failure and decreased in dehydration.

Fluid Balance. The calculated discrepancy (mL) between fluid input and fluid output recorded on a fluid balance sheet is defined as the fluid balance. Fluid input can be in the form of food or fluids but many hospitalized patients also receive additional fluids intravenously. Fluid loss from the body can occur in a number of different ways including urine, faeces, sweating, vomiting, bleeding and surgical drain output. Urine output should be greater than 0.5 mL/kg h^{-1}. *Eurovolaemia* is achieved when fluid input matches the fluid output. *Hypovolaemia* (dehydration) occurs when fluid output exceeds input and *hypervolaemia* (fluid overload) occurs when input exceeds output.

Cardiac Output, Stroke Volume, Cardiac Index, Pulmonary Artery Occlusion Pressure (PAOP). In the critical care environment invasive and non-invasive methods of performing cardiac output studies are utilized. Details of intensive care monitoring can be found in Chapter 9.

Cardiopulmonary Exercise Testing. In some patient groups it is appropriate to complete an exercise test to fully determine cardiopulmonary function. Exercise tests vary from an incremental graded exercise protocol for measuring maximum oxygen uptake, to simple walking tests which can be performed in the hospital corridor. Two of the most common methods used to assess patients with cardiorespiratory disease are the 6-minute walk test (Butland et al 1982) and the shuttle walking test (Bradley et al 1999, Revill et al 1999, Singh et al 1992) (see Chapter 6).

D = Disability

This component of the objective assessment is concerned with collecting information regarding neuro-musculoskeletal function. Any patient with a decreased level of consciousness is at risk of airway obstruction, aspiration and retention of pulmonary secretions. Alterations in mental state and consciousness can occur with hypoxia, hypercapnia, dehydration and infection. Assessment of neurological function may be required to determine the potential for respiratory compromise in progressive neuromuscular disorders such as Guillain-Barré syndrome. Appreciation of cognitive function is also important with respect to determining whether the patient is capable of consenting to physiotherapy assessment and intervention. The extent to which each aspect of disability is investigated

will be determined by the clinical environment and presentation.

Disability – Observation

General observations relating to neurological function include: Is the patient alert, appearing agitated, restless, responsive to voice, responding to pain or unresponsive? Is the patient moving? What is the quality of movement? Are there any abnormal or extraneous movements? Are both sides moving equally? Is there facial symmetry? Can the patient achieve a lip seal or swallow? Is the patient drooling? Is there obvious head trauma or evidence of surgical interventions (e.g. craniotomy, cranial incisions, external ventricular drains, intracranial pressure (ICP) monitors, high cervical or trauma collars)? Is the patient receiving any drugs (sedatives, analgesics or anaesthetics) that are likely to affect consciousness levels? Specific neurological observations may include the following.

Glasgow Coma Scale. In patients who are not sedated, consciousness is rated using the Glasgow Coma Scale (GCS) (Table 2-6). The scale rates the patient from 3 to 15 based on their best observed motor, verbal and eye responses (Teasdale & Jennett 1974). When a patient has an endotracheal tube or tracheostomy

TABLE 2-6		
The Glasgow Coma Scale: Maximum Score = 15; Minimum Score = 3		
Response	Element	Score
Eye opening	Spontaneous	4
	To speech	3
	To pain	2
	None	1
Best verbal response	Orientated	5
	Confused speech	4
	Inappropriate words	3
	Incomprehensible sounds	2
	None	1
Best motor response	Obeys commands	6
	Localizes to pain	5
	Flexion withdraw to pain	4
	Abnormal flexion (decorticate)	3
	Extension (decerebrate)	2
	None	1

(Reproduced from Teasdale & Jennett 1974, with permission)

the verbal response is classified as 'V-T' (presence of endotracheal tube).

Pupillary Response. Pupillary response is evaluated by passing a pen torch light across the open eye to determine reactivity and size of the pupil. A pin-point pupil is a sign of opiate toxicity; a fixed and dilated pupil is a sign of neurological catastrophe.

Disability – Listen

Airway patency will have been assessed during the assessment of airway early in the examination. Listen to the speech content to assess cognitive function. Is the patient confused or disoriented? Is speech intelligible? Some neurological problems result in damage to the muscles involved in producing speech leading to *dysarthria*. A dysarthric patient may also have impaired swallowing *(dysphagia)* and be at risk of aspiration. Other neurological disorders affect the ability to create speech *(expressive aphasia)* or understand speech *(receptive aphasia)*.

Disability – Feel

Several aspects of neuro-musculoskeletal assessment can be determined by feel. For example, resistance or rigidity may be felt when positioning limbs or testing movement range. The quality of resistance felt at the end of joint range should be noted. Appreciation of these factors usually accompanies specific measurement of sensation, peripheral muscle weakness and range of motion (see Disability – Measure).

Disability – Measure

In some patient presentations it will be important to complete a full neurological examination at this point in the assessment process. For example, the patient who has experienced a prolonged stay in critical care may develop reduced sensation, muscle strength, range of motion and impaired functional ability. Establishing baseline neuro-musculoskeletal characteristics will enable sensible treatment goals to be established. The patient with acute spinal cord injury will require careful charting of motor and sensory function to establish the level of neurological impairment and will influence the treatment provided. The elderly patient recovering from community-acquired pneumonia on a medical ward will need an assessment of strength

and function to determine the amount of assistance required to progress mobilization and plan discharge. The extent of neurological examination undertaken will be determined by the patient presentation.

Several other tests and measurements related to neuro-musculoskeletal disability have a direct influence on cardiorespiratory physiotherapy decision making.

Blood Glucose. Homeostatic mechanisms tightly control the concentration of glucose (sugar) in the blood to maintain a narrow range of 4.4–6.1 mmol/L. Blood glucose is measured by testing blood sampled from a finger prick or artery. Since glucose is required for brain function, a reduction in blood glucose below this level may cause a variety of neurological symptoms ranging from lethargy, muscle weakness, shaking, twitching, irritability, poor concentration and confusion. If untreated, *hypoglycaemia* may cause loss of consciousness. *Hypoglycaemia* can occur in individuals with poorly controlled diabetes; however, non-diabetic patients can also experience low blood glucose with malnutrition or binge drinking. Hyperglycaemia can cause hunger, excessive thirst and polyuria. Chronically elevated blood glucose results in damage to the eyes, kidneys and heart, poor wound healing, recurrent infections and peripheral neuropathies. Severe hyperglycaemia can result in diabetic ketoacidosis (DKA) which is a medical emergency.

Intracranial Pressure. Patients with traumatic brain injury may have an ICP monitoring device inserted into their brains. This device measures ICP or pressure inside the skull from brain tissue and cerebrospinal fluid. The normal range of ICP in the semi-recumbent position is 10–15 mmHg. Increased ICP from intracranial bleeding or brain swelling can cause secondary damage to brain tissue since the skull is a closed vault. Craniotomy is often performed to reduce the ICP by allowing the swollen brain to herniate through the skull opening. Some physiotherapy interventions may cause an increase in ICP to dangerous levels in the patient with head injury.

Functional Ability. Functional ability can be assessed using a variety of validated scales and measurement tools depending on the impairment and activity limitation (see Chapter 6). Discussion of these tools is beyond the scope of this section but may include assessment of balance or walk distance.

Quality of Life. Assessment of QOL is becoming increasingly important to determine the impact of disability on the patient and as a measure of response to treatment. QOL scales measure the effect of an illness and its management on a patient *as perceived by the patient*. Often there is little correlation between physiological measures (e.g. lung function) and QOL. A number of both generic, for example SF-36 (Ware & Sherbourne 1992), and disease-specific QOL scales are available which allow data to be gathered principally by self-report questionnaire or interview. QOL scales available for assessment of patients with respiratory or cardiovascular disease are reviewed elsewhere (Juniper et al 1999, Kinney et al 1996, Mahler 2000, Pashkow et al 1995). The choice of a QOL measure requires an evaluation of QOL scales with respect to their reliability, validity, responsiveness and appropriateness (Aaronson 1989).

E = Exposure

The final component of the structured physical assessment is concerned with physical features that have not previously been explored specifically through assessment of airway, breathing, circulation or disability. This component is termed 'exposure' since at some point full exposure of the body may be necessary. Exposure should be completed in such a way as to preserve patient dignity and comfort. This component of the assessment also involves exposure to measures of haematology, biochemistry or microbiological investigations which may also influence physiotherapy decision making.

Exposure – Observation

Skin Colour and Condition. What colour is the patient's face, chest and peripheral skin? Peripheral cyanosis (a bluish discolouration of the skin) can affect the toes, fingers and earlobes, but may also be due to poor peripheral circulation, especially in cold weather. Grey mottled skin suggests very poor peripheral perfusion and can represent a medical emergency. Jaundice, a yellow discolouration affecting the eyes, skin and mucous membranes, occurs with liver diseases

and biliary obstruction; pale skin can be a sign of anaemia. Is the skin dry, flaky or peeling? Are there any obvious skin lesions, psoriasis, rashes, ulcers or pressure areas? Appreciation of the condition of the limbs will influence physiotherapy decision making with regard to mobilization. For example, the presence of sacral or buttock pressure sores will limit the time a patient might be able to sit in a chair. Pressure sores will also affect the way in which a patient can be moved or hoisted since any shearing force on the skin in that area should be avoided and tissue viability advice sought.

Limb Exposure. Limb exposure may reveal the presence of limb deformity, amputation and the peripheral limb muscle mass. Is the muscle mass symmetrical between limbs, and between upper and lower limbs? Are there localized areas of atrophy, or generalized cachexia?

Eyes. The eyes should be examined for pallor (anaemia), redness (high haemoglobin) or jaundice. Drooping of one eyelid with enlargement of that pupil suggests Horner syndrome where there is a disturbance in the sympathetic nerve supply to that side of the head (sometimes seen in cancer of the lung).

Hands. Warm and sweaty hands with an irregular flapping tremor may be due to acute CO_2 retention. A fine tremor may be seen following nebulized bronchodilators. Weakness and wasting of the small muscles in the hands may be an early sign of an upper lobe tumour involving the brachial plexus (Pancoast tumour). Examination of the fingers may show nicotine staining from smoking. Abnormalities of the nails are common in patients with cardiorespiratory disease. For example, nail clubbing (loss of the angle between the nail bed and the nail; Fig. 2-6) is observed in a number of cardiorespiratory and gastrointestinal diseases including congenital heart disease; endocarditis; cystic fibrosis; malignant, infective and fibrotic lung disease; cirrhosis; Crohn disease and ulcerative colitis. Clubbing in patients with cystic fibrosis disappears after heart and lung or lung transplant.

Nutrition. The presence of nutritional support suggests that a patient may not be able to eat safely or has

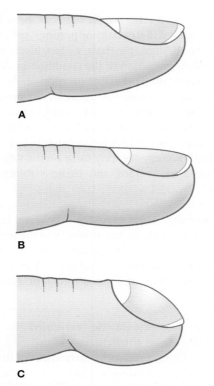

A

B

C

FIGURE 2-6 ■ Clubbing. **(A)** Normal. **(B)** Early clubbing. **(C)** Advanced clubbing.

a disturbance of gastrointestinal function. A soft, fine-bore tube inserted via the nostril to the stomach (nasogastric, NG) or jejunum (nasojejunostomy, NJ) is used to facilitate enteral feeding. A feeding tube placed directly into the stomach via the abdominal wall (percutaneous endoscopic gastrostomy, PEG) may be seen in patients who permanently require an alternative mode of delivering nutrition. A patient who does not have a functioning gastrointestinal tract will be provided with IV nutrition. Total parenteral nutrition solution (TPN) can be delivered through venous access devices but when chronically required may be delivered through a peripherally inserted central catheter (PICC line).

Abdomen. The abdomen may appear generally distended or have localized protrusions such as a hernia (protrusion of a body part through a defect in the abdominal wall). Hernias can occur at incision sites, the umbilicus or the inguinal area. Longitudinal, transverse or lateral abdominal scars or incisions may be noted. Observe any obvious rashes, erythema or cellulitis which may exist around wounds. Postoperatively, drains may be placed at any operation site to prevent the collection of fluid or blood. A stoma may be present where the ileum (ileostomy), large intestine or colon (colostomy) is drawn through and sutured to the abdominal wall to allow movement of faeces. PEG tubes to facilitate enteral feeding may be noted on the upper left quadrant of the anterior abdominal wall. Aortic pulsation is sometimes observed in the epigastric region.

Exposure – Feel

Abdominal Palpation. The abdominal compartment can be systematically palpated to incorporate the four quadrants of the abdomen (right upper quadrant, RUQ; left upper quadrant, LUQ; right lower quadrant, RLQ; and left lower quadrant, LLQ). The abdomen should be soft and non-tender on light palpation. Areas of tenderness, muscular guarding, *diastasis recti* (separation of the rectus abdominus muscles) and superficial masses may be noted. Superficial fatty tumours known as '*lipomas*' may be present on the abdominal wall which will feel soft under the skin. Ascetic fluid in the abdomen tends to cause bulges in the abdominal flank since it is affected by gravity. A hard, distended or painful abdomen will affect respiratory function. Increased resistance to diaphragm descent may inhibit tidal volume and precipitate dependent lung collapse.

Exposure – Listen

Bowel Sounds. Gastric motility can be assessed by listening to bowel sounds with a stethoscope. The preferred place to listen for bowel sounds is the right lower quadrant. Normal bowel sounds are regularly occurring gurgles and clicks. Absent bowel sounds can suggest constipation, bowel obstruction or paralytic ileus. High-pitched tinkling sounds are suggestive of bowel distension which can lead to perforation in severe cases.

Exposure – Measure

Body Weight. Respiratory function can be compromised by both obesity and severe malnourishment. The body mass index (BMI) is calculated by dividing the weight in kilograms by the square of the height in metres (kg/m^2); the normal range is 20–25 kg/m^2. BMI values below 20 represent low body weight, values of 25–30 represent high body weight, and values over 30 are classified obese. Malnourished patients have weaker respiratory muscles which are more likely to fatigue. Obesity causes an increase in residual volume and a decrease in functional residual capacity (Rubinstein et al 1990). Thus tidal breathing occurs close to closing volume. This is particularly important postoperatively, where the obese are more prone to sub-segmental lung collapse.

Laboratory Investigations. Venous blood samples can be tested to provide information regarding organ function and the concentration of certain electrolytes, enzymes, hormones and other chemicals. A list of common haematological and biochemical investigations is provided in Table 2-7. Blood, urine, sputum and other body fluids can be cultured to determine the organisms they grow and what antibiotics they are sensitive to. Interpretation of biochemical markers is important in the determination of physiotherapy decision making since abnormalities of these factors may contraindicate certain physiotherapy interventions. For example, a patient with very low platelets or a very high international normalized ratio (INR, a measure of blood coagulation) will be at high risk of bleeding should he require insertion of artificial airways or suctioning procedures. It would be considered unsafe to exercise a patient with cardiac disease who has a very low haemoglobin due to the risk of cardiac ischaemia. High serum potassium in the patient without renal failure can precipitate cardiac arrhythmias. It may not be suitable to take a patient with a severely compromised immune system (low white blood cell count) to the gymnasium, where they are at risk of exposure to pathogens which cause opportunistic infections.

USING THE INFORMATION FROM CLINICAL ASSESSMENT

Information obtained from the clinical assessment should be integrated with the physiotherapist's knowledge of disease processes and the risks and benefits of physiotherapy interventions. In this way, aspects of the clinical presentation which are amenable to physiotherapy intervention will be identified. A thorough and appropriate assessment will also identify important factors that must be considered when developing a management plan. Experienced clinicians may recognize certain features of the clinical assessment that match the pattern of clinical presentation in other patients they have treated. Pattern recognition may influence the extent of the clinical examination performed since experience will enable them to probe certain areas at the expense of others. Pattern recognition may also improve their confidence in selecting appropriate management strategies for the individual concerned. Less experienced clinicians will need to consider a number of factors in determining a management plan which may include: recognition of abnormal features in the clinical assessment; the order of relevance or urgency of the clinical presentation; which aspects of the clinical presentation can or cannot be influenced by physiotherapy interventions and which interventions have the highest likelihood of affecting more than one aspect of the clinical presentation.

DOCUMENTATION

The assessment process should be clearly documented using a concise, systematic and repeatable format to allow communication between therapists and within the broader healthcare team. Documentation should be precise, avoid jargon and use only acceptable terminology. Documentation style and content is influenced by both local and national legal and regulatory frameworks which physiotherapists must observe in terms of quality standards for record-keeping practice. A suggested documentation style for cardiorespiratory physiotherapy in the acute hospital setting is the subjective, objective, assessment, plan format, or SOAP notes. SOAP is a very common abbreviation which will have resonance for clinicians:

■ **S**ubjective: What the patient, nurses or medical staff report
■ **O**bjective: The results of physical examination or tests
■ **A**ssessment: The physiotherapist's opinion of the subjective and objective findings in respect to identification of the underlying problem. This section includes treatment delivered and evaluation (see Fig. 2-7).
■ **P**lan: Including recommendations and further actions required

TABLE 2-7
Laboratory Investigations

Investigation	Normal Value	Significance for Physiotherapy
Haemoglobin (Hb)	Men: 13–18 g/dL Women: 11.5–16 g/dL	Patients with a low Hb will look pale and may complain of dizziness, fatigue and breathlessness. A Hb of <7 requires transfusion. Mobilization/exercise should be avoided in extreme anaemia due to the risk of cardiac ischaemia.
White blood count (WBC)	4–11 × 10^9/L	High WBC indicates infection so source identification should be considered. Low WBC is characterized by low neutrophils, making patients susceptible to bacterial infections. These patients should be isolated.
Platelets (PLT)	150–400 × 10^9/L	Low platelets result in the risk of bleeding and must be considered if inserting an nasopharyngeal airway or applying manual techniques.
Haematocrit (HCT)	Men: 45% Women: 40%	Low values indicate haemorrhage and high values are observed in patients with diarrhoea.
International Normalized Ratio (INR)	0.9–1.1	High values result in bleeding risk and lower the incidence of clot formation. Patients will have higher acceptable values if taking warfarin.
Activated partial thromboplastin time (APTT)	30–40 secs	Provides information about blood clotting and is used to monitor the effects of heparin.
Sodium (Na)	135–145 mmol/L	Hypernatraemia is associated with dehydration, muscle weakness and fatigue.
Potassium (K)	3.5–5 mmol/L	Hyperkalaemia is associated with the risk of arrhythmias and sudden cardiac death.
Chloride (Cl)	95–105 mmol/L	An electrolyte needed for metabolism which maintains the body's acid-base balance. High values suggest dehydration.
Urea	2.5–6.7 mmol/L	Elevated in patients with dehydration or kidney injury (acute/chronic). Patients may present with confusion.
Creatinine	70–150 µmol/L	Like urea, high values suggest kidney dysfunction.
Magnesium (Mg)	0.65–1.0 mmol/L	Low levels result in a risk of developing arrhythmias, muscle weakness and fatigue.
Phosphate (PO$_4$)	0.8–1.4 mmol/L	Hypophosphataemia can cause symptoms of bone pain, confusion and muscle weakness. It is also necessary for optimum gastrointestinal function
C-Reactive protein (CRP)	<10 mg/L	An inflammatory marker that is part of the acute phase response to infection.
Creatine kinase (CK)	25–195 IU/L	Increased values are associated with muscle/tissue damage commonly seen following trauma, lying on a hard surface for a long time, or extreme sports (e.g. marathon running). High CKs have the potential to cause renal failure.
Lactate	0.6–2.0 mmol/L	Increased levels develop when organ hypo-perfusion occurs such as in severe hypotension.
Bilirubin	3–17 µmol/L	Mild increases suggest haemolysis. Very high levels are seen in severe liver failure and result in jaundice.
Analine transaminase (ALT)	5–35 IU/L	A biomarker of liver injury where liver function is intact.
Aspartate aminotransferase (AST)	5–35 IU/L	A biomarker of liver injury where liver function is intact.
Alkaline phosphatase (ALP)	30–150 IU/L	High levels indicate bile duct obstruction and may be elevated in pregnancy. Elevated levels are associated with active bone formation which occurs in Paget disease.
Albumin	35–50 g/L	Hypoalbuminaemia will cause general oedema due to the reduction in osmotic pressure.

Individual therapists will develop a documentation style that is consistent with local regulatory frameworks and the environment in which they work. An example of physiotherapy assessment and management documentation for a patient in the postoperative setting is provided to illustrate the SOAP format (Fig. 2-7).

EVALUATING OUTCOME

Appropriate measurement of outcome is fundamental to evaluate the effectiveness of any intervention. The method used to evaluate the outcome of intervention should directly relate to the problem identified through analysis of the clinical assessment findings. The World Health Organization (WHO) developed the International Classification of Functioning, Disability and Health (ICF) (WHO 2001) in an attempt to standardize the measurement of outcomes. Problems (and therefore goals) can be stated in terms of body structure or function (impairment), and/or in more patient-centred terms such as activity limitation and participation restriction. For example, a patient with bronchiectasis who has had recurrent admissions to hospital for chest infections over the last year may be taught an airway clearance technique for sputum clearance. In the short term the effectiveness of the intervention will be evaluated at the impairment level through change in the findings of the objective assessment (e.g. sputum volume before and after the intervention). After 12 months of using the secretion clearance technique the patient's ability to climb stairs improved (an increase in activity) and the patient was able to maintain a full-time job with a reduction in hospital admissions (reduced participation restriction). Demonstrating the effectiveness of physiotherapy management using instruments that are valid, reliable, responsive and relate to the patient's problems is increasingly required of physiotherapists by patients and funding organizations.

CONCLUSION

The goal of performing a clinical assessment within cardiorespiratory physiotherapy is to complete a process whereby the problems amenable to physiotherapy intervention are recognized. This unique process is commonly referred to as 'analysis' or clinical reasoning

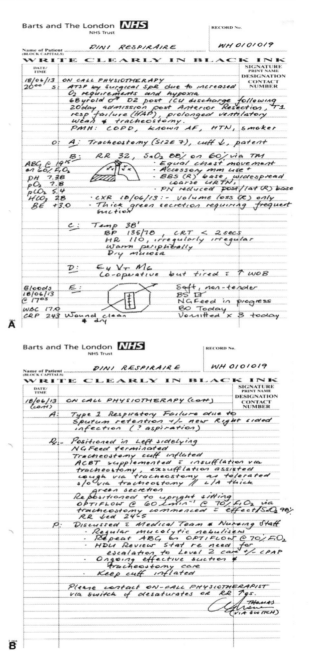

FIGURE 2-7 ■ An example of subjective, objective, assessment, plan (SOAP) notes. **(A)** contains the subjective and objective findings; **(B)** contains the assessment of the underlying problem, treatment delivered and plan for continuing management.

and requires a sound theoretical knowledge of the indications for safety, effectiveness and contra-indications of physiotherapy techniques. The quality of the analysis process is therefore dependent on the experience of the therapist and their background knowledge. Many other health professionals are capable of completing a clinical assessment, but the physiotherapist adds value to the patient journey through their unique analysis.

Of the assessment findings with reference to physical interventions. There are various models of problem analysis or clinical reasoning that the physiotherapist may adopt to assist with integration, interpretation and prioritization of the assessment findings. Regardless of the analysis model adopted it is impossible to develop an appropriate treatment plan without an accurate and appropriate assessment.

Infant and Child

INTRODUCTION

The respiratory system in children differs significantly from adults, both anatomically and physiologically (see Chapter 1). These differences have important consequences for the physiotherapy care of children in terms of respiratory assessment, treatment and choice of techniques. The principal reason for hospital admissions in children aged 0–4 years is respiratory illness, and the management of children with acute or chronic respiratory disorders has become a specialized area of respiratory physiotherapy. Most aspects of assessment will be the same as in adults (earlier in this chapter), but some specific differences will be addressed. The inexperienced physiotherapist working with children will require the support and mentorship of an experienced paediatric physiotherapist in order to develop the necessary skills.

MEDICAL NOTES

Information can be extracted from the medical notes relating to present and past medical history. When assessing a neonate, history of pregnancy, labour and delivery are relevant as well as gestational age and weight. In addition, the Apgar score at birth should be noted. This score relates to heart rate, respiratory effort, muscle tone, reflex irritability and colour and gives an indication of the degree of asphyxiation suffered by the infant at birth.

Observation Charts and Investigations

Pyrexia may indicate a possible respiratory infection.

- The core-to-peripheral temperature gradient should be noted, particularly in the critically ill

child as it is a reflection of peripheral vasoconstriction which can occur as a response to cold, hypovolaemia, sepsis or low cardiac output.

- Tachycardia may be due to sepsis or shock. It may also be caused by inadequate levels of sedation or analgesia. In preterm infants, bradycardias may be due to many causes, including retention of secretions.
- Apnoeic spells or hypoxia in the infant may indicate respiratory distress, sepsis or presence of secretions in the upper or lower respiratory tract. Short periods of apnoea may be normal in premature and newborn babies
- The trend of arterial gases and their relationship to oxygen saturation and transcutaneous oxygen should be noted, together with the degree and type of respiratory support.

COMMUNICATION

Assessment and treatment of children requires skilful age-appropriate communication with the child, the family and within the multidisciplinary team. Questions need to reflect the child's age and must take into account symptoms at rest, and when the child is running around playing or taking part in school games or sport. For example, can a baby drink a full bottle of milk or does it become breathless and start spluttering? Does a boy keep up during a game of football or is he always put in goal? Can a schoolgirl carry her books up several flights of stairs to lessons or does she have to rest at each floor? Questions are easier to answer if they relate to normal activities and how the child functions in everyday life. Many parents do not understand what is meant by the terms used to describe noisy breathing, such as 'wheezing' (Cane et al 2000) and an ability to demonstrate these sounds may be helpful.

Discussion with the Relevant Carers

Discussion with medical staff, nursing staff and the parent/carer is essential to obtain correct information about recent changes. In chronically ill children who require home physiotherapy, liaison with the primary healthcare team is essential.

When assessing the hospitalized child, information should be obtained about:

- the stability of the child's condition over the last few hours
- how well the infant tolerates handling. Does the infant become rapidly hypoxic or bradycardic?
- how long the child takes to recover from the handling episode
- whether the child is fed via the oral, NG or IV route and the timing of the last feed
- whether the child is sufficiently rested to tolerate a physiotherapy treatment.

PHYSICAL EXAMINATION

Physical examination is critical, although it will only give information about the child at rest. Nevertheless, inspection will soon reveal whether the patient is in respiratory distress with, for example, tachypnoea and/or dyspnoea. The normal RR is age dependent, and decreases with age (Table 2-8). It is important to determine whether the child can speak sentences without becoming breathless and whether accessory muscles

are being used leading to intercostal or subcostal recession. Cyanosis, if present, is fairly obvious. When reviewing a child with cystic fibrosis or bronchiectasis, it is important to inspect the sputum (colour, consistency). Palpation is good for assessing chest expansion and placing the hands on the chest will indicate, by a feeling of vibration, whether mucus is present – a method used by many parents of children with cystic fibrosis. Percussion is most useful for determining the presence of a pleural effusion (parapneumonic or empyema) indicated by dullness. Before auscultating with a stethoscope, it is worth simply listening to the child's breathing for wheeze (an expiratory sound), stridor (an inspiratory sound) or upper respiratory tract secretions heard in the throat (harsh expiratory and inspiratory sounds that are transmitted throughout the chest). The presence of a cough and its nature (dry, moist, productive, spasmodic) should be listened for. A forceful huff may also reveal abnormal sounds not obvious with quiet breathing. Finally, listening with the stethoscope may indicate abnormal sounds that can then be located to a particular area or lobe. It is always worth asking the patient to cough before listening again, as often some of the added sounds will have disappeared.

CLINICAL SIGNS

Clinical signs of respiratory distress are summarized in Box 2-1 and explained in more detail below.

Recession occurs when high negative intrathoracic pressure during inspiration pulls the soft, compliant chest wall inward. It may be sternal, subcostal or intercostal. Mild recession may be normal in preterm

TABLE 2-8			
Normal Values			
Age Group	Heart Rate Mean (Range) (beats/min)	Respiratory Rate – Range (breaths/min)	Blood Pressure Systolic/Diastolic (mmHg)
Preterm	150 (100–200)	40–60	39–59/16–36
Newborn	140 (80–200)	30–50	50–70/25–45
<2 years	130 (100–190)	20–40	87–105/53–66
>2 years	80 (60–140)	20–40	95–105/53–66
>6 years	75 (60–90)	15–30	97–112/57–71

BOX 2-1
CLINICAL SIGNS OF RESPIRATORY DISTRESS

RESPIRATORY

- Recession
  - intercostal
  - subcostal
  - sternal
- Nasal flaring
- Tachypnoea
- Expiratory grunting
- Stridor
- Cyanosis
- Abnormal breath sounds

CARDIAC

- Tachycardia/bradycardia
- Hypertension/hypotension

OTHER/GENERAL

- Neck extension
- Head bobbing
- Pallor
- Reluctance to feed
- Irritability/restlessness
- Altered conscious level
- Headache

infants but in older infants is a sign of increased respiratory effort.

Nasal flaring is a dilatation of the nostrils by the *dilatores naris* muscles and is a sign of respiratory distress in the infant. It may be a primitive response attempting to decrease airway resistance.

Tachypnoea (RR greater than 60 breaths/min) may indicate respiratory distress in infants. Normal values are listed in Table 2-8.

Grunting occurs when an infant expires against a partially closed glottis. This is an automatic response which increases functional residual capacity in an attempt to improve ventilation.

Stridor is heard in the presence of a narrowing of the upper trachea and/or larynx. This may be due to collapse of the floppy tracheal wall, inflammation or an inhaled foreign body. It is most commonly heard during inspiration, but in cases of severe narrowing it may be heard during both inspiration and expiration.

Cyanosis refers to the bluish colour of the skin and mucous membranes caused by hypoxaemia. In infants and young children it is an unreliable sign of respiratory distress as it depends on the relative amount and type of haemoglobin in the blood and the adequacy of the peripheral circulation. For the first 3–4 weeks of life, the newborn infant has an increased amount of foetal haemoglobin, which has a higher affinity for oxygen than adult haemoglobin. The result is a shift of the oxygen saturation curve to the left in infants.

Auscultation of the infant and young child is sometimes complicated by the easy transmission of sounds. In the infant who is ventilated, referred sounds such as water in the ventilator tubing may be transmitted to the chest. In the older child, secretions in the nose or throat may lead to referred sounds in both lung fields. Wheezing in the younger child or infant may be due to bronchospasm, but could also be due to retained secretions partially occluding smaller airways. It is sometimes very difficult to hear breath sounds in the spontaneously breathing preterm infant.

Cardiac manifestations of respiratory distress include an initial tachycardia and possible increase in systemic blood pressure. This changes with worsening hypoxia to bradycardia and hypotension.

Neck extension in an infant with respiratory distress may represent an attempt to reduce airway resistance.

Head bobbing occurs when infants attempt to use the sternocleidomastoid and the scalene muscles as accessory muscles of respiration. It is seen because the relatively weak neck extensors of infants are unable to stabilize the head.

Pallor is commonly seen in infants with respiratory distress and may be a sign of hypoxaemia or other problems, including anaemia.

Reluctance to feed is often associated with respiratory distress and infants may need to take frequent pauses from sucking when tachypnoeic.

Alterations in levels of consciousness should be noted. A reduction in activity may be due to neurological deficit or as a result of opiate analgesia but may also be due to hypoxia. It may be accompanied by an inability to feed or cry. Irritability and restlessness may also be indicative of a hypoxic state.

OTHER RELEVANT OBSERVATIONS

The behaviour of a child can often give important clues about their respiratory status. Agitation or irritability may be a sign of hypoxia, whilst the child in severe respiratory distress may be withdrawn and lie completely still.

It is important to note muscle tone in the infant or child with respiratory distress. A hypotonic child may have increased difficulty with breathing, coughing and expectorating, whilst hypertonia may also be associated with difficulty in clearing secretions.

Abdominal distension can cause or exacerbate respiratory distress, because the diaphragm is placed at a mechanical disadvantage. In infants this is of greater concern as the diaphragm is the primary muscle of respiration.

The Acutely Ill or Deteriorating Patient

INTRODUCTION

The first part of this chapter describes how to perform a thorough, in-depth assessment of the respiratory system. This allows the therapist to gather information to prioritize patient problems, set treatment plans and goals and also evaluate the response to physiotherapy interventions. For patients developing critical illness, however, a more rapid assessment of vital signs is required in order to ascertain clinical urgency. This section describes how to assess the acutely ill or deteriorating adult patient using the Airway, Breathing, Circulation, Disability, Exposure (A-B-C-D-E) approach. It is a logical, step-by-step process which takes into account changes in vital signs induced by critical illness. This quick and easy tool can be used in acute situations, by all clinicians regardless of their training and profession and is appropriate for all adult patient groups regardless of diagnosis.

BACKGROUND

In-hospital cardiac arrest carries a high mortality as only 10% of patients survive to leave hospital (Franklin et al 1994, Schein et al 1990). Studies show that cardiac arrest is predictable and preventable with patients showing unrecognized clinical signs of physiological deterioration several hours preceding the event (Franklin et al 1994, Schein et al 1990). This is often caused by sub-optimal ward care (McQuillan et al 1998).

Likely causes of sub-optimal ward care are 'whole systems failure' with human factors (rather than technical failure) most at fault. Cognitive errors play an important role in all adverse events (Neale et al 2001) suggesting lack of attention to clinical signs and relevance of basic bedside physiological monitoring. Less experienced staff are left with insufficient senior supervision, especially outside of normal working hours and patients admitted at the weekend have a been shown to have greater risk of death than those admitted during the week (Aylin et al 2010). Poor knowledge or application of knowledge to changes in acute physiology causes failure to recognize clinical urgency. Poor communication and failure or reluctance to seek timely advice confound these problems (Wilson et al 1999).

Initiatives across the world have addressed early identification of critical illness which has reduced mortality (Levy et al 2010). The use of the A-B-C-D-E assessment and validated 'Track and Trigger' tools (e.g. Early Warning Scores (EWS)) are promoted as they allow clinicians to quickly and accurately assess patients at high risk of deterioration and alert others to the severity of illness (National Institute for Clinical Excellence 2007, National Patient Safety Agency 2007). Using EWS also facilitates rapid re-assessment to see patients' responses to simple protocols (care bundles) and early goal-directed therapy (EGDT). This is important as EGDT (e.g. oxygen, IV antibiotics and fluids) has been shown to reduce mortality compared with standard therapy (Rivers et al 2001).

ASSESSMENT TECHNIQUE

When first approaching the patient, make a general observation of whether they look unwell. If your first impression raises any concerns it is better to call for help at this stage, to ensure it arrives quickly. It is worth noting that younger, adult patients may look well even though they have severely deranged physiology. Their compensatory mechanisms to hypotension and hypoxaemia, for example, respond more effectively than those of elderly patients. The message here is that patients may look well but the abnormal values in vital signs are important indicators of acute deterioration.

When using the A-B-C-D-E assessment it is vital that life-threatening conditions are treated and show a positive response before moving on to the next letter in the tool: for example, starting the assessment with A and the patient's airway is partially obstructed; this must be addressed before moving on to B, the next letter in the algorithm, as breathing problems cannot be treated if the airway remains obstructed. At each stage in the A-B-C-D-E assessment of the acutely ill patient use the 'look, listen and feel' approach as described earlier in this chapter.

A – Airway

The aim here is to quickly determine upper airway patency (i.e. the airway above the vocal cords) and any immediate risk of airway obstruction. Patients with an obstructed airway have a paradoxical or 'see-saw' chest movement pattern. This is an emergency and if you haven't already done so call for help immediately.

If the patient's airway is totally obstructed there will be no noise at all. If the airway is partially obstructed you may hear gurgling from either vomitus, blood or other respiratory secretions present in the oropharynx. If you hear snoring this is partial obstruction in the pharynx by the tongue or other soft tissues.

If air does not appear to be moving into or out of the chest, the first-line emergency management of complete or partial airway obstruction consists of simple skills. Suction to remove secretions in the mouth and/or place an airway opening device (e.g. an oropharyngeal airway) using the head lift–chin tilt manoeuvre taught in Basic Life Support (BLS). Once this is achieved apply oxygen by face mask. If these measures do not secure the patient's airway, then endotracheal intubation will be required by the emergency team.

B – Breathing

The aim here is to assess adequate oxygenation and ventilation. Assess the patient's general colour and look for central cyanosis. Central cyanosis causes patients lips to look blue or purple in colour, so remember 'if the lips are blue, the brain is too'. Is the patient on oxygen, and if so how much? Hypoxaemic patients must be given high concentrations of oxygen via an oxygen mask with a reservoir bag and a flow rate of 15 L/min (O'Driscoll 2008) before proceeding with the rest of the assessment. Aim for SpO_2 to be within a target range of 94–98% (British Thoracic Society 2008). Count the RR, as it is the least likely of bedside observations to have been recorded accurately (Goldhill 2001). A raised RR is the first sign of acute illness as all critically ill patients have an increased oxygen demand from elevated cellular metabolism (Goldhill et al 1999). A RR greater than 20 breaths/min means increased work of breathing, which could lead to respiratory muscle fatigue if left untreated. Look for accessory muscle activity, asymmetry and irregular breathing patterns as these also suggest increased work of breathing. A slow RR (<12 breaths/min) is a sign of respiratory depression which will cause hypercapnia and a respiratory acidosis. Either way, respiratory support should be considered, so call for senior help and refer to the critical care or medical emergency team to ensure a timely response.

If the patient cannot complete their sentences or are speaking with gasps between words, this may be a sign of acute deterioration. If there are new sounds on auscultation with a stethoscope, such as asymmetry, bronchial breathing, wheeze or crackles, this might also suggest clinically important change.

If on palpation, there is sudden asymmetry of thoracic expansion, or if there is evidence of surgical emphysema, which feels like small subcutaneous bubbles beneath the skin, then suspect a pneumothorax and recommend an urgent chest radiograph.

Emergency management of the blue and breathless patient is to give high concentrations of oxygen and/or further respiratory support such as high-flow nasal oxygen or continuous positive airway pressure (CPAP). If there are *serious* or *proven* concerns that the patient is a chronic CO_2 retainer from chronic respiratory disease, caution must be used. Recent guidelines recommend 28% oxygen aiming for target SpO_2 of 88–92% (O'Driscoll 2008). It is appropriate to assess CO_2 status with an arterial blood gas but remember even the hypoxaemic chronic CO_2 retainer will proceed to cardiac arrest if they are not protected against severe hypoxaemia. A combination of delivering a higher oxygen concentration in combination with assisted non-invasive or invasive ventilation may be necessary. Because of this referral to the critical care or emergency team is crucial.

C – Circulation

The aim here is to assess adequate perfusion (blood flow) to vital organs. Check to see if there is peripheral cyanosis (blue fingertips) as this is a sign of hypovolaemia. Note the last recorded temperature, blood pressure and heart rate. If the patient has a urinary catheter in place, check the volume and colour of the urine. Dark urine suggests that the patient is dehydrated, which may also be reflected by a low blood pressure. The kidneys are very sensitive to an SBP of less than 90 mmHg and hypotension may present as oliguria in the first instance. Untreated oliguria results in acute kidney injury which carries a significant mortality (Bernieh et al 2004). To check the urine output, look at the fluid balance chart (FBC). If there is a urinary catheter in place, urine output should be more than 30 mL/hr for 2 hours or more than 500 mL in the last 24 hours. This is easier to assess in the acute situation than estimating the patient's weight and using the formula 1 mL/kg hr^{-1}. If the patient does not have a catheter or FBC ask if they have passed urine in the last few hours or see if they have been incontinent of urine. Check the drug chart to see if the patient has received any IV fluids in the last 6 hours.

Blood pressure should be taken manually using a sphygmomanometer and stethoscope. A narrow pulse pressure (the difference between systolic and diastolic pressures) is caused by high systemic vascular resistance (vasoconstriction) and likely to be due to hypovolaemia. A wide pulse pressure is caused by a low systemic vascular resistance (vasodilatation) and sepsis should be suspected. Recording the temperature is important to assess pyrexia (>37.5°C) as well as hypopyrexia (<36°C) which is equally significant in critical illness.

If the patient feels peripherally warm, this is normal circulation. If they are cool to touch then they are cardiovascularly shut down, suggesting hypotension. Conversely if they feel hot they are cardiovascularly dilated, which is a sign of sepsis. Feel for a peripheral pulse. By doing so you will be able to assess heart rate and the quality of pulse (bounding/thready/regular/irregular). If you are unable to feel a peripheral pulse use a stethoscope placed over the heart to count the heart rate. Check the CRT, which should be less than 2 seconds. A CRT longer than 2 seconds is an indication of hypotension and hypovolaemia. 'Shock' or hypovolaemia is the most frequent cause of circulatory emergencies. Hypotension brought about by fluid loss should respond to a fluid challenge starting with 500 mL. In patients with suspected cardiac failure a small bolus of 250 mL should be attempted in the first instance.

D – Disability

The aim here is to assess neurological function. When assessing the patient's consciousness in an acutely deteriorating patient it may be easier to use the Alert-Verbal-Painful-Unresponsive (AVPU) method than the GCS (Kelly et al 2004, McNarry & Goldhill 2004). A more in-depth assessment using the GCS can be done later if necessary.

The AVPU is scored by assessing which of these descriptors fits best:

- A: Alert
- V: Drowsy, responding to *Voice*
- P: Drowsy, responding *Pain*
- U: Unresponsive.

It is important to realize that some patients may not fit into these 4 categories, especially if they have acute confusion or seem agitated. These are still important clinical signs of ill health–induced physiological deterioration.

If the patient is anything other than A (alert), examine the drug chart to see if they are on any sedatives or opiate analgesics which cause neurological depression (including the respiratory centre). It is worth noting if any reversing agents (e.g. naloxone) are prescribed. Also check the blood sugar level as hypoglycaemia and hyperglycaemia can induce changes in neurological function which can be reversed quickly and easily at the bedside.

From your assessment, if the patient is P (drowsy responding to *pain*) or U (unresponsive), this is an emergency as they will not be able to protect their airway. Immediate referral to critical care or the emergency team is essential.

If the patient is not talking in an appropriate way and not orientated to place and time or if you only hear snoring or grunting, these are signs of neurologically induced upper airway obstruction, and must be treated as an emergency.

Treatment of a disordered level of consciousness should be based around protecting the airway, providing adequate oxygenation and circulation. The patient should be nursed in the lateral recovery position, with or without an airway opening device (depending upon the situation) and given oxygen and fluids if necessary, whilst waiting for the critical care or emergency team.

E – Exposure

This will enable you to complete a full examination.

Ensuring that you maintain the patient's dignity and comfort at all times, examine under any clothing/bed covers and around the bed area for further clues. For example, in hypotension look for evidence of fluid loss, haemorrhage or any bleeding from wounds, drains etc. Check for less obvious signs of bleeding (e.g. malaena, haematemasis, haemoptysis) and other signs of fluid loss such as diarrhoea or excessive diaphoresis.

ACTIONS AND COMMUNICATION

Using the information from the acute physiology, calculate the EWS (McGinley & Pearse 2012). Local protocols will suggest the next steps and will determine the frequency of observations and level of care required. Document your findings in the patient record, but communicating these facts verbally to the relevant team(s) is of greatest importance. This can be achieved by using a communication tool such as the Situation-Background-Assessment-Recommendation (SBAR) tool, or Reason-Story-Vital Signs-Plan (RSVP) tool. Both tools are easy to remember, allowing a process to structure important conversations which require a clinician's immediate attention and action (Featherstone et al 2008, Marshall et al 2009). Com-munication tools have been shown to improve quality of clinical referral on the telephone (Marshall et al 2009), meaning that inexperienced clinicians deliver the correct information in a logical format, facilitating the appropriate and timely response.

CONCLUSION

The goal of recognizing and responding to acutely deteriorating patients is to ensure that in the early onset of critical illness, they receive the appropriate treatment and level of care. Simple-to-use assessment and communication tools will allow identification of these patients, facilitating appropriate and effective communication up the chain of command. This will ensure that these patients are managed appropriately by the right teams in the right place at the right time, enhancing patient safety.

REFERENCES

Aaronson, N.K., 1989. Quality of life assessment in clinical trials: methodological issues. Control. Clin. Trials 10 (Suppl. 4), 195S–208S.

Aylin, A., Yunus, A., Bottle, A., et al., 2010. Weekend mortality for emergency admissions: a large multicentre study. Qual. Saf. Health Care 19 (2), 213–217.

Bach, J.R., Gonclaves, M.R., Hamdan, I., Winck, J.C., 2010. Extubation of unweanable patients with neuromuscular weakness: a new management paradigm. Chest 137 (5), 1033–1039.

Bach, J.R., Saporito, L.R., 1996. Criteria for extubation and tracheostomy tube removal for patients with ventilator failure: a different approach to weaning. Chest 110 (6), 1566–1571.

Bernard, G.R., Artigas, A., Brigham, K.L., et al., 1994. The American-European Consensus Conference on ARDS: definitions, mechanisms, relevant outcomes, and clinical trial coordination. Am. J. Respir. Crit. Care Med. 149 (3 Pt 1), 818–824.

Bernieh, B., Hakim, A., Boobes, Y., et al., 2004. Outcome and predictive factors of acute renal failure in the intensive care unit. Transplant. Proc. 36 (6), 1784–1787.

Bestall, J.C., Paul, E.A., Garrod, R., et al., 1999. Usefulness of the Medical Research Council (MRC) dyspnoea scale as a measure of disability in patients with chronic obstructive pulmonary disease. Thorax 54 (7), 581–586.

Bianchi, C., Baiardi, P., 2008. Cough peak flows: standard values for children and adolescents. Am. J. Phys. Med. Rehabil. 87 (6), 461–467.

BMJ Best Practice 2014 Assessment of chest pain: differential diagnosis. <http://bestpractice.bmj.com/best-practice/monograph/301/diagnosis/differential-diagnosis.html> (accessed 19 February 2015).

Borg, G.A., 1982. Psychophysical bases of perceived exertion. Med. Sci. Sports Exerc. 14 (5), 377–381.

Bradley, J., Howard, J., Wallace, E., et al., 1999. Validity of a modified shuttle test in adult cystic fibrosis. Thorax 54 (5), 437–439.

Butland, R.J., Pang, J., Gross, E.R., et al., 1982. Two-, six-, and 12-minute walking tests in respiratory disease. Br. Med. J. 284 (6329), 1607–1608.

Cane, R.S., Ranganathan, S.C., McKenzie, S.A., 2000. What do parents of wheezy children understand by 'wheeze'? Arch. Dis. Child. 82, 327–332.

Donahoe, M., Rogers, R.M., Wilson, D.O., Pennock, B.F., 1989. Oxygen consumption of the respiratory muscles in normal and malnourished patients with chronic obstructive pulmonary disease. Am. Rev. Respir. Dis. 140 (2), 385–391.

Featherstone, P., Chalmers, T., Smith, G.B., 2008. RSVP: a system for communication of deterioration in hospital patients. Br. J. Nurs. 17 (13), 860–864.

Franklin, C., Matthew, J., 1994. Developing strategies to prevent cardiac arrest: analysing responses of physicians and nurses in the hours before the event. Crit. Care Med. 22, 244–247.

Goldhill, D.R., 2001. The critically ill: following your MEWS. QJM 94, 507–510.

Goldhill, D.R., White, S.A., Sumner, A., 1999. Physiological values and procedures in the 24 hours before ICU admission from the ward. Anaesthesia 54, 529–534.

Hengeveld, E., Banks, K., 2013. Maitland's vertebral manipulation, eighth ed. management of neuromusculoskeletal disorders – Volume 1. Churchill Livingstone. ISBN: 9780702040665.

Johnson, M.J., Oxberry, S.G., Cleland, J.G.F., Clark, A.L., 2010. Measurement of breathlessness in clinical trials in patients with chronic heart failure: the need for a standardized approach: a systematic review. Eur. J. Heart Fail. 12 (2), 137–147.

Juniper, E.F., Guyatt, G.H., Cox, F.M., et al., 1999. Development and validation of the mini asthma quality of life questionnaire. Eur. Respir. J. 14 (1), 32–38.

Kelly, C.A., Upex, A., Bateman, D.N., 2004. Comparison of consciousness level assessment in the poisoned patient using the alert/verbal/painful/unresponsive scale and the Glasgow Coma Scale. Ann. Emerg. Med. 44 (2), 108–113.

Kinney, M.R., Burfitt, S.N., Stullenbarger, E., et al., 1996. Quality of life in cardiac patient research: a meta-analysis. Nurs. Res. 45 (3), 173–180.

Lee, T.H., 2004. Chest discomfort and palpitations. In: Kasper, D.L., Braunwald, E., Fauci, A.S., et al. (Eds.), Harrison's principles of internal medicine, sixteenth ed. Part II. Cardinal manifestations and presentation of diseases. McGraw-Hill., New York, pp. 76–81.

Lee, T.H., 2012. Chapter 12 Chest discomfort. In: Longo, D.L., Fauci, A.S., Kasper, D.L., et al. (Eds.), Harrison's principles of internal medicine, eighteenth ed. Part 2. Cardinal manifestations and presentation of diseases. Section 1. Pain [electronic resource]. McGraw-Hill, New York.

Levy, M.M., Dellinger, R.P., Townsend, S.R., et al., 2010. The Surviving Sepsis Campaign: results of an international guideline-based performance improvement program targeting severe sepsis. Crit. Care Med. 38 (2), 367–374.

Mahler, D.A., 2000. How should health-related quality of life be assessed in patients with COPD? Chest 117 (Suppl. 2), 54S–57S.

Mahler, D.A., Rosiello, R.A., Harver, A., et al., 1987. Comparison of clinical dyspnea ratings and psychophysical measurements of respiratory sensation in obstructive airway disease. Am. Rev. Respir. Dis. 135 (6), 1229–1233.

Manthous, C.A., Hall, J.B., Olson, D., et al., 1995. Effect of cooling on oxygen consumption in febrile critically ill patients. Am. J. Respir. Crit. Care Med. 151 (1), 10–14.

Marshall, S., Harrison, J., Flanagan, B., 2009. The teaching of a structured tool improves clarity of inter-professional clinical communication. Qual. Saf. Health Care 18 (2), 1137–1140.

McGinley, A., Pearse, R.M., 2012. A national early warning score for acutely ill patients. BMJ, 345, e5310. doi: http://dx.doi.org/10.1136/bmj.e5310.

McNarry, A.F., Goldhill, D.R., 2004. Simple bedside assessment of consciousness: comparison of two simple assessment scales with the Glasgow Coma Scale. Anaesthesia 59 (1), 34–37.

McQuillan, P., Pilkington, S., Allan, A., et al., 1998. Confidential inquiry in to quality of care before admission to intensive care. Br. Med. J. 316 (7948), 1853–1858.

National Institute for Clinical Excellence (NICE) Guidance 50, 2007. Acutely ill patients in hospital: recognition of and response to acute illness in adults in hospital. Department of Health UK.

National Patient Safety Agency (NPSA), 2007. Recognising and responding appropriately to early signs of deterioration in hospitalised patients. Department of Health UK.

Neale, G., Woloshynowych, M., Vincent, C., 2001. Exploring the causes of adverse events in NHS hospital practice. J. R. Soc. Med. 94 (7), 322–330.

Nolan, J., Soar, J., Lockey, A., et al. (Eds.), 2011. Advanced life support, sixth ed. Resuscitation Council (UK), London.

O'Driscoll, B.R., Howard, L.S., Davidson, A.G., 2008. Guideline for the emergency oxygen uses in adult patients. British Thoracic Society. Thorax 63 (Suppl. 6), v1–v8.

Orr, A., McVean, R.J., Webb, A.K., et al., 2001. Urinary incontinence in women with cystic fibrosis is a marginalized and undertreated problem: questionnaire survey. Br. Med. J. 322 (7301), 1521.

Pashkow, P., Ades, P.A., Emery, C.F., et al., 1995. Outcome measurement in cardiac and pulmonary rehabilitation. J. Cardiopulm. Rehabil. 15 (6), 394–405.

Pickard, A., Karlen, W., Ansermino, J.M., 2011. Capillary refill time: is it still a useful clinical sign? Anesth. Analg. 113 (1), 120–123.

Revill, S.M., Morgan, M.D.L., Singh, S.J., et al., 1999. The endurance shuttle walk: a new field test for the assessment of endurance capacity in chronic obstructive pulmonary disease. Thorax 54 (3), 213–222.

Rivers, E., Nguyen, B., Havstad, S., et al., 2001. Early goal-directed therapy in the treatment of severe sepsis and septic shock. NEJM 345 (19), 1368–1377.

Robertson, L., Al-Haddad, M., 2013. Recognising the critically ill patient. Anaesth. Intens. Care Med. 14 (1), 11–14.

Rubinstein, I., Zamel, N., DuBarry, L., et al., 1990. Airflow limitation in morbidly obese, non-smoking men. Ann. Intern. Med. 112 (11), 828–832.

Schein, R.M., Hazday, N., Pena, M., et al., 1990. Clinical antecedents to in-hospital cardiopulmonary arrest. Chest 98 (6), 1388–1392.

Scottish Intercollegiate Guidelines Network, 2004. Management of urinary incontinence in primary care <www.sign.ac.uk>.

Singh, S.J., Morgan, M.D.L., Scott, S., et al., 1992. The development of the shuttle walking test of disability in patients with chronic airways obstruction. Thorax 47 (12), 1019–1024.

Smina, M., Salam, A., Khamiees, M., et al., 2003. Cough peak flows and extubation outcomes. Chest 124 (1), 262–268.

Teasdale, G., Jennett, B., 1974. Assessment of coma and impaired consciousness. Lancet 2 (7872), 81–84.

Thakar, R., Stanton, S., 2000. Management of urinary incontinence in women. Br. Med. J. 321 (7272), 1326–1331.

Thim, T., Krarup, N.H., Grove, E.L., et al., 2012. Initial assessment and treatment with the Airway, Breathing, Circulation, Disability, Exposure (ABCDE) approach. Int. J. Gen. Med. 5, 117–121.

Ware, J.E., Sherbourne, C.D., 1992. The MOS-short-form health survey (SF-36). Med. Care 30, 473–483.

Wilson, R.M., Harrison, T.M., Gibberd, R.W., Hamilton, J.D., 1999. An analysis of the causes of adverse events from the Quality in Australian Heath Care Study. Med. J. Aust. 170 (9), 411–415.

World Health Organization, 2001. International Classification of Functioning, Disability and Health <www.who.int/classifications/icf/en>.

Yorke, J., Moosavi, S.H., Shuldham, C., Jones, P.W., 2010. Quantification of dyspnoea using descriptors: development and initial testing of the Dyspnoea-12. Thorax 65 (1), 21–26.

Yorke, J., Swigris, J., Russell, A.-M., et al., 2011. Dyspnea-12 is a valid and reliable measure of breathlessness in patients with interstitial lung disease. Chest 139 (1), 159–164.

3

THORACIC IMAGING

Adults

CONOR D COLLINS ■ SUSAN J COPLEY

Paediatrics

JOY L BARBER ■ CHRISTOPHER D GEORGE

CHAPTER OUTLINE

ADULTS 84
Chest Radiography and Other Techniques 84
 Different Types of Chest Radiograph 84
 *Factors Influencing the Quality of a Chest
   Radiograph 84*
 Other Techniques 85
 Interventional Procedures 90
The Normal Chest 91
 Anatomy 91
Common Radiological Signs 95
 Consolidation 95
 Collapse (Atelectasis) 95
 Collapse of Individual Lobes 97
 Pneumothorax 99
 The Opaque Hemithorax 99
 Decreased Density of a Hemithorax 100
 Elevation of the Diaphragm 100
 Pleural Disease 101
 The Pulmonary Mass 101
 Pulmonary Nodules 101
 Cavitating Pulmonary Lesions 102
Specific Conditions 103
 The Postoperative and Critically Ill Patient 103
 Kyphoscoliosis 106
 Bronchiectasis 106
 Chronic Airflow Limitation 106

PAEDIATRICS 108
Introduction 108
Issues Particular to Paediatric Imaging 108
Modalities in Paediatric Chest Imaging 109
 Plain Chest Radiographs and Fluoroscopy 109
 Ultrasound 109
 *Computed Tomography and High-Resolution Computed
   Tomography 110*
 Magnetic Resonance Imaging 110
 Angiography and Cardiac Catheterization 110
 Barium Studies 110
 Radionuclide Studies 111
 Positron Emission Tomography 111
Basic Signs on the Plain Chest Radiograph 111
 Consolidation 111
 Collapse 112
 Pleural Fluid 112
 Pneumothorax 114
Paediatric Chest Problems 115
 Congenital Abnormalities of the Chest 115
 Neonatal Chest Problems 116
 Respiratory Tract Infections 118
 Airway Disease 120
References and Further Reading 123

Adults

CHEST RADIOGRAPHY AND OTHER TECHNIQUES

Different Types of Chest Radiograph

Chest radiography has been used as the main radiological investigation of the chest since the discovery of X-rays by Roentgen in 1895 and chest radiographs constitute 25–40% of all radiological investigations. Chest radiographs are indicated in almost any condition in which a pulmonary abnormality is suspected.

Automatic exposure devices have been developed to optimally expose the various parts of the chest. Digital image capture devices (including flat-panel detectors) have replaced conventional film radiography in most resource-rich countries. The advantage of digital or computed radiography is that it can retrieve an image of diagnostic quality from an imperfect exposure, which would result in a non-diagnostic conventional film radiograph. With the advent of picture archiving and communication systems (PACS) that enable storage and transfer of digital images, most radiology departments in the developed world are now 'filmless', with images available to view simultaneously on both local and often distant workstations.

The majority of chest radiographs are obtained in the main radiology department. The radiograph is obtained with the patient standing erect. Patients who are immobile or too ill to come to the main department have a chest radiograph performed using a mobile machine (portable film); the resulting radiograph differs from a departmental film in terms of projection, positioning and exposure, and is therefore not strictly comparable with a conventional postero-anterior (PA) view. Other types of chest radiograph are the lateral, lordotic, apical and decubitus views; these are generally taken in the main department.

Departmental radiographs are referred to as 'postero-anterior' (or PA) chest radiographs and describe the direction in which the X-ray beam traverses the patient. The patient is positioned with his anterior chest wall against the detector and his back to the X-ray tube. The arms are abducted to rotate the scapulae away from the posterior chest and the radiograph is taken during full inspiration. The tube is centred at the spinous process of the fourth thoracic vertebra. For portable films taken in an antero-posterior (AP) projection, the patient's back is against the detector and the X-ray tube is positioned at a variable distance from the patient. As the heart is placed anteriorly within the chest, it is further from the detector and is therefore magnified in an AP radiograph. The degree of magnification depends on the distance between the patient and the X-ray tube.

For a lateral radiograph the patient is turned 90 degrees, and the side of interest placed against the detector. The arms are extended forwards and the radiograph is again taken in full inspiration.

Lateral decubitus views have been used in the past for the demonstration of small pleural effusions. For this projection the patient lies horizontally with the side in question placed downwards. The detector is positioned at the back of the patient and the X-ray beam is horizontal centred at the midsternum. This provides a sensitive means of detecting small quantities of pleural fluid (50–100 mL) that cannot be identified on a frontal chest radiograph. However, ultrasonography is usually used nowadays as a reliable means of confirming the presence of small pleural effusions.

Lordotic views are sometimes used to confirm middle lobe collapse and for demonstrating a questionable apical opacity otherwise obscured by the clavicle and ribs. For this AP projection, the patient arches back so that the shoulders are touching the detector with the centring point remaining the same.

Factors Influencing the Quality of a Chest Radiograph

The quality and thus diagnostic usefulness of a chest radiograph depend critically on the conditions under which it is obtained. Of particular importance are the radiographic exposure, the projection, the orientation of the patient relative to the detector, the X-ray tube to detector distance, the depth of inspiration of the patient and the type of detector used.

The ideal chest radiograph provides an image of structures within the chest while exposing the patient to the lowest possible dose of radiation. Even at total

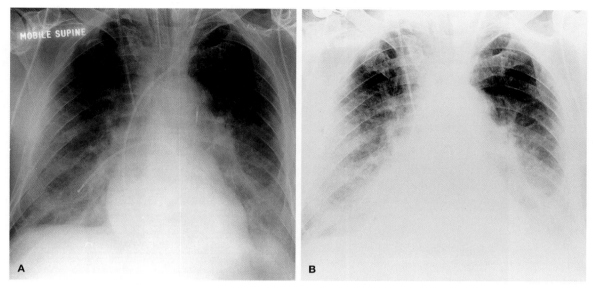

FIGURE 3-1 ■ ■ The same anteroposterior (AP) digital chest radiograph of a patient on the intensive care unit imaged on different settings. This technique has the advantage that the image can be made **(A)** darker or **(B)** lighter after it has been taken to allow better visualization of lines and tubes or lung parenchyma. Note the patient's endotracheal tube, right internal jugular central line, pulmonary artery catheter and intra-aortic balloon pump.

lung capacity with the patient erect, nearly a third of the lungs is partially obscured by the mediastinal structures, diaphragm and ribs. During exposure the X-ray beam is modified according to the structures through which it passes. The photons that have passed through the patient carry information which then must be converted into a visual form. Some of the photons emerging from the patient are aligned in a virtually parallel direction and other photons are scattered. These scattered photons degrade the final image but can be absorbed by using lead strips embedded in an aluminium sheet positioned in front of the detector. This device is known as a grid. Photons that are travelling in parallel pass through the grid to form the image on the detector.

In the intensive care setting, portable chest radiographs are often taken in less than ideal conditions. Multiple tubes, lines and dressings in conjunction with an immobile, supine patient and the use of a mobile low-kilovoltage machine often result in suboptimal radiographs. Digital techniques have largely replaced conventional 'film' radiography and an image of diagnostic quality can be retrieved from a suboptimal exposure. Similar gross over- or underexposure would

result in a non-diagnostic conventional radiograph. Manipulation of the digital image, particularly 'edge enhancement', aids the detection of linear structures such as the edge of a pneumothorax or central venous catheters (Fig. 3-1) throughout the hospital.

Other Techniques

Fluoroscopy

The patient is positioned, either standing or lying, in a screening unit allowing 'real-time' visualization of the area in question on a television monitor. The patient can be turned in any direction and this technique can help distinguish pulmonary from extrapulmonary opacities. One of the main uses of fluoroscopy is to 'screen' the diaphragm to demonstrate paralysis or abnormal movement. However, with the widespread use of computed tomography (CT) and ultrasound, the technique is now rarely used in these contexts.

Ultrasonography

High-frequency sound waves do not traverse air and the use of this technique is therefore limited for the evaluation of lung parenchyma. It is mainly used for cardiac imaging (echocardiography) and has become

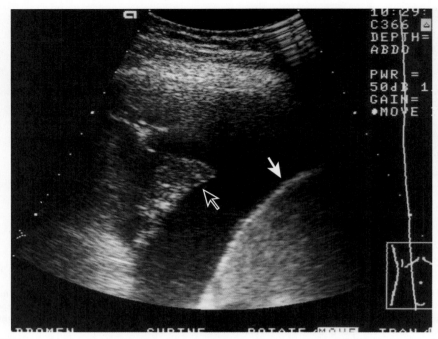

FIGURE 3-2 ■ Ultrasound of lower right hemithorax/upper abdomen demonstrating a right basal effusion with fluid interposed between collapsed right lower lobe (open arrow) and diaphragm (closed arrow).

an essential technique in the investigation of patients with valvular and ventricular function problems. Outside the heart, ultrasonography is very useful in distinguishing between fluid above the diaphragm (pleural effusion, Fig. 3-2), fluid below the diaphragm (subphrenic) and pleural thickening. Chest radiography often cannot differentiate between pleural fluid and thickening with any certainty. Ultrasound can also be used to guide the placement of a percutaneous drain into a pleural effusion or biopsy peripheral lung lesions that are in contact with the pleura. It may also be used to sample supraclavicular lymph nodes in patients with suspected lung cancer.

Computed Tomography

CT scanning depends on the same basic physical principle as conventional radiography, namely the absorption of X-rays by tissues of different densities. The basic components of a CT machine are a table on which the patient lies and a gantry through which the table slides. An X-ray tube and a series of detectors are housed within the gantry. The X-ray tube and detectors rotate around the patient. A computer is used to reconstruct the signals received by the detectors into an image. The images acquired are transverse (axial) cross-sections of the patient; however, with the advent of multi-detector CT (MDCT), coronal and sagittal reconstructions are easily acquired. In orienting the patient's right and left sides, it is the convention to view all axial CT images as if from the patient's feet.

Because of the cross-sectional nature of CT, it can accurately localize lesions seen on only one view on chest radiographs. The superior contrast resolution of CT allows superb demonstration of mediastinal anatomy (e.g. lymph nodes and vessels) (Fig. 3-3) as well as calcification within a pulmonary nodule. Highly detailed thin sections of the lung parenchyma can also be obtained, allowing the complex morphology of many interstitial lung diseases to be more accurately defined. The disadvantages of CT are its relatively high cost and increased radiation exposure to the patient compared with chest radiography. However, CT manufacturers have made significant developments to minimize dose.

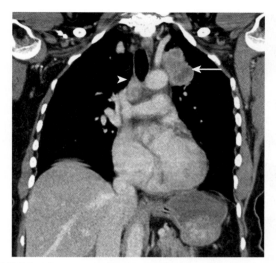

FIGURE 3-3 ◾ Coronal computed tomography (CT) image post intravenous contrast showing a lung cancer in the left upper lobe (white arrow). CT shows that the lesion is likely to be inoperable due to the enlarged contralateral lymph node adjacent to the trachea (arrowhead), which was difficult to see on chest radiography.

Whereas conventional CT scanning involves alternating table movement through the gantry with exposure, volumetric CT involves simultaneous table movement and X-ray exposure. The technique allows faster scan times, and advantages are the elimination of respiratory artefacts, minimization of motion artefacts and production of overlapping images without additional radiation exposure. Multiple rows of detectors are now commonplace in CT, so-called MDCT. The technique allows viewing of images in multiple planes (Fig. 3-4) and, due to the very fast acquisition times, is used to evaluate cardiac structures such as the coronary arteries. MDCT is also used to demonstrate pulmonary emboli, as accurate timing of a bolus of intravenous contrast allows optimal enhancement of the pulmonary arteries (Fig. 3-5).

Common Indications for CT of the Chest

1. CT scanning is used to further evaluate hilar or mediastinal masses seen or suspected on a chest radiograph.

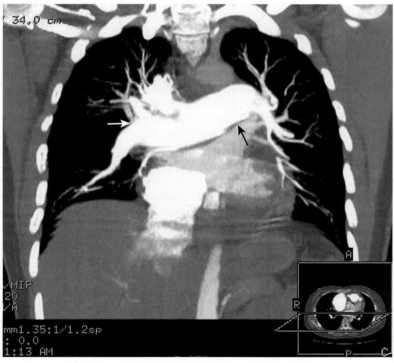

FIGURE 3-4 ◾ Example of coronal reconstruction of multidetector helical CT (MDCT) in a patient with primary pulmonary hypertension. Note the enlarged central pulmonary arteries (arrows).

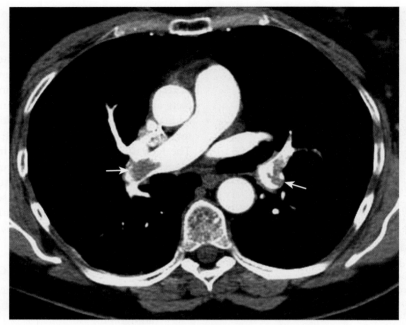

FIGURE 3-5 ■ A CT pulmonary angiogram, showing bilateral filling defects of the pulmonary arteries (arrows) consistent with bilateral pulmonary emboli.

2. Within the lungs it can be used to further define the nature of a mass or cavitating lesion not clearly seen on the chest radiograph.
3. In patients with normal chest radiographs but abnormal pulmonary function tests, thin high-resolution computed tomography (HRCT) sections of the lung may provide the first radiological evidence of parenchymal disease. This type of scanning is also very useful for assessing patients with suspected bronchiectasis.
4. CT is useful in patients with neoplasms, in assessing both their operability and their response to treatment.
5. CT is used for detection of pulmonary embolism.
6. CT is also used to guide the percutaneous needle biopsy of lung lesions or mediastinal masses.

Magnetic Resonance Imaging

The physical principles of magnetic resonance imaging (MRI) are more complex and very different from those of CT scanning. The equipment consists of a sliding table on which the patient lies within the bore of a large magnet. A combination of the intense magnetic field and a series of radiofrequency waves produces an alteration in the alignment of protons (mostly in water), resulting in the emission of different signals which are detected and subsequently analyzed for their intensity and position by a computer. The major advantages of MRI are that images may be obtained in any plane without the use of ionizing radiation. The disadvantages are its inability to produce detailed images of the lung, cost and reduced acceptability to patients because of the claustrophobic bore of the magnet. There are also important contraindications such as permanent cardiac pacemaker devices. The technique is good for imaging chest wall lesions, the great vessels (Fig. 3-6) and the heart.

Radionuclide Imaging

Ventilation–perfusion $(\dot{V}/\dot{Q})$ scanning is the commonest radionuclide study of the lungs. It is primarily used to investigate suspected pulmonary embolus. Perfusion is assessed by intravenous injection of minute particles labelled with technetium-99m, a radioactive tracer. These particles become temporarily lodged in a very small proportion of capillaries within

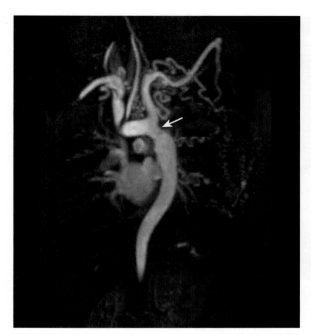

FIGURE 3-6 ■ Magnetic resonance image (MRI) of the thorax. The image shows an MR angiogram (MRA) of a coarctation of the aorta (arrow). Note the extensive arterial collaterals.

the lung and the emitted radiation is detected by a so-called gamma camera. Ventilation is assessed by the inhalation of inert gases that have also been labelled with a radioactive tracer. The ventilation and perfusion images are then compared to see if there are any areas of mismatch (Fig. 3-7). CT is often used to investigate patients with possible pulmonary embolus, as $\dot{V}/\dot{Q}$ scanning is more difficult to interpret in patients with coexisting lung disease such as asthma. In addition, the tracers have a short period of radioactivity after they are produced of a few hours and therefore scanning late at night and at weekends may be difficult.

Positron Emission Tomography

Positron emission tomography (PET) is also a form of radionuclide imaging. A detector can pinpoint where there is uptake of tracer accurately within the body. PET highlights areas that are very metabolically active, such as cancers, but also infection and inflammation. Access to this type of scanner is becoming more widespread, and it is mainly used in the chest for assessment of disease spread of lung cancer to lymph nodes and sites outside the chest (Fig. 3-8). The images may

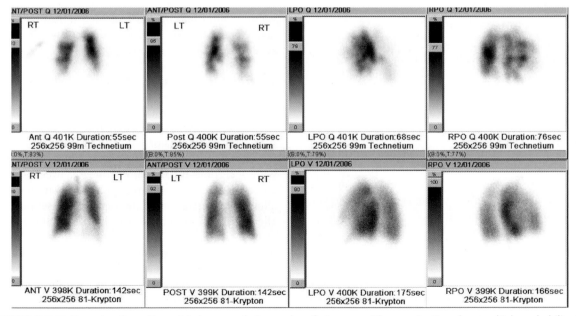

FIGURE 3-7 ■ Example of a radionuclide lung ventilation and perfusion scan. The examination shows a high probability for multiple bilateral pulmonary emboli as there are multiple perfusion abnormalities (top row of images) with no matched ventilation defects (bottom row of images), so-called mismatched defects.

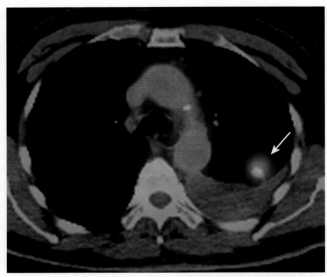

FIGURE 3-8 ■ A fused axial CT–PET scan showing increased tracer uptake in a left upper lobe pulmonary nodule due to a lung cancer (arrow). Note the left pleural effusion.

be fused with CT images (PET–CT) to give a very precise location of tumour spread.

Interventional Procedures

Percutaneous Needle Biopsy

Percutaneous needle biopsy of a pulmonary or mediastinal mass to provide a histological specimen is usually performed in patients in whom the lesion is too peripheral for bronchoscopic biopsy. Different types of needle are used and the complication rate (pneumothorax and haemoptysis) bears some relation to the site of the lesion, the size of the needle and the number of attempts to obtain tissue. Contraindications to the procedure include any patient with poor respiratory reserve unable to withstand a pneumothorax, pulmonary arterial hypertension and a previous contralateral pneumonectomy.

Pulmonary and Bronchial Arteriography, Superior Vena Cavography

Pulmonary Arteriography. This is usually undertaken in the investigation of suspected pulmonary arteriovenous malformations. It requires puncture of either the femoral vein in the groin or the antecubital vein in the elbow and the guiding of a catheter through the right side of the heart under fluoroscopy. The tip of the catheter is positioned in the main pulmonary artery or selectively placed in a smaller pulmonary artery. Contrast is then injected. Pulmonary arteriovenous malformations can be treated at the time of the arteriogram by the injection of occlusive materials (embolization).

Bronchial Arteriography. Demonstration of the bronchial arteries requires catheterization of the femoral artery and passage of a catheter into the midthoracic aorta from where the bronchial arteries are selectively catheterized. The major indication for this procedure is recurrent or life-threatening haemoptysis in patients with a chronic inflammatory disease, usually bronchiectasis. Accurate placement of the catheter not only allows demonstration of the bleeding vessel but also allows embolization to be performed simultaneously.

Superior Vena Cavography. This is performed for the evaluation of superior vena caval (SVC) obstruction and the investigation of anatomical variants. Patients with SVC compression due to tumour can be treated by the insertion of an expandable metallic mesh wire stent at the site of the SVC narrowing, thus restoring flow and relieving symptoms.

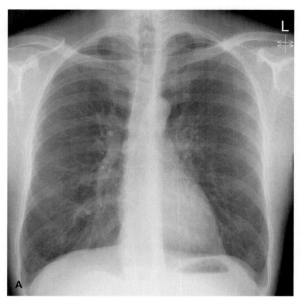 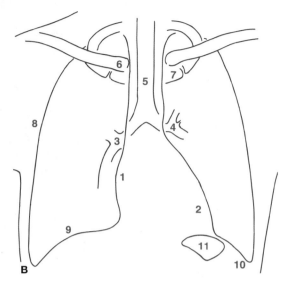

FIGURE 3-9 ■ **(A)** Normal posteroanterior (PA) chest radiograph. **(B)** Normal structures visible on a PA chest radiograph: 1, right atrium; 2, left ventricle; 3, right pulmonary artery; 4, left pulmonary artery; 5, air within trachea; 6, clavicle; 7, first rib; 8, lateral border of hemithorax; 9, right hemidiaphragm; 10, costophrenic angle; 11, gastric air bubble.

THE NORMAL CHEST

Anatomy

On the normal PA radiograph (Fig. 3-9) the following structures can be identified:

- outline of the mediastinum and heart
- the hila
- pulmonary vessels and main bronchi
- diaphragm
- soft tissues and bones of the thoracic cage.

The Heart and Mediastinum

The mediastinum consists of the organs and soft tissues in the central part of the chest. These comprise the trachea, aortic arch and great vessels, superior vena cava and oesophagus. In children the thymus gland is a prominent component. On the two-dimensional chest radiograph these structures are superimposed and cannot be clearly distinguished from each other. The mediastinum is conventionally divided into superior, anterior, middle and posterior compartments. While the boundaries of the latter three are arbitrary, it is usual to divide the mediastinum into equal thirds.

The superior mediastinum is that portion lying above the aortic arch and below the root of the neck.

The mediastinal border on the right is formed superiorly by the right brachiocephalic vein and superior vena cava. The mediastinal shadow to the left of the trachea above the aortic arch comprises the left carotid and left subclavian arteries together with the left brachiocephalic and jugular veins. On a correctly exposed chest radiograph, air in the trachea can be seen throughout its length as it descends downwards, deviating slightly to the right above the carina (where the trachea divides into the right and left main bronchi) due to displacement by the aortic arch.

The heart lies predominantly on the left within the chest, with one-third of the cardiac shadow to the right of the spine and two-thirds to the left. The density of the cardiac shadow on the left and right of the spine should be identical. The right cardiac border on a chest radiograph is formed by the right atrium. The left cardiac border is composed of the apex of the left ventricle and superiorly the left atrial appendage. The outline of the right ventricle, which is superimposed on the left ventricle, cannot be identified on a frontal radiograph. The maximum transverse diameter of the heart should be less than half the maximum transverse diameter of the thorax, as measured from the inside border of the ribs (the so-called cardiothoracic ratio).

The Hila

Hilar shadows are a complex summation of the pulmonary arteries and veins with minor contributions from other components (the main bronchi and lymph nodes). In general, the hila are of equal density and are approximately the same size. Adjacent to the left hilum, the main pulmonary artery forms a localized bulge just above the left atrial appendage and just below the aortic arch. The area between the aortic arch and the main pulmonary artery is known as the 'aorto-pulmonary window'.

The superior pulmonary veins run vertically and converge on the upper and mid-hilum on both sides. It is not possible to distinguish arteries from veins in the outer two-thirds of the lungs. The inferior pulmonary veins run obliquely in a near-horizontal plane below the lower lobe arteries to enter the left atrium beneath the carina. The hilar point is where the superior pulmonary vein on each side crosses the basal artery. This is more easily assessed on the right than on the left. Using this as an index point, the left hilum is normally 0.5–1.5 cm higher than the right one.

Abnormalities of the hilar shadows in the form of increased density or abnormal configuration are usually the result of lymph node or pulmonary artery enlargement. The detection of subtle hilar abnormalities is difficult and requires experience and knowledge of the many outlines that the hila may assume in normal individuals.

Fissures, Vessels and Segmental Bronchi Within the Lungs

Each lung is divided into lobes surrounded by visceral pleura. There are two lobes on the left (the upper and lower, separated by the major (oblique) fissure) and three on the right (the upper, middle and lower lobes which are separated by the major (oblique) and minor (horizontal or transverse) fissures). In the majority of normal subjects some or all of the minor fissure is seen on a frontal radiograph. The major fissures are only identifiable on the lateral projection. Each lobe of the lung contains a number of segments, which have their own segmental bronchi. The walls of the segmental bronchi are invisible on the chest radiograph, except when seen end-on as ring shadows measuring up to 7 mm in diameter.

The pulmonary blood vessels are responsible for the branching and linear structures within the lungs. The diameter of the blood vessels beyond the hilum varies with the position of the patient and with haemodynamic factors. In the erect position there is a gradual increase in the diameter of the vessels, travelling from apex to base. This increase in size is seen in both the arteries and veins and is abolished if the patient lies supine.

The Diaphragm

The interface between the lung and diaphragm should be sharp and, in general, the diaphragm is dome shaped with its highest point medial to the midclavicular line. The margin of the right hemidiaphragm at its highest point lies between the anterior ends of the fifth and seventh ribs. The right hemidiaphragm is usually higher than the left by up to 2 cm in the erect position. Laterally, the diaphragm dips downwards, forming a sharp angle with the chest wall known as the 'costophrenic angle'. Filling in or blunting of these angles reflects pleural disease, either fluid or thickening.

Thoracic Cage

On a high-kilovoltage chest radiograph it should be possible to identify the edges of the vertebral bodies of the dorsal spine through the heart shadow. However, a high-kilovoltage radiograph may 'burn out' the ribs, particularly the posterior portions. Because of this, the chest radiograph may be an insensitive means of demonstrating rib abnormalities, particularly fractures.

Common Anatomical Variants

The trachea lies centrally, but in the elderly may deviate markedly to the right in its lower portion due to unfolding and dilatation of the aortic arch. A small ovoid soft-tissue shadow just above the origin of the right main bronchus represents the azygos vein. This may be enlarged as a result of posture (supine position) or haemodynamic factors. It may be indistinguishable from an azygos lymph node.

Occasionally, extra fissures are seen in the lungs. The most common of these is the azygos lobe fissure;

this is seen as a fine white line running obliquely from the apex of the right lung to the azygos vein. Other accessory fissures are the superior and inferior accessory fissures, both of which are in the right lower lobe.

The surfaces of the two lungs abut each other anteriorly and posteriorly and give rise to two white lines projected over the vertebral column, known as the 'anterior and posterior junction lines', respectively. Both of these may be seen overlying the trachea – the anterior line extending from the clavicles to the left main bronchus and the posterior line lying more medially and extending above the clavicles. The azygo-oesophageal recess line is a curved line projected over the vertebral column and extending from the azygos vein to the diaphragm. It represents the interface between the right lung and right oesophageal wall.

A small 'nipple' may occasionally be seen projecting laterally from the aortic knuckle due to the left superior intercostal vein. The term 'paraspinal line' refers to the line that parallels the left and right margin of the thoracic spine. The left is thicker than the right because of the adjacent aorta.

The Lateral View

It is conventional to read the lateral film (Fig. 3-10) with the heart to the viewer's left and the dorsal spine to the right, irrespective of whether the film is labelled 'right' or 'left'. The chamber of the heart that touches the sternum is the right ventricle. Behind and above the heart lies lung, the density of which should be the same both behind the heart and behind the sternum. As the eye travels down the spine, the vertebral column should appear increasingly transradiant or 'dark' (see Fig. 3-10A); the loss of this phenomenon suggests the presence of disease in the postero-basal segments of the lower lobes. In the middle of the lateral film lie the

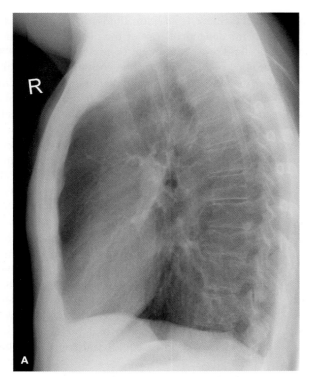

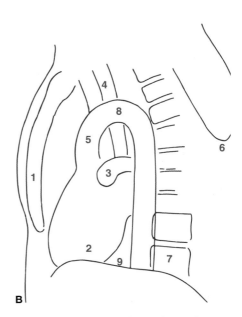

FIGURE 3-10 ■ **(A)** Normal lateral chest radiograph. **(B)** Normal structures visible on a lateral chest radiograph: 1, sternum; 2, position of left ventricle; 3, pulmonary artery; 4, air within trachea; 5, ascending aorta; 6, inferior angle of scapula; 7, dorsal vertebra; 8, aortic arch; 9, hemidiaphragm.

hilar structures with the main pulmonary artery anteriorly. The aortic arch should be easily identified, but only a variable proportion of the great vessels are visible depending on the degree of aortic unfolding. The brachiocephalic artery is most frequently identified arising anterior to the tracheal air column. The left and right brachiocephalic veins form an extrapleural bulge behind the upper sternum in about a third of individuals.

The course of the trachea is straight with a slight posterior angulation but no visible indentation from adjacent vessels. The carina is not seen on the lateral view. The posterior wall of the trachea is always visible and is known as the 'posterior tracheal stripe'.

The oblique fissures are seen as fine diagonal lines running from the upper dorsal spine to the diaphragm anteriorly. The left is more vertically oriented and is visible just behind the right. The minor fissure extends forwards horizontally from the mid-right oblique fissure. Care must be taken not to confuse rib margins with fissure lines. As the fissures undulate, two distinct fissure lines may be generated by a single fissure. The fissures should be of no more than hairline width.

The scapulae are invariably seen in the lateral view and since they are incompletely visualized, lines formed by the edge of the scapula can easily be confused with intrathoracic structures. The arms are held outstretched in front of the patient on a lateral view and these give rise to soft-tissue shadows projected over the anterior and superior mediastinum. A band-like opacity simulating pleural disease is often seen along the lower half of the anterior chest wall immediately behind the sternum. The left lung does not contact the most anterior portion of the left thoracic cavity at these levels because the heart occupies the space. This band-like opacity is known as the 'retrosternal line'.

Useful Points in Interpreting a Chest Radiograph

Documentary Information. The name of the patient and the time and date on which the radiograph was taken, particularly in relation to others in a series, should all be noted. Of particular importance is the presence of the side markers ('right' or 'left'). The radiograph should also be marked 'AP' if the anteroposterior projection was used; departmental PA films are generally not marked as such.

Radiographic Projection. A judgement as to whether a radiograph is AP or PA can be made from the following evidence.

1. The relationship of the scapulae to the lung margins (in the PA projection the scapulae are projected clear of the lungs and in AP projection they overlie the lungs).
2. The appearance of the vertebral bodies in the cervico-dorsal region. The vertebral endplates are seen more clearly in the AP projection and the laminae are more clearly seen in the PA projection.

Supine Versus Prone Position. It is important to know whether a chest radiograph was taken in the erect or supine position. In the supine position, blood flow is more evenly distributed throughout the lungs, making the upper zone vessels equal in size to those in the lower zones. This has implications in assessing the chest radiograph of a patient suspected of being in cardiac failure. In addition, fluid is distributed throughout the dependent part of the pleural space and any air–fluid levels that might be present on an erect film are impossible to detect. The position and contours of the heart, mediastinum and diaphragm are also different compared with an erect film. In the absence of any indication on the radiograph, one clue is the position of the gastric air bubble: if it is just under the left hemidiaphragm it is in the fundus and the patient is erect, whereas in the supine position air collects in the antrum of the stomach which lies centrally or slightly to the right of the vertebral column, well below the diaphragm.

Patient Rotation. The patient may be rotated around one of three axes. Axial rotation is the most common cause of unilateral transradiancy (one lung appearing darker than the other). It also distorts the mediastinal outline. The degree of rotation can be assessed by relating the medial ends of the clavicles to the spinous process of the vertebral body at the same level – they should be equidistant from the spinous processes.

Rotation about the horizontal coronal axis results in a more kyphotic or lordotic projection than normal. The main pulmonary artery and subclavian vessels may appear unduly prominent. Rotation around the horizontal sagittal axis usually leads to obvious tilt of the chest in relation to the edge of the radiograph, which is assumed to be upright.

Physical attributes of the patient, such as a kypho-scoliosis or a depressed sternum (pectus excavatum), may also distort the appearance of the thoracic cage and its contents.

State of Inspiration or Expiration. The degree of inspiration is an important consideration for the correct interpretation of a chest radiograph. A poor inspiratory effort does not necessarily imply lack of patient cooperation and may as often be related to a pathological process. At full inspiration the midpoint of the right hemidiaphragm lies between the anterior end of ribs 5–7. A shallow inspiration affects the contour of the heart and mediastinum, and may mimic the appearances of pulmonary congestion because the upper zone vessels will have the same diameter as the lower zone vessels.

Review Areas. Several areas are difficult to assess on a frontal radiograph and should be scrutinized carefully. These review areas are:

- apices
- behind the heart
- hilar regions
- bones
- lung periphery just inside the chest wall.

Detection and description of radiographic abnormalities should then be undertaken and a differential diagnosis listed based on the abnormalities detected. With experience, the structured search gives way to the rapid identification of abnormalities and a search for confirmatory radiological signs and associated abnormalities.

COMMON RADIOLOGICAL SIGNS

Consolidation

'Consolidation' is the term used to describe lung in which the air-filled spaces are replaced by the products of disease, e.g. water, pus, tumour or blood. The two most important radiological signs of consolidation are (a) an air bronchogram and (b) the silhouette sign.

TABLE 3-1	
Causes of Widespread Pulmonary Consolidation in Adults	
Fluid Transudation	**Pulmonary Oedema Due to Cardiac Failure, Renal Failure and Hepatic Failure**
Exudation	Infection, e.g. lobar pneumonia and bronchopneumonia, tuberculosis
	Acute respiratory distress syndrome (ARDS)
	Pulmonary haemorrhage due to contusion
	Pulmonary eosinophilia
Inhalation	Gastric contents
	Toxic fumes
	Oxygen toxicity
Infiltration	Lymphoma
	Adenocarcinoma

The causes of widespread consolidation may be divided into four categories (Table 3-1).

An air bronchogram is present when the airways contain air and appear as radiolucent (black) branching structures against a now white background of airless lung. The silhouette sign is present when the border of a structure is lost because the normally air-filled lung outlining the border is replaced by radio-opaque fluid or tissue. Recognition of this sign can help localize the affected area of abnormality within the chest. Thus loss of a clear right heart border is due to right middle lobe consolidation or collapse.

Localized areas of consolidation are usually due to infection. In some cases the borders of the consolidation are clearly demarcated. This usually corresponds to a fissure and the consolidation is confined to one lobe (lobar pneumonia) (Fig. 3-11). If consolidation is slow to clear with treatment, it may be secondary to partial obstruction of a lobar bronchus, such as carcinoma of the bronchus. Consolidation may also be widespread and affect both lungs (Figs 3-12, 3-13).

Collapse (Atelectasis)

'Collapse' (atelectasis) is the radiological term used when there is loss of aeration and, therefore, expansion in part or all of a lung. Collapse of a lobe or an entire lung is most frequently due to an endobronchial tumour, an inhaled foreign body or a mucous plug.

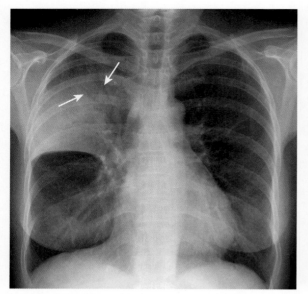

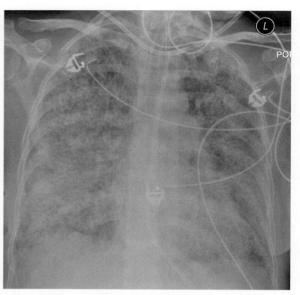

FIGURE 3-11 ■ Right upper lobe consolidation. There is increased density of the right upper lobe with air bronchograms (arrows). The cause was a right upper lobe pneumonia.

FIGURE 3-12 ■ Widespread airspace consolidation in a patient with acute respiratory distress syndrome (ARDS). The patient has a tracheostomy and nasogastric tube in situ.

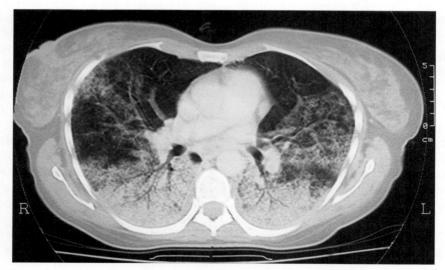

FIGURE 3-13 ■ CT scan of diffuse consolidation within apical segments of both lower lobes. Note prominent bilateral air bronchograms within consolidated lung. Infection due to *Pneumocystis carinii* and cytomegalovirus in an immunocompromised patient.

Although collapse is most often thought of as occurring at a lobar level, focal areas of pulmonary collapse at a subsegmental level occur very commonly in postoperative patients. There are many signs of lobar collapse but it is important to realize that not all these signs occur together. In addition, some non-specific signs may be present which indirectly point to the diagnosis and alert the observer to look for the more specific signs.

The most reliable and frequent finding in lobar collapse is shift of the fissures, which invariably occurs to some extent. If air stays in the collapsed lobe, the contained blood vessels remain visible and appear crowded. If there is marked volume loss, the density of the collapsed and airless lobe increases. The hila may show two types of change consisting either of gross displacement upwards or downwards, or of rearrangement of individual hilar components (i.e. vessels and airways) leading to changes in shape and prominence. Elevation of the hemidiaphragm, reflecting volume loss, is most marked in collapse of a lower lobe. The signs associated with collapse are listed in Box 3-1.

Collapse of Individual Lobes

Right Upper Lobe

On the PA radiograph there is elevation of the transverse fissure and the right hilum. If the collapse is complete, the non-aerated lobe is seen as an increased density alongside the superior mediastinum adjacent to the trachea (Fig. 3-14). On the lateral view the minor fissure moves upwards and the major fissure moves forwards. The retrosternal area becomes progressively more opaque and the anterior margin of the ascending aorta becomes effaced.

BOX 3-1
SIGNS ASSOCIATED WITH A COLLAPSED LOBE

- Increased density of the collapsed lobe
- Shift of fissures
- Silhouette sign
- Hilar shift and distortion
- Crowding of vessels and airways
- Mediastinal shift
- Crowding of the ribs
- Elevation of hemidiaphragm

Right Middle Lobe

On the PA radiograph the lateral part of the minor fissure moves down and there is blurring of the normally sharp right heart border. This may be a subtle abnormality that is easily overlooked. On the lateral view the minor fissure moves downwards and the lower half of the major fissure moves forwards, giving rise to a triangular shadow visible behind the lower sternum (Fig. 3-15).

Right Lower Lobe

On the PA view there is an increase in density overlying the medial portion of the right hemidiaphragm and the right hilum is displaced inferiorly. The right heart border usually remains sharply defined since this is in contact with the aerated right middle lobe. On the lateral view, the oblique fissure moves backwards and, with increasing collapse, there is loss of definition of the right hemidiaphragm as well as increased density overlying the lower dorsal vertebrae. Right lower lobe collapse is a mirror image of left lower lobe collapse (Fig. 3-16).

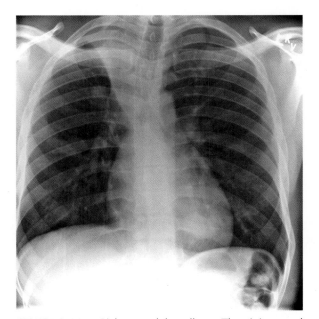

FIGURE 3-14 ■ Right upper lobe collapse. There is increased density medial to the elevated horizontal fissure. The cause was a central tumour obstructing the right upper lobe bronchus. Note the bilateral pulmonary nodules consistent with pulmonary metastases.

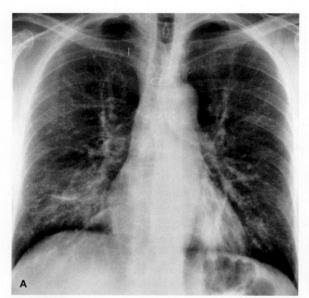

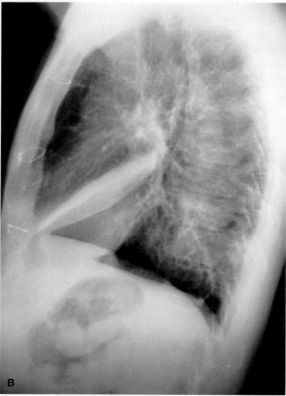

FIGURE 3-15 ■ Right middle lobe collapse in a patient post thoracotomy. **(A)** Loss of the right heart border may be subtle on the frontal film (note the patient also has some left lower lobe consolidation). **(B)** The lateral view shows the typical triangular opacity overlying the cardiac shadow.

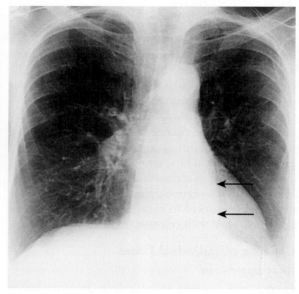

FIGURE 3-16 ■ Left lower lobe collapse. A PA radiograph shows loss of the outline of the medial portion of the left hemidiaphragm and a triangular density behind the left side of the heart (arrows). There is also volume loss of the left hemithorax and the mediastinum is deviated to the left, allowing increased visibility of the thoracic spine.

Left Upper Lobe

The main finding on the PA radiograph is of a veil-like increase in density, without a sharp margin, spreading outwards and upwards from the left hilum, which is elevated. The aortic knuckle, left hilum and left heart border may have ill-defined outlines. As volume loss increases, the collapsed lobe moves closer to the midline and the lung apex may become lucent due to hyperinflation of the apical segment of the left lower lobe. A sharp border may also return to the aortic arch. On the lateral view the oblique fissure moves upwards and forwards, remaining relatively straight and roughly parallel to the anterior chest wall (Fig. 3-17). On the PA projection, collapse (or consolidation) of the

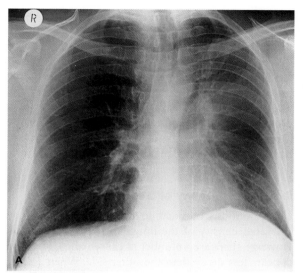

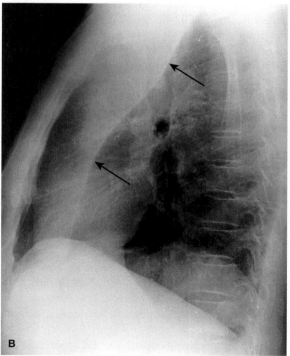

FIGURE 3-17 ■ Left upper lobe collapse. **(A)** There is a veil-like density of the left hemithorax, which obscures the outline of the aortic knuckle and left heart border superiorly. There is also volume loss on the left (the trachea is deviated to the left and the left hemidiaphragm is raised with 'peaking' centrally). **(B)** The lateral radiograph shows increased density anterior to the oblique fissure (arrows).

lingular segment of the left upper lobe should be suspected when the left cardiac border is ill defined.

Left Lower Lobe

This is most commonly seen in patients following cardiac surgery and a thoracotomy due to the retention of secretions in the left lower lobe bronchus. On the PA view there is a triangular density behind the heart with loss of the medial portion of the left hemidiaphragm (see Fig. 3-16); if the PA radiograph is underexposed, it may be impossible to see this triangular opacity. On the lateral view there is backwards displacement of the oblique fissure, and with increasing collapse there is increased density over the lower dorsal vertebrae.

Pneumothorax

When air is introduced into the pleural space, the resulting pneumothorax can be recognized radiographically. There are numerous causes of a pneumothorax but the most common include penetrating injuries (e.g. stab wound, placement of a subclavian line, post-percutaneous lung biopsy) and breaches of the visceral pleura (e.g. spontaneous rupture of a subpleural bulla or mechanical ventilation with high pressures). The cardinal radiographic sign is the visceral pleural edge: lateral to this edge no vascular shadows are visible and medial to it the collapsed lung is of higher density than the contralateral lung (Fig. 3-18). It is important to remember that in the supine position, the air of a small pneumothorax will collect anteriorly in the pleural space; thus on a portable supine chest radiograph, the pneumothorax will be visible as an area of relative translucency without a visceral pleural edge necessarily being identifiable.

If air enters the pleural space during inspiration but cannot leave on expiration (usually because of a check-valve effect of the torn flap of the visceral pleura), pressure increases rapidly and this results in a life-threatening tension pneumothorax. This can be recognized by a shift of the mediastinum to the opposite side (Fig. 3-19).

The Opaque Hemithorax

If one-half of a chest is completely opaque (a white-out) it is due either to collapse of a lung or a large pleural effusion. If there is a shift of the mediastinum

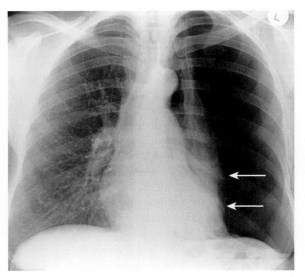

FIGURE 3-18 ■ Spontaneous pneumothorax. There is a large left-sided pneumothorax with loss of vascular markings lateral to the edge of the collapsed lung. The visceral pleural edge is visible (arrows).

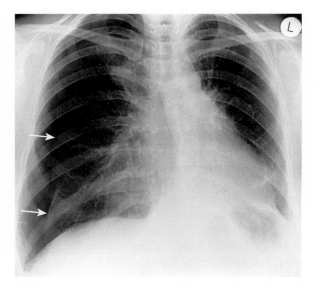

FIGURE 3-19 ■ Tension pneumothorax post thoracoscopic biopsy of a right upper zone lung nodule. The pneumothorax in Figure 3-18 involves more of the hemithorax but this pneumothorax is causing deviation of the mediastinum to the opposite side and is potentially life threatening unless treated promptly. The visceral pleural edge is visible (arrows).

to the affected side it implies that volume loss in the lung (i.e. collapse) on that side must have occurred. Where there is no shift of the mediastinum or it is shifted slightly to the side of the white-out, this is usually due to constricting pleural disease (including pleural tumour). A pleural effusion that is large enough to cause complete opacification of a hemithorax will displace the mediastinum away from the side of the white-out. Ultrasound and CT allow the distinction to be made with confidence and the latter may give further information about the underlying disease.

Decreased Density of a Hemithorax

The conditions outlined so far have all focused on increased density of the lungs on plain radiographs. However, there are a number of causes where one lung appears less dense than the other side. When a chest radiograph demonstrates greater radiolucency of one lung compared with the other, it is necessary first to determine whether this appearance is due to a pulmonary abnormality. The radiograph should be checked for patient rotation and for soft-tissue asymmetry, e.g. a mastectomy.

The pulmonary vessels are a helpful pointer to abnormalities causing a true decrease in density. In compensatory hyperinflation they are splayed apart. A search should also be made for a collapsed lobe. The vessels are considerably diminished or truncated in emphysema. CT may also be useful in elucidating the cause of a hyperlucent lung. The lungs can be seen on CT without the problem of overlying tissues and any decrease in density is more readily apparent.

Elevation of the Diaphragm

The right or left dome of the diaphragm may be elevated because it is paralyzed, pushed up or pulled up. However, there are a number of circumstances in which the diaphragm appears to be elevated without actually being so.

The radiographic evaluation of an apparently elevated diaphragm should begin with an assessment of radiograph, in particular evidence of previous surgery. Old radiographs are essential to determine whether the diaphragmatic elevation is long standing. Ultrasound will assist in determining if fluid is present above and/or below the diaphragm.

If the hemidiaphragm is paralysed, fluoroscopic or ultrasound examination is useful as it may demonstrate paradoxical movement on vigorous sniffing (instead of the diaphragm moving down, it moves up). An important proviso is that a few normal individuals show this paradoxical movement of the diaphragm on sniffing. In congenital eventration, part or all of the hemidiaphragm muscle is made up of a thin layer of fibrous tissue and it may be difficult to distinguish from paralysis even on fluoroscopy.

Pleural Disease

Because the chest radiograph is a two-dimensional image, abnormalities of the pleura and chest wall are often difficult to assess. Gross pleural abnormalities are usually obvious on a chest radiograph (Fig. 3-20), but even when there is extensive pleural pathology it may be difficult to distinguish between pleural fluid, pleural thickening (e.g. secondary to a previous inflammatory process) and a neoplasm of the pleura. In such cases, ultrasound is useful in identifying the presence of fluid. CT can readily identify the encasing and constricting nature of a mesothelioma.

The Pulmonary Mass

Most pulmonary nodules or masses are discovered by chest radiography. It is important to obtain previous examinations if at all possible. If the lesion was present previously and has not changed over a number of

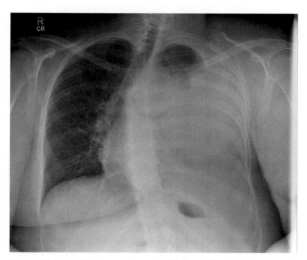

FIGURE 3-20 ■ Large pleural effusion. The left lower and mid zones are opaque due to a large left-sided pleural effusion. There is also shift of the cardiac shadow to the right. Note the absent left breast shadow due to a previous mastectomy. The cause of the pleural effusion was metastatic breast cancer.

years, it can be assumed that the lesion is benign and no further action needs to be taken. However, if the nodule was not previously present or has increased in size, further investigation is warranted.

CT (see Fig. 3-3) will detect or exclude the presence of other lesions within the lungs. The presence of calcification within a nodule, although often thought to be an indicator of benignity, will not exclude malignancy with complete certainty. In addition, CT can be used to determine the presence of hilar or mediastinal lymph node enlargement as well as direct invasion of the adjacent mediastinum or chest wall. In patients with suspected lung cancer, a cytological or histological specimen by percutaneous needle biopsy may be taken. This is usually reserved for lesions that are not accessible by bronchoscopy. It can be performed under CT or ultrasound guidance (if abutting the chest wall) but complications include pneumothorax or pulmonary haemorrhage (see other interventional techniques).

Pulmonary Nodules

A large number of conditions are characterized by multiple pulmonary nodules (Fig. 3-21). Combining the clinical information with an accurate description of the size and distribution of the nodules narrows down the list of differential diagnoses.

Metastatic deposits are by far the most common cause of multiple pulmonary nodules of varying sizes in adult patients in the United Kingdom (see Fig. 3-21), but this is not the case worldwide. In some parts of the USA, histoplasmosis is endemic and multiple lesions due to this condition may be more common than those due to malignancy. Making this important distinction may be difficult and biopsy of one lesion may be the only reliable means of distinguishing a benign from a malignant cause for the multiple nodules.

Nodules are described as 'miliary' when they are less than 5 mm in diameter and are so numerous that they cannot be counted. The crucial diagnosis to consider, even if the patient is not particularly unwell, is miliary tuberculosis, since this life-threatening disease can be readily treated (see Fig. 3-21A). If the patient is asymptomatic the differential diagnosis is more likely to lie between sarcoidosis or metastatic disease. As ever, previous radiographs showing the rate of growth of the nodules may give valuable clues to the likely nature of the disease.

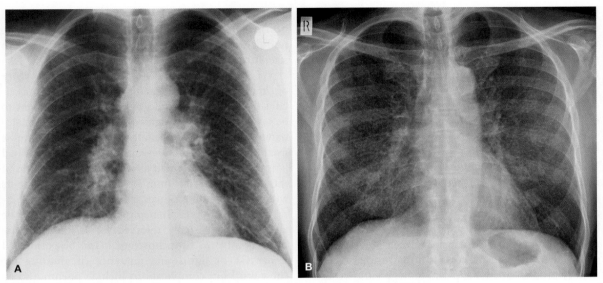

FIGURE 3-21 ■ Multiple pulmonary nodules. **(A)** Pulmonary sarcoidosis. These pulmonary nodules are small (2–3 mm) and subtle and there is bilateral hilar lymphadenopathy. **(B)** Miliary tuberculosis. These pulmonary nodules are tiny (2–3 mm) and well defined. Their appearance has been likened to millet seeds, hence the name.

Cavitating Pulmonary Lesions

The radiological definition of cavitation is a lucency representing air within a mass or an area of consolidation. The cavity may or may not contain a fluid level and is surrounded by a wall of variable thickness (Fig. 3-22).

The two most likely diagnoses in an adult presenting with a cavitating pulmonary lesion on a chest radiograph are a cancer or a lung abscess. In children, infection is the most common cause. Cavitation secondary to necrosis is well recognized in a variety of bacterial pneumonias, particularly those associated with tuberculosis, *Staphylococcus aureus,* anaerobes and *Klebsiella.* Diagnosis is usually by chest radiography in the first instance but CT is also useful for localizing the abscess and sometimes to enable percutaneous aspiration to be undertaken. It also allows assessment of the relationship of the abscess to adjacent airways so that appropriate postural drainage can be planned.

In all age groups it is important to consider tuberculosis, especially if the cavitating lesions are in the lung apices. CT may be necessary if the presence of cavitation is questionable; in addition, CT may show other features which help to narrow the differential

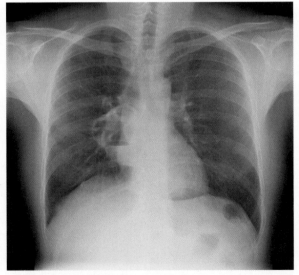

FIGURE 3-22 ■ Cavity with an air-fluid level in the right lung, projected over the hilum. The differential diagnosis would include a cavitating lung cancer or a lung abscess. In this instance, the cause was Wegener granulomatosis (renamed 'granulomatosis with polyangiitis'). Note the smaller lung nodule in the medial left lower zone.

diagnosis (e.g. pulmonary calcifications in tuberculosis, mediastinal lymph node enlargement in metastatic disease).

SPECIFIC CONDITIONS

The Postoperative and Critically Ill Patient

In the context of intensive care medicine, the portable radiograph is one of the main means of monitoring critically ill patients. However, it is a far from perfect technique as the degree of inspiration is usually poor and may vary widely on serial radiographs. In addition, evaluation of cardiac size and the lung bases is, at best, difficult. This is often compounded by the rapidly changing haemodynamic state of the patient.

To some extent the advent of digital and computed radiography has enabled more accurate assessments to be made because variations in exposure are not such a problem. For convenience it is useful to consider the various disease processes in the categories described in the following sections.

Support and Monitoring Apparatus

Careful radiographic monitoring of the position of various tubes and catheters used in the postoperative and critically ill patient is essential to decrease complications. Before evaluating the heart and lungs it is good practice to check each of these lines for proper positioning. The ideally placed central venous line ends in the superior vena cava (see Fig. 3-1). Catheters terminating in the right atrium or ventricle may cause arrhythmias or perforation. Swan–Ganz catheters used to monitor pulmonary capillary wedge pressure are ideally sited in a main or lobar pulmonary artery (see Fig. 3-1). Drugs inadvertently injected directly into the wedged catheter may cause lobar pulmonary oedema or necrosis. Both catheters (central venous pressure line and Swan–Ganz) are inserted percutaneously and therefore share certain complications. The most frequent is a pneumothorax due to puncture of the lung at the time of subclavian vein insertion. If the catheter is inserted into the mediastinum or perforates a vein or artery, there may be dramatic widening of the superior mediastinum due to haematoma. If the catheter enters the pleural space, infused fluid rapidly fills the pleural space. Catheter perforation of the right atrium or ventricle may lead to cardiac tamponade,

which may result in progressive enlargement of the heart shadow on serial radiographs.

The intra-aortic balloon pump is usually inserted via the femoral artery and is used in patients with intractable heart failure or in weaning the patient from cardiopulmonary bypass. On the frontal radiograph the tip of the catheter should be seen lying just inferior to the aortic arch (see Fig. 3-1).

A cardiac pacemaker wire is usually inserted via the external jugular, the cephalic or the femoral vein and passed under fluoroscopic control into the apex of the right ventricle. Kinks or coils of wire are undesirable and the wire should be examined carefully along its entire length.

The tip of a correctly positioned endotracheal tube (see Fig. 3-1) lies in the midtrachea, approximately 5–7 cm above the carina. This distance is needed to ensure that it does not descend into the right main stem bronchus with extension of the head and neck or ascend into the pharynx when the head and neck are flexed. If the endotracheal tube is inadvertently passed into the right main stem bronchus (the more vertical of the two main bronchi), the left lung may collapse, with a shift of the mediastinum to the left and hyperinflation of the right lung. If the endotracheal tube is positioned just below the vocal cords, the tube may retract into the pharynx, airway protection is lost and aspiration may occur. If the tube remains high in the trachea, inflation of the cuff may cause vocal cord damage. Delayed complications include focal tracheal necrosis leading ultimately to a localized stricture. It is worth noting that, even with correct positioning and cuff inflation, an endotracheal tube is not an absolute guarantee against aspiration of stomach contents into the airways.

Tracheostomy for long-term support has its own complications. A correctly placed tracheostomy tube should be parallel to the long axis of the trachea, be approximately one-half to two-thirds the diameter of the trachea and end at least 5 cm from the carina. Marked subcutaneous or mediastinal emphysema may be due to tracheal injury or a large leak around the stoma. After prolonged intubation some tracheal scarring is inevitable. Symptomatic tracheal stenosis or collapse of a short length of the trachea is less common now owing to use of low-pressure occlusion cuffs on endotracheal tubes. When positive end-expiratory pressure (PEEP) is added, the patient's tidal volume and functional residual capacity increase. This is reflected in the radiograph as increased lung aeration. PEEP may open up areas of collapse and cause radiographic clearing. However, this may be spurious as any densities present will be less obvious owing to the increased lung volume. Similarly, when the patient is weaned off PEEP, the lung volume drops and the lungs may appear to be dramatically worse. Pulmonary barotrauma (air leakage due to elevated pressure) complicates approximately 10 percent of patients on positive pressure ventilation. If air continues to leak due to continued ventilation, a tension pneumothorax may develop. The chest radiograph is often the first indicator of this potentially fatal complication.

Collapse

Following laparotomy, at least half of all patients develop some postoperative pulmonary collapse. Volume loss is most often attributed to hypoventilation and retained secretions and it is most frequent in patients with chronic bronchitis, emphysema, obesity, prolonged anaesthesia or unusually heavy analgesia. The most common radiographic manifestation is of linear densities which appear in the lower lung zones soon after surgery. Patchy, segmental or complete lobar consolidation is less common. When due to hypoventilation or large airway secretions, marked volume loss rather than dense consolidation is the usual appearance. Careful attention should be paid to unilateral elevation of the diaphragm and shifts of the minor fissure or hilar vessels. When collapse is due to multiple peripheral mucous plugs, the radiographic picture may be of pulmonary consolidation rather than volume loss. Areas of collapse tend to change rapidly and often clear with suction or physiotherapy. Postoperative collapse is not usually an infectious process, but, if not treated promptly, areas of collapse will usually become secondarily infected.

Aspiration Pneumonia

Another postoperative complication is the aspiration of gastric contents. A depressed state of consciousness and the presence of a nasogastric tube that disables the protective oesophago-gastric sphincter are the most frequent predisposing factors. An endotracheal or tracheostomy tube does not always protect the patient from aspiration. The radiographic appearance

of patchy, often bilateral, consolidation appears any time within the first 24 hours of aspiration and then progresses rapidly. In an uncomplicated case there is usually evidence of stability or regression by 72 hours, with complete clearing within 1–2 weeks. The infiltrates are usually patchy and diffuse and are most often seen at the lung bases, more commonly on the right. Complications include progression to acute respiratory distress syndrome (ARDS). Any worsening of the radiograph on the third day or thereafter should suggest the diagnosis of secondary infection.

Acute Respiratory Distress Syndrome

ARDS consists of progressive respiratory insufficiency following a major insult and can be due to a large number of factors. Over the years it has been known as 'shock lung', 'stiff lung syndrome' and 'adult hyaline membrane disease'.

At the pathophysiological level there is increased permeability of the pulmonary capillaries and the formation of platelet and fibrin microemboli. This results in alveolar oedema and haemorrhage, which can affect the entire lung. After several days, hyaline membranes form within the distal air spaces. As a general rule, symptoms occur on the second day after insult or injury, but the radiograph remains normal during the initial hours of clinical distress. Interstitial oedema is the first radiographic abnormality, which may be of a faint, hazy ground-glass appearance (Fig. 3-23), and this is followed rapidly by patchy air-space oedema. By 36–72 hours after insult, diffuse global air-space consolidation is evident. It is the timing of the radiographic changes relative to the insult and the onset of symptoms, rather than the radiological appearance alone, that suggest the diagnosis of ARDS.

Pneumonia

Pulmonary infection may occur several days after surgery. Pneumonia may complicate collapse but may result from aspiration or inhalation of infected secretions from the pharynx.

The features of consolidation have already been covered but the critically ill or postoperative patient may not show typical appearances of consolidation. Numerous factors, such as prior antibiotic therapy and coexistent heart or lung disease, may alter the radiographic features. The radiographic appearance may vary from a few ill-defined or discrete opacities to a

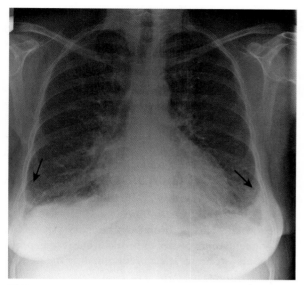

FIGURE 3-23 ■ Pulmonary oedema due to cardiac failure. There is increased opacity or 'haziness' throughout the lungs. There are small bilateral pleural effusions with blunting of both costophrenic angles and subtle septal lines (arrows; short 1–2 cm long subpleural horizontal lines) corresponding with fluid in the interstitium of the lung.

pattern of coalescence and widespread patchy consolidation. Cavity or pneumatocele (a thin-walled air-filled space) formation is not infrequent.

Extrapulmonary Air

The diagnosis of a pneumothorax is made by the identification of the thin line of the visceral pleura. Free air may also be found in the pulmonary interstitium, the mediastinum, the pericardial space and the subcutaneous tissues. In the intensive care setting, extrapulmonary air is most often due to barotrauma from mechanical ventilation or secondary to surgery or other iatrogenic procedures. Pulmonary interstitial emphysema (PIE) is difficult to recognize radiographically and is invariably due to ventilator-induced barotrauma. Unlike air bronchograms, the interstitial air is seen as black lines and streaks radiating from the hila; they do not branch or taper towards the periphery. Interstitial emphysema usually culminates in a pneumomomediastinum and this is shown on a frontal radiograph as a radiolucent band against the mediastinum bordered by the reflected mediastinal pleura. Air may outline specific structures such as the aortic arch, the descending aorta or the thymus.

Cardiac Failure

The radiographic diagnosis of early left ventricular failure is largely dependent on changes in the calibre of the pulmonary vessels in the erect patient. As the left atrial pressure rises, blood is shunted to the upper zones. This is the first and most important radiographic sign of elevated left ventricular pressure but it is important to remember that because of redistribution of blood flow in the supine position, a supine radiograph does not allow this criterion to be used.

Interstitial pulmonary oedema then follows; this is manifested by blurring of the vessel margins, a perihilar haze and a vague increased density over the lower zones. When fluid fills and distends the interlobular septa, Kerley B lines (septal lines) may be visible (see Fig. 3-23). These are best visualized in the costophrenic angles as thin white lines arising from the lateral pleural surface. As the left ventricular pressure continues to rise, multiple small, ill-defined opacities occur in the lower half of the lungs. These represent alveoli filling with fluid. Alveolar oedema may also appear as poorly defined bilateral 'butterfly' perihilar opacification. Increasing cardiac size usually accompanies cardiac failure but, if it occurs following acute myocardial infarction or an acute arrhythmia, cardiac failure may be present without an increase in cardiac size. Bilateral pleural effusions often accompany cardiac failure.

Pulmonary Embolism

The postoperative or critically ill patient has numerous risk factors for the development of deep venous thrombosis and thus pulmonary embolism. In this group, where respiratory distress is often multifactorial, the diagnosis of pulmonary embolism is extremely difficult.

Conventional radiographic findings are non-specific and include elevation of the diaphragm, collapse or segmental consolidation. A small pleural effusion may appear during the first 2 days following the embolus. It is important to recognize that a normal chest radiograph does not exclude a major pulmonary embolus; indeed, a normal radiograph in a patient with acute respiratory distress is suggestive of the diagnosis. A radionuclide perfusion scan is of use because if it is normal a pulmonary embolus can be excluded; however, this is not a practical test for a patient in an intensive care unit and the decision to treat with anti-coagulants is often made clinically.

The success of MDCT in the diagnosis of pulmonary embolism relates to its rapid scan time, volumetric data acquisition and high degree of vascular enhancement (see Fig. 3-5).

Kyphoscoliosis

Kyphoscoliosis makes assessment of the chest radiograph difficult and it is useful to reduce the distortion of thoracic contents due to the kyphoscoliosis by obtaining an oblique radiograph, positioning the patient in such a way that the spine appears at its straightest. Severe kyphoscoliosis may cause pulmonary arterial hypertension and cor pulmonale. Some congenital chest anomalies such as pulmonary agenesis (absence of a lung) and neurofibromatosis are associated with dorsal spine abnormalities. Because of the problems associated with getting a true PA and lateral view, CT scanning is often the most satisfactory method of visualizing the lungs.

Bronchiectasis

Bronchiectasis is a chronic condition characterized by local, irreversible dilatation of the bronchi, usually associated with inflammation. On a chest radiograph the findings include:

- the bronchial wall visible either as single thin lines or as parallel 'tram-lines'
- ring and curvilinear opacities which represent thickened airway walls seen end on. These tend to range in size from 8 to 20 mm, have thin (hairline) walls and may contain air–fluid levels.
- dilated airways filled with secretions giving rise to broad-band shadows some 5–10 mm wide and several centimetres long (seen end on, these dilated fluid-filled airways produce rounded or oval nodular opacities)
- overinflation throughout both lungs (particularly in cystic fibrosis)
- volume loss where bronchiectasis is localized (this may give rise to crowding of bronchi or collapse due to mucous plugging that can be severe and result in complete collapse of a lobe)
- less specific signs including consolidation, scarring and pleural thickening.

The definitive diagnosis of bronchiectasis used to be made by bronchography (injection of contrast into the bronchial airway), but this is an invasive and unpleasant procedure and has been superseded by high-resolution CT (Fig. 3-24). With this technique, thin slices are taken throughout both lungs and the findings are similar to those on the radiograph (thickened bronchial walls, bronchial dilatation, ring opacities containing air–fluid levels). Comparing the diameter of the bronchial wall with the adjacent vessel is helpful, as both should be approximately the same size. CT may also be helpful in determining the optimum position for postural drainage. Upper lobe predominance is present in early cystic fibrosis and after tubercle infection and allergic bronchopulmonary aspergillosis. The remaining causes of bronchiectasis (e.g. post-childhood infection) affect predominantly the middle and lower lobes.

Chronic Airflow Limitation

This comprises three conditions which are present simultaneously in a given patient to a greater or lesser degree: chronic bronchitis, asthma and emphysema. The first is diagnosed by the patient's history and, strictly speaking, does not have any characteristic radiological features. In asthma the chest radiograph is normal in the majority of patients between attacks, but as many as 40 percent reveal evidence of hyperinflation during an acute severe episode. In asthmatic children with recurrent infection, bronchial wall thickening occurs. Collapse of a lobe or an entire lung because of mucous plugging is another feature and may be recurrent, affecting different lobes. Complications include pneumomediastinum, which arises secondarily to PIE and pneumothorax due to rupture of a subpleural bulla. Expiratory radiographs may aid detection of a pneumothorax as well as demonstrating any air trapping secondary to bronchial occlusion.

Emphysema is a condition characterized by an increase in air spaces beyond the terminal bronchiole owing to destruction of alveolar walls. While it is strictly a pathological diagnosis, certain radiographic appearances are characteristic in more advanced cases. These include overinflation of the lungs, an alteration in the appearance of the pulmonary vessels and the presence of bullae. Overinflation results in flattening of the diaphragmatic dome (Fig. 3-25), resulting in an

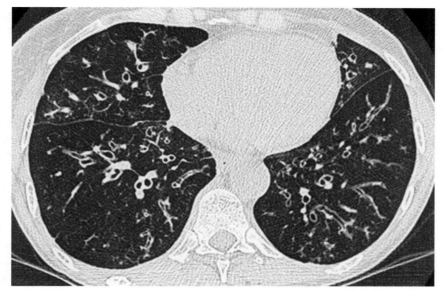

FIGURE 3-24 ■ Bronchiectasis on CT. Note the dilated, thick-walled bronchiectatic airways.

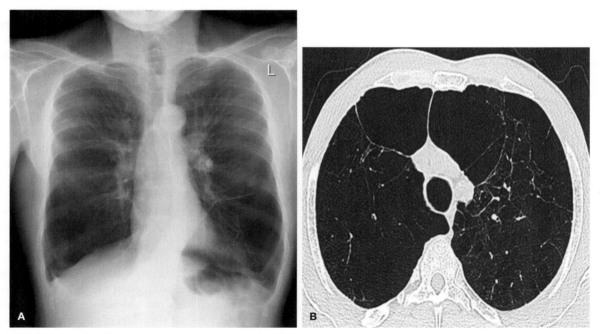

FIGURE 3-25 ■ Emphysema. **(A)** Chest radiograph. Both lungs are hyperinflated with flattening of the hemidiaphragms. **(B)** Axial CT image of the same patient showing extensive 'destruction' of the lung parenchyma, where the lungs are abnormally black.

apparently small heart and a decreased cardiothoracic ratio. The pulmonary vessels are abnormal: the smooth gradation in size of vessels from the hilum outwards is lost, with the hilar vessels being larger than normal and tapering abruptly, so-called pruning of the vessels. However, the lungs are usually unevenly involved and this is mirrored by the uneven distribution of pulmonary vessels. When emphysema is predominantly basal in distribution, there is prominent upper lobe blood diversion which should not be mistaken for evidence of left heart failure. Bullae are recognized by their translucency, their hairline walls and a distortion of adjacent pulmonary vessels. They vary greatly in size and are occasionally big enough to occupy an entire hemithorax. When large, they are an important cause of respiratory distress. Complications of bullae formation are infection and haemorrhage, which are usually manifested as the presence of an air–fluid level. Pneumothorax is another complication and occasionally may be difficult to distinguish from a large bulla.

Paediatrics

INTRODUCTION

Despite the advent of new imaging modalities such as ultrasound, CT, MRI and nuclear medicine, the plain chest radiograph remains the mainstay of paediatric chest imaging. Frequently the clinical history and examination will be augmented by a chest radiograph before a working diagnosis is made and treatment or further investigations planned.

This section aims to provide a concise and practical introduction to imaging the paediatric chest, emphasizing the importance of the plain chest radiograph but also indicating where other modalities provide additional information or allow the same information to be acquired with less use of ionizing radiation. After an introduction to imaging children, we provide an overview of imaging modalities currently available, and review important radiological signs commonly seen in paediatric chest radiographs. The final section discusses common paediatric chest problems and their radiological appearance.

The text has not been referenced extensively but a number of general references and review articles suitable for further reading are given at the end of the chapter.

ISSUES PARTICULAR TO PAEDIATRIC IMAGING

Children are not simply small adults and a range of issues need to be taken into account when performing and interpreting their imaging.

Radiation dose is a major issue in children. Children are more radiosensitive than adults and have a longer time period over which to develop complications from radiation. Estimates of dose vary between centres, but for a paediatric chest CT is in the range of 2 mSv. This is estimated to confer an additional lifetime risk of radiation-induced malignancy for a 10-year-old child of around 1/3000.

Where possible, alternative techniques such as ultrasound or MRI are used. Where radiographs are required the use of modern equipment and optimal technique, including the removal of grids and use of filters, can help to minimize dose. High-dose investigations such as nuclear medicine studies, CT and CT–PET should be performed only after careful consideration of the potential benefits of the investigation weighed against the potential risks. This benefit–risk analysis may be best undertaken within a multidisciplinary team where the viewpoints of patient, parents and all of the professional groups involved in the patient's care can be considered.

For some examinations, such as CT and MRI, the child may need to lie still for several minutes. In infants, feeding the child and wrapping them in a warm blanket can help them sleep through the scan with minimal anxiety for parent and child. Older children can often co-operate with scanning, given the right support. In some centres, children can visit the department ahead of time and play with models of the equipment, or watch videos to help familiarize themselves with the imaging machines. In those children for whom these techniques have failed, sedation can be considered.

When interpreting paediatric imaging, the observer must bear in mind the variation in normal appearance with age: for example, the change in prominence of the thymus on chest radiographs in infants. The likelihood of certain diagnoses also changes with age, with congenital causes of disease always considered in children.

MODALITIES IN PAEDIATRIC CHEST IMAGING

Plain Chest Radiographs and Fluoroscopy

Chest radiographs may be taken in the erect PA or AP position or in the supine AP position. In some circumstances, such as on the neonatal unit (NNU) where patient handling is minimized, all films are obtained in the supine AP projection. It is important that films are clearly labelled, as the appearances of some radiological signs, particularly those of pleural fluid and pneumothorax, are profoundly different in the erect and supine positions. Ideally, chest radiographs should be obtained in inspiration, using a short exposure time and with attention to technical factors so as to minimize the radiation exposure to the patient and attendants. The lateral chest radiograph necessitates a significantly higher exposure than the frontal and is not required routinely.

One of the disadvantages of conventional radiographs is that it is difficult to adequately demonstrate all soft-tissue and bony structures using the same exposure factors. The advent of digital radiography has gone some way to addressing this, as images can be manipulated after acquisition to optimize visualization of areas of interest.

Fluoroscopy and ultrasound are useful techniques for assessing diaphragmatic movements.

Ultrasound

Ultrasound is useful for examining the pleural space for fluid (Fig. 3-26). Effusions and empyemas can be located, measured and drained under ultrasound control. Because the ultrasound beam is strongly reflected by aerated lung, ultrasound is less useful for assessing lung lesions unless they are peripheral, lie

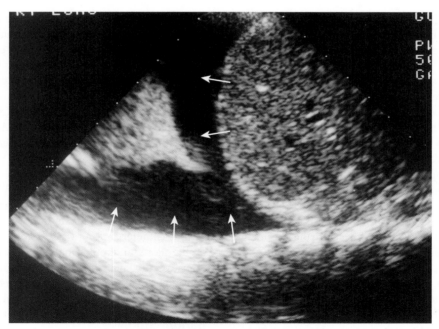

FIGURE 3-26 ■ Sagittal ultrasound of a large pleural effusion, which is poorly echogenic and appears black (white arrows). The patient's back is seen to the bottom and the liver lies to the right of the image. The effusion surrounds the partly collapsed, triangular lower lobe. *(Reproduced courtesy of Dr BJ Loveday and Dr DB Reiff.)*

against the chest wall and consist of either solid or fluid. The movement and integrity of the hemidiaphragms can be assessed using ultrasound. The disadvantage is that each hemidiaphragm can only be assessed independently and not in relationship to the other. This is important in mild hemidiaphragm paresis. Cardiac ultrasound is an extremely accurate non-invasive way of assessing congenital heart disease.

Computed Tomography and High-Resolution Computed Tomography

CT uses a narrow beam of X-rays to image the patient in 'slices'. The thickness of the slice can be varied and may be taken as a continuous spiral or as non-contiguous slices, depending on the individual scanner, region being examined and the likely pathology. Images acquired as a continuous spiral can be reconstructed to look at the area of interest in different orientations, and even in 3D. Assessment of the mediastinum and of vascular structures is facilitated by using intravascular contrast medium.

CT has better spatial resolution than MRI and can detect fine calcification, which affords it an advantage over MRI in evaluating mediastinal masses and lymphadenopathy. Bone structure, and in particular cortical change, are better imaged on CT.

Lung pathology is also best evaluated on CT. Traditionally, HRCT has been used to assess the lung. In HRCT, narrow slices 1–2 mm thick are taken at intervals through the chest. High-resolution algorithms are then used to reconstruct the data in order to maximize parenchymal detail. Slices may be taken in inspiration and expiration to look for 'air-trapping'. In young patients who cannot breath control, the expiratory view may be approximated by lying the patient on their side; the 'side down' hemithorax mimicking expiration. HRCT can be used in the diagnosis of diffuse parenchymal disease and bronchiectasis.

An alternative technique for acquiring the images is to use continuous spiral CT scanning of the chest. This has several advantages over the traditional 'stop–start' technique used in HRCT. Continuous acquisition using a modern multi-slice scanner allows images of the whole chest to be acquired in a single breath hold – significantly reducing movement artefact in children. The spiral acquisition also allows reconstruction of the data in multiple planes. The main

disadvantage of this technique is the increased radiation dose: the effective dose for a spiral CT of the chest is roughly twice that of conventional HRCT.

Magnetic Resonance Imaging

In MRI the patient lies within a strong magnetic field and is exposed to pulses of radiofrequency energy. This energy is absorbed by protons within the body. When the radiofrequency pulses are stopped, the protons return to their normal state but as they do they release energy, the magnetic resonance signal, which can be detected by coils placed around the body. Magnetic resonance signals are different for different tissues and may be altered by disease. Intravascular contrast medium for MRI is available.

MRI takes longer to acquire than CT, and is therefore prone to artefact due to respiratory and cardiac movement. These effects can be minimized by only taking images at the same point in each cardiac and respiratory cycle, a technique known as 'gating'. MRI also has lower spatial resolution.

MRI has three major advantages over CT: its superior soft-tissue contrast, its ability to acquire images in any plane and the fact that it does not use ionizing radiation. Sagittal, coronal and oblique images are of immense value in assessing mediastinal masses and in evaluating whether a paraspinal mass extends into the spinal canal.

The intravenous contrast agent gadolinium can be used in MRI to assess for tissue vascularity, and in magnetic resonance angiography (MRA) to image blood vessels and the heart. New MRA techniques are also being developed which circumvent the need for contrast.

Angiography and Cardiac Catheterization

Cardiac ultrasound and MRI/MRA have reduced the need for diagnostic conventional angiography and cardiac catheterization to assess congenital anomalies of the aorta and pulmonary vessels and congenital arteriovenous malformations. Most conventional angiography or cardiac catheterization is now performed as part of a therapeutic interventional procedure.

Barium Studies

Barium studies have a limited but very important place in the assessment of chest problems, specifically the barium swallow to evaluate extrinsic oesophageal compression by aberrant vessels or masses and the swallow/meal to assess intrinsic abnormalities such as uncoordinated swallowing, abnormal oesophageal peristalsis or gastro-oesophageal reflux that can cause aspiration. If a tracheo-oesophageal fistula is suspected, a tube oesophagram must be performed in the prone position.

There is no reliable technique for the positive diagnosis of aspiration. Recurrent aspiration may be inferred when there is severe gastro-oesophageal reflux.

Radionuclide Studies

In radionuclide studies, radiolabelled pharmaceuticals are used which distribute to specific tissues, providing quantifiable functional information which complements the anatomical information provided by other imaging modalities. The $\dot{V}/\dot{Q}$ scan uses krypton (^{81m}Kr) gas for ventilation and technetium (^{99m}Tc) labelled macroaggregates for perfusion. It detects mismatches in lung perfusion and aeration. Most ventilatory disturbances result in a corresponding reduction in perfusion, whereas if the pulmonary artery to a region is occluded (e.g. pulmonary embolus or sequestrated segment) that region remains ventilated.

The radiation burden from the $\dot{V}$ scan is less than one-fifth of a chest radiograph while the $\dot{Q}$ scan has a dose equal to less than 60 seconds of fluoroscopy.

Positron Emission Tomography

PET uses radioactive isotopes that have a short half-life, and decay by emitting a positron. The emitted positrons collide with surrounding electrons producing a pair of photons, which can be detected by the scanner. The isotope most commonly used is ^{18}F and this is incorporated with glucose to form the tracer [^{18}F]fluorodeoxyglucose (FDG). Many malignant tumours have an altered glucose metabolism that results in FDG accumulating within their cells; this increased uptake allows them to be detected.

PET provides good information on tumour activity but poor anatomical information on the location of the tumour. Hybrid CT–PET scanners perform both scans sequentially and fuse the functional information from PET with the fine anatomical CT images.

In paediatric chest imaging, PET has been used to stage and monitor malignant disease, particularly Hodgkin lymphoma, bone sarcoma and neuroblastoma. However, it is a high-dose study and is not used routinely.

BASIC SIGNS ON THE PLAIN CHEST RADIOGRAPH

Consolidation

Replacement of air in the very distal airways and alveoli by fluid or solid is called 'consolidation'. The cardinal signs of consolidation are an area of increased opacity, which may have an irregular shape, irregular margins and a non-segmental distribution and contains an air bronchogram (Fig. 3-27). The volume of the affected lung remains unchanged. If an area of consolidation abuts the mediastinum, heart or diaphragm, their clear silhouette, which is dependent upon the sharp radiological contrast between normally aerated lung (black) and solid structures (white), is lost (see Fig. 3-27). Similarly, the presence of air bronchograms within an area of consolidation can be explained by the sharp contrast between air in the

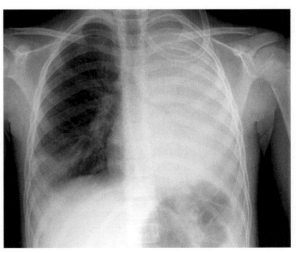

FIGURE 3-27 ■ Left lung consolidation. Mycoplasma pneumonia in a 7-year-old girl presenting with cough and fever. There is extensive consolidation in the left lung with air bronchogram and the clear outline of the left hemidiaphragm has been lost. There is also formation and focal consolidation in the lateral basal segment of the right lower lobe. (*Reproduced with permission from South & Isaacs 2012.*)

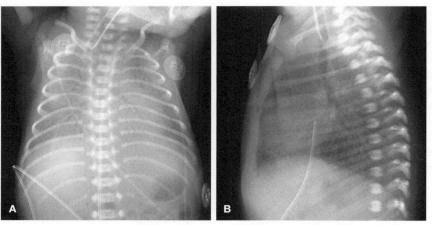

FIGURE 3-28 ■ Respiratory distress syndrome (RDS). Anteroposterior **(A)** and lateral **(B)** chest radiographs of a preterm infant with RDS. Both views show diffuse, hazy ground-glass appearance, air bronchograms, and low lung volumes. *(Reproduced with permission from Wilkins et al. 2010.)*

TABLE 3-2		
Common Causes of Consolidation in Paediatrics		
Pulmonary oedema	Cardiogenic	
	Non-cardiogenic	
Pulmonary exudate	Infection	
Blood	Traumatic contusion	
	Infarction	
Other causes	Respiratory distress syndrome (surfactant deficient disease)	
	Aspiration	
	Alveolar proteinosis	
	Lymphoma	

medium and large bronchi (black) and the surrounding non-aerated and 'solid' lung (white) (Figs 3-27, 3-28).

A variant of infective consolidation frequently seen in infants and children up to approximately 8 years of age is the 'round pneumonia'. This may mimic a mass lesion radiologically since it has well-defined borders, but the clinical picture points to an infective aetiology. While infection is the most common cause, consolidation is also caused by any pathological process in which the alveoli are filled by fluid or solid. The most common causes of consolidation in paediatric practice are listed in Table 3-2.

Collapse

When an airway is obstructed, air within the alveoli and distal airways is absorbed resulting in loss of lung volume. This may affect a lung, lobe or segment. This is manifest on the radiograph by shift of the normal fissures and crowding of airways in the collapsed lung (Figs 3-29, 3-30). If the volume loss is large there may also be mediastinal shift towards the affected side, elevation of the ipsilateral hemidiaphragm, ipsilateral rib crowding and alteration in hilar position. The collapsed lobe may or may not cause increased radio-opacity and there may be compensatory hyperinflation of unaffected lobes. If the collapsed lobe abuts on part of the diaphragm or cardiomediastinal silhouette, the clear outline of these may be lost on the radiograph, as in consolidation (see Figs 3-29, 3-30). Collapse is most often due to obstruction of a large airway by foreign body, mucous plug, tumour or extrinsic compression. Less commonly it occurs secondary to poor ventilation.

Pleural Fluid

The radiological appearance of pleural fluid is largely determined by the position of the patient. In the erect position, fluid collects at the bases and initially causes blunting of the costophrenic angles. Larger effusions cause a homogeneous opacity with a concave upper border – the meniscus. Very large effusions may cause mediastinal shift to the opposite side.

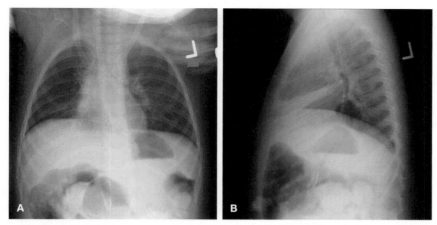

FIGURE 3-29 ■ Right middle lobe collapse. Note the 'silhouetting' of the right (atrial) heart border on the frontal radiograph **(A),** where the collapsed right middle lobe abuts the heart, and the triangular-shaped opacity on the lateral radiograph **(B)**. *(Reproduced with permission from Hutchison 2012.)*

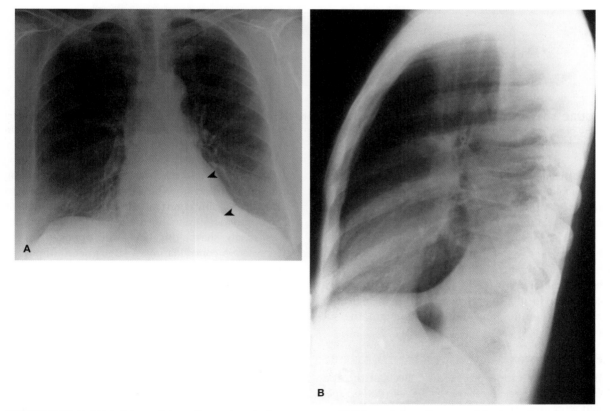

FIGURE 3-30 ■ **(A)** Left lower lobe collapse. A typical appearance of left lower lobe collapse resulting in a triangular density behind the heart (arrowheads). The contour of the medial left hemidiaphragm is lost. *(Reproduced with permission from Adam & Dixon 2008.)* **(B)** The lateral radiograph shows the collapsed left lower lobe as a wedge-shaped opacity in the lower chest posteriorly. *(Reproduced with permission from George & Gordon 1995.)*

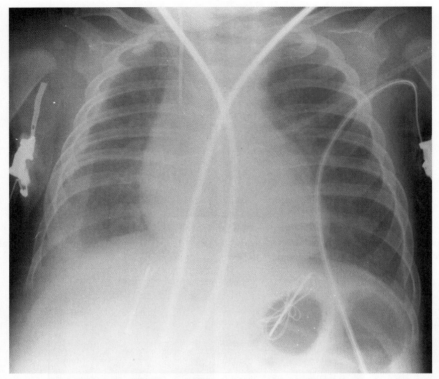

FIGURE 3-31 ■ Supine radiograph showing a pleural effusion. There is reduced transradiancy on the right and a peripheral band of soft-tissue density paralleling the chest wall with a 'step' at the position of the horizontal fissure. *(Reproduced with permission from George & Gordon 1995.)*

In the supine position, often used for neonatal and infant radiographs, an effusion causes reduced transradiancy (whiter hemithorax) of the affected side and may collect around the apex of the lung. In larger effusions a peripheral band of soft-tissue density appears between the chest wall and the lung; on the right this band has a characteristic step at the position of the horizontal fissure (Figs 3-26, 3-31). Pleural fluid may collect and loculate within fissures or between the inferior surface of the lung and the diaphragm, the 'subpulmonic' effusion.

Pneumothorax

In the erect position pleural air collects at the apex, causing increased apical transradiancy (darker apex) and absent lung markings beyond a visible lung edge. In the supine position air collects initially in the antero-inferior chest, causing quite different and often subtle signs. These include small slivers of air at the apex, around the heart and between the lung and the diaphragm. Where free air as opposed to aerated lung abuts part of the cardiomediastinal or diaphragmatic silhouette, the clarity of that border is especially sharp, this being the opposite of the effect seen in consolidation. A large pneumothorax in neonates and infants when supine may collect anteriorly and cause an increased ipsilateral transradiancy (darker hemithorax), increased sharpness of the cardiomediastinal silhouette and a deep costophrenic angle (Fig. 3-32).

A tension pneumothorax occurs when a pleural tear acts as a one-way flap valve, allowing air into the pleural space but preventing egress. The pressure within the hemithorax rises, causing mediastinal shift to the contralateral side and flattening, or even eversion, of the ipsilateral hemidiaphragm (Fig. 3-33). This is an emergency, and if clinically suspected should be treated without delaying for imaging.

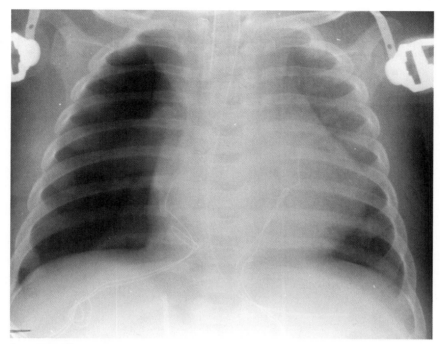

FIGURE 3-32 ■ Supine radiograph showing a postoperative right pneumothorax. There is increased transradiancy of the right hemithorax. The right heart border is very clearly defined and the right lung edge is visible. *(Reproduced with permission from George & Gordon 1995.)*

PAEDIATRIC CHEST PROBLEMS

Congenital Abnormalities of the Chest

Congenital Diaphragmatic Hernia

Large congenital diaphragmatic hernias may present as neonatal respiratory distress, although many are now diagnosed antenatally on routine antenatal ultrasound examination. They can be associated with other congenital anomalies. Most are posterior, left-sided, Bochdalek hernias. Bowel and other organs are sited in the chest and appear on the radiograph as a cystic/solid mass. The mediastinum is shifted to the contralateral side and one or both lungs may be hypoplastic (Fig. 3-34). When large, the condition carries a high mortality.

Congenital Pulmonary Airways Malformation (Congenital Cystic Adenomatoid Malformation)

This predominantly sporadic condition is caused by abnormalities of tracheobronchial branching and may affect any lobe. The hamartomatous mass of pulmonary tissue contains a proliferation of bronchial structures and may appear predominantly cystic, solid, or a combination of both. It can cause compression of the adjacent lung and mediastinal shift, impairing lung function. Appearances can mimic both congenital diaphragmatic hernia and congenital lobar emphysema. In one-fifth of cases more than one lobe is affected.

Congenital Lobar Emphysema

A focal abnormality of a lobar bronchus leads to a ball valve effect, causing air trapping and overinflation of the affected lobe. The left upper lobe is most frequently affected, followed by the right middle lobe. Initial radiographs in the first few hours of life may show an opaque mass in the region of the affected lobe. As fluid clears, the appearances are those of an overinflated lobe with compression of normal surrounding lung and mediastinal shift to the contralateral side

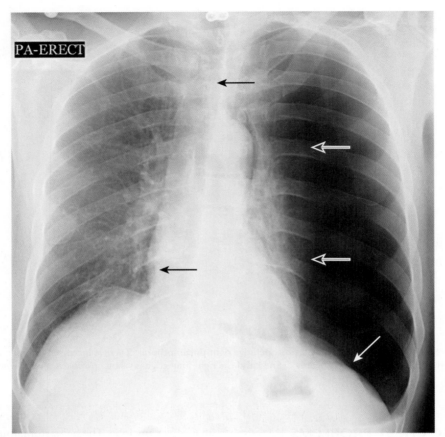

FIGURE 3-33 ■ Large left-sided tension pneumothorax. Progressive loss of air into pleural space through a one-way check-valve mechanism may cause a shift of the heart and mediastinal structures away from side of pneumothorax and lead to cardiopulmonary compromise by impairing venous return to the heart. In this patient, the left lung is almost totally collapsed (open white arrows) and there is a shift of the trachea and heart to the right (closed black arrows). The left hemidiaphragm is depressed because of the elevated left intrathoracic pressure (closed white arrow). *(Reproduced with permission from Herring 2007.)*

(Fig. 3-35). Treatment is surgical excision of the affected lobe if the neonate is in respiratory distress.

Congenital Cardiac Anomalies

There are a vast array of congenital cardiac anomalies, the most common including atrial and ventricular septal defects. The appearances seen on plain film are dependent on the specific anatomy of the anomaly; however, the contour of the heart and mediastinal vessels may appear distorted and cardiogenic oedema may be present. Children with suspected cardiac anomalies will go on to have further investigation with cardiac ultrasound +/− cross-sectional imaging.

An enlarged heart and cardiogenic oedema may also be caused by systemic overload, such as in arterio-venous malformations.

Neonatal Chest Problems

Respiratory Distress Syndrome (Surfactant-Deficient Disease)

In the normal lung, surfactant coats the surface of the alveoli, decreasing surface tension and reducing the effort of lung expansion. Surfactant deficiency is primarily seen in premature infants and results in alveolar collapse and noncompliant lungs. It is relatively common, with up to 50% of premature infants affected.

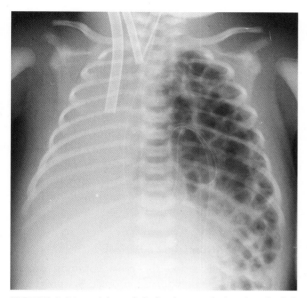

FIGURE 3-34 ■ A large left diaphragmatic hernia. The left hemithorax contains the stomach (nasogastric tube) and loops of small bowel. The mediastinum is shifted to the right. The right lung is airless and opaque because the patient is on an extracorporeal membrane oxygenator (ECMO). *(Reproduced with permission from George & Gordon 1995.)*

Clinically, it manifests as tachypnoea, cyanosis, expiratory grunting and chest wall retraction. The radiograph shows bilateral symmetrical low-volume lungs, ground-glass granularity representing collapsed alveoli and well-defined air bronchograms extending from the hilum into the peripheral lung (see Fig. 3-28). A normal chest radiograph at 6 hours of age makes the diagnosis of respiratory distress syndrome (RDS) extremely unlikely.

These neonates frequently require intermittent positive pressure ventilation which may give rise to specific complications of PIE (Fig. 3-36), bronchopulmonary dysplasia (BPD) (Fig. 3-37), pneumothorax (see Fig. 3-32) and pneumomediastinum.

PIE is caused by gas leaking from overdistended alveoli and tracking along bronchovascular sheaths. The radiographic appearance is that of a branching pattern of gas with associated bubbles affecting all or part of the lung (see Fig. 3-36).

BPD or chronic lung disease of prematurity (CLD) is seen in infants who have been on positive pressure ventilation, usually for RDS. The combination of high-pressure trauma and oxygen toxicity results in lung

FIGURE 3-35 ■ Newborn infant with congenital lobar emphysema involving the left upper lobe. Although the area is hyperlucent, lung markings can still be identified within the lesion. The overdistended left upper lobe crosses the midline (thin arrows), compresses the left lower lobe and lingula (open arrows) and causes a rightward shift of the mediastinal structures. *(Reproduced with permission from Panitch 2005.)*

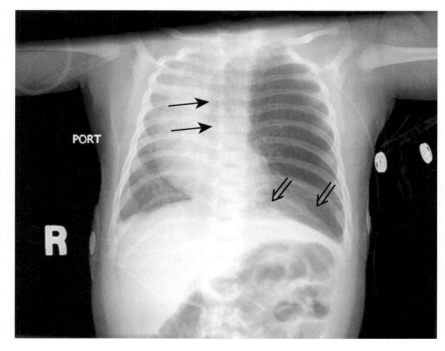

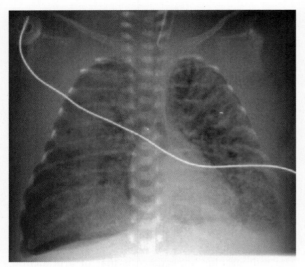

FIGURE 3-36 ■ Pulmonary interstitial emphysema (PIE). A 6-week-old girl born at 30 weeks' gestation was very difficult to ventilate. Chest radiograph shows overexpanded lungs that are seen bulging out intercostally, with the diaphragm flattened. There is also increased opacification of the lungs, due to RDS. Linearly arranged bubbly lucencies can be seen radiating from the hila, suggesting PIE secondary to high-pressure ventilation. There is also a pneumothorax seen at the base of the right lung. *(Reproduced with permission from Wilmott et al. 2012.)*

damage. The lung may pass through a number of radiological stages during the evolution of BPD. Initially there is an RDS pattern which progresses to almost complete opacification and then to a coarse pattern of linear opacities and cystic lucencies (see Fig. 3-37). The lack of adequate oxygenation in RDS may result in failure of the ductus arteriosus to close. The consequent left-to-right shunt may progress to heart failure.

Meconium Aspiration Syndrome

This is the most common cause of respiratory distress in full- or post-term neonates. The aspirated meconium causes a chemical pneumonitis and bronchial obstruction. The radiographic picture is of bilateral diffuse patchy collapse with other areas of overinflation (Fig. 3-38). Spontaneous pneumothorax, pneumomediastinum and small effusions are common but air bronchograms are rare.

Respiratory Tract Infections

Viral Infections

Viral infections generally affect the bronchi and peribronchial tissues and this is reflected in the radiological signs: symmetrical parahilar, peribronchial streaky shadowing radiating for a variable distance into the lung periphery, hilar lymphadenopathy, occasionally reticulonodular shadowing, segmental/lobar collapse and generalized overinflation secondary to narrowing of the bronchi (Fig. 3-39). Effusions are rare. Organisms commonly encountered are the respiratory syncytial virus (RSV), influenza and parainfluenza viruses, adenovirus and rhinovirus.

Bacterial and Mycoplasma Infections

In the neonatal period the most common organisms are non-haemolytic streptococci, *S. aureus* and *Escherichia coli*. Lobar consolidation is rare and more often the following signs are seen: radiating perihilar streakiness, coarse patchy parenchymal infiltrates, nodular or reticulonodular shadowing or diffuse hazy shadowing, most often basal. One important pattern to recognize is the diffuse bilateral granularity of group B haemolytic streptococcal pneumonia, which so closely mimics RDS.

In infants, bacterial infection is more often seen as lobar or patchy consolidations (see Fig. 3-27). The organisms are most commonly *Haemophilus influenzae*, *Streptococcus pneumoniae*, *S. aureus* and *Mycoplasma pneumoniae*. Pleural effusions, empyemas, abscesses and pneumatocoeles are well-recognized complications. The 'round pneumonia' is an area of infective consolidation which transiently has a rounded configuration and mimics a mass lesion. Round pneumonia is less likely to be seen in children over 8 years of age, and in this age group an alternative diagnosis should be sought for a mass-like appearance. *M. pneumoniae* infection can mimic the radiographic appearances of both bacterial and viral pneumonia; however, it is more likely than other infections to appears as unilobar reticulonodular opacification.

Tuberculosis

Tuberculosis acquired in infancy is usually manifest by unilateral hilar or paratracheal lymphadenopathy and

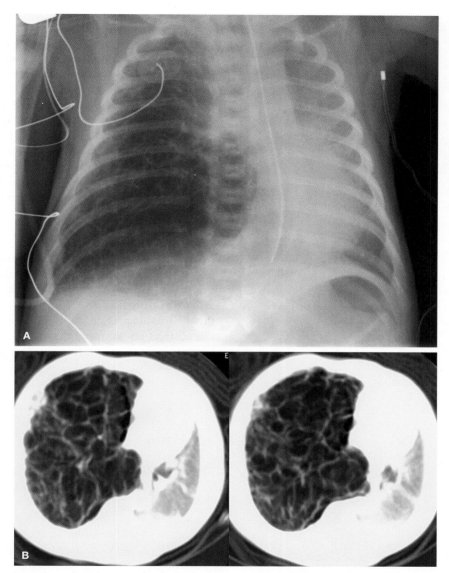

FIGURE 3-37 ■ Severe bronchopulmonary dysplasia (BPD) in an infant treated with high levels of inspired oxygen for RDS. **(A)** The chest radiograph demonstrates marked hyperexpansion of the right lung with shift of mediastinum to the left. There is a coarse pattern of linear opacities and cystic lucencies. **(B)** CT shows findings of severe BPD affecting the right lung only. *(Reproduced with permission from Hansell 2010.)*

occasionally the primary or Ghon focus is seen as an area of consolidation in the periphery of the ipsilateral lung (Fig. 3-40). Collapse is seen, usually due to compression of a bronchus by lymph nodes. Bronchopneumonic spread, with widespread areas of consolidation, occurs if either an infected node discharges into a bronchus or when host resistance is very low, facilitating spread through the airways. Miliary tuberculosis, with multiple small nodules, is caused by the haematogenous spread that occurs when an infected node discharges into the bloodstream. Cavitation is unusual in children.

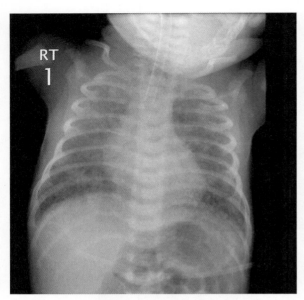

FIGURE 3-38 ■ Meconium aspiration syndrome. Ventilated infant with meconium aspiration syndrome showing typical mixed appearances of hyperinflation and patchy interstitial shadowing from atelectasis and local emphysema. *(Reproduced with permission from Stenson & Smith 2012.)*

Airway Disease

Asthma

Radiological changes are rarely seen before the age of 3 years. In chronic asthma there is generalized overinflation of the lungs with parahilar, peribronchial infiltrates but hilar lymphadenopathy is rare. Plugs of viscid mucus obstruct the airways and cause recurrent segmental or lobar collapse (see Fig. 3-30). Pneumomediastinum is a common complication but rarely requires specific treatment; pneumothorax is seen less frequently. Asthma may be triggered by gastro-oesophageal reflux and barium studies may be useful in assessing the patient.

Obstruction by Foreign Bodies

Aspirated foreign bodies most commonly lodge in the major bronchi and act like a ball valve, causing distal obstructive emphysema (Fig. 3-41). Radiographs are taken in inspiration and expiration to demonstrate the air trapping. Less commonly, the lung distal to the obstruction collapses and may become infected. Chronic aspiration of a foreign body may result in bronchiectasis.

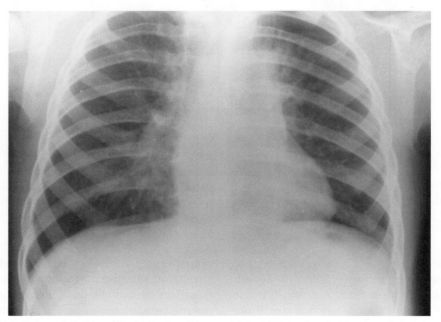

FIGURE 3-39 ■ Viral pneumonia caused by the respiratory syncytial virus (RSV). There is symmetrical perihilar and peribronchial streaky shadowing and mild hilar lymphadenopathy. *(Reproduced with permission from George & Gordon 1995.)*

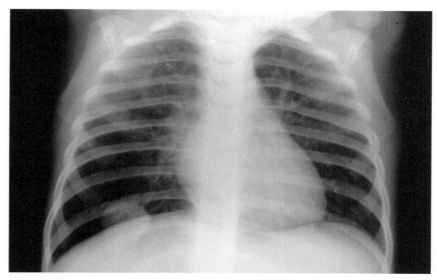

FIGURE 3-40 ■ Primary tuberculous infection. Unilateral right hilar lymphadenopathy and an area of consolidation (Ghon focus) in the ipsilateral lower zone. *(Reproduced with permission from George & Gordon 1995.)*

Cystic Fibrosis and Bronchiectasis

Cystic fibrosis is an autosomal recessive condition, causing excessively thick and viscous mucous. In the neonatal period, bowel obstruction due to meconium ileus may draw attention to the condition. In the chest the earliest signs are very similar to those of viral bronchiolitis: overinflation, focal collapse and parahilar, peribronchial infiltrates (Fig. 3-42). Recurrent infections lead to bronchiectasis, fibrosis and generalized overinflation with segmental areas of collapse. Bronchial collaterals are recruited and when these become large, haemoptysis may be a problem.

CT is very sensitive in demonstrating early changes in cystic fibrosis, and has been shown to detect regional disease before abnormalities are seen on global pulmonary function testing.

There are several signs of bronchiectasis which may be seen on CT: dilatation of the bronchus to greater than the calibre of the accompanying arteriole, non-tapering of the airways which are seen within 1 cm of the pleural surface, and thickening of the bronchiole wall; are all indicative (see Fig. 3-24). In addition to cystic fibrosis, bronchiectasis in children may also occur as a sequelae of recurrent gastro-oesophageal reflux and aspiration, foreign body aspiration and pulmonary infections such as pertussis. Rarely, it is seen in association with immune deficiency states or congenital causes such as Kartagener syndrome (primary ciliary dyskinesia).

Small Airway Disease

Inflammatory disease of the smaller airways is common and may occur following viral infection and as part of other conditions, including cystic fibrosis, asthma, recurrent aspiration, post transplantation and post chemotherapy. Inflammatory tissue narrows and obstructs the airways causing air trapping. In constrictive obliterative bronchiolitis (bronchiolitis obliterans), the small airway narrowing is irreversible due to fibrotic scar tissue. It is often idiopathic, but can occur following infection, inhalational injury, drug reactions or post transplantation. Plain radiograph changes are variable and often underestimate the extent of disease. Air trapping is best demonstrated using inspiratory and expiratory CT. Normal, healthy lung reduces in volume and appears more dense in expiration. In air trapping, the areas of affected lung remain inflated throughout expiration and appear less dense than adjacent normal lung. This retention of air during expiration helps to differentiate air trapping from other causes of 'mosaic' lung appearance, such as perfusion abnormalities (Fig. 3-43).

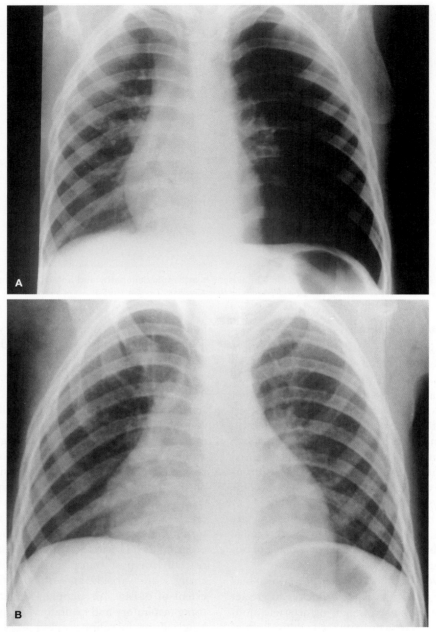

FIGURE 3-41 ■ **(A)** Aspirated foreign body lodged in the left main stem bronchus. Marked air trapping in the affected lung causing overinflation, increased transradiancy and mediastinal shift. **(B)** Same patient after bronchoscopic removal of the obstruction. *(Reproduced with permission from George & Gordon 1995.)*

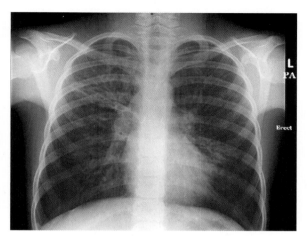

FIGURE 3-42 ■ Cystic fibrosis. Child with cystic fibrosis demonstrating classical upper lobe bronchiectasis. Note the lung overinflation and the diffuse parahilar, peribronchial infiltrates. *(Reproduced with permission from South & Isaacs 2012.)*

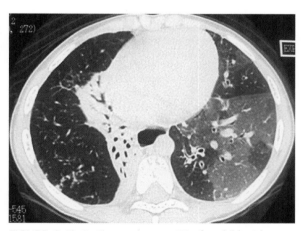

FIGURE 3-43 ■ Air-trapping on CT of a child with post-infectious bronchiolitis obliterans showing mosaic pattern, air trapping, bronchiectasis and atelectasis. The lung parenchyma takes on a 'mosaic' appearance, with segmental areas of decreased attenuation which are exaggerated on expiration, seen here in the left lung.

Swyer–James or Mcleod syndrome is an unusual form of post-infection constrictive obliterative bronchiolitis in which the affected lung fails to grow normally and remains small volume. It is usually unilateral. In these cases the plain radiograph may show the characteristic feature of unilateral hypertransradiancy caused by air trapping in the affected lung.

Acknowledgements

We would like to acknowledge the huge contribution made to the paediatric section by Professor Isky Gordon of Great Ormond Street Hospital for Sick Children, an inspiring teacher and mentor who co-authored previous editions of this chapter. We would also like to thank Dr B.J. Loveday at the Royal Surrey County Hospital, Guildford and Dr D.B. Reiff at Ashford and St Peter's Hospital for allowing us to use their radiographs as illustrations. Figures 3.30B, 3.31, 3.32, 3.34, 3.39, 3.40, 3.41 are reproduced from George C.D., Gordon I., 'Imaging the Paediatric Heart'. In: Prasad S.A., Hussey J. (Eds) Paediatric Respiratory Care: A Guide for Physiotherapists and Health Professionals. Originally published by Chapman & Hall in 1995. With kind permission from Springer Science and Business Media.

REFERENCES AND FURTHER READING

Adults

Adam, A., Dixon, A.K. (Eds.), 2008. Grainger & Allison's Diagnostic Imaging, fifth ed. Churchill Livingstone Elsevier.

Bruzzi, J.F., Munden, R.F., 2006. PET/CT imaging of lung cancer. J. Thorac. Imaging 21, 123–136.

Desai, S.R., Copley, S.J., Aziz, Z., Hansell, D.M., 2012. Thoracic Imaging (Oxford Specialist Handbooks in Radiology). Oxford University Press, Oxford. UK.

Goodman, L.R., 2007. Felson's Principles of Chest Roentgenology, third ed. W B Saunders, Philadelphia.

Hansell, D.M., et al., 2008. Fleischner Society: glossary of terms for thoracic imaging. Radiology 246, 697–722.

Hansell, D.M., Lynch, D.A., McAdams, H.P., Bankier, A.A., 2010. Imaging of Diseases of the Chest, fifth ed. Mosby Elsevier, Philadelphia.

Heitzmann, E.R., 1988. The Mediastinum: Radiologic Correlations with Anatomy and Pathology, second ed. Springer-Verlag, Berlin.

McLoud, T., Boiselle, P., 2010. Thoracic Imaging: The Requisites, second ed. Mosby Elsevier, Philadelphia.

Naidich, D.P., et al., 2007. Computed Tomography and Magnetic Resonance of the Thorax, fourth ed. Lippincott Williams & Wilkins, Philadelphia.

Paediatrics

Adam, A., Dixon, A.K. (Eds.), 2008. Grainger & Allison's Diagnostic Radiology, fifth ed. Churchill Livingstone Elsevier.

Arthur, R., 2001. The neonatal chest X-ray. Paediatr. Respir. Rev. 2, 311–323.

Copley, S.J., 2002. Application of computed tomography in childhood respiratory infections. Br. Med. Bull. 61, 263–279.

Copley, S.J., Bush, A., 2000. HRCT of paediatric lung disease. Paediatr. Respir. Rev. 1, 141–147.

De Bruyn, R., 1993. Paediatric chest. In: Cosgrove, D., Meire, H., Dewbury, K. (Eds.), Clinical Ultrasound: Abdominal and General Ultrasound, vol. 2. Churchill Livingstone, London, pp. 983–988.

Frush, D.P., 2005. Paediatric chest imaging. Radiol. Clin. North Am. 43, 253–457.

George, C.D., Gordon, I., 1995. Imaging the Paediatric Heart. In: Prasad, S.A., Hussey, J. (Eds.), Paediatric Respiratory Care. Springer Science and Business Media, Dordrecht.

Gibson, A.T., Steiner, G.M., 1997. Imaging the neonatal chest. Clin. Radiol. 52, 172–186.

Gilberto, B., Fischer, G.B., Edgar, E., et al., 2010. Post infectious bronchiolitis obliterans in children. Paediatr. Respir. Rev. 11 (4), 233–239.

Goodman, L.R., 1999. Felson's Principles of Chest Roentgenology: A Programmed Text, second ed. WB Saunders, Philadelphia.

Goodman, L.R., Putman, C.E., 1991. Intensive Care Radiology: Imaging of the Critically Ill, third ed. WB Saunders, Philadelphia.

Gordon, I., Helms, P., Fazio, F., 1981. Clinical applications of radionuclide lung scanning. Br J Radiol 54, 576–585.

Gordon, I., Matthew, D.J., Dinwiddie, R., 1987. Respiratory system. In: Gordon, I. (Ed.), Diagnostic Imaging in Paediatrics. Chapman and Hall, London, pp. 27–57.

Grainger, R.G., Allison, D.J., Dixon, A.K., 2001. Grainger and Allison's Diagnostic Radiology, A Textbook of Medical Imaging, fourth ed. Churchill Livingstone, Edinburgh.

Hansell, D., 2010. Imaging of Diseases of the Chest. Elsevier.

Hansell, D.M., Armstrong, P., Lynch, D.A., McAdams, H.P., 2005. Imaging of Diseases of the Chest, fourth ed. Elsevier Mosby, London.

Hayden, C.K., Swischuk, L.E. (Eds.), 1992. Pediatric Ultrasonography, second ed. Williams and Wilkins, Baltimore.

Heitzmann, E.R., 1988. The Mediastinum: Radiologic Correlations with Anatomy and Pathology, second ed. Springer-Verlag, Berlin.

Hendry, G.M.A., 2000. Magnetic resonance imaging of the paediatric chest. Paediatr. Respir. Rev. 1, 249–258.

Herring, W., 2007. Learning Radiology: Recognizing the Basics. Mosby Elsevier.

Hutchison, S.J., 2012. Principles of Cardiovascular Radiology. Saunders Elsevier.

Keats, T.E., Anderson, M.W., 2001. Atlas of Normal Roentgen Variants That May Simulate Disease, seventh ed. Mosby, St Louis.

Kim, O.H., Kim, W.S., Kim, M.J., et al., 2000. US (ultrasound) in the diagnosis of pediatric chest diseases. Radiographics 20, 653–671.

Lipscombe, D.J., Flower, C.D.R., Hadfield, J.W., 1981. Ultrasound of the pleura: an assessment of its clinical value. Clin. Radiol. 32, 289–290.

Newman, B., 1993. The pediatric chest. Radiol. Clin. North Am. 31, 453–719.

Panitch, H., 2005. Pediatric Pulmonology. Mosby Elsevier.

Piepsz, A., Gordon, I., Hahn, K., 1991. Paediatric nuclear medicine. Eur. J. Nucl. Med. 18, 41–66.

Reed, J.C., 2003. Chest Radiology: Plain Film Patterns and Differential Diagnoses, fifth ed. Mosby, St Louis.

Rossi, U.G., Owens, C.M., 2005. The radiology of chronic lung disease in children. Arch. Dis. Child. 90, 601–607.

Simon, G., 1975. The anterior view chest radiograph – criteria for normality derived from a basic analysis of the shadows. Clin. Radiol. 26, 429–437.

South, M., Isaacs, D. (Eds.), 2012. Practical Paediatrics, seventh ed. Churchill Livingstone Elsevier.

Stenson, B.J., Smith, C.L., 2012. Management of meconium aspiration syndrome. Paediatrics and Child Health 22 (12), 532–535.

Swischuk, L.E., 1989. Imaging of the Newborn, Infant and Young Child, third ed. Williams and Wilkins, Baltimore.

Vix, V.A., Klatte, E.C., 1970. The lateral chest radiograph in the diagnosis of hilar and mediastinal masses. Radiology 96, 307–316.

Webb, R.W., Müller, N.L., Naidich, D.P., 2001. High-Resolution CT of the Lung, third ed. Lippincott Williams & Wilkins, Philadelphia.

Wilkins, R.L., Dexter, J.R., Heuer, A.J., 2010. Clinical Assessment in Respiratory Care, sixth ed. Mosby Elsevier.

Wilmott, R.W., Boat, T.F., Bush, A., et al., 2012. Kendig and Chernick's Disorders of the Respiratory Tract in Children, eighth ed. Saunders Elsevier.

4

CARDIAC AND CARDIOVASCULAR DISEASES

ANDREW D HIRSCHHORN ▪ SEAN F MUNGOVAN ▪
DAVID A B RICHARDS

CHAPTER OUTLINE

INTRODUCTION 126

ISCHAEMIC HEART DISEASE 127
Introduction 127
Aetiology and Pathophysiology of Ischaemic Heart
Disease 127
Symptoms and Signs of Ischaemic Heart
Disease 128
Diagnosis of Ischaemic Heart Disease 128
Classification of Ischaemic Heart Disease 129
Medical Management of Ischaemic Heart
Disease 130
Physiotherapy-Specific Management of Ischaemic
Heart Disease 132

CARDIAC VALVE DISEASE 132
Introduction 132
Aetiology and Pathophysiology of Cardiac Valve
Disease 133
Symptoms and Signs of Cardiac Valve Disease 134
Diagnosis of Cardiac Valve Disease 134
Classification of Cardiac Valve Disease 136
Medical Management of Cardiac Valve
Disease 136
Physiotherapy-Specific Management of Cardiac
Valve Disease 137

CARDIOMYOPATHY 137
Introduction 137
Aetiology and Pathophysiology of
Cardiomyopathy 137
Symptoms and Signs of Cardiomyopathy 138
Diagnosis of Cardiomyopathy 138
Medical Management of Cardiomyopathy 139
Physiotherapy-Specific Management of
Cardiomyopathy 140

PERICARDIAL DISEASE 140
Introduction 140

Aetiology and Pathophysiology of Pericardial
Disease 140
Symptoms and Signs of Pericardial Disease 140
Diagnosis of Pericardial Disease 141
Classification of Pericardial Disease 141
Medical Management of Pericardial Disease 141
Physiotherapy-Specific Management of Pericardial
Disease 142

HEART FAILURE 142
Introduction 142
Aetiology and Pathophysiology of Heart
Failure 142
Symptoms and Signs of Heart Failure 143
Diagnosis of Heart Failure 144
Classification of Heart Failure 144
Medical Management of Heart Failure 145
Physiotherapy-Specific Management of Heart
Failure 146

CARDIAC ARRHYTHMIAS 147
Introduction 147
Aetiology and Pathophysiology of Cardiac
Arrhythmias 147
Symptoms and Signs of Cardiac Arrhythmias 148
Diagnosis of Cardiac Arrhythmias 148
Classification of Cardiac Arrhythmias 148
Medical Management of Cardiac Arrhythmias 148
Physiotherapy-Specific Management of Cardiac
Arrhythmias 149

GROWN-UP CONGENITAL HEART DISEASE 150
Introduction 150
Aetiology and Pathophysiology of GUCH 150
Symptoms and Signs of GUCH 150
Diagnosis of GUCH 150
Classification of GUCH 151
Medical Management of GUCH 151

125

Physiotherapy-Specific Management of GUCH 151

AORTIC DISEASE 152
Introduction 152
Aetiology and Pathophysiology of Aortic
Disease 152
Symptoms and Signs of Aortic Disease 152
Diagnosis of Aortic Disease 153
Classification of Aortic Disease 153
Medical Management of Aortic Disease 153
Physiotherapy-Specific Management of Aortic
Disease 154

PERIPHERAL ARTERY DISEASE 154
Introduction 154
Aetiology and Pathophysiology of Peripheral Artery
Disease 154
Symptoms and Signs of Peripheral Artery
Disease 154
Diagnosis of Peripheral Artery Disease 155

Classification of Peripheral Artery Disease 155
Medical Management of Peripheral Artery
Disease 155
Physiotherapy-Specific Management of Peripheral
Artery Disease 155

VENOUS THROMBOEMBOLISM 156
Introduction 156
Aetiology and Pathophysiology of Venous
Thromboembolism 156
Symptoms and Signs of Venous
Thromboembolism 157
Diagnosis of Venous Thromboembolism 157
Classification of Venous Thromboembolism 157
Medical Management of Venous
Thromboembolism 158
Physiotherapy-Specific Management of Venous
Thromboembolism 158

REFERENCES 159

INTRODUCTION

The term 'cardiovascular disease' encompasses all diseases and conditions of the heart (cardiac disease) and vascular system, both noncommunicable and communicable. The health burden of cardiovascular disease is immense; cardiovascular disease is the single largest cause of death worldwide (responsible for approximately 30% of all deaths) and one of the leading contributors to lost disability-adjusted life-years (World Health Organization 2011). The global pattern of cardiovascular disease is in constant transition. While improvements in preventative strategies and therapies for cardiovascular disease have seen a decrease in age-adjusted cardiovascular mortality in high-income regions of the world, increases in risk factors (e.g. tobacco use, unhealthy diet, physical inactivity) are contributing to a concomitant, substantial increase in cardiovascular mortality in low and middle-income regions (Gaziano & Gaziano 2012). Increasing rates of obesity, and associated conditions such as hypertension and diabetes mellitus, threaten a worsening global epidemic of noncommunicable cardiovascular disease.

This chapter describes by section some of the more common presentations of cardiac and cardiovascular disease. Our intention in writing this chapter has been to provide the student/clinician with a greater understanding of the pathophysiology and current management of these disease presentations, together with implications for the provision of physiotherapy. Brief case studies are used to place information in a clinical context. We have predominantly focused on those conditions likely to be encountered by clinicians working in hospital and cardiac rehabilitation settings. Cerebrovascular disease, including stroke, has been explicitly excluded as beyond the scope of the chapter and more suited to a text on neurological disorders/management.

An important caveat: this textbook is written predominantly for physiotherapists and is not intended as a guide to medical therapy. By virtue of length, this chapter can only serve as a summary reference for cardiac and cardiovascular disease; the reader is directed elsewhere for more comprehensive information. Reliable, contemporary sources of such information (used in research for this chapter) include: *Braunwald's Heart Disease,* currently in its ninth edition (Bonow et al 2012); the American College of Cardiology Foundation (ACCF) and American Heart Association (AHA), whose guidelines for the management of cardiovascular disease are available online at http://my.americanheart.org (American Heart Association 2014); and the European Society of Cardiology, whose guidelines are similarly available at http://www.escardio.org.

ISCHAEMIC HEART DISEASE

CASE 4-1

Mr AB is a 45-year-old computer programmer who reported severe (10/10) chest pain to his work supervisor. The supervisor immediately dialled for emergency assistance; the ambulance arrived 5 minutes later. Paramedics administered oxygen, aspirin and sublingual nitrates, and Mr AB's pain lessened from 10/10 to 7/10. A 12-lead electrocardiogram (ECG) showed changes of anterior ST-segment elevation myocardial infarction (STEMI). Mr AB was transferred to hospital for immediate coronary angiography and percutaneous coronary intervention (PCI).

Introduction

The human heart comprises a pair of functionally separate, valved muscular pumps, contained structurally as a single organ (Williams et al 1989). Composed of three major types of cardiac muscle: atrial muscle, ventricular muscle and specialized excitatory and conductive muscle fibres (Guyton & Hall 1996), the heart functions to maintain pulmonary and systemic circulation (Antoni 1989).

As with all muscle tissue, the myocardium (the cardiac muscle) requires energy to produce contractile force (Guyton & Hall 1996). Uniquely, the myocardium relies almost exclusively on oxidative metabolism for its function; even at rest the heart operates at near maximal oxygen extraction. As such, increased myocardial oxygen consumption, required during periods of increased myocardial load (e.g. increased heart rate), must be met by an increase in the supply of oxygenated blood (perfusion) (Antoni 1989).

The myocardium receives oxygenated blood via a network of epicardial arteries, known collectively as the 'coronary arteries' (Figure 1-21). The coronary arteries dilate to increase myocardial perfusion in a proportionate response to myocardial oxygen consumption or demand (Guyton and Hall 1996).

Aetiology and Pathophysiology of Ischaemic Heart Disease

Ischaemic heart disease (IHD) is characterized by a relative decrease in myocardial perfusion, such that perfusion is inadequate to meet the metabolic demands of the myocardium (Padera, Jr & Schoen 2010). As IHD is most commonly caused by atherosclerosis of the coronary arteries, the terms 'IHD', 'coronary heart disease' and 'coronary artery disease' are often used interchangeably.

Atherosclerosis is a chronic and progressive inflammatory disease of the arterial endothelium (Padera, Jr & Schoen 2010). The characteristic lesion seen in coronary atherosclerosis is the formation of atheromatous or atherosclerotic 'plaques', said plaques resulting from a combination of intimal thickening and accumulation of lipids (Padera, Jr & Schoen 2010). Advanced coronary atherosclerosis presents clinically as IHD when either: (1) expanding atheroma encroaches on the coronary artery lumen to such a degree that blood flow is impeded or (2) when acute plaque disruption leads to thrombosis and vessel occlusion (Padera, Jr & Schoen 2010).

Coronary atherosclerosis, hence IHD, is caused by a combination of predisposing risk factors. Risk factors are broadly categorized as behavioural/biological or modifiable/non-modifiable (Gaziano et al 2008). The major risk factors for IHD are presented in Table 4-1. IHD may occur in the absence of known risk factors, although for individuals with favourable levels of the major known risk factors, incidence of IHD is low. Various algorithms (e.g. The Framingham Risk Score, National Heart, Lung, and Blood Institute 2014, available online at http://www.framinghamheartstudy.org) are used to estimate risk of IHD events (and/or other cardiovascular diseases) within a given period of time, on the basis of gender, age, total and high-density

TABLE 4-1	
Major Risk Factors for Ischaemic Heart Disease	
Modifiable Factors	**Non-Modifiable Factors**
Smoking	Advanced age
Hypertension	Male gender
Diabetes mellitus	Family history of ischaemic heart disease
Dyslipidaemia	Poor socioeconomic status
Diet	Indigenous/aboriginal
Physical inactivity	
Obesity	
Social isolation	
Depression	

Adapted from Gaziano et al 2008, Morrow & Gersh 2008.

lipoprotein (HDL) cholesterol, smoking history and systolic blood pressure (SBP).

CASE 4-1 *(Continued)*

Mr AB's father had died at age 60 years with an acute myocardial infarction (AMI). His mother, brother and daughter are all well. Mr AB smoked 20 pack-years prior to his 40th birthday, but has not smoked since then. He has not had his cholesterol or blood pressure checked in recent years, and takes no regular exercise. He is 168 cm tall and weighs 86 kg (body mass index: 30 kg/m^2).

Symptoms and Signs of Ischaemic Heart Disease

The primary clinical manifestations of IHD are stable angina, unstable angina pectoris (UAP) and acute myocardial infarction (AMI). Stable angina occurs when coronary perfusion fails to meet increased metabolic demand, which may occur during exercise or tachycardia. Stable angina is 'associated with a (temporary) disturbance in myocardial function, (but) without myocardial necrosis', and typically presents as retrosternal pain/discomfort (angina pectoris) that is relieved by rest or nitrate medications (Morrow & Gersh 2008). Other symptoms of stable IHD include exertional dyspnoea and a reduced exercise capacity. Some individuals, particularly those with diabetes mellitus, may be asymptomatic.

UAP and AMI, collectively referred to as 'acute coronary syndromes', can be life-threatening and occur when physical disruption of an atherosclerotic plaque triggers thrombosis. The formation of thrombus (blood clot) within the artery leads to subtotal or total occlusion (Zakkar & Hornick 2007). UAP typically presents as frequent and prolonged episodes of retrosternal pain or discomfort, often at rest or with minimal exertion; myocardial necrosis is absent (Zakkar & Hornick 2007). AMI with myocardial necrosis occurs when thrombosis and reactive coronary arteriospasm cause prolonged (>20 minutes) myocardial ischaemia. AMI may also occur without symptoms, but typically presents as prolonged 'chest, upper extremity, jaw or epigastric discomfort/pain with exertion or rest' and/or dyspnoea, diaphoresis, nausea and syncope (Thygeson et al 2007, p. 2636).

Diagnosis of Ischaemic Heart Disease

A provisional diagnosis of IHD is normally made on the basis of risk and the presence of ischaemic symptoms. Further diagnostic tests aim to elicit whether the ischaemic symptoms relate to a gradual progression of coronary atherosclerosis, an increase in myocardial perfusion/demand mismatch (as might be precipitated by a change in activity or systemic illness), or acute thrombosis.

As noted by the American College of Cardiology (ACCF)/AHA, 'once a diagnosis of IHD is established, it is necessary in most patients to assess their risk of subsequent complications, such as AMI or death' (Finh et al 2012, p. 3102). Hence some 'diagnostic' tests are also used for risk assessment, and indeed may directly influence management.

A resting 12-lead electrocardiogram (ECG) (Box 4-1) is a first-line investigation for IHD (Sabatine & Cannon 2012). A normal ECG does not exclude IHD, however, as IHD-related ECG changes may be transient. In the absence of an acute coronary syndrome, a progressive exercise or 'stress' test with ECG monitoring (see Box 4-1) is usually conducted to confirm a provisional diagnosis of IHD.

Coronary angiography (i.e. arteriography) is used in both stable IHD and acute coronary syndromes to assess coronary artery anatomy (Popma 2012). Coronary angiography is performed by selective coronary arterial catheterization (Box 4-1). Radio-opaque dye is injected through the catheter, directly into the coronary arteries; radiographic imaging is used concurrently to map coronary anatomy and flow.

Diagnosis of Acute Myocardial Infarction

AMI is presumed, and treatment instigated, when an individual presents with prolonged and/or severe ischaemic symptoms. If the ECG shows ST-segment elevation (a typical ECG finding of AMI) in two contiguous ECG leads, the AMI is designated an ST-segment elevation myocardial infarction (STEMI); if not, a non-STEMI (NSTEMI) (Thygesen et al 2012). AMI is confirmed using blood tests for biomarkers of myocardial necrosis, most commonly cardiac troponin levels (cTnT or cTnI) (Sabatine & Cannon 2012). A rise (and subsequent fall) in these biomarkers (defined as above the 99th percentile upper reference limit)

BOX 4-1
CARDIAC INVESTIGATIONS

The 12-lead electrocardiogram (ECG): The 12-lead ECG records and depicts the electrical activity of the heart through the use of 10 surface/skin electrodes. The 'leads' record: (1) the difference in electrical activity (voltage) between electrodes in the frontal plane (the limb leads: I, II, III and augmented leads: aVR, aVL, aVF), and (2) the electrical activity towards electrodes in the sagittal plane (the precordial leads: V1 to V6), and taken together describe the pattern (waveform) of electrical activity associated with depolarization/repolarization of the myocardium. Presence/absence of the normal (P, Q, R, S, T) components of the ECG waveform, and the regularity, direction, amplitude and duration of and between these components, are used to diagnose cardiac pathology. Specific cardiac conditions produce characteristic abnormalities of the ECG waveform, and abnormalities in specific leads can be ascribed to contiguous anatomical locations, e.g. ST-segment elevation in the anterior leads (V2 to V6) is indicative of myocardial infarction of the left ventricle (Fig. 4-1).

The progressive exercise test with ECG monitoring: The progressive exercise (stress) test is used to detect evidence of myocardial ischaemia and arrhythmia during and after exercise. Patients are subjected to a progressively increasing exercise workload (usually walking on a treadmill, with staged increases in speed and gradient) while the ECG and blood pressure are monitored. The normal (healthy) response to the progressive exercise test is a progressive increase in heart rate and systolic blood pressure (SBP); ST-segment depression, T-wave inversion, and/or abnormal SBP response are indicative of myocardial ischaemia. The progressive exercise test is also used to follow the progress of individuals with known ischaemic heart disease (IHD), including after revascularization.

Cardiac catheterization: Cardiac catheterization involves the selective insertion of one or more catheters into the cardiac chambers and/or coronary arteries, usually via the femoral artery at the groin or the radial artery at the wrist. The most common indication for cardiac catheterization is to perform selective coronary angiography – to demonstrate the extent, location and morphology of arterial narrowing, and to determine the most appropriate means of revascularization (Fig. 4-2). Cardiac catheterization also allows for pressure monitoring within and across cardiac chambers (pressure gradients), e.g. to give an objective indication of the severity of aortic stenosis (see Section 2 of this chapter, Aortic Stenosis). Right heart catheterization, usually performed via the subclavian vein at the neck or the femoral vein at the groin, also allows for measurement of pulmonary artery wedge pressure, an indirect measurement of left atrial pressure (hence left ventricular function).

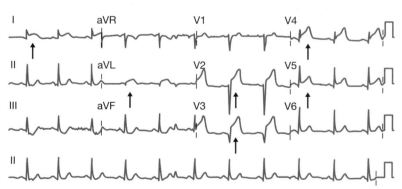

FIGURE 4-1 ■ Resting 12-lead electrocardiogram (ECG), with arrows showing anterior ST-segment elevation myocardial infarction (STEMI).

demonstrate the release of structural cardiac proteins, hence AMI (Thygesen et al 2012). Note that cardiac troponin levels will commonly be elevated after coronary revascularization (see Section 1.6.1, Coronary Revascularization), without a clear pathological mechanism and with indeterminate prognostic impact.

Classification of Ischaemic Heart Disease

IHD can be classified: (1) according to clinical manifestation; (2) anatomically, by the affected vessels and/or number thereof (e.g. left main (artery) disease, triple vessel disease); (3) according to the extent of vessel stenosis (e.g. 100%) in association with the

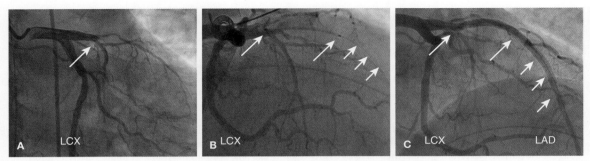

FIGURE 4-2 ■ The figure comprises three separate images of contrast injections into the left main coronary artery (top left of each frame) in the right anterior oblique projection (different craniocaudal angulation accounts for different orientation of vessels in each image). The left main coronary artery bifurcates into the left anterior descending artery (LAD) and left circumflex artery (LCX). **(A)** Thrombotic occlusion (arrow) of the LAD. The distal vessel is not seen. The LCX courses around the base of the left ventricle (from top to bottom at the left of each image) towards the lateral wall of the left ventricle. **(B)** This image was acquired after the occlusion was crossed with a guidewire (short arrows). A stent has been advanced over the guidewire. Note the radio-opaque markers (long arrows) at each end of the balloon within the stent (before balloon inflation of the stent). **C** was acquired after deployment of the stent (and withdrawal of the balloon). The obstruction of the LAD has been relieved and the distal vessel now fills with contrast.

extent of left ventricular dysfunction or (4) functionally, by the impact of IHD symptoms on physical activity (Eagle et al 2004, Luepker et al 2003). A commonly used functional classification for IHD is the Canadian Cardiovascular Society (CCS) angina grade (Campeau 1976).

Medical Management of Ischaemic Heart Disease

CASE 4-1 (Continued)

Mr AB's coronary angiogram showed thrombotic occlusion of the left anterior descending (LAD) artery, with diffuse luminal irregularities in the other large coronary arteries. The cardiologist performed balloon angioplasty and placed a drug eluting stent, after which there was normal flow down the artery. Mr AB's chest pain disappeared completely. Mr AB was placed on intravenous heparin (anticoagulant) and advised to maintain bed rest for 4 hours following arterial sheath removal. An echocardiogram 2 days later showed normal left ventricular contraction. A physiotherapist ensured that Mr AB was mobilizing safely; the clinical nurse consultant referred Mr AB to an outpatient cardiac rehabilitation programme. Discharge medications included aspirin, clopidogrel, rosuvastatin, metoprolol and ramipril.

Management of IHD is guided by clinical manifestation, the location and severity of coronary artery occlusion and the degree of functional impairment. Guidelines for the management of IHD continue to evolve with advances in diagnostic testing and IHD therapies – the reader is directed to the ACCF/AHA website (http://my.americanheart.org) for current (2014–2015) guidelines on management of patients with IHD, including coronary revascularization.

Initial medical management of the individual with known stable IHD, or at high risk of IHD, addresses modifiable risk factors. Goals of management include a reduction in the risk of cardiac events (hence improved survival) and/or improved health status (quality of life). Smoking cessation, prescribed physical activity/exercise and management of weight, hypertension and dyslipidaemia, e.g. through diet and pharmacological (medication) approaches, are effective in reducing cardiac events (Fihn et al 2012). Table 4-2 presents commonly used medications in individuals with, or at high risk of, IHD. The role of formal cardiac rehabilitation programs in secondary prevention of cardiac events is described in more detail elsewhere in Chapter 12.

Coronary Revascularization

Coronary revascularization, e.g. percutaneous coronary intervention (PCI) or coronary artery bypass

TABLE 4-2				
Commonly Used Medications in Patients with or at Risk of Ischaemic Heart Disease				
Class	Common Formulations	Action	Indication	Considerations
Anticoagulants	Heparin, enoxaparin	Prevention of fibrin clot formation	Acute coronary syndrome	Bleeding/thrombosis risk
Antiplatelet agents	Aspirin, clopidogrel	Inhibit platelet aggregation	Ischaemic heart disease, stents	Bleeding/thrombosis risk
Angiotensin-converting enzyme (ACE) inhibitors	Perindopril, ramipril	Lower blood pressure	Ischaemic heart disease, hypertension, heart failure	May cause cough, hyperlipidaemia
Angiotensin II receptor blockers (or inhibitors)	Irbesartan, olmesartan	Block activation of angiotensin	Hypertension, heart failure	May cause hyperkalaemia
β-blockers	Metoprolol, atenolol	Reduce heart rate and blood pressure	Ischaemic heart disease, heart failure	May cause fatigue, precipitate bronchospasm
Calcium channel blockers	Verapamil, diltiazem	Vasodilator	Hypertension, angina	May aggravate heart block
Diuretics	Furosemide, hydrochlorothiazide	Increase renal sodium and water excretion	Hypertension, heart failure	Hyponatraemia
Vasodilators	Glyceryl trinitrate, isosorbide mononitrate	Relax vascular smooth muscle	Prevention and treatment of angina pectoris	Headache
Digitalis preparations	Digoxin	Slow atrioventricular nodal conduction	Rate control in atrial fibrillation	Renal excretion – reduce dose in renal failure
Statins	Rosuvastatin, atorvastatin	Reduce hepatic production of cholesterol	Ischaemic heart disease, hypercholesterolaemia	May cause myalgia

graft (CABG) surgery, is generally indicated in individuals with chronic stable angina, but at high risk of cardiac events and IHD-related mortality with medical management alone (Eagle et al 2004, Morrow & Gersh 2008). Coronary revascularization is clearly indicated in individuals with acute coronary syndromes (UAP and AMI), excepting asymptomatic STEMI successfully treated with fibrinolysis and without haemodynamic instability (Morrow and Gersh 2008). The appropriateness for PCI vs CABG as the primary mode of coronary revascularization depends on the location and severity of coronary artery occlusion.

Percutaneous Coronary Intervention. PCI is an umbrella term referring to cardiac interventions performed via catheterization of peripheral arteries. In the context of IHD, PCI usually refers to the dilatation of narrowed coronary arteries by the inflation of a balloon (balloon angioplasty) and/or the placing of coronary stent(s) (see Fig. 4-2). Stents may be 'bare metal', or 'drug eluting'. Drug eluting stents reduce the risk of excessive endothelial proliferation and in-stent restenosis (compared to bare metal stents), but necessitate a longer duration of dual antiplatelet therapy. PCI is usually performed immediately after diagnostic coronary angiography in STEMI.

PCI is most commonly performed with the patient under sedation. A period of bed rest (approximately 4 hours), combined with the use of a Femostop device or digital pressure, reduces the risk of postprocedural bleeding/groin haematoma.

Coronary Artery Bypass Graft Surgery. CABG surgery refers to the surgical 'bypassing' of severely narrowed or blocked coronary arteries through the use of arterial or venous graft conduits. CABG is considered the gold standard treatment to improve survival in individuals with advanced IHD, specifically 'left main disease and triple-vessel disease (or double-vessel disease including a proximal left anterior descending (LAD) stenosis combined with left ventricular dysfunction)' (Eagle et al 2004, p. 68). CABG surgery may also be indicated over PCI for relief of disabling angina in younger and potentially more active patients.

CABG surgery is performed under general anaesthesia (usually via median sternotomy, with the heart arrested, on cardiopulmonary bypass). For comprehensive descriptions of the operative procedure, the reader is directed to Gongora & Sundt (2008) and Lemmer, Jr & Vlahakas (2010). Cardiopulmonary bypass (extracorporeal blood oxygenation) and aortic cross-clamping provide systemic and cerebral perfusion; cardioplegic solution is used to achieve cardiac arrest (i.e. the heart is stopped), thereby reducing myocardial oxygen consumption and ischaemic time.

Graft conduit may comprise *in situ* one or both internal mammary (thoracic) arteries and/or free grafts (internal mammary or radial artery or reversed long saphenous vein). Whereas *in situ* grafts require only distal anastomoses beyond coronary obstructions, free grafts are also anastomosed proximally (usually to the ascending aorta). Following revascularization, the patient is weaned from cardiopulmonary bypass and the heart is restarted.

Under some circumstances, CABG surgery may be performed 'off-pump' (off-pump coronary artery bypass, OPCAB), i.e. without the use of cardiopulmonary bypass. Purported benefits of OPCAB relate to a reduction in the adverse effects, morbidity and mortality associated with cardiopulmonary bypass (Novitzky et al 2007).

Physiotherapy-Specific Management of Ischaemic Heart Disease

Physiotherapy management of IHD primarily encompasses cardiac rehabilitation (including exercise prescription/supervision and nonpharmacological management of modifiable risk factors), and perioperative/periprocedural care for the patient undergoing revascularization (see Chapter 11). CABG surgery, for example, is associated with short-term alterations in respiratory function and exercise capacity (superimposed on IHD-related deconditioning) (Hirschhorn et al 2008, Wynne & Botti 2004). Physiotherapy treatments such as preoperative inspiratory muscle training, early postoperative mobilization and exercise prescription/supervision are effective in reducing postoperative pulmonary complications (PPCs) and accelerating the return to preoperative functional capacity (Hirschhorn et al 2008, Hulzebos et al 2006, Savci et al 2011). Nonreferral is a significant barrier to attendance at phase II (outpatient) cardiac rehabilitation (Higgins et al 2008); physiotherapists working in acute inpatient cardiology/cardiothoracic surgical settings have a role in referral to and promotion of phase II cardiac rehabilitation.

CARDIAC VALVE DISEASE

CASE 4-2

Mrs CD is a 60-year-old widow with increasing exertional dyspnoea and chest pain, and occasional presyncope. Aortic stenosis (AS) was first documented 20 years previously; Mrs CD has since had regular reviews with a cardiologist to monitor its progression. She is otherwise well and takes no regular medication.

Introduction

The four cardiac valves (left side of heart: aortic and mitral valves, right side: pulmonary and tricuspid valves Figure 1-20) control the direction and timing of blood flow within and from the heart. The term 'cardiac valve disease' encompasses a range of pathological conditions, whereby restriction to valve opening (stenosis) leads to obstruction of flow and increasing transvalvular gradient (pressure overloading) and/or inadequate valve closure (incompetence) leads to valvular regurgitation (volume overloading).

Cardiac valve diseases are generally described according to the affected valve, the type of lesion (obstruction/narrowing = stenosis, inadequate closure/insufficiency = regurgitation) and severity of lesion. This section will focus on the most common presentations of cardiac valve disease, i.e. those of the left side, with brief discussion of right-sided disease. Aetiology, pathophysiology and symptomatology are described by lesion. Unless otherwise indicated, information in this section is derived primarily from Otto & Bonow (2012), and ACCF/AHA and ESC guidelines for the management of valvular heart disease (Bonow et al 2006, Vahanian et al 2012).

Aetiology and Pathophysiology of Cardiac Valve Disease

There are various and potentially interacting aetiologies of cardiac valve disease, including congenital valve malformations, age-related degenerative changes and rheumatic disease. The predominant aetiologies vary by valve and type of lesion; the pathophysiological processes by which cardiac valve disease(s) then lead to symptomatic impairment also vary by valve/lesion (see below). Carpentier's 'pathophysiological triad' is a useful way of describing and understanding cardiac valve disease(s); this triad considers all of: (1) the *aetiology* of the disease; (2) the *lesions*, or results of the disease (e.g. leaflet thickening, commissural fusion), and (3) the *dysfunctions* that result from the lesions (e.g. restricted leaflet motion) (Carpentier et al 2010).

Aortic Stenosis

The three most common aetiologies of aortic stenosis (AS) are congenital malformation (usually a bicuspid aortic valve), age-related degenerative (aka 'calcific') changes and rheumatic disease. All result in progressive leaflet thickening and/or commissural fusion. A reduction in valve leaflet motion reduces aortic valve (left ventricular outlet) area, usually over decades; this reduced outlet area in turn leads to pressure overloading of the left ventricle. Left ventricular hypertrophy (LVH) occurs to compensate for chronic pressure overloading and initially, normal cardiac output is maintained. With time, the hypertrophic adaptation may become inadequate to maintain systolic function, and cardiac output is impaired, resulting in (pre) syncope. The hypertrophied left ventricle also has an increased perfusion demand, and is therefore at greater risk of ischaemia.

Aortic Regurgitation

Aortic regurgitation (AR) may be caused by disease of the valve leaflets, e.g. degenerative disease (often aggravated by hypertension), disease secondary to infective endocarditis, and/or disease of the wall of the aortic root, e.g. Marfan syndrome. Subsequent failure of coaptation of the aortic leaflets leads to increasing valvular insufficiency and volume overloading of the left ventricle. The left ventricle dilates (and may also hypertrophy) in response to chronic volume overloading, ultimately leading to left ventricular failure.

Mitral Stenosis

Mitral stenosis (MS) most commonly occurs as a consequence of rheumatic fever, the incidence of which has been reduced by the use of antibiotics for streptococcal infection. Rheumatic fever causes thickening, scarring and calcification of the valve leaflets, which in turn reduces the left ventricular inlet area. Left atrial and pulmonary venous pressures become elevated, leading to left atrial enlargement (which may predispose to atrial fibrillation (AF) and hence thromboembolism), pulmonary congestion and oedema. Pulmonary hypertension may lead ultimately to right-sided heart failure.

Mitral Regurgitation

Mitral regurgitation (MR) may occur secondary to abnormalities of the mitral valve leaflets themselves and/or the other components of the mitral valve apparatus, i.e. the annulus, chordae tendineae and papillary muscles. Major causes of MR are: (1) mitral valve prolapse syndrome, i.e. 'billowing' of leaflet(s) into the left atrium, a primary cardiac condition of redundant mitral valve leaflet tissue; (2) rheumatic heart disease (causing shortening, rigidity and retraction of valve leaflets); (3) IHD (causing papillary muscle dysfunction) and (4) annular dilatation (e.g. secondary to left ventricular dilatation, as in dilated cardiomyopathy (DCM)). The severity and chronicity of MR determine the pathophysiological course. In severe acute MR, left atrial and ventricular volume overload may result in simultaneous pulmonary congestion and reduced cardiac output. In chronic MR, however, compensatory left ventricular and atrial changes may allow long-term maintenance of cardiac output.

Right-Sided Cardiac Valve Disease

Right-sided cardiac valve disease is almost always related to rheumatic or congenital disease. Regurgitant disease most commonly occurs as a consequence of annular dilatation, secondary to dilatation of the right ventricle (tricuspid valve), or pulmonary hypertension (pulmonary valve). Any primary cardiac or pulmonary disease resulting in right ventricular failure and/ or pulmonary hypertension (or pulmonary artery dilatation) might thus lead to tricuspid and pulmonic regurgitation.

Symptoms and Signs of Cardiac Valve Disease

Aortic Stenosis

AS is often diagnosed before the onset of symptoms, e.g. when a routine physical examination reveals a systolic cardiac murmur (see Section 2.4, Diagnosis of Cardiac Valve Disease). Individuals with known AS, monitored over time, most commonly present with progressive exertional dyspnoea, fatigue and a reduced exercise capacity. Individuals with severe AS will often also present with angina, related to concomitant coronary atherosclerosis and/or secondary to LVH. Presyncope (a sense of dizziness or faintness) or syncopal episodes may occur, initially on exercise and ultimately at rest, when the inability to increase cardiac output leads to hypotension and reduced cerebral perfusion. Even mild symptoms may be indicative of moderate to severe AS, requiring intervention.

Aortic Regurgitation

Individuals with AR are typically asymptomatic until late in the disease course. Progressive exertional dyspnoea and orthopnoea (i.e. shortness of breath when lying flat) are the most common symptoms of severe, chronic AR; individuals with AR may also report increased awareness of the heartbeat (a 'pounding' of the heart) and angina, again secondary to LVH.

Mitral Stenosis

Notwithstanding that MS is a progressive, life-long disease, there is often a long latent period (10 to 40 years) before development of symptoms. Similarly, once present, typical symptoms of dyspnoea, fatigue and a decreased exercise tolerance may remain mild until late in the disease course. The first presenting symptom of MS is often related to AF and/or a consequent embolic event.

Mitral Regurgitation

When MR develops gradually, symptoms may be minimal until MR is of at least moderate degree. Dyspnoea and fatigue may be aggravated by the onset of AF. When severe MR develops abruptly (e.g. secondary to chordal rupture) there is usually severe dyspnoea associated with acute pulmonary oedema (APO).

Right-Sided Cardiac Valve Disease

Right-sided valve lesions usually develop gradually and may only be symptomatic (dyspnoea, fatigue, decreased exercise tolerance) late in the disease course. Tricuspid endocarditis may be associated with infective pulmonary embolism (PE). In patients with tricuspid and pulmonary regurgitation (TR, PR) secondary to lung disease, dyspnoea may be primarily due to lung disease. Abdominal bloating due to hepatic congestion is common in severe TR.

Diagnosis of Cardiac Valve Disease

CASE 4-2 (Continued)

Mrs CD's aortic valve gradient has gradually increased over the last 20 years; her most recent echocardiogram (Fig. 4-3) showed a mean systolic gradient of ≈40 mmHg (23 mmHg at baseline) and a valve area of ≈0.8 cm^2 (1.5 cm^2 at baseline). The 12-lead ECG showed sinus rhythm with changes of LVH and left atrial enlargement.

Cardiac valve disease is most commonly diagnosed (or suspected) when cardiac auscultation reveals a cardiac 'murmur', i.e. turbulent flow. The timing of murmurs (in relation to the cardiac cycle); the location(s) at which they can be heard and their pitch, duration and intensity can all be used to aid provisional diagnosis of cardiac valve disease.

Depending on the type of murmur, the patient and the (degree of) symptoms, further diagnostic testing may be indicated. Echocardiography (see Box 4-2) is the initial mode of imaging in suspected cardiac valve disease, and is recommended for all

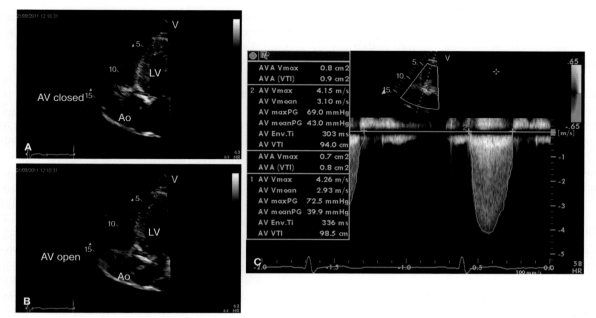

FIGURE 4-3 ▪ **A** and **B** demonstrate highly calcified aortic valve (AV) leaflets, with minimal valve leaflet movement from closed **(A),** to open **(B). (C)** This image illustrates the velocity–time integral across the aortic valve, indicating an aortic valve area of ~0.8 cm^2. *Ao,* Aortic root; *LV,* left ventricular cavity.

BOX 4-2
CARDIAC INVESTIGATIONS

Echocardiography (Connolly & Oh 2012)**:** Echocardiography refers to ultrasound examination of the heart and is used to evaluate structural, functional and haemodynamic abnormalities of the heart and great vessels. In standard non-invasive transthoracic echocardiography (TTE), an ultrasound transducer is placed sequentially at several (usually four) positions on the chest (parasternal, apical, subcostal and suprasternal) and rotated and angulated to obtain dynamic, cross-sectional, two- and/or three-dimensional images of the myocardium, cardiac valves and chambers (static echocardiography images, see Fig. 4-3). Conducted in concert with standard echocardiography, Doppler examination (comparison of frequency change between transmitted and reflected sound waves) records the direction and velocity of blood flow within the heart and great vessels, allowing for the assessments of flow patterns and pressure gradients across the cardiac valves. Colour-flow imaging or mapping, superimposed on two-dimensional echocardiographic images, provides a clear visual representation of blood flow and abnormalities thereof (e.g. regurgitation and turbulence).

In transoesophageal echocardiography (TOE) the ultrasound probe is introduced into the oesophagus and stomach, immediately adjacent to the heart. Images of the heart and great vessels may be obtained more clearly than with TTE, without interference of the subcutaneous tissue and lung.

patients with murmurs and associated cardiac signs and symptoms, and for asymptomatic patients with, e.g., holosystolic, late systolic, diastolic or continuous murmurs.

ECG is also indicated in the diagnosis and evaluation of cardiac valve disease, and may give an indication of compensatory changes in cardiac structure, e.g. increased QRS amplitude in precordial leads and augmented vector left (aVL) secondary to LVH. Chest radiography may demonstrate changes in cardiac structure (shape/size), albeit less clearly than echocardiography.

Classification of Cardiac Valve Disease

Cardiac valve disease is classified by severity (mild, moderate, severe, critical) according to qualitative and quantitative data obtained through echocardiography and/or cardiac catheterization. Such data include, for stenosis, the mean pressure gradient (mmHg) across the valve, the jet (peak systolic blood flow) velocity (m/sec), the valve area (cm^2) and the valve area index (cm^2/m^2), and for regurgitation, width of the regurgitant jet, the regurgitant volume (mL/beat) and the regurgitant fraction (%). The reader is directed to Bonow et al (2006) for a complete tabular representation of the criteria used to classify both left and right-sided cardiac valve disease.

Medical Management of Cardiac Valve Disease

CASE 4-2 (Continued)

After discussion with the cardiothoracic surgeon, Mrs CD decided to undergo aortic valve replacement (AVR) with a mechanical prosthesis, and life-long anticoagulation with warfarin. The preoperative coronary angiogram showed no significant coronary artery disease. Mrs CD was discharged to the care of her son and daughter-in-law 1 week after uncomplicated valve replacement. Her exercise capacity improved with outpatient cardiac rehabilitation; 3 months after surgery Mrs CD joined a gymnasium and was able to exercise comfortably without dyspnoea or chest pain.

Management of cardiac valve disease depends on the latter two aspects of Carpentier's pathological triad, i.e. the lesions caused by the disease and (the severity of) the resultant dysfunctions.

Aortic Stenosis

Surgical aortic valve replacement (AVR) is the recommended treatment for severe (hence even mildly) symptomatic AS. Without surgery, prognosis for patients with symptomatic AS is poor. Management of early and asymptomatic AS therefore includes patient education regarding disease progression, the need for monitoring (including approximately annual specialist review/echocardiography), and awareness of symptom development. As with CABG surgery (and indeed other cardiac valve surgery), AVR is typically performed via median sternotomy, under general anaesthetic and with cardiopulmonary bypass. Prosthetic valves may be mechanical – usually given to younger patients, but requiring life-long anticoagulation to reduce the risk of thromboembolism – or biological, potentially requiring revision usually at >10 years postimplantation. Transcatheter aortic valve implantation (TAVI), whereby a prosthetic valve is implanted percutaneously, is a recently developed alternative to AVR for patients at high risk of surgical mortality (Sinning et al 2012).

Aortic Regurgitation

As with AS, there is no specific medical management for individuals with mild to moderate AR other than regular specialist monitoring (including serial echocardiography) and, if indicated, pharmacological management of hypertension and/or cardiac arrhythmias. Surgical AVR is again the recommended treatment for symptomatic AR; patients unsuitable for surgery require pharmacological management of left ventricular dysfunction, including salt and fluid restriction, angiotensin-converting enzyme (ACE) inhibitors, digoxin and diuretics.

Mitral Stenosis

Medical management of MS involves the 'prevention of recurrent rheumatic fever, prevention and treatment of complications and monitoring of disease progression to allow intervention at the optimal timepoint'

(Otto & Bonow 2012, p. 1495). Specifically this incorporates antibiotic prophylaxis for streptococcal infection, anticoagulation in the context of *inter alia* persistent or paroxysmal AF, and annual specialist review. The recommended intervention for severe or symptomatic MS is mechanical dilatation, by percutaneous balloon mitral valvuloplasty, open surgical valvotomy or surgical mitral valve replacement.

Mitral Regurgitation

Pharmacological management to reduce afterload, i.e. systemic vasodilator therapy, is clearly indicated and potentially life-saving in patients with acute MR. Unless contraindicated by age and/or comorbidity, surgical mitral valve repair or replacement is the recommended treatment for patients with symptomatic MR (acute or chronic), or asymptomatic MR and worsening left ventricular dilatation and/or dysfunction. Repair, i.e. reconstruction of the valve, usually performed with a reinforcing annuloplasty, reduces the morbidity associated with deterioration of (biological) prosthetic valves or anticoagulation therapy (mechanical prosthetic valves).

Right-Sided Cardiac Valve Disease

TR is usually managed medically, unless associated with endocarditis, in which case surgical vegetectomy and valve repair/replacement may be required. Tricuspid valvuloplasty is often performed along with mitral valve replacement if TR is secondary to MR and pulmonary hypertension. Pulmonary valve surgery is sometimes indicated in adult patients with congenital heart disease involving the pulmonary valve.

Physiotherapy-Specific Management of Cardiac Valve Disease

As with IHD, physiotherapy management of cardiac valve disease primarily encompasses cardiac rehabilitation and perioperative care for the patient undergoing cardiac valve surgery. Patients who are hospitalized, e.g. with heart failure secondary to valve disease, yet are not candidates for surgery may require assistance with mobility and/or lower limb resistance training to prevent further deconditioning, and advice/education regarding management of dyspnoea.

CARDIOMYOPATHY

CASE 4-3

Ms XY is a 43-year-old jeweller with hypertrophic cardiomyopathy (HCM) (demonstrated on resting echocardiogram), symptoms of exertional dyspnoea (due to left ventricular outflow tract obstruction) and recurrent syncope (due to self-terminating ventricular tachycardia (VT)). Her father died suddenly at age 35 years. An elder brother has undergone septal myectomy to relieve left ventricular outflow obstruction. The surgery was successful in that the obstruction was relieved, but he died suddenly 3 months after surgery. An elder sister, who also has HCM, has been resuscitated from ventricular fibrillation (VF); she now has an implanted defibrillator, which has discharged appropriately on two occasions.

Introduction

Cardiomyopathies comprise a heterogeneous group of disease processes that affect the myocardium and are 'associated with mechanical and/or electrical dysfunction' (Maron et al 2006, p. 1809). Traditionally the term 'cardiomyopathy' was used only to describe primary diseases of the myocardium; it is now also used in the context of cardiac dysfunction associated with (and usually disproportionate to) concomitant cardiac disease, including vascular, valvular, inflammatory and other processes. This section of the chapter will focus on primary diseases of the myocardium, while acknowledging that therapy for cardiomyopathy is often similar regardless of the underlying cause.

Cardiomyopathies may be categorized by the nature of the observed structural and functional abnormalities. There are four major categories or phenotypes, being: (1) DCMs, (2) restrictive cardiomyopathies, (3) hypertrophic cardiomyopathy (HCM) and (4) arrhythmogenic right ventricular dysplasia/cardiomyopathy (ARVC) (Elliott et al 2008).

Aetiology and Pathophysiology of Cardiomyopathy

Dilated Cardiomyopathies

DCMs are characterized by dilatation of the left or both ventricular chamber(s), impaired contraction, and hence systolic dysfunction (Jefferies & Towbin 2010). These structural and functional changes occur in the absence of, or are disproportionate to, abnormal ventricular load (e.g. as might occur in MR). DCM is commonly idiopathic, but may also be related to genetic abnormalities, or occur secondary to *inter alia* cardiac toxins (e.g. chemotherapeutic agents), infection (e.g. myocarditis) and autoimmune diseases (e.g. HIV) (Hare 2012). The pathophysiological course of DCM is varied, likely due to the varied aetiology; ventricular dysfunction may be asymptomatic and self-limiting, or may progress to severe heart failure (see Section 5, Heart Failure).

Restrictive Cardiomyopathies

Restrictive cardiomyopathies are characterized by an increase in stiffness of the ventricular walls, resulting in impaired ventricular filling (diastolic dysfunction). Restrictive cardiomyopathy is most commonly caused by abnormal deposition (infiltration) of amyloid proteins in the myocardium, which results in myocardial fibrosis, e.g. secondary to amyloidosis (Hare 2012). Restrictive cardiomyopathy may also be noninfiltrative (often idiopathic or familial in origin), related to 'storage' diseases (e.g. haemochromatosis), or related to endomyocardial scarring/fibrosis (e.g. secondary to radiation therapy). Impaired ventricular filling leads to an impaired ability to augment cardiac output (e.g. during exercise), and with advancing disease, pulmonary, peripheral and visceral oedema (Hare 2012).

Hypertrophic Cardiomyopathy

HCM is a genetic cardiovascular disease, characterized by thickening of the left ventricle (LVH) in the absence of other (potentially causative) cardiac or systemic conditions (Maron et al 2003). At the macro level, variable patterns of LVH may cause mechanical impedance to left ventricular outflow (asymmetric septal hypertrophy) and displacement of the mitral valve apparatus, with consequent increases in left ventricular pressure. Decreased ventricular compliance (diastolic dysfunction) causes increased filling pressures; heart failure and pulmonary and systemic venous congestion may result. Alterations in/disorganization of myocyte architecture and contractile proteins also lead to impaired ventricular contractility, and (potentially) impaired transmission of the cardiac impulse, with the

potential for ventricular tachyarrhythmias and sudden cardiac death (SCD) (Maron 2012).

Arrhythmogenic Right Ventricular Dysplasia/Cardiomyopathy

As suggested by its name, ARVC is a cardiac disorder that predominantly affects the right ventricle. ARVC is most commonly regarded as genetically determined (Marcus et al 2010), but may also be related to non-genetic causes, e.g. congenital abnormalities and myocarditis. Progressive atrophy of the right ventricular myocardium occurs with subsequent patchy replacement with adipose and fibrous tissue (Hulot et al 2004). These structural changes interfere with: (1) myocardial contractility, with implication for the development of right ventricular dysfunction and right heart failure and (2) normal transmission of the cardiac impulse, with the potential for development of ventricular tachyarrhythmias and SCD.

Symptoms and Signs of Cardiomyopathy

Symptoms and signs of cardiomyopathy are varied, albeit primarily related to the development of progressive heart failure and/or cardiac arrhythmia (Hare 2012). Typical symptoms of DCM are those of left heart failure, e.g. dyspnoea, reduced exercise capacity and fatigue. AF may result in systemic or pulmonary emboli. Patients with restrictive cardiomyopathies may similarly present with dyspnoea, reduced exercise capacity and fatigue; symptoms of right heart failure, i.e. peripheral oedema, hepatomegaly and ascites may also occur. Patients with HCM and ARVC typically present with symptoms of cardiac arrhythmia, e.g. presyncope, dizziness, light-headedness, and/or symptoms of left/right heart failure, respectively, as the (untreated) condition progresses. The first presentation may be SCD (Hare 2012, Maron 2012). Whereas DCM, restrictive cardiomyopathies and HCM present across the lifespan, ARVC usually presents in younger individuals (teenage to <40 years) (Basso et al 2009).

Diagnosis of Cardiomyopathy

Diagnosis of cardiomyopathy typically follows the presentation of symptoms and exclusion of other structural/functional causes (through detailed personal and family history, physical examination and clinical investigation, especially ECG and echocardiography).

Exceptions are familial cardiomyopathies, including HCM, which may be diagnosed in the absence of symptoms through genetic screening and cardiac imaging (Gersh et al 2011). Endocardial biopsy and/or cardiac magnetic resonance (CMR) imaging may be used in the definitive diagnosis of ARVC (Marcus et al 2010).

Medical Management of Cardiomyopathy

Medical management of cardiomyopathy primarily encompasses surveillance, patient education regarding activity (maintenance of comfortable regular exercise while avoiding excessive exertion), guideline-directed management of heart failure (see Section 5.5, Medical Management of Heart Failure) and the management of cardiac arrhythmias, including (where indicated) the prevention of SCD (Jefferies & Towbin 2010, Wexler et al 2009). Surgery may be indicated in DCM for concomitant cardiac disease (e.g. valve repair/replacement in cardiac valve disease), or for those with non-refractory heart failure, to restore ventricular geometry and/or provide ventricular support (Hare 2012). Management of atrial arrhythmias is described in Section 6.5, Medical Management of Cardiac Arrhythmias. Figure 4-4 is a flowchart describing the management of HCM with/without left ventricular outflow tract obstruction (summarized from information presented

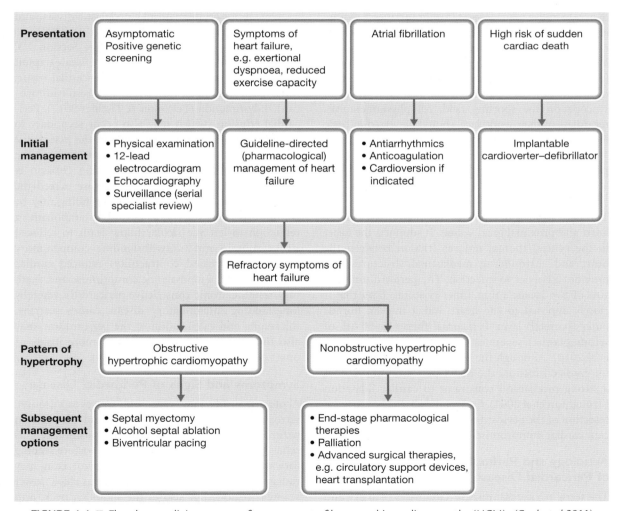

FIGURE 4-4 ■ Flowchart outlining aspects of management of hypertrophic cardiomyopathy (HCM). *(Gersh et al 2011)*

in Gersh et al 2011); surgical septal myectomy and (less commonly) percutaneous alcohol septal ablation may be warranted to relieve mechanical outflow obstruction in patients with non-refractory heart failure. Implantable cardioverter–defibrillators (see Section 6, Medical Management of Cardiac Arrhythmias) may be used prophylactically in patients with HCM and ARVC at high risk of SCD or with previous ventricular fibrillation/tachycardia (VF/VT).

Physiotherapy-Specific Management of Cardiomyopathy

The physiotherapist is unlikely to encounter the patient with primary cardiomyopathy, except: (1) in the context of perioperative management (for those patients requiring surgery or device therapy), (2) those hospitalized for management of heart failure (who may require guided in-hospital mobilization and/or respiratory care) and (3) (hopefully rarely) those with undiagnosed cardiomyopathy experiencing ventricular tachyarrythmia and syncope on the sporting field. All physiotherapists, regardless of their workplace, should be versed in basic life support and emergency contact procedures.

PERICARDIAL DISEASE

Introduction

The pericardium is a fibrous sac that envelopes the heart and proximal great vessels. It supports the heart in the central thorax, reduces friction between the heart and surrounding mediastinal structures and provides a barrier to infection. The pericardium consists of two layers: a thin, inner (visceral) layer that is closely apposed to the heart and a thicker, fibrous outer (parietal) layer. Pericardial fluid (15–50 mL of serous plasma) separates the two layers (Khandaker et al 2010). Although the pericardium is not essential for cardiac function, the intact pericardium provides a strong mechanical constraint to cardiac dilatation (Troughton et al 2004). Congenital absence or surgical resection of the pericardium does not result in significant cardiac compromise (Maisch et al 2004).

Aetiology and Pathophysiology of Pericardial Disease

The term 'pericardial disease' comprises primary and isolated conditions of the pericardial tissue (including structural anomalies), pericardial manifestations of systemic diseases and/or the accumulation of excessive fluid within the pericardial space. The four most common clinical presentations of pericardial disease are: (1) acute pericarditis, (2) pericardial effusion, (3) cardiac tamponade and (4) constrictive pericarditis (LeWinter & Tischler 2012). The aetiology of pericardial disease is variable and commonly idiopathic. Infectious causes of pericardial disease include viral agents, bacteria (notably mycobacterial tuberculosis), fungae and (rarely) parasitic agents. Noninfectious causes include pericardial injury syndromes (e.g. associated with trauma, or after AMI, cardiac intervention or cardiothoracic surgery), radiation, systemic autoimmune and auto-inflammatory diseases (e.g. systemic lupus erythematosus), neoplastic disease and some metabolic conditions (Troughton et al 2004).

Symptoms of acute pericarditis (see Section 4.3, Symptoms and Signs of Pericardial Disease) result directly from inflammation of the pericardial tissue; rarely coexistent myocarditis may also result in myocardial dysfunction (LeWinter & Tischler 2012). Pericardial effusion (which may also occur secondary to pericarditis) increases pressure within the pericardial sac; haemodynamic consequences relate to both the rate and volume of fluid accumulation (Imazio & Adler 2013). Should pericardial pressure exceed the pressure within the cardiac chambers, filling may be compromised; ultimately (as in cardiac tamponade) a reduction in left ventricular filling leads to reduced stroke volume and (notwithstanding compensatory tachycardia/increased contractility) reduced cardiac output. Acute haemodynamic compromise and death may result. Chronic constrictive pericarditis, whereby longstanding inflammatory disease causes scarring, thickening and calcification of the pericardium, may also limit cardiac filling, albeit with more insidious onset of symptoms (Maisch et al 2004).

Symptoms and Signs of Pericardial Disease

Acute pericarditis most commonly causes rapid-onset, retrosternal chest pain, often severe and 'pleuritic' in nature. Pericardial pain is typically positional; it is relieved by maintaining an upright posture/leaning forwards, and increased by lying down. Pain may radiate, characteristically to the trapezius ridge (lower scapular region) but also to the shoulder, neck, arm and upper abdomen (Khandaker et al 2010). The classical physical sign of acute pericarditis is a dynamic (i.e. inconsistent) pericardial rub, usually best heard on auscultation at the left sternal border. The 12-lead ECG usually shows diffuse ST-segment elevation in all leads excepting aVR and V1.

Pericardial effusions are often asymptomatic, particularly if small in volume and/or of insidious onset. Associated pericarditis may cause pericardial pain. Patients with large effusions or cardiac tamponade usually present with pericardial pain (from associated pericarditis) and dyspnoea, again lessened by leaning forwards (LeWinter and Tischler 2012). Patients will often report a nonspecific sense of discomfort and/or anxiety. Physical signs of large effusion/cardiac tamponade include muffled heart sounds on auscultation, an elevated jugular venous pressure (JVP) (due to restricted right heart filling), initial tachycardia and hypotension with reduced pulse pressure (Imazio & Adler 2013). The 12-lead ECG may be normal and show diffuse small voltages or 'electrical alternans' – an alternating variation in the height of the QRS complex. The classical sign of cardiac tamponade is a 'paradoxical pulse', i.e. a greater than usual drop in SBP during inspiration. Critical pericardial compression leads to progressive hypotension, hence other physical signs of reduced cardiac output/shock, including tachypnoea, diaphoresis and, ultimately, circulatory collapse.

Diagnosis of Pericardial Disease

Diagnosis of acute pericarditis is usually made on the basis of symptoms and signs, particularly the characteristic chest pain, pericardial rub and ST-segment elevation. Echocardiography (trans-thoracic (TTE), trans-oesophageal (TOE)) is used in acute pericarditis, and otherwise to determine the presence and volume of pericardial effusion and consequent compromise to cardiac filling/output. Echocardiography may also be used to guide pericardiocentesis, with a view to both diagnosis of specific aetiology and treatment of effusion/tamponade (Imazio et al 2010) (see Section 4.6, Medical Management of Pericardial Disease). Concomitant Doppler examination of the patient with cardiac tamponade shows characteristic large respiratory fluctuations in flow across tricuspid and mitral valves (Yared et al 2010).

Other diagnostic tests commonly undertaken in the patient with suspected pericardial disease include blood tests for markers of inflammation and myocardial damage (e.g. C-reactive protein, cTnT) to determine specific aetiology, cardiac computed tomography (CT) and CMR (to more clearly image the pericardium and pericardial effusion) and cardiac catheterization (to measure cardiac pressures) (LeWinter & Tischler 2012).

Classification of Pericardial Disease

Pericardial disease is classified primarily by clinical manifestation, the specific underlying aetiology (if established) and the chronicity of presentation. Pericarditis is most commonly acute and self-limiting, but may be recurrent and/or lead to chronic, restrictive disease. Pericardial effusion may further be described by volume (small, moderate, large) and whether the effusion is circumferential or localized/loculated.

Medical Management of Pericardial Disease

Initial management of acute pericarditis is directed at the diagnosis of specific aetiology, detection of effusion and alleviation of pericardial pain (Troughton et al 2004). Pericardial pain usually responds well to non-steroidal anti-inflammatory drugs (NSAIDs), e.g. ibuprofen, with/without supplementary narcotic analgesics. Corticosteroids, e.g. prednisone, may be indicated as a second-choice therapy in acute idiopathic pericarditis or for patients with systemic inflammatory disease. Patients with greater than small effusion or with a suspected cause other than idiopathic pericarditis typically require hospitalization to enable close monitoring and determination of aetiology (Khandaker et al 2010).

Subsequent management of pericardial disease is dependent on the specific aetiology, and the likelihood that associated effusion may progress to tamponade. Pharmacological treatment (e.g. antibiotic or antifungal therapy) is warranted in patients with an established infectious cause of effusion. Pericardiocentesis, i.e. drainage of the effusion, is indicated as an urgent procedure in patients considered at high risk of near-term tamponade (Khandaker et al 2010), e.g. those with suspected bacterial pericarditis, active bleeding into the pericardial space and/or acute, increasing, moderate to large effusion. Pericardiocentesis may be performed as a closed procedure, whereby a catheter is inserted percutaneously into the pericardial space under echocardiographic guidance, or as an open surgical procedure, allowing biopsy of the pericardial tissue and formation of a permanent pericardial 'window'. Chronic constrictive, and/or recurrent, severe refractory pericarditis may warrant complete surgical pericardiectomy (usually via sternotomy) (LeWinter & Tischler 2012).

Physiotherapy-Specific Management of Pericardial Disease

Patients with acute presentations of pericardial disease generally do not require specific physiotherapy intervention. Exercise prescription is generally contraindicated in active pericarditis, in part due to concerns of pain and potential haemodynamic compromise (Whaley et al 2006). Bed rest is commonly prescribed. Respiratory physiotherapy techniques that increase intrathoracic pressure, e.g. deep breathing exercises or positive pressure ventilation, may worsen haemodynamic status in patients with large effusion/tamponade (Khandaker et al 2010).

Patients with asymptomatic pericarditis of known aetiology, with less than moderate effusion and who are haemodynamically stable (e.g. with isolated ST-segment elevation early after cardiac surgery) may still benefit from gentle exercise prescription; close monitoring/supervision is recommended until signs of pericarditis have resolved. Standard postoperative physiotherapy interventions (see Section 1.7, Physiotherapy-Specific Management of Ischaemic Heart Disease) are warranted to reduce PPCs and restore premorbid functional capacity in patients undergoing surgical procedures (pericardial window, pericardiectomy).

HEART FAILURE

CASE 4-4

Mr EF is a 75-year-old retired builder with dyspnoea on mild exertion and bilateral ankle swelling. He has a previous history of cigarette smoking, alcohol abuse, obesity (body mass index: 35 kg/m), diabetes mellitus, AMI and subsequent CABG surgery. He takes no regular exercise. His blood pressure and serum cholesterol have been elevated, and he has been managed for heart failure for 5 years. Present treatment includes salt and fluid restriction (he is noncompliant), bisoprolol (to facilitate favourable left ventricular remodelling), perindopril (to optimize vascular compliance), furosemide, spironolactone, rosuvastatin and oral hypoglycaemics (to control blood sugar).

Introduction

The term 'heart failure' is used to describe those clinical syndromes where the cardiac pump is: (1) unable to maintain an adequate cardiac output to support physiological circulation (or can only do so at elevated filling pressures) and/or (2) unable to accommodate venous return (Kemp & Conte 2012). Central to the definition of heart failure is objective evidence of a structural or functional abnormality that impairs either or both ventricular ejection and filling (Yancy et al 2013). As distinct from, e.g. IHD, whereby a specific pathological process (atherosclerosis) defines the disease, heart failure as a syndrome is defined by the associated symptomatology, i.e. of pulmonary and/or systemic venous congestion (McMurray et al 2012).

Aetiology and Pathophysiology of Heart Failure

Heart failure can be conceptualized as a failure of systolic function and/or a failure of diastolic function. Systolic dysfunction implies the incapacity to maintain cardiac output due to a reduction in left ventricular ejection fraction (LVEF), aka heart failure with reduced ejection fraction (HFrEF). The aetiology of HFrEF is variable, but the most common causes are IHD and AMI (Kemp & Conte 2012). As LVEF is a function of: (1) cardiac contractility, (2) ventricular preload (defined as end-diastolic pressure) and (3) ventricular afterload, these may be used to classify the primary pathophysiological processes, or 'index events', leading to HFrEF (Table 4-3).

TABLE 4-3
Pathophysiological Processes Commonly Leading to Heart Failure

Process	Examples
Disease processes directly impairing myocardial contractility	Myocardial ischaemia, acute myocardial infarction, dilated cardiomyopathy
Disease processes increasing afterload	Systemic hypertension, aortic stenosis
Disease processes increasing preload	Aortic regurgitation, mitral regurgitation
Disease processes impairing ventricular filling	Pericardial disease, restrictive cardiomyopathy

Adapted from Macdonald 2011.

Diastolic dysfunction implies an abnormality of ventricular filling, with 'preservation' of LVEF (aka heart failure with preserved or normal ejection fraction (HFpEF/HFnlEF)). Diastolic dysfunction may occur as a result of impaired ventricular relaxation (an active, energy-dependent process) and/or increased diastolic stiffness; left ventricular systolic dysfunction and systemic vascular dysfunction may also contribute. As distinct from HFrEF, HFpEF/HFnlEF is more common in women and usually presents later in life (>65 years) (Yancy et al 2013). Hypertension, obesity, IHD and diabetes are significant risk factors for HFpEF. Diastolic dysfunction may present in isolation, e.g. in pericardial disease, but typically some degree of systolic dysfunction is also present.

It should be noted that the clinical syndrome of heart failure also encompasses the associated complex and systemic maladaptive processes that occur as a result of the primary pump failure. As described by Mann (2012a), a reduction in cardiac output and/or impaired ventricular filling leads to activation of neurohumoral mechanisms that serve to maintain cardiovascular homoeostasis in the event of volume depletion (note that volume depletion is not the problem in heart failure). These mechanisms include the sympathetic (adrenergic) nervous system (vasoconstrictor mechanism), and the renin-angiotensin-aldosterone system (fluid retentive mechanism). Sustained activation of these systems actually progressively worsens pump failure – systemic vasoconstriction, for example, increases left ventricular afterload and hence myocardial oxygen consumption.

Chronic heart failure is also commonly associated with renal impairment, given that: (1) common contributory causes of heart failure (e.g. hypertension, atherosclerosis) also affect the kidneys, and (2) the neurohumoral responses to heart failure reduce renal blood flow (Mann 2012a). Renal impairment in turn may lead to anaemia, which may worsen heart failure.

Symptoms and Signs of Heart Failure

Heart failure may present acutely, e.g. as a result of AMI, whereby myocardial necrosis results in loss of ventricular contractility. Cardiogenic shock is one severe manifestation of acute heart failure, whereby contractility is impaired to such a degree that perfusion of vital organs is acutely compromised; death may result. APO and resultant type I respiratory failure is another manifestation of acute heart failure (McMurray et al 2012).

Heart failure more typically presents as a chronic syndrome, e.g. where progressive AR leads to ventricular dilatation and remodelling. The characteristic symptoms of chronic heart failure are dyspnoea (exertional dyspnoea, orthopnoea and paroxysmal nocturnal dyspnoea), reduced exercise capacity, fatigue and fluid retention (oedema) (Greenberg & Kahn 2012). Specific symptoms and signs of left heart failure (Table 4-4) primarily relate to increased left atrial pressure, pulmonary venous congestion and pulmonary oedema. Right heart failure, usually occurring consequent to left heart failure, leads to increased right heart filling pressures, systemic venous congestion and peripheral oedema.

TABLE 4-4
Symptoms and Signs of Left and Right Heart Failure

Left Heart Failure		Right Heart Failure	
Symptoms	Signs	Symptoms	Signs
Exertional dyspnoea	Basilar lung crepitations (crackles)	Abdominal pain	Peripheral oedema
Orthopnoea	Reduced breath sounds at lung base(s)	Swollen legs	Jugular venous distension
		Nausea/loss of appetite	Hepatomegaly
Paroxysmal nocturnal dyspnoea	Tachycardia	Right upper quadrant discomfort	Ascites
Reduced exercise capacity	Tachypnoea		
Fatigue			
Palpitations			
Cough			
Wheeze			

Adapted from Greenberg & Kahn 2012.

Diagnosis of Heart Failure

CASE 4-4 (Continued)

On examination, Mr EF's blood pressure was 120/70 mmHg, and his pulse was regular at 65 beats/min. The jugular venous pressure (JVP) was elevated to the ears, and there was pulsatile hepatomegaly and ascites. There were fine crepitations at the lung bases and there was pitting oedema to the knees. The 12-lead ECG showed sinus rhythm with poor R-wave progression and QRS widening (140 msec). The echocardiogram showed severe left ventricular dilatation and severely impaired left ventricular systolic function (LVEF ≈17%) (Fig. 4-5).

A provisional diagnosis of heart failure is made on the basis of patient history (e.g. indicating a potential 'index event' and/or risk factors therefor) and physical examination. As in cardiac valve disease, echocardiography with Doppler examination is the initial mode of imaging used to determine the mechanism of heart failure and to measure LVEF (Connolly & Oh 2012). Blood tests of biomarkers for the aforementioned neurohumoral mechanisms, e.g. noradrenaline, and/or myocardial stress, e.g. brain natriuretic peptide (BNP) and N-terminal pro-BNP, may be used in the differential diagnosis of heart failure, as well as to provide prognostic information and to guide therapy (Yancy et al 2013).

Classification of Heart Failure

Heart failure can be classified according to the predisposing structural or functional pathological process. Heart failure can also be classified by the ACCF/AHA stage of disease progression and development (A–D) (Hunt 2006), and/or by the extent of symptomatic

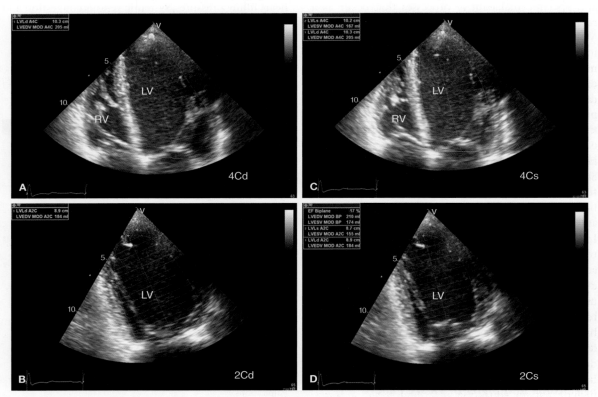

FIGURE 4-5 ■ The upper panels (A, C) are single frames from the transthoracic echocardiogram acquired from the apex (towards the top of each image) in the 4-chamber orientation. The lower panels (B, D) are single frames from the transthoracic echocardiogram acquired from the apex in the 2-chamber orientation. The left panels (A, B) were recorded at end-diastole (4Cd, 2Cd). The right panels (C, D) were recorded at end-systole (4Cs, 2Cs). LV, Left ventricle; RV, right ventricle.

TABLE 4-5

ACCF/AHA Stages of Heart Failure Disease Progression and NYHA Functional Classification

ACCF/AHA Stages of HF		NYHA Functional Classification	
A	At high risk for HF but without structural heart disease, or signs and symptoms of HF	None	
B	Structural heart disease but without signs or symptoms of HF	I	No limitation of physical activity. Ordinary physical activity does not cause symptoms of HF (symptoms with vigorous exertion).
C	Structural heart disease with prior or current symptoms of HF	I	No limitation of physical activity. Ordinary physical activity does not cause symptoms of HF.
		II	Slight limitation of physical activity. Comfortable at rest, but ordinary physical activity results in symptoms of HF (symptoms with moderate exertion).
		III	Marked limitation of physical activity. Comfortable at rest, but less than ordinary activity causes symptoms of HF (symptoms with mild exertion).
D	Refractory (end-stage) HF	IV	Unable to carry on any physical activity without symptoms of HF. Symptoms of HF at rest.

Adapted from Mann 2012b.
ACCF/AHA, American College of Cardiology/American Heart Association; *HF,* heart failure; *NYHA,* New York Heart Association.

impairment, using the New York Heart Association (NYHA) functional classification (Table 4-5) (McMurray et al 2012). LVEF has traditionally been used as a marker of the severity of heart failure (with LVEF <40% defining systolic dysfunction, 40–49% 'borderline') and has prognostic significance. As noted, however, a significant proportion of individuals with chronic heart failure have preserved (50–55%) or normal (>55%) LVEF (Yancy et al 2013).

Medical Management of Heart Failure

Initial medical management for patients at risk of, or with, early asymptomatic (chronic) heart failure addresses modifiable risk factors, e.g. hypertension, dyslipidaemia, obesity and diabetes mellitus (Mann 2012b). Commonly used medications include diuretics, ACE inhibitors, β-blockers, statins and oral hypoglycaemics (e.g. metformin). The reader is directed to Yancy et al (2013) for current recommendations on the use of specific medications as heart failure progresses. Nonpharmacological interventions include patient education regarding self-monitoring of symptoms and weight fluctuation, adherence to prescribed medication, maintenance of physical activity, and salt and fluid restriction. Cardiac rehabilitation including exercise training has been shown to reduce hospitalizations, and to improve exercise capacity and health-related quality of life, in patients with mild to moderate heart failure (Davies et al 2010).

CASE 4-4 *(Continued)*

Mr EF was admitted to hospital for 10 days, during which time strict fluid balance was maintained. His weight gradually reduced by 5 kg with additional diuretic therapy, and his oedema and ascites resolved. Mr EF's management was discussed at a combined cardiology and cardiothoracic surgical meeting, and it was agreed that implantation of a biventricular defibrillator was indicated (to optimize left ventricular systolic function and to treat malignant ventricular arrhythmias should they occur).

Mr EF was subsequently enrolled in a cardiac failure rehabilitation programme, where he was encouraged to maintain a programme of regular gentle exercise, to reduce caloric intake (to lose weight and reduce blood sugar). His 6-minute walk distance improved from 100 m to 250 m over 6 weeks, and his apnoea/hypopnoea index fell from 15/hr to 5/hr.

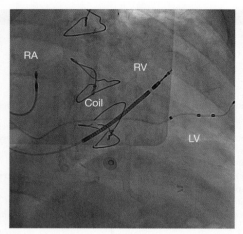

FIGURE 4-6 ■ This radiographic image shows three electrode leads within the heart. A bipolar lead is in the right atrium (RA). The lead in the right ventricle (RV) comprises bipolar pacing and recording electrodes secured by active fixation to the interventricular septum and shock coils (the proximal coil is not shown). Defibrillation shocks may be delivered between one or both of the shock coils and the defibrillator can (also not shown). The left ventricle (LV) is paced by an epicardial lead delivered to a lateral cardiac vein via the coronary sinus.

Device therapy, i.e. the surgical implantation of a biventricular pacemaker and/or implantable cardioverter-defibrillator (ICD) (Fig. 4-6), may be indicated in heart failure with severe systolic dysfunction, refractory to optimal pharmacological therapy (Krum & Driscoll 2013, Mann 2012b). Biventricular pacing, aka cardiac resynchronization therapy, synchronizes left and right ventricular contraction to improve LVEF (note that a widened QRS complex on the 12-lead ECG is indicative of dyssynchrony). Patients with reduced LVEF are also at an increased risk of potentially fatal ventricular tachyarrhythmias; an ICD will promptly diagnose and treat VF, thereby preventing SCD.

Patients with end-stage heart failure (stage D, aka 'advanced', 'end-stage' or 'refractory' heart failure), may be candidates for palliation, and/or advanced surgical therapies, e.g. cardiac transplantation, insertion of a left ventricular-assist device (VAD) (Yancy et al 2013). Temporary mechanical circulatory support devices, e.g. an extracorporeal VAD, may be used as a 'bridge to recovery' (or decision) in patients with acute, potentially reversible, heart failure.

Heart Failure Requiring Hospitalization

Patients may require hospitalization for acute decompensated heart failure, e.g. precipitated by acute myocardial ischaemia, uncontrolled hypertension, non-adherence to medications, salt and/or fluid restriction, pulmonary infection. The requirement for hospitalization is an indication of poor prognosis in patients with heretofore 'chronic' heart failure. Treatment consists of management of the underlying cause of decompensation, and optimization of medical therapy. Patients hospitalized with fluid overload may require intravenous diuretics and potentially ultrafiltration (Yancy et al 2013).

Physiotherapy-Specific Management of Heart Failure

In the inpatient setting, physiotherapists may be called upon to provide respiratory therapy for the patient with heart failure and related cough/dyspnoea. It is important to note that traditional physiotherapy treatments to aid mucociliary clearance are of little benefit in the patient with APO, but may be of use in the context of concurrent pulmonary infection. Patient education regarding management of dyspnoea (e.g. dyspnoea relief positioning, pursed-lip breathing) may also be of benefit. The application of continuous or bi-level positive airway pressure (CPAP, BiPAP) devices, to improve gas exchange in APO, may be the responsibility of the physiotherapist in some institutions. Physiotherapy management in heart failure may also encompass exercise prescription and supervision, to both limit hospitalization-related deconditioning and reduce the risk of falls. There is evolving evidence for functional electrical stimulation and lower limb resistance training to maintain exercise capacity in patients too dyspnoeic to ambulate (Smart 2013). In the outpatient setting, physiotherapy management of heart failure primarily comprises formal cardiac rehabilitation (see Chapter 12).

CARDIAC ARRHYTHMIAS

CASE 4-5

Mr GH is a 38-year-old science teacher, who presented to his cardiologist with symptoms of a 'racing heart' and associated dizziness. He was otherwise well. Physical examination and 12-lead ECG in sinus rhythm were unremarkable, the echocardiogram was normal except for mild left atrial dilatation. 24-hour ambulatory electrocardiographic monitoring (Holter monitor) indicated paroxysmal atrial fibrillation (PAF).

Introduction

The cardiac conduction system consists of specialized impulse generating (pacemaking) nodes (the sinoatrial and atrioventricular nodes) and conduction tissue (the bundle of His, left and right bundle branches and terminal Purkinje fibres (Figure 1-22) (Rubart & Zipes 2012). Coordinated contraction of the myocardium, hence maintenance of cardiac pump function, is predicated on normal function of the cardiac conduction system and unidirectional transmission of the cardiac impulse through the myocardial syncytium. The term 'cardiac arrhythmia' describes any cardiac rhythm that differs from normal sinus rhythm (i.e. that resulting from spontaneous, regular depolarization of the sinoatrial node) (Jaeger 2012).

Aetiology and Pathophysiology of Cardiac Arrhythmias

Cardiac arrhythmias may relate to: (1) a disorder of impulse generation, related to either enhanced or suppressed automaticity or triggered activity; (2) a disorder of impulse conduction (e.g. a block or delay to transmission with/without impulse 'reentry') or (3) a combination of the two (Rubart & Zipes 2012). Table 4-6 describes some of those more commonly observed cardiac arrhythmias; the range of cardiac arrhythmias with which a patient may present precludes complete discussion of their aetiology and pathophysiology in this textbook. Arrhythmias may be heritable (e.g. Wolff-Parkinson-White syndrome) or acquired, and may be associated with autonomic nervous system impairment, drugs (e.g. β-blockers), index events, e.g. ischaemia or scarring secondary to IHD/AMI, and electrolyte disturbances (commonly seen after cardiac surgery). Essentially, however, all cardiac arrhythmias

TABLE 4-6		
Common Cardiac Arrhythmias		
Arrhythmia	Common Aetiologies	Common Treatment
Supraventricular arrhythmias		
Sinus bradycardia	Sick sinus syndrome	Pacemaker, plus β-blockers
Atrial ectopic beats	May occur in normal and abnormal hearts	Treat underlying pathology if applicable
Re-entrant supraventricular tachycardia	Atrioventricular node reentry, Wolff-Parkinson-White syndrome	Radiofrequency ablation if troublesome, β-blockers
Atrial fibrillation	Hypertension, mitral valve disease	Treat underlying pathology, ± pulmonary vein isolation, digoxin, β-blockers, amiodarone
Atrial flutter	Often associated with atrial fibrillation	Cavotricuspid isthmus ablation, digoxin
Atrial tachycardia	Previous atrial surgery	Radiofrequency ablation if troublesome
Ventricular arrhythmias		
Ventricular ectopic beats	May occur in normal and abnormal hearts	Treat underlying pathology if applicable
Ventricular tachycardia	Myocardial scar, Brugada syndrome	Implanted defibrillator usually indicated
Torsade de pointes	Long QT syndrome	Implanted defibrillator indicated
Ventricular fibrillation	Acute myocardial ischaemia	Treat underlying pathology ± implanted defibrillator
Heart block		
Second-degree heart block	May be asymptomatic	Degenerative
Complete heart block	Pacemaker usually required	Degenerative, aortic root abscess

result in (variable) reductions of cardiac pump efficiency, with relatively benign through to potentially fatal consequences.

Symptoms and Signs of Cardiac Arrhythmias

Physical examination of the patient with cardiac arrhythmia is often unremarkable, although there may be evidence of pathology predisposing to arrhythmia (e.g. valvular heart disease) (Jaeger 2012). Ectopic beats (atrial or ventricular) are usually perceived as extra or missed beats. Supraventricular tachycardia usually causes rapid, regular beating, with abrupt onset and offset. AF usually causes irregular palpitations, but may be asymptomatic if the ventricular rate is neither very fast nor very slow. High-grade heart block usually causes fatigue. VT often causes sudden syncope without prodrome. Patients resuscitated from VF may have no recollection of the event.

Diagnosis of Cardiac Arrhythmias

The 12-lead ECG is the first-line investigation for the detection and differential diagnosis of cardiac arrhythmias. Paroxysmal arrhythmias, however, may not be detected on a single ECG recording. Ambulatory (portable) ECG monitors, such as Holter monitors (continuous ECG monitoring) and loop recorders (used to record an ECG in response to symptoms or an 'event'), allow for investigation outside the immediate clinical environment (Mittal et al 2011). Surgically implantable loop recorders allow for ECG monitoring over an extended (≥1 year) period of time (Miller & Zipes 2012a).

Electrophysiological studies (EPSs) (Box 4-3) allow for the monitored induction of cardiac arrhythmias, hence determination of the arrhythmic focus or circuit, and (potentially) guidance regarding therapeutic intervention.

Classification of Cardiac Arrhythmias

As with heart failure, cardiac arrhythmias can be categorized according to their pathophysiological mechanism (disorder of automaticity, etc). More commonly however, cardiac arrhythmias are categorized or described according to the origin, rate (bradyarrhythmias: <60 bpm, tachyarrhythmias: >100 bpm) and regularity or irregularity and pattern of the pathological impulse.

BOX 4-3
CARDIAC INVESTIGATIONS

Electrophysiological studies (Miller & Zipes 2012a, Ross 2011): An electrophysiological study (EPS) is performed to demonstrate conduction intervals and refractory periods within the heart. Re-entrant arrhythmias may be induced and terminated by pacing at different sites. The locations of accessory pathways and ectopic foci may be demonstrated (and treated if necessary/appropriate).

In most cases, plastic-coated multielectrode catheters are introduced percutaneously via sheaths in femoral veins, and advanced under fluoroscopic (radiographic) guidance to the heart. Separate catheters are introduced to the right atrium, the atrioventricular nodal region, the right ventricular apex and the coronary sinus. Local electrocardiograms are recorded from the various catheters in order to measure conduction intervals. Programmed stimulation is used to assess refractoriness and to initiate and terminate arrhythmias. Radiofrequency energy may be passed via the tip of an electrode catheter to ablate accessory pathways or ectopic foci (Fig. 4-7). Cryotherapy may also be employed to modify conduction.

Medical Management of Cardiac Arrhythmias

CASE 4-5 *(Continued)*

Mr GH's PAF proved refractory to a variety of medications, including metoprolol, amiodarone, flecainide and digoxin. After discussion of therapeutic options, Mr GH requested pulmonary vein isolation by radiofrequency ablation (RFA). Following pulmonary vein isolation he remained in sinus rhythm.

Management of cardiac arrhythmias potentially includes pharmacological suppression of the arrhythmia, radiofrequency ablation (RFA), cardioversion/defibrillation and surgical implantation of a permanent pacemaker (PPM) and/or ICD (Miller & Zipes 2012b). Appropriate management depends on the clinical setting, chronicity and morbid propensity of the arrhythmia. Treatment of transient AF in a hospitalized patient after CABG, for example, would differ significantly from that of chronic AF in a community-dwelling, otherwise healthy young adult.

Antiarrhythmic medications are generally indicated in patients with symptomatic arrhythmias, where medications have been demonstrated to be effective. Commonly used antiarrhythmic medications

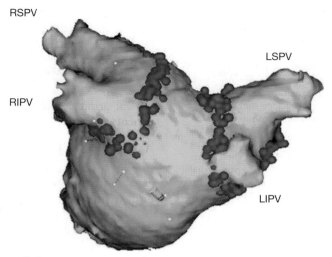

RSPV

LSPV

RIPV

LIPV

FIGURE 4-7 ■ Posterior view of left atrium (composite of CT scan and three-dimensional mapping). The red dots indicate the location of application of radiofrequency energy around right superior pulmonary vein (RSPV), right inferior pulmonary vein (RIPV), left superior pulmonary vein (LSPV) and left inferior pulmonary vein (LIPV).

TABLE 4-7
Common Antiarrhythmic Medications

Vaughan Williams Class	Common Formulations	Action
Ia,b,c	Disopyramide, lignocaine, flecainide	Sodium channel blocker
II	Metoprolol, atenolol	β-blocker
III	Amiodarone, sotalol	Potassium channel blocker
IV	Verapamil, diltiazem	Calcium channel blocker

Adapted from Miller & Zipes 2012b.

and their actions are listed in Table 4-7. Notably, these medications can also be 'proarrhythmic', hence are often only initiated in the hospital setting with cardiac telemetry. AF may predispose to atrial thromboembolism, also warranting preventive anticoagulation. RFA is most commonly used to treat supraventricular tachycardia, AF and atrial flutter refractory to antiarrhythmic medications and monomorphic VT (Miller & Zipes 2012b). Cardioversion, i.e. the delivery of a synchronized direct current (DC) 'shock' to the heart through internal or external electrodes, may be used in organized tachyarrhythmias to terminate the arrhythmia. Defibrillation via internal or external elec-trodes is used in the emergency setting to treat potentially fatal ventricular tachyarrhythmias.

Comprehensive guidelines have been published regarding the indications for surgical implantation of cardiac devices (PPMs, ICDs) (Box 4-4) (Brignole et al 2013, Epstein et al 2013). Permanent cardiac pacing is generally indicated in symptomatic sinus node dysfunction, including (often age-related) persistent sinus bradyarrhythmias, and in (irreversible) advanced second-degree or third-degree atrioventricular block. ICDs are indicated for the secondary prevention of cardiac arrest in patients with previously sustained VT or VF, and with otherwise reasonable expectation of survival >1 year. Prophylactic ICD implantation is indicated in selected patients at high risk of SCD (e.g. long QT syndrome, Brugada syndrome, cardiomyopathy with LVEF <30%).

Physiotherapy-Specific Management of Cardiac Arrhythmias

Physiotherapists have a limited role in the management of the patient with lone cardiac arrhythmia (i.e. in the absence of other structural or functional cardiac disorder). All physiotherapists, however, should be aware of the implications of cardiac arrhythmias for physical activity and exercise prescription, and be capable of applying basic cardiopulmonary resuscitation techniques in the event of cardiac arrest. Patients requiring implantation or review of a cardiac device have traditionally received advice and education regarding (short-term) restriction of shoulder/upper limb movement to minimize the risk of early lead dislodgement, although evidence for such restriction is lacking (Bavnbek et al 2010).

GROWN-UP CONGENITAL HEART DISEASE

Introduction

Grown-up congenital heart disease (GUCH) describes adult patients with congenital heart disease initially diagnosed (and managed) in infancy/childhood, and those diagnosed for the first time in adult life. The heterogeneity of congenital heart diseases, and of their related structural/functional disorders, precludes specific and comprehensive discussion of their pathophysiology here (further detail is provided in Chapter 10). Rather, this section of the chapter will discuss general principles of diagnosis and management of patients with GUCH.

Aetiology and Pathophysiology of GUCH

Congenital heart disease comprises abnormalities in cardiac structure and/or function that are present at birth, regardless of when they are diagnosed (Webb et al 2012). These abnormalities relate to alterations in the embryonic development of the cardiac and circulatory structures, commonly as a result of a genetic abnormality or underlying genetic disorder (e.g. Marfan syndrome) and/or of environmental factors (e.g. foetal alcohol syndrome) (Webb et al 2012). The aetiology of congenital heart disease is described in more detail in the paediatric section of this textbook (see Chapter 10). Advances in paediatric cardiology and cardiac surgery have led to an increased number of patients with congenital heart disease, even of great complexity, surviving into adulthood (Gatzoulis & Webb 2003).

Symptoms and Signs of GUCH

Symptoms and signs of GUCH are highly variable, and dependent on the specific structural and functional abnormality. Heart failure, cardiac arrhythmias and pulmonary and systemic hypertension are common consequences of GUCH (Baumgartner et al 2010); as such, the patient with GUCH may report symptoms including decreased exercise tolerance, dyspnoea, fatigue and/or syncope. The patient with GUCH may also experience heart disease otherwise, including IHD, cardiomyopathy and rheumatic disease.

Diagnosis of GUCH

A diagnosis of moderate or severe complex congenital heart disease is usually established in infancy/early childhood, or even prenatally. Simple forms of congenital heart disease (e.g. isolated congenital bicuspid aortic valve, isolated small atrial or ventricular septal defect (ASD, VSD)) may first be diagnosed in adulthood. Specific physical signs, e.g. a continuous cardiac murmur, cyanosis and clubbing (in the absence of known respiratory disease), and electrocardiographic abnormalities (e.g. right bundle block) are indicative of potential GUCH. Echocardiography with Doppler imaging is the first-line investigation in the diagnosis of GUCH, as well as the diagnosis of late dysfunction after childhood intervention, providing fundamental information on abnormalities of cardiac anatomy, morphology and function of cardiac chambers and valves, and the presence/severity of shunt lesions (Baumgartner et al 2010). For information on CMR, see Box 4-5. Cardiac CT provides an alternative to echocardiography in some circumstances (Baumgartner et al 2010, Warnes et al 2008).

Classification of GUCH

GUCH can be classified by the altered cardiac structure(s) (e.g. septum, mitral valve, left ventricular outflow tract) and/or resultant clinical presentation (e.g. cyanotic conditions). As noted, however, there is great variance in the structural/functional disorders associated with GUCH. The 'sequential segmental method' (Ho 2003) is a useful approach to describe (potentially complex) alterations in cardiac abnormality, whereby the arrangements and interconnections of: (1) the atrial segment, (2) the ventricular segment and (3) the arterial segment (the great arteries) are considered in turn. Using this method, an ASD could be described as 'usual atrial arrangement, concordant atrioventricular and ventriculoarterial connections, with ASD'. As heart failure is a common consequence of GUCH, the NYHA functional classification can be used to describe symptomatic impairment.

Medical Management of GUCH

Medical management of GUCH is directed at ongoing surveillance, prevention of complications (e.g. thromboembolic events, endocarditis), management of pathophysiological sequelae (e.g. heart failure, cardiac arrhythmias, pulmonary or systemic arterial hypertension), and/or interventional treatment of significant structural abnormalities (Baumgartner et al 2010). Increasingly, techniques to correct structural abnormalities (e.g. closure of simple communicating lesions – ASD, patent foramen ovale (PFO)) can be performed via cardiac catheterization (Baumgartner et al 2010, Warnes et al 2008). Open surgery via sternotomy may be required for late (primary) correction of congenital defects, or more commonly for reoperation after surgery performed in infancy or childhood. A common example of reoperation is insertion/replacement of the pulmonary valve following repair of tetralogy of Fallot. Arrhythmias are a major cause of hospitalization, morbidity and mortality in GUCH, and may warrant ablation or device therapy (Baumgartner et al 2010) (see Section 6, Medical Management of Cardiac Arrhythmias).

Physiotherapy-Specific Management of GUCH

Physiotherapists responsible for the perioperative care of patients with GUCH must consider the adaptive cardiac (re)modelling predating the surgery, and that postsurgical remodelling may be delayed and incomplete. Hence the time course (and endpoint) of recovery of postoperative functional capacity may be highly variable. Patients undergoing surgery for GUCH are commonly younger than their IHD counterparts, with fewer age- and smoking-related respiratory co-morbidities; specific, prophylactic respiratory therapy is often unwarranted.

AORTIC DISEASE

Introduction

The aorta is the largest artery in the body, arising from the heart at the aortic valve. After the coronary arteries, the next major branches are the great vessels to the brain and upper limbs. The distal aorta bifurcates into the common iliac arteries. The aorta is divided anatomically into the aortic root (which gives rise to the coronary arteries), the ascending aorta, aortic arch, descending thoracic aorta and abdominal aorta. Common to the arterial circulation, the aortic wall comprises three layers (intima, media, adventitia). The microarchitecture of these layers, however, is unique to the aorta, providing the tensile strength, elasticity and compliance required to accommodate greater haemodynamic stresses (Braverman et al 2012).

Diseases of the aorta primarily relate to atherosclerotic disease and/or physical disturbances of the aortic wall, e.g. aneurysmal disease, aortic dissection, intramural haematoma. The aorta may also (more rarely) be a focus for infectious or inflammatory disease. As the pathophysiology and management of atherosclerotic cardiovascular disease is discussed at length elsewhere in this chapter (Sections 1 and 9, Ischaemic Heart Disease and Peripheral Artery Disease), this section will focus on aneurysmal disease and aortic dissection, the most common (aortic) causes of acute morbidity and mortality.

Aetiology and Pathophysiology of Aortic Disease

An aneurysm is a (generally progressive) dilatation of the arterial wall, to >150% of 'normal' expected diameter, potentially leading to wall rupture and haemorrhage (Johnston et al 1991). Aneurysms can occur at any segment of the aorta (and indeed throughout the arterial circulation, including cerebral and visceral arteries), but most commonly affect the abdominal aorta. While the precise pathophysiology of aneurysm formation is the subject of ongoing research, it is believed that aneurysms result from a combination of: (1) degeneration of connective tissue (in the media and adventitia of the vessel wall), (2) inflammatory and immunological responses, (3) vessel wall stress and 4) molecular genetics (Braverman et al 2012). Atherosclerosis (affecting the intima of the vessel wall) is an epidemiological risk factor for aneurysm development, but is not believed to be a primary causative factor.

Pseudoaneurysms (false aneurysms) differ from true aneurysms, insofar as they describe a disruption (vs dilatation) of the arterial wall, with bleeding/haematoma contained by periarterial connective tissue (Hiratzka et al 2010). Pseudoaneurysms may occur as a result of trauma (including iatrogenic trauma), penetrating aortic ulcer or contained rupture of a (true) aortic aneurysm.

Acute aortic dissection occurs when there is rupture of the aortic intima, either as a result of a primary intimal tear or intramural haemorrhage (Erbel et al 2001). Pulsatile aortic blood flow enters the aortic wall, creating and thence propagating a 'false' aortic lumen. Dissection, usually beginning close to the aortic inlet, may progress to aortic leak or rupture, and/or may cause malperfusion of second-order vessels (the false lumen occluding the true aortic lumen) with resultant cardiac, cerebral or limb ischaemia. Retrograde dissection may cause AR and cardiac tamponade.

Aortic dissection is believed to have a similar pathophysiologic origin to that of aortic aneurysm – concomitant aortic aneurysm and inherited connective tissue disorders known to predispose to aneurysm, e.g. Marfan syndrome and Ehlers-Danlos syndrome type IV, are also associated with aortic dissection (Braverman et al 2012). Aortic dissection may also occur as a result of deceleration injuries (e.g. through motor vehicle accident) or inadvertent endothelial disruption during aortic catheterization (iatrogenic).

Symptoms and Signs of Aortic Disease

Aortic aneurysms are generally asymptomatic until such time as they expand rapidly and/or rupture. Aneurysms are therefore often detected incidentally, e.g. on radiographic examination of the chest, abdomen or lumbar spine (Aggarwal et al 2011). Abdominal aortic aneurysms may be palpable as a pulsatile epigastric or periumbilical mass (Takayama & Yamanouchi 2013). Thoracic aortic aneurysms may cause symptoms and signs of AR, e.g. murmur, and/

or relate to compression of local structures, e.g. the trachea and bronchus, causing dyspnoea, bronchospasm or cough (Braverman et al 2012). Thoracic and abdominal aneurysms may also be a focus for development of systemic thromboembolism.

A rapidly expanding aneurysm (portending rupture) or aneurysmal rupture is an emergency situation. Symptoms include severe abdominal, flank and/or back pain (abdominal aneurysm) or chest and back pain (thoracic aneurysm). Haemorrhage leads to shock, with signs of acute hypotension, loss of consciousness and collapse.

Aortic dissection most commonly causes severe, sudden-onset chest and/or back pain, often of a 'tearing' or 'stabbing' quality (Erbel et al 2001). Pain may radiate along the path of dissection. Physical signs often relate to secondary effects of the dissection, e.g. hypotension and syncope in the instance of cardiac tamponade, or neurological signs should there be compromise of the brachiocephalic and/or common carotid arteries.

Diagnosis of Aortic Disease

As previously noted, aortic aneurysms are often detected incidentally. Abdominal ultrasound, abdominal CT, and magnetic resonance aortography (MRA) may all be used in the screening/detection and serial measurement of abdominal aortic aneurysm (Aggarwal et al 2011). Similarly, TTE (aortic root, ascending aorta) and TOE (entire thoracic aorta), thoracic CT and MRA may be used to visualize thoracic aortic anatomy and to define thoracic aortic aneurysms and dissection (Hiratzka et al 2010). Multidimensional CT allows for accurate determination of cross-sectional arterial and aneurysmal diameters.

Classification of Aortic Disease

Aortic aneurysms are typically classified by the affected anatomical segment, size (maximal aortic diameter) and length of the lesion and rate of expansion. Standard tables of aortic diameter are used to define threshold criteria for presence of aneurysms as well as threshold values for intervention; an abdominal aortic diameter >3.0 cm, for example, defines an aneurysm; a diameter >5.0–5.5 cm may warrant repair. Aneurysms may also be classified by morphology; a 'fusiform' aneurysm is generally symmetric and circumferential whereas a 'saccular' aneurysm is localized to a portion of the aortic wall circumference (Braverman et al 2012).

Aortic dissections are traditionally classified anatomically using either/both of DeBakey (types I, II, III) and/or Stanford (types A, B) classification schemes, according to the origin and extension of the lesion, and specifically whether the dissection involves the ascending aorta (Erbel et al 2001). The more recent Svensson classification describes aortic dissection by the mechanism of development.

Medical Management of Aortic Disease

Management of aortic aneurysm includes imaging surveillance, therapies to reduce the risk of aneurysm expansion, and elective or urgent/emergency repair in patients at risk of/with rupture. Risk reduction includes smoking cessation and management of hypertension (thereby reducing aortic wall stress), dyslipidaemia and diabetes. Patients should receive counselling regarding appropriate lifestyle modification, including avoidance of strenuous physical activity and isometric and resistance exercise.

Abdominal aortic aneurysm repair can be performed using either open surgical or endovascular approaches. Open surgical repair involves laparotomy and direct suturing of a synthetic graft across the site of the lesion. Endovascular aneurysm repair (EVAR) involves the placement of a stented endograft within the aorta and across the site of the lesion, via the femoral arteries under fluoroscopic guidance. EVAR is less invasive, incurs a shorter hospital stay and has lower perioperative mortality than open repair; longer-term benefits over open repair are unclear (Stather et al 2013).

Ascending and aortic arch aneurysms at risk of rupture require surgical repair, usually performed via sternotomy and using cardiopulmonary bypass to maintain distal circulation (Hiratzka et al 2010). The aneurysm is resected and replaced with a synthetic (Dacron) tube-shaped graft. Depending on the position of the aneurysm, surgical repair may also involve AVR and reimplantation of the coronary arteries (modified Bentall procedure), or reconstruction of the major arch branches. Both surgical and endovascular approaches may be used to repair descending thoracic and thoracoabdominal aneurysms (Cheng et al 2010, Coady et al 2010).

Acute aortic dissection warrants urgent medical and/or surgical management (Braverman et al 2012). Patients with Stanford type A dissections, i.e. involving the ascending aorta, and/or cardiac compromise (AR, cardiac tamponade, impairment of coronary perfusion) require urgent/emergency open surgical repair, similar to that described for ascending and aortic arch aneurysms. Initial medical management of patients with stable Stanford type B dissection involves pharmacological lowering of blood pressure and reduction of cardiac contractility. Indications for subsequent surgical or endovascular repair include visceral or limb ischaemia, aortic leak and (impending) aortic rupture. Repair (prior to rupture) involves the interposition/placement of synthetic material/endograft to prevent flow into the false lumen.

Physiotherapy-Specific Management of Aortic Disease

Again, physiotherapy management of the patient with aortic aneurysm/dissection primarily encompasses perioperative/periprocedural care. Patients undergoing EVAR typically require minimal physiotherapy intervention; those undergoing surgical management, particularly via sternotomy or laparotomy, generally require postoperative respiratory care including early postoperative mobility. Preoperative workup for surgery may be limited by emergency presentation and concerns regarding the potential for aortic rupture; it is reasonable to seek medical advice before performing effort-dependent spirometry testing (Cooper 2011).

PERIPHERAL ARTERY DISEASE

Introduction

This chapter has thus far focused on central cardiovascular disease, i.e. disease of the heart and great vessels. By definition the cardiovascular system also incorporates the peripheral vasculature (arterial and venous systems), and lymphatic system. The last two sections of this chapter respectively describe commonly encountered diseases of the peripheral arterial and venous circulation (peripheral vascular diseases), i.e. peripheral artery disease (PAD) and venous thromboembolism (VTE). Whereas the term 'PAD' is often inclusive of aortic and aneurysmal disease, here we use the term exclusively to describe obstructive disorders

of blood supply to the lower and upper limbs. As well as being a primary source of impairment, PAD is strongly associated with coronary atherosclerosis and IHD, hence the risk of major cardiovascular events (Creager & Libby 2012).

Aetiology and Pathophysiology of Peripheral Artery Disease

The primary pathophysiologic processes causing PAD, as with IHD, are atherosclerosis and thromboembolism leading to vessel stenosis and/or occlusion (Tendera et al 2011). Impaired perfusion to distal tissues may cause temporary (exercise-induced) ischaemia, hence temporarily impaired function, and/or prolonged ischaemia and necrosis. Due to the similar pathophysiology, risk factors for PAD are similar to those for IHD (Tendera et al 2011). Unmodifiable risk factors include an advanced age and family history of PAD; modifiable risk factors include diabetes mellitus, smoking, hypertension, dyslipidaemia, obesity and physical inactivity.

Symptoms and Signs of Peripheral Artery Disease

PAD can be largely asymptomatic, but typically presents as intermittent claudication, i.e. exertional discomfort, pain and/or fatigue, localized to the muscles supplied by the affected vessel(s) (Wennberg 2013). Stenosis of the femoral or popliteal arteries usually presents as calf claudication; stenosis of the brachial arteries, forearm claudication. In lower limb PAD (more common than upper limb PAD), walking distance is limited. Depending on the severity and duration of PAD, there may be alterations to skin colour, temperature and integrity (e.g. delayed wound healing) (Wennberg 2013). PAD may also present more critically as either 'critical' or 'acute' limb ischaemia (CLI, ALI) whereby perfusion is severely compromised, with impending limb loss (Creager & Libby 2012). CLI presents as chronic claudication pain at rest and non-healing leg wounds/ulcers and/or gangrene. Contrariwise, ALI is defined as a 'rapid or sudden decrease in limb perfusion', secondary to e.g. thromboembolism (ACCF/AHA 2011, p. 28). ALI presents as a sudden loss of pulses and motor and sensory function (aka 'the five Ps': pain, pulselessness, pallor, paraesthesias and paralysis).

Diagnosis of Peripheral Artery Disease

Diagnosis of PAD is made on the basis of: (1) risk factors, including known atherosclerotic coronary, carotid or renal arterial disease; (2) vascular review of symptoms, including of walking impairment; (3) vascular physical examination, including auscultation of femoral arteries, peripheral pulse palpation and skin inspection and (4) non-invasive vascular clinical and laboratory tests (Creager & Libby 2012). Segmental limb pressure measurement, using a Doppler ultrasound probe to assess distal flow, is a key clinical test for PAD, and may be performed at rest or with exercise testing (e.g. treadmill). The ankle–brachial index (ABI), being the ratio of systolic ankle pressure (greater of posterior tibial and dorsalis pedis arteries) to systolic brachial artery pressure, is commonly used to both diagnose and grade lower limb PAD (an ABI <0.90 being indicative of PAD) (Tendera et al 2011). Magnetic resonance, CT and/or catheter-based angiography may be used to visualize (flow within) both the aorta and peripheral arteries (Creager & Libby 2012).

Classification of Peripheral Artery Disease

PAD can be classified according to anatomical distribution, clinical manifestation (e.g. asymptomatic, CLI, ALI) and symptomatology. Common classification systems (e.g. the Fontaine Classification and Rutherford Clinical Category) stage PAD by the pattern of claudication and presence of necrosis/gangrene (Rutherford et al 1997). Where revascularization may be indicated (see treatment, Medical Management of Peripheral Artery Disease), duplex ultrasonography and angiography are used to define the anatomic level(s) and severity of vessel stenosis/occlusion; the Trans-Atlantic Inter-Society Consensus (TASC) guidelines are then used to 'typify' vessel lesions (iliac vs femoropopliteal, types A (least severe) through D (most severe)) (Norgren et al 2007). Stenosis/occlusion in the aortoiliac region is also classified as lower limb 'inflow' disease, vs that in the common femoral artery to pedal vessels, classified as lower limb 'outflow' disease.

Medical Management of Peripheral Artery Disease

Management of asymptomatic PAD aims to reduce the risk of major cardiovascular events, reduce symptoms of claudication and preserve limb viability (Creager & Libby 2012). Initial management consists of risk factor reduction (i.e. smoking cessation, treatment of hypertension, dislipidaemia, diabetes mellitus, antiplatelet therapy). Where claudication does not result in significant functional disability, further specific therapy (beyond ongoing monitoring) is not warranted (ACCF/AHA 2011). Patients with lifestyle-limiting symptoms should undertake a supervised, intermittent walking-based exercise programme, similar to that undertaken in phase II cardiac rehabilitation; these programs have been shown to substantially improve average maximal walking distance (Watson et al 2008).

The role of pharmacotherapy in the reduction of claudication is evolving. Percutaneous intervention (angioplasty with/without stenting) is indicated for patients with lifestyle-limiting symptoms and inflow disease, and/or whose symptoms are unresponsive to exercise and pharmacotherapy. Surgical revascularization (e.g. aorto–bifemoral bypass, femoral–popliteal bypass) is indicated for patients with disabling pain and/or CLI despite maximal other therapy. ALI warrants emergency evaluation and intervention, which may include thrombolysis, surgical thrombectomy and/or revascularization. Amputation may be required in CLI/ALI if the limb/extremity is not viable (Anderson et al 2013, Tendera et al 2011).

Physiotherapy-Specific Management of Peripheral Artery Disease

As in IHD, physiotherapy management of lower limb PAD may include exercise prescription/supervision for the patient with claudication, and perioperative/periprocedural care for the patient undergoing revascularization. Patients undergoing surgical revascularization will often require aids and/or physical assistance to walk safely due to pain and deconditioning. Walking capacity is a key indicator of PAD severity and response to therapy, hence physiotherapists working in this field may be required to conduct sequential tests of walking capacity, e.g. the 6-minute walk test. In patients requiring limb/extremity amputation, physiotherapists may have a significant role in stump bandaging or casting, preparation for (and fitting of) prostheses, as well as the management of chronic or phantom limb pain.

VENOUS THROMBOEMBOLISM

Introduction

Venous diseases include *inter alia* venous thrombosis, both superficial (aka phlebitis) and deep, venous insufficiency, venous ulcers and varicosities. Along with AMI and stroke (not discussed here), VTE, comprising PE and its antecedent, deep vein thrombosis (DVT), is one of the three major cardiovascular causes of death (Goldhaber 2012). VTE is also among the leading preventable causes of death in hospitalized patients (Lee et al 2005). This section of the chapter will focus on VTE, as VTE prophylaxis is considered a key indication for physiotherapy intervention in hospitalized patients, particularly those with underlying cardiorespiratory disease.

Aetiology and Pathophysiology of Venous Thromboembolism

VTE refers to the disease process whereby thrombi (blood clots) form abnormally within the venous circulation. VTE occurs as a result of 'Virchow's triad', i.e. a combination of: (1) abnormalities of blood flow (venous stasis), (2) blood vessel endothelial damage (providing a focus for thrombus formation) and (3) blood clotting (hypercoagulability) (Riedel 2001). Thrombi initially aggregate in areas of abnormal blood flow, e.g. veins subject to external compression. Influenced by the balance between thrombogenic stimuli

and protective and therapeutic mechanisms, thrombi may resolve spontaneously without becoming symptomatic, extend to cause venous outflow obstruction, and/or embolize to the pulmonary circulation (Ozaki & Bartholomew 2012).

The two most common clinical manifestations of VTE are DVT and PE.

Deep Vein Thrombosis

DVT most commonly occurs in the lower extremities (calf and thigh), but may also occur in the upper extremities. Risk factors for DVT (and hence PE) can be categorized as 'chronic predisposing factors', and 'acute provoking factors' (Table 4-8) (Ho et al 2005). The primary pathophysiological concern associated with DVT is embolization; however, DVT of itself can also result in peripheral vascular compromise, infection and venous gangrene. 'Post-thrombotic syndrome' is a chronic complication of DVT, damage to the venous valves resulting in regurgitant venous flow/ venous pooling (Kearon 2003).

Pulmonary Embolism

PE occurs when thrombus detaches from the site of formation, and moves centrally through the venous and right-sided heart circulation to 'lodge' in the pulmonary arterial circulation. Consequent effects relate to the size of the embolic fragment(s), the degree and chronicity of pulmonary circulatory obstruction, and

TABLE 4-8		
Risk Factors for Venous Thromboembolism		
Acute Provoking	**Chronic Predisposing (Modifiable)**	**Chronic Predisposing (Non-Modifiable)**
Recent (or current) hospitalization	Obesity	Advanced age
Surgery (especially lower limb arthroplasty, major abdominal/pelvic surgery)	Metabolic syndrome	Arterial disease (including ischaemic heart disease)
Trauma or fracture of lower limb/pelvis	Smoking	Cancer (chemotherapy)
Long-distance travel	Hypertension	Leg paralysis
Insertion of intravascular device (e.g. cardiac device, central venous catheter)	Dyslipidaemia	Personal or familial history of venous thromboembolism
		Heart failure
		Chronic obstructive pulmonary disease
		Pregnancy
		Oestrogen therapy
		Primary hypercoagulable states (thrombophilia)
		Acquired thrombotic disorders

the underlying health/cardiopulmonary reserve of the patient. So-called 'submassive' and/or 'non-massive' PE, where a lesser degree of pulmonary vasculature is obstructed, may result in impaired gas exchange due to increased alveolar dead space and ventilation–perfusion mismatching. Pulmonary infarction may occur, more commonly in individuals with pre-existing cardiopulmonary disease.

'Massive' PE has severe haemodynamic as well as respiratory consequences. Pulmonary vascular resistance is increased both as a result of substantive obstruction(s) to the pulmonary vascular bed and (to a lesser extent) the release of vasoconstrictive neurohumeral agents. A significant increase in right ventricular afterload results in right ventricular dysfunction and dilatation. Right ventricular dilatation may flatten the interventricular septum and cause left ventricular dysfunction (with compromise of coronary and systemic circulation). Severe right ventricular dilatation may lead to right ventricular infarction and death. Arterial hypoxaemia occurs as a result of ventilation–perfusion mismatch (both overperfusion of unembolized areas of the lung, and persistent perfusion of areas of collapse/infarction).

While the majority of PEs lodge in lower order pulmonary vessels, massive emboli, e.g. lodging in the bifurcation of the pulmonary artery, may lead to circulatory failure and sudden death.

Symptoms and Signs of Venous Thromboembolism

Deep Vein Thrombosis

DVT is often asymptomatic. Symptoms of DVT, including local pain and tenderness, erythema, and swelling of the affected limb, are indicative of proximal vein involvement and increased risk of PE (Ho et al 2005). Post-thrombotic syndrome, occurring in approximately 20–30% of patients with DVT, has symptoms including chronic leg ulcers, local pain and swelling, these latter typically aggravated by dependent postures (e.g. prolonged standing/walking) (Kearon 2003).

Pulmonary Embolism

While PE may also be asymptomatic, common symptoms and signs of PE include acute onset dyspnoea, tachypnoea, pleuritic or atypical chest pain, haemoptysis/cough, tachycardia and syncope (Riedel 2001). Approximately 10% of patients with symptomatic PE will die within 1 hour of symptom onset (Kearon 2003).

Diagnosis of Venous Thromboembolism

Clinical diagnosis of VTE usually incorporates the use of 'pretest' probability models, non-invasive and/or radiological investigations, and D-dimer assays (i.e. blood tests for products of fibrinolysis – present in VTE) (Lee et al 2005).

Pretest probability models, e.g. the Wells score, are used to provide an *a priori* estimate of DVT risk (low, moderate, high) on the basis of clinical features (Wells et al 1997). An individual with entire leg swelling, tenderness along the deep vein system, and following recent surgery (with no likely alternative diagnosis) would, for example, be classified as high probability for DVT. Duplex compression ultrasonography (Box 4-6) is the front-line investigation for clinically suspected DVT, but may be less accurate in asymptomatic patients and those with isolated calf DVT (Turpie et al 2002). Blood tests for fibrin D-dimer are useful to exclude DVT (and PE) in patients with low pretest probability (Ho et al 2005).

Pretest probability models, e.g. the revised Geneva score (Torbicki et al 2008), are also used to provide an estimate of PE risk. Computed tomographic pulmonary angiography (CTPA) (see Box 4-6) has replaced invasive (catheter-based) pulmonary angiography as the gold-standard test for definitive diagnosis/exclusion of PE (Goldhaber 2012), but still involves the use of intravenous contrast with attendant risks. Ventilation–perfusion scanning is an alternative investigation for PE but is difficult to interpret in individuals with concomitant lung disease.

Classification of Venous Thromboembolism

DVT is typically described according to the anatomical location(s) and (length of) extension of thrombus/thrombi. 'Proximal' (vs distal) lower limb DVT implies that a thrombus involves the popliteal and/or more proximal veins, and is associated with a higher incidence of PE. PEs are variously described by: (1) the number and anatomical location of thrombi (e.g. a 'saddle' thrombus, located at the bifurcation of the

BOX 4-6
CARDIOVASCULAR INVESTIGATIONS

Duplex compression ultrasonography: Duplex compression ultrasonography uses the same principles as echocardiography, i.e. the combined use of non-invasive ultrasound transmission/reflection and Doppler examination, in this case to image and detect flow in the peripheral veins. Typically performed at the bedside, duplex ultrasonography involves the sequential examination of all, or discrete segments of, the lower and/or upper extremities. The inability to fully compress the lumen of a venous segment with gentle pressure from the ultrasound probe is indicative of local thrombosis. A negative test does not rule out pulmonary embolism (PE), e.g. following complete embolization of deep vein thrombosis (DVT).

Computed tomographic pulmonary angiography (CTPA) (Mos et al 2012): Computed tomography (CT) relies on the same basic physiological principle as conventional radiography, namely the absorption of X-rays by tissues of differing densities. As with cardiac magnetic resonance (CMR) imaging, for CTPA the patient lies on a table within a rotating gantry, in this case housing an X-ray tube and detectors. Intravenous contrast is used to define the pulmonary vasculature; a computer then constructs images of the thorax (including of the pulmonary vasculature) from sequential radiographic images. PE is diagnosed on the basis of 'interruption to contrast material in the pulmonary veins' (Mos et al 2012, p. 139); comparative (right : left) ventricular size also provides important prognostic information. Newer 'multirow-detector', helical (or spiral) CT enables the derivation of multiplanar, high-definition images, reducing the time needed for image acquisition to seconds (and hence reducing movement artefact and radiation exposure).

pulmonary artery), (2) the degree of pulmonary vascular obstruction, (3) the chronicity of thrombus and symptom development and 4) the estimated risk of PE-related early death (a function of clinical markers, e.g. shock, and markers of right ventricular dysfunction/myocardial injury). The terms 'massive', 'submassive' and 'non-massive' are often used to classify PE by degree of pulmonary vascular obstruction, but are considered ambiguous (Jaff et al 2011).

Medical Management of Venous Thromboembolism

Medical management of VTE incorporates both prophylaxis in at-risk individuals and treatment for those with diagnosed VTE (Goldhaber 2012). Clinical practice guidelines have been published for the prevention of VTE in *inter alia* Australian hospitals (National Health and Medical Research Council 2009); said guidelines provide evidence-based recommendations for the use of pharmacological and mechanical thromboprophylactic agents (e.g. low–molecular-weight heparin (LMWH), graduated compression stockings, sequential pneumatic compression devices). These agents address blood coagulability and venous stasis respectively.

Treatment of diagnosed DVT aims to: (1) prevent extension, including the risk of embolization; (2) prevent recurrence of DVT and post-thrombotic syndrome and (3) relieve symptoms. Anticoagulation, initially with LMWH, thence warfarin (target INR 2.0 to 3.0), is the primary therapy for DVT; note that LMWH does not directly dissolve the thrombus but does prevent further formation/extension, thereby facilitating endogenous fibrinolysis. Insertion of a vena caval filter may be indicated to prevent PE in patients for whom anticoagulation is contraindicated (e.g. those at high risk of haemorrhage). Catheter or surgical thrombolysis/embolectomy may be warranted in patients with acute extensive proximal DVT and/or profound circulatory compromise.

Treatment of diagnosed PE is symptom- and risk-dependent (Jaff et al 2011, Torbicki et al 2008). Patients with acute haemodynamic and/or respiratory compromise may require intensive cardiorespiratory care (mechanical ventilation/vasopressors) pending definitive PE therapy. Again, anticoagulation with LMWH or unfractionated heparin is the mainstay of treatment. Thrombolysis and embolectomy (surgical or percutaneous) may be warranted in patients with massive PE to reduce pulmonary vascular obstruction and right ventricular dysfunction; potential benefits of thrombolysis, however, must be weighed against risks of bleeding complications, e.g. intracranial haemorrhage. Long-term anticoagulation (≥3–6 months) with warfarin and/or LMWH reduces the risk of DVT/PE recurrence.

Physiotherapy-Specific Management of Venous Thromboembolism

Physiotherapists have an important role in VTE prophylaxis and detection in hospitalized patients, particularly those whose conditions predispose to immobility and/or VTE (e.g. hip/knee arthroplasty, major abdominal surgery, stroke). Routine assessment, e.g. of patients having undergone joint arthroplasty, should include physical assessment of the lower limb; often the first report of DVT symptoms will be made during physiotherapy-supervised exercise or mobility.

Traditionally, physiotherapists have prescribed lower limb range-of-motion (bed) exercises (e.g. calf pumps) for DVT prevention in patients on bed rest; there is sound mechanistic sense for these to reduce venous stasis, but limited published evidence of benefit. Ensuring adequate fitting and/or compliance with mechanical thromboprophylactic devices is often the physiotherapist's responsibility. Early mobility of surgical and critically ill patients has significant respiratory and functional benefits, and can only reduce VTE risk. Of note, in patients receiving anticoagulation for acute DVT, early exercise/mobility (as opposed to bed rest) reduces short-term risk of PE, new or progression of DVT, and post-thrombotic symptoms (Aissaoui et al 2009, Liu et al 2015).

REFERENCES

Aggarwal, S., Qamar, A., Sharma, V., Sharma, A., 2011. Abdominal aortic aneurysm: a comprehensive review. Exp. Clin. Cardio. 16 (1), 11–15.

Aissaoui, N., Martins, E., Mouly, S., et al., 2009. A meta-analysis of bed rest versus early ambulation in the management of pulmonary embolism, deep vein thrombosis, or both. Int. J. Cardiol. 137, 37–41.

American College of Cardiology Foundation/American Heart Association 2011, 'ACCF/AHA pocket guidelines November 2011: Management of patients with peripheral artery disease (lower extremity, renal, mesenteric and abdominal aortic', viewed 15 January 2014, <http://www.cardiosource.org/~/media/Files/Science%20and%20Quality/Guidelines/Pocket%20Guides/2011_PAD_PktGuide.ashx>.

American Heart Association 2014, 'My American Heart For Professionals', viewed 15 January 2014, <http://my.americanheart.org/professional/index.jsp/>.

Anderson, J.L., Halperin, J.L., Albert, N.M., et al., 2013. Management of patients with peripheral artery disease (compilation of 2005 and 2011 ACCF/AHA guideline recommendations): a report of the American College of Cardiology Foundation/American Heart Association Task Force on Practice Guidelines. Circulation 127, 1425–1443.

Williams, P.L., Warwick, R., Dyson, M., Bannister, L.H. (Eds.), 1989. Angiology. In: Gray's Anatomy, thirty-seventh ed. Churchill Livingstone, New York, pp. 661–821.

Antoni, H., 1989. Function of the heart. In: Schmidt, R.F., Thews, G. (Eds.), Human Physiology, second ed. Springer-Verlag, Berlin, pp. 439–479.

Basso, C., Corrado, D., Marcus, F.I., et al., 2009. Arrhythmogenic right ventricular cardiomyopathy. Lancet 373, 1289–1300.

Baumgartner, H., Bonhoeffer, P., De Groot, N.M.S., et al., 2010. ESC guidelines for the management of grown up congenital heart disease (new version 2010). Eur. Heart J. 31, 2915–2957.

Bavnbek, K., Ahsan, S.Y., Sanders, J., et al., 2010. Wound management and restrictive arm movement following cardiac device implantation: evidence for practice? Eur. J. Cardiovasc. Nurs. 9 (2), 85–91.

Bonow, R.O., Mann, D.L., Zipes, D.P., Libby, P. (Eds.), 2012. Braunwald's Heart Disease: A Textbook of Cardiovascular Medicine. Saunders Elsevier, Philadelphia.

Bonow, R.O., Carabello, B.A., Chatterjee, K., et al., 2006. ACC/AHA 2006 guidelines for the management of patients with valvular heart disease: a report of the American College of Cardiology/American Heart Association Task Force on Practice Guidelines. Circulation 114, e84–e231.

Braverman, A.C., Thompson, R.W., Sanchez, L.A., 2012. Diseases of the aorta. In: Bonow, R.O., Mann, D.L., Zipes, D.P., Libby, P. (Eds.), Braunwald's Heart Disease: A Textbook of Cardiovascular Medicine. Saunders Elsevier, Philadelphia, pp. 1309–1337.

Brignole, M., Auricchio, A., Baron-Esquivias, G., et al., 2013. 2013 ESC guidelines on cardiac pacing and cardiac resynchronization therapy. Europace 15, 1070–1118.

Campeau, L., 1976. Letter: grading of angina pectoris. Circulation 54 (3), 522–523.

Carpentier, A., Adams, D.H., Filsoufi, F., 2010. Carpentier's Reconstructive Valve Surgery: From VALVE analysis to Valve Reconstruction. Saunders Elsevier, Maryland Heights, Missouri.

Cheng, D., Martin, J., Shennib, H., et al., 2010. Endovascular aortic repair versus open surgical repair for descending thoracic aortic disease: a systematic review and meta-analysis of comparative studies. J. Am. Coll. Cardiol. 55 (10), 986–1001.

Coady, M.A., Ikonomidis, J.S., Cheung, A.T., et al., 2010. Surgical management of descending thoracic aortic disease: open and endovascular approaches: a scientific statement from the American Heart Association. Circulation 121, 2780–2804.

Connolly, H.M., Oh, J.K., 2012. Echocardiography. In: Bonow, R.O., Mann, D.L., Zipes, D.P., Libby, P. (Eds.), Braunwald's Heart Disease: A Textbook of Cardiovascular Medicine. Saunders Elsevier, Philadelphia, pp. 200–276.

Cooper, B.G., 2011. An update on contraindications for lung function testing. Thorax 66, 714–723.

Creager, M.A., Libby, P., 2012. Peripheral artery diseases. In: Bonow, R.O., Mann, D.L., Zipes, D.P., Libby, P. (Eds.), Braunwald's Heart Disease: A Textbook of Cardiovascular Medicine. Saunders Elsevier, Philadelphia, pp. 1338–1358.

Davies, E.J., Moxham, T., Rees, K., et al., 2010. Exercise based rehabilitation for heart failure. Cochrane Database Syst. Rev. (4), CD003331.

Eagle, K.A., Guyton, R.A., Davidoff, R., et al., 2004. ACC/AHA 2004 guideline update for coronary artery bypass graft surgery: a report of the American College of Cardiology/American Heart

Association Task Force on Practice Guidelines (Committee to Update the 1999 Guidelines for Coronary Artery Bypass Graft Surgery). Circulation 110 (14), e340–e437.

Elliott, P., Andersson, B., Arbustini, E., et al., 2008. Classification of the cardiomyopathies: a position statement from the European Society of Cardiology Working Group on Myocardial and Pericardial Diseases. Eur. Heart J. 29, 270–276.

Epstein, A.E., DiMarco, J.P., Ellenbogen, K.A., et al., 2013. 2012 ACCF/AHA/HRS focused update into the ACCF/AHA/HRS 2008 guidelines for device-based therapy of cardiac rhythm abnormalities: a report of the American College of Cardiology Foundation/American Heart Association Task Force on Practice Guidelines and the Heart Rhythm Society. Circulation 127, e283–e352.

Erbel, R., Alfonso, F., Boileau, C., et al., 2001. Diagnosis and management of aortic dissection: recommendations of the Task Force on Aortic Dissection, European Society of Cardiology. Eur. Heart J. 22, 1642–1681.

Fihn, S.D., Gardin, J.M., Abrams, J., et al., 2012. Guidelines for the diagnosis and management of patients with stable ischemic heart disease: executive summary. A report of the American College of Cardiology Foundation/American Heart Association Task Force on Practice Guidelines, and the American College of Physician, American Association for Thoracic Surgery, Preventative Cardiovascular Nurses Association, Society for Cardiovascular Angiography and Interventions and Society of Thoracic Surgeons 2012. Circulation 126, 3097–3137.

Gatzoulis, M.A., Webb, G.D., 2003. Adults with congenital heart disease: a growing population. In: Gatzoulis, M.A., Webb, G.D., Daubeney, P.E.F. (Eds.), Diagnosis and Management of Adult Congenital Heart Disease. Churchill Livingstone, Philadelphia, pp. 2–4.

Gaziano, J.M., Manson, J.E., Ridker, P.M., 2008. Primary and secondary prevention of coronary heart disease. In: Libby, P., Bonow, R.O., Zipes, D.P., Mann, D.L. (Eds.), Braunwald's Heart Disease: A Textbook of Cardiovascular Medicine, eighth ed. Saunders Elsevier, Philadelphia, pp. 1119–1148.

Gaziano, T.A., Gaziano, J.M., 2012. Global burden of cardiovascular disease. In: Bonow, R.O., Mann, D.L., Zipes, D.P., Libby, P. (Eds.), Braunwald's Heart Disease: A Textbook of Cardiovascular Medicine. Saunders Elsevier, Philadelphia, pp. 1–20.

Gersh, B.J., Maron, B.J., Bonow, R.O., et al., 2011. 2011 ACCF/AHA guideline for the diagnosis and treatment of hypertrophic cardiomyopathy: executive summary. Circulation 124, 2761–2796.

Goldhaber, S.Z., 2012. Pulmonary embolism. In: Bonow, R.O., Mann, D.L., Zipes, D.P., Libby, P. (Eds.), Braunwald's Heart Disease: A Textbook of Cardiovascular Medicine. Saunders Elsevier, Philadelphia, pp. 1679–1695.

Gongora, E., Sundt, T.M., 2008. Myocardial Revascularization with Cardiopulmonary Bypass. In: Cohn, L. (Ed.), Cardiac Surgery in the Adult, third ed. McGraw-Hill, New York, pp. 599–632.

Greenberg, B., Kahn, A.M., 2012. Clinical assessment of heart failure. In: Bonow, R.O., Mann, D.L., Zipes, D.P., Libby, P. (Eds.), Braunwald's Heart Disease: A Textbook of Cardiovascular Medicine. Saunders Elsevier, Philadelphia, pp. 505–516.

Guyton, A.C., Hall, J.E., 1996. Heart muscle; the heart as a pump. In: Guyton, A.C., Hall, J.E. (Eds.), Textbook of Medical Physiology, ninth ed. W.B. Saunders Company, Philadelphia, pp. 107–119.

Hare, J.M., 2012. The dilated, restricted and infiltrative cardiomyopathies. In: Bonow, R.O., Mann, D.L., Zipes, D.P., Libby, P. (Eds.), Braunwald's Heart Disease: A Textbook of Cardiovascular Medicine. Saunders Elsevier, Philadelphia, pp. 1561–1581.

Higgins, R.O., Murphy, B.M., Goble, A.J., et al., 2008. Cardiac rehabilitation program attendance after coronary artery bypass surgery: overcoming the barriers. Med. J. Aust. 188 (12), 712–714.

Hiratzka, L.F., Bakris, G.L., Beckman, J.A., et al., 2010. 2010 ACCF/AHA/AATS/ACR/ASA/SCA/SCAI/SIR/STS/SVM Guidelines for the diagnosis and management of patients with thoracic aortic disease. Circulation 121, e266–e369.

Hirschhorn, A.D., Richards, D., Mungovan, S.F., et al., 2008. Supervised moderate intensity exercise improves distance walked at hospital discharge following coronary artery bypass graft surgery – a randomised, controlled trial. Heart Lung Circ. 17 (2), 129–138.

Ho, S.Y., 2003. Cardiac morphology and nomenclature. In: Gatzoulis, M.A., Webb, G.D., Daubeney, P.E.F. (Eds.), Diagnosis and Management of Adult Congenital Heart Disease. Churchill Livingstone, Philadelphia, pp. 5–13.

Ho, W.K., Hankey, G.J., Lee, C.H., Eikelboom, J.W., 2005. Venous thromboembolism: diagnosis and management of deep vein thrombosis. Med. J. Aust. 182 (9), 476–481.

Hulot, J.S., Jouven, X., Empana, J.P., et al., 2004. Natural history and risk stratification of arrhythmogenic right ventricular dysplasia/cardiomyopathy. Circulation 1110, 1879–1884.

Hulzebos, E.H.J., Helders, P.J.M., Favie, N.J., et al., 2006. Preoperative intensive inspiratory muscle training to prevent postoperative pulmonary complications in high-risk patients undergoing CABG surgery – a randomized clinical trial. J. Am. Med. Assoc. 296 (15), 1851–1857.

Hundley, W.G., Bluemke, D.A., Finn, J.P., et al., 2010. ACCF/ACR/AHA/NASCI/SCMR 2010 expert consensus document on cardiovascular magnetic resonance: a report of the American College of Cardiology Task Force on Expert Consensus Documents. Circulation 121, 2462–2508.

Hunt, S.A., 2006. ACC/AHA guidelines: A-, B-, C-, and D-based approach to chronic heart failure therapy. Eur. Heart J. Suppl. 8, e3–e5.

Imazio, M., Adler, Y., 2013. Management of pericardial effusion. Eur. Heart J. 34, 1186–1197.

Imazio, M., Mayosi, B.M., Brucato, A., Adler, Y., 2010. Pericardial effusion triage. Int. J. Cardiol. 145 (2), 403–404.

Jaeger, F.J. 2012, 'Cardiac arrhythmias', Cleveland Clinic Center for Continuing Education, viewed 15 January 2014, <http://www.clevelandclinicmeded.com/medicalpubs/diseasemanagement/cardiology/cardiac-arrhythmias/>.

Jaff, M.R., McMurtry, S., Archer, S.L., et al., 2011. Management of massive and submassive pulmonary embolism, iliofemoral deep vein thrombosis, and chronic thromboembolic pulmonary hypertension: a scientific statement from the American Heart Association. Circulation 123, 1788–1830.

Jefferies, J.L., Towbin, J.A., 2010. Dilated cardiomyopathy. Lancet 375, 752–762.

Johnston, K.W., Rutherford, R.B., Tilson, M.D., et al., 1991. Suggested standards for reporting on arterial aneurysms. J. Vasc. Surg. 13 (3), 452–458.

Kearon, C., 2003. Natural history of venous thromboembolism. Circulation 107, 22–30.

Kemp, C.D., Conte, J.V., 2012. The pathophysiology of heart failure. Cardiovasc. Pathol. 21, 365–371.

Khandaker, M.H., Espinosa, R.E., Nishimura, R.A., et al., 2010. Pericardial disease: diagnosis and management. Mayo Clin. Proc. 85 (6), 572–593.

Krum, H., Driscoll, A., 2013. Management of heart failure. Med. J. Aust. 199 (5), 174–178.

Kwong, R.Y., 2012. Cardiovascular magnetic resonance imaging. In: Bonow, R.O., Mann, D.L., Zipes, D.P., Libby, P. (Eds.), Braunwald's Heart Disease: A Textbook of Cardiovascular Medicine. Saunders Elsevier, Philadelphia, pp. 340–361.

Lee, C.H., Hankey, G.J., Ho, W.K., Eikelboom, J.W., 2005. Venous thromboembolism: diagnosis and management of pulmonary embolism. Med. J. Aust. 182 (11), 569–574.

Lemmer, J.H. Jr., Vlahakes, G.J., 2010. Operative Management. In: Lemmer, J.H., Jr., Vlahakes, G.J. (Eds.), Handbook of patient care in cardiac surgery, seventh ed. Lippincott Williams & Wilkins, Philadelphia, pp. 33–80.

LeWinter, W.M., Tischler, M.D., 2012. Pericardial diseases. In: Bonow, R.O., Mann, D.L., Zipes, D.P., Libby, P. (Eds.), Braunwald's heart disease: a textbook of cardiovascular medicine. Saunders Elsevier, Philadelphia, pp. 1651–1671.

Liu, Z., Tao, X., Chen, Y., et al., 2015. Bed rest versus early ambulation with standard anticoagulation in the management of deep vein thrombosis: a meta-analysis. PLoS ONE 10, e0121388.

Luepker, R.V., Apple, F.S., Christenson, R.H., et al., 2003. Case definitions for acute coronary heart disease in epidemiology and clinical research studies: a statement from the AHA Council on Epidemiology and Prevention; AHA Statistics Committee; World Heart Federation Council on Epidemiology and Prevention; the European Society of Cardiology Working Group on Epidemiology and Prevention; Centers for Disease Control and Prevention; and the National Heart, Lung, and Blood Institute. Circulation 108 (20), 2543–2549.

Macdonald, P., 2011. Pathophysiology of cardiac failure. In: Thompson, P.L. (Ed.), Coronary care manual, second ed. Elsevier Australia, Sydney, pp. 88–96.

Maisch, B., Seferovic, P.M., Ristic, A.D., et al., 2004. Guidelines on the diagnosis and management of pericardial diseases. Eur. Heart J. 25 (7), 1–28.

Mann, D.L., 2012a. Pathophysiology of heart failure. In: Bonow, R.O., Mann, D.L., Zipes, D.P., Libby, P. (Eds.), Braunwald's heart disease: a textbook of cardiovascular medicine. Saunders Elsevier, Philadelphia, pp. 487–504.

Mann, D.L., 2012b. Management of heart failure patients with reduced ejection fraction. In: Bonow, R.O., Mann, D.L., Zipes, D.P., Libby, P. (Eds.), Braunwald's heart disease: a textbook of cardiovascular medicine. Saunders Elsevier, Philadelphia, pp. 543–577.

Marcus, F.I., McKenna, W.J., Sherrill, D., et al., 2010. Diagnosis of arrhythmogenic right ventricular cardiomyopathy/dysplasia. Eur. Heart J. 31, 806–814.

Maron, B.J., 2012. Hypertrophic cardiomyopathy. In: Bonow, R.O., Mann, D.L., Zipes, D.P., Libby, P. (Eds.), Braunwald's heart disease: a textbook of cardiovascular medicine. Saunders Elsevier, Philadelphia, pp. 1582–1594.

Maron, B.J., McKenna, W.J., Danielson, G.K., et al., 2003. American College of Cardiology/European Society of Cardiology clinical expert consensus document on hypertrophic cardiomyopathy. Eur. Heart J. 24, 1965–1991.

Maron, B.J., Towbin, J.A., Thiene, G., et al., 2006. Contemporary definitions and classifications of the cardiomyopathies. Circulation 113, 1807–1816.

McMurray, J.J.V., Adamopoulos, S., Anker, S.D., et al., 2012. ESC guidelines for the diagnosis and treatment of acute and chronic heart failure 2012. Eur. Heart J. 33, 1787–1847.

Miller, J.M., Zipes, D.P., 2012a. Diagnosis of cardiac arrhythmias. In: Bonow, R.O., Mann, D.L., Zipes, D.P., Libby, P. (Eds.), Braunwald's Heart Disease: a Textbook of Cardiovascular Medicine. Saunders Elsevier, Philadelphia, pp. 687–709.

Miller, J.M., Zipes, D.P., 2012b. Therapy for cardiac arrhythmias. In: Bonow, R.O., Mann, D.L., Zipes, D.P., Libby, P. (Eds.), Braunwald's Heart Disease: A Textbook of Cardiovascular Medicine. Saunders Elsevier, Philadelphia, pp. 710–744.

Mittal, S., Movsowitz, C., Steinberg, J.S., 2011. Ambulatory external electrocardiographic monitoring. J. Am. Coll. Cardiol. 58, 1741–1749.

Morrow, D.A., Gersh, B.J., 2008. Chronic coronary artery disease. In: Libby, P., Bonow, R.O., Zipes, D.P., Mann, D.L. (Eds.), Braunwald's Heart Disease: A Textbook of Cardiovascular Medicine, eighth ed. Saunders Elsevier, Philadelphia, pp. 1353–1418.

Mos, I.C.M., Klok, F.A., Kroft, L.J.M., et al., 2012. Imaging tests in the diagnosis of pulmonary embolism. Semin. Respir. Crit. Care Med. 33, 138–143.

National Health and Medical Research Council, 2009. Clinical Practice Guideline for the Prevention of Venous Thromboembolism (Deep Vein Thrombosis and Pulmonary Embolism) in Patients Admitted to Australian Hospitals. National Health and Medical Research Council, Melbourne.

National Heart, Lung, and Blood Institute, Boston University 2014, Framingham Heart Study, viewed 15 January 2014, <http://www.framinghamheartstudy.org/>.

Norgren, L., Hiatt, W.R., Dormandy, J.A., et al., 2007. Inter-society consensus for the management of peripheral arterial disease (TASC II). J. Vasc. Surg. 45, s5–s67.

Novitzky, D., Shroyer, A.L., Collins, J.F., et al., 2007. A study design to assess the safety and efficacy of on-pump versus off-pump coronary bypass grafting: the ROOBY trial. Clin. Trials 4 (1), 81–91.

Otto, C.M., Bonow, R.O., 2012. Valvular heart disease. In: Bonow, R.O., Mann, D.L., Zipes, D.P., Libby, P. (Eds.), Braunwald's Heart Disease: A Textbook of Cardiovascular Medicine. Saunders Elsevier, Philadelphia, pp. 1468–1539.

Ozaki, A., Bartholomew, J.R. 2012, Pulmonary embolism, Cleveland Clinic Center for Continuing Education, viewed 15 January 2014,

<http://www.clevelandclinicmeded.com/medicalpubs/disease management/cardiology/venous-thromboembolism/>.

Padera, R.F. Jr., Schoen, F.J., 2010. Pathology of cardiac surgery. In: Cohn, L.H. (Ed.), Cardiac Surgery in the Adult, third ed. McGraw-Hill Education, New York, pp. 111–178.

Popma, J.J., 2012. Coronary arteriography. In: Bonow, R.O., Mann, D.L., Zipes, D.P., Libby, P. (Eds.), Braunwald's Heart Disease: A Textbook of Cardiovascular Medicine. Saunders, Philadelphia, pp. 406–440.

Riedel, M., 2001. Acute pulmonary embolism 1: pathophysiology, clinical presentation, and diagnosis. Heart 85, 229–240.

Ross, D.L., 2011. Catheter ablation of arrhythmias. In: Thompson, P.L. (Ed.), Coronary Care Manual, second ed. Churchill Livingstone, Sydney, pp. 406–416.

Rubart, M., Zipes, D.P., 2012. Genesis of cardiac arrhythmias: electrophysiologic considerations. In: Bonow, R.O., Mann, D.L., Zipes, D.P., Libby, P. (Eds.), Braunwald's Heart Disease: A Textbook of Cardiovascular Medicine. Saunders, Philadelphia, pp. 653–686.

Rutherford, R.B., Baker, J.D., Ernst, C., et al., 1997. Recommended standards for reports dealing with lower extremity ischemia: revised version. J. Vasc. Surg. 26 (3), 517–538.

Sabatine, M.S., Cannon, C.P., 2012. Approach to the patient with chest pain. In: Bonow, R.O., Mann, D.L., Zipes, D.P., Libby, P. (Eds.), Braunwald's Heart Disease: A Textbook of Cardiovascular Medicine. Saunders, Philadelphia, pp. 1076–1086.

Savci, S., Degirmenci, B., Saglam, M., et al., 2011. Short-term effects of inspiratory muscle training in coronary artery bypass graft surgery: a randomized controlled trial. Scand. Cardiovasc. J. 45, 286–293.

Sinning, J.-M., Werner, N., Nickenig, G., Grbe, E., 2012. Transcatheter aortic valve implantation: the evidence. Heart 98, iv65–iv72.

Smart, N.A., 2013. How do cardiorespiratory fitness improvements vary with physical training modality in heart failure patients? A quantitative guide. Exp. Clin. Cardio. 18, e21–e25.

Stather, P.W., Sidloff, D., Dattani, N., et al., 2013. Systematic review and meta-analysis of the early and late outcomes of open and endovascular repair of abdominal aortic aneurysm. Br. J. Surg. 100, 863–872.

Swerdlow, C.D., Hayes, D.L., Zipes, D.P., 2012. Pacemakers and implantable cardioverter-defibrillators. In: Bonow, R.O., Mann, D.L., Zipes, D.P., Libby, P. (Eds.), Braunwald's Heart Disease: A Textbook of Cardiovascular Medicine. Saunders, Philadelphia, pp. 745–770.

Takayama, T., Yamanouchi, D., 2013. Aneurysmal disease: the abdominal aorta. Surg. Clin. North Am. 93, 877–891.

Tendera, M., Aboyans, V., Bartelink, M., et al., 2011. ESC Guidelines on the diagnosis and treatment of peripheral artery diseases. Eur. Heart J. 32, 2851–2906.

Thygesen, K., Alpert, J.S., White, H.D., et al., 2007. Universal definition of myocardial infarction. Circulation 116 (22), 2634–2653.

Thygeson, K., Aplpert, J.S., Jaffe, A.S., et al., 2012. Third universal definition of myocardial infarction. Circulation 126, 2020–2035.

Torbicki, A., Perrier, A., Konstantinides, S., et al., 2008. Guidelines on the diagnosis and management of acute pulmonary embolism. Eur. Heart J. 29, 2276–2315.

Troughton, R.W., Asher, C.R., Klein, A.L., 2004. Pericarditis. Lancet 363, 717–727.

Turpie, A.G.G., Chin, B.S.P., Lip, G.Y.H., 2002. Venous thromboembolism: pathophysiology, clinical features, and prevention. Br. Med. J. 325, 887–890.

Vahanian, A., Alfieri, O., Andreotti, F., et al., 2012. Guidelines on the management of valvular heart disease (version 2012). Eur. Heart J. 33, 2451–2496.

Warnes, C.A., Williams, R.G., Bashore, T.M., et al., 2008. ACC/AHA 2008 guidelines for the management of adults with congenital heart disease. Circulation 118, e714–e833.

Watson, L., Ellis, B., Leng, G.C., 2008. Exercise for intermittent claudication. Cochrane Database Syst. Rev. (4), CD000990.

Webb, G.D., Smallhorn, J.F., Therrien, J., Redington, A.N., 2012. Congenital heart disease. In: Bonow, R.O., Mann, D.L., Zipes, D.P., Libby, P. (Eds.), Braunwald's Heart Disease: A Textbook of Cardiovascular Medicine. Saunders, Philadelphia, pp. 1411–1467.

Wells, P.S., Anderson, D.R., Bormanis, J., et al., 1997. Value of assessment of pretest probability of deep-vein thrombosis in clinical management. Lancet 350 (9094), 1795–1798.

Wennberg, P.W., 2013. Approach to the patient with peripheral arterial disease. Circulation 128, 2241–2250.

Wexler, R., Elton, T., Pleister, A., Feldman, D., 2009. Cardiomyopathy: an overview. Am. Fam. Physician 79 (9), 778–784.

Whaley, M.H., Brubaker, P.H., Otto, R. (Eds.), 2006. Exercise Prescription Modifications for Cardiac Patients. In: ACSM's Guidelines for Exercise Testing and Prescription, seventh ed. Lippincott Williams & Wilkins, Philadelphia, pp. 174–204.

World Health Organization, 2011. Global Status Report on Noncommunicable Diseases 2010. World Health Organization, Geneva.

Wynne, R., Botti, M., 2004. Postoperative pulmonary dysfunction in adults after cardiac surgery with cardiopulmonary bypass: clinical significance and implications for practice. Am. J. Crit. Care 13 (5), 384–393.

Yancy, C.W., Jessup, M., Bozkurt, B., et al. 2013, '2013 ACCF/AHA Guideline for the management of heart failure: a report of the American College of Cardiology Foundation/American Heart Association Task Force of Practice Guidelines', Circulation viewed 15 January 2014, <http://circ.ahajournals.org/content/early/2013/06/03/CIR.0b013e31829e8776.citation>.

Yared, K., Baggish, A.L., Picard, M.H., et al., 2010. Multimodality imaging of pericardial diseases. JACC Cardiovasc. Imaging 3 (6), 650–660.

Zakkar, M., Hornick, P., 2007. Surgery for coronary artery disease. Surgery 25 (5), 231–237.

5

RESPIRATORY DISEASES

ANNE E HOLLAND ■ JENNIFER A ALISON
with a contribution from

ALEX HARVEY ■ MANDY JONES
(Dysfunctional Breathing)

■ ■ ■ ■ ■ ■ ■ ■ ■ ■ ■ ■ ■ ■ ■ ■ ■ ■

CHAPTER OUTLINE

CHRONIC OBSTRUCTIVE PULMONARY
DISEASE 164
Aetiology 164
Pathophysiology 164
Clinical Features 167
Diagnosis/Investigations 168
Co-Morbid Conditions 168
Medical Management 168
Physiotherapy Management 169

BRONCHIECTASIS 170
Aetiology 170
Pathophysiology 170
Clinical Features 170
Diagnosis and Investigations 171
Medical Management 171
Physiotherapy Management 172

CYSTIC FIBROSIS 172
Aetiology 172
Pathophysiology 173
Clinical Features 173
Diagnosis and Investigations 174
Medical Management 174
Physiotherapy Management 175

INTERSTITIAL LUNG DISEASE 177
Clinical Features 178
Pathophysiology 178
Diagnosis and Investigations 178

Medical Management 178
Physiotherapy Management 179

PULMONARY ARTERIAL HYPERTENSION 179
Aetiology 179
Clinical Features 180
Pathophysiology 180
Diagnosis and Investigations 180
Medical Management 181
Physiotherapy Management 181

ASTHMA 182
Aetiology 182
Pathophysiology 182
Clinical Features 182
Diagnosis/Investigations 182
Medical Management 182
Physiotherapy Management 184

DYSFUNCTIONAL BREATHING 185
Carbon Dioxide Theory 185
Effects of Hypocapnia 185
Aetiology of Dysfunctional Breathing 186
Diagnosis of Dysfunctional Breathing 186
Management of Dysfunctional Breathing 186
Compensatory Breath Holds 187
Rescue Techniques 188
Dysfunctional Breathing and Speech 188
Dysfunctional Breathing and Exercise 188

REFERENCES 188

This chapter provides an overview of the clinical features, pathophysiology and management of some of the common respiratory conditions that are treated by physiotherapists.

CHRONIC OBSTRUCTIVE PULMONARY DISEASE

Chronic obstructive pulmonary disease (COPD) is a disease characterized by persistent airflow limitation that is usually progressive. COPD previously has been used as an umbrella term for the combination of chronic bronchitis and emphysema but COPD is now considered a disease entity in its own right (GOLD 2015). Previous terminology for COPD has been 'chronic obstructive airways disease (COAD)', 'chronic obstructive lung disease (COLD)' and 'chronic airflow limitation (CAL)'.

COPD is an increasing cause of morbidity and mortality, and is projected to be the fourth leading cause of death worldwide by 2030 (Mathers & Loncar 2006). The increase is related to the expanding epidemic of smoking and the impact of ageing. The prevalence of COPD is difficult to determine due to the under-diagnosis but in some countries, reported prevalence is as high as 20% of those aged over 60 years (Menezes et al 2005). COPD is more prevalent in smokers than non-smokers (see Aetiology) and those aged over 40 years, and higher in men than women, although in developed countries, the prevalence is almost equal in men and women, reflecting the changing pattern in cigarette smoking (Mannino et al 2002). However, it is important to note that there is a substantial prevalence of COPD (i.e. 3–11%) in people who have never smoked (Buist et al 2007).

The economic burden of COPD is high, with costs increasing with increasing disease severity. These costs are not only related to the direct healthcare costs but also to the lost productivity due to poor health and carer burden.

Aetiology

The most common cause of COPD is cigarette smoking. However, smoking other types of tobacco, passive smoking, inhalation of organic and inorganic dusts, chemical agents, fumes from the burning of biomass fuels (as might occur in cooking over open fires in a confined space) and outdoor air pollution

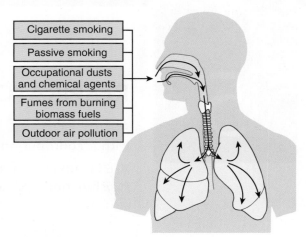

FIGURE 5-1 ■ Predisposing factors for chronic obstructive pulmonary disease (COPD).

increase the risk of developing COPD (Fig. 5-1), as do childhood respiratory infections and long-standing asthma. Foetal and childhood exposure to smoke and low socio-economic status are also risk factors for COPD. Alpha-1 antitrypsin deficiency, a genetically inherited disorder that occurs in a small percentage of the world's population, is associated with the development of early onset emphysema, with or without a smoking history.

Pathophysiology

The inhalation of noxious particles causes lung inflammation and results in the following changes within the lungs:

1. Mucous gland hypertrophy with consequent increased mucus production
2. Destruction of ciliated epithelial cells in the airway walls (Fig. 5-2)
3. Chronic inflammatory changes and associated small airway fibrosis with consequent narrowing in the small airways
4. Increase in bronchial smooth muscle (Chung 2005)
5. Loss of alveolar walls with consequent destruction of associated capillary beds (Fig. 5-3).

The pathophysiological changes in the mucus secreting glands and the destruction of cilia in the airways result in increased sputum production and reduced mucociliary clearance. Chronic cough and sputum expectoration as a consequence of these changes are indicative of chronic bronchitis, for which the following clinical definition is used: sputum expectoration on most days for at least 3 months of the year over 2 successive years.

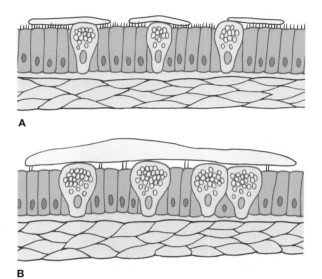

A

B

FIGURE 5-2 ■ Bronchial mucosa in chronic bronchitis. **(A)** Normal bronchial mucosa. **(B)** Bronchial mucosa showing enlarged mucus secreting glands and loss of ciliated epithelial cells.

The loss of alveolar walls is indicative of emphysema, for which the following anatomical definition is used: enlargement of the air spaces distal to the terminal bronchiole, with destruction of their walls.

Consequences of the Pathological Changes

1. Airflow limitation and lung hyperinflation

The changes in lung pathology, illustrated in Figure 5-4, lead to airflow limitation, which results in a reduction of expired gas and consequent gas trapping, causing lung hyperinflation. Hyperinflation alters the mechanics of breathing, placing the diaphragm in a more shortened, low flat position (Fig. 5-5) which reduces its contribution to ventilation. The consequences of hyperinflation become more evident during exertion when ventilation increases by increases in tidal volume and respiratory rate, the latter requiring increased inspiratory and expiratory flow rates. The increased flow rates reduce the time for expiration which, in the presence of expiratory flow limitation, results in further hyperinflation during exercise (i.e. dynamic hyperinflation). Dynamic hyperinflation further impacts on the mechanics of breathing, causing an increased sensation of dyspnoea (O'Donnell 2001) (Fig. 5-6).

2. Gas exchange abnormalities

Gas exchange abnormalities arise from alveolar and capillary bed destruction, leading to increased

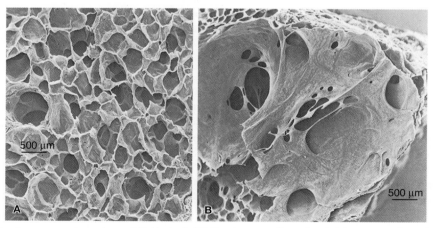

A 500 μm

B 500 μm

FIGURE 5-3 ■ Emphysematous lung tissue. **(A)** Normal. **(B)** Emphysema. *(Reproduced with permission from Thibodeau, G., Patton, K.T., 2008. Structure and Function of the Body, thirteenth ed. Mosby.)*

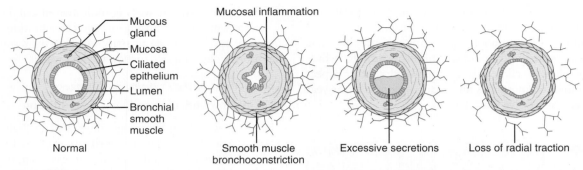

FIGURE 5-4 ■ Causes of increased resistance to the flow of expiratory air. Schematic representation of a normal airway and causes of airway narrowing: airway inflammation, smooth muscle bronchoconstriction, mucus hypersecretion and loss of radial traction due to alveolar destruction. The latter results in the airways being more compressible during expiration. *(Adapted with permission from Ellis, E., Alison, J. (Eds.), 1992. Key Issues in Cardiorespiratory Physiotherapy, Butterworth-Heinemann, Oxford.)*

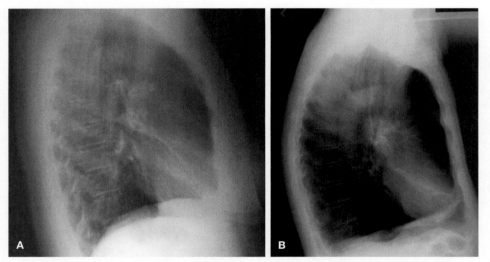

FIGURE 5-5 ■ Chest radiograph in emphysema. **(A)** Normal. **(B)** Emphysema. *(Reproduced with permission from Davies, A., Moores, C., 2010. The Respiratory System: Basic Science and Clinical Conditions, 2e, Churchill Livingstone (A), and Goldman, L., Ausiello, D.A., 2008. Cecil Medicine, twenty-third ed. Saunders (B).)*

physiological dead space (i.e. a high dead space to tidal volume ratio (V_D/V_T)) and ventilation–perfusion $(\dot{V}/\dot{Q})$ mismatch. During exertion, the high V_D/V_T means that there is an increased requirement for ventilation for a given level of carbon dioxide production, while the $\dot{V}/\dot{Q}$ mismatch results in oxygen desaturation which may further increase ventilatory demand and the sensation of dyspnoea (O'Donnell 2001).

3. Dyspnoea

Both the altered mechanics of breathing due to hyperinflation and the gas exchange abnormalities contribute to dyspnoea. People with mild disease only experience dyspnoea at high levels of exertion, whereas those with moderate to severe COPD may become dyspnoeic during everyday tasks. More about dyspnoea and breathlessness can be found in Chapter 12.

4. Reduced exercise tolerance

These physiological impairments such as airflow limitation, dynamic hyperinflation, altered mechanics of breathing and gas exchange abnormalities (O'Donnell 2001) contribute to ventilatory constraints

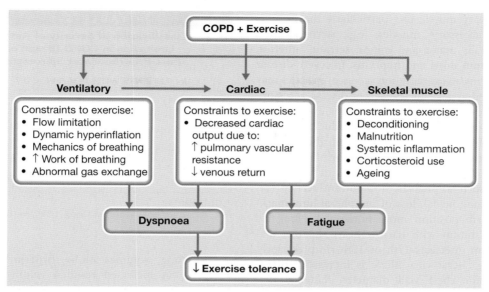

FIGURE 5-6 ■ Ventilatory constraints to exercise and reduction in exercise tolerance in people with chronic obstructive pulmonary disease (COPD). *(Reproduced with permission from Alison, J.A., McKeough, Z.J., 2010. Exercise and quality of life in COPD. In: Preedy, V.R., Watson, R.R. (Eds.), Handbook of Disease Burdens and Quality of Life Measures. Springer, New York.)*

to exercise (see Fig. 5-6) and a reduction in exercise tolerance in people with COPD compared to age-matched healthy individuals (Watz et al 2009). Dyspnoea, related to these physiological impairments, is often the symptom that limits exercise; however, skeletal muscle deconditioning due to the vicious cycle of dyspnoea limiting exercise participation is also an important contribution to reduced exercise tolerance.

5. Skeletal muscle dysfunction

People with COPD may have skeletal muscle dysfunction most likely due to deconditioning related to inactivity caused by exertional dyspnoea ('Skeletal muscle dysfunction in COPD. A statement of the American Thoracic Society and European Respiratory Society' 1999). Besides deconditioning, other factors such as malnutrition, skeletal muscle myopathy, low levels of anabolic hormones, systemic inflammation, corticosteroid use, ageing, increased lactic acid production and hypoxia may contribute to skeletal muscle dysfunction ('Key concepts and advances in pulmonary rehabilitation. A statement of the American Thoracic Society and European Respiratory Society' 2013; Spruit et al 2013) (see Fig. 5-6).

6. Reduced cardiac output

Cardiac output may be reduced due to a reduction in right ventricular stroke volume as a consequence of increased pulmonary vascular resistance from hypoxic vasoconstriction and/or loss of capillary bed and vascular restructuring. A reduced right heart pre-load from decreased venous return consequent to hyperinflation may also reduce cardiac output (Sietsema 2001). During exercise, such reductions in cardiac output may limit blood supply, and thus oxygen availability, to the exercising muscles, with early onset of lactic acidosis (Casaburi et al 1991) adding to the constraints to exercise in COPD (see Fig. 5-6).

Clinical Features

The main symptoms of COPD are progressive dyspnoea, cough and sputum. On examination a person with COPD may have the following signs depending on disease severity. The more severe the disease the more obvious the following signs will be:

■ Barrel chest, where the antero-posterior diameter of the chest wall is enlarged (like a barrel) due to hyperinflation.

- Accessory muscle use, particularly the inspiratory accessory muscles, e.g. sternomastoid, pectoralis major and minor, serratus anterior, latissimus dorsi and trapezius. In severe disease or during an exacerbation accessory muscles may be used at rest. In less severe disease accessory muscle use may only occur during exercise. The accessory muscles are recruited due to the diaphragm being less available to contribute to ventilation as a consequence of hyperinflation.
- Chest radiograph showing signs of hyperinflation such as increased radiotranslucency (i.e. dark lung fields), loss of peripheral lung markings, rib position more horizontal, elongated mediastinum with narrow heart shadow; diaphragm intersects 11th or 12th rib posteriorly. In the lateral view, there is increased antero-posterior chest wall diameter, flattened diaphragm and more air in space between sternum and heart shadow (see Fig. 5-5).
- Decreased breath sounds on auscultation due to loss of alveoli and hyperinflation. There may be coarse crackles if sputum is present in the airways.
- Reduced functional exercise capacity measured by a reduced distance walked in either the 6-minute walk test or incremental shuttle walk test compared to predicted. See Chapter 6 for field walking tests.
- Oxygen desaturation during exercise. In severe disease oxygen saturation may be low at rest.

Diagnosis/Investigations

The following aid in the diagnosis of COPD.

- Symptoms of dyspnoea, chronic cough and/or sputum production
- History of exposure to tobacco smoke, noxious fumes, occupational dusts and chemicals
- Older age
- Lung function tests
  Spirometry: forced expiratory volume in 1 second (FEV_1) to forced vital capacity (FVC) ratio <0.7 indicating airway obstruction, combined with the following FEV_1 percentage predicted to indicate disease severity (Table 5-1). See section of pulmonary function testing in Chapter 1, Measuring Lung Volumes and Capacities.

TABLE 5-1		
Classification of Severity of Airflow Limitation in COPD (Based on Post-Bronchodilator Spirometry)		
IN PATIENTS WITH FEV_1/FVC < 0.7		
GOLD Stage*		
GOLD 1	Mild	$FEV_1 \geq 80\%$ predicted
GOLD 2	Moderate	$50\% \leq FEV_1 < 80\%$ predicted
GOLD 3	Severe	$30\% \leq FEV_1 < 50\%$ predicted
GOLD 4	Very severe	$FEV_1 < 30\%$ predicted

*(GOLD, 2015)
FEV_1, Forced expiratory volume in 1 second; *FVC*, forced vital capacity.

- Lung volumes show hyperinflation with an increased residual volume (RV) and functional residual capacity (FRC), and an increased RV to total lung capacity (TLC) ratio above predicted (see Chapter 1).
- Transfer factor for carbon monoxide (TLCO) is often reduced due to the loss of surface area for gas exchange as a consequence of destruction of the alveolar walls and associated capillary bed.
- Chest radiograph showing signs of hyperinflation as discussed (see Fig. 5-5).

Co-Morbid Conditions

COPD may be associated with other conditions due to smoking being a common risk factor, e.g. ischaemic heart disease, lung cancer and hypertension. Other common co-morbid conditions include bronchiectasis (O'Brien et al 2000, Patel et al 2004), heart failure, diabetes, osteoporosis, anxiety and/or depressive disorders (Key concepts in pulmonary rehabilitation 2013).

Medical Management

Smoking Cessation

Therapies to aid smoking cessation include behavioural counselling, nicotine replacement therapy and oral pharmacological agents. People with COPD who have recently quit smoking show improvements in lung function, respiratory symptoms and functional and mental status within the first 3 months of quitting (Tashkin et al 2011).

Vaccinations

People with COPD are advised to have an influenza vaccination, which reduces frequency of COPD exacerbations (Poole et al 2000), and also a pneumococcal vaccination.

Medications

Medications for people with COPD include inhaled short- and long-acting bronchodilators, inhaled corticosteroids and antibiotics during an acute infective exacerbation. Inhaler technique should be checked and corrected if necessary (see the section on inhaled medications in Chapter 7).

Surgical Interventions

Lung volume reduction surgery has been offered to people with COPD who meet specific criteria (Criner et al 2011). More recently, bronchoscopic lung volume reduction using valves, stents or steam (Shah et al 2011, Snell et al 2012) have been trialled. For a few patients with very severe COPD, lung transplantation may be considered.

Oxygen Therapy

Long-term continuous oxygen therapy may be appropriate to manage hypoxaemia (with or without right heart failure) in people with severe COPD. Continuous oxygen therapy for at least 15 hours per day has been shown to prolong life (Qaseem et al 2011). (See the section on oxygen therapy in Chapter 7.)

Ventilatory Support

Non-invasive ventilation (NIV) may be used in some patients with chronic respiratory failure, obstructive sleep apnoea or during an acute exacerbation (Chapter 7).

Physiotherapy Management

Pulmonary Rehabilitation

There is high level evidence from large randomized controlled trials and systematic reviews that pulmonary rehabilitation reduces dyspnoea, improves exercise capacity and quality of life and reduces hospital admissions and length of stay (Puhan et al 2009, Ries

et al 2007). Pulmonary rehabilitation after a hospital admission for an exacerbation of COPD reduced readmission to 14%, compared with 57% if no pulmonary rehabilitation was provided (Puhan et al 2009). See Chapter 12 for information on pulmonary rehabilitation.

Breathing Exercises

Various forms of breathing exercises such as pursed-lip breathing, diaphragmatic breathing, Pranayama yoga breathing and computer feedback to slow respiratory rate have been trialled in COPD. The proposed mechanism of action is that by slowing respiratory rate and increasing time for expiration, more gas will be exhaled, which may reduce hyperinflation, thus reducing dyspnoea and improving exercise capacity. A recent Cochrane review (Holland et al 2012b) concluded that breathing exercises may improve functional exercise capacity in those people with COPD unable to undertake exercise training, but did not provide additional benefit to exercise training. In addition, the effect of breathing exercises on dyspnoea was inconsistent. Currently there is not strong evidence for breathing exercises in COPD.

Airway Clearance

Airway clearance techniques (ACTs) (see Chapter 7) may be used to aid secretion clearance in people with COPD. During periods of stable COPD, there is some evidence that ACTs may reduce hospitalizations and improve quality of life (Osadnik et al 2012). During an acute exacerbation, ACTs have been shown to reduce the likelihood of requiring ventilatory support (via NIV or intubation) as well as reducing hospital length of stay (Osadnik et al 2012). ACTs that include some form of positive expiratory pressure (PEP) appear to be more effective.

Management during an Exacerbation

An exacerbation of COPD is characterized by a change in baseline dyspnoea, cough and/or sputum production that is beyond normal day-to-day variability and is acute in onset. During a hospital admission for an exacerbation of COPD, physiotherapy techniques to aid secretion clearance may be instituted if the patient has excessive secretions or difficulty clearing secretions (see Chapter 7). NIV may be used in respiratory failure to avoid intubation. While in hospital, early mobilization and promotion of physical activity should be part of patient management to reduce further deconditioning (Pitta et al 2006).

BRONCHIECTASIS

'Bronchiectasis' is the term used for the permanent abnormal dilatation of one or more bronchi (Barker 2002, Chang & Bilton 2008). While bronchiectasis is a feature of cystic fibrosis (CF), this section will be confined to non-CF bronchiectasis. Details on CF are outlined later in this chapter.

Aetiology

The major known causes of bronchiectasis are damage to the airways due to severe lower respiratory tract infections related to pneumonia, whooping cough or measles (usually in childhood) (Chang et al 2008, Eastham et al 2004, Karakoc et al 2009, Singleton et al 2000); immunodeficiencies which affect the respiratory system (Li et al 2005, Shoemark et al 2007); inhaled foreign bodies; gastric aspiration; primary ciliary dyskinesia; tuberculosis and allergic bronchopulmonary aspergillosis (Shoemark et al 2007). Bronchiectasis has also been associated as a secondary manifestation of primary lung diseases such as COPD (O'Brien et al 2000, Patel et al 2004), sarcoidosis (Lewis et al 2002) and bronchiolitis obliterans (Chang et al 1998). However, in more than half the cases the underlying cause of bronchiectasis is not identified (Pasteur et al 2010, Shoemark et al 2007).

The true prevalence of bronchiectasis is unknown, due in part to the lack of simple and inexpensive methods of diagnosis (Weycker et al 2005). Prevalence of bronchiectasis is higher in developing countries (Habesoglu et al 2011) and in the indigenous populations of affluent countries (Chang et al 2008, Edwards et al 2003, Singleton et al 2000). There is a perception that the prevalence of bronchiectasis is declining with antibiotics for childhood respiratory infections and immunization for measles and whooping cough. However, the prevalence rate in people aged 60 and over is increasing, probably due to improved diagnosis (Seitz et al 2012). There is also evidence of an increase

in the global burden of bronchiectasis with increasing hospitalizations (Seitz et al 2010) and mortality rates (Roberts & Hubbard 2010).

Pathophysiology

The inflammatory processes related to acute or chronic lung infection damage the cilia, which enables bacteria to remain in the airway and colonize the mucus. These microorganisms stimulate a host inflammatory response which further inhibits ciliary function, damages the elastic and muscular tissue of the bronchial walls and stimulates mucus production (Cole 1997) (Fig. 5-7). The loss of elastic and muscular tissue in the airway wall leads to a dilatation of the bronchi. A vicious cycle ensues where clearance of bronchial secretion from these dilated bronchi is impaired and secretions often become chronically infected, producing a persistent host inflammatory response which results in a progressive destructive lung disease. Depending upon the aetiology, bronchiectasis can be localized to a specific lung region or can be widespread.

Clinical Features

Symptoms vary according to disease severity, with some people being totally asymptomatic and others, with severe disease, having a cough productive of large amounts of purulent sputum which is sometimes bloodstained. Severe exacerbations may be accompanied by chest pain, breathlessness and fevers. The signs are non-specific and include auscultation findings of

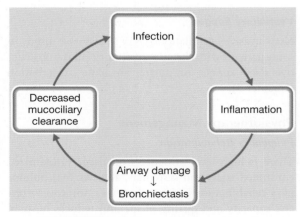

FIGURE 5-7 ■ Vicious cycle of bronchiectasis.

localized or widespread inspiratory and expiratory crackles with occasional wheezing. Clubbing of fingers and/or toes may occur in severe disease. In some cases of more severe disease, exercise tolerance may be reduced.

Diagnosis and Investigations

- High-resolution computed tomography (HRCT) scanning is the most definitive method of diagnosing bronchiectasis (Smith and Flower 1996). Findings on HRCT show one or more abnormally dilated bronchi (see Chapter 3). Such findings, with associated symptoms of chronic productive cough and recurrent lower respiratory tract infections, are indicative of bronchiectasis.
- Chest radiograph is an insensitive method for evaluating bronchiectasis, detecting less than 50% of patients with bronchiectasis (Currie et al 1987). The chest radiograph may be normal or there may be signs of thickened bronchial walls (tramlining), crowding of vessels with loss of volume and cyst-like shadows with fluid levels.

Investigations to aid with management:

- Sputum specimens are analyzed to identify the micro-organisms and their sensitivity to antibiotics. The most common bacteria found in bronchiectatic sputum are *Haemophilus influenzae*, *Streptococcus pneumoniae* and *Pseudomonas aeruginosa*. The latter is found in patients with diffuse bronchiectasis and associated with accelerated lung disease (Evans et al 1996).
- Lung function tests are used to assess severity of airflow obstruction and the degree of reversibility.

Investigations to identify possible underlying aetiology include:

- bronchoscopy if a foreign body or tumour is suspected
- serum immunoglobulins to detect hypogammaglobinaemia
- *Aspergillus* precipitins and serum total immunoglobulin E (IgE) levels to diagnose allergic bronchopulmonary aspergillosis
- gene mutation analysis in people with idiopathic bronchiectasis to exclude some of the more benign mutations of CF (Pasteur et al 2000)

- electron microscopy of the cilia if the diagnosis of primary ciliary dyskinesia is being considered (Ferkol & Leigh 2006).

Diagnosing the cause of bronchiectasis may help to define a specific approach to treatment.

Medical Management

Antibiotics are fundamental to treating infective exacerbations and controlling the severity of bronchiectasis. The choice of antibiotic will be determined by the sensitivity of micro-organisms grown in sputum culture. Antibiotics can be given orally, nebulized or intravenously. The route and frequency of delivery will be determined by the severity of the disease (Pasteur et al 2010, Wurzel et al 2011). Oral antibiotics may be given as prophylaxis for occasional infective exacerbations or continuously for repeated severe infections. Patients with severe disease and persistent purulent sputum who repeatedly relapse following a short course of antibiotics may be maintained on long-term oral antibiotics. Nebulized antibiotics may be used for patients with severe bronchiectasis whose disease is progressive and difficult to control (Currie 1997). Intravenous antibiotics may be used for severe disease, patients who fail to respond to oral antibiotics and those chronically infected with *P. aeruginosa*.

Bronchodilators may be prescribed if there is some demonstrable reversibility of airflow obstruction (Hassan et al 1999).

Hypertonic saline (4–7%) has been shown to increase the ciliary transportability of bronchiectatic sputum, probably through its action of altering mucus rheology and improving the hydration of the airway surface (Wills and Greenstone 2006). Short-term studies of inhaled nebulized hypertonic saline in bronchiectasis have shown reduced mucus viscosity, increased expectorated sputum, improved ease of expectoration and improved lung function (Kellett et al 2005). Longer-term studies of hypertonic saline, while demonstrating improved lung function, reduction in positive sputum cultures and improved quality of life, showed no differences in these outcomes compared to inhaling isotonic saline (Nicolson et al 2012). (See the section on inhalation therapy in Chapter 7.)

Mannitol is a naturally occurring sugar alcohol which when inhaled improves mucus clearance both acutely and over 24 hours in bronchiectasis (Daviskas & Rubin 2013). The proposed mechanism of action is that mannitol creates an osmotic gradient that draws water into the airway lumen, which improves hydration and alters the rheology of the mucus, enhancing mucociliary clearance and cough effectiveness (Daviskas & Rubin 2013).

Vaccination with both influenza and pneumococcal vaccines are recommended (Chang et al 2007a, 2007b).

Surgical resection may be considered only if the bronchiectasis is localized, but there are no randomized controlled trials to compare surgical versus conservative treatment in the decision-making process (Corless & Warburton 2000). In very severe widespread bronchiectasis with respiratory failure, lung transplantation may be considered.

Physiotherapy Management

Physiotherapy interventions may help in the treatment of excess bronchial secretions and reduced exercise tolerance.

Excess Bronchial Secretions

ACTs such as active cycle of breathing techniques (ACBT), postural drainage and PEP therapy (see Chapter 7) are commonly used to aid secretion clearance; however, there are limited studies of the effectiveness of such techniques in bronchiectasis (Lee et al 2013). The choice of ACTs will depend on the physiotherapy assessment, the disease severity, patient preference and the ability of the patient to use the ACT independently (Pasteur et al 2010). If an available HRCT scan indicates specific areas of bronchiectasis, these areas should be the target of the ACT. Any prescribed ACT should be re-evaluated for effectiveness over time. In some cases, a diagnosis of bronchiectasis may be confirmed in the absence of a daily sputum production. Such patients may be taught an ACT to be used during acute exacerbations of pulmonary infection (Pasteur et al 2010). The frequency of use of ACTs will vary among individuals and may be increased during episodes of superimposed infection.

During an acute exacerbation of pulmonary infection, patients may be hospitalized. The patient will probably be expectorating an increased amount of more purulent sputum and may be febrile, dehydrated and breathless. Haemoptysis is not uncommon and pleuritic chest pain may be present. ACTs, and possibly hypertonic saline, can be used to aid secretion clearance. If bronchodilators are prescribed, these should be taken before chest physiotherapy to aid secretion clearance. NIV (see Chapter 7) may be indicated if the patient is in respiratory failure.

Exercise Training

While there are only a few studies evaluating the effects of exercise training in bronchiectasis (Mandal et al 2012, Newall et al 2005), the principles of preventing deconditioning and improving exercise capacity and quality of life apply to bronchiectasis as in other chronic lung diseases. Thus exercise should be encouraged and in some cases pulmonary rehabilitation (see Chapter 12) may be beneficial. Limited evidence suggests that inspiratory muscle training (IMT) may improve exercise endurance and quality of life (Bradley et al 2002).

CYSTIC FIBROSIS

CF is the most common life-limiting inherited disease in Caucasian populations. It is a multi-system disorder of the exocrine glands, characterized by recurrent respiratory infections, pancreatic insufficiency and malnutrition. It is the most common cause of suppurative lung disease in children and young adults (de Abreau e Silva and Dodge 1995).

When CF was first recognized in the late 1930's, 70% of babies with the disease died within the first year of life (Andersen 1938). Life expectancy for those with CF has improved dramatically, with survival now approaching 50 years (Dodge et al 2007). Improvements have been attributed to earlier diagnosis, improved management in infancy, advances in nutritional management, improved ACTs, better antibiotics and comprehensive care at specialized CF centres (Bell et al 2008).

Aetiology

CF is caused by mutations in a single gene called the 'cystic fibrosis transmembrane conductance regulator (CFTR)'. The CFTR acts as a chloride channel in airway epithelial cells. Defects in the CFTR result in decreased secretion of chloride and water by airway epithelial cells, which leads to dehydrated mucus (Koch & Hoiby 1993). However, the CFTR may also have other functions including regulation of endosomal pH and adenosine triphosphate (ATP) transport and it may act as a receptor site for binding, endocytosing and clearing bacteria (Jaffe & Bush 2001).

Pathophysiology

CF is a systemic disease affecting a range of organs including the respiratory tract, gastrointestinal tract, genitourinary tract and hepatobiliary tree. Obstruction of exocrine ducts by viscous secretions plays a role in the pathogenesis of most of these manifestations. Ninety percent of the mortality and most of the morbidity is attributable to respiratory manifestations of CF (Ratjen & Doring 2003).

Most studies indicate that babies born with CF have normal lungs at birth (Boucher 2004, Hodson 2000, Jaffe & Bush 2001). Pathological changes develop rapidly, with inflammatory markers demonstrated in the lungs of babies as young as 4 weeks even before the onset of infection (Khan et al 1995). Alterations in electrolyte transport give rise to a decrease in height of the periciliary liquid layer and formation of mucous plaques and plugs, which are adherent to the airway surface (Boucher 2004). These factors diminish the efficiency of ciliary-dependent mucus clearance. The formation of thickened mucous plaques provides an ideal environment for proliferation of bacterial microorganisms and the CF airway becomes chronically infected (Boucher 2004). *Staphylococcus aureus* is most common early in life, however by adulthood 80–90% of patients will be colonized with *P. aeruginosa* (Robinson 2001, Wilson & Kotsimbos 2004), which is associated with faster deterioration in lung function. In some centres acquisition of *Burkholderia cepacia* has resulted in rapid decline and death in previously healthy patients, resulting in increased attention to infection control strategies in all centres (Doull 2001).

Clinical Features

Respiratory Features

The majority of older children and adults have a cough productive of sputum. Breathlessness on exertion is common, along with reduced exercise capacity and diminished physical activity compared to age-matched peers (Rasekaba et al 2013). The clinical course is generally marked by acute exacerbations of lung disease occurring on a background of chronic airway infection. Acute exacerbations are characterized by a constellation of respiratory and systemic

---

BOX 5-1

A DEFINITION OF AN ACUTE EXACERBATION OF CYSTIC FIBROSIS

An acute exacerbation may defined as the presence of ≥4 out of 12 signs and symptoms of a respiratory exacerbation:

- Change in sputum production
- New or increased haemoptysis
- Increased cough
- Increased dyspnoea
- Malaise
- Fatigue or lethargy
- Fever
- Anorexia or weight loss
- Sinus pain or tenderness
- Changes in sinus discharge
- Loss of appetite
- >10% (of best over the previous 6 months) deterioration in lung function

(Bradley et al 2001).

---

signs and symptoms (Box 5-1). Massive haemoptysis, defined as 300–500 mL over 24 hours, occurs in 5–7% of patients with CF (Porter et al 1983) and may be life-threatening. Minor haemoptysis, involving blood streaking of expectorated mucus, is far more common and is a frequent feature of exacerbations. Pneumothorax occurs in 5–8% of patients with CF. Incidence increases with age; 16–18% of patients over 18 years will experience a pneumothorax (Flume 2003).

Non-Respiratory Features

As CF is a multi-system disorder, non-respiratory features are also important. Pancreatic insufficiency, causing maldigestion and malabsorption of fats and proteins, occurs in 90% of people with CF by 1 year of age (Orenstein et al 2002). Inadequate nutritional status is linked to poor survival (Liou et al 2001). CF-related diabetes mellitus occurs in up to 50% of patients aged over 30 years (Lanng et al 1995) and it increases in incidence and severity during pulmonary exacerbations (Orenstein et al 2002). Recurrent episodes of distal intestinal obstruction occur in 3.5% of patients with CF as a result of excessively viscid intestinal secretions. A high incidence of gastro-oesophageal reflux has also been reported in CF (Ledson et al 1998), which may contribute to deterioration in respiratory function, particularly in infants (Button et al 2003). It is estimated that 17% of children and 24% of adults with CF have clinically significant liver disease.

Musculoskeletal Dysfunction

The prevalence of spinal pain in CF ranges from 43–94% (Botton et al 2003, Festini et al 2004, Flume et al 2009, Hayes et al 2011, Kelemen et al 2012, Parasa & Maffulli 1999, Ravilly et al 1996a, 1996b, Sawicki et al 2008, Sermet-Gaudelus et al 2009, Stenekes et al 2009) and prevalence of chest pain from 16–64% (Festini et al 2004, Hayes et al 2011, Kelemen et al 2012, Koh et al 2005b, Ravilly et al 1996b, Sermet-Gaudelus et al 2009). CF arthropathy affects up to 9% of patients, resulting in joint pain, long bone pain, arthralgia and joint effusions, particularly during exacerbations (Botton et al 2003). Joint pain has also been reported in association with some antibiotic treatments. The prevalence of osteoporosis in adults with CF is 23.5% and osteopenia 38% (Paccou et al 2010). Increased rates of long bone, rib and vertebral fractures have been reported (Hind et al 2008). Presence of musculoskeletal pain in CF is associated with worse quality of life, increased respiratory symptoms, sleep disturbance, anxiety and depression (Chastain & Cook 2000, Eksterowicz 2000, Festini et al 2004, Flume et al 2009, Kelemen et al 2012, Koh et al 2005a, Ravilly et al 1996b, Sawicki et al 2008, Sermet-Gaudelus et al 2009, Stenekes et al 2009).

Diagnosis and Investigations

Newborn Screening

In many countries screening for CF occurs shortly after birth, by measurement of immunoreactive trypsin in a dry blood heelstick sample. This is followed by genetic testing for the most common CFTR mutations if required. The results of a large randomized controlled trial of newborn screening for CF reported improved height, weight and head circumference in a screened group compared with a non-screened group (Farrell et al 2001) as well as higher cognitive function (Koscik et al 2004), which may be due to an earlier and more aggressive approach to treatment.

Other Diagnostic Methods

Not all countries have adopted newborn screening and some diagnoses are made by other methods. In newborns, gastrointestinal abnormalities are often the earliest feature. Failure to pass meconium (meconium ileus) occurs in 10–15% of cases (Park & Grand 1981). Young children with CF may also present with failure to thrive due to pancreatic insufficiency and malabsorption. Occasionally older children present having been managed for other respiratory conditions such as asthma. In adulthood a late diagnosis may be made when the patient presents with infertility. Diagnosis is made on the basis of clinical findings supported by two positive sweat test results (Orenstein et al 2002). The results can be confirmed by genetic testing for two disease-causing CFTR mutations. In difficult cases the nasal potential difference can be used to directly measure the defects in electrolyte transport across the epithelium (Knowles et al 1995).

Monitoring

The progress of CF lung disease is monitored by serial measurements of spirometry in all patients with CF who are old enough to perform the procedure, as FEV_1 is an important predictor of survival (Kerem et al 1992). Measures of height and weight are also routinely monitored at clinic visits, along with more sophisticated measures of nutritional status as required. Sputum samples are also obtained regularly where possible (Bell et al 2008).

Medical Management

The mainstays of therapy in CF are antibiotic treatment, inhaled therapies, nutritional support and airway clearance. Patients with more severe disease may be considered for NIV and lung transplantation. It is generally accepted that outcomes are better when people with CF are treated in a specialist centre with a multi-disciplinary team which includes physiotherapy (Mahadeva et al 1998). Shared care arrangements, for example between specialist centres and regional centres, may also occur (Bell et al 2008).

Antibiotic Treatment

It is routine practice to treat acute exacerbations of CF lung disease with intravenous antibiotics appropriate to the infecting organism (Orenstein et al 2002). Treatment lasts for 10–14 days and can be given in hospital or at home, depending on the condition of the patient (Hodson 2000). Eradication therapy for *P. aeruginosa* is also common, where antibiotics are given upon the first detection of the organism with the aim of eliminating it from culture, with generally high success rates (Jones 2005). Macrolides are a long-term treatment for CF that have both antibiotic and anti-inflammatory properties, resulting in improvement in clinical status and preserved pulmonary function (Equi et al 2002, Saiman et al 2003).

Inhaled Therapies

Human recombinant dornase alfa (recombinant human deoxyribonuclease, rhDNase) decreases the viscoelasticity of airway secretions and aids expectoration. Two large-scale trials have shown benefits in lung function and number of exacerbations in those treated with once daily rhDNase compared with placebo in individuals with mild to moderate lung disease (Fuchs et al 1994, Quan et al 2001). Nebulized hypertonic saline has been used to draw fluid to the airway surface and improve mucociliary clearance. A large trial in adults with CF has shown improvement in lung function and reduction in exacerbations when hypertonic saline was inhaled twice daily for 48 weeks (Elkins et al 2006b). Some antibiotics may also be given via inhalation.

Nutritional Support

Pancreatic enzyme supplementation is required to ensure adequate fat absorption in 85% of patients with CF (Hodson 2000). Most patients also require fat-soluble vitamin supplementation and pharmacologic acid suppression. If adequate nutritional status cannot be maintained with these strategies, high-calorie oral supplements are given and some patients may require nocturnal gastrostomy or jejunostomy feeding (Orenstein et al 2002).

End Stage Disease

Lung transplantation confers a survival advantage for people with CF and early referral should be considered, especially in women with CF where survival time is less than that of men (McIntyre 2013). NIV is effective for patients developing respiratory failure, either nocturnally or as a bridge to transplantation (Hodson et al 1991, Young et al 2008). Expert symptom management, delivered with the assistance of a palliative care service, may be indicated to alleviate distressing breathlessness or other symptoms. It is important to offer palliation even if the patient is listed for transplantation.

Physiotherapy Management

Airway Clearance Techniques

ACTs are integral to CF care across the lifespan. Short-term beneficial effects on mucus transport have been documented (van der Schans et al 2003) and one uncontrolled study showed a detrimental effect on lung function when ACTs were withdrawn (Desmond et al 1983). Although this evidence base is not extensive, ACTs are considered to be such an integral component of CF care that it is unlikely that further trials will be conducted using a non-ACT comparison.

A variety of ACTs have been used in CF and details of their application can be found in Chapter 7. Several systematic reviews note that no single ACT is superior, nor is one approach suitable for all patients (Elkins et al 2006a, McKoy et al 2012, Morrison & Agnew 2009), such that treatments should be individualized. However, there are some general considerations for ACTs in CF that are outlined in the following sections.

Infants and Young Children. A number of studies have demonstrated provocation of gastro-oesophageal reflux during head-down tilted postural drainage in infants, children and adolescents with CF (Button et al 1997, 1998, Vandenplas et al 1991). A long-term study has shown that infants with CF who performed postural drainage with a head-down tilt had significantly worse lung function and more radiological changes at 5 years compared with those who did not use head-down tilt (Button et al 2003). As a result, modified postural drainage without head-down positioning is recommended for infants and young children who cannot actively participate in therapy. More recently there have been reports of more active forms of airway clearance for infants and young children, such as infant PEP, assisted autogenic drainage (Lannefors et al 2004), play and age-appropriate daily physical activity (Dennersten et al 2009).

Airway Clearance Techniques in Complex Patients. ACTs may need to be modified or withheld in the presence of haemoptysis (Wilson & Kotsimbos 2004). If haemoptysis is scant (<5 mL) it has been suggested that ACTs should continue, but avoid high pressure

PEP therapy and head-down tilt, and reduce the force of coughing (Flume et al 2010). Recurrent episodes of scant haemoptysis may not require modification to ACTs. With mild to moderate haemoptysis (<250 mL in 24 hours), cease manual techniques, positive pressure and positions involving head-down tilt. ACTs including active cycle of breathing, autogenic drainage (Flume et al 2010) and gentle huffing and coughing can be considered. For massive haemoptysis (>250 mL in 24 hours), position in high sidelying with bleeding side down (Thomas 2003) and cease ACT until active bleeding has resolved (Flume et al 2010).

Patients with pneumothoraxes may also require modification of their airway clearance regimen (Haworth et al 2000). Positive pressure ACTs should be ceased until cleared by the medical team. If the pneumothorax has been drained, consider cessation or reduction in positive pressure therapies while draining and for 48 hours afterwards, to avoid pleural fistula and risk of recurrence (Flume et al 2010). Gentle coughing and huffing can continue.

Exercise as Airway Clearance. In adults with CF, reduced mechanical impedance of sputum is reported with treadmill walking but not cycle exercise, and both forms of exercise improved ease of expectoration (Dwyer et al 2011). A transient increase in FEV_1 and peak expiratory flow rate following exercise has also been demonstrated in CF (Bilton et al 1992, Loughlin et al 1981, Macfarlane & Heaf 1990). This may facilitate the clearance of secretions and improve ventilation. Some people with mild lung disease and good lung function use exercise together with forced expiration (huffing), coughing and expectoration as standalone airway clearance therapy. Others with more extensive lung disease and larger volumes of sputum use exercise as an adjunct to a formal airway clearance therapy regimen.

INHALATION THERAPY. Physiotherapists play an important role in optimizing inhalation therapy. A slower breathing pattern results in more peripheral deposition of the inhaled medication, improved homogeneity of the deposition pattern and increased overall drug deposition (Laube et al 2000). For this reason physiotherapists often combine inhalation therapy with ACTs such as the ACBT or autogenic drainage (see Chapter 7). Changes in body position

(e.g. inhalations in sidelying) may also be used, although there is currently little evidence that this gives rise to changes in deposition of inhaled medications in CF lungs. The combination of PEP with inhalation therapy (most commonly hypertonic or isotonic saline) reduces total treatment time and thus minimizes treatment burden, although this practice has also been little studied.

MAXIMISING EXERCISE CAPACITY. Exercise training is a critical component of treatment for CF. Exercise capacity is a good predictor of survival in children and adults with CF (Nixon et al 1992, Pianosi et al 2005) and those with better physical fitness have better quality of life. Structured exercise programs for people with CF improve fitness, preserve lung function or slow the rate of pulmonary decline and maintain bone mineral density (Bradley & Moran 2008, Elbasan et al 2012, Hebestreit et al 2010, Hulzebos et al 2011, Paranjape et al 2012, Shoemaker et al 2008, Tejero Garcia et al 2011). It is recommended that all patients should be encouraged to exercise several times per week (Yankaskas et al 2004). Exercise training in CF should follow the well-established principles outlined in Chapter 12. Because of the importance of good infection control to long-term outcomes in CF (see Infection Control), group exercise classes are not recommended.

MANAGEMENT OF MUSCULOSKELETAL COMPLICATIONS. A physiotherapy approach including spinal joint mobilization, massage, muscle strengthening and postural advice has been shown to reduce pain and improve respiratory symptoms in CF (Lee et al 2009, Sandsund et al 2011). Weightbearing exercise should be encouraged to maximize bone health, especially during childhood and adolescence.

PREGNANCY AND CONTINENCE. As a result of increased survival, pregnancy in women with CF is more common. Pregnancy has physiological impacts on the respiratory, cardiac and musculoskeletal systems, which may in turn impact upon a woman's ability to undertake the airway clearance and exercise regimens that are required to maintain good health. A regular airway clearance routine is advised throughout pregnancy. Regular physiotherapy review is required and modifications to usual ACT routines may be needed (e.g. use of upright sitting postures). Modifications to exercise training should also be planned to maintain an appropriate level of physical activity throughout pregnancy.

The prevalence of urinary incontinence in girls and women with CF is significantly higher than age-matched peers, ranging from 22–74% (Browne et al 2009, Cornacchia et al 2001, Moran et al 2003, Nixon et al 2002, Orr et al 2001, Vella et al 2009, White et al 2000). Urinary incontinence may also be more prevalent in men with CF than their healthy peers, although less data are available (Browne et al 2009, Burge et al 2011, Gumery et al 2002). In CF, urinary incontinence is associated with high levels of anxiety and depression and poor quality of life (Gumery et al 2002, Nankivell et al 2010). While the cause of urinary incontinence in CF is not known, it is clear that symptoms are often experienced in association with ACTs and repetitive coughing. Pelvic floor muscle training effectively improves continence in women in the general population (Dumoulin & Hay-Smith 2010). Physiotherapists should screen for continence and offer pelvic floor muscle training as appropriate.

PHYSIOTHERAPY IN END STAGE DISEASE. Sputum clearance may provide important symptomatic relief and it may be appropriate to continue ACTs even during palliation, depending on the patient's wishes. Minimizing the work of breathing during airway clearance is an important consideration. Some patients will require more passive techniques such as percussion or thoracic compressions. NIV may also be useful to unload the respiratory muscles, relieve dyspnoea or as an adjunct to airway clearance (Sands et al 2011). Symptom management with soft-tissue massage and positioning should also be considered.

INFECTION CONTROL. Because respiratory tract infections have a critical impact on morbidity and mortality in CF (Ledson et al 2002), segregation and cohorting of patients according to respiratory organisms are now routinely practised ('Cystic fibrosis Australia, infection control and hygiene guidelines' 2000, 'Cystic Fibrosis Foundation. Infection control recommendations for patients with cystic fibrosis' 2001). Patients with different organisms should not carry out airway clearance or exercise in the same room. In many centres, no patient with CF may carry out treatment in the same room as another, regardless of colonizing organisms. Physiotherapists should be aware of each patient's colonizing organisms and their local infection control requirements. Patients with CF should never share airway clearance equipment and physiotherapists should use good hand hygiene.

INTERSTITIAL LUNG DISEASE

The interstitial lung diseases (ILDs) are a group of over 200 conditions which affect the lung interstitium. They are characterized by varying combinations of interstitial inflammation and fibrosis, a restrictive ventilatory pattern (see Chapter 1), impaired gas exchange, dyspnoea on exertion and reduced exercise capacity (Harris-Eze et al 1996, Hansen & Wasserman 1996). While some ILDs occur as a result of a known exposure (most often dust, drugs or allergens), the majority have no known cause (Box 5-2). Idiopathic pulmonary

---

BOX 5-2
CLASSIFICATION OF INTERSTITIAL LUNG DISEASES

INTERSTITIAL LUNG DISEASE OF KNOWN CAUSE

- Hypersensitivity pneumonitis – e.g. bird fancier's lung, other allergen exposure
- Pneumoconiosis – e.g. asbestosis, silicosis
- Drug induced – e.g. amiodarone, chemotherapeutic agents

INTERSTITIAL LUNG DISEASES OF UNKNOWN CAUSE

- Major idiopathic interstitial pneumonias
  - Idiopathic pulmonary fibrosis
  - Idiopathic nonspecific interstitial pneumonia
  - Respiratory bronchiolitis – interstitial lung disease
  - Desquamative interstitial pneumonia
  - Cryptogenic organizing pneumonia
  - Acute interstitial pneumonia
- Rare idiopathic interstitial pneumonias
  - Idiopathic lymphoid interstitial pneumonia
  - Idiopathic pleuroparenchymal fibroelastosis
- Unclassifiable idiopathic interstitial pneumonias
- Interstitial lung disease associated with connective tissue disease
  - e.g. Rheumatoid arthritis, scleroderma
- Granulomatous interstitial lung disease
  - e.g. Sarcoidosis
- Other interstitial lung disease, including
  - Lymphangioleiomyomatosis
  - Pulmonary Langerhans cell hystiocytosis
  - Eosinophilic pneumonias

Adapted from Ryu et al 2007 and Travis et al 2013.

fibrosis (IPF) is the most common form of ILD, accounting for 25–35% of cases (Ryu et al 2007). It is associated with the worst prognosis, with a median survival of 3–5 years (Mapel et al 1998). However, the clinical course varies widely and some patients with IPF will experience long periods of stability, while others will have frequent exacerbations or a rapid decline (Ley et al 2011).

Clinical Features

Dyspnoea on exertion is a prominent feature of the ILDs. Where disease is rapidly progressive, as in some patients with IPF, dyspnoea can be profound and distressing even on minimal activity. A dry persistent cough is also characteristic of the ILDs. Auscultation may reveal bilateral 'Velcro' crackles which occur throughout inspiration, particularly in IPF, although they may also be heard in other ILDs such as asbestosis and sarcoidosis (Cottin & Cordier 2012). Finger clubbing occurs in some patients and is a predictor of mortality in patients with combined pulmonary fibrosis and emphysema syndrome (Kishaba et al 2012).

Pathophysiology

The interstitium is the lung tissue between the alveolar epithelium and capillary endothelium. IPF is considered to be a disease of aberrant wound healing (Selman et al 2001), where an excessive response to injury results in thickening of the interstitium and impairment of gas exchange. In other ILDs, such as hypersensitivity pneumonitis, inflammation may contribute to interstitial thickening (Bradley et al 2008). Destruction of the pulmonary capillary bed may also occur, contributing to $\dot{V}/\dot{Q}$ mismatch and oxygen diffusion limitation (Agusti et al 1991). Circulatory limitation results from pulmonary capillary destruction and vasoconstriction, leading to pulmonary hypertension and cardiac dysfunction in some patients (Hansen & Wasserman 1996). As a result of the restrictive ventilatory pattern, rapid, shallow breathing is common in the ILDs, which worsens on exercise and as the disease progresses (Javaheri & Sicilian 1992). Ventilatory limitation to exercise may occur, although it is not a major contributor to exercise limitation in most patients (Harris-Eze et al 1996). Peripheral muscle dysfunction limits exercise capacity and

contributes up to 20% of the variance in peak oxygen uptake (Nishiyama et al 2005). This may be a result of physical deconditioning (Markovitz & Cooper 1998) or myopathy induced by common treatments such as corticosteroids and immunosuppressants (Nici et al 2006).

Diagnosis and Investigations

Obtaining an accurate diagnosis of the type of ILD is challenging but important, as it affects both estimation of prognosis and eligibility for treatment. A detailed clinical history and blood tests are used to assess for environmental and occupational exposures, presence of connective tissue disease or drug-related ILD. Spirometry characteristically shows a restrictive ventilatory pattern, and diffusing capacity for carbon monoxide is reduced. A high-resolution CT scan is required to make a diagnosis ('Idiopathic pulmonary fibrosis: The diagnosis and management of suspected idiopathic pulmonary fibrosis' 2013). In some cases a surgical lung biopsy is required to confirm that histological features are consistent with the clinical and radiological features. In IPF, it is recommended that diagnosis is made by a multi-disciplinary team consisting of a respiratory physician, radiologist and (when required) a pathologist (Travis et al 2013).

Medical Management

There is no conclusive evidence for any pharmacological management to increase survival in people with IPF (Raghu et al 2011, 'Idiopathic pulmonary fibrosis: The diagnosis and management of suspected idiopathic pulmonary fibrosis' 2013). However pirfenidone, an anti-fibrotic and anti-inflammatory agent, has been approved for use in some countries on the basis of trials showing a slowing of the decline in FVC (Noble et al 2011, Taniguchi et al 2010). There are many clinical trials underway and new treatment options for IPF are likely in the future. At present, supportive care plays a very important role in IPF management, particularly referral for pulmonary rehabilitation, oxygen therapy, and lung transplantation (Raghu et al 2011, 'Idiopathic pulmonary fibrosis: The diagnosis and management of suspected idiopathic pulmonary fibrosis' 2013). Management of co-morbidities may also have an important impact on long-term outcomes in IPF (Collard et al 2012), including treatment of gastro-oesophageal reflux, cardiovascular disease and mood disorders.

In other ILDs, treatment will depend on the underlying cause. For patients with hypersensitivity pneumonitis (e.g. 'bird fancier's lung'), removal of the antigen is essential and prednisolone may be required in some cases. Prednisolone may also be used to treat sarcoidosis if there is evidence of progressive disease or extra-pulmonary involvement. Immunosuppressive therapy may be used in connective tissue disease and scleroderma lung, depending on the severity or progression of disease. In some ILDs there may be no appropriate pharmacological management (Bradley et al 2008).

Physiotherapy Management

Pulmonary rehabilitation improves exercise capacity, symptoms and quality of life in people with ILD (Holland & Hill 2008) and it is recommended in international guidelines for IPF management (Raghu et al 2011, 'Idiopathic pulmonary fibrosis: The diagnosis and management of suspected idiopathic pulmonary fibrosis' 2013). Existing studies have used exercise training protocols developed for people with COPD (Holland et al 2008, Nishiyama et al 2008) and this approach appears to be safe and effective. However, modifications may be necessary for some patients with ILD. Profound exercise-induced desaturation and pulmonary hypertension are common, particularly in IPF (Glaser et al 2009, Lama et al 2003); as a result, high-flow oxygen therapy may be required during exercise. Where adherence to the exercise protocol is limited by distressing dyspnoea, an interval training approach may be useful. Close supervision during exercise is often required.

As the ILDs are a diverse group of chronic lung conditions, physiotherapists should be aware of special considerations for rehabilitation in some diagnostic groups. In IPF, referral to pulmonary rehabilitation early in the disease course may be required to attain larger and more sustained benefits, whereas those with other types of ILDs may attain benefits regardless of disease severity (Holland et al 2012a). Early referral to pulmonary rehabilitation should therefore be encouraged, particularly in IPF. Some patients with ILD may be listed for lung transplantation and physiotherapists should consider how best to optimize physical condition while on the waiting list, particularly peripheral muscle strength. For patients with connective tissue–related ILD, joint pathology and pain must be considered when establishing an exercise programme (Garin et al 2009) and low-impact training programs may be required (McNamara et al 2013).

Physiotherapists may also be required to treat patients who are admitted to hospital with an acute exacerbation of IPF. Acute exacerbations are defined as acute, clinically significant deteriorations of unidentifiable cause in patients with underlying IPF (Collard et al 2007). Patients with an acute exacerbation have a worsening of symptoms over 30 days or less, new bilateral radiographic opacities and the absence of infection or any other identifiable cause (Collard et al 2007). While physiotherapy will not impact on the underlying cause or clinical course of an acute exacerbation, there may be an important role in addressing the negative sequelae, including physical deconditioning related to inactivity and the effects of high-dose corticosteroid therapy on peripheral muscle (Raghu et al 2011). Physiotherapy assessment and treatment should follow the usual principles for patients with an acute respiratory illness (Chapter 2) and may address oxygenation, mobilization and rehabilitation as appropriate during the recovery phase.

PULMONARY ARTERIAL HYPERTENSION

Pulmonary hypertension is defined as an increase in the resting mean pulmonary arterial pressure to at least 25 mmHg on right heart catheterization (Galie et al 2009a). Pulmonary arterial hypertension (PAH) refers to a specific category of pulmonary hypertension (Group 1, Box 5-3). PAH has underlying pathophysiology that distinguishes it from other forms of pulmonary hypertension such as those arising due to left heart disease or lung disease, and has different treatment options.

Aetiology

In some people, PAH occurs without a family history of the disease or an identified risk factor (idiopathic PAH). A germline mutation in the bone morphogenetic protein receptor type 2 (BMPR2) gene has been linked to PAH in 70% of those with heritable disease, with other mutations detected in smaller numbers of

BOX 5-3
CLINICAL CLASSIFICATION OF PULMONARY HYPERTENSION

1. **Pulmonary arterial hypertension (PAH)**
   a. Idiopathic PAH
   b. Heritable PAH
   c. Drug and toxin induced PAH
   d. Associated with connective tissue disease, HIV infection, portal hypertension, congenital heart disease, schistosomiasis, chronic haemolytic anaemia
   e. Persistent pulmonary hypertension of the newborn
1'. **Pulmonary veno-occlusive disease (PVOD) and/or pulmonary capillary haemangiomatosis (PCH)**
2. **Pulmonary hypertension owing to left heart disease**
   a. Systolic dysfunction
   b. Diastolic dysfunction
   c. Valvular disease
3. **Pulmonary hypertension owing to lung diseases and/or hypoxia**
   a. Chronic obstructive pulmonary disease
   b. Interstitial lung disease
   c. Other pulmonary diseases with a mixed obstructive and restrictive pattern
   d. Sleep disordered breathing
   e. Alveolar hypoventilation disorders
   f. Chronic exposure to high altitude
   g. Developmental abnormalities
4. **Chronic thromboembolic pulmonary hypertension (CTEPH)**
5. **Pulmonary hypertension with unclear multifactorial mechanisms**
   a. Haematologic disorders – myeloproliferative disorders, splenectomy
   b. Systemic disorders – e.g. sarcoidosis, pulmonary Langerhans cell histiocytosis
   c. Metabolic disorders – glycogen storage disease, Gaucher disease, thyroid disorders
   d. Others – tumoural obstruction, fibrosing mediastinitis, chronic renal failure on dialysis (Simonneau et al 2009)

patients. Ingestion of some appetite suppressants is a known risk factor for developing PAH. In connective tissue disease PAH is seen in 7–12% of patients and it has also been reported in mixed connective tissue disease, systemic lupus erythematosus, rheumatoid arthritis, Sjögren syndrome and polymyositis. It is a rare but well-documented complication of HIV infection. Portopulmonary hypertension may be seen in advanced liver disease. In congenital heart disease, presence of a systemic-to-pulmonary shunt frequently results in development of pulmonary vascular disease

and PAH. Eisenmenger syndrome, where development of PAH results in reversal of the shunt and central cyanosis, is the most advanced form of PAH associated with congenital heart disease (Simonneau et al 2009).

Clinical Features

Dyspnoea is the presenting symptom in many people with PAH. However, a range of other symptoms can occur, including fatigue, dizziness, chest discomfort, chest pain, palpitations, cough, pre-syncope, syncope, lower limb oedema and abdominal distension. The non-specific nature of these symptoms may contribute to the delay in diagnosis experienced by many patients with PAH (Brown et al 2011). Without treatment the prognosis for people with PAH is extremely poor, with death usually resulting from right heart failure.

Pathophysiology

In PAH, endothelial dysfunction in the pulmonary arterial circulation results in vasoconstriction, remodelling of the vessel walls, inflammation and thrombosis. This leads to increased pulmonary vascular resistance, elevated pulmonary artery pressures and increased right ventricular afterload. Over time, right ventricular hypertrophy and dilatation result in right heart failure, with impairment of stroke volume and a reduction in systemic oxygen delivery (Galie et al 2009a).

During exercise pulmonary blood flow is increased, which may result in further elevation in pulmonary artery pressures due to reduced distensibility and size of the pulmonary vascular bed. The dilated right ventricle does not contract efficiently and as a result has limited capacity to increase stroke volume (Holverda et al 2006). The elevation in heart rate with exercise is also reduced (Provencher et al 2006). As a result, cardiac output may be insufficient to meet the demands of exercise. Abnormalities in gas exchange, ventilatory responses and systemic endothelial function may also contribute to exercise limitation (Fowler et al 2012). There is also increasing evidence of peripheral muscle dysfunction in people with PAH, which may contribute to ongoing reductions in exercise capacity even when pulmonary haemodynamics have stabilized or improved on medical therapy (Mainguy et al 2010b).

Diagnosis and Investigations

An echocardiogram is useful to estimate pulmonary arterial systolic pressure in patients with suspected

PAH. However, a definitive diagnosis can only be made with right heart catheterization, which allows direct evaluation of the pulmonary vasculature and can rule out left heart dysfunction or pulmonary venous hypertension. Right heart catheterization is mandatory if PAH-specific therapies are being considered, due to the potential for harm if they are used in non–group 1 PAH patients (see Box 5-3). Right heart catheterization also allows a more accurate assessment of disease severity and response to treatment.

Because elevated pulmonary artery pressures can occur due to a variety of underlying conditions (see Box 5-3), other investigations may be required to rule out alternative diagnoses. For instance, HRCT may be used to screen for ILD, or sleep studies to rule out obstructive sleep apnoea. Elevated levels of brain natriuretic peptide in peripheral blood (>150 pg/mL) correlate with poor survival (Fijalkowska et al 2006); however, this marker is also elevated in pulmonary hypertension due to left heart disease, so it is not diagnostic. The 6-minute walk distance has a strong relationship to survival in PAH (Benza et al 2010). It is commonly used to evaluate functional performance, screen for exercise-induced oxyhaemoglobin desaturation and document response to therapy.

Medical Management

The development of PAH-specific therapies has transformed the outlook for people with PAH, with many patients now able to achieve clinical stability and improvements in life expectancy. Three classes of medications, acting on three different pathways, have been approved for use in PAH. Endothelin receptor antagonists, phosphodiesterase type-5 inhibitors and prostanoids act via different pathways to improve symptoms, exercise capacity and pulmonary haemodynamics. A meta-analysis of 23 randomized controlled trials has shown 43% decrease in mortality for patients treated with PAH-specific therapies (Galie et al 2009b). Combination therapy with more than one PAH-specific therapy may be used in patients who are not responding to monotherapy. Calcium channel blockers may be useful in a small group of patients with PAH who respond favourably to acute vasodilator testing at the time of right heart catheterization. Anticoagulation, diuretics and oxygen therapy may be used in appropriate patients. Lung transplantation may be offered to those with advanced disease who are not responding to medical therapy (Galie et al 2009b).

Physiotherapy Management

Patients who are stable on PAH-specific therapies may benefit from supervised exercise training to improve exercise capacity and quality of life. A number of studies have shown that endurance and resistance training can be undertaken safely in this group, without evidence of disease progression. Although the initial programs were conducted in the inpatient setting with intensive monitoring (Mereles et al 2006), more recent studies show that similar benefits can be obtained with exercise training conducted entirely in the outpatient setting (de Man et al 2009, Fox et al 2011, Mainguy et al 2010a). The improvements in exercise capacity were accompanied by increased capillarization and oxidative enzyme activity in the quadriceps (de Man et al 2009), suggesting that peripheral muscle changes are an important contributor to outcomes.

People with PAH may report symptoms such as chest pain, palpitations or dizziness during exercise. A study of exercise training in 183 people with a variety of causes of pulmonary hypertension reported that seven individuals (4%) experienced pre-syncope or syncope during the course of the programme (Grunig et al 2012). Because the symptoms characteristic of PAH may not be detected by the usual symptom monitoring scales used during pulmonary rehabilitation (Nici et al 2006), physiotherapists should closely monitor people with PAH during exercise, as well as provide detailed education regarding self-monitoring and which symptoms should be avoided.

There are some special considerations for rehabilitation in PAH. A recent history of syncope on exertion is a contraindication to exercise training (Mainguy et al 2010a, Mereles et al 2006). To date, exercise training trials in PAH have only included participants who are stable on PAH-specific therapies and as a result, rehabilitation should only be considered in this group. Most trials of exercise training for people with PAH have used low- to moderate-intensity exercise prescriptions (de Man et al 2009, Fox et al 2011, Mereles et al 2006); however, a more recent study showed that treadmill training at 70–80% of heart rate reserve was well tolerated in female patients with moderate severity disease (Grunig et al 2012), suggesting that some patients with PAH may tolerate an exercise prescription similar to that generally used in pulmonary rehabilitation (Chapter 12). However, at present there is little information to guide exercise prescription in this group.

ASTHMA

Asthma is characterized by hyperreactive airways that respond to various stimuli by widespread inflammation and airway narrowing, which is often reversible either spontaneously or with treatment. The prevalence of asthma is estimated at approximately 300 million people of all ages worldwide (Global strategy for asthma management and prevention: GINA www.ginasthma.org http://www.ginasthma.org/local/uploads/files/GINA_Report_2015_Aug11.pdf) and is a major cause of disability and health resource utilization for those affected (Global strategy for asthma management and prevention: GINA www.ginasthma.org http://www.ginasthma.org/local/uploads/files/GINA_Report_2015_Aug11.pdf).

Aetiology

Asthma commonly begins in childhood but can occur at any age. There is often a predisposition to asthma if parents or close relatives are asthmatic or atopic. Environmental factors can trigger an attack of asthma, including allergens such as house dust mite; furred animals (dogs, cats, etc.); pollens and moulds and chemical irritants such as tobacco smoke, air pollution or inhaled chemicals. In addition, exercise (especially running in cold air), respiratory tract infections and some foods and drinks can also be triggers.

Pathophysiology

The mechanisms by which asthma occurs are complex and still under debate due to the variety of triggers for an attack of asthma. In asthma triggered by allergens, the antigen–antibody reaction causes the mast cells in the airways to degranulate, releasing substances that decrease cyclic adenosine monophosphate (AMP) in the bronchial smooth muscle, resulting in contraction (bronchoconstriction), and increase capillary permeability and inflammation. Mucous glands may be hypertrophied, releasing thick sticky mucus that can lead to mucous plugging of small airways.

Inflammatory cells (eosinophils) in the mucus may give the appearance of infection due to yellow colour.

Consequences of the Pathological Changes

The pathophysiological changes of bronchoconstriction, airway inflammation and mucous secretion lead to narrowed airways and mucous plugging and result in the following clinical signs and symptoms.

Clinical Features

Symptoms of asthma include recurrent episodes of wheezing, cough, breathlessness and chest tightness. Signs during an attack of asthma are wheeze on auscultation, obstructive pattern on spirometry, hyperinflation on chest X-ray, and use of accessory inspiratory muscles of breathing. Children with asthma often have atopic (allergic) features such as eczema, food allergies, hay fever or urticaria.

Diagnosis/Investigations

A clinical diagnosis of asthma is based on episodic symptoms of wheeze, chest tightness, breathlessness and cough, especially if such symptoms occur after exposure to an allergen and there is a strong positive family history of asthma and atopy. Reversal of symptoms and improved spirometry (less obstruction) after the inhalation of a bronchodilator medication aids with diagnosis. There are various challenge tests to measure airway responsiveness, which help to establish a diagnosis of asthma, including inhaled methacholine or histamine, inhaled mannitol or an exercise challenge test.

Medical Management

While there is no known cure for asthma, medications are largely effective in controlling asthma (Table 5-2). Thus drug therapy is the mainstay of medical management and is broadly divided into long-term 'controller' medications and short-term 'reliever' medications or combined therapy in which controller and reliever drugs are combined in one medication. The 'controller' drugs are mostly corticosteroids that reduce airway inflammation and chromones such as sodium cromglycate and nedocromil sodium that inhibit mast cell degranulation. The 'reliever' drugs are bronchodilators such as β_2-adrenergic agonists (e.g. salbutamol)

TABLE 5-2

Examples of Current Asthma (and COPD) Medications

RELIEVERS

Drug Class	Drug Name	Brand Names	Device	Device Colour
Inhaled short-acting β2 agonist bronchodilators	Salbutamol	Ventolin	MDI/nebules	Blue
		Airomir	MDI/Autohaler	Blue
		Asmol	MDI	Blue
		Epaq	MDI	Blue
	Terbutaline	Bricanyl	Turbuhaler	Blue
Inhaled short-acting anticholinergic bronchodilators	Ipratropium bromide	Apoven	MDI	Green
		Atrovent	MDI/nebules	Green
		Ipratrin		Green
Combination	Salbutamol and ipratropium bromide	Combivent	MDI	Green

PREVENTERS

Drug Class	Drug Name	Brand Names	Device	Device Colour
Inhaled corticosteroids	Beclomethasone	Qvar	MDI/Autohaler	Brown
	Budesonide	Pulmicort	Turbuhaler	Brown
	Fluticasone	Flixotide	MDI/Accuhaler	Orange
	Ciclesonide	Alvesco	MDI	Red
Non-steroidal inhaled anti-inflammatories	Sodium cromoglycate	Intal (Forte)	MDI	Purple
	Nedocromil sodium	Tilade	MDI	Yellow
Leukotriene receptor agonists	Montelukast sodium	Singulair	Tablet	
		Accolate	Tablet	
		Zafirlukast	Tablet	
Oral/parenteral steroids	Prednisolone	Panafcort	Tablet	
		PredMix	Liquid	

SYMPTOM CONTROLLERS

Drug Class	Drug Name	Brand Names	Device	Device Colour
Inhaled long-acting β2 agonist bronchodilators	Salmeterol	Serevent	MDI/Accuhaler	Green
	Eformoterol	Oxis	Turbuhaler	Green
	Eformoterol	Foradile	Aerolizer	Pale blue
	Indacaterol	OnBrez	Breezhaler	White and blue
For COPD only				
Inhaled long-acting anticholinergic bronchodilators	Tiotropium	Spiriva	Handihaler	Green and grey

COMBINATION MEDICATIONS

Drug Class	Drug Name	Brand Names	Device	Device Colour
Combination long-acting bronchodilators + corticosteroid	Fluticasone + salmeterol	Seretide	MDI/Accuhaler	Purple
	Budesonide + eformoterol	Symbicort	Turbuhaler	Red and white

COPD, Chronic obstructive pulmonary disease; *MDI*, metered dose inhaler.

that act to relax the bronchial smooth muscle. Combined therapy usually consists of a corticosteroid and a β_2 agonist. Most asthma medications are given via metered dose inhalers that deliver the drug directly to the lungs, thus largely avoiding systemic side effects. In addition, several nations have developed 'Asthma Management Plans' to promote maximal asthma control, patient self-efficacy and reduced morbidity from asthma and reliever medication use. The National Asthma Council of Australia has published one such plan that can be found at http://www.nationalasthma.org.au. This includes written *action plans* that aim to help those with asthma and/or their carers take early action to prevent or reduce the severity of an asthma attack (http://www.nationalasthma.org.au/health-professionals/asthma-action-plans). These online educational tools also include useful information related to using asthma (and COPD) medications, including videos of the correct inhaler technique (http://www.nationalasthma.org.au/understanding-asthma/using-your-medicines-correctly). Many of these resources are translated into other languages, including Arabic, Chinese, Greek, Italian, Turkish and Vietnamese.

Physiotherapy Management

The role of physiotherapy in the management of asthma has varied considerably over the years as the role of health professionals has changed and evidence for and against particular interventions has grown.

Education

Physiotherapists may play a key role in education about the condition and how to take inhaled medications; however, in many developed countries specific asthma educators perform this role (Fig. 5-8).

Exercise

Exercise can induce an attack of asthma (exercise-induced asthma or EIA). The proposed mechanism of EIA is that heat and water loss from the airways due to higher ventilation required for exercise changes the osmolarity within the airway and induces mast cell degranulation with release of mediators that cause bronchoconstriction. Asthmatic children with moderate to severe asthma have low levels of physical activity (Welsh et al 2004) and reduced aerobic capacity,

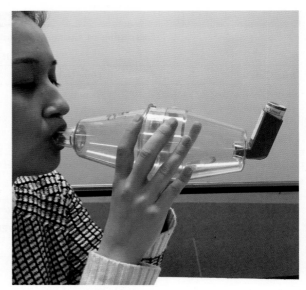

FIGURE 5-8 ■ Asthma patient using an inhaler with a spacer.

endurance time, and cardiac function (Alioglu et al 2007), particularly those who are obese or overweight, but this is certainly not the case for all asthmatic children. Physical inactivity in adults with asthma has been associated with poorer lung function, greater healthcare utilization and decreased quality of life (Avallone & McLeish 2013).

Physiotherapists may play a role in the exercise training of people with asthma. The aim of exercise training is to increase aerobic capacity so that the ventilation is lower for a given level of exercise after training, thus reducing the stimulus for EIA (Hallstrand et al 2000). It is important to note that higher aerobic capacity does not eliminate the potential for EIA (Thio et al 1996), only that a higher relative intensity of exercise can be achieved before the same level of ventilatory stimulus occurs. A Cochrane systematic review (Carson et al 2013) found that exercise training in people with asthma was well tolerated, improved aerobic capacity and had positive effects on health-related quality of life. Prior to exercise, the presence of bronchoconstriction should be determined and exercise should not proceed if airway obstruction persists after inhalation of a bronchodilator medication. Even if there are no symptoms of asthma, medications to block EIA may need to be given prior to exercise training.

Breathing Techniques

There is growing evidence for the role of breathing exercises in the management of asthma. Mechanistically, asthma may be associated with hyperventilation that reduces carbon dioxide levels leading to hypocapnia, which has been implicated as a contributor to bronchoconstriction (Laffey et al 2002, van den Elshout et al 1991). Breathing exercises that reduce hyperventilation and increase levels of carbon dioxide may aid in controlling asthma symptoms. A number of methods of breathing exercises have been developed such as the Papworth method (Holloway & West 2007), Buteyko method (Bruton & Lewith 2005, Burgess et al 2011) and yoga breathing (Burgess et al 2011, Singh et al 1990). There is some evidence from a Cochrane systematic review (Freitas et al 2013) that breathing exercises may have positive effects on asthma symptoms and asthma quality of life scores.

DYSFUNCTIONAL BREATHING

Dysfunctional breathing/hyperventilation syndrome (DB/HVS) is a respiratory disorder, psychologically or physiologically based, involving breathing too deeply and/or too rapidly (hyperventilation) (Brashear 1983), or erratic breathing interspersed with breath holding or sighing (dysfunctional breathing) (Morgan 2002). Hyperventilation is defined as a state of alveolar ventilation in excess of metabolic requirements, leading to a decreased arterial partial pressure of carbon dioxide ($PaCO_2$) (Malmberg et al 2000) and respiratory alkalosis. If sustained, these physiological changes may result in a wide range of clinical symptoms which characterize DB/HVS (Hornsveld & Garssen 1997). In many patients, DB/HVS is not a continuously symptomatic state but a syndrome of episodic symptoms which occur with or without recognizable provocation (Magarian 1982). However, where chronic hyperventilation ensues, it is suggested that the central respiratory control centres become more sensitive and trigger breathing at a lower level of $PaCO_2$, perpetuating a hypocapnic state (low $PaCO_2$) (Magarian 1982). Not all patients with DB/HVS present with hyperventilation and hypocapnia. As such, the term 'dysfunctional breathing' encompasses a complex set of behaviour and symptoms with no obvious physiological explanation (Morgan 2002). Either way, DB/HVS can result in significant patient morbidity and an array of symptoms including breathlessness, chest tightness, dizziness, tremor and paraesthesia. The presence of these symptoms can themselves result in anxiety, which can provoke further breathing irregularity.

Carbon Dioxide Theory

Breathing in excess of the body's metabolic requirement produces low $PaCO_2$ (hypocapnia). If sustained, hypocapnia results in respiratory alkalosis, which is associated with a wide range of symptoms (Fig. 5-9). It has been hypothesized that over time, the central chemoreceptors 'reset' to trigger at lower levels of CO_2 perpetuating the problem of over-breathing (hyperventilation). However, not all patients with DB hyperventilate.

Effects of Hypocapnia

Hypocapnia is associated with the following physiological responses:

- cerebral artery vasoconstriction
  - dizziness or syncope
- coronary artery vasoconstriction
  - chest pain
- increased motor and sensory nerve cell membrane irritability
  - paraesthesia
  - anaesthesia

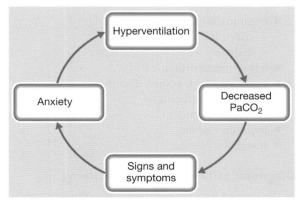

FIGURE 5-9 ■ Vicious cycle of hyperventilation.

■ sympathetic nervous system dominance
  ■ increased heart rate
  ■ palpitations
  ■ increased respiratory frequency
■ reduced oxygen delivery (Bohr effect)
■ imbalanced magnesium and calcium ratio
  ■ tetany.

Aetiology of Dysfunctional Breathing

DB may develop secondary to causes of multiple origins:

■ respiratory disease
  ■ asthma
  ■ pleurisy
  ■ pneumonia
■ psychiatric disease
■ pain
■ pharmacology and drugs
  ■ alcohol
  ■ nicotine
  ■ cocaine
  ■ aspirin
  ■ caffeine
■ psychological problems
  ■ anxiety or panic
  ■ depression
  ■ phobias
  ■ emotional response
■ physiological issues
  ■ altitude
  ■ pyrexia
  ■ pregnancy
  ■ hormones
■ organic disorders
  ■ anaemia
  ■ diabetes
■ left ventricular failure
■ central nervous system disorders
■ pulmonary embolus
■ vestibular disorder
■ hyperthyroidism
■ metabolic disease.

Diagnosis of Dysfunctional Breathing

In the general adult population, the estimated prevalence of DB/HVS is 9.5% (Thomas et al 2005).

However, as the mechanisms underpinning DB/HVS are poorly understood, the diagnosis of DB/HVS often occurs late, with the patient having undergone extensive negative investigations under various other medical specialities (Gardner 2004). As the predominant symptoms are often unexplained breathlessness and 'air hunger' (50–90% of individuals with DB/HVS; Brashear 1983), these patients often present to the respiratory physician. However, the diversity of the clinical signs and symptoms makes diagnosis extremely difficult.

Because of these difficulties, there is a concern that diagnosed cases merely represent the tip of a 'clinical iceberg' with many patients' symptoms going unrecognized and consequently untreated.

Diagnosis is made based on several assessment criteria:

■ subjective assessment
■ observation
  ■ apical breathing pattern
  ■ signs of air hunger
  ■ repeated sighs, yawns, sniffs, coughs
■ difficulty with speech or voice projection
■ personality
■ emotional state
■ validated assessment tool
  ■ Nijmegen questionnaire (>23 is positive for HVS/DB) (Fig. 5-10).

Management of Dysfunctional Breathing

Breathing exercises are recommended as a first-line treatment for DB/HVS, but other treatment techniques including pharmacological interventions and education are also advocated (Bott et al 2009). The overall aim of breathing exercises is to reduce respiratory frequency and depth of breathing (tidal volume) to match alveolar ventilation to metabolic demand (Bott et al 2009). Breathing exercises include several different approaches including Buteyko breathing and yoga breathing. Most commonly, patients are taught breathing control (relaxed diaphragmatic breathing using the lower part of the chest) in either sidelying, supine or sitting positions, with or without the use of visual and proprioceptive feedback. Breathing control encourages patients to gradually alter their breathing pattern, with the ultimate goal to restore and maintain

Nijmegen questionnaire

A score of over 23 out of 64 suggests a positive diagnosis of hyperventilation syndrome.

	Never 0	Rarely 1	Sometimes 2	Often 3	Very often 4
Chest pain					
Feeling tense					
Blurred vision					
Dizzy spells					
Feeling confused					
Faster or deeper breathing					
Short of breath					
Tight feelings in chest					
Bloated feelings in stomach					
Tingling fingers					
Unable to breathe deeply					
Stiff fingers or arms					
Tight feelings around mouth					
Cold hands or feet					
Palpitations					
Feelings of anxiety					

FIGURE 5-10 ■ Nijmegen questionnaire.

a normal breathing pattern and to reprogramme the respiratory centre to trigger inspiration at a higher level of carbon dioxide (Innocenti & Troup 2008; Bott et al 2009).

In addition, patients are taught how to effectively manage their speech by reading out loud, using punctuation to guide breathing points. Exercise is encouraged, using synchronized paced breathing to aid normalization of respiratory pattern and encourage activity without anxiety. Relaxation techniques may also be of benefit to some patients. Education to provide a physiological basis for symptoms experienced by the patient is also important; early onset symptom recognition will empower effective self-management in patients with DB.

These techniques may be consolidated by an individualized home programme tailored for each individual patient's needs (Innocenti & Troup 2008).

Compensatory Breath Holds

Additional breathing control techniques such as the use of short breath holds following sighing/yawning, may also be useful in the management of DB/HVS to aid patients to normalize their breathing patterns. These compensatory breath holds should *not* be preceded by a deep inspiration and should be followed by a period of diaphragmatic breathing control. The rationale for this exercise is that the period of breath holding will gradually allow CO_2 to rise and allow patients to gradually tolerate the symptoms of air hunger and dyspnoea.

Rescue Techniques

Rescue techniques can be taught to patients to help manage an acute attack of symptoms. These include:

- positions of ease, e.g. forward-lean sitting with arms supported
- breathing into hands cupped over nose and mouth to rebreathe CO_2
- use of a fan to blow air across the nose and mouth to help reduce the sensation of breathlessness

Dysfunctional Breathing and Speech

Patients with DB/HVS often have difficulty speaking at length and report increased breathlessness and poor voice projection. This may be secondary to forgetting to pause for breath during speech or speaking to the end of exhalation followed by a gasping inhalation. Management strategies include encouraging the patient to read out loud, using punctuation to allow time for effective breathing. When in conversation, patients are encouraged to slow down their speech and incorporate regular pauses for breathing, particularly expiration. Inspiration at low lung volumes may assist this process.

Dysfunctional Breathing and Exercise

Exercise may aid the normalization of breathing, as many patients automatically revert to a diaphragmatic breathing pattern on exertion. If patients find exercise difficult, walking slowly using paced breathing control with pulsed oximetry (to reassure the patient that oxygenation is well maintained) may be helpful.

It is important to educate patients of expected changes they may experience on exertion:

- increased minute ventilation due to increased consumption
- loss of rest phase after exhalation
- upper chest involvement
- switching from nose to mouth breathing
- breathlessness not harmful.

REFERENCES

Agusti, A.G., Roca, J., Gea, J., et al., 1991. Mechanisms of gas-exchange impairment in idiopathic pulmonary fibrosis. Am. Rev. Respir. Dis. 143, 219–225.

Alioglu, B., Ertugrul, T., Unal, M., 2007. Cardiopulmonary responses of asthmatic children to exercise: analysis of systolic and diastolic cardiac function. Pediatr. Pulmonol. 42, 283–289.

Andersen, D.H., 1938. Cystic fibrosis of the pancreas and its relation to celiac disease. Am. J. Dis. Child. 56, 344–399.

Avallone, K.M., McLeish, A.C., 2013. Asthma and aerobic exercise: a review of the empirical literature. J. Asthma 50 (2), 109–116.

Barker, A.F., 2002. Bronchiectasis. N. Engl. J. Med. 346, 1383–1393.

Bell, S.C., Robinson, P.J., Fitzgerald, D.A. 2008. *Cystic fibrosis standards of care Australia* [Online]. Available: http://www.thoracic.org.au/imagesDB/wysiwyg/CF_standardsofcare_Australia_2008.pdf [Accessed July 14 2013].

Benza, R.L., Miller, D.P., Gomberg-Maitland, M., et al., 2010. Predicting survival in pulmonary arterial hypertension: insights from the registry to evaluate early and long-term pulmonary arterial hypertension disease management (reveal). Circulation 122, 164–172.

Bilton, D., Dodd, M.E., Abbot, J.V., Webb, A.K., 1992. The benefits of exercise combined with physiotherapy in the treatment of adults with cystic fibrosis. Respir. Med. 86, 507–511.

Bott, J., Blumenthal, S., Buxton, M., et al., 2009. Guidelines for the physiotherapy management of the adult, medical, spontaneously breathing patient. Thorax 64 (Suppl. I), i1–i51.

Botton, E., Saraux, A., Laselve, H., et al., 2003. Musculoskeletal manifestations in cystic fibrosis. Joint Bone Spine 70, 327–335.

Boucher, R.C., 2004. New concepts of the pathogenesis of cystic fibrosis lung disease. Eur. Respir. J. 23, 146–158.

Bradley, B., Branley, H.M., Egan, J.J., et al., 2008. Interstitial lung disease guideline: the British Thoracic Society in collaboration with the Thoracic Society of Australia and New Zealand and the Irish Thoracic Society. Thorax 63 (Suppl. 5), v1–v58.

Bradley, J., McAlister, O., Elborn, S., 2001. Pulmonary function, inflammation, exercise capacity and quality of life in cystic fibrosis. Eur. Respir. J. 17, 712–715.

Bradley, J., Moran, F. 2008. Physical training for cystic fibrosis. Cochrane Database Syst. Rev. (1) CD002768.

Bradley, J., Moran, F., Greenstone, M. 2002. Physical training for bronchiectasis. Cochrane Database Syst. Rev. (3) CD002166.

Brashear, R.E., 1983. Hyperventilation syndrome. Lung 161, 257–273.

Brown, L.M., Chen, H., Halpern, S., et al., 2011. Delay in recognition of pulmonary arterial hypertension: factors identified from the reveal registry. Chest 140, 19–26.

Browne, W.J., Wood, C.J., Desai, M., Weller, P.H., 2009. Urinary incontinence in 9–16 year olds with cystic fibrosis compared to other respiratory conditions and a normal group. J. Cyst. Fibros. 8, 50–57.

Bruton, A., Lewith, G.T., 2005. The Buteyko breathing technique for asthma: a review. Complement. Ther. Med. 13 (1), 41–46.

Buist, A.S., McBurnie, M.A., Vollmer, W.M., et al., 2007. International variation in the prevalence of COPD (the BOLD study): a population-based prevalence study. Lancet 370, 741–750.

Burge, A.T., Holland, A.E., Sherburn, M., et al., 2011. Prevalence and impact of incontinence in adult men with cystic fibrosis. Respirology 16, 57.

Burgess, J., Ekanayake, B., Lowe, A., et al., 2011. Systematic review of the effectiveness of breathing retraining in asthma management. Expert Rev. Respir. Med. 5 (6), 789–807.

Button, B.M., Heine, R.G., Catto-Smith, A.G., et al., 2003. Chest physiotherapy in infants with cystic fibrosis: to tip or not? A five-year study. Pediatr. Pulmonol. 35, 208–213.

Button, B.M., Heine, R.G., Catto-Smith, A.G., Phelan, P.D., 1998. Postural drainage in cystic fibrosis: is there a link with gastro-oesophageal reflux? J. Paediatr. Child Health 34, 330–334.

Button, B.M., Heine, R.G., Catto-Smith, A.G., et al., 1997. Postural drainage and gastro-oesophageal reflux in infants with cystic fibrosis. Arch. Dis. Child. 76, 148–150.

Carson, K.V., Chandratilleke, M.G., Picot, J., et al., 2013. Physical training for asthma. Cochrane Database Syst. Rev. (9), CD001116.

Casaburi, R., Patessio, A., Ioli, F., et al., 1991. Reductions in exercise lactic acidosis and ventilation as a result of exercise training in patients with obstructive lung disease. Am. Rev. Respir. Dis. 143, 9–18.

Chang, A.B., Bilton, D., 2008. Exacerbations in cystic fibrosis: 4–non-cystic fibrosis bronchiectasis. Thorax 63, 269–276.

Chang, A.B., Grimwood, K., Maguire, G., et al., 2008. Management of bronchiectasis and chronic suppurative lung disease in indigenous children and adults from rural and remote Australian communities. Med. J. Aust. 189, 386–393.

Chang, A.B., Masel, J.P., Masters, B., 1998. Post-infectious bronchiolitis obliterans: clinical, radiological and pulmonary function sequelae. Pediatr. Radiol. 28, 23–29.

Chang, C.C., Morris, P.S., Chang, A.B., 2007a. Influenza vaccine for children and adults with bronchiectasis. Cochrane Database Syst. Rev. (3), CD006218.

Chang, C.C., Singleton, R.J., Morris, P.S., Chang, A.B., 2007b. Pneumococcal vaccines for children and adults with bronchiectasis. Cochrane Database Syst. Rev. (2), CD006316.

Chastain, D.C., Cook, A.J., 2000. Chronic pain in CF: associated beliefs and behaviours. Pediatr. Pulmonol. Suppl. 20, 116–117.

Chung, K.F., 2005. The role of airway smooth muscle in the pathogenesis of airway wall remodeling in chronic obstructive pulmonary disease. Proc. Am. Thorac. Soc. 2, 347–354, discussion 371-2.

Cole, P., 1997. The damaging role of bacteria in chronic lung infection. J. Antimicrob. Chemother. 40 (Suppl. A), 5–10.

Collard, H.R., Moore, B.B., Flaherty, K.R., et al., 2007. Acute exacerbations of idiopathic pulmonary fibrosis. Am. J. Respir. Crit. Care Med. 176, 636–643.

Collard, H.R., Ward, A.J., Lanes, S., et al., 2012. Burden of illness in idiopathic pulmonary fibrosis. J. Med. Econ. 15, 829–835.

Corless, J.A., Warburton, C.J., 2000. Surgery vs non-surgical treatment for bronchiectasis. Cochrane Database Syst. Rev. (4), CD002180.

Cornacchia, M., Zenorini, A., Perobelli, S., et al., 2001. Prevalence of urinary incontinence in women with cystic fibrosis. BJU Int. 88, 44–48.

Cottin, V., Cordier, J.F., 2012. Velcro crackles: the key for early diagnosis of idiopathic pulmonary fibrosis? Eur. Respir. J. 40, 519–521.

Criner, G.J., Cordova, F., Sternberg, A.L., Martinez, F.J., 2011. The National Emphysema Treatment Trial (Nett) Part II: lessons learned about lung volume reduction surgery. Am. J. Respir. Crit. Care Med. 184, 881–893.

Currie, D.C., 1997. Nebulisers for bronchiectasis. Thorax 52 (Suppl. 2), S72–S74.

Currie, D.C., Cooke, J.C., Morgan, A.D., et al., 1987. Interpretation of bronchograms and chest radiographs in patients with chronic sputum production. Thorax 42, 278–284.

Cystic fibrosis Australia, infection control and hygiene guidelines. 2000.

Cystic fibrosis foundation. Infection control recommendations for patients with cystic fibrosis. 2001.

Daviskas, E., Rubin, B.K., 2013. Effect of inhaled dry powder mannitol on mucus and its clearance. Expert Rev. Respir. Med. 7, 65–75.

De Abreau E Silva, F.A., Dodge, J.A. 1995. Guidelines for the diagnosis and management of cystic fibrosis. WHO Human Genetics Program.

De Man, F.S., Handoko, M.L., Groepenhoff, H., et al., 2009. Effects of exercise training in patients with idiopathic pulmonary arterial hypertension. Eur. Respir. J. 34, 669–675.

Dennersten, U., Lannefors, L., Hoglund, P., et al., 2009. Lung function in the aging Swedish cystic fibrosis population. Respir. Med. 103, 1076–1082.

Desmond, K.J., Schwenk, W.F., Thomas, E., et al., 1983. Immediate and long-term effects of chest physiotherapy in patients with cystic fibrosis. J. Paediatr. 103, 538–542.

Dodge, J.A., Lewis, P.A., Stanton, M., Wilsher, J., 2007. Cystic fibrosis mortality and survival in the UK: 1947-2003. Eur. Respir. J. 29, 522–526.

Doull, I.J., 2001. Recent advances in cystic fibrosis. Arch. Dis. Child. 85, 62–66.

Dumoulin, C., Hay-Smith, J., 2010. Pelvic floor muscle training versus no treatment, or inactive control treatments, for urinary incontinence in women. Cochrane Database Syst. Rev. (1), CD005654.

Dwyer, T.J., Alison, J.A., McKeough, Z.J., et al., 2011. Effects of exercise on respiratory flow and sputum properties in patients with cystic fibrosis. Chest 139, 870–877.

Eastham, K.M., Fall, A.J., Mitchell, L., Spencer, D.A., 2004. The need to redefine non-cystic fibrosis bronchiectasis in childhood. Thorax 59, 324–327.

Edwards, E.A., Asher, M.I., Byrnes, C.A., 2003. Paediatric bronchiectasis in the twenty-first century: experience of a tertiary children's hospital in New Zealand. J. Paediatr. Child Health 39, 111–117.

Eksterowicz, N., 2000. Pain management in cystic fibrosis. Paediatr. Pulmonol. (Suppl. 20), 114–115.

Elbasan, B., Tunali, N., Duzgun, I., Ozcelik, U., 2012. Effects of chest physiotherapy and aerobic exercise training on physical fitness in young children with cystic fibrosis. Ital. J. Pediatr. 38, 2.

Elkins, M.R., Jones, A., Van Der Schans, C., 2006a. Positive expiratory pressure physiotherapy for airway clearance in people with cystic fibrosis. Cochrane Database Syst. Rev. (2), CD003147.

Elkins, M.R., Robinson, M., Rose, B.R., et al., 2006b. A controlled trial of long-term inhaled hypertonic saline in patients with cystic fibrosis. N. Engl. J. Med. 354, 229–240.

Equi, A., Balfour-Lynn, I.M., Bush, A., Rosenthal, M., 2002. Long term azithromycin in children with cystic fibrosis: a randomised, placebo-controlled crossover trial. Lancet 360, 978–984.

Evans, S.A., Turner, S.M., Bosch, B.J., et al., 1996. Lung function in bronchiectasis: the influence of pseudomonas aeruginosa. Eur. Respir. J. 9, 1601–1604.

Farrell, P.M., Kosorok, M.R., Rock, M.J., et al., 2001. Early diagnosis of cystic fibrosis through neonatal screening prevents severe malnutrition and improves long-term growth. Wisconsin Cystic Fibrosis Neonatal Screening Study Group. Pediatrics 107, 1–13.

Ferkol, T., Leigh, M., 2006. Primary ciliary dyskinesia and newborn respiratory distress. Semin. Perinatol. 30, 335–340.

Festini, F., Ballarin, S., Codamo, T., et al., 2004. Prevalence of pain in adults with cystic fibrosis. J. Cyst. Fibros. 3, 51–57.

Fijalkowska, A., Kurzyna, M., Torbicki, A., et al., 2006. Serum n-terminal brain natriuretic peptide as a prognostic parameter in patients with pulmonary hypertension. Chest 129, 1313–1321.

Flume, P.A., 2003. Pneumothorax in cystic fibrosis. Chest 123, 217–221.

Flume, P.A., Ciolino, J., Gray, S., Lester, M.K., 2009. Patient-reported pain and impaired sleep quality in adult patients with cystic fibrosis. J. Cyst. Fibros. 8, 321–325.

Flume, P.A., Mogayzel, P.J. Jr., Robinson, K.A., et al., 2010. Cystic fibrosis pulmonary guidelines: pulmonary complications: hemoptysis and pneumothorax. Am. J. Respir. Crit. Care Med. 182, 298–306.

Fowler, R.M., Gain, K.R., Gabbay, E., 2012. Exercise intolerance in pulmonary arterial hypertension. Pulm. Med. 2012, 359204.

Fox, B.D., Kassirer, M., Weiss, I., et al., 2011. Ambulatory rehabilitation improves exercise capacity in patients with pulmonary hypertension. J. Card. Fail. 17, 196–200.

Freitas, D.A., Holloway, E.A., Bruno, S.S., et al., 2013. Breathing exercises for adults with asthma. Cochrane Database Syst. Rev. (10), CD001277.

Fuchs, H.J., Borowitz, D.S., Christiansen, D.H., et al., 1994. Effect of aerosolized recombinant human DNase on exacerbations of respiratory symptoms and on pulmonary function in patients with cystic fibrosis. The pulmozyme study group. N. Engl. J. Med. 331, 637–642.

Galie, N., Hoeper, M.M., Humbert, M., et al., 2009a. Guidelines for the diagnosis and treatment of pulmonary hypertension: the Task Force for the Diagnosis and Treatment of Pulmonary Hypertension of the European Society of Cardiology (esc) and the European Respiratory Society (ers), endorsed by the International Society of Heart and Lung Transplantation (ishlt). Eur. Heart J. 30, 2493–2537.

Galie, N., Manes, A., Negro, L., et al., 2009b. A meta-analysis of randomized controlled trials in pulmonary arterial hypertension. Eur. Heart J. 30, 394–403.

Gardner, W.N., 2004. Hyperventilation. Am. J. Respir. Crit. Care Med. 170, 105–108.

Garin, M.C., Highland, K.B., Silver, R.M., Strange, C., 2009. Limitations to the 6-minute walk test in interstitial lung disease and pulmonary hypertension in scleroderma. J. Rheumatol. 36, 330–336.

Glaser, S., Noga, O., Koch, B., et al., 2009. Impact of pulmonary hypertension on gas exchange and exercise capacity in patients with pulmonary fibrosis. Respir. Med. 103, 317–324.

Global strategy for the diagnosis, management, and prevention of chronic obstructive pulmonary disease (GOLD), updated 2015. Available from <www.goldcopd.org>, accessed 2/12/2013.

Grunig, E., Lichtblau, M., Ehlken, N., et al., 2012. Safety and efficacy of exercise training in various forms of pulmonary hypertension. Eur. Respir. J. 40, 84–92.

Gumery, L., Hodgson, G., Humphries, N., et al., 2002. The prevalence of urinary incontinence in the adult male population of a regional cystic fibrosis centre. J. Cyst. Fibros. 1, S173.

Habesoglu, M.A., Ugurlu, A.O., Eyuboglu, F.O., 2011. Clinical, radiologic, and functional evaluation of 304 patients with bronchiectasis. Ann. Thorac. Med. 6, 131–136.

Hallstrand, T.S., Bates, P.W., Schoene, R.B., 2000. Aerobic conditioning in mild asthma decreases the hyperpnea of exercise and improves exercise and ventilatory capacity. Chest 118, 1460–1469.

Hansen, J.E., Wasserman, K., 1996. Pathophysiology of activity limitation in patients with interstitial lung disease. Chest 109, 1566–1576.

Harris-Eze, A.O., Sridhar, G., Clemens, R.E., et al., 1996. Role of hypoxemia and pulmonary mechanics in exercise limitation in interstitial lung disease. Am. J. Respir. Crit. Care Med. 154, 994–1001.

Hassan, J.A., Saadiah, S., Roslan, H., Zainudin, B.M., 1999. Bronchodilator response to inhaled beta-2 agonist and anticholinergic drugs in patients with bronchiectasis. Respirology 4, 423–426.

Haworth, C.S., Dodd, M.E., Atkins, M., et al., 2000. Pneumothorax in adults with cystic fibrosis dependent on nasal intermittent positive pressure ventilation (nippv): a management dilemma. Thorax 55, 620–622.

Hayes, M., Yaster, M., Haythornthwaite, J.A., et al., 2011. Pain is a common problem affecting clinical outcomes in adults with cystic fibrosis. Chest 140, 1598–1603.

Hebestreit, H., Kieser, S., Junge, S., et al., 2010. Long-term effects of a partially supervised conditioning programme in cystic fibrosis. Eur. Respir. J. 35, 578–583.

Hind, K., Truscott, J.G., Conway, S.P., 2008. Exercise during childhood and adolescence: a prophylaxis against cystic fibrosis-related low bone mineral density? Exercise for bone health in children with cystic fibrosis. J. Cyst. Fibros. 7, 270–276.

Hodson, M.E., 2000. Treatment of cystic fibrosis in the adult. Respiration 67, 595–607.

Hodson, M.E., Madden, B.P., Steven, M.H., et al., 1991. Non-invasive mechanical ventilation for cystic fibrosis patients: a potential bridge to transplantation. Eur. Respir. J. 4, 524–527.

Holland, A., Hill, C., 2008. Physical training for interstitial lung disease. Cochrane Database Syst. Rev. (4), CD006322.

Holland, A.E., Hill, C.J., Conron, M., et al., 2008. Short term improvement in exercise capacity and symptoms following exercise training in interstitial lung disease. Thorax 63, 549–554.

Holland, A.E., Hill, C.J., Glaspole, I., et al., 2012a. Predictors of benefit following pulmonary rehabilitation for interstitial lung disease. Respir. Med. 106, 429–435.

Holland, A.E., Hill, C.J., Jones, A.Y., McDonald, C.F., 2012b. Breathing exercises for chronic obstructive pulmonary disease. Cochrane Database Syst. Rev. (10), CD008250.

Holloway, E.A., West, R.J., 2007. Integrated breathing and relaxation training (the Papworth method) for adults with asthma in primary care: a randomised controlled trial. Thorax 62 (12), 1039–1042.

Holverda, S., Gan, C.T., Marcus, J.T., et al., 2006. Impaired stroke volume response to exercise in pulmonary arterial hypertension. J. Am. Coll. Cardiol. 47, 1732–1733.

Hornsveld, H., Garssen, B., 1997. Hyperventilation syndrome: an elegant but scientifically untenable concept. Neth. J. Med. 50, 13–20.

Hulzebos, H., Snieder, H., Van Der Et, J., et al., 2011. High-intensity interval training in an adolescent with cystic fibrosis: a physiological perspective. Physiother. Theory Pract. 27, 231–237. [Epub 2010 Jul 22].

Innocenti, D.M., Troup, F., 2008. Hyperventilation. In: Pryor, J.A., Prasad, S.A. (Eds.), Physiotherapy for Respiratory and Cardiac Problems, fourth ed. Churchill Livingstone, Edinburgh.

Jaffe, A., Bush, A., 2001. Cystic fibrosis: review of the decade. Monaldi Arch. Chest Dis. 56, 240–247.

Javaheri, S., Sicilian, L., 1992. Lung function, breathing pattern, and gas exchange in interstitial lung disease. Thorax 47, 93–97.

Jones, A.M., 2005. Eradication therapy for early pseudomonas aeruginosa infection in CF: many questions still unanswered. Eur. Respir. J. 26, 373–375.

Karakoc, G.B., Inal, A., Yilmaz, M., et al., 2009. Exhaled breath condensate MMP-9 levels in children with bronchiectasis. Pediatr. Pulmonol. 44, 1010–1016.

Kelemen, L., Lee, A.L., Button, B.M., et al., 2012. Pain impacts on quality of life and interferes with treatment in adults with cystic fibrosis. Physiother. Res. Int. 17 (3), 132–141.

Kellett, F., Redfern, J., Niven, R.M., 2005. Evaluation of nebulised hypertonic saline (7%) as an adjunct to physiotherapy in patients with stable bronchiectasis. Respir. Med. 99, 27–31.

Kerem, E., Reisman, J., Corey, M., et al., 1992. Prediction of mortality in patients with cystic fibrosis. N. Engl. J. Med. 326, 1187–1191.

Spruit, M.A., Singh, S.J., Garvey, C., et al., 2013. An official American Thoracic Society/European Respiratory Society statement: key concepts and advances in pulmonary rehabilitation. Am. J. Respir. Crit. Care Med. 188, e13–e64.

Khan, T.Z., Wagener, J.S., Bost, T., et al., 1995. Early pulmonary inflammation in infants with cystic fibrosis. Am. J. Respir. Crit. Care Med. 151, 1075–1082.

Kishaba, T., Shimaoka, Y., Fukuyama, H., et al., 2012. A cohort study of mortality predictors and characteristics of patients with combined pulmonary fibrosis and emphysema. BMJ open 2.

Knowles, M.R., Paradiso, A.M., Boucher, R.C., 1995. In vivo nasal potential difference: techniques and protocols for assessing efficacy of gene transfer in cystic fibrosis. Hum. Gene Ther. 6, 445–455.

Koch, C., Hoiby, N., 1993. Pathogenesis of cystic fibrosis. Lancet 341, 1065–1069.

Koh, J.L., Harrison, D., Palermo, T.M., et al., 2005a. Assessment of acute and chronic pain symptoms in children with cystic fibrosis. Pediatr. Pulmonol. 40, 330–335.

Koh, J.L., Harrison, D., Palermo, T.M., et al., 2005b. Assessment of acute and chronic pain symptoms in children with cystic fibrosis. Pediatr. Pulmonol. 40, 330–335.

Koscik, R.L., Farrell, P.M., Kosorok, M.R., et al., 2004. Cognitive function of children with cystic fibrosis: deleterious effect of early malnutrition. Pediatrics 113, 1549–1558.

Laffey, J.G., Kavanagh, B.P., 2002. Hypocapnia. N. Engl. J. Med. 347 (1), 43–53.

Lama, V.N., Flaherty, K.R., Toews, G.B., et al., 2003. Prognostic value of desaturation during a 6-minute walk test in idiopathic interstitial pneumonia. Am. J. Respir. Crit. Care Med. 168, 1084–1090.

Lannefors, L., Button, B.M., McIlwaine, M., 2004. Physiotherapy in infants and young children with cystic fibrosis: current practice and future developments. J. R. Soc. Med. 97 (Suppl. 44), 8–25.

Lanng, S., Hansen, A., Thorsteinsson, B., et al., 1995. Glucose tolerance in patients with cystic fibrosis: five year prospective study. BMJ 311, 655–659.

Laube, B.L., Jashnani, R., Dalby, R.N., Zeitlin, P.L., 2000. Targeting aerosol deposition in patients with cystic fibrosis: effects of alterations in particle size and inspiratory flow rate. Chest 118, 1069–1076.

Ledson, M.J., Gallagher, M.J., Jackson, M., et al., 2002. Outcome of Burkholderia cepacia colonisation in an adult cystic fibrosis centre. Thorax 57, 142–145.

Ledson, M.J., Tran, J., Walshaw, M.J., 1998. Prevalence and mechanisms of gastro-oesophageal reflux in adult cystic fibrosis patients. J. R. Soc. Med. 91, 7–9.

Lee, A., Holdsworth, M., Holland, A., Button, B., 2009. The immediate effect of musculoskeletal physiotherapy techniques and massage on pain and ease of breathing in adults with cystic fibrosis. J. Cyst. Fibros. 8, 79–81.

Lee, A.L., Burge, A., Holland, A.E., 2013. Airway clearance techniques for bronchiectasis. Cochrane Database Syst. Rev. (5), CD008351.

Lewis, M.M., Mortelliti, M.P., Yeager, H. Jr., Tsou, E., 2002. Clinical bronchiectasis complicating pulmonary sarcoidosis: case series of seven patients. Sarcoidosis Vasc. Diffuse Lung Dis. 19, 154–159.

Ley, B., Collard, H.R., King, T.E. Jr., 2011. Clinical course and prediction of survival in idiopathic pulmonary fibrosis. Am. J. Respir. Crit. Care Med. 183, 431–440.

Li, A.M., Sonnappa, S., Lex, C., et al., 2005. Non-CF bronchiectasis: does knowing the aetiology lead to changes in management? Eur. Respir. J. 26, 8–14.

Liou, T.G., Adler, F.R., Fitzsimmons, S.C., et al., 2001. Predictive 5-year survivorship model of cystic fibrosis. Am. J. Epidemiol. 153, 345–352.

Loughlin, G.M., Cota, K.A., Taussig, L.M., 1981. The relationship between flow transients and bronchial lability in cystic fibrosis. Chest 79, 206–210.

Macfarlane, P.I., Heaf, D., 1990. Changes in airflow obstruction and oxygen saturation in response to exercise and bronchodilators in cystic fibrosis. Pediatr. Pulmonol. 8, 4–11.

Magarian, G.J., 1982. Hyperventilation syndromes: infrequently recognised common expressions of anxiety and stress. Medicine 61 (4), 219–236.

Mahadeva, R., Webb, K., Westerbeek, R.C., et al., 1998. Clinical outcome in relation to care in centres specialising in cystic fibrosis: cross sectional study. BMJ 316, 1771–1775.

Mainguy, V., Maltais, F., Saey, D., et al., 2010a. Effects of a rehabilitation program on skeletal muscle function in idiopathic pulmonary arterial hypertension. J Cardiopulm. Rehabil. Prev. 30, 319–323.

Mainguy, V., Maltais, F., Saey, D., et al., 2010b. Peripheral muscle dysfunction in idiopathic pulmonary arterial hypertension. Thorax 65, 113–117.

Malmberg, L.P., Tamminen, K., Sovijarvi, A.R.A., 2000. Orthostatic increases of respiratory gas exchange in hyperventilation syndrome. Thorax 55, 295–310.

Mandal, P., Sidhu, M.K., Kope, L., et al., 2012. A pilot study of pulmonary rehabilitation and chest physiotherapy versus chest physiotherapy alone in bronchiectasis. Respir. Med. 106, 1647–1654.

Mannino, D.M., Homa, D.M., Akinbami, L.J., et al., 2002. Chronic obstructive pulmonary disease surveillance: United States, 1971-2000. Morb. Mortal. Wkly Rep. Surveill. Summ. 51, 1–16.

Mapel, D.W., Hunt, W.C., Utton, R., et al., 1998. Idiopathic pulmonary fibrosis: survival in population based and hospital based cohorts. Thorax 53, 469–476.

Markovitz, G.H., Cooper, C.B., 1998. Exercise and interstitial lung disease. Curr. Opin. Pulm. Med. 4, 272–280.

Mathers, C.D., Loncar, D., 2006. Projections of global mortality and burden of disease from 2002 to 2030. PLoS Med. 3, e442.

McIntyre, K., 2013. Gender and survival in cystic fibrosis. Curr. Opin. Pulm. Med. 19, 692–697.

McKoy, N.A., Saldanha, I.J., Odelola, O.A., Robinson, K.A., 2012. Active cycle of breathing technique for cystic fibrosis. Cochrane Database Syst. Rev. (12), CD007862.

McNamara, R.J., McKeough, Z.J., McKenzie, D.K., Alison, J.A., 2013. Water-based exercise in COPD with physical comorbidities: a randomised controlled trial. Eur. Respir. J. 41, 1284–1291.

Menezes, A.M., Perez-Padilla, R., Jardim, J.R., et al., 2005. Chronic obstructive pulmonary disease in five Latin American cities (the Platino study): a prevalence study. Lancet 366, 1875–1881.

Mereles, D., Ehlken, N., Kreuscher, S., et al., 2006. Exercise and respiratory training improve exercise capacity and quality of life in patients with severe chronic pulmonary hypertension. Circulation 114, 1482–1489.

Moran, F., Bradley, J.M., Boyle, L., Elborn, J.S., 2003. Incontinence in adult females with cystic fibrosis: a Northern Ireland survey. Int. J. Clin. Pract. 57, 182–183.

Morgan, M.D.L., 2002. Dysfunctional breathing in asthma: is it common, identifiable and correctable? Thorax 57 (Suppl. II), ii31–ii35.

Morrison, L., Agnew, J., 2009. Oscillating devices for airway clearance in people with cystic fibrosis. Cochrane Database Syst. Rev. (1), CD006842.

Nankivell, G., Caldwell, P., Follett, J., 2010. Urinary incontinence in adolescent females with cystic fibrosis. Paediatr. Respir. Rev. 11, 95–99.

National Clinical Guideline Centre, 2013. Idiopathic pulmonary fibrosis: The diagnosis and management of suspected idiopathic pulmonary fibrosis. National Institute for Health and Care Excellence (NICE), London, p. (Clinical guideline; no. 163).

Newall, C., Stockley, R.A., Hill, S.L., 2005. Exercise training and inspiratory muscle training in patients with bronchiectasis. Thorax 60, 943–948.

Nici, L., Donner, C., Wouters, E., et al., 2006. American Thoracic Society/European Respiratory Society statement on pulmonary rehabilitation. Am. J. Respir. Crit. Care Med. 173, 1390–1413.

Nicolson, C.H., Stirling, R.G., Borg, B.M., et al., 2012. The long term effect of inhaled hypertonic saline 6% in non-cystic fibrosis bronchiectasis. Respir. Med. 106, 661–667.

Nishiyama, O., Kondoh, Y., Kimura, T., et al., 2008. Effects of pulmonary rehabilitation in patients with idiopathic pulmonary fibrosis. Respirology 13, 394–399.

Nishiyama, O., Taniguchi, H., Kondoh, Y., et al., 2005. Quadriceps weakness is related to exercise capacity in idiopathic pulmonary fibrosis. Chest 127, 2028–2033.

Nixon, G.M., Glazner, J.A., Martin, J.M., Sawyer, S.M., 2002. Urinary incontinence in female adolescents with cystic fibrosis. Pediatrics 110, e22.

Nixon, P.A., Orenstein, D.M., Kelsey, S.F., Doershuk, C.F., 1992. The prognostic value of exercise testing in patients with cystic fibrosis. N. Engl. J. Med. 327, 1785–1788.

Noble, P.W., Albera, C., Bradford, W.Z., et al., 2011. Pirfenidone in patients with idiopathic pulmonary fibrosis (capacity): two randomised trials. Lancet 377, 1760–1769.

O'Brien, C., Guest, P.J., Hill, S.L., Stockley, R.A., 2000. Physiological and radiological characterisation of patients diagnosed with chronic obstructive pulmonary disease in primary care. Thorax 55, 635–642.

O'Donnell, D.E., 2001. Ventilatory limitations in chronic obstructive pulmonary disease. Med. Sci. Sports Exerc. 3, S647–S655.

Orenstein, D.M., Winnie, G.B., Altman, H., 2002. Cystic fibrosis: a 2002 update. J. Pediatr. 140, 156–164.

Orr, A., McVean, R.J., Webb, A.K., Dodd, M.E., 2001. Questionnaire survey of urinary incontinence in women with cystic fibrosis. BMJ 322, 1521.

Osadnik, C.R., McDonald, C.F., Jones, A.P., Holland, A.E., 2012. Airway clearance techniques for chronic obstructive pulmonary disease. Cochrane Database Syst. Rev. (3), CD008328.

Paccou, J., Zeboulon, N., Combescure, C., et al., 2010. The prevalence of osteoporosis, osteopenia, and fractures among adults with cystic fibrosis: a systematic literature review with meta-analysis. Calcif. Tissue Int. 86, 1–7.

Paranjape, S., Barnes, L., Carson, K., et al., 2012. Exercise improves lung function and habitual activity in children with cystic fibrosis. J. Cyst. Fibros. 11, 18–23. [Epub 2011 Sep 3].

Parasa, R.B., Maffulli, N., 1999. Musculoskeletal involvement in cystic fibrosis. Bull. Hosp. Jt Dis. 58, 37–44.

Park, R.W., Grand, R.J., 1981. Gastrointestinal manifestations of cystic fibrosis: a review. Gastroenterology 81, 1143–1161.

Pasteur, M.C., Bilton, D., Hill, A.T., 2010. British Thoracic Society guideline for non-CF bronchiectasis. Thorax 65 (Suppl. 1), i1–i58.

Pasteur, M.C., Helliwell, S.M., Houghton, S.J., et al., 2000. An investigation into causative factors in patients with bronchiectasis. Am. J. Respir. Crit. Care Med. 162, 1277–1284.

Patel, I.S., Vlahos, I., Wilkinson, T.M., et al., 2004. Bronchiectasis, exacerbation indices, and inflammation in chronic obstructive pulmonary disease. Am. J. Respir. Crit. Care Med. 170, 400–407.

Pianosi, P., Leblanc, J., Almudevar, A., 2005. Peak oxygen uptake and mortality in children with cystic fibrosis. Thorax 60, 50–54.

Pitta, F., Troosters, T., Probst, V.S., et al., 2006. Physical activity and hospitalization for exacerbation of COPD. Chest 129, 536–544.

Poole, P.J., Chacko, E., Wood-Baker, R.W., Cates, C.J., 2000. Influenza vaccine for patients with chronic obstructive pulmonary disease. Cochrane Database Syst. Rev. (4), CD002733.

Porter, D.K., Van Every, M.J., Anthracite, R.F., Mack, J.W. Jr., 1983. Massive hemoptysis in cystic fibrosis. Arch. Intern. Med. 143, 287–290.

Provencher, S., Chemla, D., Herve, P., et al., 2006. Heart rate responses during the 6-minute walk test in pulmonary arterial hypertension. Eur. Respir. J. 27, 114–120.

Puhan, M., Scharplatz, M., Troosters, T., et al., 2009. Pulmonary rehabilitation following exacerbations of chronic obstructive pulmonary disease. Cochrane Database Syst. Rev. (1), CD005305.

Qaseem, A., Wilt, T.J., Weinberger, S.E., et al., 2011. Diagnosis and management of stable chronic obstructive pulmonary disease: a clinical practice guideline update from the American College of Physicians, American College of Chest Physicians, American Thoracic Society, and European Respiratory Society. Ann. Intern. Med. 155 (3), 179–191.

Quan, J.M., Tiddens, H.A., Sy, J.P., et al., 2001. A two-year randomized, placebo-controlled trial of dornase alfa in young patients with cystic fibrosis with mild lung function abnormalities. J. Pediatr. 139, 813–820.

Raghu, G., Collard, H.R., Egan, J.J., et al., 2011. An official ATS/ERS/JRS/ALAT statement: idiopathic pulmonary fibrosis: evidence-based guidelines for diagnosis and management. Am. J. Respir. Crit. Care Med. 183, 788–824.

Rasekaba, T.M., Button, B.M., Wilson, J.W., Holland, A.E., 2013. Reduced physical activity associated with work and transport in adults with cystic fibrosis. J. Cyst. Fibros. 12, 229–233.

Ratjen, F., Doring, G., 2003. Cystic fibrosis. Lancet 361, 681–689.

Ravilly, S., Robinson, W., Suresh, S., et al., 1996a. Chronic pain in cystic fibrosis. Pediatrics 98, 741–747.

Ravilly, S., Robinson, W., Suresh, S., et al., 1996b. Chronic pain in cystic fibrosis. Pediatrics 98, 741–747.

Ries, A.L., Bauldoff, G.S., Carlin, B.W., et al., 2007. Pulmonary rehabilitation: joint ACCP/AACVPR evidence-based clinical practice guidelines. Chest 131, 4S–42S.

Roberts, H.J., Hubbard, R., 2010. Trends in bronchiectasis mortality in England and Wales. Respir. Med. 104, 981–985.

Robinson, P., 2001. Cystic fibrosis. Thorax 56, 237–241.

Ryu, J.H., Daniels, C.E., Hartman, T.E., Yi, E.S., 2007. Diagnosis of interstitial lung diseases. Mayo Clin. Proc. 82, 976–986.

Saiman, L., Marshall, B.C., Mayer-Hamblett, N., et al., 2003. Azithromycin in patients with cystic fibrosis chronically infected with pseudomonas aeruginosa: a randomized controlled trial. JAMA 290, 1749–1756.

Sands, D., Repetto, T., Dupont, L.J., et al., 2011. End of life care for patients with cystic fibrosis. J. Cyst. Fibros. 10 (Suppl. 2), S37–S44.

Sandsund, C.A., Roughton, M., Hodson, M.E., Pryor, J.A., 2011. Musculoskeletal techniques for clinically stable adults with cystic fibrosis: a preliminary randomised controlled trial. Physiotherapy 97, 209–217.

Sawicki, G.S., Sellers, D.E., Robinson, W.M., 2008. Self-reported physical and psychological symptom burden in adults with cystic fibrosis. J. Pain Symptom Manage. 35, 372–380.

Seitz, A.E., Olivier, K.N., Adjemian, J., et al., 2012. Trends in bronchiectasis among Medicare beneficiaries in the United States, 2000 to 2007. Chest 142, 432–439.

Seitz, A.E., Olivier, K.N., Steiner, C.A., et al., 2010. Trends and burden of bronchiectasis-associated hospitalizations in the United States, 1993-2006. Chest 138, 944–949.

Selman, M., King, T.E., Pardo, A., 2001. Idiopathic pulmonary fibrosis: prevailing and evolving hypotheses about its pathogenesis and implications for therapy. Ann. Intern. Med. 134, 136–151.

Sermet-Gaudelus, I., De Villartay, P., De Dreuzy, P., et al., 2009. Pain in children and adults with cystic fibrosis: a comparative study. J. Pain Symptom Manage. 38, 281–290.

Shah, P.L., Slebos, D.J., Cardoso, P.F., et al., 2011. Bronchoscopic lung-volume reduction with exhale airway stents for emphysema (ease trial): randomised, sham-controlled, multicentre trial. Lancet 378, 997–1005.

Shoemaker, M., Hurt, H., Arndt, L., 2008. The evidence regarding exercise training in the management of cystic fibrosis: a systematic review. Cardiopulm Phys. Ther. J. 19, 75–83.

Shoemark, A., Ozerovitch, L., Wilson, R., 2007. Aetiology in adult patients with bronchiectasis. Respir. Med. 101, 1163–1170.

Sietsema, K., 2001. Cardiovascular limitations in chronic pulmonary disease. Med. Sci. Sports Exerc. 33, S656–S661.

Simonneau, G., Robbins, I.M., Beghetti, M., et al., 2009. Updated clinical classification of pulmonary hypertension. J. Am. Coll. Cardiol. 54, S43–S54.

Singh, V., Wisniewski, A., Britton, J., Tattersfield, A., 1990. Effect of yoga breathing exercises (pranayama) on airway reactivity in subjects with asthma. Lancet 335 (8702), 1381–1383.

Singleton, R., Morris, A., Redding, G., et al., 2000. Bronchiectasis in Alaska Native children: causes and clinical courses. Pediatr. Pulmonol. 29, 182–187.

1999. Skeletal muscle dysfunction in chronic obstructive pulmonary disease: a statement of the American Thoracic Society and European Respiratory Society. Am. J. Respir. Crit. Care Med. 159, S1–S40.

Smith, I.E., Flower, C.D., 1996. Review article: imaging in bronchiectasis. Br. J. Radiol. 69, 589–593.

Snell, G., Herth, F.J., Hopkins, P., et al., 2012. Bronchoscopic thermal vapour ablation therapy in the management of heterogeneous emphysema. Eur. Respir. J. 39, 1326–1333.

Stenekes, S.J., Hughes, A., Gregoire, M.C., et al., 2009. Frequency and self-management of pain, dyspnea, and cough in cystic fibrosis. J. Pain Symptom Manage. 38, 837–848.

Taniguchi, H., Ebina, M., Kondoh, Y., et al., 2010. Pirfenidone in idiopathic pulmonary fibrosis. Eur. Respir. J. 35, 821–829.

Tashkin, D.P., Rennard, S., Taylor Hays, J., et al., 2011. Lung function and respiratory symptoms in a 1-year randomized smoking cessation trial of varenicline in COPD patients. Respir. Med. 105, 1682–1690.

Tejero Garcia, S., Giraldez Sanchez, M., Cejudo, P., et al., 2011. Bone health, daily physical activity, and exercise tolerance in patients with cystic fibrosis. Chest 140, 475–481. [Epub 2011 Feb 3].

Thio, B.J., Nagelkerke, A.F., Ketel, A.G., et al., 1996. Exercise-induced asthma and cardiovascular fitness in asthmatic children. Thorax 51, 207–209.

Thomas, S.R., 2003. The pulmonary physician in critical care. Illustrative case 1: cystic fibrosis. Thorax 58, 357–360.

Thomas, M., McKinley, R.K., Freeman, E., et al., 2005. The prevalence of dysfunctional breathing in adults in the community with and without asthma. Prim. Care Respir. J. 14, 78–82.

Travis, W.D., Costabel, U., Hansell, D.M., et al., 2013. An official American Thoracic Society/European Respiratory Society statement: update of the international multidisciplinary classification of the idiopathic interstitial pneumonias. Am. J. Respir. Crit. Care Med. 188, 733–748.

van den Elshout, F.J., van Herwaarden, C.L., Folgering, H.T., 1991. Effects of hypercapnia and hypocapnia on respiratory resistance in normal and asthmatic subjects. Thorax 46 (1), 28–32.

Van Der Schans, C., Prasad, A., Main, E., 2003. Chest physiotherapy compared to no chest physiotherapy for cystic fibrosis. Cochrane Database Syst. Rev. 3, 3.

Vandenplas, Y., Diericx, A., Blecker, U., et al., 1991. Esophageal pH monitoring data during chest physiotherapy. J. Pediatr. Gastroenterol. Nutr. 13, 23–26.

Vella, M., Cartwright, R., Cardozo, L., et al., 2009. Prevalence of incontinence and incontinence-specific quality of life impairment in women with cystic fibrosis. Neurourol. Urodyn. 28, 986–989.

Watz, H., Waschki, B., Meyer, T., Magnussen, H., 2009. Physical activity in patients with COPD. Eur. Respir. J. 33, 262–272.

Welsh, L., Roberts, R.G.D., Kemp, J.G., 2004. Fitness and physical activity in children with asthma. Sports Med. 34, 861–870.

Weycker, D., Edelsberg, J., Oster, G., Tino, G., 2005. Prevalence and economic burden of bronchiectasis. Clin. Pulm. Med. 12, 205–209.

White, D., Stiller, K., Roney, F., 2000. The prevalence and severity of symptoms of incontinence in adult cystic fibrosis patients. Physiother. Theory Pract. 16, 35–42.

Wills, P., Greenstone, M., 2006. Inhaled hyperosmolar agents for bronchiectasis. Cochrane Database Syst. Rev. (2), CD002996.

Wilson, J.W., Kotsimbos, A.T.C., 2004. The management of cystic fibrosis. In: Muers, M.A. (Ed.), Respiratory Diseases. Oxford University Press, Oxford.

Wurzel, D., Marchant, J.M., Yerkovich, S.T., et al., 2011. Short courses of antibiotics for children and adults with bronchiectasis. Cochrane Database Syst. Rev. (6), CD008695.

Yankaskas, J.R., Marshall, B.C., Sufian, B., et al., 2004. Cystic fibrosis adult care: consensus conference report. Chest 125, 1S–39S.

Young, A.C., Wilson, J.W., Kotsimbos, T.C., Naughton, M.T., 2008. Randomised placebo controlled trial of non-invasive ventilation for hypercapnia in cystic fibrosis. Thorax 63, 72–77.

6

OUTCOME MEASUREMENT IN CARDIORESPIRATORY PHYSIOTHERAPY PRACTICE

SELINA M PARRY ■ LINDA DENEHY
with contributions from

CLAIRE E BALDWIN ■ BRONWEN CONNOLLY
(ICU)

ELIZABETH H SKINNER
(Health-Related Quality of Life)

SALLY J SINGH
(Field Walking Tests)

SARAH RAND ■ CRAIG A WILLIAMS
(Paediatrics)

CHAPTER OUTLINE

INTRODUCTION 196

INTERNATIONAL CLASSIFICATION OF FUNCTIONING FRAMEWORK 196

SELECTION OF AN OUTCOME MEASURE 196
What is an Outcome Measure? 196
What Determines the Choice of an Outcome Measure? 196

MEASUREMENT OF IMPAIRMENT AT BODY STRUCTURE/FUNCTIONS LEVEL 198
Respiratory Outcome Measures 198
Measurement of Muscle 199
Muscle Mass 199
Muscle Strength 202

MEASUREMENT OF ACTIVITY LIMITATIONS 211
Measures of Physical Function and Mobility in the ICU Setting 211
Other Measures of Mobility and Activities of Daily Living in Acute Care 217
Exercise Testing 218
Field Walking Tests 221
Physical Activity 223

MEASUREMENT OF PARTICIPATION RESTRICTION 226
Quality of Life 226
Why Health-Related Quality of Life? 227
Summary 239

REFERENCES 240

INTRODUCTION

Cardiorespiratory physiotherapists work closely with patients across the continuum of recovery including: critical care, acute hospitalization, community and rehabilitation programs. As outlined in Chapter 2, the key to effective physiotherapy management of a patient is the accurate identification of the patient's problems, in particular those which are amenable to physiotherapy intervention.

Physiotherapy cardiorespiratory problems commonly encountered include:

- impaired airway clearance
- dyspnoea
- decreased exercise tolerance/decreased mobility levels
- reduced lung volume
- impaired gas exchange
- airflow limitation
- respiratory muscle dysfunction.

Physiotherapists provide respiratory and/or rehabilitation strategies to address the identified physiotherapy-amenable problems. In order to determine treatment efficacy, it is important that an appropriate clinical outcome measure is selected which is sensitive and able to detect a 'true' change as a result of the physiotherapist's intervention. It is useful to consider outcome measures which can be utilized in the short, medium and long term and which can be mapped within the domains of the International Classification of Functioning (ICF) framework: impairment, activity limitation and participation restriction. There are a number of factors which influence the choice of an outcome measure. This chapter aims to provide a concise and practical introduction to outcome measures which may be utilized in cardiorespiratory physiotherapy practice to evaluate impairment, activity limitation and participation restriction. The focus is largely on the adult population; however, paediatric considerations are discussed briefly within this chapter.

INTERNATIONAL CLASSIFICATION OF FUNCTIONING FRAMEWORK

The ICF disability and health framework provides a versatile and multi-dimensional framework upon which outcome measures can be conceptualized at an individual, institutional and social level (World Health Organization 2001). Within a specific health condition three domains can be evaluated which include:

(1) body functions and structures – impairments
(2) activities – capability and restrictions in function
(3) participation – capability and restriction particularly considering social, recreation, work (within the wider community and societal setting).

Applied to the measurement of muscle strength and function in critically ill patients for example, muscle weakness would be classified as impairment at the body function and structure level, while functional mobility and activities of daily living (ADLs) are classified as activity limitations.

SELECTION OF AN OUTCOME MEASURE

What is an Outcome Measure?

A physiotherapy outcome measure is 'a test or scale administered and interpreted by physiotherapists that has been shown to measure accurately a particular attribute of interest to patients and therapists and is expected to be influenced by intervention' (Mayo et al 1994).

What Determines the Choice of an Outcome Measure?

There are five main considerations when selecting an outcome measure for use in clinical and research practice to evaluate patient related outcomes:

1. **What is the purpose? What construct are you measuring?** This considers where the measure maps within the ICF framework (i.e. impairment, activity limitation or participation restriction).
2. **Measurement properties** – Examination of the reliability, validity and responsiveness of an outcome measure (see Table 6-1 for more information).

	TABLE 6-1	
	Measurement Properties of Outcome Measures/Instruments	
Measurement Property	**Type**	**Definition**
Reliability *Ability of an instrument to obtain accurate results which are free from measurement error*	1. Internal consistency	■ Measure of homogeneity of items (i.e. to what extent do the items measure consistently?). ■ Cronbach's alpha (a correlation coefficient) is used to measure the internal reliability of instruments and subscales (Cronbach 1951) and should exceed 0.7 (DeVellis 2003).
	2. Test retest	■ Measure of instrument stability over time, as an individual's test score should not change each time the instrument is administered in the absence of change (Portney and Watkins 2009). ■ Also often termed *'reproducibility'* (Portney and Watkins 2009).
	3. Inter-rater	■ Measure of ability of an instrument to obtain accurate results which are free from measurement error when the instrument is repeated by different assessors (i.e. do different assessors obtain the same result assuming there has been no change in the patient's status between tests?) (Portney and Watkins 2009). ■ Also often termed *'repeatability'*.
	4. Intra-rater	■ Measure of ability of an instrument to obtain accurate results which are free from measurement error when the same assessor repeats the testing (Portney and Watkins 2009).
Validity *Determines the ability of an instrument to measure what it is intended to measure*	5. Content	■ Defined as the degree to which the content of an instrument is an adequate reflection of the construct to be measured (Mokkink et al 2010).
	6. Construct	■ Defined as the degree to which the scores of an instrument are consistent with hypotheses, based on the assumption that the instrument validly measures the construct to be measured (Mokkink et al 2010). Construct validity can be examined by assessing convergent and discriminative validity with respect to a previously developed validated instrument (concurrent validity); comparing instrument scores to known construct differences between groups using receiver operating characteristics (ROC) analysis and/or factor analysis (Portney and Watkins 2009).
	7. Criterion	■ Defined as the ability of an instrument to measure as expected against an external criterion, usually the gold standard. ■ In absence of a gold standard comparator it may be called 'concurrent validity'. This can be either convergent (e.g. scores agree where the same constructs are expected to be measured, or related scales) or divergent (e.g. scores do not agree on constructs that appear to be different) (Portney and Watkins 2009).
	8. Predictive	■ Another form of criterion validity and is present when the instrument scores predict other variables or outcomes as expected (e.g. the ability to predict change scores or outcomes as expected, e.g. the ability to predict changes in patient's health status or other health outcomes such as complications, resource consumption or mortality) (Portney and Watkins 2009).
Responsiveness		■ Refers to the ability of an instrument to detect a true change in the score obtained which is statistically or clinically meaningful over time. This is a critical measurement property in the context of clinical and research practice and selecting an instrument that is not responsive to change in specific populations may mean that change is not detected with intervention. ■ *Minimal important difference (MID) or minimal clinical important difference (MCID)* defines the minimum change at which observed change is considered clinically meaningful for patients and/or clinicians (Portney and Watkins 2009). ■ There are two main methods used to determine MID: 1) anchor-based approach, which takes into consideration the patient's perception of change using anchors such as 'much worse' and 'much better' in a scale such as the global rating of change scale and 2) distribution-based approach, for example calculation of the effect size standardized using a measure of variability (Ferreira and Herbert 2008).

3. **Clinical Utility** – Practical considerations such as resources/equipment required, testing space and costs, as well as the expertise and time required to accurately perform the outcome measure (Fitzpatrick et al 1998).

4. **Sensitivity/Clinical Applicability** – The floor and ceiling effects of a test need to be considered (percentage of occasions where participants scored the lowest or highest score possible for a test, respectively) relative to the time point at which the measurement is being performed within the specific patient population that is being evaluated.

5. **Patient/Environmental Considerations** – Factors such as patient alertness, delirium, medical acuity, environmental setting constraints (i.e. there will be a difference between the critical care and outpatient rehabilitation setting). Consideration of the patient's ability to understand and follow commands in performance within a specific outcome measure may also be impacted by the age of the patient (neonate/paediatric versus adult) and cognitive capability. It is also important to consider whether familiarization with a test may impact the patient's performance with a test. For example, ensuring a patient understands the concept of pacing in the shuttle walk test if evaluating functional capacity.

When selecting the most appropriate measure to evaluate efficacy of an intervention and to determine change over time, clinicians and researchers need to consider whether the measurement properties of the measure of interest have been established. Table 6-1 provides an outline of the measurement properties, which are important to consider when selecting an outcome measure. Measures developed for one setting or patient population should only be extrapolated with caution to other populations (Portney et al 2009). The COnsensus-based Standards for the selection of health Measurement INstruments (COSMIN) and its scoring system have been recently developed to standardize the assessment of the methodological quality of studies reporting measurement properties (Mokkink et al 2010). Box 6-1 outlines practical points to consider when choosing an outcome measure.

BOX 6-1
CONSIDERATIONS IN CHOOSING AN OUTCOME MEASURE

- Decide what construct/parameter you want to measure, i.e. muscle strength.
- Use the International Classification of Functioning framework to map outcome measures within the categories of impairment, activity limitation and participation restriction.
- Consider the following in the choice of an outcome measure
  - Practicalities of undertaking the test
  - Training and resources/costs required
  - Has your outcome measure been examined in your population of interest?
  - What are the measurement properties of your test, i.e. reliability, validity, responsiveness?
  - Is your test sensitive to detect a 'true' change at the time points of testing you have selected?

MEASUREMENT OF IMPAIRMENT AT BODY STRUCTURE/FUNCTIONS LEVEL

Respiratory Outcome Measures

Impaired Airway Clearance/Low Lung Volumes and Breathlessness

There are a variety of outcome measures which are used in clinical practice to determine the efficacy of an intervention aimed at assisting either airway clearance or addressing low lung volumes/ventilation deficiencies. These measures are the assessment asterisks which assist the therapist in identifying the primary physiotherapy problem/s for the patient and guide the appropriate selection of an intervention.

Auscultation is routinely used in clinical practice to assess lung sounds as part of objective assessment and can also be used post intervention particularly, since it is easy, rapid, non-invasive and cost-effective to reassess changes in lung sounds. The reliability of auscultation between assessors is limited, with no difference based on the level of clinical expertise (Brooks et al 1995, Marques et al 2006). Vital signs, in particular changes in respiratory rate and oxygen saturation as measured using pulse oximetry, can also be used post intervention (Marques et al 2006). The ability to tolerate a treatment intervention is particularly important in the paediatric population, with a predominant focus on evaluation of trends and changes in vital signs to guide intervention dosage and progression. Arterial blood gases are considered the gold standard for determining the patient's arterial oxygen saturation, as they provide detailed and highly accurate information. The limitation with use of arterial blood gases is that it involves an invasive technique, and is often not commonly assessed as part of a physiotherapy treatment in the ward setting. In the intensive care unit (ICU) setting, arterial blood gases are routinely evaluated to determine management efficacy due to the accessibility of readings, with most patients having an arterial line and direct access point for arterial blood to be collected. Sputum expectoration can be quantified in terms of the volume or weight of sputum produced (Marques et al 2006). Spirometry is primarily utilized in the diagnosis of the severity of lung disease. It is also utilized to evaluate change in lung volume status preintervention and postintervention, particularly when measuring vital capacity in individuals with neuromuscular dysfunction such as spinal cord injury or Guillain-Barré syndrome. The American Thoracic Society (ATS) guidelines provide detailed information on the standardization of spirometry testing (Miller et al 2005).

Dyspnoea

Dyspnoea is defined as the subjective experience of feeling breathless, and is a particularly important measure to evaluate in patients with lung disease. There are a variety of different dyspnoea scales, including the Baseline Dyspnea Index and the modified Medical Research Council (mMRC) Dyspnoea Scale, which have been developed to evaluate the level of breathlessness. Readers are encouraged to refer to the ATS statement on dyspnoea for further information which recommends evaluation in the following domains: (1) sensory-perceptual, (2) affective and (3) disability (Parshall et al 2012).

See Box 6-2 for a suggested respiratory impairment based outcome measures for common physiotherapy problems.

Measurement of Muscle

Muscle mass is a passive non-volitional outcome which enables quantification of muscle morphology, and may relate to measurement of muscle strength and

---

> **BOX 6-2**
> ### ASSESSMENT OF IMPAIRMENT – RESPIRATORY OUTCOME MEASURES
>
> **IMPAIRED AIRWAY CLEARANCE**
> - Sputum expectoration – quantity in terms of volume/weight
> - Auscultation
> - Sputum expectoration may result in improvement in ventilation; therefore may see changes in vital signs particularly pulse oximetry, respiratory rate
> - Imaging such as chest radiography, arterial blood gases
>
> **LOW LUNG VOLUMES**
> - Auscultation
> - Vital signs – pulse oximetry, respiratory rate
> - Spirometry – particularly in individuals with neuromuscular dysfunction such as spinal cord injury or neuromuscular diseases monitoring of vital capacity can provide a measure of overall lung volume status
> - Imaging such as chest radiography, arterial blood gases
>
> **DYSPNOEA**
> - Borg dyspnoea scale
> - Baseline Dyspnoea Index
> - mMRC breathlessness scale
> - Vital signs – particularly respiratory rate
>
> In the longer term for these problems, it is important to consider the other aspects of the ICF framework – activity limitation and participation restriction.
>
> ICF, International Classification of Functioning; MRC, Medical Research Council.

---

functional outcomes. However, muscle strength provides greater detail on the patient's level of impairment, as it is a dynamic measure. Measurement of muscle strength requires patients to be alert and able to cooperate with testing, which is in contrast to measurement of muscle mass, which can be quantified using non-volitional methods (Parry et al 2015).

Muscle Mass

Definitions

Muscle mass is defined as 'the measurement of the size of a specific muscle or total body composition' (Heymsfield et al 2005). Some common ways of monitoring changes in muscle mass clinically at the bedside over time include: neuromuscular ultrasound imaging, body composition analysis and use of anthropometric measures of limb girth.

Neuromuscular Ultrasound Imaging

Ultrasound has gained popularity in recent years as a non-volitional tool for measuring properties of muscle structure such as muscle cross-sectional area or muscle mass in the cardiorespiratory population (Parry et al 2015c, Puthucheary et al 2013, Seymour et al 2009, Thomaes et al 2012) and also changes in muscle quality (echogenicity) (Parry et al 2015c, Puthucheary et al 2015). Neuromuscular ultrasound imaging is cost effective, portable to the bedside and quick to set up, and basic measurements (e.g. thickness) can be made from images in real-time. With adequate training, ultrasonography can be used by non-specialist clinicians to undertake image acquisition and analysis. This has been demonstrated in healthy and critically ill studies where novice assessors (<3 hours training) were compared with established experts in the field (Cartwright et al 2013, Sarwal et al 2014). Furthermore, ultrasonography appears to be a valid and reliable alternative to the 'gold standard' of magnetic resonance imaging (Reeves et al 2004b), with recent improvements in ultrasound technology producing muscle images of much greater resolution, therefore making ultrasonography a valuable tool for clinical and research purposes (Delaney et al 2010, Reeves et al 2004a).

Specific details for measurement techniques vary according to the individual muscle group under examination, but it is important to maintain a standardized approach to ensure accurate and reliable images, especially if monitoring change over sequential time points. Units of measurement depend on the muscle property being analyzed, for example mm^2 for cross-sectional area or arbitrary units (based on pixel count) for echogenicity. Typically real-time images are captured and stored for off-line measuring using dedicated imaging ultrasonography software for analysis.

Muscle groups that have been imaged in research studies have primarily evaluated: biceps brachia, forearm extensors, tibialis anterior and the quadriceps. The quadriceps is extremely important for function and performance of daily activities such as walking, standing from a chair, going up and down stairs and

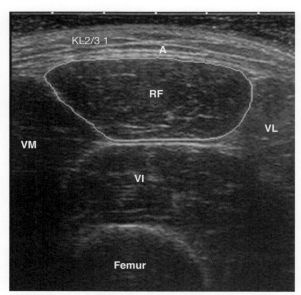

FIGURE 6-1 ■ Neuromuscular ultrasound image. *A*, subcutaneous tissue; *RF*, rectus femoris; *VI*, vastus intermedius; *VL*, vastus lateralis; *VM*, vastus medialis.

running. It has thus been the most commonly imaged muscle (rectus femoris in particular) and quantification of cross-sectional area favoured (Fig. 6-1). Neuromuscular ultrasound imaging has been shown to have high inter-rater and inter-session reliability and concurrent validity against measures of muscle strength and function, and is responsive to change over time within individuals with critical illness and chronic diseases such as chronic obstructive pulmonary disease (COPD) (Table 6-2). Ultrasound imaging is an attractive modality, particularly in the acutely ill who may be unable to undertake volitional assessment of strength and/or function. This is a rapidly growing area of research and clinical interest within individuals with cardiorespiratory impairment and in the future may be a core outcome measure for evaluation of changes in muscle quantity and quality.

Body Composition Analysis

Bioimpedance spectroscopy enables bedside quantification of body water and mass compartments including fat-free and fat mass measurements (Baldwin et al 2012). Prediction equations and algorithms have been developed for some populations (Earthman et al

TABLE 6-2
Measurement of Impairment – Muscle Mass (Quadriceps)

Patient Population	Reliability, Measurement Error	Validity	Responsiveness
COPD	Yes Excellent reproducibility for quadriceps thickness and CSA (Menon et al 2012) Excellent reliability between novice and experienced assessors for rectus femoris CSA (Hammond et al 2014)	Yes CSA valid with/for: quadriceps strength (Hammond et al 2014, Seymour et al 2009), MRC dyspnoea scale (Seymour et al 2009) Lower quadriceps CSA was predictive of readmission and mortality in individuals with acute COPD exacerbation (Greening et al 2015)	Yes Responsive to resistance training for quadriceps thickness and CSA (Menon et al 2012)
ILD	X	Yes CSA valid with/for: moderate correlation with knee extensor strength in advanced ILD (Mendes et al 2015)	X
CVD	Yes Excellent test-retest reliability for measurement of muscle thickness (Thomaes et al 2012)	Yes Rectus femoris thickness valid with/for: computed tomography and muscle strength (Thomaes et al 2012)	X
Lung Cancer	X	X	X
ICU	Yes Excellent intra-rater reliability for measurement of muscle thickness (Baldwin and Bersten 2014) Excellent intra- and inter-rater reliability for Heckmatt qualitative analysis of muscle echointensity (Grimm et al 2013)	Yes Rectus femoris CSA/thickness valid with/for: extensor muscle strength, moderate to excellent correlation with muscle strength (Baldwin and Bersten 2014, Campbell et al 1995), negative correlation with ICU LOS (Gruther et al 2008) Rectus femoris/vastus intermedius quality changes (echointensity) valid with/for: muscle strength and physical function (Parry et al 2015) and muscle biopsy (Puthucheary et al 2015)	Yes Measures of muscle quantity (muscle thickness/cross sectional area) are sensitive to change over time in the ICU setting (Puthucheary et al 2013, Reid et al 2004)

COPD, Chronic obstructive pulmonary disease; CSA, cross sectional area; CVD, cardiovascular disease; ICU, intensive care unit; ILD, interstitial lung disease ; LOS, length of stay; MRC, Medical Research Council.

2007), with the majority of the research undertaken in oncological and healthy patient populations. If none are available then it is recommended that the raw data be utilized within the first instance. There are challenges with using bioimpedance spectroscopy in the cardiorespiratory physiotherapy setting, which need to be taken into consideration prior to implementation into practice. These include cost of purchasing a machine and disposable electrode tabs, which are required for each patient at each testing time; fluid status and ability to obtain an accurate height and weight measurement, which can be particularly prob-lematic within the acute/critical care setting. However, because it is non-invasive, quick to use and non-volitional, further research is required to examine the potential role for bioimpedance spectroscopy in evaluating outcomes in individuals with cardiorespiratory ailments.

Anthropometry

Anthropometric circumference measurements are not recommended as a primary end point in clinical and research physiotherapy practice. Circumference measurements were shown not to be sensitive to change

BOX 6-3
ASSESSMENT OF
IMPAIRMENT – MUSCLE MASS

■ Ultrasonography is a promising non-volitional tool for evaluation of muscle mass (quantity) and changes in muscle quality (echogenicity) particularly in critical care.
■ Greater research is required to determine the validity/ prognostic capability and responsiveness in relation to physiotherapy interventions.
■ Anthropometry is not recommended for use in clinical/ research practice to evaluate changes in muscle mass.

over time during the critical care admission period (Campbell et al 1995, Reid et al 2004) and the utility of this tool as a measure of muscle mass is questionable. Non-critical care studies have demonstrated that circumference measurements are unreliable and under-represent the actual amount of muscle wasting that may develop (Duffin 1977, Nicholas et al 1976, Young et al 1980). Factors such as oedema can also impact the accuracy and validity of circumference measurements, which are common secondary sequelae that occur in individuals with critical illness.

See Box 6-3 for assessment of impairment related to muscle mass.

Muscle Strength

Definitions

Muscle strength is defined as the maximal force that can be generated by a specific muscle or muscle group. It can be measured by isometric or dynamic means (concentric or eccentric movement of an external load) and is expressed in kilograms or newtons (1 kg = 9.81 N). A 'maximal voluntary contraction' specifically refers to the maximal isometric force that can be volitionally generated, i.e. through effort, as measured by the gold standard of dynamometry. Strength can be differentiated from related measures of muscle performance, such as muscle power (work done over a specific period of time) and torque (measure of the tendency of a force to produce rotation). Furthermore, muscle strength is influenced by contractile properties of the muscle such as fibre length, type, cross-sectional area, and pennation angle (Lieber 2010).

Volitional and Non-Volitional Assessment of Muscle Strength

Muscle strength can be assessed using either volitional (effort-dependent) or non-volitional (effort-independent) methods. Volitional techniques are appealing for a variety of clinical and practical reasons. Typically they are available to use at the patient's bedside; are quick, relatively easy and simple to perform; often require little or no additional equipment and can be conducted by a variety of different healthcare professionals. In order to perform volitional assessments of muscle strength, patients must be awake, cooperative and motivated to participate in testing in order to ensure their true maximum effort is measured. This is important for obtaining accurate, reliable and valid results of baseline parameters and recording change over time. This can be challenging in some environments; for example within the critical care setting where factors such as pain, use of sedation or opiate medications, presence of invasive lines or attachments and patient fatigue may impede assessment. It is therefore crucial that procedures to assess awakening and attention are undertaken prior to testing to promote optimal conditions (Fig. 6-2). It is also important that clinicians are vigilant during testing to avoid discrepancies in patient posture, the test position and therapist handling when performing volitional assessments.

A number of different screening tools can be used to establish if patients are appropriate to take part in volitional strength assessments. These tools have been used in research trials and clinical practice and include the Glasgow Coma Scale (Teasdale et al 1974), the Richmond Agitation-Sedation Scale (Sessler et al 2002), the Attention Screening Examination (part of the Confusion Assessment Method for the ICU (CAM-ICU)) (Ely et al 2001) and finally subjective responses to a range of simple commands (De Jonghe et al 2002). In addition, delirium is a common problem in the acutely unwell, particularly in critically ill patients, affecting 50–80% of the ICU population (Ouimet et al 2007, Spronk et al 2009). In a landmark study of 821 patients admitted to ICU the incidence of delirium was 74%, occurred mainly in the first 10 days after admission and was associated with worse global cognition and executive function at 3 and 12 months (Pandharipande et al 2013). Routine screening for delirium

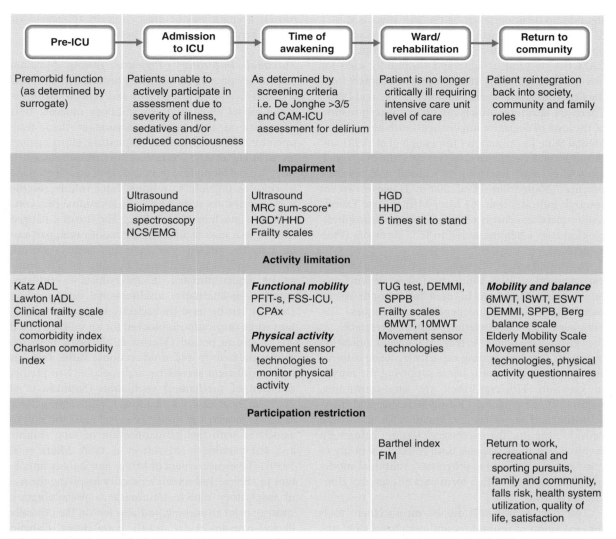

Pre-ICU	Admission to ICU	Time of awakening	Ward/ rehabilitation	Return to community
Premorbid function (as determined by surrogate)	Patients unable to actively participate in assessment due to severity of illness, sedatives and/or reduced consciousness	As determined by screening criteria i.e. De Jonghe >3/5 and CAM-ICU assessment for delirium	Patient is no longer critically ill requiring intensive care unit level of care	Patient reintegration back into society, community and family roles
Impairment				
	Ultrasound Bioimpedance spectroscopy NCS/EMG	Ultrasound MRC sum-score* HGD*/HHD Frailty scales	HGD HHD 5 times sit to stand	
Activity limitation				
Katz ADL Lawton IADL Clinical frailty scale Functional comorbidity index Charlson comorbidity index		*Functional mobility* PFIT-s, FSS-ICU, CPAx *Physical activity* Movement sensor technologies to monitor physical activity	TUG test, DEMMI, SPPB Frailty scales 6MWT, 10MWT Movement sensor technologies	*Mobility and balance* 6MWT, ISWT, ESWT DEMMI, SPPB, Berg balance scale Elderly Mobility Scale Movement sensor technologies, physical activity questionnaires
Participation restriction				
			Barthel index FIM	Return to work, recreational and sporting pursuits, family and community, falls risk, health system utilization, quality of life, satisfaction

FIGURE 6-2 ■ Suggested schematic guide to mapping of outcome measures within the International Classification of Functioning (ICF) framework. *6MWT*, 6-Minute walk test; *10MWT*, 10-metre walk test; *ADL*, activity of daily living; *CAM-ICU*, Confusion Assessment Method-ICU; *CPAx*, Chelsea Critical Care Physical Assessment Tool; *DEMMI*, De Morton Mobility Index; *EMG*, electromyography; *ESWT*, endurance shuttle walk test; *FIM*, Functional Independence Measure; *FSS-ICU*, Functional Status Score for the Intensive Care Unit; *HGD*, handgrip dynamometry; *HHD*, hand-held dynamometry; *IADL*, independence in ADLs; *ICU*, intensive care unit; *IMS*, ICU Mobility Scale; *ISWT*, incremental shuttle walk test; *MRC*, Medical Research Council; *NCS*, nerve conduction study; *PFIT-s*, Physical Function Intensive care Test-scored; *SPPB*, Short Physical Performance Battery; *TUG*, Timed Up and Go Test. *Methods for clinically diagnosing the presence of intensive care unit acquired weakness (ICU-AW) on awakening. *(Figure 2 from Parry, S., Granger, C.L., Berney, S., et al., 2015. Assessment of impairment and activity limitations in the critically ill: a systematic review of measurement instruments and their clinimetric properties. Intensive Care Med. 41 (5), 744–762. With kind permission from Springer Science and Business Media.)*

should also be undertaken, as this can affect accuracy of test results and patients' ability to participate in physical and neuro-cognitive rehabilitation. The CAM-ICU is valid, reliable and commonly used for this purpose (Ely et al 2001), and was adapted from the Confusion Assessment Method (Inouye et al 1990). There are also tools which can enable determination of the level of cognitive impairment, such as the Mini-Mental State Examination (Tombaugh et al 1992) and the Montreal Cognitive Assessment (MoCA), which are widely used screening in clinical and research practice (Nasreddine et al 2005). However, recent research indicates that the Mini-Mental State Examination correlates poorly with more robust neurophysiological tests when measured in ICU survivors (Pfoh et al 2015).

In the absence of sufficient patient alertness, participation or the ability to follow instructions, non-volitional tests can be used for strength assessment. These effort-independent techniques (i.e. peripheral nerve stimulation) can be preferable, as they give a more objective, reliable and valid indication of muscle force-generating capacity by using external stimulation of the motor nerve supplying the muscle in question. However, they are time-consuming, require trained personnel for performance and interpretation and are often not practical for use at the bedside due to the necessary testing equipment involved. For these reasons, until the clinical utility of non-volitional measures progresses, volitional modes of assessment more often form part of everyday clinical assessment.

This next section will discuss measurement tools for evaluation of respiratory and peripheral strength.

Respiratory Muscle Strength Measurement

Standardized testing of the respiratory muscles has been well documented and includes tests of both inspiratory and expiratory strength and endurance, and electrophysiological methods to assess the integrity of the respiratory neuromotor components (ATS/European Respiratory Society (ERS) 2002). The most commonly used tests in the acute/critical care setting are those for inspiratory muscle strength (described in the following section), endurance with pressure time product, diaphragm electromyography and phrenic nerve conduction. Non-invasive tests of inspiratory muscle strength may be most clinically applicable for physiotherapists to use at the bedside.

Maximal Inspiratory Pressure Testing. Maximal inspiratory pressure (Pi_{max}/MIP) testing is a volitional test that is simple to perform and reflects a coordinated global effort of the inspiratory muscles. It is quantified as the negative pressure at the airway opening during a maximal inspiratory effort against an occluded airway. The maximum pressure sustained for 1 second should be recorded from an effort made as close as possible to residual lung volume, as the trans-respiratory system pressure at residual may contribute as much as 30% to Pi_{max}. The use of a flanged mouthpiece may facilitate good mouth seal, particularly in the presence of neuromuscular weakness. Patients should be positioned upright. As MIP tends to be underestimated in mechanically ventilated patients, an alternative unidirectional valve method (MIP_{uni}) can be used that selectively permits exhalation while inspiration is blocked for an uninterrupted 20–25 second period (Marini et al 1986). Both the single manoeuvre and unidirectional valve methods have insufficient sensitivity and specificity to predict duration of mechanical ventilation (Supinski et al 2011) or readiness for weaning (Tobin 2006). They also have similar test limitations, including difficulties associated with the standardization of lung volume and test variability (Marini et al 1986, Multz et al 1990). The measurement of MIP is particularly important in clinical and research practice involving the use of inspiratory muscle training as a prehabilitation strategy prior to surgery, and also within the critically ill and neuromuscular disease populations (Cahalin et al 2013, Elkins et al 2015, Tamplin et al 2014, Valkenet et al 2011).

Phrenic Nerve Stimulation. The main non-volitional measurement of respiratory muscle strength is either trans-diaphragmatic pressure (Pdi) or pressure at the airway/tracheal opening in response to phrenic nerve stimulation. Measurements specifically reflect diaphragm contractility/force, independent of central nervous system influences. Phrenic nerve stimulation has been examined in the critically ill and has predominantly been limited to research studies with a bilateral anterior magnetic approach (Cattapan et al

2003, Demoule et al 2013, Hermans et al 2010, Jaber et al 2011, Laghi et al 2003). Limitations to more widespread use include equipment costs, the need for technical expertise and lack of agreement on standardized stimulation protocols.

Peripheral Muscle Strength Measurement

Like respiratory muscle strength, peripheral muscle strength can be assessed by volitional and non-volitional means, and can be used to evaluate and monitor change in presentation. Volitional assessment typically involves manual muscle testing and/or hand-held or portable dynamometry, while non-volitional tests involve motor nerve stimulation.

Manual Muscle Strength Testing. Manual muscle strength testing is most commonly utilized in the critical care setting from a clinical and research perspective (Parry et al 2015). The advantage of manual muscle strength testing is that it requires no additional equipment, is low cost and can be performed within the environment of critical care – with lines, attachments and changing medical stability. Manual muscle strength testing is the mainstay for the diagnosis of ICU-acquired weakness (ICU-AW) (Fan et al 2014, Parry et al 2015). The value of a formal diagnosis of ICU-AW includes the potential for a prompt course of treatment, or risk stratification of patients to early inpatient rehabilitation.

Manual muscle strength testing using the Medical Research Council Sum-score (MRC-SS) is currently recommended for the clinical diagnosis of ICU-AW (Gosselink et al 2008). A score of <48/60 is considered indicative of ICU-AW (De Jonghe et al 2002) and scores <36/60 are classified as severe ICU-AW (Hermans et al 2012). The MRC-SS involves assessment of six muscle groups bilaterally and has traditionally been scored out of 60 using the six-point scoring system (Kleyweg et al 1991) (Table 6-3). A new collapsed four-point scoring system has been developed (Vanhoutte et al 2012) and has recently been validated within the critical care setting (Parry et al 2015a) (see Table 6-3). Excellent inter-rater reliability for has been established for raw MRC-SS's in the ICU population (Connolly et al 2013, Fan et al 2010, Hermans et al 2012, Hough et al 2011) (Table 6-4). However, there is considerable variability in the

TABLE 6-3

Manual Muscle Testing: Muscle Groups Assessed and Scoring Systems

Muscle Groups Assessed	6-Point Medical Research Council Strength Grading (Kleyweg et al 1991)	Modified 4-Point Grading (Vanhoutte et al 2012)
Shoulder abduction	0 – no visible contraction	0 – paralysis
Elbow flexion	1 – visible contraction but no limb movement	1 – severe weakness
Wrist extension	2 – active movement with gravity eliminated	
Hip flexion	3 – active movement against gravity	2 – slight weakness
Knee extension	4 – active movement against gravity and resistance	
Ankle dorsiflexion	5 – active movement against full resistance/ normal power	3 – normal strength

agreement of a diagnosis of ICU-AW (MRC-SS <48/60) when examined with the six-point scoring system, being poor to good when diagnosed in the ICU (Connolly et al 2013, Hermans et al 2012, Hough et al 2011) and almost perfect after ICU discharge (Hough et al 2011). While a standard worldwide approach has not been adopted for muscle strength testing, the two common techniques are: (1) isometric: at one point in range and (2) through-range of movement (Elliott et al 2011). Yet these two techniques are not comparable and thus cannot be used interchangeably (Parry et al 2015a). The isometric technique is preferred, as it has the highest level of reliability and agreement for the diagnosis of ICU-AW (Parry et al 2015a). Clear step-by-step guidelines for the isometric technique in the critically ill have been described in the literature (Ciesla et al 2011). A diagnosis of ICU-AW (<48/60) has limited clinical predictive value for ICU or hospital length of stay, or mortality, while preserved muscle strength (>48/60) may predict a more favourable outcome (Connolly et al 2013). One study of surgical ICU patients reported that for each 1-unit increase in

TABLE 6-4
Summary of Volitional Measures of Peripheral Skeletal Muscle Strength for Patients in the Intensive Care Unit

Outcome Measure	Content	Scoring	Reliability	Validity and Responsiveness	Comments
Medical Research Council Sum-score (MRC-SS)	Evaluation of 6 muscle groups bilaterally	Calculate raw score and use to diagnose ICU-AW: <48 out of 60 on six-point scale for diagnosis of ICU-AW, <24 out of 36 (to be reconfirmed) on four-point scale for diagnosis of ICU-AW (Parry et al 2015)	**6-point scale** Excellent inter-rater in stable GBS patients (ICC = 0.96) (Kleyweg et al 1991) Excellent inter-rater in ICU patients (ICC range 0.78–0.99) (Connolly et al 2013, Fan et al 2010, Hermans et al 2012, Hough et al 2011) Best inter-rater reliability with an isometric versus through-range technique (Parry et al 2015) **Agreement for ICU-AW diagnosis** Poor to good in the ICU (Kappa range from 0.26–0.68) (Connolly et al 2013, Hermans et al 2012, Hough et al 2011) Excellent after ICU discharge (Kappa = 1.0) (Hough et al 2011) **4-point scale** Excellent inter-rater reliability (isometric ICC = 0.90; through-range ICC = 0.94) (Parry et al 2015)	**6-point scale validity** Conflicting findings for prediction of ICU and hospital mortality (Ali et al 2008, Connolly et al 2013, Sharshar et al 2009) Lower MRC score or Dx of ICU-AW associated with longer ICU and hospital LOS, mortality and poorer functional outcomes (Ali et al 2008, Connolly et al 2013, Hermans et al 2014) **Responsiveness** Greater variability in grades 4 and 5 using Oxford scale (Hermans et al 2012) **Normative values** Yes – considered normal strength if above cut-off of 48 out of 60 **4-point scale validity** Moderate correlation between diagnosis of ICU-AW and mechanical ventilation hours, physical function and discharge to home (Parry et al 2015)	**Equipment** Nil additional equipment required **Feasibility** Stringent training in testing procedure is important for accuracy Can take up to 30 minutes to perform with very weak patients **Limitations** Need alert and cooperative patients

TABLE 6-4
Summary of Volitional Measures of Peripheral Skeletal Muscle Strength for Patients in the Intensive Care Unit (Continued)

Outcome Measure	Content	Scoring	Reliability	Validity and Responsiveness	Comments
Handgrip dynamometry (HGD)	Dynamometer in second handle position, patient upright/seated, elbow flexed to 90 degrees, wrist neutral (Fess 1992) Peak isometric force recorded (best of three efforts)	Calculate peak force (kg or lb) and use to diagnose ICU-AW	Excellent inter-rater and test-retest in ICU patients (ICC range 0.85–0.97) (Baldwin et al 2013, Hermans et al 2012, Parry et al 2015)	**Validity** Inconsistent associations between HGD and mortality and LOS (Ali et al 2008, Lee et al 2012) Good to excellent correlation with MRC and MIP (Fan et al 2014) **Responsiveness** High diagnostic accuracy for diagnosis of ICU-AW using gender specific cut-off values (Ali et al 2008, Parry et al 2015) Large % minimal detectable difference in ICU patients to ensure change in score not just due to chance (Baldwin et al 2013) **Normative values** Yes (Bohannon et al 2006, Massy-Westropp et al 2004)	**Equipment** HGD **Feasibility** Quick (<5 minutes) and simple screening tool for ICU-AW (recommended first tier of assessment, (Parry et al 2015) Little expertise and training required **Limitations** Need alert and cooperative patients Not suitable for very weak patients **Other** Published guidelines for testing methodology (Fess 1992) Consider hand dominance when interpreting results Ensure dynamometer is calibrated

Continued on following page

TABLE 6-4

Summary of Volitional Measures of Peripheral Skeletal Muscle Strength for Patients in the Intensive Care Unit (Continued)

Outcome Measure	Content	Scoring	Reliability	Validity and Responsiveness	Comments
Handheld dynamometry (HHD)	Positioning for various muscle groups described in detail (Vanpee et al 2011) Peak isometric force recorded (best of three efforts)	Calculate peak force (kg or lb)	Good to excellent inter-rater in ICU patients (ICC range 0.71–0.96) (Baldwin et al 2013, Vanpee et al 2011) Excellent test-retest for knee extension but poor for elbow flexion (ICC range 0.423–0.857) (ICC range 0.89–0.92) (Baldwin et al 2013)	**Validity** Not established against fixed dynamometers in the critically ill **Responsiveness** Large % minimal detectable difference in ICU patients to ensure change in score not just due to chance (Baldwin et al 2013)	**Equipment** Dynamometer **Feasibility** Quick and simple test Low cost compared to non-volitional testing equipment **Limitations** Need alert and cooperative patients Assessor needs to be strong enough to counter the force generated by the patient Need at least antigravity strength to be tested (Vanpee et al 2011) **Other** Positioning for testing not always standardized (Baldwin et al 2013, Vanpee et al 2011) Ensure dynamometer is calibrated

Dx, Diagnosis; *GBS*, Guillain-Barré syndrome; *ICC*, intra-class correlation coefficient; *ICU*, intensive care unit; *ICU-AW*, intensive care unit–acquired weakness; *LOS*, length of stay; *MIP*, maximal inspiratory pressure; *MRC*, Medical Research Council; *PFIT*, physical function in intensive care test.

strength there was a 5% relative decrease in the odds of mortality (Lee et al 2012). Further research is required to determine the responsiveness and predictive utility of MRC-SS testing in the ICU setting. The ordinal nature of the MRC-SS scale limits its sensitivity, particularly at the higher grades (4–5), which results in a ceiling effect (Baldwin et al 2013, Hermans et al 2012). Small degrees of weakness may remain subclinical and undiagnosed with manual muscle testing. Dynamometry has been recommended as an alternative for the objective evaluation of muscle strength in individuals with at least antigravity strength (Vanpee et al 2011).

Dynamometry. Dynamometers (force gauges) can be classified as fixed/isokinetic or portable/hand-held, with various devices in existence to enable the measurement of different muscle actions. In terms of measurement parameters, fixed dynamometry such as the Cybex dynamometer (laboratory based) is the gold standard for the measurement of maximal voluntary contractions and can measure the widest range of impairments, including isometric and isokinetic force, and related variables such as power, torque and velocity (Stark et al 2011). This form of testing has limited clinical utility within the clinical hospital and outpatient community settings due to the expertise, cost, and maintenance associated with these devices and is primarily used in research studies. Portable handheld dynamometers are increasingly being adopted into clinical practice for objective measurement of muscle strength (Robles et al 2011, Vanpee et al 2014).

Handgrip Dynamometry. Dynamometry of handgrip strength has been considered to be an indicator of general health and has been evaluated in the critical care, acute and community setting (Baldwin et al 2013, Jakobsen et al 2010, Trutschnigg et al 2008). Handgrip dynamometry has the advantage that it is less time-consuming, has lower costs/maintenance required and can be used easily in the clinical setting due to its portability compared to fixed dynamometry described earlier. There are both standardized guidelines for handgrip dynamometry from the American Society of Hand Therapists (Fess 1992) as well as published normative reference values in the paediatric, adolescent and adult population for comparison when examining changes in strength over time (Bohannon et al 2006, Massy-Westropp et al 2004, Mathiowetz et al 1985, Mathiowetz et al 1986, McQuiddy et al 2015, Rauch et al 2002).

The patient set up for assessment of handgrip strength testing is given in Figure 6-3:

- sitting as upright as possible
- shoulder adducted and in neutral rotation
- elbow flexed to 90 degrees
- forearm and wrist in neutral position
- zero to 30 degrees wrist extension
- Jamar dynamometer set to second handle position.

It is recommended that patients are allowed to generate their maximum peak force over a 3-second duration with a minimum of 60 seconds rest in between three sets. In individuals with critical illness it has been shown that their time to peak force generation is significantly longer, and that this patient group should be provided a minimum of 6 seconds to generate maximum peak force (Baldwin et al 2013). There has been variation in the analysis – some studies examine the highest score recorded of three attempts while others report the mean of three scores. Dynamometry of handgrip strength has been recommended as an alternative screening tool for the diagnosis of ICU-AW, as it is directly related to the MRC-SS, with ICU-AW diagnosed at a cut-off level of 11 kg for males and 7 kg for females (Ali et al 2008, Parry et al 2015a).

Dynamometry for handgrip is distinctly different to dynamometry used to measure peripheral muscle groups. Hand-held dynamometry should be assessed using a 'make test', whereby the examiner holds the dynamometer steady, matching the resistance the patient exerts against it (Bohannon 1988). In contrast, a 'break' test means that the examiner pushes the dynamometer as hard as they can until the patient is forced to move their limb joint due to their muscular force being overcome by the therapist's resistance (Bohannon 1988). In addition to the previously described limitations for volitional strength testing, one of the main limitations of portable dynamometry is the reliance on the examiner to provide sufficient resistance at the upper limits of force generation. Accordingly, dynamometry appears to be most reliable in the range of mild to moderate weakness around

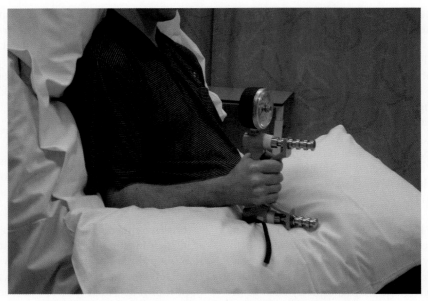

FIGURE 6-3 ■ Patient set-up for assessment of handgrip strength testing.

MRC grades 3–4 (Baldwin et al 2013). It also cannot be used in individuals who do not have at least anti-gravity strength (grade 3). Hand-held dynamometry has been utilized in a variety of cardiorespiratory populations. including patients with COPD and critical illness (Robles et al 2011, Vanpee et al 2014).

Functional Strength Testing. Strength testing can also be evaluated through observation and evaluation of functional tasks such as sit to stand. Observational evaluation is commonly utilized in infants and toddlers, as the reliability and repeatability of dynamometry or manual muscle strength testing can be limited by the child's cognitive and language development in order to be able to understand the task. Observational evaluation can include assessment of their ability to perform different movements against gravity at developmental milestones; i.e. whether a 6-month-old baby can sit unsupported, or an 8-month-old infant can push themselves onto their knees and crawl (Pountney 2007). There are a wide array of neurodevelopmental tools which are used within the paediatric setting, including the Alberta Infant Motor Scale, Movement Assessment of Infants and Peabody Developmental Motor Scales (Darrah et al 1998, Spittle et al 2008).

Other functional strength tests have been developed, including the Five Times Sit to Stand Test, which is a measure of functional lower limb strength (Bohannon et al 2010). This test requires individuals to stand up and sit down five times as quickly as they can with information on the time (seconds) and level of assistance recorded (Bohannon et al 2010). Normative values for this test have been developed within the adult population (Bohannon 2006).

Peripheral Nerve Stimulation. Non-volitional force measurements can be made in response to electrical or magnetic stimulation of peripheral motor nerves. However, the range of muscles which can be evaluated by non-volitional methods is restricted to select groups, in part due to the anatomical location of most peripheral nerves, and that a particular nerve may innervate several individual muscles. Furthermore, these techniques can be costly and time consuming, requiring specialist equipment and skilled personnel for their implementation and interpretation, and hence they are most commonly used in the research setting. Contraindications to magnetic stimulation include presence of pacemakers and/or metallic objects in the field and it is advisable to avoid the technique

BOX 6-4
EVALUATION OF IMPAIRMENT – MUSCLE STRENGTH

- Screening for the presence of intensive care unit-acquired weakness (ICU-AW) is recommended using a two-tier approach: 1) handgrip dynamometry using cut-off scores developed by Ali 2008 and colleagues (<7 kg for females and <11 kg for males) and then 2) thorough manual muscle strength testing using an isometric approach.
- In the clinical setting, portable hand-held dynamometry is recommended for evaluation of peripheral muscle strength.
- The gold standard for volitional strength testing is isokinetic/fixed dynamometry testing within the laboratory setting.
- In the paediatric population if unable to perform objective strength evaluation such as dynamometry, can observe movements and functional activities relative to developmental milestones to understand the level of impairment in muscle strength.
- In clinical practice, recommend portable dynamometry to provide an objective measure of muscle strength – in paediatric/adolescent and adult populations.
- In the absence of access to equipment, manual strength testing is recommended, but rigorous screening for suitability of the patient to undertake testing and training of assessors is recommended to minimize variability in testing procedure.
- Normative values are available for dynamometry testing across the lifespan.
- Non-volitional muscle stimulation is primarily reserved for research purposes.

during pregnancy (Man et al 2004). Examples of non-volitional assessment of muscle force are measurement of adductor pollicis with ulnar nerve stimulation, quadriceps via femoral nerve stimulation and ankle dorsiflexors using peroneal nerve stimulation.

See Box 6-4 for evaluation of impairment related to muscle strength.

MEASUREMENT OF ACTIVITY LIMITATIONS

The World Health Organization defines activity limitations as the 'difficulty encountered by an individual in executing a task or action' (World Health Organization 2001). As physiotherapists the primary outcome we are often interested in is physical functional ability, which will be the focus of this section of the chapter. It is also important to consider activity limitations in terms of cognitive, mental and psychological outcome measures. Outcome measures used to evaluate these constructs need to be reliable, valid and responsive within the patient population of interest. It is not recommended to extrapolate findings from one patient cohort to another, i.e. critical care to the outpatient heart failure clinic.

The measurement of function is complex, containing information about task completion (cognition), coordination, processing of visual information and central motor drive and the activation of signalling pathways from the motor cortex to the muscle (Sherwood 2004).

Measures of Physical Function and Mobility in the ICU Setting

A range of different tools are available which evaluate physical function with six specifically developed for the ICU setting, including the Physical Function in Intensive Care Test-scored (PFIT-s), the Functional Status Score for the Intensive Care Unit (FSS-ICU), the ICU Mobility Scale, the Surgical ICU Optimal Mobilisation Score, the Chelsea Critical Care Physiotherapy Assessment Tool and the Perme Mobility Scale (Table 6-5) (Parry et al 2015). The recommended tools based on current research evidence include: PFIT-s (Denehy et al 2013, Nordon-Craft et al 2014, Parry et al 2015b), FSS-ICU (Thrush et al 2012, Parry et al 2015b, Zanni et al 2010) and the Chelsea Critical Care Physiotherapy Assessment Tool (Corner et al 2013, Corner et al 2014), as these measures have the most robust clinimetric properties (Parry et al 2015).

The PFIT-s encompasses domains that reflect clinically important aspects of physical function – strength, endurance/exercise capacity and functional ability (Parry et al 2015, Denehy et al 2013). The minimal clinically important difference has been determined as >1.5 points out of 10 (Denehy et al 2013). The PFIT-s can also be used to prescribe exercise intensity (Berney et al 2012). For example, time spent marching on the spot was used to assess gait endurance and for exercise training with participants initially recommended to

Text continued on p. 217

TABLE 6-5

Example Functional Assessment Tools for Use in Cardiorespiratory Patients Across the Continuum

Outcome Measure	Content	Scoring	Reliability	Validity and Responsiveness	Comments
PHYSICAL FUNCTION IN THE ICU					
Physical Function in ICU Test-scored (PFIT-s) (Denehy et al 2013)	Physical function battery test. Four domains: 1) STS assistance level 2) shoulder flexion strength 3) knee extensor strength 4) marching-on-the-spot cadence	Interval score out of 10. MCID is 1.5 out of 10 (can also be scored ordinal out of 12)	Excellent inter-rater reliability (ICC 0.996–1.00) (Skinner et al 2009)	Valid, responsive to change and predictive of key outcomes. PFIT-s has moderate convergent validity with TUG-test (r = −0.60), 6MWT (r = 0.41) and MRC-SS (rho = 0.49). Higher admission PFIT-s predict of MRC-SS ≥48, increased likelihood of discharge home, reduced likelihood of discharge to rehabilitation and reduced hospital LOS (Denehy et al 2013, Parry et al 2015). **Responsiveness** ESI for PFIT-s was 0.82 – representing a large responsiveness to change. **Normal range** No defined cut-off value for what is considered normal	**Equipment** Stopwatch/clock (for measuring cadence). **Feasibility** Safe and inexpensive test with high clinical utility. Quick to administer and minimal training required to perform the testing. **Limitations** Small floor effect on ICU awakening and at ICU discharge (Nordon-Craft et al. 2014 Parry et al 2015). **Other** Can be used to prescribe exercise intensity (Berney et al 2012)
Functional status score in the ICU (FSS-ICU) (Zanni et al 2010)	Assessment of physical function based on five tasks 1) rolling 2) supine to sit transfer 3) unsupported sitting 4) sit to stand 5) ambulation	Scored from 0–35 using 7-point scoring system of FIM from 1 (total dependence) to 7 (complete independence)	No published data	Discriminates between discharge settings and documents functional improvements of patients in a LTACH setting (Thrush, 2012). Moderate validity between FSS-ICU and muscle strength on awakening (Parry et al 2015). **Responsiveness** Limited information on the responsiveness of FSS-ICU, small effect size (ES = 0.25) reported in one study involving chronically critically ill patients (Thrush et al 2012) and in one study within the ICU setting (ES = 0.46) (Parry et al 2015)	**Equipment** None required. **Feasibility** Quick to administer and involves assessment of functional tasks routinely evaluated in rehabilitation practice. **Limitations** Greater clinimetric analysis of this outcome is required

TABLE 6-5
Example Functional Assessment Tools for Use in Cardiorespiratory Patients Across the Continuum (Continued)

Outcome Measure	Content	Scoring	Reliability	Validity and Responsiveness	Comments
PHYSICAL FUNCTION IN THE ICU					
Chelsea Critical Care Physical Assessment Tool (CPAx) (Corner, Wood et al. 2013, Corner, Soni et al. 2014)	Battery test Includes assessment of: ■ respiratory function ■ cough ■ bed mobility ■ supine to SOEOB ■ dynamic sitting ■ standing balance ■ sit to stand ■ transfer bed to chair ■ stepping ■ grip strength	Discrete scores provided for each component assessed ranging from 0–5 with overall score out of 50	Excellent inter-rater reliability (Corner et al 2013)	Valid with/for: moderate correlation with mechanical ventilation duration, muscle strength Good to excellent correlation with SF-36 physical function domain, higher scores correlated with discharge to home (Corner et al 2013, Corner et al 2014)	**Equipment** Peak cough flow measurement such as spirometer Grip dynamometer **Feasibility** Components evaluated are part of routine physiotherapy assessment, which is advantageous **Limitations:** Multiple components to testing – potentially more time-consuming **Other** Can be used to facilitate direction of rehabilitation in specific areas of impairment relative to each domain score
Perme Mobility Scale (Nawa et al 2014)	Assessment of mobility Consists of 15 items across seven categories: mental status, potential mobility barriers, functional strength, bed mobility, transfers, gait and endurance	Score ranges from 0–32 with maximum range of 2–4 points for each of the 15 items A higher score indicates few mobility barriers and minimal assistance required for mobility activities	Excellent inter-rater reliability for overall score in one study	No published data	**Equipment** None required **Feasibility** <2 minutes to complete scoring **Limitations** Limited clinimetric data currently established
ICU mobility scale (IMS) (Hodgson, Berney et al. 2013)	Assessment of physical function Consists of 11 levels ranging from 0 (lying in bed) to 10 (walking independently without a gait aid)	Ordinal 11-point scale	Excellent inter-rater agreement (weighted kappa 0.92–0.98) comparing physiotherapist (both junior and senior) and nursing staff	No published data	**Equipment** None required **Feasibility** Quick to evaluate at the bedside taking <1 minute **Limitations** Limited clinimetric data currently established

Continued on following page

TABLE 6-5

Example Functional Assessment Tools for Use in Cardiorespiratory Patients Across the Continuum (Continued)

Outcome Measure	Content	Scoring	Reliability	Validity and Responsiveness	Comments
PHYSICAL FUNCTION IN THE ICU					
Surgical ICU optimal mobility scale (SOMS) (Kasotakis et al 2012)	Scoring system used to determine optimal mobility level for surgical patients Five levels included: 0 – no activity 1 – PROM, upright in bed 2 – sitting up 3 – standing 4 – ambulating	Nominal classification of mobility in the surgical ICU Patients scored on one of four levels with algorithm for which level patient is appropriate	Excellent inter-rater reliability reported in one study (kappa = 0.80)	SOMS predictive of in-hospital mortality, and correlation with ICU and hospital LOS	**Equipment** None required **Feasibility** Quick to administer **Limitations:** Only developed for the surgical population
MOBILITY MEASURES FOR THE ICU OR ACUTE HOSPITAL WARD					
De Morton Mobility Index (DEMMI) (de Morton et al 2008)	Assessment of 15 functional mobility tasks within the domains of ■ bed mobility ■ chair mobility ■ static balance ■ walking ■ dynamic balance	Raw ordinal score is converted to an interval score from 0–100 MCID is 10 out of 100	High intra-rater and inter-rater reliability (de Morton et al 2011)	Excellent convergent (Barthel index and hierarchical assessment of balance and mobility), construct and discriminant validity (de Morton et al 2011) Low scores are associated with discharge to inpatient rehabilitation rather than home	**Equipment** Bed/plinth, chair, pen **Feasibility** Does not require formal training; quick to administer (<10 minutes) Website resource available www.demmi.org.au **Other** Negligible floor/ceiling effect in the acute setting Has not been evaluated in the ICU setting Also validated in the rehabilitation and community settings

TABLE 6-5

Example Functional Assessment Tools for Use in Cardiorespiratory Patients Across the Continuum *(Continued)*

Outcome Measure	Content	Scoring	Reliability	Validity and Responsiveness	Comments
MOBILITY MEASURES FOR THE ICU OR ACUTE HOSPITAL WARD					
Elderly mobility scale (Smith 1994)	Assessment of physical function of seven tasks ■ lying to sitting ■ sitting to lying ■ sit to stand ■ static standing ■ gait independence ■ timed 6-metre walk ■ functional reach test	Ordinal score from 0–20	Excellent inter-rater reliability (rho = 0.88) Excellent intra-rater reliability	Validated against the modified Rivermead mobility index, Barthel index, FIM and functional ambulation classification (Prosser and Canby 1997, Smith 1994) Scores <10 indicate dependence in mobility Scores 10–13 indicate borderline safety with mobility Scores ≥14 indicate likely independence with mobility	**Equipment** Stopwatch and distance marker for 6-metre walk (excludes distance for acceleration and deceleration) Tape measure for functional reach **Feasibility** Quick to administer (5 minutes) **Other** Functional reach component may predict falls risk Designed for frail older patients in acute medical or community settings
ACTIVITIES OF DAILY LIVING					
Functional independence measure (FIM)	Assessment of functional independence in adults 18 Items	Individual items rated from 1 (total dependence) to 7 (complete independence) to a total score/126			**Feasibility** Requires training for reliable use

Continued on following page

TABLE 6-5

Example Functional Assessment Tools for Use in Cardiorespiratory Patients Across the Continuum *(Continued)*

Outcome Measure	Content	Scoring	Reliability	Validity and Responsiveness	Comments
ACTIVITIES OF DAILY LIVING					
WeeFIM (Msall et al 1993, Ottenbacher et al 1996).	Adapted from adult version FIM. Designed for use in assessing functional independence in children aged 6 months to 8 years (Msall et al 1993, Ottenbacher et al 1996). 18 items – three main domains (self care, mobility and cognition are assessed) either by interviewing parents or observing a child's performance of a task to criterion standards (Msall et al 1993, Ottenbacher et al 1996).	Individual items rated from 1 (total dependence) to 7 (complete independence) to provide a total score out of 126 with a minimum score of 18 (Msall et al 1993, Ottenbacher et al 1996).	Excellent reliability demonstrated both for direct observation and also by interview of parent (Sperle et al 1997)	**Normative values** Available in a **US paediatric population** (Msall et al 1994)	**Feasibility** Requires training for reliable use. Predominantly investigated in children with developmental delay or neurological impairment such as traumatic brain injury or cerebral palsy

6MWT, 6-Minute walk test; *ADLs*, activities of daily living; *ESI*, effect size index; *FIM*, functional independence measure; *ICC*, intra-class correlation coefficient; *ICU*, intensive care unit; *LOS*, length of stay; *LTACH*, long-term acute care hospital; *MCID*, minimum clinical important difference; *MRC-SS*, Medical Research Council Sum-score; *PROM*, passive range of movement; *SF-36*, Short-Form 36; *SOEOB*, sit over edge of bed; *STS*, Sit To Stand; *TUG*, Timed Up and Go.

march on the spot for at least 70% of the time that they achieved on their first test (Berney et al 2012), in accordance with the guidelines for exercise training published by the American College of Sports Medicine (American College of Sports Medicine 2000). The FSS-ICU involves assessment of five functional tasks (rolling, supine to sit transfers, unsupported sitting, sit to stand transfers and ambulation). The five tasks are scored on a seven-point scoring system from the Functional Independence Measure (Parry et al 2015b, Zanni et al 2010). Higher scores present better function and total scores range from 0 to 35 (Zanni et al 2010). The FSS-ICU was originally developed for use in the ICU setting; one recent study reported on the validity and responsiveness of the FSS-ICU in the ICU setting (Parry et al 2015b). The Chelsea Critical Care Physiotherapy Assessment Tool, also known as the 'CPAx', involves evaluation of 10 commonly assessed physical and respiratory measures, including grip strength, standing balance, respiratory function and cough. Higher scores represent better function, and total scores range from 0 to 50. It has been shown to be reliable, valid and responsive to change over time (Corner et al 2013, Corner et al 2014).

The measurement of mobility milestones such as the duration of unsupported sitting on the edge of the bed, number of days to first sit out of bed, maximum distance ambulated and percentage of patients who sit out of bed prior to ICU discharge (Adler et al 2012) may be appropriate to use as either measures of process/quality control within an ICU, or in research studies. They are not objective measures, which enable determination of responsiveness to an intervention such as physiotherapy and rehabilitation, and thus validated measures such as the PFIT-s or FSS-ICU are recommended for clinical practice.

Other Measures of Mobility and Activities of Daily Living in Acute Care

Aside from measures of physical function/functional mobility that have been specifically developed for use in the critically ill, there are a range of other general mobility measures and measures of ADLs that have been used in the acute setting with varying degrees of acceptability (see Table 6-5). The De Morton Mobility Index (DEMMI) assesses patients' level of independence with tasks ranging from bed mobility (bridge, roll onto side, lying to sitting) to higher-level dynamic balance (pick up pen from floor, walk four steps backwards, jump) (de Morton et al 2008). A raw score is converted to an interval score out of 100, with high scores representing better function. The minimal clinically important difference is 10 points on the 100-point scale (de Morton et al 2011a). The DEMMI is highly reliable, requires minimal training to use and has been validated in older medical patients in the acute setting, rehabilitation and the community (de Morton et al 2011a, de Morton et al 2011b). This means that it can be used across the spectrum of acute illness to recovery, with baseline testing most appropriate from the time of ICU discharge due to a potential floor effect in the ICU.

Alternatively, the Elderly Mobility Scale, which assesses tasks from lying to sitting to a timed 6-metre walk, has been tested for reliability and validity in elderly inpatients (Prosser et al 1997, Smith 1994). Scores >14/20 have been associated with an increased likelihood of a patient being discharged home, and low scores (<10) with increased falls risk and the likelihood of a high level of mobility and ADL assistance requirements. A measure developed specifically for use in the acute neurological setting and then later modified for acute orthopaedic patients is the Acute Care Index Of Function that assesses tasks ranging from bed mobility to wheelchair mobility and stair climbing (Roach et al 1998a, Roach et al 1998b, Van Dillen et al 1988). Although tested for reliability and validity, this scale has limited use to date in the ICU (Bissett et al 2015). Other functional tests that have been used in the acute hospital setting are the timed Five Times Sit to Stand test, the Timed Up and Go test, Berg balance scale, functional ambulation classification and field walking tests such as 2-minute and 6-minute walk. Other ADL measures that may be appropriate to use in the acute and community setting for evaluation of the cardiorespiratory patient include: the Functional Independence Measure (FIM), Barthel index, Katz ADL index and the Glittre ADL index, (Elliott et al 2011).

There is a paediatric version called the 'Functional Independence Measure for Children', also known as the 'WeeFIM', which is designed to measure severity of disability and changes in functional ability of children from 6 months to 8 years (Msall et al 1993, Ottenbacher et al 1996). It is an 18-item functional measure which can be completed by direct observation or interviewing the primary caregiver/parent (Msall et al 1993, Ottenbacher et al 1996). It has been shown to have robust measurement properties in the paediatric population (Ottenbacher et al 1996, Sperle et al 1997). The Paediatric Evaluation of Disability Inventory (PEDI) is another common outcome measure which provides more detailed information on the use of environmental modifications and assistive equipment, and is more time-consuming to perform compared to the WeeFIM (Haley et al 1992, Ottenbacher et al 1996). Predominantly, measurement of activity limitation is linked with neurodevelopmental milestone achievement and thus neurodevelopmental measures such as Alberta Infant Motor Scale, Movement Assessment of Infants and Peabody developmental motor scales may be used in neonates and paediatric populations (Darrah et al 1998, Spittle et al 2008).

Exercise Testing

The main reasons for implementing a systematic clinical exercise-testing programme include:

1. diagnosis
2. determination of the severity and functional effects of the disease
3. prognosis
4. assessment for suitability of treatment, i.e. surgery, transplantation, supplemental oxygen therapy
5. determination of efficacy of therapeutic intervention
6. outcome variable for clinical trials
7. motivation and measurable goals to improve fitness
8. quantification of exercise rehabilitative training intensity
9. development of knowledge and understanding of the disease.

A cardiopulmonary exercise test (CPET or CPEX) is the 'gold standard' measure for evaluation of functional capacity/'fitness'. The main outcome of interest is maximal oxygen uptake (VO_{2max}), which represents the maximal rate at which oxygen can be transported, consumed and utilized during whole body exercise. Cardiopulmonary exercise testing involves a patient exercising incrementally to a submaximal or maximal exertion level on an ergometer (arm, treadmill or cycle, with cycle ergometry being the most commonly used in clinical practice). It is also possible to utilize a test which is discontinuous, meaning after the completion of each stage, the patient is given a defined rest period before the next incremental stage is attempted. Typically a CPET will last between 6 and 12 minutes. The CPET needs to be performed in a dedicated clinical laboratory, with expert trained assessors to monitor the patient closely during testing and interpret the results of testing. Equipment and measurement includes: cycle ergometry, 12-lead ECG, non-invasive blood pressure cuffed monitoring, measurement of VO_2 and volume of carbon dioxide (VCO_2) through a mask and pulse oximetry to monitor oxygen saturation levels. There are several guidelines for adult and paediatric exercise tests published and readers are referred to these for more detailed information on CPET (ATS/ACCP 2003).

The determination of VO_{2max} requires that at the cessation of the test (volitional exhaustion), the participant's oxygen consumption is no longer increasing linearly and exhibits a plateau. In practice, either because the testing team have not motivated the patient to the point of volitional exhaustion or the patient is unwilling to push himself or herself to exhaustion, the oxygen consumption can be linear, still be increasing or can even be decreasing. Due to the lack of a plateau, often the term 'peak VO_2' (or VO_{2peak}) is used. In an attempt to verify a 'maximal' effort, secondary criteria from the CPET are often used to validate the VO_{2max} test. These criteria include heart rate >195 beats/min (cycle ergometer) or >200 beats/min (treadmill), respiratory exchange ratio (RER) >1.00 and blood lactate accumulation >4.0 mmol/L.

In healthy children these secondary criteria have been called into question, due to their unreliability, resulting in the acceptance of sub-maximal peak VO_2 values or incorrectly rejecting a true VO_{2max} measurement. Peak heart rate for children during cycle ergometry has been reported as 195 beats/min and for children during treadmill exercise as 200 beats/min (Rowland 1996) but should be taken only as guides. The traditional calculation of '220 bpm – age' which is used commonly in adults is not applicable to children.

Maximal heart rate is genetically predetermined and the maximal heart rate achieved by children and adolescents is independent of age. In addition, in contrast to adults in whom maximal heart rate decreases with age, the maximal heart rate remains relatively stable at around 190 beats/min in children and adolescents (Bongers et al 2012).

Additionally, the accumulation of blood lactate for the same relative intensity is generally lower in children than in adults. During the initial stages of a progressive incremental exercise for the determination of peak VO_2 blood lactate levels do not significantly increase above resting values of 1–2 mmol/L. As the test progresses, a point is reached where blood lactate begins to increase rapidly with a subsequent steep rise until exhaustion. There is considerable variation in the post exercise blood lactates of children and adolescents, with values of peak VO_2 ranging from less than 4.0 mmol/L to more than 13.0 mmol/L using the same protocol, sampling and assay techniques (Williams et al 1990). Some paediatric exercise testing laboratories recommend post exercise blood lactates of 6 to 9 mmol/L as a criterion of peak VO_2 being accepted as a maximal index of aerobic fitness (Cumming et al 1980). However, blood lactate levels are highly influenced by methodological variations, e.g. mode of exercise, exercise protocols and site of sampling, and this practice should be discouraged. Blood lactate sampling is currently not routinely used in clinical paediatric exercise testing laboratories.

A recent study in patients with cystic fibrosis (Saynor et al 2013) determined that the only method by which a physiotherapist and their team can be confident that a maximal value has been attained is the conduction of a subsequent exercise bout [10 minutes later] following the completion of the initial incremental test. By following this method there is a greater confidence that the maximal limits of the oxygen transport chain have been reached and therefore the ensuing interpretation of the data is more secure.

A CPET is beneficial within the clinical setting because it can determine the mechanisms of the limitation of the oxygen transport chain and its association to exercise tolerance and quality of life. Although VO_{2max} is the variable most commonly reported, there is a wealth of submaximal data that might be of interest to the physiotherapist and their clinical teams (see

Table 6-6 for definitions). Additionally, the opportunity to be able to measure other variables during cycle or treadmill testing, e.g., electrocardiography (ECG), blood pressure, oxygen saturation, cardiac output and oxygen extraction, increases the capability of investigating the exercise limitations of the cardiac, pulmonary and muscular systems. For a comprehensive review of the utility of CPET, readers are referred to Wasserman et al (2005).

Recently a test known as the steep ramp test (SRT) has been validated in a healthy school aged population group and in a clinical setting with young cystic fibrosis patients (Bongers et al 2013). The SRT is seen as a possible replacement for the CPET where maximal testing is contraindicated or the equipment required is not available. The advantages of the SRT compared to a CPET include the shorter duration protocol ($\approx$2–3 minutes), lower cost, as only a cycle ergometer is required, and minimal training required by staff to conduct this test. The main outcome variable is peak work rate measured in watts. Bongers et al (2013) argue that paediatric patients with chronic diseases might better tolerate this test, as it places a smaller burden on the cardiopulmonary system. While some norm referenced values and comparative values to CPET scores have been produced, this test is still in its infancy and requires greater consideration for reliability and validity across clinical groups. While the SRT is an inexpensive and quick test to operate, it is a relatively blunt tool to assess functional change in a clinical setting. Originally designed as a method to determine and readjust training work rates in adult chronic heart failure patients, the reliance on only one outcome variable that the detection of casual factors related to increased or decreased work rate cannot be ascertained within the test protocol.

Criteria to Determine a Maximal Exercise Test. Not all individuals tested will show a levelling off of VO_2 during the test. Therefore it has been suggested to assume a maximal effort if at least one of the following criteria is met during an exercise test:

1. The patient achieves predicted peak VO_2 and/or predicted maximal work rate (ATS/ACCP 2003). The equations to predict $VO2_{peak}$ and maximal work rate are test, gender and age specific.

TABLE 6-6

Physiological Measurements during a CPET to Assess Function

Symbol	Measurement	Function
VO_{2max}	Aerobic fitness	Maximal rate of transport, consumption and utilization of oxygen as evidenced by a failure of oxygen to increase despite an increasing work rate
VO_{2peak}	Aerobic fitness (this term often used in the paediatric literature because of the failure of the majority of young people to provide criteria for a VO_{2max} test)	Highest VO_2 achieved during a 'presumed' maximal effort which may or may not be equal to VO_{2max}
WR_{max}	Maximal work rate	The maximal power output in watts (W)
V_E	Minute ventilation	The volume of air exhaled each minute as a product of the tidal volume and breathing frequency
VCO_2	Volume of carbon dioxide	The volume of CO_2 produced
V_T	Tidal volume	Volume of expired air per breath
b_f	Breathing frequency	Frequency of heart beat usually per minute
RER	Respiratory exchange ratio	The ratio of the volume of carbon dioxide produced divided by the volume of oxygen consumed provides an indicator of the pulmonary exchange of the two gases across differing physiological and metabolic conditions.
$\Delta VO_2/\Delta WR$	Aerobic contribution of work	The VO_2^- work rate relationship reflects how much oxygen is utilized relative to the quantity of performed external work. Typically this is 10 mL/min W^{-1}
GET	Gaseous exchange threshold	A non-invasive estimation of the lactate threshold and maker for increasing blood lactate above resting baseline values

CPET, Cardiopulmonary exercise test.

2. The patient reaches a maximal heart rate (HR) at or above predicted peak HR (ATS/ACCP 2003).
3. Peak ventilation approaches or exceeds (estimated) maximal voluntary ventilation (MVV) (ATS/ACCP 2003).
4. Maximal RER during exercise exceeds 1.03 (cycle ergometry) or 1.0 (treadmill) in children and adolescents (Rowland 1996). In adults, a RER above 1.05 is usually considered an indicator of a maximal effort (Nes et al 2012).
5. A rating of 9–10 on a 0–10 Borg scale for perceived exertion or 17 or above on a 6–20 scale (ATS/ACCP 2003, Nes et al. 2012), 6–8 rating on The OMNI rate of perceived exertion.

Reasons to Terminate a Test

1. if the child is unable to continue for any reason
2. participant requests to stop
3. if arterial oxygen saturation (SaO_2) falls >10% below baseline
4. extreme shortness of breath
5. struggling to keep pace or rhythm
6. complaining of chest pain
7. abnormal ECG changes
8. excessive rise in BP
9. signs of poor perfusion: light headedness, confusion, ataxia, pallor, cyanosis or cold and clammy skin
10. failure of HR to increase with increased exercise intensity.

The ATS/European Respiratory Society (ERS) guidelines outline the importance of selecting the most appropriative normative reference values to ensure accurate interpretation of a patient's test results (ATS 2003). The reference values are also different depending on whether the testing is conducted

TABLE 6-7

Functional Exercise Testing Normative Values for Healthy Children

Test	Normative Values
V_E/VCO_2 at peak exercise	Children 11.1 ± 0.4 years: F, 28.7 ± 2.2; M, 27.9 ± 2.4 (Armstrong et al 1997)
V_E/VO_2 at peak exercise	Children 11.1 ± 0.4 years: F, 29.5 ± 3.; M, 29.8 ± 3.2 Children ≅ 11 years: F, 39.22 ± 3.35; M, 35.29 ± 1.72 (Rowland and Cunningham 1997) Children ≅ 14 years: F, 39.37 ± 3.88; M, 34.05 ± 2.58
$\Delta V_E/\Delta VCO_2$	F, −0.64 × age + 38 (SEE 4.0); M, −0.64 × age + 38 (SEE 3.6) (Ten Harkel et al 2011)
$\Delta VO_2/\Delta WR$ slope	F, 9.3 mL/min W^{-1} (SD 1.0); M, 9.9 mL/min W^{-1} (SD 0.9) (Ten Harkel et al 2011)
Maximum voluntary ventilation (MVV)	Children 27.7 × FEV_1 = 8.8 × predicted FEV_1 (Stein et al 2003)

F, Female; FEV_1, forced expiratory volume in 1 second; M, male; SD, standard deviation; SEE, standard error of estimate; VCO_2, volume of carbon dioxide; V_E, ventilation; VO_2, volume of oxygen; WR, work rate.

using a cycle or treadmill ergometer, and thus needs to be taken into consideration when selecting the most appropriate normative values for comparison. More recently a reference set of data of normal values for parameters measured during cardiopulmonary exercise testing have been developed for the paediatric and adolescent population (8–18 years) (Ten Harkel et al 2011). Normative values are summarized for paediatrics in Table 6-7. The adoption of guidelines such as ATS/American College of Clinical Pharmacy (ACCP) and ERS is critical to ensure high-quality exercise testing in both research and clinical practice.

Field Walking Tests

Field walking tests are commonly utilized at the time of hospital discharge or in the community setting to evaluate a patient's exercise/functional capacity. There is limited utility in using field walking tests earlier in the hospitalization, i.e. when the patient is acutely or critically unwell, as the patient will not have sufficient cardiorespiratory and musculoskeletal reserve to perform the field walking tests.

Field walking tests are valuable but still an under-utilized tool for clinical assessments; this is surprising, given that clinical examination and static tests, e.g. lung function, have been shown to be poor predictors of exercise performance. Most organizations such as Cystic Fibrosis Society, American Heart Association, United States National Asthma Education Program, ATS and ERS have published guidelines on the use of exercise testing in the diagnosis and/or treatment of disease in their respective patient groups. The ATS and ERS guidelines are recommended as a key resource for readers to refer to as a guide (Holland et al 2014).

Field walking tests are widely used in rehabilitation programmes, as they require little equipment and are relatively straightforward to perform for both the assessor and the patient. In more sophisticated centres, CPETs may be conducted. The three field walking tests described below can elicit a VO_{2peak} and peak heart rate similar to laboratory testing involving cardiopulmonary exercise testing (Holland et al 2014). Therefore it is important to be aware of the absolute and relative contraindications for exercise testing. Patients should rest for at least 15 minutes before commencing an exercise test. If a patient is on long-term oxygen therapy, oxygen should be given at their standard flow rate or as directed by the physician. Field walking tests are performed to identify an individual's exercise capacity, factors limiting exercise performance (musculoskeletal limitations, subjective fatigue and dyspnoea) and to evaluate treatment efficacy.

The three most commonly reported/described field walking tests are:

1. 6-minute walk test (6MWT)
2. incremental shuttle walk test (ISWT)
3. endurance shuttle walk test (ESWT).

The 6-minute walk test is the most commonly reported field walking test and is used in individuals with chronic respiratory diseases including COPD, critical care, lung cancer, transplantation and cardiac conditions.

Within the paediatric/adolescent population there are two other tests which are commonly assessed (particularly in cystic fibrosis):

4. modified shuttle walk test (MSWT)
5. step/stair climbing test.

Each of these tests will be briefly described. Readers are encouraged to refer to the ATS/ERS technical standards for performance of field walking tests (Holland et al 2014) and associated systematic review on the measurement properties of the tests (Singh et al 2014) for more detail.

6-Minute Walk Test. The 6MWT is a **self-paced** test of functional capacity. The test requires an individual to cover as much ground as possible over 6 minutes, being allowed to stop and rest if required. The 6-minute walk distance (6MWD) in metres is recorded. The course must be 30 m long, and unobstructed and on flat ground (no inclination); instructions and encouragement should be standardized as per the published guidelines (Holland et al 2014). Patients are required to perform two measures with a minimum of 30 minutes between tests, and the 'best' value is reported. There are 18 published sets of reference equations for the 6MWD in healthy adults (Holland et al 2014, Singh et al 2014). There is wide variation in predicted 6MWD generated by different reference equations; therefore it is recommended that reference equations generated and verified within your country and local population are applied where possible (Holland et al 2014, Singh et al 2014). The ATS/ERS technical standards recommends a minimal important difference (MID) for the 6MWD in chronic lung disease of 30 metres; we can be confident that the MID lies between 25 and 33 metres (Holland et al 2014, Singh et al 2014). More recently the MID has been defined in lung cancer (22–42 metres) (Granger et al 2015) and in critical care (20–30 metres) (Chan et al 2015).

Incremental Shuttle Walk Test. The ISWT is an **externally paced** exercise test, which is controlled by a series of prerecorded audio signals. The test has 12 levels, starting at a very slow speed of walking, with 20 seconds to complete each 10-m length, increasing gradually at the end of each minute. The maximum

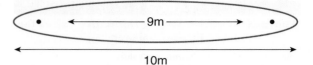

FIGURE 6-4 ■ Incremental shuttle walk test course.

duration of the test is 20 minutes. The test is conducted around a 10-metre course (Fig. 6-4), identified by two markers which are placed 0.5 m from each other, representing an elliptical course, and avoiding abrupt changes in directions. The test can be terminated by the patient if they develop intolerable symptoms or by the assessor if the patient fails to reach the marker in the time allowed. The total distance in metres is recorded. The ISWT is incremental in nature and has been shown to have a strong relationship with performance on laboratory-based tests such as a CPET. Similar to the 6MWT, two measures need to be performed with a minimum of 30 minutes between tests performed on the same day. The MID for the ISWT has been reported as 47.5 m in one study within individuals with COPD (Singh et al 2008; Singh et al 2014). Three papers have described reference values for the ISWT: two from South America and one from the United Kingdom (Singh et al 2014). There is a need for the development of reference equations for the ISWT and ESWT across different countries.

Endurance Shuttle Walk Test. The ESWT is an endurance field walking test where patients are asked to walk for as long as they can at the preset speed; it is another **externally paced** field test. It is performed over the same course as the ISWT, i.e. 10-metre distance is marked out with cones 0.5 metres from each end. There are 16 predefined speeds available (1.78–6 km/h) and the most appropriate speed is selected based upon performance on the ISWT, and usually is in the range of 70–85% of the maximum performance, with a maximum time of 20 minutes for the test. The ESWT is considered to be a companion test to the IWST, and can only be performed after an ISWT has been undertaken, and thus ESWT only needs to be performed once. The speed of walking and total time in minutes is recorded. The MID for ESWT in chronic respiratory diseases has been defined as 4.5 minutes (Eaton et al 2006).

Modified Shuttle Walk Test. The MSWT is an **externally paced** test, which is controlled by a series of prerecorded audio signals. The set up for this test is the same as the ISWT described (over a 10-metre course), except that there are 15 levels, with the speed of the test progressively increasing, with the patient moving from walking to running. It has been most extensively evaluated in paediatric and adolescent children with cystic fibrosis (Bradley et al 2000, Cox et al 2006, Radtke et al 2009, Selvadurai et al 2003). It has been shown to be a reliable, repeatable and sensitive measure of functional capacity in this patient population. The MSWT has been shown to be responsive to the effect of hospitalization for intravenous antibiotics and for supportive therapy management including airway clearance techniques (Bradley et al 2000, Cox et al 2006, Selvadurai et al 2003).

Step Test. Step tests such as the 3-minute step test has been used in the cystic fibrosis and lung transplantation population (Aurora et al 2001, Balfour-Lynn et al 1998, Radtke et al 2009). The testing requires the individuals to step up and down on a step 15 centimetres in height, with the stepping pace externally paced. It is usual during a stepping test to record heart rate and oxygen saturation (Aurora et al 2001, Balfour-Lynn et al 1998) but it would be more difficult although not impossible to assess ventilatory variables using a portable oxygen and carbon dioxide analyzer. By administering an incremental stepping rate, some of the criticisms of self-paced tests were removed (Prasad et al 2000). Nonetheless, step tests are submaximal in intensity, as patients can find it difficult to reach the maximal limits of the cardiopulmonary system. Another weakness of the test is that work rate cannot be quantified accurately due to the differing resultants of stepping height (leg length), body mass and work rate and its sensitivity to detect clinical changes has been questioned (Narang et al 2003).

The choice of field walking test is dictated by facilities, equipment and staff skills and availability. It is important to consider the type of training regimen offered within the programme, to examine the meas-urable impact of the programme the test conventionally matches the training programme, so for example it is likely that a cycle-based training regime will show greater benefit using a cycle-based exercise test compared to a walking-based test. Overall, endurance tests, either walking or cycling, tend to be more responsive to rehabilitation than incremental exercise tests. A summary of the clinimetric properties of these tests is provided in Table 6-8.

Physical Activity

Physical activity, its definition and general description is discussed in Chapter 12. There are a variety of methods available to measure physical activity in the clinical setting. These include objective movement sensors, such as accelerometers or pedometers, which detect and record movement (Westerterp 2009), and subjective patient-reported measures, such as questionnaires, which ask the participant to recall their engagement in physical activity (Westerterp 2009). Questionnaires are advantageous in that they are quick, inexpensive, associated with minimal participant burden and feasible to implement on a large scale. There are a number of different questionnaires available for use; however, there is no consensus as to which is the best questionnaire for use in clinical practice or in different specific populations.

The Physical Activity Scale for the Elderly (PASE) is a questionnaire which asks the participant to recall their level of physical activity over the previous 7 days (Washburn et al 1993). This questionnaire was originally developed in a population of healthy community-dwelling older adults in the United States (Washburn et al 1993) and since then has been widely used across many patient groups (Forsén et al 2010), including people with cancer. The PASE has well-established clinimetric properties in the healthy elderly population: moderate criterion validity with doubly labelled water analysis ($r = 0.68$) (Schuit 1997); fair convergent validity with accelerometry ($r = 0.49$) (Washburn 1999) and excellent test-retest reliability ($r = 0.84$) (Washburn et al 1993). Other physical activity questionnaires include the Godin Exercise Leisure Time Questionnaire (Godin et al 1985b, Godin et al 1985a) and the International Physical Activity Questionnaire (IPAQ) (Craig et al 2003).

TABLE 6-8

Field Walking Tests – Reliability, Validity and Responsiveness Within Different Cardiorespiratory Populations

Population	6MWD			ISWT			ESWT		
	Reliability	Validity	Responsiveness	Reliability	Validity	Responsiveness	Reliability	Validity	Responsiveness
COPD	Yes Reliable for distance and SpO_2, requires repeat tests 6MWD is not accurate when performed in the home setting	Yes Valid with/for: CPET, physical activity, FEV_1, dyspnoea, HR-QoL, mortality, hospitalization	Yes Responsive to: pulmonary rehabilitation, pharmaceutical interventions	Yes Reliable for distance and SpO_2, requires repeat tests	Yes Valid with/for: CPET, quadriceps strength, physical activity, RFTs, mortality, hospitalization	Yes Responsive to: pulmonary rehabilitation, oxygen, bronchodilators Floor effect Greater desaturation than observed in 6MWD	Yes Reliable for distance and SpO_2, requires repeat tests	X	Yes Most responsive to pulmonary rehabilitation, oxygen therapy, and bronchodilators
ILD	Yes Reliable for distance, requires repeat tests	Yes Valid with/for: CPET, physical activity, dyspnoea, mortality, HR-QoL, DLCO	Yes Responsive to pulmonary rehabilitation	X	X	X	X	X	X
Cystic fibrosis	Yes Reliable for distance and SpO_2	Yes Valid with/for: CPET, physical activity, FEV_1	X	X	Relatively unknown (one study: no association with survival)	X	X	X	X
PAH	Yes	Yes Valid with/for: CPET, physical activity, HR-QoL, mortality	Yes Responsive to: drugs	X	X	X	X	X	X
Lung Cancer	X	Yes Valid with/for: mortality, postoperative outcomes, HR-QoL, radiation pneumonitis	X	X	Yes Valid with/for: CPET, mortality, postoperative outcomes, strength	X	X	Relatively unknown (one study: poor with CPET)	X

CVD	Yes Reliable for distance in cardiac surgery and heart failure populations	Yes Valid with/for: peak heart rate during 6MWT and during cycle-exercise at ventilatory threshold, mortality, HR-QoL	Yes Responsive to change in clinical status following cardiac rehabilitation	Yes Reliable in cardiac surgery population and cardiovascular disease	Yes Valid with/for: CPET	Yes Responsive to change in clinical status	X	X	X
ICU	Yes Reliable for distance	Yes Valid with/for: TUG test, balance (BBS), HR-QoL, mortality, hospitalization	Yes Responsive to changes in HR-QoL (SF-36 PF domain), and patient report of change in function (global rating of change)	X	X	X	X	X	X

6WMD, 6-Minute walk distance; 6WMT, 6-minute walk test; BBS, Berg balance scale; COPD, chronic obstructive pulmonary disease; CPET, cardiopulmonary exercise test; CVD, cardiovascular disease; DLCO, diffusing capacity of lungs for carbon monoxide; ESWT, endurance shuttle walk test; FEV₁, forced expiratory volume in 1 second; HR-QoL, health-related quality of life; ILD, interstitial lung disease; ISWT, incremental shuttle walk test; PAH, pulmonary arterial hypertension; PF, physical function; RFT, respiratory function tests; SF-36, Short-Form 36; SpO₂, oxyhaemoglobin saturation; TUG, Timed Up and Go.

Motion sensors provide information on the body's physical movement. During physical activity the body is propelled forwards with a certain acceleration; this is caused by muscular activity and results in energy expenditure (Vanhees et al 2005). For this reason accelerometers and pedometers have been widely used as a surrogate measure of energy expenditure, and thus level of physical activity. Accelerometers measure acceleration in one, two or three planes. Tri-axial accelerometers measure acceleration in the vertical, medial-lateral and anterior–posterior planes. Accelerometers provide information on an individual's physical activity intensity and distance travelled. Outcomes are often reported in steps or accelerations per minute. Pedometers are the most basic form of motion sensors. Pedometers act with a spring mechanism which detects vertical motion and thus gives an estimation of step count in a set time period (Vanhees et al 2005). The distance an individual has walked can be estimated by multiplying their step length with the measured step count. The gold standard for measurement of physical activity is direct calorimetry, which measures energy expenditure due to the physical activity performed (Vanhees et al 2005).

There is increasing interest in the use of technology through smart phone applications, movement sensor technologies and use of activity monitoring to capture real-time data on an individual's level of activity and how this may impact their participation restriction but also prognostication of future outcomes and risk of re-hospitalization. This is a rapidly growing area for future research and clinical practice.

See Box 6-5 for a summary of methods of activity limitations measurement.

MEASUREMENT OF PARTICIPATION RESTRICTION

The World Health Organization has defined participation restriction as a 'problem experienced by an individual in involvement in life situations' (World Health Organization 2001) and tells us about the level of disability experienced by an individual. For the purposes of this chapter we will primarily focus on health-related quality of life measures within individuals with cardiorespiratory impairment/s.

> **BOX 6-5**
> **SUMMARY – ACTIVITY LIMITATIONS**
>
> ■ In the ICU recommend measures: PFIT-s, FSS-ICU and/or CPAx.
> ■ Ward/hospital setting: variety of different outcome measures are available, therefore need to consider most appropriate for population of interest.
> ■ CPET is the gold standard for evaluation of exercise capacity.
> ■ Field walking tests – recommended for clinical practice. If perform 6MWT must repeat test twice.
> ■ Physical activity can be measured using activity monitors and/or questionnaires such as the PASE or IPAQ.
>
> ---
>
> *6MWT*, 6-Minute Walk Test; *CPAx*, Chelsea Critical Care Physical Assessment Tool; *CPET*, cardiopulmonary exercise test; *FSS-ICU*, Functional Status Score for the Intensive Care Unit; *ICU*, intensive care unit; *IPAQ*, International Physical Activity Questionnaire; *PASE*, Physical Activity Scale for the Elderly; *PFIT-s*, Physical Function in Intensive Care Test-scored.

Quality of Life

Quality of life has been defined by the World Health Organization (WHO) as:

'… an individual's perceptions of their positions in life in the context of the culture and value system in which they live and in relation to their goals, expectations, standards and concerns. It is a broad ranging concept affected in a complex way by the person's physical health, psychological state, level of independence, social relationships, and their relationship to salient features of their environment' (1993).

Although quality of life is an all-encompassing concept, health-related quality of life is commonly used in the evaluation of healthcare, pertains to the characteristics of life that are affected by one's health (Hawthorne 2007) and falls under participation restriction category within the ICF framework. Most individuals with a perspective on health-related quality of life (HR-QoL) readily agree that to measure quality of life, patients should report their perception of their ability to participate in daily activities that are construed as necessary and important to a fulfilling life. However, it is difficult to characterize exactly how this is or should be measured and this is evident where authors have used terms such as 'quality of life', 'health status' and 'functional status' interchangeably (Kerridge et al 1994). Within this chapter, 'HR-QoL' is used as an umbrella term to denote aspects of health status including (but not limited to) physical functioning, social and family functioning, anxiety, sleep quality, cognitive functioning, communication, role limitations, emotional functioning and psychological well-being, pain, fatigue and health transition. The single feature common to these diverse concepts measured as HR-QoL is that these aspects of health are usually measured by self-report and are designed and accepted to encapsulate the patient's perception of their own health state, rather than the health system or healthcare provider's perception of the patient health state. There is limited general consensus as to which dimensions of health are the most important to measure, although generic instruments cover at least physical, mental and social health, and somatic perceptions (Hawthorne & Richardson 2001, Schipper et al 1996). The selection of conceptual dimensions for a health status or HR-QoL instrument is a difficult process; for example, the construction of the Medical Outcomes Study 36-item Short-Form Health Survey (SF-36) necessitated the selection of eight dimensions from 40 physical and mental health concepts (Ware et al 1993).

Why Health-Related Quality of Life?

Patient-reported outcomes are increasingly emphasized in the context of healthcare delivery and their importance should not be underestimated, although quality of life should be considered as one of a body of outcome measures, including other psychological and physical impairments such as functional exercise capacity, physical function and comorbid illnesses such as depression, anxiety, sleep and activity restriction scales.

Health-Related Quality of Life Outcome Measures

There are many instruments available for the measurement of HR-QoL, and they can be categorized into four main areas: generic (designed for general populations); disease-specific (for use in particular populations); dimension-specific (for use with common symptoms or sequelae) or utility measures (Garratt

et al 2002). It is impractical to give an overview of all of the instruments available to measure HR-QoL, as, for example, a recent systematic review reported that 10 generic and 13 disease-specific instruments have been identified for use in patient care and research of people with COPD alone (Weldam et al 2013). Disease-specific measures are more commonly used than generic measures and Tables 6-9 and 6-10 give an overview of the most robust and/or commonly used generic and disease-specific HR-QoL measures in cardiorespiratory physiotherapy. It is common to find smaller, niche populations using generic measures in disease-specific populations where the populations are discrete and disease-specific measures have not been developed or validated, e.g. people with atrial fibrillation (Thrall et al 2006). It should also be noted that some instruments have different forms, for example, the Short-Form 36 (e.g. SF-12); the Assessment of Quality of Life (e.g. AQoL-8D) and the WHO Quality of Life-BREF (e.g. WHOQOL-100) have one or more different versions (either shorter or longer). For the purpose of this chapter, the most commonly used questionnaire is presented.

Psychometric Properties of HR-QoL Instruments

Accurate measurement of HR-QoL relies on the psychometric and measurement properties of the instruments. Outcomes after illness can be examined in the context of the healthy population, the healthy age and sex-matched population and other disease populations. Once an understanding of community health is gained, this allows more effective comparison between community groups and disease populations. Additionally, it is of interest to review the specific HR-QoL outcomes in different populations in order to note whether HR-QoL outcomes differ for specific diagnostic or clinical groups and where the HR-QoL deficits are most profound. This information may help with service delivery or policy decisions and prioritization and is particularly important, as HR-QoL norms may vary internationally (Table 6-11).

Adult – Disease-Specific

Different instruments may be more or less appropriate to use for reporting health profiles in different population settings; therefore head-to-head comparison of

Text continued on p. 238

TABLE 6-9

Generic Measures of HR-QoL

Results May Vary According to Population

Outcome Measure	Time to Complete (Minutes)	Content/Mode of Administration	Scoring/ Interpretation	Validity	Reliability	Responsiveness: Sensitivity	Minimal Important Difference	Measures Health Utility? Normative Data?	Widely Used?
Medical Outcomes Study 36-item Short-Form Health Survey (SF-36) (Ware & Sherbourne 1992, Ware et al 1994, Ware et al 1993)	10–20	Items: 36 Domains: 8 (Physical functioning, role limitation (physical, emotional), bodily pain, vitality, general health, social functioning, mental health) Mode: Interview/ self-administered	Scoring: By domain and component summary scores (physical and mental) Domains: Version 1: 0 (worst health) to 100 (optimal health) Version 2 and summary scores (norm-based): mean (SD) 50 (10) where 50 = population mean	Content: Yes Construct: Yes Criterion: Yes Predictive: Yes Can predict mortality in patients undergoing coronary bypass and hospitalization/ mortality in heart failure	IC: Yes TR: Yes Highest internal consistency of generic measures	Responsiveness: Yes Sensitivity: Yes	MID: Version 1 5 points MID: Version 2 2–3 points MID: COPD 8–12.5 points MID: chronic disease 10–25 points	Yes (mapped) Extensive normative data	Yes
EuroQoL 5D questionnaire (EuroQoL 1990, Kind 1996) EuroQoL 5D-5L (Herdman et al 2011)	5	Items: 5 Domains: 5 (Anxiety/depression, pain/discomfort, mobility, self-care, usual activities Visual analogue scale EQ-5D: 3 response options to each item EQ-5D-5L: 5 response options to each item Mode: Self-administered/ interview	Scoring: −0.59 (worst health) to 1.00 (best health) VAS: 0 (worst state) to 100 (best state)	Content: Yes Construct: Moderate Criterion: Yes Predictive: Some content validity established by the EuroQoL group Construct validity in acute coronary syndrome Some evidence of validity for 5D-5L in cardiovascular disease, COPD, asthma, diabetes	IC: Yes TR: Yes Good test re-test reliability in general population Acceptable in heart failure Good reliability in rheumatoid arthritis patients	Responsiveness: Moderate Sensitivity: No 5D-5L may have better sensitivity EQ-5D limited by ceiling effect	MID: 0.074 (range −0.011 to 0.140) 0.09–0.10 for all cancers, 0.07–0.08 for lung cancer VAS 7–10 (using FACT-G quintiles)	Yes Value method: TTO Widespread normative data (especially European)	Yes

Sickness Impact Profile (Bergner et al 1981, Bergner et al 1976a, Bergner et al 1976b, Carter et al 1976, Gilson et al 1975, Pollard et al 1976)	35	Items: 136 Domains: 2 major (physical and psychosocial) including 12 categories (alertness behaviour, ambulation, body care/movement, communication, eating, emotional behaviour, home management, mobility, recreation/ pastime, sleep and rest, social interaction, work Mode: Interview/ self-administered	Scoring: 0 – 100 (percentage) where 0 = best HR-QoL and 100 = worst HR-QoL Percentage determined by calculating the sum of the scale values of all questions and dividing by 136 (e.g. an average) which is then converted to a percentage	Content: Yes Construct: Moderate Criterion: Yes Predictive: Yes Some evidence of validity in COPD and patients with lung volume reduction surgery	IC: Yes TR: Yes Reliable in patients with COPD	Responsiveness: Yes Sensitivity: Not discriminative of mild/ moderate cases of COPD (better in severe COPD, FEV_1 <50%)	MID: Physical domain 5 points Psychological domain: 8–11 points	No Some normative data	Yes
Nottingham Health Profile (Hunt et al 1985)	10	Part 1 Items: 38 Domains: 6 (emotional reactions, energy, pain, physical mobility, social isolation, sleep) Part 2 Activities of daily life: 7 (occupation, housework, social activity, home life, sex life, hobbies, holidays) Mode: Interview/ self-administered	Scoring: No overall score Dimension scores range from 0 to 100 (where 0 = best health state and 100 = worst health state)	Content: Moderate Construct: Yes Criterion: Yes Predictive: Not established Adequate construct validity in COPD and asthma	IC: Yes TR: Yes	Responsiveness: Yes Sensitivity: Yes	MID: Not described	No Some normative data	Yes

Continued on following page

TABLE 6-9

Generic Measures of HR-QoL (Continued)

Results May Vary According to Population (Continued)

Outcome Measure	Time to Complete (Minutes)	Content/Mode of Administration	Scoring/ Interpretation	Validity	Reliability	Responsiveness: Sensitivity	Minimal Important Difference	Measures Health Utility? Normative Data?	Widely Used?
COOP-WONCA Charts (Landgraf and Nelson 1992, Nelson et al 1987)	5	Items: 6 Domains: 6 (physical fitness, emotional feelings, daily activities, social activities, change in health, overall health, pain) Mode: Interview/ self-administered	Scoring: 5 point Likert scale of 1 = no impairment to 5 = most impaired Calculation of a total sum score is not required	Content: Yes Construct: Yes Criterion: Yes Predictive: Yes	IC: Moderate TR: Yes Poor reproducibility in COPD (2-month gap)	Responsiveness: Yes Sensitivity: Moderate	MID: Effect size greater than 0.2	No Some normative data	Moderate
WHOQOL-BREF (WHO 1998)	10–15	Items: 26 Domains: 4 (physical, psychological, social relationships, environment) Mode: Interview/ self-administered	Domain scores range from 0 (worst possible health state) to 100 (best possible health state) Scoring: 5 point Likert scale; mean scores then multiplied by 4 to calculate raw domain scores, which are then transferred to 0–100 scale	Content: Yes Construct: Yes Criterion: Moderate Predictive: Moderate Comparable validity to SGRQ in COPD	IC: Yes TR: Yes	Responsiveness: Yes Sensitivity: Yes	MID: Not described	No Extensive normative data	Moderate

Instrument		Items/Domains/Mode	Scoring	Validity	Reliability	Responsiveness/Sensitivity	MID	Normative/Value method	Rating
Assessment of Quality of Life (Hawthorne et al 2000a, Hawthorne et al 2000b, Hawthorne et al 1999) Also known as AQoL-4D	5	Items: 15 Domains: 5 (illness, independent living, physical senses, social relationships, psychological well-being) Items 1–3 (illness domain) don't count towards calculation of health utility Mode: Self-administered/Interview	Scoring: −0.04 (worst health) to 1.00 (best health) Scales: 0 to 9 (where 0 = good health and 9 = worst possible health)	Content: Yes Construct: Yes Criterion: Yes Predictive: Yes	IC: Yes TR: Yes	Responsiveness: Moderate Sensitivity: Yes	MID: 0.06	Yes Value method: TTO Some normative data (particularly Australian)	Moderate
Canadian Health Utilities Index (HUI) Instruments (1, 2, 3) (Feeny et al 1995, Feeny et al 2002, Torrance et al 1995)	3–8	Items: 7/8 (HUI 2/3) Domains: 8 (vision, hearing, speech, ambulation, dexterity, emotion, cognition, pain) Mode: Interview/self-administration	Scoring: −0.36 (worst health) to 1.00 (best health) Algorithm used to calculate utility scores based on health status classifications	Content: Yes Construct: Moderate Criterion: Yes Predictive: Yes Validity in heart failure	IC: Yes TR: Yes	Responsiveness: Yes Sensitivity: Moderate	MID: 0.02–0.04	Yes Value method: VAS/SG Extensive normative data	Yes
QWB (Kaplan et al 1996)	7–18	Items: 30 Domains: 4 (mobility/confinement, physical activity, social activity, symptoms/medical problems) Mode: Interview	Scoring: 0.00 (worst health) to 1.00 (best health)	Content: Low Construct: Low Criterion: Moderate Predictive: No	IC: Yes TR: Yes	Responsiveness: No Sensitivity: Moderate Perhaps these properties in cystic fibrosis but not COPD	MID: Not described	Yes Value method: VAS Normative data	Moderate

Continued on following page

Outcome Measure	Time to Complete (Minutes)	Content/Mode of Administration	Scoring/ Interpretation	Validity	Reliability	Responsiveness: Sensitivity	Minimal Important Difference	Measures Health Utility? Normative Data?	Widely Used?
15-D (Sintonen 1994, Sintonen 1995, Sintonen 2001)	5–10	Items: 15 Domains: 15 (mobility, vision, hearing, breathing, sleeping, eating, speech, excretion, usual activities, mental function, discomfort and symptoms, depression, distress, vitality, sexual activity Mode: Self-administration/ interview	Scoring: +0.11 (worst health) to 1.00 (best health) Each domain scored on 5 ordinal levels where 1 = best function and 5 = worst function	Content: Yes Construct: Yes Criterion: Yes Predictive: Moderate	IC: Yes TR: Yes Test-retest reliability better than EQ-5D in COPD	Responsiveness: Yes Sensitivity: More sensitive than EQ-5D in ICU	MID: 0.02–0.03 (multiple myeloma)	Yes Value method: VAS Normative data	No
Short-Form 6D (Brazier et al 2002, Brazier et al 1998)	5	Items: 11 Domains: 7 (physical functioning, role limitation (physical, emotional), bodily pain, vitality, social functioning, mental health) Mode: Interview/ self-administered	Scoring: +0.30 (worst health) to 1.00 (best health)	Content: Yes Construct: Yes Criterion: Yes Predictive: No	IC: No TR: Yes	Responsiveness: Yes Sensitivity: Yes	MID: 0.03–0.041	Yes Value method: SG Yes	Moderate

COOP-WONCA, Dartmouth Primary Care Cooperative Information Project/World Organization of Colleges, Academies and Academic Associations of General Practitioners/Family Physicians; *COPD*, chronic obstructive pulmonary disease; *EQ-5D*, Euro-Qol 5 dimensions; *FEV₁*, forced expiratory volume (1 second); *IC*, internal consistency; *MID*, minimal important difference; *QWB*, quality of well-being scale; *SD*, standard deviation; *SG*, standard gamble; *SGRQ*, St George's Respiratory Questionnaire; *TR*, test-retest reliability; *TTO*, time trade-off; *VAS*, visual analogue scale; *WHOQOL-BREF*, World Health Organization Quality of Life-BREF.

TABLE 6-10

Disease-Specific Measures of HRQoL

Outcome Measure	Population	Time to Complete (Minutes)	Content/Mode of Administration	Scoring	Validity	Reliability	Responsiveness and Sensitivity	MID	Widely Used?
					RESPIRATORY				
The St. George's Respiratory Questionnaire (SGRQ) (Jones et al 1991, Jones et al 1992)	Chronic respiratory disease (including bronchiectasis, asthma and chronic bronchitis) IPF-specific version (SGRQ-I)	10–15	Assesses effects of chronic disease on health and well-being Items = 50 Domains = 3 (symptoms, activity and impacts) Mode: Supervised self-administration	Total score: 0 = best health state to 100 worst health state (each domain also scored 0–100) Section I: 5-point Likert scale Sections II and III: Dichotomous (yes/no) Each item and domain has a different weight	Content: Moderate Construct: Moderate Criterion: Yes Predictive: Yes (can predict disease progression, survival, complications) Correlates with presence of cough; sputum; wheeze and moderate correlation with 6MWT	IC: Yes TR: Yes	Responsiveness: Yes (symptoms most responsive to change) Sensitivity: Yes Sensitivity superior to CRQ in moderate to severe COPD	MID: 4 units (threshold)	Yes

Continued on following page

TABLE 6-10
Disease-Specific Measures of HRQoL (Continued)

RESPIRATORY

Outcome Measure	Population	Time to Complete (Minutes)	Content/Mode of Administration	Scoring	Validity	Reliability	Responsiveness and Sensitivity	MID	Widely Used?
Chronic Respiratory Questionnaire (CRQ) (Guyatt et al 1987)	Chronic respiratory disease (COPD)	15 (interview) 15–25 self-administration	Assesses effect of COPD on a person's life. Items = 20 Domains = 4 (dyspnoea, fatigue, emotional function and mastery) Dyspnoea individualized to each person (select the 5 activities most relevant to them) Mode: Interview; self-administration	Items in each section are scored on a 7 point modified Likert scale, from 1 (most severe) to 7 (no impairment) Can present total score (not recommended by developers) and subscores on domains (item scores summed to provide domain scores; or mean scores)	Content: Moderate Construct: Yes Criterion: Yes Predictive: Yes Factor analysis confirmed domain structure of CRQ but not SGRQ CRQ scores differ in patients with relapse of pulmonary condition to those without and may predict mortality	IC: Yes TR: Yes High reproducibility	Responsiveness: Yes (total and emotions score most responsive to change) Sensitivity: Yes Self-administered more responsive More responsive than the SGRQ, SF-36, HUI after rehabilitation in chronic lung disease	MID: 0.5 per question on the 7-point scale; 1.0 reflects a moderate change; 1.5 represents a large change Important difference in total score is 10 points	Yes

CARDIOTHORACIC

Instrument	Condition	Time	Description	Scoring	Validity	Reliability	Responsiveness	MID	
The Minnesota Living with Heart Failure Questionnaire (MLHFQ) (Rector et al 1987a, Rector et al 1987b) Current evidence primarily supports the use of the MLHFQ in heart failure although there is emerging evidence for the KCCQ.	Heart failure	5–10	Assesses patient perception of the effects of heart failure in their lives and the medical intervention received over the last month Items: 21 Domains: 3 (physical (8 items), emotional (5 items) and other (8 items)) Mode: Self-administration/ interview	Items are scored on a 6-point (0 to 5) Likert scale where 0 = best QoL and 5 = worst QoL Total score ranges from 0–105 points (summed total of item scores) where 0 = best health state and 105 = worst health state. Physical domain scores 0–40; emotional domain scores 0–25	Content: Yes Construct: Yes Criterion: Moderate Predictive: Yes Excellent correlation with the CHFQ Good correlation between the physical subscale of the MLHFQ and the physical items of the SF-36. Correlation with hospital admissions, ED visits and mortality	IC: Yes TR: Yes Good test-retest reliability in patients on Pimobendan Test-retest reliability higher than CHFQ	Responsiveness: Yes Sensitivity: Yes MLHFQ has detected change with ionotropes, ACE inhibitors and exercise training Sensitive to patients with different severities of CHF	MID: 5 points on total score	Yes
Chronic Heart Failure Questionnaire (CHFQ) (Guyatt et al 1989)	Heart failure	10–15	Assesses effects of heart failure on a person's life Items: 16 Domains: 3 (dyspnoea (5 items), fatigue (4 items), emotional (7 items). Mode: Interview	Items are scored on a 7-point (1 to 7) Likert scale where 1 = worst health state and 7 = best health state Total scores range from 16–112 where 16 = worst health state and 112 = best health state	Content: Yes Construct: Low Criterion: Yes Predictive: Yes Some concerns with the construct validity Correlates highly with the 6MWT	IC: Yes TR: Yes	Responsiveness: Yes Sensitivity: Yes Sensitive to patients with different severities of CHF	MID: 1 to 2 points	Moderate

Continued on following page

TABLE 6-10
Disease-Specific Measures of HRQoL (Continued)

CANCER

Outcome Measure	Population	Time to Complete (Minutes)	Content/Mode of Administration	Scoring	Validity	Reliability	Responsiveness and Sensitivity	MID	Widely Used?
European Organization for Research and Treatment of Cancer Quality of Life Questionnaire (Core-30) (EORTC QLQ-C30) (Aaronson et al 1993) Supplementary respiratory-specific: (Lung cancer): LC-13 (Bergman et al 1994) (Not designed to use alone but in conjunction with EORTC QLQ-C30	Cancer Lung cancer	10 5	C30 is the core questionnaire used in conjunction with supplemental questionnaires per tumour stream *Core* Items: 30 Domains: 9 (functional scales: physical, role, cognitive, emotional, social; symptom scales: fatigue, pain, nausea, vomiting; global health status; quality of life scale) *Lung cancer* Items: 13 Domains: 2 (lung-cancer related symptoms, treatment side effects) Mode: Self-administration/ interview	Items are scored on a modified Likert scale 1 (not at all) to 4 (very much) or 1 (very poor) to 7 (excellent) Subscale scores transformed into 0 (worst health state) to 100 (best health state) Symptom score scores range from 0 (best symptom state) to 100 (worst symptom state) Summation of subscale scores not recommended	*Core:* Content: Moderate Construct: Yes Criterion: Yes Predictive: Yes *Lung cancer:* Content: Yes Construct: Yes Criterion: Yes Predictive: Yes Only evidence of content validity from original validation Some of the scales have been found to predict survival in lung cancer and mesothelioma	*Core:* IC: Yes TR: Yes *Lung cancer:* IC: Yes TR: Yes	*Core:* Responsiveness: Yes Sensitivity: Yes *Lung cancer:* Responsiveness: Yes Sensitivity: Yes	In people with lung cancer based on performance status: MID (improvement): physical function (9 points); role (14 points); social (5 points); global health status (9 points); fatigue (14 points); pain (15 points) MID (deterioration): physical (4 points); role (5 points); social (7 points); global health status (4 points); fatigue (6 points); pain (3 points)	Yes

Measure	Condition			Description	Scoring	Validity	Reliability	Responsiveness	MID	
Functional Assessment of Cancer Therapy (FACT) series G – general (Cella et al 1993) L – lung (Cella et al 1995)	Cancer	5	8	*General:* Items: 27 Domains: 4 (physical, social/family, emotional, functional well-being) *Lung:* Items: 36 Domains: 5 (physical, social/family, emotional, functional well-being AND lung cancer subscale (symptoms, cognitive function, regret of smoking)) Mode: Self administration/ interview	Items are scored on a five point Likert scale from 0 (not at all) to 4 (very much) Subscale scores are summed to provide a total score (0 worst QoL to 135 QoL best QoL). Can also score as TOI, which is the sum of the physical, functional and lung cancer subscales	*General:* Content: Yes Construct: Yes Criterion: Yes Predictive: No *Lung:* Content: Yes Construct: Yes Criterion: Yes Predictive: No More evidence of content validation than EORTC QLQ-C30	*General:* IC: Yes TR: Yes *Lung:* IC: Yes TR: Yes Evidence is more substantial for IC and TR for the FACT-G than the EORTC QLQ-C30	*General:* Responsiveness: Yes Sensitivity: Yes *Lung:* Responsiveness: Yes Sensitivity: Yes	MID: FACT-G 5–6 points FACT-L 6–7 points; 2–3 points on the lung cancer subscale	Yes

6MWT, 6-Minute walk test; *ACE*, angiotensin-converting enzyme; *CHF*, chronic heart failure; *COPD*, chronic obstructive pulmonary disease; *ED*, emergency department; *HUI*, health utilities index; *IC*, internal consistency; *IPF*, Interstitial Pulmonary Fibrosis; *KCCQ*, Kansas City Cardiomyopathy Questionnaire; *MID*, minimal important difference; *QoL*, quality of life; *SF-36*, Short-Form 36; *TOI*, Trial Outcome Index; *TR*, test-retest reliability.

	TABLE 6-11										
	Example International Overall and Healthy Population Normative Data, Mean (SD), SF-36, for Median Age 60										
	n	PF	RP	BP	GH	SF	V	RE	MH	PCS	MCS
Australian Norms[†]	18,468	83 (24)	80 (35)	77 (25)	72 (20)	85 (23)	65 (20)	83 (32)	76 (17)	49.8 (10)	50.1 (10)
Australian Norms[‡]	9,922*	89 (0.3)	89 (0.5)	85 (0.4)	79 (0.3)	90 (0.3)	70 (0.3)	88 (0.5)	79 (0.2)	53.1 (0.1)	51.7 (0.1)
Chinese Norms[§]	1,688	82 (20)	81 (34)	82 (20)	57 (20)	83 (18)	52 (21)	84 (32)	60 (23)	1.2 X	X
UK Norms 1999[¶]	8,889	88 (20)	87 (22)	79 (23)	71 (20)	83 (23)	58 (20)	86 (22)	72 (18)	X	X
UK Norms 1993[¶]	6,506	93 (13)	91 (23)	86 (18)	79 (16)	91 (16)	64 (18)	86 (29)	75 (16)	X	X
Canadian Norms**	9,411	86 (20)	82 (33)	76 (23)	77 (18)	86 (20)	66 (18)	84 (32)	78 (15)	50.5 (9)	51.7 (9)
US Norms[††]	2,474	84 (23)	81 (34)	75 (24)	72 (20)	83 (23)	61 (21)	81 (33)	74 (18)	X	X
German Norms[‡‡]	2,000	71 (26)	70 (40)	63 (27)	59 (18)	85 (22)	60 (19)	87 (30)	73 (17)	44.8 (10)	53.2 (8)
Swiss Norms[§§]	X	71 (25)	55 (42)	X	62 (21)	X	55 (19)	61 (42)	X	42 (12)	47 (11)

BP, Bodily pain; *GH,* general health; *MCS,* mental component summary, *MH,* mental health; *PCS,* physical component summary; *PF,* physical functioning; *RE,* role emotional; *RP,* role physical; *SD,* standard deviation; *SF,* social functioning; *SF-36,* Short-Form 36; *V,* vitality; *X,* not reported.
*Mean (standard error).
[†]Persons unstandardized values (ABS 1997).
[‡]Persons with no serious physical conditions (ABS 1997).
[§]Hangzhou population (Li et al 2003).
[¶]SF-36 V2 (Jenkinson et al 1999).
[¶]Persons not reporting longstanding illness (Jenkinson et al 1993), SF-36V1, cited in (Eddleston et al 2000).
**Age and sex standardized scores (Hopman et al 2000).
[††]Overall US norms (Ware et al 1993).
[‡‡]In German (Ellert & Bellach 1999), cited in (Graf et al 2003).
[§§](Perneger et al 1995) cited in (Merlani et al 2007).

instruments in specific populations has been recommended (Brazier et al 1999). The two most widely used and robust measures in each of the following major disease areas are presented in Table 6-10: respiratory disease, cardiac disease and oncology. In patients with coronary revascularization, the Euro-QoL 5 Dimensions (EQ-5D) or SF-36 have been recommended, with the most disease-specific evidence for the Seattle Angina Questionnaire (SAQ) (Mackintosh et al 2010). The mini-Asthma Quality of Life Questionnaire (mini-AQLQ) has been recommended to be used as an asthma-specific instrument in conjunction with the EQ-5D in people with asthma (Gibbons &

Fitzpatrick 2009). There are few disease-specific tools available to measure HR-QoL in surgical populations and the ones that exist (such as the Gastrointestinal Quality of Life Index (GIQLI) (Barkun et al 1992) have limited evidence for their measurement properties. Disease-specific oncology HR-QOL measures for surgery relating to cancer exist and can be sourced using the core questionnaires presented in Table 6-10. There are no population-specific HR-QoL questionnaires for older populations and generic HR-QoLs are used mostly in this population, with the most common instrument of choice the SF-36 (Hickey et al 2005). There are some disease-specific measures that exist for different medical conditions, such as obesity (the Impact of Weight on Quality of Life-Lite (IWQOL-Lite)) (Kolotkin and Crosby 2002, Kolotkin et al 2001), although again there is limited evidence for their measurement properties. The most commonly used measure of HR-QoL in patients with renal failure or renal disease is the SF-36 (Liem et al 2007, Spiegel et al 2008). Several disease-specific quality of life measures have been developed for people with renal failure or renal disease. The most robust of these is the Kidney Disease Quality of Life (KDQOL); however, at 80 items, the questionnaire is significantly longer than the SF-36 and there is more evidence for the use of the SF-36 in this population (Gibbons and Fitzpatrick 2010). Finally, there is no published population-specific quality of life measure developed for people with critical illness or who have been admitted to ICU. The most commonly used measures in this population have again been generic measures, specifically SF-36, EQ-5D, sickness impact profile (SIP) and Nottingham Health Profile (NHP) with a significant recent increase in the EQ-5D (Dowdy et al 2005, Oeyen et al 2010, Winters et al 2010), despite it having not been validated in this population. The SF-36 is well validated in the ICU population (Chrispin et al 1997, Heyland et al 2000, Khoudri et al 2007, Wehler et al 2003) and is recommended for use in the ICU, along with the EQ-5D (Angus and Carlet 2003). The AQoL is also a candidate for use in the ICU, with recent evidence supporting its clinimetric properties in this population (Skinner et al 2013).

Paediatric HR-QoL Measures

There are both generic and disease specific HR-QoL measures available for use in clinical and research practice. Generic measures include the Paediatric Quality of Life Inventory and the Child Health Questionnaire (Varni et al 2001, Waters et al 2000), which are less sensitive to changes that are important to a particular disease such as cystic fibrosis and respiratory symptoms. There are a number of disease-specific questionnaires which have been developed, including the Cystic Fibrosis Questionnaire – revised, and the Cystic Fibrosis Quality of Life measures (Gee et al 2000, Quittner et al 2005). These questionnaires can often be either self-report or parental report, depending on the language and cognitive developmental ability of the child/adolescent.

Other Considerations

Method of Administration. It should be noted that in some instruments, results can vary in the measurement of HR-QoL depending on the mode of administration selected (Bennett et al 2003, Buskirk and Stein 2008, Lyons et al 1999, Wilson et al 1995). For example, different modes include self-administration, interview (face-to-face), interview (telephone), postal self-administration or parental report (for paediatric population). Physiotherapists should weigh up the relative merits of maximizing response rates by selecting different administration methods against the relative disadvantage of reducing the reliability of the data.

Proxy Respondents. The use of proxy respondents (i.e. respondents answering questions on behalf of the individual, such as a family member) is the last significant discussion point pertaining to the measurement of HR-QoL. Proxy responses cannot be considered interchangeable with individual responses for many of the generic measures, such as the SIP (De Bruin et al 1992), although the degree of error in proxy estimation may be a function of the instrument. For example, in the case of the SF-36 in critical illness, although agreement between patient and proxy was reported to be good to excellent, clinically significant differences between proxy and patient estimation occurred in five of eight domains (Hofhuis et al 2003). Data from the European Organization for Research and Treatment of Cancer Quality of Life Questionnaire C30 (EORTC QLQ-C30) demonstrates mixed results depending on the domains. It is recommended that patient response data is sought where possible.

See Box 6-6 for a summary of measurement of participation restriction.

Summary

Physiotherapists utilize outcome measures in clinical and research practice to determine the efficacy of a particular intervention aimed at improving the patient's well-being and general health. The choice of outcome measure will depend on: the instrument's measurement properties, clinical utility and patient/environmental factors. Outcome measures should be mapped within the ICF framework to measures of impairment, activity limitation and participation restriction.

BOX 6-6
MEASUREMENT OF PARTICIPATION RESTRICTION

■ Patient-reported outcomes are integral to healthcare and health-related quality of life measures the patient perception of how their health state affects their life (participation restriction).

■ HR-QoL can be measured using generic or disease-specific instruments and should be measured from the individual.

■ The optimal generic measures in cardiorespiratory populations are SF-36, EQ-5D and AQoL, and in paediatrics the Paediatric Quality of Life Inventory Generic and Child Health Questionnaire.

■ The Chronic Respiratory Questionnaire, the St. George's Respiratory Questionnaire, the Chronic Heart Failure Questionnaire, the Minnesota Living with Heart Failure Questionnaire, The European Organization for Research and Treatment of Cancer Quality of Life Questionnaire (Core-30) and the Functional Assessment of Cancer Therapy are the most robust disease-specific tools for cardiorespiratory populations. There are also two commonly utilized cystic fibrosis specific questionnaires: Cystic Fibrosis Questionnaire Revised and Cystic Fibrosis Quality of Life Measure.

AQoL, Assessment Quality of Life; *EQ-5D*, Euroquol-5 dimensions; *HR-QoL*, health-related quality of life; *SF-36*, Short-Form 36.

REFERENCES

Aaronson, N.K., Ahmedzai, S., Bergman, B., et al., 1993. The European Organization for Research and Treatment of Cancer QLQ-C30: a quality-of-life instrument for use in international clinical trials in oncology. J. Natl Cancer Inst. 85, 365–376.

ABS, 1997. 1995 National Health Survey: SF-36 population norms, Australia. Australian Bureau of Statistics, Canberra.

Adler, J., Malone, D., 2012. Early mobilization in the intensive care unit: a systematic review. Cardiopulm. Phys. Ther. J. 23, 5–13.

Ali, N., O'Brien, J., Hoffmann, S., et al., 2008. Acquired weakness, handgrip strength, and mortality in critically ill patients. Am. J. Respir. Crit. Care Med. 178, 261–268.

American College of Sports Medicine, 2000. Guidelines for exercise testing and prescription. Williams and Wilkins, Philadelphia.

American Thoracic Society/American College of Chest Physicians, 2003. Statement of cardiopulmonary exercise testing. Am. J. Respir. Crit. Care. Med. 167, 211–277.

American Thoracic Society / European Respiratory Society, 2002. ATS/ERS statement on respiratory muscle testing. Am. J. Respir. Crit. Care. Med. 166, 518–624.

Angus, D.C., Carlet, J., 2003. Surviving intensive care: a report from the 2002 Brussels Roundtable. Intensive Care Med. 29, 368–377.

Armstrong, N., Kirby, B.J., McManus, A.M., Welsman, J.R., 1997. Prepubescents' ventilatory responses to exercise with reference to sex and body size. Chest 112 (6), 1554–1560.

ATS/ACCP Statement on Cardiopulmonary Exercise Testing, 2003. American Thoracic Society/American College of Chest Physicians. Am. J. Respir. Crit. Care Med. 167 (2), 211–277.

Aurora, P., Prasad, S., Balfour-Lynn, I., et al., 2001. Exercise tolerance in children with cystic fibrosis undergoing lung transplantation assessment. Eur. Respir. J. 18, 293–297.

Baldwin, C.E., Bersten, A.D., 2014. Alterations in respiratory and limb muscle strength and size in patients with sepsis who are mechanically ventilated. Phys. Ther. 94 (1), 68–82.

Baldwin, C., Paratz, J., Bersten, A., 2012. Body composition analysis in critically ill survivors: a comparison of bioelectrical impedance spectroscopy devices. J. Parenter. Enteral Nutr. 36, 306–315.

Baldwin, C., Paratz, J., Bersten, A., 2013. Muscle strength assessment in critically ill patients with handheld dynamometry: an investigation of reliability, minimal detectable change, and time to peak force generation. J. Crit. Care 28, 77–86.

Balfour-Lynn, I., Prasad, S., Laverty, A., et al., 1998. A step in the right direction: assessing exercise tolerance in cystic fibrosis. Pediatr. Pulmonol. 25, 278–284.

Barkun, J.S., Barkun, A.N., Sampalis, J.S., et al., 1992. Randomised controlled trial of laparoscopic versus mini cholecystectomy. The McGill Gallstone Treatment Group. Lancet 340, 1116–1119.

Bennett, S.J., Oldridge, N.B., Eckert, G.J., et al., 2003. Comparison of quality of life measures in heart failure. Nurs. Res. 52, 207–216.

Bergman, B., Aaronson, N.K., Ahmedzai, S., et al., 1994. The EORTC QLQ-LC13: a modular supplement to the EORTC Core Quality of Life Questionnaire (QLQ-C30) for use in lung cancer clinical trials. EORTC Study Group on Quality of Life. Eur. J. Cancer 30A, 635–642.

Bergner, M., Bobbitt, R.A., Carter, W.B., Gilson, B.S., 1981. The Sickness Impact Profile: development and final revision of a health status measure. Med. Care 19, 787–805.

Bergner, M., Bobbitt, R.A., Kressel, S., et al., 1976a. The sickness impact profile: conceptual formulation and methodology for the development of a health status measure. Int. J. Health Serv. 6, 393–415.

Bergner, M., Bobbitt, R.A., Pollard, W.E., et al., 1976b. The sickness impact profile: validation of a health status measure. Med. Care 14, 57–67.

Berney, S., Haines, K., Skinner, E.H., et al., 2012. Safety and feasibility of an exercise prescription approach to rehabilitation across the continuum of care for survivors of critical illness. Phys. Ther. 92, 1524–1535.

Bissett, B., Green, M., Marzano, V., et al., 2015. Reliability and utility of the Acute Care Index of Function in intensive care patients: An observational study. Heart Lung [Epub ahead of print].

Bohannon, R., 1988. Make tests and break tests of elbow flexor muscle strength. Phys. Ther. 68, 193–194.

Bohannon, R.W., 2006. Reference values for the five-repetition sit-to-stand test: a descriptive meta-analysis of data from elders. Percept. Mot. Skills 103, 215–222.

Bohannon, R., Bubela, D., Magasi, S., et al., 2010. Sit-to-stand test: performance and determinants across the age-span. Isokinet. Exerc. Sci. 18, 235–240.

Bohannon, R., Peolsson, A., Massy-Westropp, N., et al., 2006. Reference values for adult grip strength measured with a Jamar dynamometer: a descriptive meta-analysis. Physiotherapy 92, 11–15.

Bongers, B., de Vries, S., Helders, P., et al., 2013. The steep ramp test in healthy children and adolescents: reliability and validity. Med. Sci. Sports Exerc. 42, 366–371.

Bongers, B.C., Hulzebos, H.J., van Brussel, M., Takken, T. Pediatric norms for cardiopulmonary exercise testing 2012.

Bradley, J., Howard, J., Wallace, E., et al., 2000. Reliability, repeatability and sensitivity of the modified shuttle test in adult cystic fibrosis. Chest 117, 1666–1671.

Brazier, J., Deverill, M., Green, C., et al., 1999. A review of the use of health status measures in economic evaluation. Health Technol. Assess. 3, i–iv, 1–164.

Brazier, J., Roberts, J., Deverill, M., 2002. The estimation of a preference-based measure of health from the SF-36. J. Health Econ. 21, 271–292.

Brazier, J., Usherwood, T., Harper, R., Thomas, K., 1998. Deriving a preference based single index from the UK SF-36 health survey. J. Clin. Epidemiol. 51, 1115–1128.

Brooks, D., Thomas, J., 1995. Interrater reliability of auscultation of breath sounds among physical therapists. Phys. Ther. 75, 1082–1088.

Buskirk, T.D., Stein, K.D., 2008. Telephone vs. mail survey gives different SF-36 quality-of-life scores among cancer survivors. J. Clin. Epidemiol. 61, 1049–1055.

Cahalin, L., Arena, R., Guazzi, M., et al., 2013. Inspiratory muscle training in heart disease and heart failure: a review of the literature with a focus on method of training and outcomes. Expert Rev. Cardiovasc. Ther. 11, 161–177.

Campbell, I., Watt, T., Withers, D., et al., 1995. Muscle thickness, measured with ultrasound, may be an indicator of lean tissue wasting in multiple organ failure in the presence of edema. Am. J. Clin. Nutr. 62, 533–539.

Carter, W.B., Bobbitt, R.A., Bergner, M., Gilson, B.S., 1976. Validation of an interval scaling: the sickness impact profile. Health Serv. Res. 11, 516–528.

Cartwright, M., Demar, S., Griffin, L., et al., 2013. Validity and reliability of nerve and muscle ultrasound. Muscle Nerve 47, 515–521.

Cattapan, S., Laghu, F., Tobin, M., 2003. Can diaphragmatic contractility be assessed by airway twitch pressure in mechanically ventilated patients? Thorax 58, 58–62.

Cella, D.F., Tulsky, D.S., Gray, G., et al., 1993. The Functional Assessment of Cancer Therapy scale: development and validation of the general measure. J. Clin. Oncol. 11, 570–579.

Cella, D.F., Bonomi, A.E., Lloyd, S.R., et al., 1995. Reliability and validity of the Functional Assessment of Cancer Therapy-Lung (FACT-L) quality of life instrument. Lung Cancer 12, 199–220.

Chan, K., Pfoh, E., Denehy, L., et al., 2015. Construct validity and minimal important difference of 6-minute walk distance in survivors of acute respiratory failure. Chest 147, 1316–1326.

Chrispin, P.S., Scotton, H., Rogers, J., et al., 1997. Short Form 36 in the intensive care unit: assessment of acceptability, reliability and validity of the questionnaire. Anaesthesia 52, 15–23.

Ciesla, N., Dinglas, V., Fan, E., et al., 2011. Manual muscle testing: a method of measuring extremity muscle strength applied to critically ill patients. J. Vis. Exp. 12, 2632.

Connolly, B., Jones, G., Curtis, A., et al., 2013. Clinical predictive value of manual muscle strength testing during critical illness: an observational cohort study. Crit. Care 17, R229.

Corner, E., Soni, N., Handy, H., et al., 2014. Construct validity of the Chelsea Critical Care Physical Assessment Tool: an observational study of recovery from critical illness. Crit. Care 18, R55.

Corner, E., Wood, H., Englebretsen, C., et al., 2013. The Chelsea Critical Care Physical Assessment Tool (CPAx): validation of an innovative new tool to measure physical morbidity in the general adult critical care population – an observational proof-of-concept pilot study. Physiotherapy 99, 33–41.

Cox, N., Follett, J., McKay, K., 2006. Modified shuttle test performance in hospitalized children and adolescents with cystic fibrosis. J. Cyst. Fibros. 5, 165–170.

Craig, C.L., Marshall, A.L., Sjostrom, M., et al., 2003. International physical activity questionnaire: 12-country reliability and validity. Med. Sci. Sports Exerc. 35, 1381–1395.

Cronbach, L.J., 1951. Coefficient alpha and the internal structure of tests. Psychometrika 16 (3), 297–334.

Cumming, G.R., Hastman, C., McCort, J., McCullough, S., 1980. High serum lactates do occur in young children after maximal work. Int. J. Sports Med. 1, 66–69.

Darrah, J., Piper, M., Watt, M., 1998. Assessment of gross motor skills of at-risk infants: predictive validity of the Alberta Infant Motor Scale. Dev. Med. Child Neurol. 40, 485–491.

De Bruin, A.F., De Witte, L.P., Stevens, F., Diederiks, J.P., 1992. Sickness Impact Profile: the state of the art of a generic functional status measure. Soc. Sci. Med. 35, 1003–1014.

De Jonghe, B., Sharshar, T., Lefaucheur, J.P., et al., 2002. Paresis acquired in the intensive care unit: a prospective multicenter study. J. Am. Med. Assoc. 288, 2859–2867.

de Morton, N., Brusco, N., Wood, L., et al., 2011a. The de Morton Mobility Index (DEMMI) provides a valid measure for measuring and monitoring the mobility of patients making the transition from hospital to the community: an observational study. J. Physiother. 57, 109–116.

de Morton, N., Davidson, M., Keating, J., 2008. The de Morton Mobility index (DEMMI): an essential index for an ageing world. Health Qual. Life Outcomes 6, 63.

Delaney, S., Worsley, P., Warner, M., et al., 2010. Assessing contractile ability of the quadriceps muscle using ultrasound imaging. Muscle Nerve 42, 530–538.

Demoule, A., Jung, B., Prodanovic, H., et al., 2013. Diaphragm dysfunction on admission to intensive care unit: prevalence, risk factors, and prognostic impact – a prospective study. Am. J. Respir. Crit. Care. Med. 188, 213–219.

Denehy, L., de Morton, N., Skinner, E., et al., 2013. A physical function test for use in the intensive care unit: validity, responsiveness, and predictive utility of the physical function ICU test (scored). Phys. Ther. 93 (12), 1636–1645.

DeVellis, R.F., 2003. Scale Development: Theory and Applications, second ed. Sage Publications, Newbury Park: CA.

Dowdy, D.W., Eid, M.P., Sedrakyan, A., et al., 2005. Quality of life in adult survivors of critical illness: a systematic review of the literature. Intensive Care Med. 31, 611–620.

Duffin, D., 1977. Knee strength and function following meniscectomy. Physiotherapy 63 (11), 362–363.

Earthman, C., Traughber, D., Dobratz, J., et al., 2007. Bioimpedance spectroscopy for clinical assessment of fluid distribution and body cell mass. Nutr. Clin. Pract. 22, 389–405.

Eaton, T., Young, P., Nicol, K., et al., 2006. The endurance shuttle walking test: a responsive measure in pulmonary rehabilitation for COPD patients. Chron. Respir. Dis. 3, 3–9.

Eddleston, J.M., White, P., Guthrie, E., 2000. Survival, morbidity, and quality of life after discharge from intensive care. Crit. Care Med. 28, 2293–2299.

Elkins, M., Dentice, R., 2015. Inspiratory muscle training facilitates weaning from mechanical ventilation among patients in the intensive care unit: a systematic review. J. Physiother. 61, 125–134.

Ellert, U., Bellach, B.M., 1999. [The SF-36 in the Federal Health Survey – description of a current normal sample]. Gesundheitswesen 61 Spec No, S184–S190.

Elliott, D., Denehy, L., Berney, S., et al., 2011. Assessing physical function and activity for survivors of a critical illness: a review of instruments. Aust. Crit. Care 24, 155–166.

Ely, E., Margolin, R., Francis, J., et al., 2001. Evaluation of delirium in critically ill patients: validation of the Confusion Assessment Method for the Intensive Care Unit (CAM-ICU). Crit. Care Med. 29, 1370–1379.

EuroQoL, 1990. EuroQol – a new facility for the measurement of health-related quality of life. Health Policy (New York) 16, 199–208.

Fan, E., Cheek, F., Chlan, L., et al., 2014. An official American Thoracic Society clinical practice guideline: the diagnosis of intensive care unit-acquired weakness in adults. Am. J. Respir. Crit. Care. Med. 190, 1437–1446.

Fan, E., Ciesla, N.D., Truong, A.D., et al., 2010. Inter-rater reliability of manual muscle strength testing in ICU survivors and simulated patients. Intensive Care Med. 36, 1038–1043.

Fan, E., Dowdy, D., Colantuoni, E., et al., 2014. Physical complications in acute lung injury survivors: a 2-year longitudinal prospective study. Crit. Care Med. 42 (4), 849–859.

Feeny, D., Furlong, W., Boyle, M., Torrance, G.W., 1995. Multiattribute health status classification systems. Health Utilities Index. Pharmacoeconomics 7, 490–502.

Feeny, D., Furlong, W., Torrance, G.W., et al., 2002. Multiattribute and single-attribute utility functions for the health utilities index mark 3 system. Med. Care 40, 113–128.

Ferreira, M.L., Herbert, R.D., 2008. What does 'clinically important' really mean? Aust. J. Physiother. 54, 229–230.

Fess, E., 1992. In Clinical Assessment Recommendations, Chicago, American Society of Hand Therapists.

Fitzpatrick, R., Davey, C., Buxton, M., et al., 1998. Evaluating patient-based outcome measures for use in clinical trials. Health Technol. Assess. 2, 1–74.

Forsén, L., Loland, N.W., Vuillemin, A., et al., 2010. Self-administered physical activity questionnaires for the elderly: a systematic review of measurement properties. Sports Med. 40, 601–623.

Garratt, A., Schmidt, L., Mackintosh, A., Fitzpatrick, R., 2002. Quality of life measurement: bibliographic study of patient assessed health outcome measures. Br. Med. J. 324, 1417.

Gee, L., Abbott, J., Conway, S., et al., 2000. Development of a disease specific health related quality of life measure for adults and adolescents with cystic fibrosis. Thorax 55, 946–954.

Gibbons, E., Fitzpatrick, R., 2009. A structured review of patient-reported outcome measures for people with asthma: an update. In: Group, P-r O.M. (Ed.). University of Oxford, Oxford.

Gibbons, E., Fitzpatrick, R., 2010. A structured review of patient-reported outcome measures for adults with chronic kidney disease. In: Group, P-r O.M. (Ed.). University of Oxford.

Gilson, B.S., Gilson, J.S., Bergner, M., et al., 1975. The sickness impact profile. Development of an outcome measure of health care. Am. J. Public Health 65, 1304–1310.

Godin, G., Jobin, J., Bouillon, J., 1985a. Assessment of leisure-time exercise behavior by self-report – a validity study. Med. Sci. Sports Exerc. 17, 285.

Godin, G., Shephard, R.J., 1985b. A simple method to assess exercise behavior in the community. Can. J. Appl. Sport Sci. 10, 141–146.

Gosselink, R., Bott, J., Johnson, M., et al., 2008. Physiotherapy for adult patients with critical illness: recommendations of the European respiratory society and European society of intensive care medicine task force on physiotherapy for critically ill patients. Intensive Care Med. 34, 1188–1199.

Graf, J., Koch, M., Dujardin, R., et al., 2003. Health-related quality of life before, 1 month after, and 9 months after intensive care in medical cardiovascular and pulmonary patients. Crit. Care Med. 31 (8), 2163–2169.

Granger, C., Holland, A., Gordon, I., et al., 2015. Minimal important difference of the six-minute walk distance in lung cancer. Chron. Respir. Dis. 12, 146–154.

Greening, N.J., Harvey-Dunstan, T.C., Chaplin, E.J., et al., 2015. Bedside Assessment of Quadriceps Muscle by Ultrasound after Admission for Acute Exacerbations of Chronic Respiratory Disease. Am. J. Respir. Crit. Care Med. 192 (7), 810–816. doi:10.1164/rccm.201503-0535OC.

Grimm, A., Teschner, U., Porzelius, C., et al., 2013. Muscle ultrasound for early assessment of critical illness neuromyopathy in severe sepsis. Crit. Care 17 (5), R227.

Gruther, W., Benesch, T., Zorn, C., et al., 2008. Muscle wasting in intensive care patients: ultrasound observation of the M. quadriceps femoris muscle layer. J. Rehabil. Med. 40 (3), 185–189.

Guyatt, G.H., Berman, L.B., Townsend, M., et al., 1987. A measure of quality of life for clinical trials in chronic lung disease. Thorax 42, 773–778.

Guyatt, G.H., Nogradi, S., Halcrow, S., et al., 1989. Development and testing of a new measure of health status for clinical trials in heart failure. J. Gen. Intern. Med. 4, 101–107.

Haley, S., Coster, W., Ludlow, L., et al. 1992. Pediatric Evaluation of Disability Inventory: Development, Standardization and Administration Manual, Boston, MA.

Hammond, K., Mampilly, J., Laghi, F., et al., 2014. Validity and reliability of rectus femoris ultrasound measurements: comparison of curved-array and linear-array transducers. J. Rehabil. Res. Dev. 51 (7), 1155–1164.

Hawthorne, G., 2007. Measuring the value of health-related quality of life. In: Ritsner, M.S., Awad, A.G. (Eds.), Quality of Life Impairment in Schizophrenia, Mood and Anxiety Disorders. Springer.

Hawthorne, G., Richardson, J., 2001. Measuring the value of program outcomes: a review of multiattribute utility measures. Expert Rev. Pharmacoecon. Outcomes Res. 1, 215–228.

Hawthorne, G., Richardson, J., Day, N., 2000a. Using the Assessment of Quality of Life (AQoL) Instrument Version 1.0. Technical Report twelfth ed. Centre for Health Program Evaluation, Melbourne, Victoria, Australia.

Hawthorne, G., Richardson, J., Day, N., et al., 2000b. Construction and utility scaling of the Assessment of Quality of Life (AQoL) instrument. Centre for Health Program Evaluation, Melbourne.

Hawthorne, G., Richardson, J., Osborne, R., 1999. The Assessment of Quality of Life (AQoL) instrument: a psychometric measure of health-related quality of life. Qual. Life Res. 8, 209–224.

Herdman, M., Gudex, C., Lloyd, A., et al., 2011. Development and preliminary testing of the new five-level version of EQ-5D (EQ-5D-5L). Qual. Life Res. 20, 1727–1736.

Hermans, G., Agten, A., Testelman, D., et al., 2010. Increased duration of mechanical ventilation is associated with decreased diaphragmatic force: a prospective observational study. Crit. Care 14, R127.

Hermans, G., Clerckx, B., Vanhullebusch, T., et al., 2012. Interobserver agreement of Medical Research Council Sum-score and handgrip strength in the intensive care unit. Muscle Nerve 45, 18–25.

Hermans, G., Van Mechelen, H., Clerckx, B., et al., 2014. Acute outcomes and 1-year mortality of intensive care unit-acquired weakness: a cohort study and propensity-matched analysis. Am. J. Respir. Crit. Care. Med. 190 (4), 410–420.

Heymsfield, S., Lohman, T., Wang, Z., et al., 2005. Human Body Composition. Human Kinetics, United States.

Heyland, D.K., Hopman, W., Coo, H., et al., 2000. Long-term health-related quality of life in survivors of sepsis. Short Form 36: A valid and reliable measure of health-related quality of life. Crit. Care Med. 28, 3599–3605.

Hickey, A., Barker, M., McGee, H., O'boyle, C., 2005. Measuring health-related quality of life in older patient populations: a review of current approaches. Pharmacoeconomics 23, 971–993.

Hodgson, C., Berney, S., Haines, K., et al., 2013. Development of a mobility scale for use in a multicentre Australia and New Zealand: trial of early activity and mobilisation in ICU. Am. J. Respir. Crit. Care. Med. 187, A1323.

Hofhuis, J., Hautvast, J.L., Schrijvers, A.J., Bakker, J., 2003. Quality of life on admission to the intensive care: can we query the relatives? Intensive Care Med. 29, 974–979.

Holland, A., Spruit, M.A., Troosters, T., et al., 2014. An official European Respiratory Society/American Thoracic Society technical standard: field walking tests in chronic respiratory disease. Eur. Respir. J. 44 (6), 1428–1446. doi:10.1183/0903196.00150314.

Hopman, W.M., Towheed, T., Anastassiades, T., et al., 2000. Canadian normative data for the SF-36 health survey. Canadian Multicentre Osteoporosis Study Research Group. Can. Med. Assoc. J. 163, 265–271.

Hough, C., Lieu, B., Caldwell, E., 2011. Manual muscle strength testing of critically ill patients: feasibility and interobserver agreement. Crit. Care 15, R43.

Hunt, S.M., McEwen, J., McKenna, S.P., 1985. Measuring health status: a new tool for clinicians and epidemiologists. J. R. Coll. Gen. Pract. 35, 185–188.

Inouye, S., van Dyck, C., Alessi, C., et al., 1990. Clarifying confusion: the confusion assessment method – a new method for detection of delirium. Ann. Intern. Med. 113, 941–948.

Jaber, S., Petrof, B., Jung, B., et al., 2011. Rapidly progressive diaphragmatic weakness and injury during mechanical ventilation in humans. Am. J. Respir. Crit. Care. Med. 183, 364–371.

Jakobsen, L., Rask, I., Kondrup, J., 2010. Validation of handgrip strength and endurance as a measure of physical function and quality of life in healthy subjects and patients. Nutrition 26, 542–550.

Jenkinson, C., Coulter, A., Wright, L., 1993. Short form 36 (SF36) health survey questionnaire: normative data for adults of working age. Br. Med. J. 306, 1437–1440.

Jenkinson, C., Stewart-Brown, S., Petersen, S., Paice, C., 1999. Assessment of the SF-36 version 2 in the United Kingdom. J. Epidemiol. Community Health 53, 46–50.

Jones, P.W., Quirk, F.H., Baveystock, C.M., 1991. The St George's Respiratory Questionnaire. Respir. Med. 85 (Suppl. B), 25–31, discussion 33–37.

Jones, P.W., Quirk, F.H., Baveystock, C.M., Littlejohns, P., 1992. A self-complete measure of health status for chronic airflow limitation. The St. George's Respiratory Questionnaire. Am. Rev. Respir. Dis. 145, 1321–1327.

Kaplan, R., Ganiats, T., Sieber, W., Anderson, J.P., 1996. The Quality of Well-being Scale. Medical Outcomes Trust Bulletin 2–3.

Kasotakis, G., Schmidt, U., Perry, D., et al., 2012. The surgical intensive care unit optimal mobility score predicts mortality and length of stay. Crit. Care Med. 40 (4), 1122–1128.

Kerridge, R., Brooks, R., Hillman, K., 1994. Quality of life after intensive care. In: Vincent, J.L. (Ed.), Yearbook of Intensive Care and Emergency Medicine. Springer, New York.

Khoudri, I., Ali Zeggwagh, A., Abidi, K., et al., 2007. Measurement properties of the Short Form 36 and health-related quality of life after intensive care in Morocco. Acta Anaesthesiol. Scand. 51, 189–197.

Kind, P., 1996. The EuroQoL instrument: an index of health-related quality of life. In: Spilker, B. (Ed.), Quality of Life and Pharmacoeconomics in Clinical Trials, second ed. Lippincott-Raven Publishers, Philadelphia.

Kleyweg, R., Van der Meché, F., Schmitz, P., 1991. Interobserver agreement in the assessment of muscle strength and functional abilities in Guillain-Barré syndrome. Muscle Nerve 14, 1103–1109.

Kolotkin, R.L., Crosby, R.D., 2002. Psychometric evaluation of the impact of weight on quality of life-lite questionnaire (IWQOL-lite) in a community sample. Qual. Life Res. 11, 157–171.

Kolotkin, R.L., Crosby, R.D., Kosloski, K.D., Williams, G.R., 2001. Development of a brief measure to assess quality of life in obesity. Obes. Res. 9, 102–111.

Laghi, F., Cattapan, S., Jurban, A., et al., 2003. Is weaning failure caused by low frequency fatigue of the diaphragm? Am. J. Respir. Crit. Care. Med. 167, 120–127.

Landgraf, J.M., Nelson, E.C., 1992. Summary of the WONCA/COOP International Health Assessment Field Trial. The Dartmouth COOP Primary Care Network. Aust. Fam. Physician 21, 255–257, 260–262, 266–269.

Lee, J., Waak, K., Grosse-Sundrup, M., et al., 2012. Global muscle strength but not grip strength predicts mortality and length of stay in a general population in a surgical intensive care unit. Phys. Ther. 92, 1546–1555.

Li, L., Wang, H.M., Shen, Y., 2003. Chinese SF-36 Health Survey: translation, cultural adaptation, validation, and normalisation. J. Epidemiol. Community Health 57, 259–263.

Liem, Y.S., Bosch, J.L., Arends, L.R., et al., 2007. Quality of life assessed with the Medical Outcomes Study Short Form 36-Item Health Survey of patients on renal replacement therapy: a systematic review and meta-analysis. Value Health 10, 390–397.

Lyons, R.A., Wareham, K., Lucas, M., et al., 1999. SF-36 scores vary by method of administration: implications for study design. J. Public Health (Bangkok) 21, 41–45.

Man, W., Moxham, J., Polkey, M., 2004. Magnetic stimulation for the measurement of respiratory and skeletal muscle function. Eur. Respir. J. 24, 846–860.

Marini, J., Smith, T., Lamb, V., 1986. Estimation of inspiratory muscle strength in mechanically ventilated patients: the measurement of maximal inspiratory pressure. J. Crit. Care 1, 32–38.

Marques, A., Bruton, A., Barney, A., 2006. Clinically useful outcome measures for physiotherapy airway clearance techniques: a review. Phys. Ther. Rev. 11, 299–307.

Massy-Westropp, N., Rankin, W., Ahem, M., et al., 2004. Measuring grip strength in normal adults: reference ranges and a comparison of electronic and hydraulic instruments. J. Hand Surg. [Am] 29, 514–519.

Mathiowetz, V., Kashman, N., Volland, G., et al., 1985. Grip and pinch strength: normative data for adults. Arch. Phys. Med. Rehabil. 66, 69–74.

Mathiowetz, V., Wiemer, D., Federman, S., 1986. Grip and pinch strength: norms for 6 to 19 year olds. Am. J. Occup. Ther. 40, 705–711.

Mayo, N., Cole, B., Dowler, J., et al., 1994. Use of outcome measures in physiotherapy: Survey of current practice. Canadian Journal of Rehabilitation 81, 82.

McQuiddy, V., Scheerer, C., Lavalley, R., et al., 2015. Normative values for grip and pinch strength for 6 to 19-Year-Olds. Arch. Phys. Med. Rehabil. 96 (9), 1627–1633. In Press Corrected Proof.

Mendes, P., Wickerson, L., Helm, D., et al. 2015 Skeletal muscle atrophy in advanced interstitial lung disease Respirology E-pub ahead of print.

Menon, M., Houchen, L., Harrison, S., et al., 2012. Ultrasound assessment of lower limb muscle mass in response to resistance training in COPD. Respir. Res. 13, 119.

Merlani, P., Chenaud, C., Mariotti, N., Ricou, B., 2007. Long-term outcome of elderly patients requiring intensive care admission for abdominal pathologies: survival and quality of life. Acta Anaesthesiol. Scand. 51, 530–537.

Miller, M., Hankinson, J., Brusasco, V., et al., 2005. Series 'ATS/ERS task force: standardisation of lung function testing' – standardisation of spirometry. Eur. Respir. J. 26, 319–338.

Mokkink, L., Terwee, C., Patrick, D., et al., 2010. The COSMIN checklist for assessing the methodological quality of studies on measurement properties of health status measurement instruments: an international Delphi study. Qual. Life Res. 19, 539–549.

Msall, M., DiGaudio, K., Duffy, L., 1993. Use of functional assessment in children with developmental disabilities. In: Granger, C., Gresham, G. (Eds.), Physical Medicine and Rehabilitation Clinics of North America, vol. 4. New Developments in Functional Assessment. WB Saunders, Philadelphia.

Msall, M., DiGuadio, K., Duffy, L., et al., 1994. WeeFIM: normative sample of an instrument for tracking functional independence in children. Clin. Pediatr. (Phila) 33, 431–438.

Multz, A., Aldrich, T., Prezant, D., et al., 1990. Maximal inspiratory pressure is not a reliable test of inspiratory muscle strength in mechanically ventilated patients. Am. Rev. Respir. Dis. 142, 529–532.

Narang, I., Pike, S., Rosenthal, M., et al., 2003. Three-minute step test to assess exercise capacity in children with cystic fibrosis with mild lung disease. Pediatr. Pulmonol. 35 (2), 108–113.

Nasreddine, Z., Phillips, N., Bedirian, V., et al., 2005. The Montreal Cognitive Assessment, MoCA: a brief screening tool for mild cognitive impairment. J. Am. Geriatr. Soc. 53, 695–699.

Nawa, R., Lettvin, C., Winkelman, C., et al., 2014. Initial inter-rater reliability for a novel measure of patient mobility in a cardiovascular ICU. J. Crit. Care 29 (3), 475.e471–475.e475.

Nelson, E., Wasson, J., Kirk, J., et al., 1987. Assessment of function in routine clinical practice: description of the COOP Chart method and preliminary findings. J. Chronic Dis. 40 (Suppl. 1), 55S–69S.

Nes, B.M., Janszky, I., Aspenes, S.T., et al., 2012. Exercise patterns and peak oxygen uptake in a healthy population: the HUNT study. Med. Sci. Sports Exerc. 44 (10), 1881–1889.

Nicholas, J., Taylor, F., Buckingham, R., et al., 1976. Measurement of circumference of the knee with ordinary tape measure. Ann. Rheum. Dis. 35, 282–284.

Nordon-Craft, A., Schenkman, M., Edbrooke, L., et al., 2014. The physical function intensive care test: implementation in survivors of critical illness. Phys. Ther. 94 (10), 1499–1507.

Oeyen, S.G., Vandijck, D.M., Benoit, D.D., et al., 2010. Quality of life after intensive care: a systematic review of the literature. Crit. Care Med. 38, 2386–2400.

Ottenbacher, K., Taylor, E., Msall, M., et al., 1996. The stability and equivalence reliability of the Functional Independence Measure for children (WeeFIM). Dev. Med. Child Neurol. 38, 907–916.

Ouimet, S., Kavanagh, B.P., Gottfried, S.B., et al., 2007. Incidence, risk factors and consequences of ICU delirium. Intensive Care Med. 33, 66–73.

Pandharipande, P., Girard, T., Jackson, J., et al., 2013. Long-term cognitive impairment after critical illness. NEJM 369, 1306–1316.

Parry, S., Berney, S., Granger, C., et al., 2015a. A new two-tier strength assessment approach to the diagnosis of weakness in intensive care: an observational study. Crit. Care 19, 52.

Parry, S., Denehy, L., Beach, L., et al., 2015b. Functional outcomes in ICU: what should we be using? An observational study. Crit. Care 19, 127. Accepted – published online 29 March 2015.

Parry, S., El-Ansary, D., Cartwright, M., et al., 2015c. Ultrasonography in the intensive care setting can be used to detect changes in the quality and quantity of muscle and is related to muscle strength and function. J. Crit. Care [Epub Ahead of Print].

Parry, S., Granger, C.L., Berney, S., et al., 2015d. Assessment of impairment and activity limitations in the critically ill: a systematic review of measurement instruments and their clinimetric properties. Intensive Care Med. 41 (5), 744–762. Accepted – in press. Volume 41, Issue 5 / May, 2015, Pages 744–762.

Parshall, M., Schwartzstein, R., Adams, L.K., et al., 2012. An official American Thoracic Society statement: update on the mechanisms, assessment and management of dyspnea. Am. J. Respir. Crit. Care. Med. 185, 435–452.

Perneger, T.V., Leplege, A., Etter, J.F., Rougemont, A., 1995. Validation of a French-language version of the MOS 36-Item Short Form Health Survey (SF-36) in young healthy adults. J. Clin. Epidemiol. 48, 1051–1060.

Pfoh, E.R., Chan, K., Dinglas, V., et al., 2015. Cognitive screening among acute respiratory failure survivors: a cross-sectional evaluation of the Mini-Mental State Evaluation. Crit. Care 19 (1), 220. doi:10.1186/s13054-015-0934-5.

Pollard, W.E., Bobbitt, R.A., Bergner, M., et al., 1976. The Sickness Impact Profile: reliability of a health status measure. Med. Care 14, 146–155.

Portney, L., Watkins, M., 2009. Foundations of Clinical Research, Applications to Practice. Appleton and Lange, Connecticut.

Pountney, T., 2007. Physiotherapy for Children. Butterworth-Heinemann/Elsevier, Edinburgh; New York.

Prasad, S.A., Randall, S.D., Balfour-Lynn, I.M., 2000. Fifteen-count breathlessness score: an objective measure for children. Pediatr. Pulmonol. 30, 56–62.

Prosser, L., Canby, A., 1997. Further validation of the Elderly Mobility Scale for measurement of mobility of hospitalised elderly people. Clin. Rehabil. 11, 338–343.

Puthucheary, Z., Phadke, R., Rawal, J., et al., 2015. Qualitative ultrasound in acute critical illness muscle wasting. Crit. Care Med. 43 (8), 1603–1611. [Epub Ahead of Print].

Puthucheary, Z., Rawal, J., McPhail, M., et al., 2013. Acute skeletal muscle wasting in critical illness. JAMA 310, 1591–1600.

Quittner, A., Buu, A., Messer, M., et al., 2005. Development and validation of the cystic fibrosis questionnaire in the United States: a health-related quality of life measure for cystic fibrosis. Chest 128, 2347–2354.

Radtke, T., Stevens, D., Benden, C., et al., 2009. Clinical exercise testing in children and adolescents with cystic fibrosis. Pediatr. Phys. Ther. 21, 275–281.

Rauch, F., Neu, C., Wassmer, G., et al., 2002. Muscle analysis by measurement of maximal isometric grip force: new reference data and clinical applications in pediatrics. Pediatr. Res. 51, 505–510.

Rector, T.S., Francis, G.S., Cohn, J.N., 1987a. Patients' self-assessment of their congestive heart failure. Part 1 Patient perceived dysfunction and its poor correlation with maximal exercise tests. Heart Fail. 192–196.

Rector, T.S., Kubo, S.H., Cohn, J.N., 1987b. Patients' self assessment of their congestive heart failure. Part 2: Contentreliability and validity of a new measure, the Minnesota Living with Heart Failure Questionnaire. Heart Fail. 198–209.

Reeves, N., Maganaris, C., Narici, M., 2004a. Ultrasonographic assessment of skeletal muscle size. Eur. J. Appl. Physiol. 91, 116–118.

Reeves, N.D., Maganaris, C.N., Narici, M.V., 2004b. Ultrasonographic assessment of human skeletal muscle size. Eur. J. Appl. Physiol. 91, 116–118.

Reid, C.L., Campbell, I.T., Little, R.A., 2004. Muscle wasting and energy balance in critical illness. Clin. Nutr. 23, 273–280.

Roach, K., Ally, D., Finnerty, B., et al., 1998a. The relationship between duration of physical therapy services in the acute setting and change in functional status in patients with lower-extremity orthopaedic problems. Phys. Ther. 78, 19–24.

Roach, K., Van Dillen, L., 1998b. Development of an acute care index of functional status for patients with neurologic impairment. Phys. Ther. 68, 1102–1108.

Robles, P., Mathur, S., Janaudis-Fereira, T., et al., 2011. Measurement of peripheral muscle strength in individuals with chronic obstructive pulmonary disease: a systematic review. J. Cardiopulm. Rehabil. Prev. 31, 11–24.

Rowland, T.W., 1996. Developmental Exercise Physiology. Human Kinetics, Champaign, IL.

Rowland, T.W., Cunningham, L.N., 1997. Development of ventilatory responses to exercise in normal white children: a longitudinal study. Chest 111 (2), 327–332.

Sarwal, A., Parry, S., Berry, M., et al., 2014. Inter-observer reliability of quantitative muscle ultrasound analysis in the critically ill population. J. Ultrasound Med. 34, 1191-1200.

Saynor, Z., Barker, A., Oades, P., et al., 2013. A protocol to determine valid VO_{2max} in young cystic fibrosis patients. J. Sci. Med. Sports 16, 539–544.

Schipper, H., Clinch, J.J., Olweny, C.L.M., 1996. Quality of life studies: definitions and conceptual issues. In: Spilker, B. (Ed.), Quality of Life and Pharmacoeconomics in Clinical Trials. Lippincott-Raven, Philadelphia.

Schuit, A.J., 1997. Validity of the Physical Activity Scale for the Elderly (PASE): according to energy expenditure assessed by the doubly labeled water method. J. Clin. Epidemiol. 50, 541–546.

Selvadurai, H., Cooper, P., Meyers, N., et al., 2003. Validation of shuttle tests in children with cystic fibrosis. Pediatr. Pulmonol. 35, 133–138.

Sessler, C., Gosnell, M., Grap, M., et al., 2002. The Richmond Agitation-Sedation Scale: validity and reliability in adult intensive care unit patients. Am. J. Respir. Crit. Care Med. 166, 1338–1344.

Seymour, J., Ward, K., Sidhu, P., et al., 2009. Ultrasound measurement of rectus femoris cross-sectional area and the relationship with quadriceps strength in COPD. Thorax 64, 418–423.

Sharshar, T., Bastuji-Garin, S., Stevens, R., et al., 2009. Presence and severity of intensive care unit-acquired paresis at time of awakening are associated with increased intensive care unit and hospital mortality. Crit. Care Med. 37 (12), 3047–3053.

Sherwood, L., 2004. Human Physiology: From Cells to Systems, 5th ed. Thomson Brooks/Cole Learning, Belmont CA.

Singh, S.J., Jones, P.W., Evans, R., Morgan, M.D., 2008. Minimum clinically important improvement for the incremental shuttle walking test. Thorax 63 (9), 775–777.

Singh, S., Puhan, M., Andrianopoulos, V., et al., 2014. An official systematic review of the European Respiratory Society/American Thoracic Society: measurement properties of field walking tests in chronic respiratory disease. Eur. Respir. J. 44, 1447–1478.

Sintonen, H., 1994. The 15D-measure of health-related quality of lfie. I. Reliability, validity, and sensitivity of its health state descriptive system. National Centre for Health Program Evaluation, Melbourne.

Sintonen, H., 1995. The 15D-measure of health-related quality of life. II. Feasibility, reliability and validity of its valuation system. National Centre for Health Program Evaluation, Melbourne.

Sintonen, H., 2001. The 15D instrument of health-related quality of life: properties and applications. Ann. Med. 33, 328–336.

Skinner, E., Berney, S., Warrillow, S., et al., 2009. Development of a physical function outcome measure (PFIT) and a pilot exercise training protocol for use in intensive care. Crit. Care Resusc. 11, 110–115.

Skinner, E.H., Denehy, L., Warrillow, S., Hawthorne, G., 2013. Comparison of the measurement properties of the AQoL and SF-6D in critical illness. Crit. Care. Resusc. 15, 205–212.

Smith, R., 1994. Validation and reliability of the Elderly Mobility Scale. Physiotherapy 80, 744–747.

Sperle, P., Ottenbacher, K., Braun, S., et al., 1997. Equivalence reliability of the Functional Independence Measure for Children (WeeFIM) administration methods. Am. J. Occup. Ther. 51, 35–41.

Spiegel, B.M., Melmed, G., Robbins, S., Esrailian, E., 2008. Biomarkers and health-related quality of life in end-stage renal disease: a systematic review. Clin. J. Am. Soc. Nephrol. 3, 1759–1768.

Spittle, A., Doyle, L., Boyd, R., 2008. A systematic review of the clinimetric properties of neuromotor assessments for preterm infants during the first year of life. Dev. Med. Child Neurol. 50, 254–266.

Spronk, P.E., Riekerk, B., Hofhuis, J., et al., 2009. Occurrence of delirium is severely underestimated in the ICU during daily care. Intensive Care Med. 35, 1276–1280.

Stark, T., Walker, B., Phillips, J., et al., 2011. Hand-held dynamometry correlation with the gold standard isokinetic dynamometry: a systematic review. Phys. Med. Rehabil. 3, 472–479.

Stein, R., Selvadurai, H., Coates, A., et al., 2003. Determination of maximal voluntary ventilation in children with cystic fibrosis. Pediatr. Pulmonol. 35 (6), 467–471.

Supinski, G., Callahan, L.A., 2011. Correlation of MIP to Pdi twitch pressure in mechanically ventilated ICU patients. Am. J. Respir. Crit. Care. Med. 183, A4253.

Tamplin, J., Berlowitz, D., 2014. A systematic review and meta-analysis of the effects of respiratory muscle training on pulmonary function in tetraplegia. Spinal Cord 52, 175–180.

Teasdale, G., Jennett, B., 1974. Assessment of coma and impaired consciousness. A practical scale. Lancet 2, 81–84.

Ten Harkel, A., Takken, T., Van Osch-Gevers, M., et al., 2011. Normal values for cardiopulmonary exercise testing in children. Eur. J. Cardiovasc. Prev. Rehabil. 18, 48–54.

Thomaes, T., Thomis, M., Onkelinx, S., et al., 2012. Reliability and validity of the ultrasound technique to measure the rectus femoris muscle diameter in older CAD-patients. BMC Med. Imaging 12, 7.

Thrall, G., Lane, D., Carroll, D., Lip, G.Y., 2006. Quality of life in patients with atrial fibrillation: a systematic review. Am. J. Med. 119, 448.e1–448.e19.

Thrush, A., Rozek, M., Dekerlegand, J., 2012. The clinical utility of the Functional Status Score for the Intensive Care Unit (FSS-ICU) at a long-term acute care hospital: a prospective cohort study. Phys. Ther. 92, 1536–1545.

Tobin, M., 2006. Principles and Practice of Mechanical Ventilation. McGraw-Hill, New York.

Tombaugh, T., McIntyre, N., 1992. The Mini-Mental State Examination: a comprehensive review. J. Am. Geriatr. Soc. 40, 922–935.

Torrance, G.W., Furlong, W., Feeny, D., Boyle, M., 1995. Multi-attribute preference functions. Health Utilities Index. Pharmacoeconomics 7, 503–520.

Trutschnigg, B., Kilgour, R., Reinglas, J., et al., 2008. Precision and reliability of strength (Jamar vs. Biodex handgrip) and body composition (dual-energy X-ray absortiometry vs. bioimpedance analysis) measurements in advanced cancer patients. Appl. Physiol. Nutr. Metab. 33, 1232–1239.

Valkenet, K., van de Port, I., Dronkers, J., et al., 2011. The effects of preoperative exercise therapy on postoperative outcome: a systematic review. Clin. Rehabil. 25, 99–111.

Van Dillen, L., Roach, K., 1988. Reliability and validity of the acute care index of function for patients with neurologic impairment. Phys. Ther. 68 (7), 1098–1101.

Vanhees, L., Lefevre, J., Philippaerts, R., et al., 2005. How to assess physical activity? How to assess physical fitness? Eur. J. Cardiovasc. Prev. Rehabil. 12, 102–114.

Vanhoutte, E., Faber, C., van Nes, S., et al., 2012. Modifying the medical research council grading system through Rasch analyses. Brain 135, 1639–1649.

Vanpee, G., Hermans, G., Segers, J., et al., 2014. Assessment of limb muscle strength in critically ill patients: a systematic review. Crit. Care Med. 42, 701–711.

Vanpee, G., Segers, J., Wouters, P., et al., 2011. Inter-observer agreement of hand-held dynamometry in critically ill patients. Am. J. Respir. Crit. Care Med. 183.

Varni, J., Seid, M., Kurtin, P., 2001. PedsQL 4.0: reliability and validity of the pediatric quality of life inventory version 4.0 generic core scales in healthy and patient populations. Med. Care 39, 800–812.

Ware, J.E., Kosinski, M., Keller, S., 1994. Physical and Mental Health Summary Scales: A User's Manual. MA The Health Institute, New England Medical Centre, Boston.

Ware, J.E., Jr., Sherbourne, C.D., 1992. The MOS 36-item short-form health survey (SF-36). I. Conceptual framework and item selection. Med. Care 30, 473–483.

Ware, J.E., Snow, K.K., Kosinski, M., Gandek, B., 1993. SF-36 Health Survey: Manual and interpretation guide. MA The Health Institute, New England Medical Centre, Boston.

Washburn, R., Smith, K., Jette, A., et al., 1993. The Physical Activity Scale for the Elderly (PASE): development and evaluation. J. Clin. Epidemiol. 46, 153–162.

Washburn, R.A., 1999. Physical Activity Scale for the Elderly (PASE): the relationship with activity measured by a portable accelerometer. J. Sports Med. Phys. Fitness 39, 336–340.

Wasserman, K., Hansen, J., Sue, D., et al., 2005. Principles of Exercise Testing and Interpretation. Lippincott Williams & Wilkins, Philadelphia.

Waters, E., Salmon, L., Wake, M., et al., 2000. The Child Health Questionnaire in Australia: reliability, validity and population means. Aust. N. Z. J. Public Health 24, 207–210.

Wehler, M., Geise, A., Hadzionerovic, D., et al., 2003. Health-related quality-of-life of patients with multiple organ dysfunction: individual changes and comparison with normative population. Crit. Care Med. 31, 1094–1101.

Westerterp, K., 2009. Assessment of physical activity: a critical appraisal. Eur. J. Appl. Physiol. 105, 823–828.

Williams, J.R., Armstrong, N., Kirby, B.J., 1990. The 4 mM blood lactate level as an index of exercise performance in 11–13 year old children. J. Sports Sci. 8 (2), 139–147.

Wilson, J.R., Rayos, G., Yeoh, T.K., et al., 1995. Dissociation between exertional symptoms and circulatory function in patients with heart failure. Circulation 92, 47–53.

Winters, B.D., Eberlein, M., Leung, J., et al., 2010. Long-term mortality and quality of life in sepsis: a systematic review. Crit. Care Med. 38, 1276–1283.

World Health Organization, 2001. International Classification of Functioning, Disability and Health. World Health Organization, Geneva, Switzerland.

WHO, 1993. Study protocol for the World Health Organization project to develop a Quality of Life assessment instrument (WHOQOL). Qual. Life Res. 2, 153–159.

WHO, 1998. Development of the World Health Organization WHOQOL-BREF quality of life assessment. The WHOQOL Group. Phychol. Med. 28, 551–558.

Young, A., Hughes, A., Russell, P., et al., 1980. Measurement of quadriceps muscle wasting by ultrasonography. Rheumatol. Rehabil. XIX, 141–148.

Zanni, J.M., Korupolu, R., Fan, E., et al., 2010. Rehabilitation therapy and outcomes in acute respiratory failure: an observational pilot project. J. Crit. Care 25 (2), 254–262.

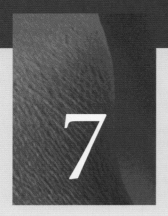

7

PHYSIOTHERAPY INTERVENTIONS

ELEANOR MAIN

with contributions from

SUE BERNEY ■ LINDA DENEHY
(Manual and Ventilator Hyperinflation)

MICHELLE CHATWIN
(Mechanical Insufflation/Exsufflation and Assisted Cough,
Intrapulmonary Percussive Ventilation (IPV))

MARK R ELKINS
(Inhalation Therapy)

DANIEL FLUNT ■ AMANDA J PIPER
(Non-Invasive Ventilation)

ANNEMARIE L LEE ■ BREDGE MCCARREN ■
HARRIET SHANNON ■ SARAH RAND
(Airway Clearance Techniques)

ROSEMARY MOORE
(Oxygen Therapy)

BARBARA A WEBBER
(Glossopharyngeal Breathing)

MARIE T WILLIAMS
(Techniques for Improving Dyspnoea)

■ ■ ■ ■ ■ ■ ■ ■ ■ ■ ■ ■ ■ ■ ■ ■

CHAPTER OUTLINE

AIRWAY CLEARANCE TECHNIQUES 250
  Theoretical Rationales for Secretion Clearance
    Interventions 252
  Airway Clearance Strategies for Babies and
    Children 253

Traditional and Manual Airway Clearance
Techniques 255
  Postural Drainage and Modified Postural
    Drainage 255
  Manual Techniques 258

Suction 265
Independently Performed Airway Clearance
Techniques 266
  Breathing Techniques 266
  Device-Dependent Techniques 274
  Machine-Dependent Techniques 284
Exercise and Pulmonary Rehabilitation for Airway
Clearance 291
Adjunctive Techniques 292

TECHNIQUES FOR IMPROVING LUNG
VOLUMES 292
Intermittent Positive Pressure Breathing 292
  Preparation of the Apparatus 294
  Treatment of the Patient 295
  Contraindications for IPPB 296
Non-Invasive Ventilation 296
  Introduction 296
  What is Non-Invasive Ventilation? 296
  Indications for Non-Invasive Ventilation 297
  Practical Issues in the Application of Non-Invasive
    Ventilation 302
Incentive Spirometry 308
Manual and Ventilator Hyperinflation 310
  Manual Hyperinflation Procedure 311
Glossopharyngeal Breathing 313

TECHNIQUES FOR IMPROVING GAS
EXCHANGE 317
Positioning and Mobilization 317
  To Improve Oxygen Transport in Acute
    Cardiopulmonary Dysfunction 320
  To Improve Oxygen Transport in Post-Acute and
    Chronic Cardiopulmonary Dysfunction 324
  Summary 325
Oxygen Therapy 325
  Introduction 325
  Oxygen Therapy in the Acute Setting 326

INHALATION THERAPY 334
Hypertonic Saline 335
  Mechanisms of Action 336
  Evidence About Efficacy 336
  Interaction with Physiotherapy 337

Mannitol 337
  Mechanisms of Action 338
  Evidence about Efficacy 338
  Interaction with Physiotherapy 339
Dornase Alpha 339
  Mechanisms of Action 339
  Evidence about Efficacy 339
  Interaction with Physiotherapy 340
Bronchodilators 340
Structuring an Airway Clearance Session 341
  Order of Interventions 341
  Combining Interventions 341

TECHNIQUES FOR IMPROVING DYSPNOEA 342
Differences between Shortness of Breath and
Dyspnoea 342
Mechanisms Underpinning Dyspnoea 343
Assessment of Dyspnoea 345
Management Strategies for Dyspnoea 346
Inspiratory Muscle Training 348
Breathing Control 350

TECHNIQUES FOR IMPROVING
DYSFUNCTIONAL BREATHING 355
Manual Therapy Techniques for Musculoskeletal
Dysfunction 355
  Subjective Assessment 358
  Physical Assessment: Posture 359
  Physical Assessment: Range of Motion 359
  Physiotherapy Management 360
  Postural Correction and Motor Control Training 361
  Mobilization Techniques 361
  Muscle-Lengthening Techniques 362
  Taping 362
  Muscle Retraining (Strength and Endurance) 364
  Neural Tissue Techniques 365
  Summary 365
Neurophysiological Facilitation of Respiration 366
  Neural Control 367
  Respiratory Muscles 368
  Neurophysiological Facilitatory Stimuli 372
  Clinical Application 377
References 377

Airway Clearance Techniques

Airway clearance techniques (ACTs) are used to facilitate mucociliary clearance (MCC) and aid in the removal of retained secretions. Under normal circumstances the MCC mechanism is extremely effective and efficient. However, the pathophysiology of many respiratory diseases and the effects of anaesthesia and surgical procedures may result in excess sputum production and/or impairment of the inherent biological mechanisms responsible for removing secretions. ACTs may be indicated for short-term use or over a longer duration.

Postural drainage (PD) and breathing techniques have been described in the literature for more than a century as airway clearance strategies for people with difficulty clearing excessive pulmonary secretions. However, it is only in the last 40 years that a number of different airway clearance devices have been developed and marketed internationally, and that serious efforts have been made to evaluate the scientific evidence for airway clearance interventions. The global evolution of different ACTs has resulted in invention, modification, retention or rejection of different methods. Certain ACTs have strong geographical dominance, usually as a consequence of the origin of the technique or marketing in that country, rather than as a result of best evidence.

Airway clearance strategies may involve singular and focused interventions for the purpose of removing secretions and improving lung recruitment and gas exchange in patients with atelectasis. Strategies may also involve indirect or adjunctive interventions that facilitate or enhance effective airway clearance at different ages or stages of the disease process, for example inhalation therapy, exercise, oxygen therapy or non-invasive ventilation (NIV). Underpinning these numerous ACTs are a clutch of theoretical pulmonary physiology principles which lend them credibility. Among these are: 'interdependence', 'pendelluft', 'equal pressure point (EPP)', 'hysteresis', 'collateral ventilation', 'altered rheology' and 'two-phase gas liquid flow interactions'. The aim is to optimize care by selecting any one or a combination of these in responding intelligently and sensitively to individual and changing patient requirements during their lifetime.

The fact remains that at present, a robust evidence base does not yet exist and much of clinical airway clearance practice for physiotherapists remains in the domain of clinical expertise. The paucity of evidence is partly explained by the relatively immature research machinery in allied health care internationally, but is also partly to do with inadequate or inappropriate research designs. Although there have been improvements in the design, quality and rigour of research conducted in airway clearance strategies, these have not yet resulted in clarity for clinical practice. Ironically, in this field of research, even the gold-standard long-term randomised controlled trial (RCT) may be an inappropriate research design. This is because it does not account for the unpredictable behaviour of participants who cannot easily be (and are not usually) blinded to the airway clearance treatment they are allocated (Main et al 2015).

People with chronic lung conditions can develop strong preferences for the way they undertake their daily airway clearance treatments. Significant participant dropouts in four recent long-term airway clearance studies have exposed unanticipated but fundamental shortcomings in the standard RCT trial design in airway clearance physiotherapy studies (McIlwaine et al 2010, 2013, Pryor et al 2010b, Sontag et al 2010). Strong patient preference, lack of blinding and the requirement for effortful and demanding participation over long intervals are likely to continue jeopardizing research into the best airway clearance strategies for patients with chronic lung disease (Main 2013). Researchers must begin to address these problems more imaginatively in future clinical trial designs if any progress is to be made in identifying clinically effective airway clearance strategies (Brewin & Bradley 1989).

The best evidence from a plethora of early, underpowered, typically short-term studies, crossover design and 1–14 days in length, has been synthesized in five Cochrane reviews related to ACTs for cystic fibrosis (CF), published between 2000 and 2011 (Elkins et al 2006a, Main et al 2005, McKoy et al 2012, Morrison & Agnew 2009, Warnock et al 2013). All conclude that there is currently insufficient evidence to suggest superiority of any one technique over another. The earliest of these reviews, recently updated, compared airway clearance to no treatment in people with CF. The review included 96 participants in 8 crossover studies (6 of which were single treatments and 2 of which involved 2 and 4 treatments respectively), and concluded that there was some evidence that airway clearance increased mucus transport rate. There was insufficient evidence to indicate any long-term effects (Warnock et al 2013).

Selection and prescription of the most optimal ACT will be influenced by the underlying airway pathophysiology contributing to sputum retention in the individual patient (Holland et al 2003, Holland & Button 2006). The selected technique should be associated with maximal clearance of airway secretions and minimal risk of adverse events, including exacerbation of the underlying pathophysiology (Hill et al 2010) or aggravation of comorbidities or other symptoms.

There is rarely a single, preferred ACT for any given condition. The use of conventional chest physiotherapy (gravity-assisted drainage, manual techniques, coughing) in CF compared to no treatment has been associated with short-term improvements in sputum expectoration, although the benefits in the long-term are unknown (Warnock et al 2013). In patients experiencing an acute exacerbation of chronic obstructive pulmonary disease (COPD), short-term airway clearance therapy reduced both the need for additional ventilatory support and length of hospital stay compared to no treatment (Osadnik et al 2012). It may also improve mucus expectoration and lung function in non-CF bronchiectasis (Lee et al 2013). It is not known whether techniques improve symptoms or quality of life in the long term. Comparisons of 'conventional chest physiotherapy', positive expiratory pressure (PEP), breathing techniques and oscillating PEP (OPEP) to other ACTs in CF found no evidence that any technique was superior to another in physiological effects and patient-reported outcomes (Elkins et al 2006a, Main et al 2005, McKoy et al 2012, Morrison & Agnew 2009).

The overall effectiveness of any chosen ACT will also be influenced by patient related factors; of particular importance is compliance with treatment. Patient satisfaction, motivation and perceived efficacy are intimately related to adherence (Lapin 2000).

These have been identified as factors when patients choose independent techniques (Elkins et al 2006a, Lewis et al 2012). Patient preference may be influenced not only by relief of symptoms but by the adaptability of techniques into lifestyle and the degree of treatment burden on the patient and/or carer, particularly in individuals who require long-term treatment. The choice of technique should also be within the capabilities of the patient, with respect to their age and current clinical state. Patient response to techniques may differ depending on the stage of their condition; therefore regular review of technique effectiveness, quality of treatment and patient response will provide guidance in airway clearance prescription and identify the need for modification or correction in both short- and long-term use. For some patients, combining techniques may improve treatment outcomes, for example the use of additional support, such as NIV for patients who are acutely unwell or experiencing respiratory failure secondary to sputum retention. The ease with which this can be incorporated into an existing routine may influence technique selection.

Almost 50% of adults and around 30% of children with CF admit that they do not undertake airway clearance as recommended, and these figures are likely to be similar for non-CF bronchiectasis (O'Donohoe & Fullen 2014, Myers 2009). The reasons for poor compliance with airway clearance strategies or cough suppression may be numerous and multifactorial, including burden of care, lack of time or confidence in the treatment, but may also include secondary complications of the disease, for example urinary stress incontinence in females with chronic respiratory disease (Browne et al 2009, Nankivell et al 2010, Rees et al 2013). In these cases, airway clearance modalities which incorporate breathing control (BC) and avoidance of the high pressures associated with Valsalva manoeuvres could be recommended. Or, for example, patients with advanced respiratory disease may have significantly deranged spinal and thoracic musculoskeletal functional anatomy as a result of chronic air-trapping, hyperinflated chest walls, flattened diaphragms and overuse of accessory muscles (Laurin et al 2012). Typically this manifests in a barrel-shaped chest and forwards protracted shoulders, which not only ultimately increase the work of breathing but also create circumstances in which musculoskeletal pain can further exacerbate restricted or splinted chest wall movement.

Treatment options available to patients may also be determined by therapists' skills and the equipment available within a healthcare service. The patient's resources and the social acceptability of some techniques may also be relevant. The need for meticulous cleaning of devices to minimize the risk of infection will influence patient safety and may be a key factor.

The prescription of techniques will depend on the patient's clinical state. All prescriptions must be realistic and complemented by general physical activity or exercise which will enhance the effects of airway clearance therapy. In general, airway clearance strategies will be changed and adapted during the course of a chronic illness, generally progressing from techniques that are dependent on the assistance of a parent or healthcare practitioner in early life, to self-administered techniques that can be performed independently and portably if necessary in later life.

There are few contraindications or adverse events related to ACTs. The scope and spectrum of techniques available allow for significant modifications to care which avoid individual issues that arise. For example, manual techniques may be contraindicated in the presence of unstable rib fractures, but alternatives, including PEP therapy or breathing techniques are available.

Theoretical Rationales for Secretion Clearance Interventions

There are three main physiological mechanisms by which physiotherapy ACTs may assist with secretion clearance. These are:

- increase in expiratory flow
- oscillation of airflow
- increasing lung volumes.

The physiological effect of an increase in expiratory flow occurring during some physiotherapy interventions is explained by the two-phase gas-liquid flow mechanism. Two-phase gas-liquid flow explains the interaction of liquid (airway secretions) and gas (air) within a conduit (airway) (Zhao et al 2013). The theory of fluid mechanics defines two flow patterns that can be applied to physiotherapy secretion clear-ance interventions. The first pattern is mist flow, which occurs when very fast expiratory flow rate shears the secretions off the wall of the airway in small particles (mist) towards the oropharynx. The second pattern is annular flow when the increase in the expiratory flow rate moves secretions which line the airway in a wave-like pattern towards the oropharynx (Leith 1985).

Cough is the only intervention that may achieve mist flow (Leith 1977). Cough is the backup mechanism for impaired MCC. The supramaximal transient expiratory flow rates of 12 L/s in 30–50 ms bursts (Knudson et al 1974) are proposed to mobilize secretions within the upper central airways (from sixth or seventh generation) (Leith 1968). This critical level of supramaximal flow occurs due to the high intrathoracic pressures, large inspired volumes and the dynamic compression of the airways that occurs during coughing. Therefore for an effective cough, patients are required to be able to inspire large volumes, create high intrathoracic pressure (through effective contraction of abdominal and expiratory accessory muscles), have closure of the glottis and have airways that dynamically narrow but do not collapse.

There needs to be a critical volume of secretions within the airway for cough to be effective (King et al 1985). Cough has been proven effective in radio aerosol clearance of both excessive (37.5 ± SE 7.9 g) (Hasani et al 1994a) and small (9.1 ± SE 2.0 g) volumes of secretions (Hasani et al 1994b). However, in healthy individuals and in asymptomatic smokers, cough did not improve clearance (Bennett et al 1990, 1992; Kamishima et al 1983).

Cough has also been shown to mobilize secretions from more distal (away from oropharynx) airways (Hasani et al 1994a, 1991). The smaller relative resistance of the peripheral airways is inadequate for generating the supramaximal flows required for mist flow but is high enough to mobilize secretions through annular flow. For this mechanism to be effective, there is a requirement for a critical volume of secretions, and a critical depth and stickiness of secretions and a need for an expiratory bias to airflow. This critical level of expiratory bias to airflow occurs when peak expiratory flow rate (PEF) during any secretion clearance technique is at least 10% faster than the peak inspiratory flow rate (PIF) or PEF:PIF >1.1 (Kim et al 1986a, 1986b, 1987; Sackner and Kim, 1987).

In addition to cough, physiotherapy secretion clearance interventions including huff from both high and low lung volumes, chest wall vibrations and OPEP (Flutter device) have been shown to generate PEF which is at least 10% faster than PIF in stable patients with CF (McCarren & Alison 2006b). Improvements in radio-aerosol clearance of mucus have been shown to occur with huff from high lung volumes (van der Schans et al 1990) and huff from low lung volumes during the forced expiration technique (Hasani et al 1994a).

The potential physiological effects of oscillating air flow during secretion clearance physiotherapy interventions are threefold:

- increase in expiratory flow rate (King et al 1983)
- mechanical stimulation of ciliated epithelial cells of the airway due to oscillation of the airway or chest wall which may stimulate cilial beat (Sanderson et al 1988, 1990)
- alter the rheology of the mucus, which may facilitate MCC (King et al 1983).

The oscillation of airflow (Fig. 7-1) can be created by intermittent positive pressure applied to the chest wall manually (i.e. percussion and vibration) or to the airways mechanically (i.e. intrapulmonary percussive ventilation (IPV)), or by applying intermittent resistance to airflow at the mouth (i.e. oscillatory PEP devices). The range of oscillation frequency shown to be effective for secretion movement is 3–17 Hz (cycles per second) with optimal clearance at 13 Hz (Gross et al 1985, King et al 1983).

The physiological effects of increasing lung volumes may improve secretion clearance via two potential mechanisms. The increase of volume of air within the airways due to an increase in positive back-pressure within the airways may dilate narrowed or floppy airways to increase flow within these airways (Langenderfer 1998). If the patient has floppy airways which close with forced expiration, the positive back-pressure within these smaller airways may maintain airway patency and thus increase the expiratory flow (Zach & Oberwaldner 1987). In addition, this positive back-pressure may open collateral ventilation channels between the ventilated and non-ventilated airspaces, distal to the mucus obstruction (Menkes & Traystman 1977) to get air behind secretions obstructing the small airways. This would increase the pressure and airflow behind the secretions to move the secretions towards the oropharynx (Langenderfer 1998). The positive back-pressure is caused by applying resistance to expiratory flow at the mouth (i.e. PEP devices). The second proposed mechanism of increasing lung volumes is by increasing functional residual capacity (FRC) to greater than closing capacity (Fig. 1-13). This may open non-ventilated airspaces, to enable airflow and the mucociliary mechanism to clear secretions towards the oropharynx. This increase in FRC may occur with positioning, breathing exercises or continuous positive airway pressure (CPAP), to name a few.

Airway Clearance Strategies for Babies and Children

ACTs for infants and young children with mucous hypersecretion have a weak evidence base and can be

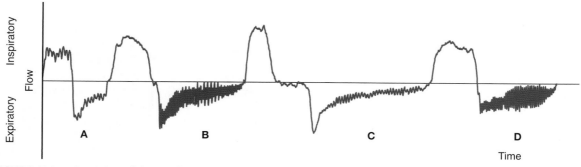

FIGURE 7-1 ■ Examples of the oscillation of airflow that occur in a patient with cystic fibrosis during **(A)** percussion, **(B)** vibration, **(C)** acapella and **(D)** flutter respectively.

challenging to perform. The majority of the evidence to support the use of ACTs in infants and young children is from the CF population and in general, ACTs have been adapted from techniques developed for older patients with chronic sputum retention (Lannefors et al 2004). The limited evidence on ACTs in infants and young children with non-CF bronchiectasis comes from consensus statements, and assumptions about benefit are extrapolated from assumptions about common symptomology between the conditions (Barbato et al 2009). Age-related physiological and pathophysiological differences between children and adults, such as differences in airway mucus composition, respiratory mechanics and lung development exist (see Chapter 1). These along with other unique aspects of development such as gastro-oesophageal reflux (GOR) and behavioural challenges are also important considerations when initiating ACTs in this age group (Schechter 2007).

The international uptake of newborn screening for CF early in the millennium was relatively slow but became far more widely implemented from 2007. The USA, UK, Ireland, France, Italy, Spain, Austria, Poland and the Czech Republic now have CF newborn screening programs either regionally or nationally, as do Australia and New Zealand (Massie & Clements 2005, Southern et al 2007). This has resulted in the emergence of a novel cohort of infants in these countries who may have a diagnosis of CF but may have few, if any, overt respiratory symptoms (Prasad et al 2008).

This cohort has quite reasonably created some uncertainty about the role of traditional routine daily chest physiotherapy when parents are not able to observe or appreciate any palpable benefit from an intervention that is not always popular (Prasad et al 2008).

The uncertainty arises because a number of studies have suggested that despite an apparent lack of symptoms in babies with CF, there are demonstrable changes on CT, and bronchoalveolar lavage (BAL) studies have shown the presence of inflammatory markers and bacterial and viral pathogens (Armstrong et al 1995, Khan et al 1995, Rosenfeld et al 2001).

Recent evidence suggests that with current care in the UK, the reductions in lung function observed in these infants at 3 months of age have largely resolved by 1 year of age and these benefits are maintained at 2 years (Nguyen et al 2014). The infants who participated in this longitudinal cohort were receiving a variety of physiotherapy and airway clearance interventions, ranging from modified postural drainage and percussion (mPD&P) once or twice daily, to exercise and mPD&P, to infant PEP. In the absence of firm evidence, the UK consensus guidelines currently recommend the early establishment of a physiotherapy regimen of advice and education for parents, physical activity, exercise and ACTs (Prasad et al 2008). The most commonly used ACTs for infants and young children who have a chronic respiratory disorder (with increased airway secretions) are mPD&P, infant PEP, assisted autogenic drainage (AAD) and bubble PEP (Fig. 7-2) (Main et al 2015). Usually after 4 years of age, other ACTs can be added. These will be covered in more detail within relevant sections of this chapter.

For infants and young children, regular physical activity and focused exercise training is important not just for airway clearance but for the many other benefits they provide. Physical activity is possible even with an infant; for example, floor play sessions with the addition of exercise sessions, playing on a gym ball (Fig. 7-3), trampolining (Fig. 7-4) or swimming for example.

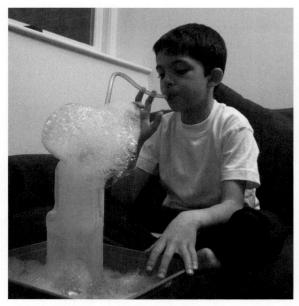

FIGURE 7-2 ■ Using bubble positive expiratory pressure (PEP).

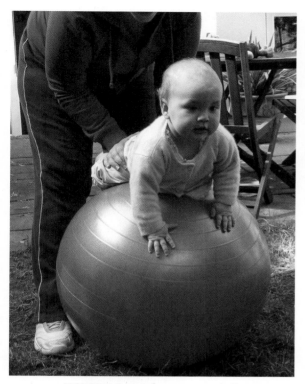

FIGURE 7-3 ▪ Infant on a gym ball.

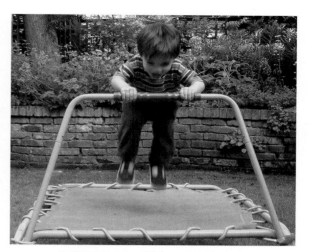

FIGURE 7-4 ▪ Child on a trampoline.

TRADITIONAL AND MANUAL AIRWAY CLEARANCE TECHNIQUES

Postural Drainage and Modified Postural Drainage

PD was one of the first ACTs described for people with chronic respiratory disease and appeared to be a successful airway clearance strategy in single case studies of patients with bronchiectasis over a century ago (Ewart 1901). Nelson (1934) described the use of positioning for draining secretions based on the anatomy of the bronchial tree (see Fig. 1-2). The recognized positions (Thoracic Society 1950) are shown in Figures 7-5 through 7-15 and described in Table 7-1. PD is achieved by placing individuals in specific recumbent or semi-recumbent positions that enable gravity to move mucus from peripheral airways in selected lung segments to more central airways for expectoration (Eaton et al 2007, Ewart 1901, Lannefors et al 2004, Sutton et al 1983, Webber et al 1986). Some standard

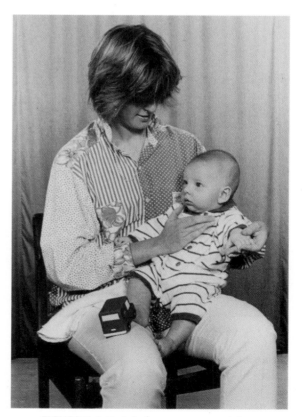

FIGURE 7-5 ▪ Apical segments upper lobes.

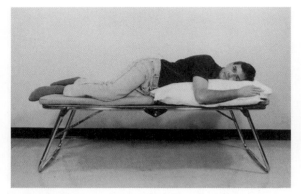

FIGURE 7-6 ▪ Posterior segment right upper lobe.

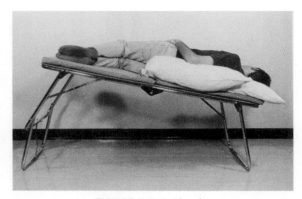

FIGURE 7-9 ▪ Lingula.

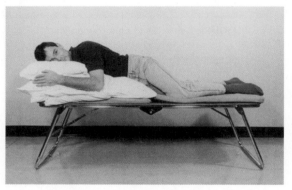

FIGURE 7-7 ▪ Posterior segment left upper lobe.

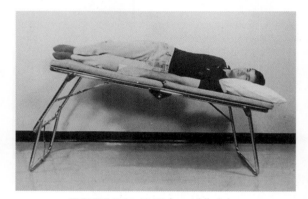

FIGURE 7-10 ▪ Right middle lobe.

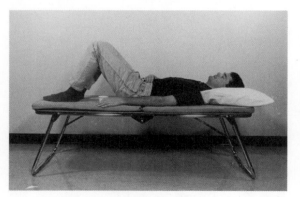

FIGURE 7-8 ▪ Anterior segments upper lobes.

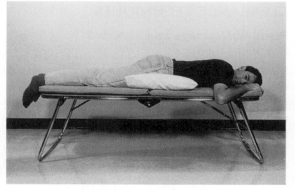

FIGURE 7-11 ▪ Apical segments lower lobes.

PD positions incorporate a head-down tilt of approximately 30°, where the head is lower than the thorax.

The use of gravity-assisted positioning, including a head-down tip, has traditionally been a component of airway clearance in babies and children. This position prompted concerns that GOR, and therefore potentially pulmonary micro-aspiration, might be exacerbated in some adult patients and particularly in infants and young children with CF. Evidence suggests that GOR is more common in infants and children

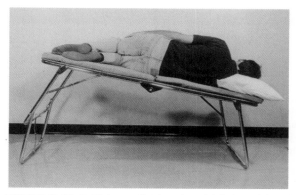

FIGURE 7-12 ■ Right medial basal and left lateral basal segments lower lobes.

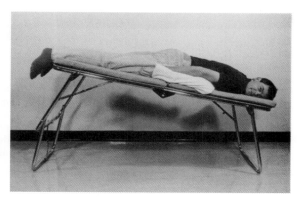

FIGURE 7-15 ■ Posterior basal segments lower lobes.

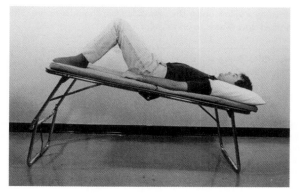

FIGURE 7-13 ■ Anterior and anteromedial basal segments.

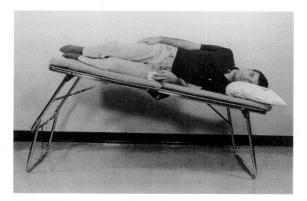

FIGURE 7-14 ■ Lateral basal segment right lower lobe.

with CF, and is twice as common in people with chronic respiratory disease including bronchiectasis, than in a healthy population (Cecins et al 1999).

An early study compared the effects of standard PD with an alternative called 'modified PD (mPD)', which used horizontal positions instead of head-down tilt in 20 infants with CF. Significantly more episodes of GOR (p <0.05) were seen with PD than with mPD, particularly during supine and prone positioning (Button et al 2004). Another study in adults who were significant sputum producers also suggested mPD was as useful as standard PD and was preferred by patients (Cecins et al 1999). Despite the risk of GOR, standard PD remains a very useful tool in the ACT armament. Two studies have demonstrated that PD is more effective than OPEP or ACBT alone in terms of volume of secretions cleared, and appeared to hint that gravity-assisted positions are more helpful than sitting upright for ACTs, but may not require the head-down tilt (Cecins et al 1999, Eaton et al 2007). While PD may be of significant benefit to some, others continue to find it uncomfortable and time consuming, and it may increase symptoms of breathlessness (Currie et al 1986). It is inappropriate to use the head-down tipped positions immediately following meals and in the presence of cardiac failure, severe hypertension, cerebral oedema, aortic and cerebral aneurysms, severe haemoptysis, abdominal distension, GOR and after recent surgery or trauma to the head or neck. A head-down tip should never be used in children with raised intracranial pressure or in preterm infants because of the risk of periventricular haemorrhage. Abdominal distension places the diaphragm at a mechanical disadvantage and a head-down tilt is likely to exacerbate this further.

In patients with CF the upper lobes and perihilar and apical segments of the lower lobes are frequently

	Lung segments (refer to Fig. 1-4)		
Upper lobe	S^1	Right apical segments	Sitting upright
	S^2	Right posterior segment	Lying on the left side horizontally turned 45° on to the face, resting against a pillow, with another supporting the head
	S^{1+2}	Left apicoposterior segment	Sitting upright or lying on the right side turned 45° on to the face, with three pillows arranged to lift the shoulders 30 cm from the horizontal
	S^3	Anterior segments	Lying supine with the knees flexed
Lingula	S^4	Superior segment	Both segments: lying supine with the body a quarter turned to the right maintained by a pillow under the left side from shoulder to hip. The chest is tilted downwards to an angle of 15°
	S^5	Inferior segment	
Middle lobe	S^4	Lateral segment	Both segments: lying supine with the body a quarter turned to the left maintained by a pillow under the right side from shoulder to hip. The chest is tilted downwards to an angle of 15°
	S^5	Medial segment	
Lower lobe	S^6	Apical segment	Lying prone with a pillow under the abdomen
	S^7	Right medial basal (cardiac) segment	Lying on the right side with the chest tilted downwards to an angle of 20°
	S^8	Right anterior basal segment	Lying supine with the knees flexed and the chest tilted downwards to an angle of 20°
	S^{7+8}	Left anteromedial basal segment	Lying supine with the knees flexed and the chest tilted downwards to an angle of 20° or lying on the left side with the chest tilted downwards to an angle of 20°
	S^9	Lateral basal segments	Lying on the opposite side with the chest tilted downwards to an angle of 20°
	S^{10}	Posterior basal segments	Lying prone with a pillow under the hips and the chest tilted downwards to an angle of 20°

TABLE 7-1

Gravity-Assisted Drainage Positions

Patient positions are shown in Figures 7-5 through 7-15.

the most severely affected, although the cause is unknown (Tomashefski et al 1986) and positions other than sitting may be indicated only occasionally. It appears that for a significant minority of patients with GOR, standard PD may contribute to clinically significant exacerbation of GOR (Button et al 2004), and for these patients, mPD or alternative airway clearance strategies may be advisable. Modified PD is now used more commonly than PD in the care of children and infants with CF and non-CF bronchiectasis. When PD or mPD clearly enhance airway clearance in individual patients and there are no contraindications or side effects, they should be encouraged. If severely affected patients find PD or mPD useful during an exacerbation, the concurrent use of intermittent positive pressure breathing (IPPB) or NIV may help to overcome the increased breathlessness with the additional benefits of PEP therapy for secretion management (Bott et al 2009).

Manual Techniques

There are a number of techniques that physiotherapists may use for the management of cardiorespiratory patients to assist with secretion clearance. Manual techniques are amongst the longest standing airway clearance strategies, and involve the external application of forces to the chest wall to facilitate secretion clearance.

These techniques include percussion (chest clapping), chest wall vibrations or shaking (rhythmical chest wall compressions during expiration with fast or slow oscillations, respectively), chest compressions (usually applied as overpressure at the end of expiration to assist cough, support expiratory manoeuvres, or reduce air trapping) and rib springing. These techniques are typically used to both loosen secretions as well as to reduce fatigue or increase effectiveness of particular techniques. Percussion and vibration are the more popular interventions, whereas there is less evidence on shaking, chest compression and rib springing.

There has been considerable research investigating the effects of these treatment interventions in combination with other treatment modalities in a wide variety of clinical scenarios involving medical, surgical and intubated and ventilated patients. The emphasis of the research has been evaluating the effects of the interventions on secretion clearance. The quality of most of this research is low, for a wide variety of reasons including methodology and measurement issues or inadequate sample size to name a few. Despite this, both of these interventions still continue to be used by physiotherapists, in specific patient groups, for example, those in intensive care (Stiller et al 1990, Chaboyer et al 2004, Jones et al 1992, King & Morrell, 1992) and in patients with excessive secretions (McCarren et al 2003, Samuels et al 1995).

There is no strong current evidence to either support or reject the use of manual techniques (percussion and vibration) over other airway clearance interventions (Elkins et al 2006a, Lee et al 2013, Main et al 2005, McKoy et al 2012, Robinson et al 2010).

There is some evidence for the physiological effects of percussion and vibration on secretion clearance. During both of these manual interventions, an intermittent positive pressure is applied to the chest wall. This positive pressure is transmitted through the lungs to the airways, resulting in a physiological increase and oscillation of the expiratory flow (McCarren & Alison 2006b). Both the increase and oscillation of the expiratory flow are proposed to assist with secretion clearance. While both of these interventions do not achieve the optimal increase and oscillation of airflow when compared to other interventions, perhaps the combined effects are the most appropriate intervention in some patients.

In addition, there are some clinical situations where patients are unable to use more independent treatment strategies. Manual treatments are passive and require an assistant; therefore these treatments may be more appropriate in patients who are unable to manage their own treatment, i.e. in patients who are unconscious, heavily sedated, too young or fatigued.

Finally, the patient's preference and adherence is another key factor in treatment selection. The research into preference is inconclusive. Patient preference for treatment interventions vary, with no one prominent intervention (McKoy et al 2012, Morrison & Agnew 2009, Robinson et al 2010). Therefore patients may prefer to use percussion and vibration in assisting with secretion clearance.

In self-ventilating patients, evidence has routinely shown that a combination of PD or mPD and percussion or vibrations have been as useful as other ACTs in terms of airway clearance strategies (Main et al 2005, Mazzocco et al 1985, McIlwaine et al 2010, Sontag et al 2010). Both fast and slow percussion have been shown to improve sputum production significantly when used in addition to PD and forced expiration techniques (FETs) (Gallon 1991). However, manual techniques have also commonly been the least preferred ACT in research studies, largely because they involve dependence on a carer to deliver the treatment, which can be uncomfortable, inconvenient or embarrassing and socially limiting (McIlwaine et al 2010, Sontag et al 2010).

Historically PD and percussion were the mainstay of ACTs in CF care, but in the last four decades a number of newer and more independent airway clearance strategies have been developed which are more active and allow patients to be more self-reliant in their daily routine (Rand et al 2013). There may still be a significant role for PD and percussion in sputum producing babies and infants with CF or non-CF bronchiectasis, or in patients with severe disease who may find it helpful in conjunction with oxygen or positive pressure supplementation.

Chest Percussion/Clapping

Percussion is the relaxed rhythmical tapping of the chest wall, by flexion and extension of the wrist on the patient's chest wall, usually using cupped hands (Fig. 7-16). For adults, two hands are generally used, but one hand may also be appropriate for self-percussion. Percussion with one hand is used for small children and babies (see Fig. 7-16). In neonates and preterm infants 'tenting', using the first two or three fingers of one hand with slight elevation of the middle finger, or

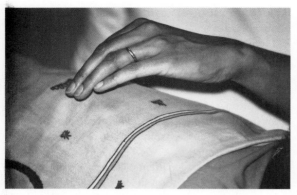

FIGURE 7-16 ■ Single-handed percussion.

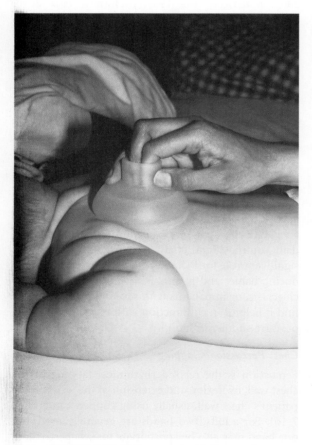

FIGURE 7-17 ■ Percussion with face mask.

a soft round paediatric face mask may be more appropriate (Fig. 7-17) (Tudehope & Bagley 1980).

Percussion is applied over the specific segment being treated during tidal breathing or thoracic expansion exercises (TEEs). The range of the frequency of percussion is 4.6–8.5 Hz (claps per second) in healthy individuals and patients with CF (Blazey et al 1998, McCarren & Alison 2006b). The use of percussion has been shown to increase the efficiency of PD (Gallon 1991), thereby decreasing treatment time.

Alternatively, it may be applied using a mechanical percussor, with both methods effective (Bauer et al 1994). The application of force to the chest wall creates changes in the intrapleural pressure which are transmitted through the thoracic cage and assist in dislodging secretions from the airway wall. Other techniques such as gravity-assisted drainage and ACBT can be applied concurrently to facilitate further clearance.

Percussion may result in the increased clearance of secretions. During percussion the resultant physiological effects are an oscillation of airflow and increase in expiratory flow (McCarren & Alison, 2006b). The oscillation of airflow reflects the frequency of the application of percussion and may facilitate secretion clearance by stimulating cilial beat and/or changing sputum viscosity. The PEF of 0.83 L/s during percussion is significantly greater than during tidal breathing in patients with CF. However, neither this PEF nor the PEF:PIF 0.99 results in annular flow of secretions to the oropharynx and will not be adequate to assist with secretion clearance. The oscillation of airflow of percussion is within the physiological range to assist with secretion clearance (4.6–8.5 Hz), and to optimize the effectiveness of percussion, physiotherapists should aim to percuss using frequencies towards the upper end of this range.

Overall there have been very few reports on adverse effects due to the application of percussion. A number of systematic reviews reported no adverse events in patients with bronchiectasis, stable chronic obstructive airway disease and CF (Lee et al 2013, McKoy et al 2012, Osadnik et al 2012, Warnock et al 2013). The few reports of adverse effects during percussion occured during acute exacerbations. Average desaturation of 7.5% (MacDonnell et al 1986) and small increases in airway obstruction (decrease in forced expiratory volume in 1 second (FEV_1)) occurred in patients with

BOX 7-1
KEY POINTS FOR PERFORMING PERCUSSION/CHEST CLAPPING

- Common patient positions: gravity-assisted drainage (traditional or modified), side lying
- A sheet or layer of clothing over the chest wall area minimizes sensory stimulation of the skin.
- Patient is instructed to breathe at tidal volumes during the procedure.
- Rhythmical flexion and extension of the wrist should be applied to the patient's chest wall.
- For spontaneously breathing patients, this technique should be followed by expiratory manoeuvres, such as forced expiration technique (FET) or coughing to clear secretions.
- The duration of the technique will depend on the clinical presentation of the patient and sputum volume.

CF and COPD (Campbell et al 1975, Wollmer et al 1985). Premedication with bronchodilator therapy may reduce this effect, but if adverse responses persist, percussion should be avoided. There are no known reports of adverse events during percussion in intubated and ventilated patients. Physiotherapists should continually monitor oxygen saturation, consider the use of bronchodilators prior to treatment and keep the duration of percussion to less than 5 minutes in patients with an acute exacerbation (Hill et al 2010, Tang et al 2010).

The force of percussion should be based on patient feedback and adapted to suit their needs. It should not be uncomfortable or painful, nor too vigorous. Key points for applying the technique are outlined in Box 7-1.

Vibrations/Chest Shaking and Compression

Chest wall vibrations involve the application of fine oscillatory movements combined with chest wall compression, initiated at the end of inspiration and applied throughout expiration (Fig. 7-19). The vibrations, applied by a physiotherapist's hands and fingers, should be of sufficient intensity to compress the rib cage and increase expiratory flow, while being comfortable for the patient. Both the compressive and oscillatory forces applied during vibration are transmitted through the lung to the airways (McCarren et al 2006b). These are clinically useful techniques, but

at present, chest wall vibrations remain relatively poorly defined and vary considerably between practitioners and institutions. The terms 'chest vibrations', 'compressions', 'shaking' and 'expiratory flow increase techniques' have been used variously in the literature (Almeida et al 2005, Marti et al 2013, Sutton et al 1985, Wong et al 2003).

The compressions and oscillations applied during chest wall vibrations are believed to aid secretion clearance via a number of physiological mechanisms, including increasing annular flow via the two-phase gas–liquid flow mechanism, to move secretions towards the large airways for removal by suction or cough (Kim et al 1987, King 1998, McCarren & Alison 2006, Ntoumenopoulos 2005, van der Schans et al 1999, Wanner 1984). Chest wall vibrations have been shown to generate a PEF:PIF >1.1, which is likely to optimize conditions for secretion clearance (Gregson et al 2012, McCarren & Alison 2006). If able to, patients are instructed to take deep breaths (TEEs) to use the augmented effect of airflow on secretion movement. The rationale is that the resultant increase in PEF will assist in moving secretions to the oropharynx (Kim et al 1987a, McCarren & Alison 2006a).

A significant contributor to increasing expiratory flow during vibration is lung recoil following maximal inspiration. When well timed, both the compressive and oscillatory forces applied to the chest wall during vibration augment the effects of lung recoil to increase the expiratory flow of vibration (Gregson et al 2012, McCarren & Alison 2006b). Combining both the compression and oscillation during vibration optimizes the increase in expiratory flow. To optimize the effectiveness of vibration on secretion clearance, the patient should inspire slowly or be manually hyperinflated to a maximal safe volume before a rapid extrathoracic compressive force is applied at the beginning of expiration, followed by fine oscillatory compressions until expiration is complete (Gregson et al 2012).

In children, there is a strong linear relationship between the maximum force applied during chest wall vibrations and the age of the child, most likely reflecting modification of techniques to accommodate changes in chest wall compliance (Gregson et al 2007). However, the maximum force applied during physiotherapy can vary substantially between physiotherapists. Similarly, there is marked variability in the

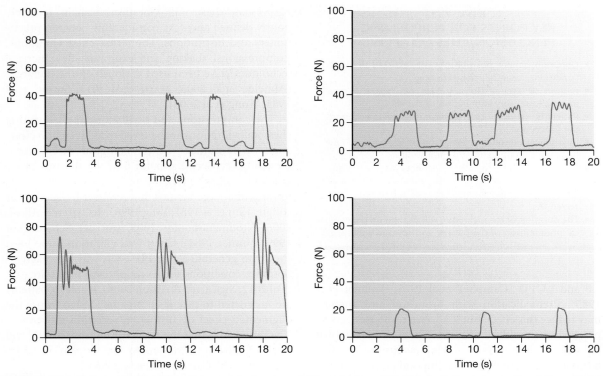

FIGURE 7-18 ■ Force–time profiles of chest wall vibrations delivered by four different physiotherapists to four infants (5–14 months). The patterns are repeatable within each treatment but vary considerably between therapists with respect to magnitude and duration of vibration, and amplitude, number and frequency of oscillations.

pattern of force–time profiles between physiotherapists with respect to the duration of vibration and amplitude, number and frequency of oscillations. Figure 7-18 illustrates the style of force profiles delivered to four infants, all aged between 5 and 14 months by four different physiotherapists. By contrast, there is remarkable consistency within and between each physiotherapist's treatment sessions (Gregson et al 2007, Shannon et al 2009). The clinical consequences for such variation in treatment profiles remain unclear.

In children, evidence suggests that chest wall vibrations applied to mechanically ventilated patients increase both peak expiratory flow and the peak expiratory-to-inspiratory flow ratio bias (PEF:PIF ratio) over and above the changes that would occur when using manual lung inflations alone (Gregson et al 2012, Shannon et al 2015). Chest wall vibrations also appear to be used much more frequently in intubated and ventilated children than percussion, probably because the glottis is held open by the endotracheal tube, facilitating rapid expiratory flow during vibrations that improve mucus clearance.

In children who are not intubated, vibrations can be applied effectively when reflex glottic closure does not occur and when the respiratory rate is normal or near normal (30–40 breaths/min). If infants are breathing very rapidly, the expiratory phase is so short that vibrations are more difficult to perform.

Published mean oscillation rate (±SD mean) during chest wall vibrations have varied in the literature from 5.5 (±0.8) Hz in healthy individuals to 8.4 (±0.4) Hz in patients with CF (McCarren & Alison 2006b, McCarren et al 2006a, 2006b), and 3.4–11 Hz in ventilated children (Gregson et al 2007). The upper end of this oscillation frequency is within the physiological range that may assist with secretion clearance by changing mucus rheology.

There are no known reports of any adverse events during the application of vibration. However, routine treatments should be avoided as they may have

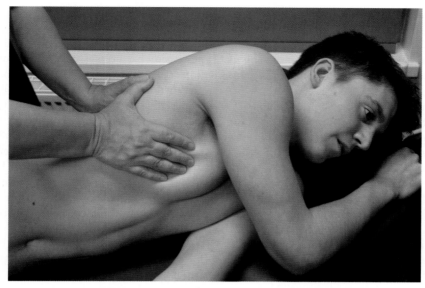

FIGURE 7-19 ■ Performing chest wall vibrations.

potentially detrimental effects (Horiuchi et al 1997, Krause & Hoehn 2000, Stiller 2000). In children with dietary deficiencies, liver disease, bone mineral deficiency (e.g. rickets) or coagulopathies, manual techniques should be applied with caution. Manual techniques may not be appropriate in extremely premature infants, and specific issues related to this group of patients are covered in Chapter 10. Ideally treatment should occur before feeds or adequate time allowed following a feed to avoid problems associated with vomiting and aspiration.

Vibrations are often applied with similar concurrent techniques to percussion to gain more effect. Key points for applying vibrations are outlined in Box 7-2.

Shaking, Chest Compression and Rib Springing

Physiotherapists may also use these three other manual interventions. Shaking is similar to vibration except that the oscillation component has a larger amplitude and slower frequency. Shaking is also used to clear secretions.

Controlled compression of the chest wall may be applied by the physiotherapist as gentle pressure throughout exhalation to enhance expiratory flow. It may be applied in patients with respiratory disease and sputum retention or postoperative patients or following thoracic trauma in those whom chest vibrations

---

BOX 7-2
KEY POINTS FOR PERFORMING VIBRATIONS

- Common patient positions: gravity-assisted drainage (traditional or modified), side lying
- A layer of towel or clothing over the chest wall area may be necessary to minimize sensory stimulation of the skin.
- Physiotherapist's hands are placed on the patient's chest wall.
- Patient is instructed to inspire deeply and slowly if spontaneously breathing.
- During expiration, a vibratory action is applied in the direction of the normal movement of the ribs and is transmitted through the chest using body weight.
- The vibration may use large amplitude movement (chest shaking) or fine amplitude movement (chest vibrations).
- For spontaneously breathing patients, this technique is often applied following TEEs as part of the ACBT, with vibrations followed by expiratory manoeuvres, such as forced expiration technique (FET) or coughing to clear secretions

---

and shaking is not appropriate, but controlled compression during huffing would facilitate secretion clearance. It has been applied in mechanically ventilated patients (Guimarães et al 2013). Chest compression (overpressure at the end of expiration) can also applied to the chest wall, over either the sternum or lower margins of the lateral chest wall. Chest compression is proposed to facilitate the effectiveness of huffing of coughing to aid with secretion clearance. This is commonly used in postoperative patients or patients who are fatigued.

Alternatively, rib springing may be applied in paralyzed patients, where an overpressure is applied at the end of expiration to encourage inspiration. Rib springing has been described as compression of the chest wall, continued throughout the latter phase of expiration, and followed by overpressure applied at the end of the breath out. The subsequent quick release of the hands is used to increase inspiratory volume. The proposed theoretical rationale for this intervention is that the stretch of the inspiratory intercostal muscles results in contraction, which aids inspiration. This technique is most appropriate in patients who are unconscious or heavily sedated. There is limited anecdotal evidence that these techniques are used but there is no evidence on the efficacy of these interventions.

In conclusion, manual techniques are useful in patients who prefer these techniques or are unable to participate in the independent treatment of their impairments. For most patients the evidence suggests that adherence is better if self-administered techniques are used (Bott et al 2009). There is physiological justification for the use of vibration and percussion to assist with secretion clearance. Until there is more high-quality research with definitive answers about the effectiveness of these interventions we are reliant upon patient preference and the physiological rationale to aid our decisions on treatment selection.

Clinical Application and Evidence for Manual Techniques. Chest percussion may be a beneficial addition to gravity-assisted drainage to increase sputum expectoration in patients with copious secretions (Gallon 1992) but may be less effective in patients with COPD with fewer secretions (Sutton et al 1985, Van der Schans et al 1986). In patients with clinically stable CF, it offers little additional benefit beyond TEEs (Webber et al 1985), but in patients with non-CF bronchiectasis, secretion clearance may be increased (Mazzocco et al 1985). When applied as a long-term treatment strategy for patients with an acute exacerbation of COPD (AECOPD), no gain in quality of life was achieved compared to ACBT alone (Cross et al 2012).

For patients with COPD who are acutely unwell, percussion has been associated with oxygen desaturation (Connors et al 1980) and increased airflow obstruction (Campbell et al 1975, Wollmer et al 1985). These side effects may be related to sputum volume, with no adverse events reported in CF (Pryor et al 1979) or non-CF bronchiectasis (Gallon 1992, Mazzocco et al 1985). To minimize side effects, it may be important to incorporate periods of BC with percussion in patients who are acutely unwell. Oxygen saturation levels should be monitored during the procedure for any patient who is considered at risk of developing hypoxaemia during the treatment.

The effects of vibrations appear to be selective, with little benefit over conventional chest physiotherapy in patients with COPD (Mohsenifar et al 1985) and in patients with non-CF bronchiectasis or chronic bronchitis (Sutton et al 1985).

A comparison of OPEP devices (Flutter and Acapella) and manual techniques showed that although the OPEP devices produced higher oscillation frequencies than chest wall vibration and percussion in 18 young adults with CF, chest wall vibration produced greater expiratory flow rates and a higher PEF:PIF ratio (McCarren & Alison 2006b). Theoretically, the higher PEF during vibration compared to the other physiotherapy interventions would promote secretion clearance, and the frequency of vibration oscillations was within the range demonstrated to increase mucus transport. This evidence supports the physiological rationale for the use of vibration to aid secretion clearance. In patients who are unable to huff or cough effectively, vibrations may be an alternative technique to clear secretions (McCarren & Alison, 2006a).

In infants and small children who are not yet old enough to cooperate with more active techniques, chest percussion or vibrations are often used. These techniques may be indicated in patients who are unable self-manage their airway clearance, which may include patients with neuromuscular weakness, intellectually or cognitively impaired patients or those who are acutely unwell and/or too fatigued to complete independent techniques which have higher energy requirements effectively. While there is little indication for chest percussion or vibrations in postoperative or

BOX 7-3
CONTRAINDICATIONS AND PRECAUTIONS FOR MANUAL TECHNIQUES

- Severe haemoptysis or risk of further haemoptysis during or after the technique
- Lung contusion
- Thoracic cage/sternum/rib fractures
- Diagnosis of osteoporosis/osteogenesis imperfecta/ osteomyelitis of thorax or other bone diseases (metastatic bone cancer) which are associated with brittle or extremely fragile bone as the technique may increase the risk of rib pathology
- Coagulopathy or thrombocytopaenia (e.g. platelet count <150 × 109/L)
- Acute pain (secondary to surgery or pleuritic pain) which may be exacerbated with manual techniques
- Conditions in which skin integrity is lost (secondary to surgery, burns, wounds, skin flaps or grafts)
- Worsening bronchospasm accompanied by shortness of breath
- Suspected or known active pulmonary tuberculosis due to risk of further spread
- Subcutaneous emphysema
- Recently placed transvenous or subcutaneous pacemaker
- Severe hypoxaemia
- Pulmonary oedema
- Pre-term infants, particularly if combined with head-down tilt positioning (gravity-assisted drainage)

chest trauma patients, these techniques may be applied in combination with other techniques in patients in intensive care to enhance secretion movement. Manual techniques are not well tolerated by all patients, and the precautions and contraindications to be considered are outlined in Box 7-3.

Suction

Suction techniques may be required either via the nasopharyngeal, oropharyngeal or endotracheal routes, depending on whether there is an artificial airway in situ. Airway suction for intubated adults is described in Chapter 9 and for children, including the non-intubated infant and small child, see Chapter 10. Suction is required occasionally in the non-intubated adult who has retained secretions, usually via the nasopharynx.

Adverse effects have been reported and include hypoxaemia, mechanical trauma, apnoea, bronchospasm, pneumothorax, atelectasis, cardiac arrhythmias and even death on rare occasions (Clark et al 1990, 1999; Czarnik et al 1991; Kerem et al 1990; Shah et al 1992; Singer et al 1994; Stone & Turner 1989; Wood 1998). Practice varies widely among centres and where available, local suction guidelines should be utilised to ensure safe practice (Sole et al 2003).

Nasotracheal suction is a means of stimulating a cough, but is an unpleasant procedure for the patient and should be performed only when absolutely necessary. The indication for suction is the inability to cough effectively and expectorate when airway secretions are retained. It may be necessary, for example, when an acute exacerbation of chronic bronchitis has led to carbon dioxide narcosis and respiratory failure, or in neurological disorders, postoperative complications or laryngeal dysfunction. Before airway suction is undertaken it is important that the procedure is explained carefully to the patient.

It is also important to be aware of the possibility of causing laryngeal spasm (Sykes et al 1976) or vagal nerve stimulation, which may lead to cardiac arrhythmias (Jacob in Oh, 1990). Nasopharyngeal suction is contraindicated when there is stridor or severe bronchospasm, and in patients with head injuries when there is a leak of cerebrospinal fluid into the nasal passages. Retention of secretions may be a problem in patients with respiratory muscle paralysis, but there is usually no benefit in using airway suction in an attempt to stimulate an effective cough. It is the lack of volume of air that prevents clearance of secretions in these patients and techniques such as mechanical insufflation/exsufflation, assisted cough, IPPB, glossopharyngeal breathing (GPB) and gravity-assisted positioning should be considered.

Airway suction causes damage to the tracheal epithelium and this can be minimized by the appropriate choice of catheter and careful technique (Brazier 1999). A flexible catheter of suitable size, usually 12 FG in adults, should be lubricated with a water-soluble jelly and gently passed through the nasal passage so that it curves down into the pharynx. Occasionally a cough may be stimulated when the catheter reaches the pharynx and suction can then be applied, the secretions aspirated and the catheter withdrawn. More often it is necessary to pass the catheter between the vocal cords and into the trachea to stimulate coughing. The catheter is less likely to enter the oesophagus if the neck is extended, and if the patient is able to cooperate it is often helpful if they can put their tongue out. The catheter should be inserted during the inspiratory phase and if it passes into the trachea, will stimulate vigorous coughing. When suction is applied, the vacuum pressure should be kept as low as possible, usually within 60–150 mmHg (8.0–20 kPa), although this will vary depending on the viscosity of the mucus. A built-in fingertip control or Y-connector is recommended to allow a more gradual build-up of suction pressure than is possible by the release of a kinked catheter tube.

Oxygen should always be available during the suction procedure and the patient observed for signs of hypoxia. If it has been difficult to insert the catheter and the patient looks cyanosed, instead of withdrawing the catheter from the trachea, suction should be stopped and oxygen administered until the patient's colour has improved. Suction can then be restarted. Suction can be performed in adults who are being nursed in the sitting position, but comatose patients should be suctioned in side lying to avoid the possibility of aspiration if vomiting occurs.

The nasopharyngeal suctioning clinical practice guidelines of the American Association for Respiratory Care (AARC) (updated 2004) provide useful evidence-based points on the technique (Brooks et al 2001, Guideline 1992).

Oropharyngeal suction through an airway is an alternative method if suction is necessary. An oropharyngeal airway is a plastic tube shaped to fit the curved palate. It is inserted with its tip directed towards the roof of the mouth and is then rotated so that the tip lies over the back of the tongue. Portable suction units are available for domiciliary use and for patients in transit. They may be powered manually, by mains electricity or by battery.

Provided suction is carried out carefully and oxygen is always available, it is a valuable technique and may avoid the need for more invasive procedures such as bronchoscopy, endotracheal intubation or mini-tracheotomy. However, it should not be undertaken until every attempt to achieve effective coughing has failed.

INDEPENDENTLY PERFORMED AIRWAY CLEARANCE TECHNIQUES

Breathing Techniques

Active Cycle of Breathing Techniques

ACBT is an airway clearance strategy renamed to clarify the directed breathing and FETs first described in the literature in 1979 (Pryor et al 1979, Pryor & Webber 1979). The purpose of this technique is to produce dynamic compression and collapse of the airways downstream of the EPP, creating a 'pinch point' and increased turbulent airflow. It consists of three distinct breathing cycles performed in sequence: BC, TEEs and FETs. The cycle can be repeated and the length of each component can be adapted to individual need (Fig. 7-20). It can be used across many ages and across all stages of disease. Each component of this technique plays a key role in the movement of secretions.

Breathing Control. BC is tidal volume breathing at a patient's own respiratory rate and volume. The person is encouraged to breath with the lower chest, using a diaphragmatic breathing pattern, with relaxation of the upper chest and shoulders. It may be facilitated by placing either the patient's or the physiotherapist's hand over the diaphragm to encourage lower breathing and upper chest relaxation. It allows recovery from fatigue, oxygen desaturation or signs of bronchospasm, and relieves breathlessness which may be generated during more active components of the cycle (Pryor et al 1990). The duration will depend upon the patient's rate of recovery.

Thoracic Expansion Exercises. TEEs are deep breathing exercises (DBEs) with an emphasis on slow, controlled inspiration through the nose. Inspiration is active, with larger than normal volume breaths which are often combined with a 3-second end inspiratory breath hold, with the glottis open, prior to passive expiration. The active and deeper volume inspiration is believed to facilitate collateral channel ventilation, with air flowing through the interbronchial pathways of Martin, the bronchoalveolar communications of Lambert and the interalveolar pores of Kohn (Menkes & Traystman 1977) to areas peripheral to retained secretions (see Fig. 1-11).

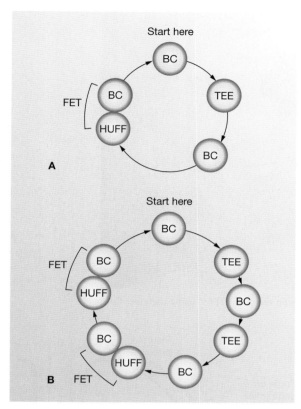

FIGURE 7-20 ■ Options for applying the active cycle of breathing techniques (ACBT) according to patient requirements, illustrating the technique's flexibility. *BC,* breathing control; *FET,* forced expiration technique; *TEE,* thoracic expansion exercise. **(A)** For patients with secretions but little airway hyperreactivity, one set of TEEs may be immediately followed by FET. **(B)** For a patient with bronchospasm and mucus plugging in whom secretions loosen slowly, multiple sets of TEE may be necessary, interspersed with a period of BC prior to FET.

This increase in airflow is enhanced by the breath hold to compensate for asynchronous ventilation, which may be present in patients with respiratory conditions or in collapsed airways due to secretions following surgery. During inspiration, unobstructed, healthy lung units will fill more rapidly while obstructed, diseased units fill more slowly. Slower units partially receive their inspired volume via collateral channels from more rapidly ventilating units, through *Pendelluft flow* (Mead et al 1970). The effectiveness of TEE is also explained by alveolar interdependence (Mead et al 1970). During inspiration, expanding alveoli exert forces on adjacent alveoli, encouraging recruitment of lung units (due to elasticity of the lung interstitium). The high lung volumes achieved during TEEs generate greater expanding forces between alveoli compared to tidal volumes and assist in re-expanding lung tissue (Fig. 7-21).

The number of TEEs is often limited to three or four, with a pause for a period of BC. This minimizes hyperventilation or fatigue in patients who become breathless during the technique, which may occur after too many consecutive breaths. Alternatively, a patient may take a tidal volume breath in between each TEE or may eliminate the breath hold. This technique can be facilitated by proprioceptive feedback, with the patients' or the physiotherapists' hands placed on the area of chest wall where movement is to be encouraged (Fig. 7-22; chest wall feedback). This has been associated with increased chest wall movement and ventilation (Tucker et al 1999).

Sometimes an additional increase in lung volume can be achieved by using a 'sniff' manoeuvre at the end of a deep inspiration. This manoeuvre may not be

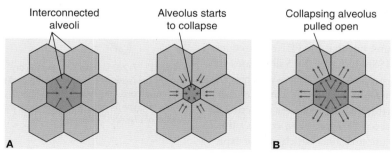

FIGURE 7-21 ■ Alveolar interdependence. **(A)** If an alveolus starts to collapse, the surrounding alveoli are stretched or pulled inwards towards it. **(B)** Then the walls of surrounding alveoli recoil, pulling the collapsed alveolus open by exerting these expanding forces on it.

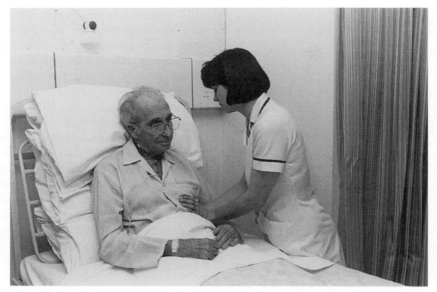

FIGURE 7-22 ■ Patient performing thoracic expansion exercises (TEEs) using therapist feedback.

appropriate in patients who are hyperinflated, but for surgical patients who need further motivation to increase their lung volume, it may be a useful technique.

Forced Expiration Technique. The FETs are the principle component of ACBT. They are a combination of one to two forced expirations (huffs) and BC. Huffing from low lung volumes will move peripherally situated secretions towards the mouth, where a high lung volume huff or cough can be used to clear them from the upper airways. A series of coughs can clear bronchial secretions, but clinically a single continuous huff down to the same lung volume is as effective and less exhausting. Hasani et al compared cough with the FET and concluded that both were equally effective in clearing lung secretions, but that the FET required less effort (Hasani et al 1994a). Figure 7-23 illustrates the pressure within and around the airways, which is the basis for forced expiration as an ACT (West & Luks 2015). In this picture, the pleural pressure is +20 cmH$_2$O and the lung elastic recoil pressure is +5 cmH$_2$O, both of which are the driving pressures which enable expiratory flow. Alveolar pressure is the sum of both pressures, which is 25 cmH$_2$O. Airway pressure falls along the airway from the alveolus down towards the mouth

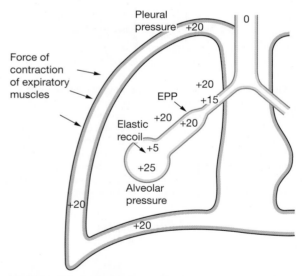

FIGURE 7-23 ■ Forced expiratory manoeuvre: huff or cough; pressure differences within and around the airway and the equal pressure point. *EPP,* Equal pressure point. *(Pryor 1991. In Pryor JA (ed) Respiratory care, p 84. Reproduced with permission of Elsevier, Edinburgh).*

(0 cmH$_2$O) during expiration. As the pressure falls, at some point the airway pressure equals the pleural pressure, which is known as the equal pressure point (EPP). Proximal to this point, towards the mouth, airway pressure falls below the pleural pressure, resulting in dynamic compression and a narrowed airway. This is an important part of the clearance mechanism of either a huff or cough. At lung volumes above FRC, the EPPs are located in lobar or segmental bronchi (Macklem 1974). As lung volume decreases during a forced expiratory manoeuvre, the EPPs move distally into the smaller more peripheral airways. This phenomenon can be utilized by the patient to assist airway clearance during the FET.

In people with chronic lung disease and reduced elastic recoil pressure, the driving pressure during a forced expiration is less; therefore the EPP will occur earlier in the phase of expiration and in smaller airways than normal. The shift in this EPP into the smaller airways, which are more compliant, may result in premature airway collapse if the force used during the technique is excessive. A huff is not an explosive manoeuvre. To be maximally effective, the length of the huff and the force of contraction of the expiratory muscles should encourage maximal expiratory airflow while minimizing airway collapse.

The position of the EPP within the airways is also dependent on lung volumes with smaller volumes moving the EPP towards the alveoli during expiration. To mobilize peripheral secretions, it is more effective to commence huffing from low to mid-lung volumes. To huff from a low to mid-lung volume, a small to medium-sized breath is inhaled, and with the mouth and glottis open, expiration should be long enough to loosen secretions from more peripherally situated airways, but not long enough to induce unnecessary paroxysmal cough.

The mean transpulmonary pressure during voluntary coughing is greater than during a forced expiration. This results in greater compression and narrowing of the airways, which limits airflow and reduces the efficiency of bronchial clearance. The greater airway compression may render coughing less effective in patients with conditions prone to premature airway collapse (Langlands 1967). In 1989, Freitag et al demonstrated an oscillatory movement, 'hidden' vibrations, of the airway walls in addition to the squeezing action produced by the forced expiratory manoeuvre (Freitag et al 1989). The viscosity of mucus is shear-dependent (Lopez-Vidriero & Reid 1978) and the shear forces generated during a huff should reduce mucus viscosity (Selsby & Jones 1990). This, together with the high flow of a forced expiratory manoeuvre, would also be expected to aid mucus clearance and the expectoration of sputum.

While it forms part of the ACBT, the forced expiratory manoeuvres are probably the most effective part of chest physiotherapy (van der Schans 1997). For this reason, this technique is often applied as part of other ACTs. For example, in the tetraplegic patient, clearance of secretions from the upper airways is difficult because maximum lung volume cannot be achieved and the EPPs will therefore never reach the largest airways (Morgan et al 1986). Secretions can be cleared from the smaller airways but accumulate in the larger upper airways. The use of positive airway pressure ventilation or GPB may assist clearance from the upper airways. Or, on occasion, gravity-assisted positions may be indicated; for example, if a patient has a lung abscess.

The second part of the FET is BC following one to two huffs. This recovery phase is important to minimize the increase in airflow obstruction or fatigue. The duration of the pause will depend on the patient, but a patient with fatigue, bronchospasm or unstable airways may require a longer rest period.

To encourage glottis opening a peak flow mouthpiece or similar piece of tubing may be used during the huff to provide audible feedback and improve technique efficacy (Fig. 7-24). This may be helpful when instructing children or patients with an impaired technique. Manual support during huffing may be provided, particularly for those using the technique following surgery or in patients exhibiting respiratory muscle weakness (Sivasothy et al 2001). To generate sufficient expiratory pressures during huffing, an upright position may need to be adopted to optimize expiratory flow and pressure (Badr et al 2002, Elkins et al 2005).

Clinical Application and Evidence for ACBT. ACBT is a flexible technique, with the repetition and order of each component adaptable to individual patient needs (see Fig. 7-20). It is often prescribed for patients with respiratory conditions with excess secretions. It may

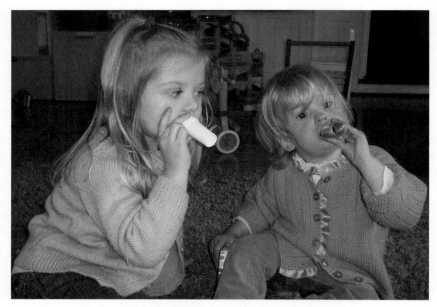

FIGURE 7-24 ▪ Learning to huff.

also be used in those with sputum retention following thoracic trauma or surgery. Such patients as well as those with minimal breathlessness will benefit from the breath hold, but its inclusion should be based on observation of a patient's respiratory rate and work of breathing.

For many patients using this technique, ACBT has been applied effectively in the upright seated position, but can also be combined with other devices, positioning, including gravity-assisted drainage (with head-down tilt or modified) (Cecins et al 1999), to further facilitate secretion clearance. Other concurrent techniques include manual techniques (chest percussion or vibrations) or inhalation therapy, if there is an indication that the inclusion of these techniques may further assist the clearance of secretions. The prescription and duration of a treatment session may be based on whether an effective huff is sounding dry and non-productive or if a patient is becoming fatigued and further performance will render the technique ineffective. For some patients, shorter sessions with fewer cycles may be necessary, but with a greater frequency.

ACBT has been found to be an effective technique for clearing secretions in patients with CF (Pryor & Webber 1979, Webber et al 1986, Wilson et al 1985). A Cochrane systematic review, comparing the clinical effectiveness of ACBT with other airway clearance therapies in CF, included 18 studies involving 375 participants. Sixteen of these studies involved an intervention period of 1 week or less (13 were single-treatment studies). There was insufficient evidence to suggest that ACBT was superior to any other ACT. ACBT was found to be comparable to other therapies in terms of patient preference, lung function, sputum weight, oxygen saturation and number of pulmonary exacerbations (McKoy et al 2012), and on lung function, exercise capacity and quality of life in the long-term (Pryor et al 2010a). In patients with non-CF bronchiectasis who are stable or acutely unwell, ACBT offers similar benefit in terms of sputum volume, with no greater risk of desaturation or increased obstruction (Patterson et al 2005, 2007, Syed et al 2009).

In patients with COPD, ACBT increases clearance in those with both copious secretions (Hasani et al 1994a) and minimal secretions (Hasani et al 1994b, van der Schans et al 1990), although it may be less effective in patients with a high level of hyperinflation (van der Schans et al 1990). Overall, patients often prefer this technique due to its independence, flexibility and lack of need for specialist equipment.

Autogenic Drainage and Assisted Autogenic Drainage

Autogenic drainage (AD) is an independently performed breathing technique developed in Belgium during the 1960's. It aims to achieve high expiratory flow from sequentially different lung volumes to assist with ventilation and airway clearance from peripheral to central airways in a variety of clinical conditions (Dab & Alexander 1979, Fink 2007). Unlike ACBT, however, AD is a three-phased regimen; Chevaillier originally described these as 'unstick', 'collect' and 'evacuate', using controlled breathing to maximize expiratory flow while minimizing airway closure, starting with low volume breathing at expiratory reserve volumes (Chevaillier 2009, Schöni 1989).

The rationale for the AD technique is the generation of shearing forces induced by airflow at different lung volumes to loosen and mobilize secretions (Fig. 7-25). The aim is to achieve the highest possible expiratory airflow while avoiding dynamic airway collapse, and with the absence of forced expiration or FET, may be a useful technique for patients who have a significant degree of pressure-dependent airway collapse (Schöni 1989). The speed of the expiratory flow reduces the adhesion of mucus, shears secretions from bronchial walls and transports them from the peripheral to proximal airways (Chevaillier 1984). When secretions are heard or felt, cough is suppressed but a series of higher volume breaths are taken, again without cough. The final phase involves large volume breaths near vital capacity (VC), before FET or huffs are used to clear secretions. The key points and suggested instructions for the stages of AD are outlined in Table 7-2.

The duration of each phase will depend on the efficacy of airflow to mobilize secretions, while the overall duration of AD will be influenced by the volume and viscosity of secretions. Drainage should be done thoroughly and it is an appropriate technique for patients with obstructive and restrictive pulmonary diseases with excess secretions. In those with greater loss of elastic recoil, more control during expiration may be required to avoid airway collapse (Agostini & Knowles 2007). While it is flexible and allows the patient to be independent, it is a complex treatment strategy which may be technically difficult for some patients. It requires patience and cooperation and takes time for the patient to learn and utilize feedback to adequately perform the technique.

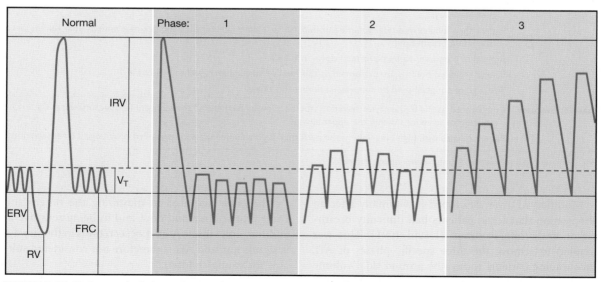

FIGURE 7-25 ■ Autogenic drainage (AD), Belgian method. Phases of AD shown on a spirogram of a healthy individual. Phase 1: unstick; phase 2: collect; phase 3: evacuate. *ERV*, Expiratory reserve volume; *FRC*, functional residual capacity; *IRV*, inspiratory reserve volume; *RV*, residual volume; *V_T*, tidal volume (IRV + V_T + ERV = vital capacity). *(Schöni 1989. Reproduced with permission of the Journal of the Royal Society of Medicine).*

	TABLE 7-2
	Phases and Patient Instructions for Autogenic Drainage
Phase	**Patient Instructions and Rationale**
Preparation	
Patient position	Options for patient position: upright sitting, side lying, supine
Other	If required, inhalers or nebulizers may be used prior to commencing the technique.
Phase 1: Unstick	Patient slowly inspires through the nose, followed by a 2 to 3 second breath hold. This warms and humidifies the inspired air and minimizes airflow turbulence
	Patient exhales with an open mouth and glottis, down to ERV. To encourage technique accuracy, an analogy for a patient would be to steam up a mirror or glasses during expiration.
	Patient then inhales with mid-tidal lung volumes (around 1.5 to 2 times greater than the size of a normal tidal volume) with a breath hold. Slow inspiration and breath holds minimize ventilation asynchronism to allow more even filling of lung units.
	Exhalation is performed down into ERV, with the upper airway open, a similar technique to sighing. The amount of force used during expiration should be controlled.
	While exhaling through the nose is preferable, expiring through the mouth may enhance auditory feedback to help the patient locate secretions.
	Tactile feedback of secretions vibrating in the chest may be felt on the chest wall, with high frequency of vibrations indicating movement of peripheral secretions.
	Several repeated breaths are performed at this level of lung volumes within this phase.
	The urge to cough should be suppressed during this phase.
	Key points: The time period spent in inspiration and expiration should be similar. The aim is to achieve the highest possible expiratory airflow while keeping resistance low and avoiding bronchospasm and dynamic collapse. This allows mucus to travel the furthest distance over a longer expiration, with movement of the equal pressure point into the peripheral airways to mobilize distal secretions
Phase 2: Collect	Commenced as the frequency of secretion vibration lowers, indicating that secretions are moving into more central airways.
	Patient then inhales mid-tidal volume (around 1.5 to 2 times greater than the size of a normal tidal volume) into IRV with a breath hold.
	Expiration continues to be performed down into ERV.
	Several repeated breaths are performed at this level of lung volumes within this phase.
	The urge to cough should be suppressed during this phase.
Phase 3: Evacuate	Commenced as the frequency of secretion vibration lowers further and the auditory feedback indicates the position of secretions within the upper airway.
	Patient inhales with high lung volumes to perform a high volume huff and controlled coughing to clear secretions.

ERV, Expiratory reserve volume; *IRV*, inspiratory reserve volume.

Modified AD was developed in Germany after an observation that some patients had difficulty breathing at lower lung volumes (David 1991). This was adapted to remove the three specific phases of AD, encouraging patients to breathe around tidal volume with a breath hold of 2–3 seconds at end inspiration. Expiration is a relaxed but faster process, down to both normal expiratory levels and expiratory reserve volume (Fig. 7-26) (Schöni 1989).

The effort required in mastering the ranges and control of volume and flow, and in being sensitive to auditory and vibratory cues of secretions in the airways is significant, and AD is therefore not considered suitable for young children.

AAD is an adaptation of AD for infants and young children not yet capable of carrying out the technique independently and requires the assistance of a parent or carer (Lannefors et al 2004). The aim of AAD is also

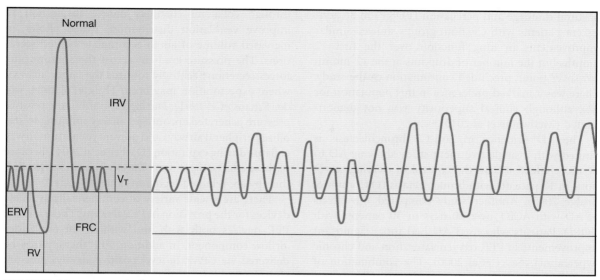

FIGURE 7-26 ■ Autogenic drainage (AD), German method. AD shown on a spirogram of a normal person. The method is not divided into separate phases. *ERV,* Expiratory reserve volume; *FRC,* functional residual capacity; *IRV,* inspiratory reserve volume; *RV,* residual volume; V_T, tidal volume (IRV + V_T + ERV = vital capacity). *(David 1991. In: Pryor JA (ed) Respiratory care, p 69. Reproduced with permission of Elsevier, Edinburgh.)*

to achieve an optimal expiratory flow progressively through all generations of bronchi without causing dynamic airway collapse. In infants, AAD is achieved by the therapist or trained carer placing their hands over the child's chest and, using the child's own breathing pattern, manually increasing the expiratory flow velocity by gentle external compression. In theory this prolongs expiration towards residual volume (Lannefors et al 2004). A small single study has suggested that GOR is not provoked during AAD treatment (Van Ginderdeuren et al 2003). There is currently no objective evidence to support any airway clearance benefits of AAD in infants and young children. For some infants, assisted AD may be combined with controlled bouncing, with the gentle up-and-down movement on a Swiss or gym ball encouraging patient relaxation while enhancing expiratory flow.

The choice of method for applying AD, with or without modification or assistance should be based on the option that elicits the best patient outcomes (Lapin 2002).

Clinical Application and Evidence for Autogenic Drainage. Short-term studies in children and adults

with CF have shown AD to be equivalent to Flutter in terms of lung function, but less effective in reducing sputum viscoelasticity (App et al 1998). It was also more effective than cough alone, but produced less sputum and was less likely to elicit bronchospasm than high pressure PEP (Pfleger et al 1992). It was also equivalent to PD in terms of sputum yield, but less likely to elicit desaturation (Giles et al 1995). A 2-day crossover study comparing AD with ACBT concluded that AD was as effective as ACBT but cleared sputum faster (Miller et al 1995).

Another short-term study found that sputum yield from AD could be significantly increased if preceded by saline inhalation delivered by nebulizer or IPV (Van Ginderdeuren et al 2008). In some patients with CF, greater sputum expectoration was achieved with AD compared to PEP therapy (Lindemann et al 1990).

A longer-term study over 12 months in the UK, comparing ACBT, Flutter, PEP, RC-Cornet and AD, suggested clinical equivalence between methods in terms of all the outcomes measured including quality of life and lung function (Pryor et al 2010a).

In addition, a Canadian 24-month crossover study published in the same year compared AD with postural drainage and percussion (PD&P) in 36 adolescent patients with CF. Both groups showed similar improvements in lung function over the first 12 months but the number of dropouts at the 12-month crossover point, precluded continuation of the study. There was a marked preference in this population for AD, although clinical superiority was not demonstrated (McIlwaine et al 2010).

The AD evidence in non-CF bronchiectasis is limited with a single treatment study showing AD to be more effective than the control in clearing secretions in 13 patients with bronchiectasis (O'Connor & Bridge 2005). Another study compared the effects of AD with ACBT over 20 days in 30 patients with COPD. Patients who used AD had more significant improvements in PEF, oxygen saturation and chronic hypercapnia (Savci et al 2000). The combination of controlled breathing to reduce airway collapse and high PEFs might therefore be an important ACT choice for patients with non-CF bronchiectasis for whom air trapping, desaturation or bronchial reactivity are known features.

Device-Dependent Techniques

Positive Expiratory Pressure and Infant PEP Therapy

The use of IPPB specifically for secretion management by physiotherapists only emerged in the mid 1960s, but it is still used in many clinical settings today. The PEP mask, developed in Denmark in the late 1970s, was one of the earliest portable PEP secretion clearance devices which remains widely used in Scandinavia, Europe and Canada.

The use of PEP for secretion management may be beneficial in a number of respects. PEP therapy involves the patient breathing out against a flow or threshold-limited resistance in order to produce positive airway pressure. PEP devices usually incorporate a one-way valve allowing unrestricted (or supported) inspiration and a resistance to expiration either through a resistor valve or via an orifice, which may be varied depending on individual requirements.

PEP therapy is applied using a face mask or mouthpiece via the one-way valve. The physiological rationale of PEP therapy is that in the presence of small airway obstruction caused by secretion retention, PEP therapy promotes airflow past the obstruction or through collateral channels during inspiration to improve ventilation distribution, which allows an increased volume of air to accumulate behind secretions. The pressure gradient across the sputum plug forces secretions centrally towards the larger airways, where expectoration may occur (Falk et al 1984, van der Schans et al 1991). During expiration, the positive pressure generated encourages airway splinting to stabilize peripheral airways and prevent premature airway collapse during expiration (Darbee et al 2004). Because of these effects, the most common indications for PEP therapy are retained secretions and atelectasis.

There are a wide variety of commercially available devices for the provision of PEP therapy. These include PEP devices both with and without an oscillatory airflow component. In addition, PEP therapy may be delivered via CPAP, bi-level positive airways pressure (BiPAP), and intermittent positive pressure ventilation (IPPV) devices. There are also devices that provide pressure throughout the breathing cycle with percussive airway oscillations, such as IPV.

A commonly applied PEP therapy system consists of a close-fitting mask and a one-way valve to which expiratory resistors are attached (Fig. 7-27). Alternatively, a mouthpiece with holes of varying diameters (PariPEP) to apply expiratory resistance or a Thera-PEP may be used (Fig. 7-28), with no difference in pressures generated between the different interfaces. A manometer is placed in parallel with the resistor to determine the correct pressure generated during initial therapy instruction.

During PEP therapy, the individual is required to perform a controlled expiration against the resistance, aimed at maintaining typical expiratory pressures at the mouth between 10–20 cmH$_2$O (aiming for 15 cmH$_2$O). Inserting a manometer into the circuit can provide both a useful monitor for the therapist and a very useful feedback mechanism for the patient. This form of therapy, involving slightly elevated tidal volume inspiration, and slightly active expiration against the resistance, is termed 'low-PEP'. The resistor that gives a stable pressure level of 10–20 cmH$_2$O during the middle of expiration with optimal expiratory flow which can be replicated is the one which should be selected (Elkins et al 2006a, Falk & Andersen, 1991).

For low-pressure PEP therapy, common instructions for the technique are outlined in Box 7-4.

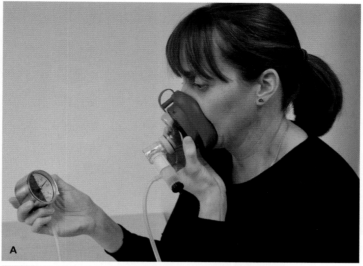

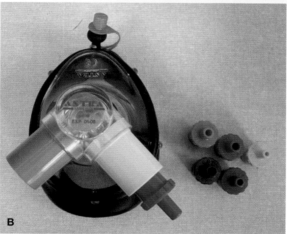

FIGURE 7-27 ■ **(A)** Using the positive expiratory pressure (PEP) mask. **(B)** A PEP device with mask attachment. *(Astra PEP, Astra Tech, Stonehouse, UK; **B** is reproduced with permission from Flude et al. (2012)).*

PEP therapy is an independent technique which can be combined with other airway clearance options, including positioning and inhalation therapy, and is beneficial for those patients with unstable or compliant airways. It is suitable for patients who are clinically stable or experiencing an acute exacerbation of their respiratory condition at varying levels of disease severity. PEP therapy can also be used in patients of all ages from infancy to older age.

Infant PEP is usually delivered via an appropriately sized face mask which is held in place over the infant's

nose and mouth by the parent/carer and is usually performed in combination with some physical activity; for example, sitting and bouncing on a gym ball (Fig. 7-29). This is because infants are unable to change the size of their breath on command, and the additional activity will result in natural modulation of lung volumes. The mechanism of action of infant PEP is therefore different to that of PEP therapy for older children and adults. Infant PEP is primarily aimed at changing the ventilation distribution in infant's lungs while also creating the positive expiratory airways

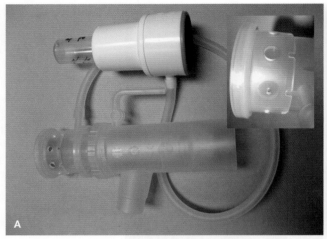

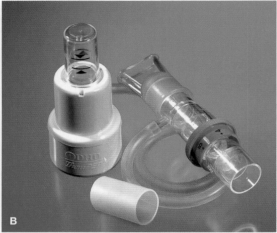

FIGURE 7-28 ■ Mouthpiece positive expiratory pressure (PEP). **(A)** PariPEP device. A pressure monitor is at right. **(B)** TheraPEP device. (*A, Pari Respiratory Equipment, Midlothian, Virginia, USA. Reproduced with permission from Marks (2007). B, Courtesy Smiths Medical, Rockland, MA. Reproduced with permission from Cameron & Monroe (2011)).*

BOX 7-4
KEY POINTS WHEN USING
POSITIVE EXPIRATORY PRESSURE
(PEP) THERAPY

■ Common patient position: seated comfortably, leaning forwards with elbows supported on a table
■ Mask positioned firmly over the nose and mouth, creating an effective seal
  ■ Alternatively, a mouthpiece with a nose clip during training purposes (for patients in whom loss of upper airway flow is high) may be used.
■ Patient inspires with slightly larger than tidal volume breath through the mask/mouthpiece.
■ Slightly active expiration is then performed through the PEP mask/mouthpiece for at least 3 seconds, maintaining a steady PEP of 10–20 cmH$_2$O
■ This is repeated consecutively for approximately 6–12 breaths, without losing the seal of the mask/mouthpiece. The number of breaths will depend on the rate of secretion mobilization and volume, fatigue and dyspnoea levels.
■ Cycles of tidal volume breaths are followed by one or more sets of forced expiration technique (FET) followed by coughing if required to further mobilize secretions.
■ The number of cycles may typically range from 6 to 12, before most secretions have been cleared. This, and the frequency of treatment will depend on symptoms and sputum volume, which will vary according to the patient's condition and clinical status.

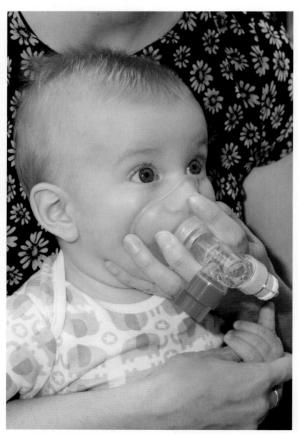

FIGURE 7-29 ■ Applying infant positive expiratory pressure (PEP).

pressures to assist in splinting open the airways on expiration. These mechanisms facilitate changes in ventilation distribution and potentially clearance of secretions. The generation of specific airways pressures is not the focus of treatment when using infant PEP, as infants have poorly developed collateral ventilation. A pressure manometer is therefore not required in the infant PEP circuit.

PEP therapy via a mask or mouthpiece can be used for anyone over the age of about 4 years, as long they are able to follow instructions (see Fig. 7-27). PEP therapy requires an awareness of breath size, as individuals are advised to inspire a volume of air that is slightly larger than a tidal volume breath at rest. An inspiratory hold just before breathing out is also recommended, to allow for the physiological mechanisms of pendelluft flow, interdependence and collateral ventilation to take place.

There are clinical precautions which may influence the choice of this technique outlined in Box 7-5.

Clinical Application and Evidence for PEP Therapy.
PEP therapy is recommended for patients with an AECOPD (NICE guidelines for COPD, 2010), CF (UK standards of care for CF) and non-CF bronchiectasis (Murray et al 2009, Pasteur et al 2010).

There are a number of single intervention or very short-term studies that have shown PEP to be as effective as other ACTs (Braggion et al 1995, Falk et al 1984, Lannefors et al 2004, West, K. et al 2010). Short-term improvements in both central and peripheral radio aerosol clearance were found with both PEP with FET and ACBT with gravity-assisted drainage when compared to control by Mortensen et al (1991).

In a number of long-term studies by a Canadian research group, involving patients with CF, PEP was reported to be superior to PD and percussion (McIlwaine et al 1997), OPEP via the Flutter device (McIlwaine et al 2001) and high-frequency chest wall oscillation (HFCWO) (McIlwaine et al 2013). The last study compared the use of HFCWO vest therapy to PEP therapy in 107 individuals with CF. PEP therapy required a shorter treatment time and the group using PEP had significantly fewer pulmonary exacerbations (1.14 versus 2.0) and a significantly longer time to first pulmonary exacerbation (220 versus 115 days).

These findings have not yet translated into unequivocal guidance in favour of PEP by the Cochrane systematic review of PEP therapy for CF (Elkins et al 2006a). In this review, there were no significant differences between PEP and other ACTs in single treatments or treatments undertaken for <3 months in terms of FEV_1. Longer-term studies had equivocal or conflicting results regarding effects of PEP on FEV_1. However, in studies with an ACT intervention period exceeding 1 month, any measures of participant preference were always in favour of PEP (Elkins et al 2006a). Both PEP and OPEP (Flutter) had equivalent effects on lung function, exercise capacity and quality of life over the course of 1 year (Pryor et al 2010a).

In patients with an acute exacerbation of CF, PEP is equally effective in sputum expectoration compared to conventional chest physiotherapy and was identified by patients to be equally tolerable (Braggion et al 1995).

The evidence for PEP in patients with bronchiectasis is limited. In a recent Cochrane review evaluating ACTs for non-CF bronchiectasis, there were no studies evaluating non-oscillatory PEP devices (Lee et al 2015). In postoperative patients, PEP therapy is not

---

BOX 7-5

CLINICAL PRECAUTIONS FOR POSITIVE EXPIRATORY PRESSURE (PEP) THERAPY

- Undrained pneumothorax or drained pneumothorax, due to risk of barotrauma
- Post lung lobectomy or lung transplantation, due to the risk of pneumothorax or compromise to the anastomosis
- Haemodynamic instability or severe cardiovascular disease due to the application of positive pressure to the thorax, although with low pressure PEP, the risk is minimal
- Undrained empyema or lung abscess, due to the risk of sudden release of large volume of loculated fluid
- Active haemoptysis due to the risk of inducing excessive bleeding with the technique
- Inability to tolerate due to increased work of breathing
- Sinusitis
- Facial fractures or surgery, particularly in the selection of a mask interface
- Middle ear infection, due to the risk of increased pressure within the Eustachian tubes during the technique

routinely applied to manage postoperative pulmonary complications (PPC), and there appears to be no additional benefit of combining PEP therapy with other physiotherapy approaches following thoracic surgery or abdominal surgery (Orman & Westerdahl 2010).

A randomized trial of patients who had undergone cardiac surgery reported significantly increased oxygenation in those individuals who had PEP therapy in the first 2 postoperative days compared with control patients who only performed deep breaths (Urell et al 2011).

In patients with chronic bronchitis, long-term use of PEP therapy was associated with reduced mucus production and fewer exacerbations (Christensen et al 1990). Those with AECOPD characterized by excess secretions had a reduced need for NIV with PEP therapy compared to control (Bellone et al 2002). A Cochrane review investigating the immediate, short-term and long-term effects of ACTs for COPD included 28 studies in the review. In general, all ACTs were associated with a reduced need for ventilator assistance and reduced hospital length of stay in patients with AECOPD. However, the magnitude of benefit from PEP-based ACTs appeared to be greater than for non-PEP ACTs (Osadnik et al 2012). This was not corroborated in a recent multicentre RCT in Australia by the same author. This trial compared usual care (including physical exercise) with or without additional PEP therapy on symptoms, quality of life and incidence of re-exacerbation in 92 patients with AECOPD and a productive cough. No significant differences were found between the control and intervention groups in any of the outcome measures, and the authors concluded that PEP therapy demonstrated negligible additional benefit on short-term (8 weeks) or long-term (6 months) outcomes following discharge when used during AECOPD (Osadnik et al 2014).

Finally, twice daily infant PEP was compared to twice daily mPD in 26 newborns with CF in an RCT over 12 months (Costantini et al 2001). Oxygen saturations were significantly higher in the PEP group compared to the PD group (98.1% vs 96.7%, p <0.05) and the incidence of GOR was about 20% in both groups, which was similar to that occurring naturally in infants with CF (Heine et al 1998). The authors concluded that infant PEP was safe and effective, and there was greater preference for it over mPD.

HiPEP. A variation of PEP therapy is high-pressure PEP (HiPEP) (Oberwaldner et al 1986). It applies the same tidal volume breath sequence as low-PEP, but patients also perform a forced expiratory manoeuvre through the PEP mask, with pressures of 40–120 cmH_2O typically generated. The target pressures for HiPEP are calculated during spirometry, such that the target resistance would generate a pressure that allows the patient to produce a forced vital capacity (FVC) that is greater than the FVC produced without PEP. HiPEP is not used as commonly in clinical practice as low-pressure PEP. The rationale behind the technique is that the application of PEP during a forced manoeuvre helps to prevent dynamic airway collapse in patients who have unstable airways during forced expiration. The splinting of the airways during a forced expiration manoeuvre allows the patient to expire a volume greater than their usual FVC. As the EPP develops later in expiration and more peripherally within the airways, it facilitates more peripheral secretion clearance.

Suggested instructions for using HiPEP are given in Box 7-6. Assessment for the technique involves the patient performing FVC manoeuvres through the

---

BOX 7-6

KEY POINTS WHEN USING HIGH-PRESSURE POSITIVE EXPIRATORY PRESSURE (HIPEP) THERAPY

- Common patient position: upright sitting, with the elbows leaning on the table and with the shoulders close to the neck to support the lung apices
- Mask positioned firmly over the nose and mouth, creating an effective seal
- Patient inspires with slightly larger than tidal volume breath through the mask.
- Slightly active expiration is then performed through the positive expiratory pressure (PEP) mask for at least 3 seconds, maintaining a steady PEP of 10–25 cmH_2O.
- This cycle of inspiration and expiration is repeated 8–10 times.
- Patient then inspires to total lung capacity followed by a forced expiratory manoeuvre against resistance down to low lung volumes (residual volume), with pressures between 25–120 cmH_2O generated.
- This is followed by coughing at low lung volumes to expectorate secretions.
- The sequence of breathing manoeuvres may be repeated until no further sputum is produced.

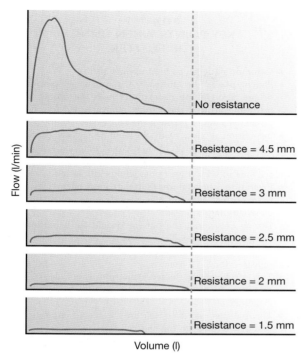

FIGURE 7-30 ■ High-pressure positive expiratory pressure (HiPEP). Maximum expiratory flow–volume curves obtained without resistance (top curve) and with each of the different PEP mask expiratory resistors. In this example, the resistor of choice for treatment is the 2-mm aperture, as it demonstrates a maximal forced vital capacity (FVC), good plateau formation and no curvilinearity at the end of flow.

mask which is attached to a spirometer (Oberwaldner et al 1986). The shape of the expiratory flow volume curves are used to select the appropriate resistor for the PEP mask. The most appropriate one is chosen on the basis of maximal homogeneity, with an expiration exceeding the patient's normal FVC and demonstrates constant expiratory flow (no evidence of airway obstruction) (Oberwaldner et al 1991) (Fig. 7-30). Care should be taken with this technique, as an incorrect resistance may lead to deterioration in lung function and ineffective airway clearance.

Clinical Application and Evidence for HiPEP. Short- and long-term improvements in lung function secondary to greater sputum clearance were found in patients using the technique during an acute exacerba-

tion of CF and when stable (Oberwaldner et al 1986, 1991). Compared to AD, a greater volume of sputum was cleared with HiPEP (Pfleger et al 1992). This independent technique may also be effective in patients with other respiratory conditions in whom stabilization of airways during forced expiration and coughing is required. It does require the generation of large respiratory forces, and this may be difficult for patients with higher dyspnoea or fatigue levels.

Inspiratory Resistance-Positive Expiratory Pressure (IR-PEP). This technique is achieved by placing a resistor into the inspiratory port of a PEP mask to provide resistance to both inspiration and expiration. The patient breathes in and out against a resistance, slowing the inspiratory rate and allowing inspiration to be more even. It may be used in patients with an underlying respiratory disease and concurrent asthma, in the event that asthma induces airway instability. The effects of IR-PEP have been explored in patients undergoing surgery (Olsen et al 1999, Westerdahl et al 2001). Although the technique was not as effective as CPAP therapy (Olsen et al 1999), it was equivalent to standard PEP therapy (Ingwersen et al 1993).

Oscillating PEP Therapy Including Bubble PEP

OPEP therapy devices offer the combination of PEP with high-frequency oscillations within the airways during the expiratory phase of the breathing cycle to facilitate secretions clearance. They are similar to the PEP device in that they involve breathing against an expiratory resistance, but the resistance is intermittent or interrupted by a ball valve, lever or collapsible tubing, such that oscillations of variable frequency (depending on device or use), are transmitted to the airways during the expiratory cycle. The PEP component encourages airflow behind secretions, oscillation induces vibrations within the airway wall to displace secretions into the airway lumen and the repeated accelerations of expiratory airflow favour movement of secretions from the peripheral to the central airways (App et al 1998). There are three main devices used to provide OPEP: the Flutter, the Acapella and the RC-Cornet. Bottle or bubble PEP is also a form of OPEP therapy. There are a number of other devices that provide theoretically similar effects; for example, the Aerobika, Lung Flute and Quake.

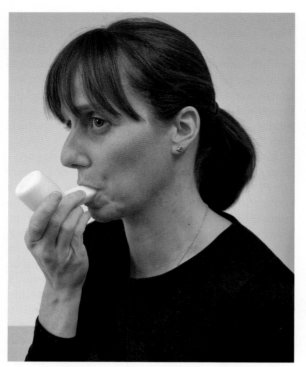

FIGURE 7-31 ■ Using the Flutter device.

The Flutter Device. The Flutter is a small, pipe-shaped, handheld device with a mouthpiece, a perforated cover which encases a stainless steel ball resting in a circular cone (Fig. 7-31). During expiration, the high-density ball rolls up and down the cone, creating interruptions in expiratory flow and generating PEP within the range of 18–35 cmH₂O (Altaus 2009). An oscillatory vibration of the air within the airways is also generated which shear secretions from the airways and alter sputum rheology, reducing the viscoelasticity of the secretions (App et al 1998). The frequency of oscillations mimic cilial beat frequency and are determined by the angle at which the device is held (Lindemann 1992). Suggested instructions for the Flutter are outlined in Box 7-7.

The device is commonly used in an upright seated position (see Fig. 7-31), but can applied in other positions, provided that effective oscillation can be achieved. The number of breaths per cycle and the number of cycles will depend on the volume of secretions and the levels of fatigue and dyspnoea of the patient.

Flutter therapy is not associated with adverse events in patients with COPD (Bellone et al 2002). The clinical precautions for the use of OPEP therapy are similar to those described for PEP therapy, with the addition of an increased risk of early, uncontrolled coughing in patients with hyperreactive airways.

Clinical Application and Evidence for the Flutter. In patients with CF, there is single-treatment evidence that Flutter is as effective as AD in terms of sputum volume and spirometry, but the frequencies and amplitudes of applied oscillations in the Flutter additionally decreased mucus viscoelasticity, theoretically improving MCC and cough clearance of secretions (App et al 1998).

A Cochrane systematic review updated in 2006 included four studies that all incorporated the Flutter OPEP device (Elkins et al 2006a). Two of these, conducted over 4 weeks or less, found no differences in outcomes. One of these was a 2-week study comparing PEP vs Flutter (van Winden et al 1998); the other was 4 weeks of PEP vs PD vs Flutter (Padman et al 1999). In the remaining two studies which lasted at least 12 months, comparisons between PEP and Flutter resulted in conflicting advice: one in favour of PEP in adolescents with CF (McIlwaine et al 2001) and the other in favour of Flutter in adults with CF (Newbold et al 2005).

McIlwaine found that lung function began to decline after 9 months of therapy with the Flutter compared to the PEP mask (McIlwaine et al 2001). The authors hypothesized that this decline may have been a result of the continuation of expiration into the expiratory reserve volume with the Flutter, which may result in airway closure; an effect which is not apparent with PEP therapy. The decline was also potentially attributable to patient age, with Flutter being a more technically difficult technique for younger children included in this study (McIlwaine et al 2001). Patient age, their technique and the duration of expiration may be important considerations when selecting this device.

Another long-term study published since this Cochrane review found no significant differences in outcomes between ACBT, AD, PEP and the two OPEP devices, Flutter and RC-Cornet (Pryor et al 2010b). In patients with exacerbation of CF, the Flutter was as effective as conventional chest physiotherapy (Gondor et al 1999, Homnick et al 1998) and may be more effective in improving sputum expectoration in some patients (Konstan et al 1994).

In non-CF bronchiectasis, the only OPEP devices that have appeared in the literature to date are the Flutter and Acapella devices, which appear to have similar performance characteristics (Volsko et al 2003). In patients with non-CF bronchiectasis, the Flutter improved secretion transport and reduced viscosity more than PEP therapy (Ramos et al 2009, Tambascio et al 2011). A very recent systematic review of OPEP devices for non-CF bronchiectasis included seven studies, all with relatively small sample sizes, representing 146 participants. Five of these studies were single treatment studies (Eaton et al 2007, Figueiredo et al 2012, Guimarães et al 2012, Naraparaju et al 2010, Patterson et al 2005), and the remaining two were conducted over 4 weeks (Thompson et al 2002) and 6 months, respectively (Murray et al 2009). The review suggested that in stable non-CF bronchiectasis, OPEP therapy was associated with improvements in sputum expectoration and quality of life measures compared to no treatment. Compared to other ACTs,

the effects in terms of sputum expectoration, lung function, gas exchange and symptoms were equivalent (Lee et al 2015). Flutter was as well tolerated and was preferred by patients (Eaton et al 2007).

In patients with copious sputum production secondary to COPD, the Flutter was equally effective in terms of lung function and oxygen saturation as gravity-assisted drainage and percussion (Ambrosino et al 1995) and more effective in terms of sputum expectoration (Bellone et al 2000). It was also found to reduce hyperinflation more effectively than PD and slow expiration (Guimarães et al 2012).

In patients following thoracic surgery, the addition of a Flutter into the postoperative routine offers no advantage in sputum clearance (Chatham et al 1993). For this reason, it is rarely applied for patients after surgery in the absence of any history of respiratory disease or prior use of the technique.

RC-Cornet. Based on similar physiological principles, the RC-Cornet consists of a mouthpiece, a curved tube, a valve hose and a sound damper (Fig. 7-32). Expiration through the tube creates an increasing pressure within the hose until it is sufficient to cause the hose end to open, allowing air to flow through the device, creating a PEP and oscillatory vibrations within the airways. The pressure and flow rate can be adjusted by rotating the mouthpiece in the tube. Suggestions for using the RC-Cornet are outlined in Box 7-8. It has the

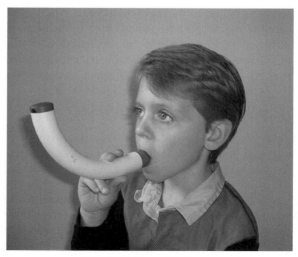

FIGURE 7-32 ■ RC-Cornet.

advantage of being position-independent with the flow, pressure and frequency of oscillations adjusted to suit the individual patient.

Evidence for the RC-Cornet. In patients with severe COPD, the addition of regular use of the RC-Cornet reduced the need for antibiotics and improved lung function over a two-year period when combined with drug therapy (Cegla et al 2002). In patients with COPD, it is as effective as the Flutter in terms of sputum expectoration and improving dyspnoea and is accepted by patients (Cegla et al 1997). When compared to the Acapella in patients with bronchiectasis, increased sputum volume was achieved with the RC-Cornet and was preferred by patients (Shabari et al 2011). In children with CF when used over the long term, it demonstrated equivalent improvements compared to PEP therapy (Main et al 2006).

Acapella. The Acapella (Fig. 7-33) is also a flow-operated oscillatory device which uses a counter-weighted plug and magnet to create airflow oscillations, which are produced by breathing and reforming the magnetic attraction by the plug as it intermittently occludes air passing through the device. The frequency/resistance dial allows adjustments to the expiratory pressure and the frequency of oscillations. It has the option of adjusting the flow pressure and frequency

of the oscillations for each individual patient and may be used with a mouthpiece or mask with a nebulizer in situ.

Inspiration can occur through the nose or mouth, with a short inspiratory hold and a more active exhalation through the device. This is followed by huffing and coughing as required to facilitate secretion removal, with the similar prescription described for the Flutter applicable to the Acapella. Compared to the Flutter, the Acapella produces more effective oscillations at lower airflows and a wider range of PEP. This may broaden its application to patients with low expiratory flows due to severe airflow obstruction or airway instability, age or size, which may increase its capacity to stabilize airways during expiration (Volsko et al 2003). The Acapella is flexible in the positions in which it can be used (options include sitting, side lying or gravity-assisted drainage positions).

Evidence for Clinical Application of the Acapella. In patients with non-CF bronchiectasis, a 3-month trial of regular Acapella was associated with improvement in sputum volume and patient-reported outcomes of cough and health-related quality of life (HRQoL) and exercise capacity compared to no treatment (Murray et al 2009). In this same patient group, Acapella offered comparable benefit to ACBT or other ACTs in those in a stable disease state (Patterson et al 2005) and when acutely unwell (Patterson et al 2007). Sputum expectoration was greater with the Acapella compared to a threshold inspiratory muscle training (IMT) device applied as an ACT, suggesting that the oscillatory effect of the Acapella and enhanced expiratory flow are of significant benefit (Naraparaju et al 2010).

When prescribed for children during an acute exacerbation of CF, patients were equally compliant with PEP mask and Acapella, with similar effects on lung function, sputum expectoration and satisfaction between the devices (West, K. et al 2010).

Bubble Pep or Bottle Pep. For older infants under the age of 4 who no longer tolerate infant PEP but who are unable to progress to other forms of ACT, 'bubble PEP' may be a useful OPEP bridging ACT. Bottle or bubble PEP is an alternative method to administer low pressure OPEP therapy. It is a threshold resistor type of PEP in that the expiratory pressure remains constant once the tubing diameter is ≥8 mm, independent of tube length (Mestriner et al 2009). It is a simple improvised device that can be constructed using easily accessible and low-cost equipment in the home or hospital setting. It consists of a length of smooth bore rubber tubing and a plastic bottle (1–2 L in size) that is approximately half filled with water.

The child is instructed to inhale through their nose or around the tube in their mouth using slightly active tidal volume breathing and expire through the tube into the column of water, with the number of breaths and cycles similar to that described for the Flutter. Blowing through the tubing creates bubbles in the bottle. The height of water in the bottle (approximately 10 cm above the bottom of the flexible tube) provides the threshold resistance to expiration and the bubbling effect produces an oscillatory effect in the airways (Fig. 7-34).

This is a fun way of engaging younger children in a secretion management technique which provides feedback and can be combined with more traditional ACTs such as ACBT. The addition of liquid detergent and a small quantity of food colouring adds to the novelty of the treatment for young children (see Fig. 7-2). There is no published evidence to support the use of bubble PEP in CF or non-CF bronchiectasis.

The equipment for bottle PEP should be thoroughly cleaned after each use. The water should be discarded immediately following treatment and the equipment cleaned. Fresh water should be used for each treatment session, with the bottle and tubing changed regularly.

While it is a good technique for children, it is also relevant to some adults with sputum retention secondary to respiratory disease due to the low cost compared to other modes of PEP therapy. Although it offers no additional benefit to standard preoperative and postoperative physiotherapy in surgical patients (Campbell et al 1986), it may be useful in selected patients in whom other techniques to facilitate secretion clearance are less effective. It is not appropriate for confused patients or those with other cognitive impairment due to the risk of inhaling water during inspiration (aspiration).

The Shaker Classic or Shaker Deluxe. The Shaker Classic and Shaker Deluxe devices are similar to the Flutter. They also contains a high-density stainless steel ball enclosed in a small cone, but have a detachable mouthpiece, making them easier to use in positions other than sitting.

The Quake. The Quake does not rely on an oscillating valve, but uses a manually turned cylinder that fits within another cylinder (Fig. 7-35). Airflow only occurs when the slots within the two cylinders correspond. Airflow is interrupted at regular intervals as the patient turns the crank. The rate at which the device is cranked will determine the frequency of flow interruption. For this reason, it may be a useful device in patients who are limited in generating high expiratory flow rates.

The Lung Flute. The Lung Flute (Fig. 7-36) uses low-frequency acoustic wave technology to facilitate

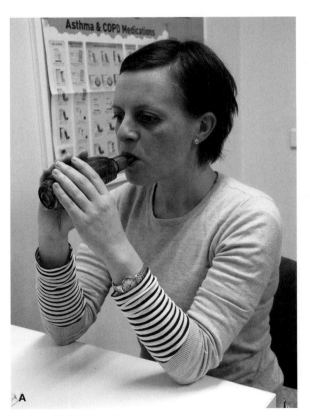

FIGURE 7-33 ■ **(A)** Using the Acapella.
Continued on following page

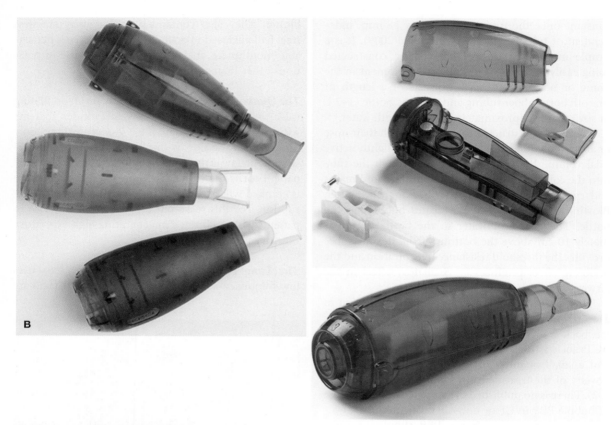

FIGURE 7-33, cont'd ▪ **(B)** Positive expiratory pressure (PEP) devices: TheraPEP and Acapella. *(Reproduced with permission from Frownfelter & Dean (2006)).*

secretion clearance. Expiration through the mouth-piece over a reed within the horn of the lung flute generates an acoustic wave that travels into the lower airways to facilitate secretion transport.

Machine-Dependent Techniques

Non-Invasive Ventilation for Airway Clearance

Non-Invasive Ventilation (NIV) as a technique to improve lung volumes is covered later in this chapter (Non-Invasive Ventilation p. 296). However, NIV is sometimes used to enhance airway clearance. PEP therapy may be combined with positive inspiratory pressure (PIP) delivered via NIV as CPAP, BiPAP and IPPV devices. These options are usually not used as primary ACTs but are reserved for patients who have very severe disease, hypoxia, inspiratory muscle

weakness or dyspnoea, and are therefore less able to perform airway clearance easily without assistance. They can be very useful adjuncts to other ACTs, especially when people have difficulty expectorating (Fauroux et al 1999, Flight et al 2012, Holland et al 2003, Moran et al 2009, Young et al 2008).

There is some evidence that NIV might slow or reverse the decline in lung function in people with advanced CF, and that it is more effective in conjunction with oxygen than oxygen alone for advanced disease (Gozal 1997, Moran et al 2009). There is also some evidence of improvement in functional capacity, lung function, respiratory rate and oxygen saturation when children or young adults with CF and pulmonary impairment undertake treadmill walking with NIV (Lima et al 2014).

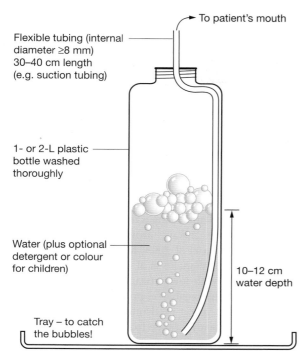

Flexible tubing (internal diameter ≥8 mm) 30–40 cm length (e.g. suction tubing)

To patient's mouth

1- or 2-L plastic bottle washed thoroughly

Water (plus optional detergent or colour for children)

10–12 cm water depth

Tray – to catch the bubbles!

FIGURE 7-34 ■ Setup and equipment required for bottle/bubble positive expiratory pressure (PEP).

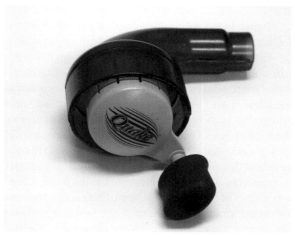

FIGURE 7-35 ■ Quake.

Devices that combine elements of both positive and negative pressure throughout the breathing cycle with or without airway oscillations, such as IPV, may also be useful in airway clearance, but are less commonly used (Paneroni et al 2011). There is no evidence that

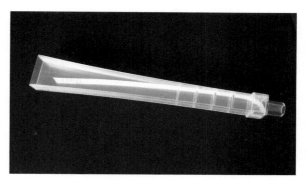

FIGURE 7-36 ■ Lung Flute.

cough assist devices are of any benefit in either CF or non-CF bronchiectasis. The pathophysiology of these diseases, which does not typically include respiratory muscle weakness, suggests this form of treatment is unlikely to be helpful except perhaps at end-stage disease, when fatigue and weakness may be important features (Sivasothy et al 2001).

Mechanical Insufflation/Exsufflation and Assisted Cough

A mechanical insufflator/exsufflator uses positive pressure to deliver a maximal lung inhalation followed by an abrupt switch to negative pressure to the upper airway. The rapid change from positive to negative pressure is aimed at simulating the airflow changes that occur during a cough, thereby assisting sputum clearance. In 1953, various portable devices were manufactured to deliver mechanical insufflation/exsufflation (e.g. OEM Cof-flater portable cough machine, St Louis, MO USA). The most commonly used mechanical insufflator/exsufflator devices today include; CoughAssist and CoughAssist E70 (Philips-Respironics, Pittsburgh Murrysville, USA); NIPPY Clearway (B & D Electromedical, Warwickshire, England) and Pegaso (Dimla Italia, Bologna, Italy).

These devices can produce expiratory airflows of greater than 160 L/min (marketing literature). Initial investigations showed mechanical insufflation/exsufflation to be effective at removing inhaled foreign bodies from anesthetized dogs (Bickerman 1954). Barach and Beck demonstrated clinical and radiographic improvement in 92 of 103 acutely ill patients with respiratory tract infections with the use of mechanical insufflation/exsufflation (Beck & Barach 1954). This included 72 patients with bronchopulmonary lung disease and 27 with skeletal or neuromuscular disease; however, it was more effective in patients with neuromuscular disease. The cardiovascular effects of mechanical insufflation/exsufflation were evaluated by Beck and Scarrone (1956); they found patients demonstrated an increase in mean heart rate by 17 beats per minute, and an increase in systolic blood pressure of 8 mmHg. They also found an increase in cardiac output (CO) by 2.1 L/min and echocardiograph changes reflective of rotation of the heart during normal coughing (Beck & Scarrone 1956).

Although pneumothorax is a potential risk from mechanical insufflation/exsufflation, there has only been one report of 2 patients with neuromuscular disease who developed pneumothoraxes (Suri et al 2008). The authors could not conclude that mechanical insufflation/exsufflation was the sole factor in causing pneumothorax, as there were other risk factors for pneumothorax in these patients, including the use of NIV and the presence of scoliosis. As the aim of mechanical insufflation/exsufflation is to clear a large amount of secretions from the upper airways, there is a risk of mobilizing large mucus plugs into the central airways where they may result in airways obstruction. Where appropriate, suitable emergency equipment (e.g. resuscitation bag and suction) should be available when using this device.

Mechanical insufflation/exsufflation has been shown to increase peak cough flow (PCF) in patients with neuromuscular disease (Bach 2003, Chatwin et al 2003, Mustfa et al 2003, Sancho et al 2004, Sivasothy et al 2001); an increase in PCF is thought to improve the efficacy of the cough and thus assist in secretion removal. Mustfa et al (2003) and Sancho et al (2004) found a significant improvement from baseline PCF with mechanical insufflation/exsufflation for both bulbar and non-bulbar motor neurone disease patients, although non-bulbar patients had the greatest change in PCF with mechanical insufflation/exsufflation.

Mechanical insufflation/exsufflation has also been effective at preventing intubation or mini-tracheostomy (Vianello et al 2005) and decreases treatment time (Chatwin & Simonds 2009) in patients with neuromuscular disease. When mechanical insufflation/exsufflation has been combined with non-invasive ventilation and applied as a protocolized treatment when arterial oxygen saturation decreases below 95% on room air, extubation of patients with severe ventilator impairment is possible (Bach et al 2010; Chatwin et al 2011, 2013; Goncalves et al 2012). This protocolized approach has increased survival in patients with neuromuscular disease when compared to a non-protocolized approach (Bach et al 1997, Gomez-Merino & Bach 2002). Mechanical insufflation/exsufflation has not been shown to be effective in patients with COPD (Sivasothy et al 2001, Winck et al 2004).

Patients who are novices to the device may not tolerate high pressure changes initially. Very high pressures also cause leakage around the mask. Some authors (Chatwin et al 2003, Miske et al 2004, Sivasothy et al 2001, Vianello et al 2005) have reported a good outcome with low pressures. One study (Miske et al 2004) in the paediatric population (age range 3 months to 28.6 years) used median pressures of $+30$ to -30 cmH$_2$O with a range from $+15$ to $+40$ cmH$_2$O (for insufflation and -20 to -50 cmH$_2$O for exsufflation). However, once the patient has acclimatized to the settings they are often using higher pressures (Bach 1993, 1994; Bach et al 1993, 2000, 2002; Chatwin et al 2011; Tzeng & Bach 2000).

Higher pressures are required as patients become weaker; they require more assistance from the machine. In order to generate these higher airflows, higher pressures are required. One study found in a paediatric population who were instructed to receive passive insufflation and exsufflation at pressures of $+40$ and -40 cmH$_2$O produced peak expiratory flows of greater than 100 L/min (Fauroux et al 2008). Fauroux et al also found that there was a pressure discrepancy between the pressure recorded on the CoughAssist compared to the pressure measured at the mask. There was a drop of 5–15 cmH$_2$O depending on the pressure set on the machine. The higher the targeted pressure the greater the discrepancy. Newer machines like the CoughAssist E70 and NIPPY Clearway measure more accurately and are able to achieve higher pressures than earlier devices.

Historically, mechanical insufflation/exsufflation devices are often used in automatic mode (Bach 1993, 1994; Bach et al 1993, 2000, 2002; Tzeng & Bach 2000), enabling the device to be used in the domiciliary environment without a trained professional. In this mode, the device swings between a set negative and positive pressure, and will hold in insufflation for a set period before switching to exsufflation for a set time (the movement in manual mode should be one sweeping movement with no pauses between insufflation and exsufflation), and then pause. The patient learns to coordinate their cough when the device switches to exsufflation. When setting up the device, instruct the patient that a deep breath is coming and tell them to cough as they feel the negative pressure. More recent devices, for example, CoughAssist E70 and NIPPY Clearway, have advanced triggering features allowing the patient to trigger the insufflation for a timed hold. Devices now have software that enables the therapist to work out natural timings for insufflation and exsufflation based on the patient's 'natural' cough profile. However, at present there is no evidence to prove that this is better than a therapist setting the insufflation and exsufflation times manually. Patients may well need longer insufflation/exsufflation times than the patient's 'natural' cough to enhance cough efficacy.

The newer mechanical insufflation/exsufflation devices also have the ability to add vibrations onto the insufflation, exsufflation or both. At time of writing there is no evidence to say this function mobilizes more secretions. The interruption with vibration of the expiratory flow may even decrease peak expiratory airflow.

CoughAssist E70 and NIPPY Clearway both have vibrations optionally superimposed on insufflation and exsufflation (Fig. 7-37). The patient initially acclimatizes to the device in manual mode, usually with a full face mask. To set up, start the insufflation (positive) pressure at 15–20 cmH$_2$O and increase the insufflation pressure to give a passive inspiration to total lung capacity (TLC). Initially start with the exsufflation (negative) pressure the same as the insufflation pressure; then increase the negative pressure to 10–20 cmH$_2$O greater than the positive pressure. The best indicator of efficacy is an increase in the audible sound of the cough (Szeinberg et al 1988).

Intrapulmonary Percussive Ventilation (IPV)

In some areas of Europe and the USA, IPV has been used as a method of airway clearance at home and within hospitals. The IPV device was developed in 1979 by Forrest M. Bird (Percussionaire Corporation, Sandpoint, Idaho, USA). The IPV device consists of a high-pressure flow generator, a valve for flow

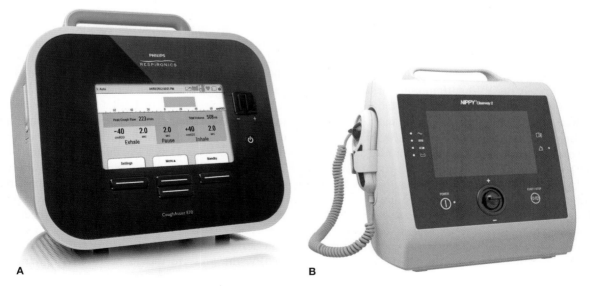

FIGURE 7-37 ■ Mechanical insufflator/exsufflator devices. **(A)** CoughAssist E70 (Philips-Respironics, Pittsburgh Murrysville, USA). **(B)** NIPPY Clearway 2 (B & D Electromedical, Warwickshire, England).

interruption and a breathing circuit with nebulizer that can be attached to a face mask, mouthpiece or catheter mount. IPV is actually a modified method of IPPB which superimposes high-frequency mini bursts of air (50–550 cycles per minute) on the individual's intrinsic breathing pattern; all this creates an internal vibration (percussion) within the lungs. Internal or external vibration of the chest is hypothesized to promote clearance of sputum from the peripheral bronchial tree (Fink & Mahlmeister 2002). IPV may provide ventilatory support in patients with neuromuscular disease (Chatwin et al 2004) and in patients with COPD (Nava et al 2006). IPV devices include the Percussionaire range (Percussionaire Corporation, Sandpoint, Idaho, USA); the IMP II (Breas, Mölnlycke, Sweden) and the Pegaso (Dimla Italia, Bologna, Italy).

IPV has been evaluated in tracheostomized patients with Duchenne muscular dystrophy (DMD) and compared to physiotherapy consisting of the forced expiration technique and manually assisted coughing (Toussaint et al 2003). Sputum clearance was collected with a mucus trap and sputum weight was calculated. The patient group was split into DMD patients who were hypersecretive and those who were normosecretive; it was concluded that IPV enhanced peripheral bronchial secretion clearance in hypersecretive DMD patients compared to conventional physiotherapy.

Clini et al (2006) investigated the effects of IPV on tracheostomized patients who were weaning from mechanical ventilation in the intensive care unit (ICU). Their patient group (n = 46) received 15 days of two 1-hour physiotherapy sessions per day with one group (n = 24) receiving IPV for 10 minutes prior to physiotherapy sessions. They assessed arterial blood gases (ABGs), the partial pressure of oxygen in arterial blood to the fraction of inspired oxygen ($PaO_2:FiO_2$) ratio and maximal expiratory pressure every fifth day during the 15-day period (Clini et al 2006). At 15 days, the IPV group had a significantly better $PaO_2:FiO_2$ ratio and higher maximal expiratory pressure. At follow-up this group also had a lower incidence of pneumonia, indicating IPV may have a role in decreasing the amount of atelectasis in long-term weaning patients.

Vargas et al (2005) investigated COPD patients with an acute respiratory exacerbation and mild respiratory acidosis. Again, one group received standard treatment (oxygen, bronchodilators, steroids and anti-

biotic) and the other standard treatment with the addition of IPV (30 minutes twice a day). Patients who received IPV were discharged home earlier 6.8 ± 1 days versus 7.9 ± 1.3 days p < 0.05. IPV also helped avoid further deterioration of pH <7.35 that required NIV (IPV 0/16 patients; standard treatment alone 6/17 patients). The authors postulated that the IPV group may have benefited from improved secretion removal but acknowledge that this is speculative, because sputum quantity was not measured in this study.

Previous studies have also investigated sputum mobilization in CF patients, by comparing the use of IPV to other modes of airway clearance, e.g. PD and percussion, high-frequency chest wall compression (HFCFC) and the Flutter device (Newhouse et al 1998, Scherer et al 1998, Varekojis et al 2003). These studies have shown IPV to be equal in efficacy to the other methods of airway clearance in sputum mobilization when the amount of sputum produced was assessed by dry weight. There was also no increased benefit in the use of IPV in patients with bronchiectasis when compared to chest physical therapy that consisted of a combination of forced expiration, PD, percussion and vibration (Paneroni et al 2011). However, patients reported a lower level of dyspnoea with the IPV treatment compared to the chest physical therapy session.

Importantly, IPV has a role in removal of secretions in patients with both restrictive and obstructive respiratory disease. In preliminary safety studies investigating the physiological affects of IPV (Nava et al 2006) and investigating sputum removal (Toussaint et al 2003), some starting settings can be suggested. For patients who need increased ventilatory support, start with a working pressure of 1.2–1.4 mbar and increase rapidly until vibrations can be felt when palpating the chest wall. Start with a low-frequency 100–200 c/min; this will ensure adequate ventilatory support. For patients with the ability to spontaneously breathe, one can start with a lower pressure of 1.0 mbar and increase rapidly until vibrations can be felt when palpating the chest wall. Starting with a higher frequency is possible (200–350 c/min) if one is aiming for secretion clearance alone. Once the patient has acclimatized to IPV, the pressure should be titrated upward to provide sufficient ventilation and/or vibration to the chest wall. Also consider adjusting the frequency to optimize secretion clearance. Inverting the inspiratory to expiratory (I:E) ratio will assist ventilatory support, i.e. 2:1 (Toussaint et al 2003) (Fig. 7-38). IPV can be used in conjunction with AD to assist in clearance of peripheral secretions. When treating patients with neuromuscular weakness, it may also be necessary to apply manually assisted coughs to clear secretions from the main airway.

High-Frequency Chest Wall Oscillation

HFCWO (also known as HFCWC or high-frequency chest compression (HFCC)), is administered by an inflatable vest that fits snugly over the thorax and is attached to an air pulse generating compressor which delivers intermittent positive pressure airflow into the jacket. The rapid inflation and deflation of the jacket creates airway oscillations at the chest wall at frequencies of 5–25 Hz (Fig. 7-39).

The hypothesis is that mucus clearance is enhanced as a consequence of this airflow oscillation and vibration of the airway walls. The proposed mechanism is that increased mucus–airflow interaction leads to increased cough-like shear forces and decreased mucus viscoelasticity (King et al 1983, Tomkiewicz et al 1994). Furthermore, HFCWO supposedly creates an expiratory bias to airflow, promoting movement of mucus towards the mouth, and may also enhance ciliary activity (Chang et al 1988, Freitag et al 1989, Hansen et al 1994, King et al 1984, 1990).

Early short-term evidence for this technique suggested HFCWO was as effective as other ACTs for patients with CF (Darbee et al 2005, Oermann et al 2001, Warwick & Hansen 1991). Some studies demonstrated a significant increase in sputum clearance after HFCWO in comparison with baseline or control, but no significant difference in efficacy between HFCWO and other ACTs, including PD&P, PEP and high-frequency oral oscillation (HFOO) (Braggion et al 1995, Scherer et al 1998).

Potential benefits in airway clearance with HFCWO were also reported in other conditions including asthma, COPD, neuromuscular disease, postoperative patients and those requiring long-term ventilatory support (Allan et al 2003, Chiappetta & Beckerman 1995, Perry et al 1998, Wen et al 1996, Whitman et al 1993).

Other studies comparing HFCWO with PD&P demonstrated significantly more sputum clearance with HFCWO over PD&P (Hansen & Warwick 1990, Kluft et al 1996). However, more recent studies have suggested HFCWO clears significantly fewer secretions than other techniques in an infective exacerbation (Osman et al 2010), and importantly, could increase the frequency of exacerbations and shorten the time to an exacerbation when compared with PEP therapy over the long term (McIlwaine et al 2013).

Different studies have used different protocols in the application of HFCWO (Arens et al 1994, Braggion et al 1995, Darbee et al 2005, Kluft et al 1996, Oermann et al 2001, Stites et al 2006, Varekojis et al 2003, Warwick & Hansen 1991, Warwick et al 2004). Most commonly, a total treatment time of 30 minutes covering six frequencies between 6 Hz and 25 Hz has been used, and standard manufacturers' guidelines suggest 10–30 minutes of total treatment time. Early animal studies found 13 Hz to be an optimum treatment frequency (Gross et al 1985, King et al 1983) and some manufacturers suggest 10 minutes each at 10, 12 and 14 Hz. However, more recently it has been recommended that an individual 'tuning' method should be used to identify optimum treatment frequencies, which vary among individuals and according to the waveform of the machine used (Milla et al 2006).

In non-CF bronchiectasis, a recent Turkish cross-over study comparing 5 days of HFCWO with 5 days of PD, vibration and percussion in patients with primary ciliary dyskinesia (PCD) found no differences between these airway clearance strategies (Gokdemir et al 2014). Another Italian study compared HFCWO with a variety of other airway clearance strategies and a control group who had no intervention over 15 days. Both HFCWO and the other ACTs performed better than the control group for all outcomes measures. Some improvements in dyspnoea were reported in the HFCWO group but the heterogeneous ACT comparison group makes this outcome difficult to interpret (Nicolini et al 2013). Improvements in dyspnoea were also reported in an American study involving four consecutive HFCWO treatments for patients during an acute exacerbation (Mahajan et al 2011).

HFCWO is widely used in the USA, where it is considered an attractive and cost effective alternative to PD&P, which requires an assistant. However, in the

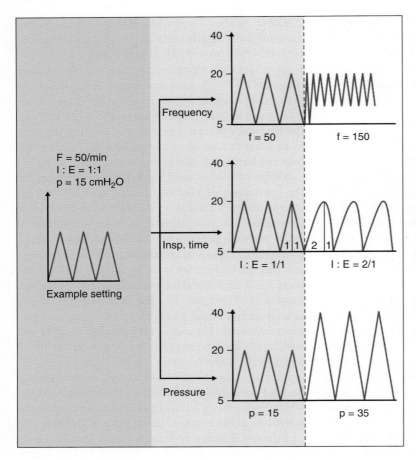

F = 50/min
I : E = 1:1
p = 15 cmH₂O

Example setting

FIGURE 7-38 ■ This simplified diagram shows example intrapulmonary percussive ventilation (IPV) settings in the left panel. The middle panel shows the example settings separated for oscillation frequency, inspiratory time (Insp. time) and pressure. The right panel shows the effect of the changes made to the settings. Continuous positive pressure (CPAP) of 5 cmH₂O is present with all settings (Toussaint et al 2012). As the frequency is increased the CPAP effect appears, and the greater the bias for secretion mobilization. By inverting the inspiratory to expiratory (I : E) ratio and increasing the pressure the greater the ventilatory support to the patient. *F*, Frequency; *p*, pressure. *(Reproduced with permission from Dr Michel Toussaint.)*

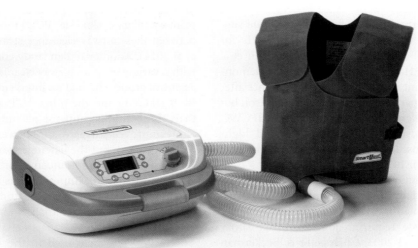

FIGURE 7-39 ■ High-frequency chest wall oscillation (HFCWO) vest system. *(SmartVest courtesy of Electromed Inc.)*

UK and Europe where other independently performed techniques are the mainstay of care for airway clearance, HFCWO is not used as extensively.

EXERCISE AND PULMONARY REHABILITATION FOR AIRWAY CLEARANCE

Physical activity and exercise have become key components in the management of individuals with CF in particular and increasingly in patients with non-CF bronchiectasis. Exercise is hypothesized to enhance MCC through a number of physiological pathways (Rand et al 2013). A Cochrane systematic review concluded that the addition of exercise to airway clearance significantly improves lung function compared to airway clearance treatment alone in individuals with CF (Bradley & Moran 2008). In people with CF, the combination of an ACT and exercise programme led to a reduction in the decline in lung function when compared with airway clearance and usual physical activities (Schneiderman-Walker et al 2000).

The physiological mechanisms by which exercise acts on MCC remains unclear but may be due to the increase in ventilatory demand during exercise, which is met by increases in tidal volume and respiratory flow (Dwyer et al 2011a). This increase in ventilation and PEF has the potential to increase mechanical clearance of secretions from the airways. It is proposed that if PEF is greater than the PIF during exercise, the annular flow of mucus towards the oropharynx may be augmented through two-phase gas–liquid flow (Kim et al 1986b).

Moderate intensity exercise may also increase the water content of mucus in people with CF, as it inhibits the sodium conductance in luminal nasal respiratory epithelium, potentially further explaining benefits in terms of ease of expectoration (Hebestreit et al 2001). An increase in airway surface hydration occurs following exercise due to the creation of an osmotic stimulus associated with high levels of ventilation (Daviskas et al 1995). The increase in ventilation may also have the potential to affect mucus rheology due to the associated shear forces, which have been shown to reduce mucus viscoelasticity (App et al 1998). The physical body movements associated with exercise may have an additional effect on mucus rheology.

A 3-day crossover study investigated the effects of a single bout of moderate intensity exercise (treadmill or cycle exercise) in 14 adults with CF on ventilation, PEF, expiratory flow bias ratio (PEF:PIF), sputum properties and subjective ease of expectoration (Dwyer et al 2011a). There was a subjective improvement in ease of expectoration during both treadmill and cycle exercise. The ventilation, PEF and PEF:PIF were all significantly higher during both treadmill and cycle exercise compared to baseline measurements with a trend towards the highest values during cycle exercise. The PEF:PIF ratio did not meet the >1.10 threshold believed to be necessary for the promotion of annular flow from the airways to the oropharynx, and authors hypothesized that expiratory airflow bias did not contribute to the ease of expectoration reported by the participants. There were significant changes in sputum mechanical impedance following treadmill exercise compared with the control group, suggesting perhaps that the body oscillations associated with running (rather than cycling) may have reduced sputum viscoelasticity, in a similar way to other oscillatory PEP devices (App et al 1998).

In another small study comparing the effects of treadmill exercise with PEP and OPEP in adults with CF, treadmill exercise produced a PEF:PIF of only 0.9 while OPEP produced a PEF:PIF of 1.13, considered sufficient to mobilize secretions proximally (Kim et al 1987). Both the treadmill and OPEP significantly reduced mucus viscoelasticity. Further research is required to fully confirm the physiological effects of exercise in CF but it appears that exercise in CF has the potential to affect airway clearance in addition to the well-documented improvements in fitness, HRQoL and positive effects on lung function.

Pulmonary rehabilitation refers to a multidisciplinary package of care that may be offered to people with chronic lung disease and usually includes patient education, exercise training, psychosocial support, and nutritional intervention and evaluation for oxygen supplementation (Ries et al 2007, ZuWallack & Hedges 2008). There is reasonable evidence to show that exercise and/or pulmonary rehabilitation are both safe and effective in CF and non-CF bronchiectasis, and have positive benefits in terms of improving dyspnoea, fatigue, exercise tolerance, peripheral muscle dysfunction and quality of life, which may be enhanced by the addition of IMT (Bradley & Moran 2008, Bradley et al 2002, Newall et al 2005).

Although the exercise training component of pulmonary rehabilitation is not considered to be an ACT in its own right, it may play a useful role in supplementing airway clearance in some individuals, especially if adherence to their normal ACT is poor (Lannefors & Wollmer 1992). However, it appears that pulmonary rehabilitation in isolation is not as effective as physiotherapy and should not replace it as an airway clearance strategy, particularly in people who produce moderate to large amounts of sputum (Bilton et al 1992, Salh et al 1989). Nonetheless, if exercise prescription is well calibrated for individuals, there is an expectation that tidal lung volumes during activity would increase significantly, and may enhance expiratory airflow to mobilize secretions and promote clearance of these from the smaller airways. This may be enhanced if patients are encouraged to cough and clear their chest during exercise and activity or regular and timed FETs are included throughout exercise to optimize this. During exacerbations, dyspnoea may preclude exercise as an effective form of airway clearance and may need adapting, either with supplemental oxygen or with NIV (Bott et al 2009).

ADJUNCTIVE TECHNIQUES

Management of Stress Incontinence

Many people with chronic respiratory disease who require ACTs have stress incontinence of urine and sometimes faeces. Urinary incontinence, the involuntary loss of urine, is associated with adverse effects on quality of life (National Institute for Health and Clinical Excellence 2006). The prevalence of urinary incontinence in the population as a whole increases with increasing age up to 46% in women and 34% in men aged over 80 years (Scottish Intercollegiate Guidelines Network 2004). The prevalence associated with chronic lung disease is known to be higher and at an earlier age; for example in people with CF, incontinence in women ranges from 38% to 68% (Cornacchia et al 2001, Orr et al 2001, White et al 2000); in men is 16% (Gumery et al 2005) and in children from 14% to 33% (Moraes et al 2002, Prasad et al 2006).

Urinary incontinence frequently reduces adherence to an ACT and often causes embarrassment. During assessment (see Chapter 2), the physiotherapist should include questions to identify this problem, even in young girls with chronic respiratory disorders. Voluntary contraction of the pelvic floor muscles just before and throughout a cough or huff, known as 'The Knack', can be used to reduce stress-related leakage of urine. This manoeuvre, performed by consciously contracting the pelvic floor muscle prior to cough and then maintaining the contraction during the cough can reduce urinary leakage by 98.2% with a medium cough, and 73.3% with a deep cough, after a week of training (Miller et al 1998). If this technique does not lead to a clinically significant reduction in leakage, referral to a physiotherapist specializing in continence therapy should be considered.

Acknowledgements

Thanks to Jennifer Pryor and Ammani Prasad for their sections taken from *Physiotherapy Techniques*, 4th edition, and to Caroline Nicolson and Narelle Cox for their suggestions on content.

Techniques for Improving Lung Volumes

INTERMITTENT POSITIVE PRESSURE BREATHING

Intermittent positive pressure breathing (IPPB) is the maintenance of a positive airway pressure throughout inspiration, with airway pressure returning to atmospheric pressure during expiration. The AARC has developed clinical practice guidelines for the use of IPPB as a hyperinflation and aerosol delivery technique (AARC 2003). The literature on IPPB has been reviewed by Bott et al (1992) and Denehy & Berney (2001). The use of IPPB has a place in the management of patients with reduced lung volumes and the rationale for using IPPB should be based on its known physiological effects, the availability of other treatment modalities, the condition of the patient and the current research knowledge base. The Bird ventilator (Fig. 7-40) is a pressure-cycled device convenient to use for providing IPPB as an adjunct to physiotherapy in the spontaneously breathing patient.

IPPB has been shown to augment tidal volume (Stiller et al 1992, Sukumalchantra et al 1965) and when using an IPPB device in the completely relaxed individual, the work of breathing during inspiration approaches zero (Ayres et al 1963). These two effects may assist in the clearance of bronchial secretions when more simple ACTs alone are not effective, for example in the semi-comatose patient with chronic bronchitis and sputum retention (Pavia et al 1988), the postoperative patient or in a patient with neuromuscular disease and a chest infection. The reduction in the work of breathing can be used with effect in the exhausted patient with acute severe asthma, but there is no evidence that the effect of bronchodilators delivered by IPPB is greater than from a nebulizer alone (Webber et al 1974).

Ideally the IPPB device for use with physiotherapy should be portable and have simple controls. Other important features include a positive pressure range of 0–35 cmH$_2$O and a sensitive patient 'trigger' for the inspiratory phase, which requires minimal effort. Fully automatic control is unpleasant for most patients and unnecessary for physiotherapy. A hand triggering device is useful to test the ventilator and nebulizer. In addition, ability to modify the inspiratory gas flow rate is useful. Optimal distribution of gas to the more peripheral airways is achieved at relatively slow flow rates, but if the patient is very short of breath and has a fast respiratory rate, a slow inspiratory phase may be unacceptable. It is often useful to alter the flow control several times during a single treatment session, providing slow breaths when attempting to mobilize peripheral secretions, and a faster flow rate when a patient is recovering his breath after expectoration. Some IPPB ventilators do not require flow rate adjustment because automatic variable flow is provided with each breath. This feature is known as 'flow sensitivity' and means that the flow of the inspired gas adapts to the resistance of the individual's airways.

An efficient nebulizer in the circuit is necessary to humidify the driving gas and, when appropriate, to deliver bronchodilator drugs. When driven by oxygen, air must be entrained by the apparatus to provide an air/oxygen mixture for the patient. The use of 100% oxygen for a patient is very rare and potentially dangerous. When air is not entrained through the apparatus, the flow rate control must be regulated to provide an adequate flow to the patient.

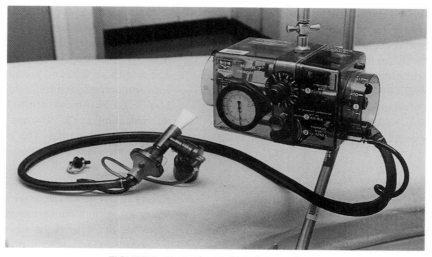

FIGURE 7-40 ■ The Bird Mark 7 ventilator.

When IPPB (such as the Bird ventilator) is driven by oxygen and the air-mix control is in use, the percentage of oxygen delivered to the patient is approximately 45% (Starke et al 1979). This percentage will be considerably higher than the controlled percentage delivered by an appropriate Venturi mask, for example to a patient with chronic bronchitis. This higher percentage is rarely dangerous during treatment because the patient's ventilation is assisted and the removal of secretions as a result of treatment is likely to lead subsequently to an improvement in ABG tensions (Gormezano & Branthwaite 1972).

It has been suggested that a few patients become more drowsy during or after IPPB as a result of the high percentage of oxygen received. Starke et al (1979) showed that increased drowsiness caused by hypercapnia occurred whether oxygen or air was the driving gas for IPPB and that the deterioration was dependent on inappropriate settings of the ventilator. The pressure and flow controls must be set to provide an adequate tidal volume, this being particularly important when treating patients with a rigid thoracic cage (Starke et al 1979). Occasionally, IPPB may be powered by Entonox (a mix of oxygen and nitrous oxide) and in this case the air-mix control would need to be in the position to provide 100% of the driving gas with no additional air entrained.

To prevent cross-infection, it is essential for each patient to have his own breathing circuit, which consists of tubing, nebulizer, exhalation valve and a mouthpiece or mask. The majority of patients prefer to use a mouthpiece, but a face mask is required when treating confused patients. A flanged mouthpiece (Fig. 7-41) is useful for patients who have difficulty making an airtight seal around the mouthpiece.

The type of breathing circuit used will depend on local infection control guidelines. The circuits can be autoclavable, non-disposable but non-autoclavable, or disposable. Many countries use single patient disposable circuits.

Preparation of the Apparatus

1. Normal saline solution or the drug to be nebulized (3–4 mL in total) is inserted into the nebulizer chamber.
2. The breathing circuit is connected to the IPPB ventilator and the ventilator connected to the

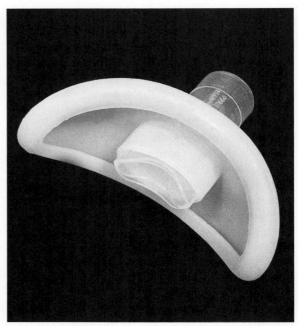

FIGURE 7-41 ■ Flange mouthpiece for use with intermittent positive pressure breathing (IPPB).

driving gas source. It can be used from an oxygen or air cylinder if piped compressed gas is unavailable.
3. If there is an air-mix control, this should be in the position for entrainment of air.
4. If there is an automatic control (expiratory timer), this should be turned off to allow the patient to 'trigger' the machine at his desired rate.
5. The sensitivity, flow and pressure controls are set appropriately for the individual. With the Bird Mark 7, the sensitivity control is usually adjusted to a low number (5–7) where minimal inspiratory effort is required. The pressure and flow controls are adjusted to provide regular assisted ventilation without discomfort. A patient with a rigid ribcage will require a higher pressure setting to obtain an adequate tidal volume than someone with a more mobile ribcage. When adjusting the settings for a new patient, it may be easiest to start with a pressure at approximately 12 cmH$_2$O and the flow at about '10';

then gradually increase the pressure and reduce the flow until the pattern of breathing is the most appropriate for the individual. Some IPPB devices do not have numbered markings, but after finding the most effective settings for a patient during one treatment, it is useful to note the positions of the controls in order to use these as a starting point at the next treatment. The controls to be set on the Bennett PR-1 are the nebulizer, sensitivity and pressure.

6. Before starting a treatment, the hand triggering device is operated to check that there are no leaks in the breathing circuit and that the nebulizer is functioning well.

Treatment of the Patient

The position in which IPPB is used depends on the indication for treatment. It may be used in side lying, high side lying or the sitting position. The patient should be positioned comfortably and encouraged to relax the upper chest and shoulder girdle.

After the purpose of the IPPB treatment has been explained, the patient is asked to close his lips firmly around the mouthpiece and then to make a slight inspiratory effort, which will trigger the device into inspiratory flow. The patient should then relax throughout inspiration, allowing his lungs to be inflated. When the pre-set pressure is reached at the mouth the ventilator cycles into expiration; the patient should remain relaxed and let the air out quietly.

If the patient attempts to assist inspiration there will be a delay in reaching the cycling pressure. A delay will also occur if there is a leak around the mouthpiece, at any of the circuit connections or from the patient's nose. A nose clip may be required until the patient becomes familiar with the technique.

Observation of the manometer on the ventilator should allow detection of any faults in the patient's technique. At the start of inspiration the needle should swing minimally to a negative pressure and then swing smoothly up to the positive pressure set, before cutting out into expiration and returning to zero. A larger negative swing at the beginning of inspiration shows that the patient is making an unnecessary effort in triggering the device. If the patient makes an active effort throughout inspiration, the needle will rise very slowly to the inspiratory set pressure and if they attempt to start expiration before the pre-set pressure is reached, the needle will rise sharply above the set pressure and then cut out into expiration.

When IPPB is taught correctly the work of breathing is relieved, but if the patient is allowed to assist either inspiration or expiration there may be an increase in the work of breathing.

A short pause between completion of expiration and the next inspiration avoids hyperventilation and possible dizziness. Occasionally children using IPPB tend to swallow air during treatment. It is important to observe the size of the abdomen before and during IPPB to recognize signs of abdominal distension and discontinue treatment if this occurs.

When IPPB is used to relieve the work of breathing while delivering bronchodilator therapy, for example in the acute severe asthmatic patient, it may be helpful for the physiotherapist to hold the breathing circuit to allow the patient to relax the shoulders and arms as much as possible.

A facemask for IPPB may be used for drowsy or confused patients or those with facial weakness unable to make an airtight seal at the mouth. When using IPPB to assist in mobilizing secretions, the patient should be appropriately positioned to assist loosening and mobilization of secretions, for example in side lying. The patient's jaw should be elevated and the mask held firmly over the face, ensuring an airtight fit. Chest shaking during the expiratory phase may be used to assist in mobilizing secretions. In a drowsy patient it may be necessary to stimulate coughing using nasotracheal suction if spontaneous coughing is not stimulated by IPPB and chest shaking.

In medical patients with retained secretions and poor respiratory reserve, IPPB may be useful both to mobilize secretions and to relieve the effort of breathing following expectoration. The flow control on a Bird ventilator should be adjusted to give a slow, comfortable breath to mobilize secretions, but following the exertion of expectoration there may be an increase in respiratory requirements, which may necessitate increasing the flow and possibly reducing the pressure until the breathing effort and pattern return to normal or baseline.

IPPB may be used in patients with chest wall deformity, for example kyphoscoliosis (Sinha &

Bergofsky 1972), when there is difficulty with clearing secretions during an infective episode. To achieve an adequate increase in ventilation in patients with a rigid ribcage, the pressure setting needs to be higher than for a more mobile ribcage.

Occasionally, in postoperative patients, IPPB is the adjunct of choice when the patient is unable to augment tidal volume adequately during treatment. In these patients, in contrast to the relaxed technique normally used with IPPB, thoracic expansion may be actively encouraged during the inspiratory phase.

Contraindications for IPPB

- Pneumothorax
- Large bullae
- Lung abscess, as the size of the air space may increase
- Severe haemoptysis, as treatment is inappropriate until the bleeding has lessened
- Postoperative air leak, unless the advantages of IPPB would outweigh the possibility of increasing the air leak during treatment
- Bronchial tumour in the proximal airways; air may flow past the tumour during inspiration and may be trapped on expiration as the airways narrow. There would be no contraindication if the tumour were situated peripherally.

NON-INVASIVE VENTILATION

Introduction

Since the late 1990s, there has been a rapid growth in the use of NIV for managing respiratory failure in both the acute and chronic setting. A solid rationale underlies its use in hypoventilation syndromes and there is good clinical evidence for its effectiveness in an expanding range of acute clinical situations. However, NIV is frequently underutilized or misused by healthcare personnel unfamiliar with the technique or who lack an understanding of the appropriate indications for its use. In many centres, physiotherapists have become key players in implementing this therapy (Piper & Moran 2006, Simonelli et al 2013, Zuffo et al 2012), often using it as an adjunct to other physiotherapeutic techniques (Garrod et al 2000, Holland et al 2003, Menadue et al 2009). Even if not directly involved

in the assessment and setup of NIV, physiotherapists are involved in treating individuals using this therapy (Moran et al 2005). Therefore understanding the theoretical and practical aspects of NIV are now core requirements of any physiotherapist involved in the management of patients with acute or chronic respiratory failure.

This section will outline the basics of NIV, the indications and limitations of its use, and the role it can play in augmenting currently established physiotherapy techniques.

What Is Non-Invasive Ventilation?

NIV is a technique whereby positive pressure is applied to the airways and lungs without the need for an endotracheal or tracheostomy tube with the aim of providing ventilatory assistance. Irrespective of the setting, the goals of therapy are to improve gas exchange, assist inspiratory efforts, reduce the work of breathing and alleviate symptoms related to respiratory insufficiency.

Over the past few years, there have been significant advancements in the technology routinely available to deliver NIV both in the hospital and home settings. Different devices may provide a single level of pressure (CPAP), two levels of pressure (pressure preset or bi-level ventilatory support) or volume support (volume pre-set) ventilation, with the latter two device types often referred to collectively as 'non-invasive positive pressure ventilation (NPPV)'. Although CPAP does not actively assist inspiration, it is frequently included under the umbrella term 'NIV' and has often been used in patients with acute hypoxaemic respiratory failure (Duggal et al 2013, Vital et al 2013) or in the postoperative setting (Squadrone et al 2005). Pressure and volume pre-set modes of ventilation each have advantages and limitations. Pressure preset ventilation is more comfortable for the patient, while volume preset ventilation provides a more reliable tidal volume delivery in the situation of changing chest wall mechanics or airway resistance. There is no strong evidence that one type of ventilatory support is superior to another in either the acute (Girault et al 1997) or chronic (Tuggey & Elliott 2005) setting. However, pressure pre-set devices, primarily bi-level ventilators, have become more widely used due to simplicity and comfort. More recently, dual modes of ventilatory support have been developed whereby the device adjusts the level of pressure support within a pre-set range in order to achieve a 'target' tidal set by the clinician (Windisch & Storre 2012). While this mode is now available on most portable home ventilator devices, there is again little evidence at present to suggest that patient outcomes are better with volume-targeted pressure support compared to standard bi-level therapy for routine clinical use (Crescimanno et al 2011, Murphy et al 2012, Oscroft et al 2010, Storre et al 2006). Rather, success with NIV depends upon the clinician's understanding of the underlying pathological processes that have contributed to the patient's respiratory deterioration, and choosing a machine and mode of ventilatory support which best meets the respiratory needs of the patient.

Indications for Non-Invasive Ventilation

Chronic Respiratory Failure

To best understand how and when NIV works in patients with chronic hypercapnia, it is important to first appreciate the mechanisms by which abnormal sleep-breathing contributes to the development of awake respiratory failure.

Sleep is associated with a number of normal physiological changes in breathing. These include a reduction in ventilatory drive, reduced output to the postural muscles with resulting increases in upper airway resistance, and decreased ventilatory responses to hypoxia and hypercapnia. These changes are more marked during rapid eye movement (REM) sleep than in non-REM sleep. In addition, during REM sleep there is an active inhibition of postural muscle activity so that ventilation becomes heavily reliant on diaphragmatic activity. These changes during sleep are of minor significance for individuals in whom the respiratory system is normal, although the development of upper airway obstruction is not uncommon in the general population. However, for those with preexisting diaphragmatic weakness, altered chest wall mechanics or severe lung disease, sleep-associated changes in breathing, ventilation and gas exchange can become quite profound (Becker et al 1999).

When the diaphragm is weak (e.g. neuromuscular disorders) or at a mechanical disadvantage (e.g. chest wall deformity or severe lung disease), adequate

ventilation during wakefulness and non-REM sleep can be achieved by recruiting other inspiratory and accessory muscles. However, in REM sleep, postural muscle activity is lost, resulting in a reduction in minute ventilation and deteriorating gas exchange (Arnulf et al 2000). The ability to arouse from sleep in response to these alterations in breathing provides some defence, as transient wakefulness permits the reemergence of accessory muscle activity and restoration of ventilation, albeit briefly. However, repeated arousal from sleep produces sleep fragmentation, which in itself can alter respiratory drive and arousal thresholds, so that eventually more extreme changes in blood gases must occur before the arousal response is activated.

Consequently, nocturnal hypoventilation first becomes apparent in REM sleep (Bye et al 1990, Ragette et al 2002). However, as REM sleep takes up only a relatively small proportion of total sleep time, patients with REM hypoventilation, even if severe, may remain clinically stable for months or even years before daytime hypercapnia develops. However, with ageing, weight gain or the development of an intercurrent illness such as a chest infection, more severe sleep-disordered breathing occurs, extending the period of hypoventilation throughout sleep and eventually into wakefulness as well (Fig. 7-42). Once nocturnal hypoventilation develops, daytime hypercapnia is likely to evolve within the next 12–24 months (Ward et al 2005). Consequently, it is crucial to identify patients with nocturnal hypoventilation early and treat them appropriately with nocturnal NIV in order to prevent the complications associated with an acute respiratory crisis (Box 7-9).

In addition to nocturnal hypoventilation, upper airway obstruction and central apnoeas in both non-REM and REM sleep can also be present in these patients. Distinguishing the type of sleep-disordered breathing occurring in an individual is clinically helpful in determining the most appropriate mode of ventilatory support and settings to use to correct these nocturnal events and reverse daytime hypercapnia.

Assessing 'At-Risk' Patients

A high degree of clinical vigilance and monitoring needs to be undertaken in patients with disorders known to be associated with hypoventilation during

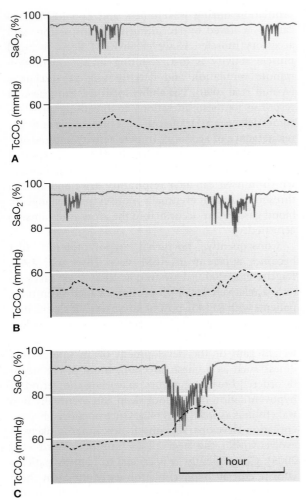

A

B

C

1 hour

FIGURE 7-42 ■ Serial recordings of oxygen saturation (SaO_2) (solid line) and transcutaneous carbon dioxide ($TcCO_2$) (dotted line) from a patient with Duchenne muscular dystrophy (DMD) showing progressive nocturnal respiratory failure. **(A)** Mild sleep-disordered breathing, with modest falls in SaO_2. **(B)** Eight months later, more substantial oxygen desaturation was apparent during rapid eye movement (REM) sleep, with rises in carbon dioxide. **(C)** Severe REM desaturation occurs. This was accompanied by large rises in transcutaneous CO_2, with failure of CO_2 to return to baseline values between periods of abnormal breathing. Over the same period, awake arterial CO_2 had risen from 40 to 45 mmHg (5.3 to 6.0 kPa), with no change in inspiratory muscle pressures.

BOX 7-9

COMMON CONDITIONS WHERE NOCTURNAL HYPERCAPNIC RESPIRATORY FAILURE IS LIKELY TO OCCUR

Neuromuscular	Myopathies
	■ Duchenne muscular dystrophy
	■ Acid maltase deficiency
	Neuropathies
	■ Poliomyelitis
	■ Motor neurone disease
	■ Bilateral phrenic nerve palsy
Chest wall	Kyphoscoliosis
	Thoracoplasty
	Obesity hypoventilation syndrome
Impaired ventilatory control	Brainstem injury
	Primary alveolar hypoventilation
Airway obstruction	Severe obstructive sleep apnoea
Lung disease	Chronic obstructive pulmonary disease
	Cystic fibrosis
	Bronchiectasis

---

sleep. Even when overt daytime respiratory failure is present, this may not be clinically apparent, as patients often report few symptoms, reflecting the insidious way in which chronic respiratory failure can develop. Consequently, specific questions regarding sleep and daytime symptoms related to nocturnal hypoventilation need to be included in the routine clinical evaluation of these patients. Attention should be paid to daytime sleepiness, sleep quality, snoring, morning headaches and exertional dyspnoea, as well as to the frequency of chest infections, cough ability and exercise tolerance. Strong use of the accessory respiratory muscles at rest, including the sternomastoid and abdominal muscles, should raise the possibility that respiratory function may worsen during sleep and prompt the initiation of objective monitoring of respiratory function and gas exchange.

In 'at-risk' individuals, daytime respiratory function should be monitored to determine the timing of more invasive or complex measures such as ABGs or overnight sleep studies. Although measures such as VC and respiratory muscle strength are not sensitive enough to identify sleep hypoventilation in COPD patients and those with morbid obesity, these simple measures are useful in those with neuromuscular disorders. These tests can be readily carried out at the bedside, in the patient's home or during clinic visits. Where facial or buccal muscle weakness is present, face mask spirometry (Banerjee et al 2013) or sniff nasal inspiratory pressure (Morgan et al 2005) may be used in place of mouthpiece techniques. A low VC, a significant fall in VC from sitting to supine (>20%) or a maximum inspiratory mouth pressure less than 30 cmH$_2$O have all be shown to be indicators of possible sleep hypoventilation (Bye et al 1990, Ragette et al 2002). In a study of patients with primary myopathies such as Duchenne, congenital and limb girdle muscular dystrophy, a supine VC <60% of predicted predisposed the patient to REM hypoventilation (Ragette et al 2002). When the supine VC fell below 40% of predicted, continuous sleep hypoventilation was likely, and once supine VC was below 30% of predicted, the patient was highly likely to have daytime respiratory failure (Ragette et al 2002).

In addition, measuring and monitoring expiratory muscle strength and cough strength are key aspects of respiratory function that need to be undertaken in conjunction with nocturnal ventilation assessment in patients with neuromuscular disorders to ensure the timely introduction of airway clearance and chest wall mobility techniques. It is generally recommended that lung inflation techniques such as lung volume recruitment manoeuvers are commenced when VC falls below 2.0 L (Kang & Bach 2000), and assisted coughing techniques are begun when PCF values are less than 270 L/min (McKim et al 2011).

Although daytime indices are helpful in identifying patients who are at risk of sleep hypoventilation prior to the development of awake hypercapnia, they cannot specifically identify the presence or severity of nocturnal hypoventilation. This requires more detailed sleep investigations. NIV is usually commenced when symptoms of hypoventilation are present, once daytime hypercapnia (partial pressure of arterial carbon dioxide (PaCO$_2$) >45 mmHg) develops or if nocturnal hypoventilation is present demonstrated by sustained falls in oxygen saturation below 88% (Consensus Conference Report 1999) or rises in transcutaneous carbon dioxide >10 mmHg from wakefulness or a peak CO$_2$ >47 mmHg for more than 50% of the night (Wallgren-Pettersson et al 2004).

Acute Respiratory Failure

NIV has emerged as a valuable and effective treatment option for patients with acute respiratory failure. It avoids the complications of endotracheal intubation, is more comfortable for the patient, allowing speech and swallowing, and avoids the need for sedation and immobilization. Therapy does not have to be confined to the ICU or emergency department and NIV is now increasingly used on general medical or surgical wards (Lightowler et al 2003, Plant et al 2000, Ward & Horobin 2012). The use of NIV is supported by high-level evidence in patients with severe exacerbations of COPD or acute cardiogenic pulmonary oedema, avoiding the need for intubation and reducing morbidity and mortality (Ram et al 2004, Vital et al 2013). Although evidence for the use of NIV in other causes of acute respiratory conditions is less robust (Lim et al 2012) or controversial (Confalonieri et al 1999, Ferrer et al 2003), it appears that this therapy is being increasingly used in these situations (Walkey & Wiener 2013). This is of some concern as the need for invasive ventilation following a trial of NIV (i.e. NIV failure) has been shown to be associated with a higher mortality rate in both COPD (Chandra et al 2012) and non-COPD populations (Walkey & Wiener 2013). Higher rates of NIV failure are more likely to be seen in patients without underlying COPD or cardiac disease (Carrillo et al 2012a, Walkey & Wiener 2013), highlighting the importance of appropriate patient selection when using this technique and the need to monitor response to therapy in order to intervene early if no improvement occurs.

Assessing the Need for Non-Invasive Ventilation

NIV should be considered when patients develop signs of incipient respiratory failure such as severe dyspnoea, paradoxical breathing, accessory muscle use or deteriorating gas exchange which is not responding to usual medical intervention. A successful outcome depends to a significant extent on the ability of NIV to rapidly correct acidosis, decrease CO$_2$ or improve oxygenation, reduce respiratory rate and relieve respiratory distress (Confalonieri et al 2005, Lightowler et al 2003). This in turn will be influenced by the tolerance of the patient to the mask, the ability to minimize mouth–mask leaks and to coordinate patient breathing with the ventilator (Di Marco et al 2011). When assessing the suitability of a patient for NIV, the indications for therapy and the presence any contraindications or precautions need to be carefully considered (Box 7-10). Decisions also need to take into account the experience and expertise of the staff available to set up and manage the NIV equipment and the type of monitoring required. Whether the patient is managed in an intensive care, high dependency or ward environment will be influenced by local policy and staffing, as well as the likelihood of NIV success. Even though NIV is a highly effective technique in patients with COPD or heart failure, therapy failure occurs even in these populations and arrangements for escalation of care or institution of a more palliative treatment approach need to made at the time NIV is initiated (Roberts et al 2008).

At present there are four indications for the use of NIV in the acute setting which are supported by a high level of evidence from good quality randomized trials and meta-analyses.

Chronic Obstructive Pulmonary Disease. The strongest evidence for NIV and where it is most commonly used in the acute setting is for acute exacerbations of COPD (Ram et al 2004, Walkey & Wiener 2013). In the majority of studies reported, bi-level ventilation has been used. Compared to usual medical care, NIV significantly reduces the need for intubation and mortality while diminishing complications related to therapy and the length of hospital stay (Ram et al 2004). Data from the US obtained from 7.5 million hospitalizations for acute exacerbations of COPD from 1998 to 2008 showed a progressive increase in the use of NIV as initial respiratory support along with a decline in invasive ventilation use and mortality rates over this time period (Chandra et al 2012). However, the timing of intervention is important in achieving clinical benefits. The result of commencing therapy too early is that NIV is no more effective than usual care and may not be well tolerated (Keenan et al 2003), while waiting until severe respiratory acidosis has developed significantly increases the likelihood of treatment failure (Confalonieri et al 2005, Ram et al 2004).

Cardiogenic Pulmonary Oedema. A number of randomized trials have been undertaken evaluating CPAP and bi-level ventilation in patients presenting with acute pulmonary oedema. Both therapies are more effective than oxygen therapy in reducing the need for intubation and in reducing mortality, although the latter outcome has been shown in smaller studies only (Vital et al 2013). CPAP has been recommended as the first therapy option due to more robust evidence for its effectiveness and safety, lower cost and greater simplicity of titration (Vital et al 2013). However, bi-level support may be more effective in patients presenting with hypercapnia or who fail to respond to CPAP (Nava et al 2003).

The potential mechanisms by which CPAP may improve the patient's clinical status include improving FRC, reducing breathing effort (Lenique et al 1997), augmenting CO (Baratz et al 1992) and reducing left ventricular afterload (Naughton et al 1995). Since bi-level ventilation provides the benefits of CPAP

BOX 7-10

INDICATIONS AND CONTRAINDICATIONS TO NON-INVASIVE VENTILATION (NIV) IN THE ACUTE SETTING

Indications

Respiratory acidosis (pH <7.35 with $PaCO_2$ >45 mmHg) or hypoxaemia (PaO_2/FiO_2 <200)

Use of accessory muscles or presence of abdominal paradox

Dyspnoea

Manageable secretions

Contraindications

Severe hypoxaemia

Respiratory arrest, extreme acidosis (pH <7.2)

Haemodynamic or cardiac instability

Multiple organ failure

Agitation, encephalopathic, uncooperative patient

High risk of aspiration: vomiting, gastro-intestinal bleeding

Inability to fit mask due to facial trauma, burns

Untreated pneumothorax

Recent airway or gastro-intestinal surgery

FiO_2, Fraction of inspired oxygen; $PaCO_2$, partial pressure of carbon dioxide in arterial blood; PaO_2, partial pressure of oxygen in arterial blood.

through the use of an end expiratory positive airway pressure (EPAP) in addition to inspiratory augmentation through pressure support/inspiratory positive airway pressure (IPAP), this ventilatory mode is considered a better option when patients continue to experience high work of breathing or hypercapnia.

Weaning and Post Extubation Respiratory Failure. A meta-analysis of randomized trials comparing early extubation onto NIV to conventional weaning approaches in patients who fail spontaneous breathing trials found that NIV reduced the risk of death and ventilator-acquired pneumonia (Burns et al 2010). However, these benefits were only apparent in patients with COPD. In contrast, the routine use of NIV following extubation has not been shown to confer any benefits over oxygen therapy alone (Jiang et al 1999). Similarly, the application of NIV once respiratory distress or failure is already established post extubation does not alter the rate of re-intubation or length of ICU or hospital stay (Esteban et al 2004, Keenan et al 2002). On the other hand, identifying patients at high risk for developing respiratory failure post extubation such as those with underlying cardiorespiratory disease or hypercapnia, and extubating to NIV is more successful in preventing reintubation (Ferrer et al 2006, 2009) and risk of death (Ferrer et al 2009) than standard care.

Immunocompromised Patients. Immunocompromised patients have a poor outcome if they develop pulmonary infiltrates and acute hypoxemic respiratory failure. Early use of NIV in these patients has been shown to reduce intubation rates, complications and mortality compared to standard care (Antonelli et al 2000, Hilbert et al 2001). These benefits are likely a consequence of avoiding intubation and the infectious complications arising from this. CPAP has also been used successfully in this group (Principi et al 2004).

Evidence for Other Indications. A number of small studies suggest a possible role for NIV in the management of severe asthma and data have shown that it is being increasingly used in clinical practice (Walkey & Wiener 2013). However, a recent Cochrane review concluded there was insufficient evidence for the routine use of therapy for this indication at present

(Lim et al 2012). Randomized trials of NIV for acute respiratory failure in patients with neuromuscular disease, chest wall deformity or obesity hypoventilation have not been undertaken. However, the effectiveness of long-term NIV in these individuals and the high morbidity and mortality arising from endotracheal ventilation in these groups means that a trial of NIV is frequently used as first-line therapy (Flandreau et al 2011). Using the same protocol for commencing NIV, Carrillo et al (2012b) found that treatment success, length of hospital stay and survival in patients with acute hypercapnic obesity hypoventilation syndrome was as good as or better than patients with COPD, in whom there is strong evidence for NIV use.

NIV has been widely used to prevent or treat respiratory complications arising from cardiac, abdominal and thoracic surgery (Auriant et al 2001, Joris et al 1997, Pasquina et al 2004, Perrin et al 2007, Squadrone et al 2005, Zarbock et al 2009). A meta-analysis which included five studies of positive pressure use in the postoperative period found a significantly reduced risk of re-intubation and incidence of pneumonia, reduced length of hospital stay and increased hospital survival compared to standard therapy (Glossop et al 2012). In four of these studies, CPAP was used. Careful patient selection to exclude contraindications to positive pressure including the potential impact of high inspiratory pressures on the integrity of anastomoses must be considered.

At present there is only low to moderate quality data available regarding the use of NIV in blunt chest wall trauma (Duggal et al 2013, Keenan et al 2011). If therapy is to be used it needs to be commenced early in the course of the injury before acute respiratory distress occurs (Duggal et al 2013). Success rates with NIV in acute lung injury and adult respiratory distress syndrome are very low, and therefore this approach is not routinely recommended for this circumstance (Agarwal et al 2006).

In clinical practice, NIV is frequently implemented as a therapy ceiling in patients with do-not-intubate directives (Roberts et al 2008). Patients with COPD or congestive heart failure who develop respiratory failure have a relatively high likelihood of surviving to discharge if NIV is used, in contrast to low hospital survival rates in those with pneumonia or cancer

(Levy et al 2004). A recent randomized trial in patients with end-stage cancer and breathlessness demonstrated that NIV reduced dyspnoea more rapidly than oxygen therapy (Nava et al 2013). The greatest benefit was seen after the first hour and in those with hypercapnia.

Practical Issues in the Application of Non-Invasive Ventilation

Interfaces

NIV is only successful if the patient is compliant with therapy and wears the mask. Mask intolerance may account for up to 30% of NIV failures in the acute setting (Antonaglia et al 2011). A variety of interfaces are available for NIV, including nasal masks and pillows, oral masks, oronasal masks, total face masks, helmets and mouthpieces (Fig. 7-43). Advances in mask design have meant a greater degree of comfort and choice for the patient and therapist.

While successful outcomes in acute respiratory failure have been reported with both nasal or oronasal masks (Kwok et al 2003), an oronasal is generally preferred in the acute setting (Crimi et al 2010) to better control mouth leaks and ensure the effective delivery of ventilatory support. However, skin damage and necrosis is not uncommon, especially with oronasal masks. Substantial pressure on the nasal bridge where there is little subcutaneous tissue can impair skin perfusion, create tissue hypoxia and eventually lead to tissue damage. The total face mask was introduced to eliminate pressure over the nasal bridge. Several studies have shown that total face masks and oronasal masks achieve similar improvements in gas exchange and clinical outcomes, although the total face mask tends to be associated with greater intolerance (Cuvelier et al 2009, Ozsancak et al 2011). However, it is a useful alternative for patients developing nasal bridge ulceration, those intolerant of the oronasal mask, or those failing to respond to oronasal mask ventilation. The helmet is a newer interface that encloses the entire head of the patient and is sealed at the neck. Although it can be useful for patients intolerant of other interfaces, changes to settings may be needed to reduce patient–ventilator asynchrony that can arise with this interface (Navalesi et al 2007, Racca et al 2009).

In a daytime study looking at various interfaces in patients with chronic hypercapnic respiratory failure,

the nasal mask was best tolerated, although oronasal and nasal pillow interfaces were associated with significantly lower $PaCO_2$ levels (Navalesi et al 2000). During sleep, oronasal and nasal masks were shown to be equally effective in delivering NIV (Willson et al 2004). With improvements in mask design and comfort, increasing numbers of patients are favouring oronasal masks for home ventilation (Garner et al 2013).

Often overlooked is the impact mask design can have on the effectiveness of ventilatory support. Ventilators designed specifically for non-invasive applications generally operate using a single circuit with an expiratory port placed either within the mask itself or close to the mask at the end of the ventilator circuit. Bench studies have demonstrated that positioning of exhalation vents within the mask generate less CO_2 rebreathing than when the expiratory ports are placed at the mask-circuit connection (Schettino et al 2003).

The choice of interfaces for children and especially infants is far more restricted. Mask fitting can be a particular challenge for those with facial deformity, where skin damage, discomfort or mask leak may limit the willingness of the child or parents to continue with therapy (Ramirez et al 2012). In choosing a mask, it is important to ensure dead space is minimized and sufficient carbon dioxide washout is occurring. Clinicians also need to consider the growth of facial structures in children, with a number of studies reporting maxillary retrusion or facial flattening arising from the long-term use of mask therapy (Fauroux et al 2005, Villa et al 2002). This may resolve to some extent by alternating or changing mask types (Ramirez et al 2012).

Initiating and Monitoring Therapy

After identifying that the patient is suitable for NIV, an appropriate ventilator and interface needs to be chosen and initial settings selected. These choices will be guided by the goals of ventilation for the individual and their clinical presentation.

In the acute setting, IPAP and EPAP settings of 10 cmH_2O and 5 cmH_2O, respectively, are often chosen as initial settings and then adjusted upward to relieve dyspnoea, reduce respiratory rate below 25 bpm, and improve gas exchange. In those with COPD exacerbations, the EPAP is set to counterbalance intrinsic positive end expiratory pressure (PEEP) and improve

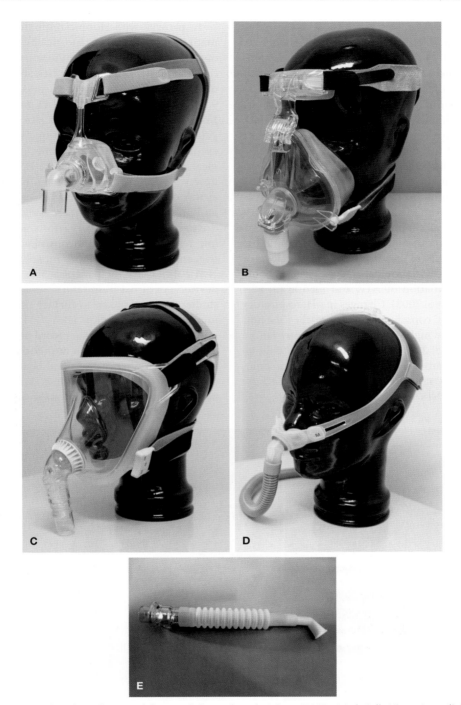

FIGURE 7-43 ■ Examples of interfaces used for NIV. **(A)** Nasal mask: Mirage FX (ResMed, Bella Vista, Australia). **(B)** Oronasal mask: ComfortGel Full Face Mask (Philips Respironics, Murrysville, PA, USA). **(C)** Total face mask: FitLife (Philips Respironics, Murrysville, Penn. USA). **(D)** Nasal pillows: Swift FX (ResMed, Bella Vista, Australia). **(E)** Mouthpiece with Whisper Swivel II expiratory port and tapered silicone tube (Philips Respironics, Murrysville, PA, USA).

inspiratory triggering, with settings of 4–6 cmH$_2$O generally required. Patients with concurrent obesity (Gursel et al 2011) or heart failure and hypercapnia (Bihari & Bersten 2012) may do better with slightly higher EPAP. Adjustments to other settings, such as pressurization time or inspiratory trigger levels, are undertaken to improve synchronization and comfort. For postoperative respiratory failure and cardiogenic pulmonary oedema, CPAP around 10 cmH$_2$O of pressure has generally been used.

Monitoring in the acute setting is crucial to identify early any deterioration in the patient's clinical situation and to uncover any technical problems with NIV so that prompt and appropriate action can be taken. Clinical evaluation should include oxygen saturation, respiratory rate, blood pressure, heart rate and level of consciousness. ABGs should be repeated 1–2 hours following the initiation of NIV, and then again at 4 hours (Roberts et al 2008). Changes in pH, respiratory rate and level of consciousness within the first few hours of NIV are highly predictive of therapy failure (Confalonieri et al 2005). Delays in intubation following NIV failure are associated with poorer outcomes (Esteban et al 2004, Wood et al 1998), highlighting the need to identify NIV non-responders early.

In patients with chronic respiratory failure, acclimatization to the mask and machine can be carried out during the day, with monitoring of oxygen saturation and ideally CO$_2$, either end-tidally or transcutaneously (Fig. 7-44). Again low pressures, commonly IPAP 9–10 cmH$_2$O and EPAP 4 cmH$_2$O, are trialled initially. Inspiratory pressure increases are then based on patient tolerance and saturation, with the aim of eventually achieving tidal volumes of 6–10 mL/kg of ideal body weight (Berry et al 2010). EPAP is adjusted upward to improve triggering and prevent any upper airway obstruction which may appear during sleep. A backup rate is used when there is reduced inspiratory drive and absent inspiratory efforts, an inappropriately low respiratory rate or inconsistency in inspiratory triggering due to respiratory muscle weakness (Berry et al 2010). Once the patient is able to sleep with the device, nocturnal respiratory monitoring or sleep studies are undertaken to further titrate settings and improve synchronization (Box 7-11). Newer devices provide in-built software to record parameters important in acute and long-term monitoring of the patient, including compliance, leaks and tidal volume (Contal et al 2012). Evaluation of these signals can provide useful information about the quality of ventilation and

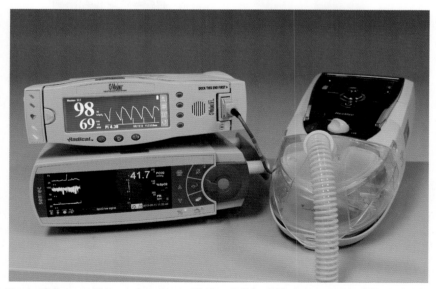

FIGURE 7-44 ■ Monitoring set up for non-invasive ventilation (NIV) trials. Oximeter (top left) and transcutaneous carbon dioxide monitor (bottom left) used to measure the physiological response to non-invasive ventilatory support. An active integrated humidifier (on right side) is attached between the bi-level ventilator and the patient via a single limb tube.

BOX 7-11

STEPS IN INITIATING NON-INVASIVE VENTILATION (NIV) THERAPY FOR HOME VENTILATORY SUPPORT

■ Introduce the patient slowly to the equipment and all its parts.

■ Ensure the mask fits comfortably and that the patient can experience the mask on their face without the ventilator connected.

■ Allow the patient the opportunity to feel the operation of the machine through the mask on their hand or cheek before applying it over their nose or mouth.

■ Permit the patient the opportunity to practice breathing with the ventilator, either holding the mask in place or allowing them to hold it in place before applying the straps.

■ Adjust settings initially for comfort and establish whether the patient can relax comfortably in a sleeping posture.

■ Provide opportunities for the patient to feed back any discomfort or uncertainty with regard to the use of the equipment.

■ Assess and adjust the performance of the ventilator during an afternoon nap to optimize gas exchange and patient comfort.

■ Progress to an overnight monitoring to optimize gas exchange and sleep quality.

BOX 7-12

PHYSIOTHERAPY IN THE MANAGEMENT OF NON-INVASIVE VENTILATION (NIV)

Assessment of the patient with chronic respiratory failure
  Identification of symptoms of sleep-disordered breathing
  Pulmonary function testing including respiratory muscle strength
  Exercise tolerance (e.g. 6-minute walking test, shuttle test)
  Level of dyspnoea during daily activities
  Cough strength
Initiating therapy
  Choice of device and setting
  Acclimatizing the patient to mask and machine
  Education of patient and family regarding therapy
  Monitoring response to therapy
Discharge planning
  Training patient and/or caregivers in the care and operation of equipment
  Development of a home exercise programme
  Need for oxygen or ventilatory support required during activities
  Need for NIV as an adjunct to training
  Assist in the development of emergency care plans
  Training in lung volume recruitment and appropriate airway clearance techniques (if needed)
Follow-up
  Monitoring of the patient's clinical status
  Troubleshooting problems: technical problems versus changes in clinical condition
  Change in ventilator type or set up with disease progression

---

identify potential problems contributing to suboptimal therapy (Rabec et al 2009). Once the patient is discharged home using ventilatory support, a programme of regular review and monitoring clinical status and equipment needs to be arranged (Piper 2010). How often these reviews are scheduled and where will depend on the severity, stage and progression of the patient's disorder, ease of transport, compliance with therapy, response to treatment and comorbid issues (Box 7-12).

Humidification

The high flow rates delivered by NIV can produce drying of the airways, especially in the presence of leak (Richards et al 1996). This can lead to changes in ciliary activity, mucous secretion and increased nasal resistance (Esquinas Rodriguez et al 2011, Wood et al 2000). The need for humidification is influenced by number of factors, including the interface used, the ambient temperature, the degree of leak present and the level of pressure used (Esquinas Rodriguez et al 2011, Holland et al 2007).

In the acute setting, heated humidifiers are preferable to heat moisture exchangers as the latter have been shown to increase dead space and work of breathing (Lellouche et al 2002), producing a higher $PaCO_2$ despite significant increases in minute ventilation (Jaber et al 2002). In a small study of hypercapnic patients undergoing home bi-level ventilation, compliance with therapy, reduction in $PaCO_2$ and side effects were similar with heated humidification and heat moisture exchangers. However, less throat dryness was reported with heated humidification. At study completion, the majority of patients expressed a preference of heated humidifiers for long-term use (Nava et al 2008).

Oxygen Therapy

Supplemental oxygen is commonly required during NIV, especially in the acute setting. With many of the portable NIV-specific ventilators, oxygen is entrained either into the ventilator tubing or into a port on the mask itself. The actual FiO_2 delivered will vary depending on a complex interaction of several factors including the oxygen injection site, ventilator settings, the type of leak port, unintentional leaks and the oxygen flow rate used (Dai et al 2013, Storre et al 2014). In practice, the oxygen flow rate used is adjusted to achieve an oxygen saturation >90%. Portable pulse dose oxygen concentrators should not be used with nocturnal NIV (Lobato et al 2011).

Adverse Effects

A number of complications and adverse side-effects can arise during attempts to establish patients on NIV (Carron et al 2013). For the most part these are minor, with serious complications only rarely encountered. Nevertheless, identifying potential problems arising from NIV and undertaking strategies to minimize or prevent these occurring will improve patient safety.

The most common complications associated with NIV relate to the interface. Pressure areas occur when there is excessive pressure on the skin for a prolonged period. Artificial skin or gel pads applied to the nasal bridge can provide some protection. Changing to a different style of mask or alternating between interfaces to avoid sustained pressure on the same area will also help. Care needs to be taken to use an appropriately fitting mask and not to overtighten the head straps. Air leak from around the mask or through the mouth (with nasal interfaces) is inevitable with NIV. Although ventilators designed for NIV have some leak-compensating capabilities, significant leak can reduce effective ventilation and lead to poorer patient outcomes. In the acute setting, high leak is a major factor generating patient–ventilator asynchrony and discomfort (Vignaux et al 2009), which can lead to reduced tolerance of NIV and subsequently its failure (Carlucci et al 2001). During long-term home ventilation, leak during sleep can cause inadequate ventilatory support and asynchrony, with the latter being associated with poorer nocturnal gas exchange (Fanfulla et al 2007), reduced sleep quality (Guo et al 2007) and worsening morning dyspnoea when NIV is removed (Adler et al 2012).

The more serious complications arising from NIV include aspiration of gastric contents (Kohlenberg et al 2010), abdominal distension, which if severe can compromise respiratory function and render NIV intolerable, and barotrauma. In some disorders such as CF and COPD, subpleural cysts may be present, increasing the possibility of rupture due to or coincident with the use of positive pressure therapy. Patients with DMD have also been reported to have an increased risk of spontaneous pneumothorax (Simonds 2004). Although this risk is small, it is potentially life threatening for a patient with limited respiratory reserve. Clinicians and patients should be aware of the potential for this occurring, promptly investigating any sudden shortness of breath or chest pain.

Airway Clearance and Non-Invasive Ventilation

Respiratory physiotherapists may become involved in the management of patients using NIV in various capacities (Moran et al 2005, Piper & Moran 2006, Simonelli et al 2013, Ward & Horobin 2012, Zuffo et al 2012). This can include assessing patients for NIV, implementing the technique, reviewing patients once established on therapy and troubleshooting problems, or using NIV as an adjunct to other physiotherapy techniques (see Box 7-12).

In the acute setting, one of the most common causes of NIV failure is the inability to clear secretions effectively (Carlucci et al 2001). While there is currently limited published data confirming the efficacy of various ACTs during acute NIV use, the practice is widespread (Moran et al 2005). In a recent Brazilian study, CPAP or bi-level support was used as an adjunct to chest physiotherapy in 19% of intensive care patients with the aim of resolving atelectasis and normalizing lung function (Yamauchi et al 2012). Several small randomized trials in the acute setting have shown that the addition of ACTs such as ACBTs (Inal-Ince et al 2004), PEP (Bellone et al 2002) and IPV (Antonaglia et al 2006) to patients receiving NIV provided some benefits, including reduced length of time NIV was required and length of ICU admission.

NIV may also be used as a stand-alone method to aid in secretion removal, especially in patients who complain of fatigue, who desaturate with chest therapy or who are poorly tolerant of treatment. In patients with CF, the use of NIV during chest physiotherapy sessions has been shown to reduce the adverse effects of reduced respiratory muscle performance and oxygen desaturation that can occur during spontaneous breathing in patients with severe disease (Fauroux et al 1999, Holland et al 2003). For the breathless patient who is unable to lie flat, use of NIV may permit the use of PD positions that would otherwise not be tolerated (Piper et al 1992). In patients with muscle weakness and poor cough, mask ventilation may be used to assist deep breathing and mobilization of secretions, although in these circumstances breath stacking and mechanical insufflation/exsufflation are likely to be more effective (Chatwin et al 2003). Tidal volumes or inspiratory pressure settings may be increased during physiotherapy sessions to aid chest wall expansion and assist the mobilization of secretions (Piper & Moran 2006).

Non-Invasive Ventilation as an Adjunct to Exercise

People with chronic respiratory failure frequently have a ventilatory limitation to exercise. Severe exertional breathlessness limits physical activity and is a significant barrier to achieving an intensity of exercise training that produces physiological and clinical benefits. In some studies of patients with chronic respiratory failure, NIV used at night only has been associated with improvements in daytime exercise endurance and physical activity without the patient undergoing a specific training intervention (Fuschillo et al 2003, Murphy et al 2012, Schonhofer et al 2008, Young et al 2008). In patients with COPD, several randomized trials have shown that the addition of nocturnal NIV to a formal pulmonary rehabilitation programme augments improvements in exercise tolerance and HRQoL achieved with pulmonary rehabilitation alone (Duiverman et al 2008, 2011; Garrod et al 2000). Finally, there is a growing body of literature showing that the use of NIV during exercise training (treadmill or cycling) produces significantly greater improvements in dyspnoea, functional capacity, quality of life and physiological adaptations to physical training than unsupported training or oxygen therapy in patients with COPD and restrictive chest wall disorders (Borel et al 2008, Borghi-Silva et al 2010, Johnson

et al 2002, Toledo et al 2007, van 't Hul et al 2006) (Fig. 7-45).

Possible mechanisms underlying the benefits of NIV as an adjunct to exercise training include respiratory muscle unloading or rest (Kyroussis et al 2000), improved breathing pattern reducing dynamic hyperinflation (Diaz et al 2002, van 't Hul et al 2004) and improved peripheral muscle blood flow (Borghi-Silva et al 2009). Several practical aspects of this technique are crucial in achieving a positive outcome. Patients must be carefully selected, as there is a variable response to NIV-assisted exercise, with only around 50% of individuals improving exercise tolerance (Borel et al 2008, van 't Hul et al 2004). Benefits are most likely to be seen in patients with more severe disease, weaker inspiratory muscles (van 't Hul et al 2004), and more severe obstructive (Bianchi et al 2002) or restrictive (Borel et al 2008) lung mechanics. Therapists also need to consider the performance characteristics of the NIV device used and the settings chosen. The motor of the device must be able to meet the high ventilatory demands of the patient during exercise, with adequate inspiratory triggering and pressurization key characteristics of an appropriate device (Piper & Menadue 2009). While relatively low levels of pressure support (10–15 cmH$_2$O) may be sufficient for some COPD patients during treadmill or cycling training (Johnson et al 2002, van 't Hul et al 2006) and in patients with acute respiratory failure (Menadue et al 2010a), pressure support levels closer to 20–25 cmH$_2$O are often needed for patients with chest wall disorders (Borel et al 2008, Menadue et al 2010b) or during ground walking (Dreher et al 2007, Menadue et al 2009). Acclimatization and a short trial of therapy can help identify those individuals most likely to benefit from NIV-assisted training (Piper & Menadue 2009).

Conclusion

NIV is a technique which is becoming increasingly used to manage both chronic and acute respiratory failure. Evidence for the effectiveness of this technique in a wide range of clinical situations has seen it become an integral part of the respiratory management of patients with respiratory failure. Respiratory physiotherapists need to acquire knowledge and skills in the appropriate use of NIV in order to effectively manage individuals undergoing this therapy.

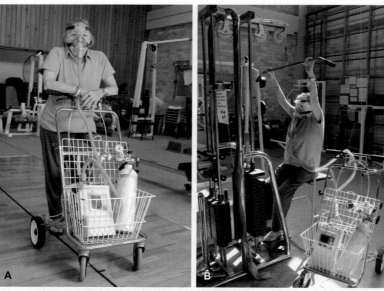

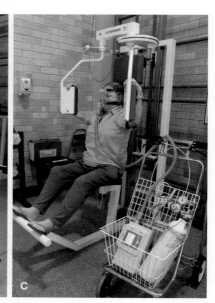

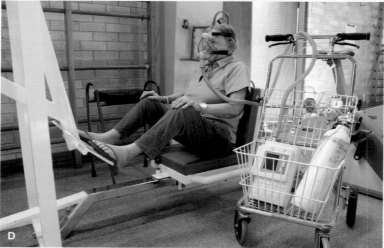

FIGURE 7-45 ■ Patient with severe chronic obstructive pulmonary disease (COPD) and very limited exercise tolerance on oxygen alone shown using non-invasive ventilation (NIV) (with internal battery) during exercise training. The device has been set up in spontaneous mode with supplemental oxygen entrained into the ventilator circuit. The patient is able to exercise at a sufficient intensity to achieve peripheral conditioning. Her circuit training includes: **(A)** Ground walking with rollator trolley. **(B)** Latissimus dorsi pull-down machine. **(C)** Chest butterfly machine and **(D)** Leg press machine.

INCENTIVE SPIROMETRY

Significant upper abdominal and cardiac surgeries have always been associated with an increased risk of PPCs including atelectasis, pleural effusion and pneumonia. Although there is some debate about the defi-

nition of PPC and therefore the perceived incidence of this pathology (Wynne & Botti 2004), there appears to be consensus that they are exacerbated by factors such as internal mammary artery dissection, cardiac bypass and general anaesthesia (Wynne & Botti 2004). The presence of PPCs increases healthcare costs (Pasquina et al 2003) and is negatively linked to hospital length of stay, morbidity and mortality (Haeffener et al 2008). National Cardiovascular Outcomes Research (NICOR 2011) has identified an increasing incidence of cardiac surgery in higher-risk patient groups, and consequently there may be an increased likelihood of PPCs. It therefore remains important to identify effective management strategies.

Historically, a variety of chest physiotherapy techniques have been used with the aim of lowering the risk of PPCs in the post–cardiac surgery population (Brasher et al 2003, Reeve & Ewan 2005). It has been suggested that by using 'therapeutic manoeuvres that increase lung volume' the risk and severity of such complications can be reduced (Restrepo et al 2011). The incentive spirometer has been available since the 1970s in various formats, but the evidence for its benefits remains inconclusive. Despite this, it is a low-cost intervention and continues to be used in many postoperative units in many countries around the world.

The device is activated by the patient's inspiratory effort. When a slow, deep inspiration is performed with the lips sealed around the mouthpiece (Fig. 7-46),

the ongoing inspiration is motivated by visual feedback, for example a ball rising to a pre-set marker. The patient aims to generate a predetermined flow or to achieve a pre-set volume and is encouraged to hold at full inspiration for 2–3 seconds. A short, sharp inspiration can activate the flow-generated incentive spirometry (IS) devices with little increase in tidal volume, but with a volume-dependent device an increase in tidal volume must be achieved before the pre-set level can be reached. The increased work of breathing required should be considered in patients at risk of inspiratory muscle fatigue and in patients with severely impaired respiratory muscle function. Spirometers with a low imposed work of breathing should be considered, if appropriate for these groups, and in some postoperative patients (Weindler & Kiefer 2001).

In 2014, an updated Cochrane review concluded that there was low-quality evidence with respect to effectiveness of IS for prevention of PPCs in patients after upper abdominal surgery (do Nascimento Junior 2014). They included 12 studies with a total of 1834 participants. This review suggested an urgent need to conduct well-designed trials with high methodological

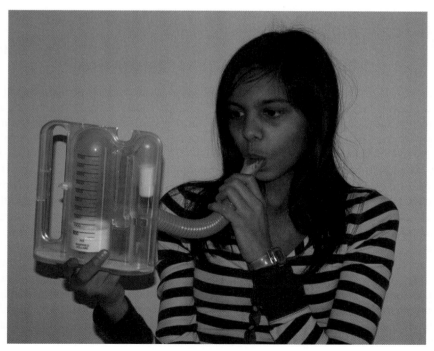

FIGURE 7-46 ■ Using an incentive spirometer (Voldyne).

rigour in this field, in order to define any benefit from the use of IS regarding mortality. Four trials (152 patients) compared the effects of IS with no respiratory treatment. There was no statistically significant difference between the participants receiving IS and those who had no respiratory treatment for clinical complications (relative risk (RR) 0.59, 95% confidence interval (CI) 0.30 to 1.18). Two trials (194 patients) compared IS with DBEs. There were no statistically significant differences between the participants receiving IS and those receiving DBEs in the meta-analysis for respiratory failure (RR 0.67, 95% CI 0.04 to 10.50). Two trials (946 patients) compared IS with other chest physiotherapy. There were no statistically significant differences between the participants receiving IS compared to those receiving physiotherapy in the risk of developing a PPC. There was no evidence that IS is effective in the prevention of pulmonary complications.

Similarly, in 2012 an updated Cochrane review concluded there is no evidence of benefit from IS in reducing pulmonary complications after coronary artery bypass graft (Freitas 2012). This update included 592 participants from seven studies (two new and one that had been excluded in the previous review in 2007). There was no evidence of a difference between groups in the incidence of any pulmonary complications and functional capacity between treatment with IS and treatment with physical therapy, positive pressure breathing techniques (including CPAP, BiPAP and IPPB; ACBTs or preoperative patient education. Patients treated with IS had worse pulmonary function and arterial oxygenation compared with positive pressure breathing. Based on these studies there was no improvement in the muscle strength between groups who received IS demonstrated by maximal inspiratory pressure and maximal expiratory pressure.

Haeffener et al (2008) found that a protocol of IS with the addition of EPAP had a positive effect on respiratory muscle strength, pulmonary function and 6-minute walk test (6MWT) distance at 1-month follow-up. They also found a significant reduction in hospital length of stay and rates of postoperative pneumonia in their intervention group. The sample sizes were small (17 in each group) and did not reach the original recruitment target. Yánez-Brage et al (2009) found that preoperative physiotherapy, including the

provision of an incentive spirometer for those in the intervention group, resulted in a significantly lower incidence of atelectasis. The number needed to treat was five patients to avoid one episode of atelectasis. Their sample size was 263.

A systematic review by Overend et al (2001) examined the use of IS for the prevention of PPCs. The authors concluded that the evidence does not support the use of IS for decreasing the incidence of PPCs following cardiac or upper abdominal surgery. Gosselink et al (2000) undertook a randomized controlled trial to investigate the additional effect of IS to chest physiotherapy in the prevention of PPCs following thoracic surgery for lung and oesophageal resections. The addition of IS to physiotherapy did not further reduce either pulmonary complications or hospital stay. However, a systematic review for the American College of Physicians on strategies to reduce PPCs following non-cardiothoracic surgery (Lawrence et al 2006) concluded that any type of lung expansion intervention is better than no prophylaxis. With significant advances in anaesthesia and surgery (including the increasing use of minimally invasive surgery) early postoperative mobilization may be the treatment of choice for the majority of patients who are able.

MANUAL AND VENTILATOR HYPERINFLATION

The goals of respiratory physiotherapy management in the ICU are to promote secretion clearance, optimize oxygenation, improve lung volume and prevent respiratory complications (Denehy and Berney 2006). Mechanical ventilation results in an increased ventilation–perfusion ($\dot{V}/\dot{Q}$) mismatch; reduction in FRC; reduced surfactant and impaired mucociliary transport. These factors increase the likelihood of developing atelectasis and retaining secretions, leading to an increased risk of developing nosocomial pneumonia (Garrard et al 1995). The techniques of manual or ventilator hyperinflation (VHI) may be indicated to mobilize and assist clearance of excess bronchial secretions and to reinflate areas of lung collapse in the intubated patient.

Manual hyperinflation (MHI) was first described more than half a century ago as a technique involving the delivery of a slow inspiration, an inspiratory pause and then a rapid expiration (Clement & Hübsch 1968). Several studies have examined the effects of MHI on secretion clearance, oxygenation and pulmonary compliance (Berney and Denehy 2002; Berney et al 2004; Choi et al 2005; Hodgson et al 2000; Maa et al 2005; Paratz et al 2002; Patman et al 2000; Savian et al 2006). MHI may improve pulmonary compliance, arterial oxygenation and clearance of airway secretions, and may therefore benefit intubated and mechanically ventilated critically ill patients (Paulus et al 2008).

The technique used for VHI was first described in 2002 (Berney and Denehy 2002). A recent systematic review (Anderson et al 2015) examining the evidence of both MHI and VHI concluded the two techniques have similar effects on secretion clearance, dynamic and static pulmonary compliance and oxygenation, and that neither technique has a detrimental effect on cardiovascular stability. However, there was a high risk of bias evident in the four included studies. Skills training for physiotherapists is important and a manometer in the circuit is very helpful for monitoring airway pressures.

Hyperinflations are indicated to prevent and treat atelectasis, promote the removal of retained secretions and improve pulmonary compliance. The precautions and contraindications are to be found in Box 7-13. Techniques and equipment requirements for each of MHI and VHI are described in the following sections.

Manual Hyperinflation Procedure

The procedure for manual hyperinflation involves disconnecting the patient from the ventilator and attaching a manual resuscitation bag through which a large inspiratory volume (1.5–4 times the baseline tidal volume) is delivered to the patient (McCarren & Chow 1996; Singer 1994) to achieve peak inspiratory pressures of no more than 40 cmH$_2$O (Rothen et al 1993), followed by a rapid unobstructed expiration at a high peak flow rate (Fig. 7-47). The technique involves three components:

Slow even inspiration: This involves an increase in tidal volume over three seconds, resulting in a more laminar gas flow to promote even distribution of ventilation.

Inspiratory pause: A 3-second hold is performed at maximum volume to facilitate recruitment of poorly ventilated alveoli.

BOX 7-13
PRECAUTIONS AND CONTRAINDICATIONS FOR LUNG HYPERINFLATION

Precautions for hyperinflation include:
- Cardiovascular instability requiring high levels of vasopressor/inotropic support
- Presence of an intra-aortic balloon pump
- Presence of extracorporeal membrane oxygenation (ECMO) (Hyperinflation treatment should be discussed with intensive care unit (ICU) consultant prior to treatment.)
- History of obstructive airways disease
- Increased intracranial pressure (ICP) (If a patient with elevated ICP develops pulmonary collapse a discussion with ICU consultant regarding the institution of hyperinflation should occur prior to any treatment being provided.)
- External ventricular drainage (EVD) in situ.

Contraindications for hyperinflation include:
- Patients ventilated on lung protective strategy (i.e. 4–6 mL/kg, 10–15 cmH$_2$O positive end-expiratory pressure (PEEP)); for example, those with acute respiratory distress syndrome (ARDS)
- Severe pneumonia
- Pulmonary contusions
- Undrained pneumothorax
- Acute bronchospasm
- Thoracic surgery with lung resection
- Patients who are ventilated for an exacerbation of obstructive pulmonary disease with prolonged expiration and elevated intrinsic PEEP
- Presence of inflated gastric or oesophageal balloons.

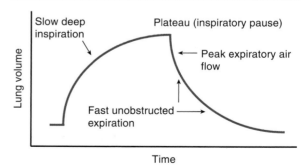

FIGURE 7-47 ▪ Manual hyperinflation (MHI) involves a slow deep inspiration, inspiratory pause and unobstructed expiration. The slow deep inspiration increases tidal volume with the pause to allow filling of alveoli with slow time constants. The rapid, unobstructed expiratory phase enhances mucociliary flow. The technique has been compared to a cough where a deep inspiratory effort is followed by a very rapid expulsive flow of air.

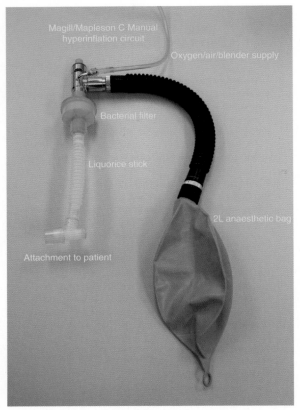

FIGURE 7-48 ■ An example of a manual hyperinflation (MHI) circuit: a Magill circuit with specific parts of the circuit labelled.

Expiratory phase: this is rapid and unobstructed to enhance MCC. Research suggests that the expiratory flow rate needs to exceed inspiratory flow by 10% to aid secretion clearance, with a velocity of more than 1000 cm/sec (referred to as 'two-way gas–liquid flow') (Maxwell and Ellis 2003).

MHI equipment:

- Manual resuscitation bag (e.g. Magill: Mapelson C, Laerdal circuits) (Fig. 7-48)
- Oxygen supply/mixer (to entrain oxygen and also green oxygen tubing)
- Liquorice stick (catheter mount) and bacterial filter
- Infection control measures: apron, gloves, protective eye wear (optional)
- PEEP valve (optional)

MHI technique:

- Position patient to target lung area for treatment.
- Attach circuit to oxygen flow metre and set flow at 10–12 L/min for Mapleson C or 14 L/min for Laerdal.
- Check bagging circuit (expiratory valve completely open, ensure no tears or holes in the bag).
- Explain technique to the patient.
- Disconnect patient from ventilator, attach bagging circuit via the liquorice stick (catheter mount) to the endotracheal tube.
- Allow bag to inflate fully.
- Once the bag is fully inflated, slowly compress the bag, timed to coincide with patient inspiration, over a period of 3 seconds until the bag is fully compressed.
- Maintain compression for 3 seconds.
- Monitor cardiovascular stability throughout.
- Release the expiratory valve quickly (flicking motion) keeping bag compressed with other hand.
- A cough reflex may be triggered (if secretions heard, suction if appropriate).
- Dosage: 6 sets of 6 breaths, head-down tilt if required (Berney et al 2004)
- Reconnect the patient to the ventilator and ensure correct ventilation mode/settings.

VHI technique:

- Position the patient to target lung area for treatment.
- Change ventilator to a volume-controlled mode (pressure-related volume control/synchronized intermittent mandatory ventilation (PRVC SIMV) or synchronized intermittent mandatory ventilation/volume cycled ventilation (SIMV VCV)).
- Change alarm limits, increase tidal volume limit to >2 L.
- Reduce ventilator flow rate to around 20 L/min and rate to 6 breath/min.
- Increase the inspiratory time up to 5 seconds, add a 2-second pause; use a square wave form.
- Gradually increase tidal volume in 200-mL increments to a PIP of 40–45 cmH$_2$O delivering around 6 breaths per minute.

- Monitor cardiovascular stability throughout.
- Suction as appropriate.
- Dosage: 6 sets of 6 breaths (Berney et al 2004)
- Return the patient to both their ventilator settings and alarm settings when finished with VHI.

VHI is generally performed in VCV mode but can also be performed in pressure cycled modes. If hyperinflating in a pressure cycled mode, gradually titrate inspiratory pressure to generate greater tidal volumes and PIP of 40 cmH$_2$O. VHI has been shown to be as effective as MHI for sputum clearance and improving lung compliance (Berney and Denehy 2002). The technique of hyperinflation is often combined with gravity assisted drainage to further enhance MCC (Berney et al 2004).

Despite its less frequent use, VHI has some potential advantages over MHI, largely related to the avoidance of ventilator disconnection. These include maintenance of a PEEP, decreased infection risk and accurate control of ventilation parameters. Patients requiring higher levels of PEEP (>10 cmH$_2$O) may benefit more from VHI than MHI, as disconnecting the patient from the ventilator would cause a drop in PEEP and potential de-recruitment (Hodgson et al 1999). VHI allows constant monitoring and maintenance of airway pressures and flow profiles which is advantageous when gas trapping is of concern.

GLOSSOPHARYNGEAL BREATHING

GPB is a technique useful in patients with a reduced VC resulting from respiratory muscle weakness or paralysis. Although its original use was in rehabilitation of patients with poliomyelitis, it can be invaluable when taught to people with tetraplegia (Alvarez et al 1981, Bach 2012, Bach & Alba 1990, Bianchi et al 2004) and in many people with neuromuscular diseases (Bach 1995, Bach et al 2007, Baydur et al 1990). Another more recent use of GPB is for breath-hold divers to prolong their period of time under water (Lindholm & Nyren 2005, Walterspacher et al 2011).

GPB was first described by Dail (1951) when patients with poliomyelitis were observed to be gulping air into their lungs. It was this gulping action that gave the technique the name 'frog breathing'. GPB is a form of positive pressure ventilation produced by the patient's voluntary muscles where boluses of air are forced into the lungs. It is essential to understand that GPB is *not* swallowing air into the stomach, but gulping air into the lungs.

Paralyzed patients dependent on a mechanical ventilator are sometimes able to use GPB continuously, other than during sleep, to substitute the mechanical ventilation. GPB is very useful in patients who are able to breathe spontaneously, but whose power to cough and clear secretions is inadequate. The technique also enables these patients to shout to attract attention and to help to maintain or improve lung and chest wall compliance (Bach et al 1987, Dail et al 1955). For patients dependent on a ventilator, either noninvasively or via a tracheostomy, GPB can be lifesaving (Bach 1995) in an emergency if the ventilator becomes disconnected or if there should be a power failure, and can increase the feeling of independence (Make et al 1998). The medical uses of GPB are summarized in Box 7-14.

With severe bulbar dysfunction it is not possible to do GPB, but with some weakness of the oropharyngeal muscles it can often be achieved. The technique is contraindicated in patients with obstructive airways disease where the positive pressure could increase air trapping. It is also contraindicated in cardiac failure, where the long inspiratory period with high intrathoracic pressure could decrease venous return, causing a fall in blood pressure.

With GPB the 'breath in' is a series of pumping strokes produced by action of the lips, tongue, soft palate, pharynx and larynx. Air is held in the chest by

---

BOX 7-14
USES OF GLOSSOPHARYNGEAL BREATHING

Where the lungs are normal, but the respiratory muscles are weak or paralysed:
- To produce a more effective cough
  - to avoid chest infections
  - to treat chest infections
  - to assist in weaning from a tracheostomy
- To make the voice louder
- To maintain or improve lung and chest wall compliance
- To be a substitute for mechanical ventilation
- To provide security if ventilator dependent

the larynx, which acts as a valve as the mouth is opened for the next gulp. Expiration occurs by normal elastic recoil of the lungs and ribcage.

Before starting to teach GPB, it may be helpful for the patient to experience the feeling of inflating the chest by using an intermittent positive pressure ventilator with a mouthpiece. After inflating the lungs, the mouthpiece is removed and the patient should try and hold all the air in the lungs with the mouth open, avoiding escape of air through the larynx or nose. A teaching video is available that may help both patient and physiotherapist when learning or teaching GPB (Webber & Higgens 1999).

Each gulp of air is made up of three stages (Box 7-15). The first and most important stage (Box 7-16 and Fig. 7-49A) in learning GPB is the enlargement of the mouth and throat cavity by depressing the tracheal and laryngeal cartilages. The tongue should remain flat with the tip touching the inside of the lower teeth. Using a torch, the physiotherapist should be able to see the uvula when this is correct. The patient may find it helpful to watch the movement in a mirror and possibly by feeling the cartilages with their fingers. An exercise that often helps to initiate movement of the

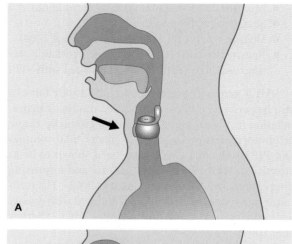

A

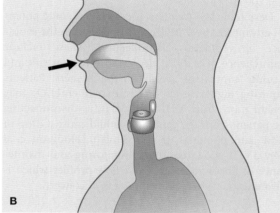

B

BOX 7-15
THREE STAGES FOR EACH GULP IN GLOSSOPHARYNGEAL BREATHING (FIG. 7-49)

A. Enlarge throat cavity.
B. Hold throat open and close lips.
C. Let floor of mouth rise to normal position while air is pumped through larynx.

BOX 7-16
STAGE 1 (FIG. 7-49A)

1. Enlargement of throat cavity
   Depress cartilages
   Tongue flat
   Uvula visible
2. Hold this open position for 3–5 seconds.
3. Progress to starting with closed mouth – open mouth, jaw and throat at the same time – hold open.
4. Take deep breath – hold it – open mouth, jaw and throat.

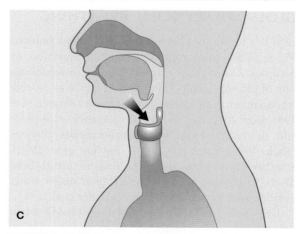

C

FIGURE 7-49 ■ (A, B and C) The stages of glossopharyngeal breathing (GPB). See Box 7.15.

BOX 7-17
STAGE 2 (FIG. 7-49B)

1. With throat open, close lips to trap air in throat.
2. Check that tongue position and open throat are maintained while opening and closing lips. Do not let jaw rise.

BOX 7-18
STAGE 3 (FIG. 7-49C)

After opening throat (stage 1) and trapping air with lips (stage 2):
   Let floor of mouth, tongue and cartilages rise to the normal position while air is pumped through the larynx.

cartilages is for the physiotherapist to place a finger horizontally under the chin back against the trachea and give pressure in an upwards direction resisting downward movement of the base of the tongue. To emphasize the downward cartilage movement, practice should progress to holding the throat in this open position for 3–5 seconds.

When this movement has been achieved, stages 2 and 3 are added to complete the cycle (Box 7-17 and Fig. 7-49B, Box 7-18 and Fig. 7-49C). The cycle should be practised slowly at first and then gradually speeded up until the movement flows. It is important to avoid stages 2 and 3 being done simultaneously. The air has to be trapped in the throat in stage 2 before the jaw and cartilages are allowed to rise in stage 3. It is *essential* to maintain the lowered jaw during stage 2.

The next stage is to take a maximum breath in and, while holding this breath, to add several glossopharyngeal gulps, to augment the VC. A 'normal' breath must *not* be taken before each gulp.

When correct, the patient will feel the chest filling with air and the physiotherapist can test the 'GPB VC' by putting a mouthpiece attached to the expiratory limb of a Wright respirometer (Mark 8 or 14) in the patient's mouth before exhalation.

The respirometer can be used to measure the volume per gulp. VC is measured, then VC + 5 or 10 gulps. The VC is subtracted from the total VC + gulps and this volume is divided by the number of gulps to give the average volume per gulp. The patient will require less effort and reach maximum capacity more quickly if a large volume gulp is achieved. The volume per gulp is directly related to the amount of downward movement of the cartilages. A study by Kelleher & Parida (1957) reported a group of patients in whom the average volume per gulp varied from 25 to 120 mL and when teaching GPB an attempt should be made to achieve at least 80 mL per gulp. Peak cough flow (PCF) is sometimes used to assess GPB, a measurement being made at VC and then another measurement after VC + gulps. This gives an indication of effectiveness of the gulps taken, but the measurement of volumes is more useful.

If GPB were being used continuously as a substitute for normal tidal breathing, approximately 6–8 gulps would be taken before breathing out. When used for clearance of secretions, 10–25 gulps may be required to obtain a maximal VC. Volumes of 2.5–3.0 L can be achieved and the expiratory flow produced is sufficient to mobilize secretions (Make et al 1998).

GPB would normally be taught with the patient in a comfortable sitting position, but for patients following cervical spinal cord injury, a supine position would be more appropriate, in that their FVC is significantly greater in this position than in the sitting position (Baydur et al 2001, Ben-Dov et al 2009). It will reduce the added difficulties of orthostatic/postural hypotension while trying to learn GPB. When mastered by any patient, GPB should be practised in positions useful to clear bronchial secretions. After filling the chest to capacity, the patient signals to the physiotherapist, who compresses the chest as the air is let out. The patient may have sufficient muscle power to apply compression, or carers can be taught to give assistance.

GPB is learnt easily by some patients, but others need time and patience to acquire this skill. Although frequent self-practice can be helpful in the learning stages, it is recommended to ensure correct opening of the throat (stage 1) before letting the patient proceed to stages 2 and 3. It can be tiring to learn GPB and therefore short frequent sessions are most effective. Once learnt, it is *not* tiring to use the technique.

There are reasons why a person may fail to achieve GPB initially. The soft palate may not be closing, so air passes out through the nose instead of into the trachea. This can often be corrected by asking the patient to take several gulps while the nose is alternately pinched

BOX 7-19
STAGES WITH NASAL
GLOSSOPHARYNGEAL BREATHING

1. Take a deep breath through the nose, flaring the nostrils, and hold the air in the lungs.
2. Depress cartilages and tongue and try to flare nostrils at the same time.
3. Let cartilages rise to normal position as air is forced through the larynx.
4. Repeat 2 and 3 until lungs are full.

closed for two gulps and released for two gulps. When the nose is held closed, the patient will feel pressure inside the mouth and throat and possibly in the ears. GPB should then be repeated without the nose being pinched and the patient should attempt to reproduce the same feeling of pressure with every gulp. Occasionally patients have very poor soft palate control and will need to wear a nose clip. Exercises to improve soft palate control may be helpful.

A few patients who find it difficult to stop air leaking through the nose achieve GPB by taking the gulps through the nose while keeping the mouth shut. Other people prefer to do nasal GPB, as it is less obtrusive and the gulps of air have more humidification from the nasal mucosa. It is important initially to teach the stages using the mouth technique in order to observe the tongue position. The stages for nasal GPB are shown in Box 7-19.

Another problem that may be found during the learning stages of GPB is weakness of the vocal cords. If the cords are unable to hold the air in the lungs, the VC is decreased after attempting some gulps. This can be tested by asking the patient to take a very deep breath using intermittent positive pressure by mouthpiece and then, with the mouthpiece removed, he should say 'ah, ah, ah…' in short staccato bursts during expiration. If all the 'ahs' run into a continuous sound, the cords are failing to shut off the flow of air under pressure. To strengthen the cords, the patient can start to take a volume of air just greater than his VC and practise the 'ah, ah' sounds. When this is achieved, the volume of air can be gradually increased and the expiration exercises repeated.

GPB is a valuable technique to consider when treating tetraplegics with a VC of less than 2 L. Instruction can begin when the patient has reached a stable condition, but it is inappropriate in the acute phase or during an acute chest infection. When successfully learnt, it is invaluable during a period of chest infection to assist in the clearance of secretions, and even more so if combined with other techniques such as manual assisted coughs. A study of patients with cervical spinal cord injuries (C4–C8) demonstrated that 20 of 25 patients could do GPB successfully, improving lung function and chest expansion (Nygren-Bonnier et al 2009b). If a high-level spinal cord injury is managed with non-invasive IPPV (NIV), GPB can be taught and provides security in case of ventilator failure (Bach 2012).

In patients with Duchenne muscular dystrophy (DMD) and other neuromuscular diseases it would often be easiest to teach GPB as a 'normal' part of treatment, before deterioration in respiratory muscle function and difficulty in clearing secretions occur. If it is taught to boys with DMD around the age of 10–12 years it can be used when the first problems of chest infection arise. Patients who have not been taught have undergone tracheotomy for respiratory failure which could have been avoided using GPB (Bach et al 2007). This is true of any of the progressive neuromuscular conditions that inevitably end up in respiratory failure due to weakening respiratory musculature and function. Patients with DMD often learn to do GPB by copying other patients, but it is important for the physiotherapist to assess and enhance their technique using spirometry and teaching effective assisted coughing prior to the occurrence of an emergency situation.

A study was undertaken to evaluate if children with spinal muscular atrophy (SMA) type II would be able to learn GPB. Five of 11 children were able to learn the technique and four showed improvements in lung function and chest expansion (Nygren-Bonnier et al 2009a).

GPB has been of benefit to patients with motor neurone disease (Bereiter 2001) by making the voice more audible and providing an effective cough. In multiple sclerosis, GPB has achieved improvement in speech, respiratory function and more effective clearance of secretions (Aldridge 2005, Johansson et al 2012).

It is possible to teach GPB to patients with an uncuffed tracheostomy tube if there is a dressing providing an effective seal around the tube to avoid air leaks and some form of plug to the tube. A one-way valve, for example a Passy–Muir valve, fitted between the tracheostomy tube and the ventilator tubing acts as a plug, preventing air from escaping into the ventilator tubing, but allowing it to enter the lungs. If a ventilator-dependent patient has a one-way valve in situ and can do GPB, it gives a great sense of security should a ventilator tube become kinked or disconnected. Before starting to learn GPB, it is essential that patients who are entirely ventilator-dependent learn to use intermittent positive pressure by mouthpiece. It gives them a reliable respiratory support during the learning stages. While increasing the period of time using GPB, it is important to ensure that normal blood gases are maintained. Patients usually take 6–8 gulps per breath, 10–12 times per minute, to provide a normal minute volume. When learning to build up their endurance they may experience a sense of desperate need for air, but by taking a larger number of gulps (perhaps 20 or 25) at high speed, this feeling can be relieved and the normal pattern resumed.

To learn GPB requires commitment from both patient and physiotherapist and, if taught as an outpatient, tuition sessions at least weekly are recommended to maintain motivation. Filming the patient on video to give visual feedback is sometimes a useful teaching tool. GPB can be a much more versatile breathing technique than using a mechanical insufflator/exsufflator. It requires no equipment and in addition to making coughing more effective, for many patients it gives confidence when away from the home ventilator allowing greater independence and improved quality of life. When a patient learns the technique successfully the physiotherapist gains confidence and sees the benefits it can give. Bach (1992) wrote that although potentially extremely useful, GPB is rarely used because there are few healthcare professionals familiar with the technique. Many patients would benefit if physiotherapists familiarized themselves with the technique and included it as a treatment option when indicated. The guidelines for physiotherapy management of the neuromuscular patient suggest including GPB more widely in their rehabilitation plan (BTS/ACPRC 2009).

Acknowledgments

Barbara Webber would like to thank two physiotherapists for their helpful advice: Michelle Chatwin and Sophie Nawarski.

Techniques for Improving Gas Exchange

POSITIONING AND MOBILIZATION

Optimal cardiopulmonary function and gas exchange reflect the optimal matching of oxygen demand and supply (Dantzker 1983, Weber et al 1983). Oxygen delivery and oxygen consumption based on demand are essential components of the oxygen transport system. The components of oxygen delivery ($\dot{D}O_2$) are arterial oxygen content and cardiac output (CO), and the components of oxygen consumption ($\dot{V}O_2$) are the arteriovenous oxygen content difference and CO. In health, $\dot{D}O_2$ is approximately four times greater than $\dot{V}O_2$ at rest, so there is considerable oxygen reserve that is drawn upon during times of increased metabolic demand such as exercise, stress, illness and repair. Because of the large reserve, $\dot{V}O_2$ is thought to be normally supply-independent. This reserve capacity, however, becomes compromised secondary to acute and chronic pathological conditions. In patients who are critically ill with $\dot{D}O_2$ severely compromised, $\dot{V}O_2$ may be supply-dependent until $\dot{D}O_2$ reaches a critical threshold, i.e. the level at which metabolic demands are met (Phang & Russell 1993). Below this critical threshold, patients are increasingly dependent on anaerobic metabolism reflected by increased minute ventilation, respiratory exchange ratio and serum lactate levels.

The efficiency with which oxygen is transported from the atmosphere along the steps of the oxygen transport pathway to the tissues determines the efficiency of oxygen transport overall (Fig. 7-50). The steps in the oxygen transport pathway include ventilation of the alveoli, diffusion of oxygen across the alveolar capillary membrane, perfusion of the lungs, biochemical reaction of oxygen with the blood, affinity

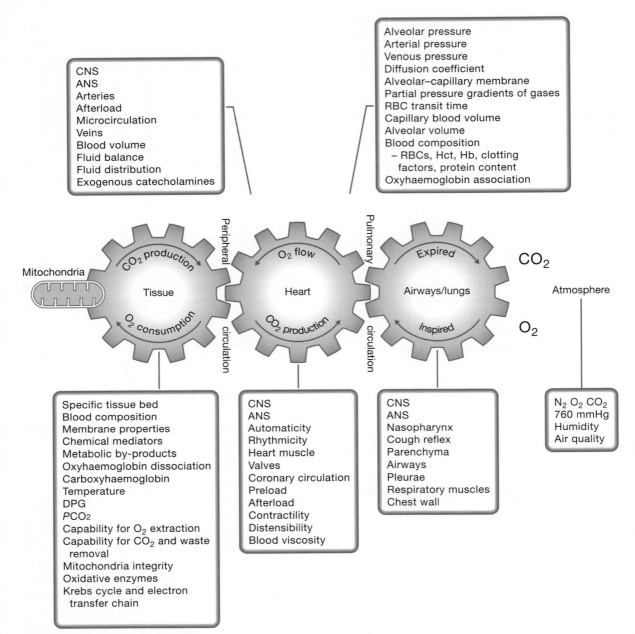

FIGURE 7-50 ■ A scheme of the components of ventilatory–cardiovascular–metabolic coupling underlying oxygen transport. *ANS*, Autonomic nervous system; *CNS*, central nervous system; *CO₂*, carbon dioxide; *DPG*, diphosphoglycerate; *Hct*, haematocrit; *Hb*, haemoglobin; *N₂*, nitrogen; *O₂*, oxygen; *PCO₂*, pressure of carbon dioxide; *RBC*, red blood cell. *(Modified from Wasserman et al 1987).*

of oxygen with haemoglobin, CO, integrity of the peripheral circulation and oxygen extraction at the tissue level critical (Wasserman et al 1987). At rest, the demand for oxygen reflects basal metabolic requirements. Metabolic demand changes normally in response to gravitational (positional), exercise and psychological stressors. When one or more steps in the oxygen transport pathway are impaired secondary to cardiopulmonary dysfunction, oxygen demand at rest and in response to stressors can be increased significantly. Impairment of one step in the pathway may be compensated by other steps, thereby maintaining normal gas exchange and arterial oxygenation. With severe impairment involving several steps, arterial oxygenation may be reduced, the work of the heart and lungs increased, tissue oxygenation impaired and, in the most extreme situation, multiorgan system failure may ensue.

While the oxygen transport pathway ensures that an adequate supply of oxygen meets the demands of the working tissues, the carbon dioxide pathway ensures that carbon dioxide, a primary by-product of metabolism, is eliminated. This pathway is basically the reverse of the oxygen transport pathway in that carbon dioxide is transported from the tissues, via the circulation, to the lungs for elimination. Carbon dioxide is a highly diffusible gas and is readily eliminated from the body. However, carbon dioxide retention is a hallmark of diseases in which the ventilatory muscle pump is operating inefficiently or the normal elastic recoil of the lung parenchyma is lost.

Cardiopulmonary dysfunction, in which oxygen transport is threatened or impaired, results from four principal factors:

- the underlying disease pathophysiology
- bed rest/recumbency and restricted mobility
- extrinsic factors imposed by the patient's medical care
- intrinsic factors relating to the patient (Box 7-20) (Dean 1994a, Dean & Ross 1992a).

An analysis of the factors that contribute to cardiopulmonary dysfunction provides the basis for assessment and prescribing the parameters of positioning and mobilization to enhance oxygen transport for a given patient. In some cases, e.g. low haemoglobin, the

---

BOX 7-20

FACTORS CONTRIBUTING TO CARDIOPULMONARY DYSFUNCTION, I.E. FACTORS THAT COMPROMISE OR THREATEN OXYGEN TRANSPORT

- *Cardiopulmonary pathophysiology*
  Acute
  Chronic
    Primary
    Secondary
  Acute and chronic
  Bed rest/recumbency and restricted mobility
- *Extrinsic factors*
  Reduced arousal
  Surgical procedures
  Incisions
  Dressings and bindings
  Casts/splinting devices/traction
  Invasive lines/catheters
  Monitoring equipment
  Medications
  Intubation
  Mechanical ventilation
  Suctioning
  Pain

Anxiety
Hospital admission
- *Intrinsic factors*
  Age
  Gender
  Ethnicity
  Congenital abnormalities
  Smoking history
  Occupation
  Air quality
  Obesity
  Nutritional deficits
  Deformity
  Fluid and electrolyte balance
  Conditioning level
  Impaired immunity
  Anaemia/polycythaemia
  Thyroid abnormalities
  Multisystem complications
  Previous medical and surgical history

Adapted from Dean 1993, Dean and Ross 1992a and Ross and Dean 1992.

underlying impairment of oxygen transport cannot be affected directly by physical intervention. However, mobilization and exercise can improve aerobic capacity in patients with anaemia, a factor not directly modifiable by physiotherapy interventions, by increasing the efficiency of other steps in the oxygen transport pathway (Williams 1995). Further, even though some factors are not directly modifiable by physiotherapy interventions, they influence treatment outcome and thus need to be considered when planning, modifying and progressing treatment. Fluid imbalance, for example, is the result of many factors, including reduced muscle activity (Koomans & Boer 1997). Physiotherapy that incorporates body position and exercise challenges may have a profound effect on fluid balance by maintaining fluid balance between the intravascular and extravascular compartments.

Ageing and weight deserve special consideration. Patients who are older have progressively lower lung function, and oxygen transport reserve capacity overall (Rossi et al 1996). These changes predispose this population to complications. In addition, obesity often complicates the clinical picture of patients: the heavier the patient, the greater the risk. Body positioning and mobilization are particularly important in offsetting the deleterious effects of being recumbent with the added physical burden of adipose tissue surrounding the chest wall (Beck 1998).

In children, positioning may be used to optimize respiratory function. The supine position has been shown to be the least beneficial, while prone positioning has been shown to improve respiratory function, decrease GOR (Blumenthal & Lealman 1982) and reduce energy expenditure (Brackbill et al 1973). It is often used in closely monitored infants with respiratory problems in a hospital setting (Casadro-Flores et al 2002), but parents should be advised against using this position when babies are sleeping unattended because of its association with sudden infant death (Southall & Samuels 1992).

Patterns of regional ventilation in infants differ significantly from adults (Davies et al 1985), with ventilation in infants and small children being preferentially distributed to the uppermost regions of the lungs. In acutely ill children with unilateral lung disease, care should be taken if positioning the child with the affected lung uppermost, as this may cause rapid deterioration of respiratory status. Spontaneously breathing newborn infants are better oxygenated when tilted slightly head up (Thoresen et al 1988) and show a drop in PaO_2 if placed flat or tilted head down.

It is suggested that the redistribution of ventilation, which occurs with a change in body position, results in optimized ventilation to specific lung regions and localized improvement in airway patency. This may result in enhanced secretion clearance from these regions, which are not necessarily those positioned in such a way to allow gravitational drainage (Lannefors & Wollmer 1992).

To Improve Oxygen Transport in Acute Cardiopulmonary Dysfunction

Positioning and mobilization have profound acute effects on cardiovascular and cardiopulmonary function and hence on the up-regulation of oxygen transport capacity (Table 7-3). These effects translate into improved gas exchange overall and reductions in the fraction of inspired oxygen, pharmacological and ventilatory support (Burns & Jones 1975; Dean 2006b, 2006c; Svanberg 1957). Mobilization and exercise are the most potent interventions to optimize oxygen transport and aerobic capacity. Patients decondition rapidly when gravitational and exercise stressors are removed. It is particularly important to offset these effects in patients with a history of prolonged debility before admission, and elderly patients (Sevransky & Haponik 2003). Failure to extubate is associated with prolonged hospital stay and, in turn, healthcare cost (Seymour et al 2004).

This may be particularly important for patients with neuromuscular conditions who are weak and at high risk of aspiration (Vianello et al 2000). While the objective of optimizing conditioning may initially appear a premature priority given the status of patients who are severely ill in the ICU, cough strength that can be correlated to general body strength, or the converse, a weak cough related to general debility, can be predictive of extubation outcome (Khamiees et al 2001). Being able to tolerate a spontaneous breathing trial is key to eventual weaning. Furthermore, maintaining spontaneous breathing may help minimize sedation and improve cardiopulmonary function in some patients; for example, patients with acute lung injury and receiving airway pressure-released ventilation

TABLE 7-3
Acute Effects of Upright Positioning and Mobilization on Oxygen Transport

Systemic Response	STIMULUS	
	Positioning (Supine to Upright)	Mobilization
Cardiopulmonary	↑ Total lung capacity	↑ Alveolar ventilation
	↑ Tidal volume	↑ Tidal volume
	↑ Vital capacity	↑ Breathing frequency
	↑ Functioning residual capacity	↑ A–aO_2 gradient
	↑ Residual volume	↑ Pulmonary arteriovenous shunt
	↑ Expiratory reserve volume	↓ V̇/Q̇ matching
	↑ Forced expiratory volume	↑ Distension and recruitment of lung units with low ventilation
	↑ Forced expiratory flow	and low perfusion
	↑ Lung compliance	↑ Mobilization of secretions
	↓ Airway resistance	↑ Pulmonary lymphatic drainage
	↓ Airway closure	↑ Surfactant production and distribution
	↑ PaO_2	
	↑ AP diameter of chest	
	↓ Lateral diameter of ribcage and abdomen	
	Altered pulmonary blood flow distribution	
	↓ Work of breathing	
	↑ Diaphragmatic excursion	
	↑ Mobilization of secretions	
Cardiovascular	↑ Total blood volume	↑ Cardiac output
	↓ Central blood volume	↑ Stroke volume and heart rate
	↓ Central venous pressure	↑ Oxygen binding in blood
	↓ Pulmonary vascular congestion	↑ Oxygen dissociation and extraction at the tissue level
	↑ Lymphatic drainage	
	↓ Work of the heart	

Adapted from Dean and Ross (1992a) and Imle and Klemic (1989).

AP, Anteroposterior; A–aO_2, alveolar–arterial oxygen gradient; PaO_2, partial pressure of oxygen in arterial blood; V̇/Q̇, alveolar-ventilation perfusion; ↓, decreases; ↑, increases.

(Putensen et al 2001). Weaning needs to be tailored to each patient and should not be unnecessarily prolonged (Nevins & Epstein 2001).

Positioning

The distributions of ventilation (V̇), perfusion (Q̇) and ventilation and perfusion matching in the lungs are primarily influenced by gravity and therefore body position (Clauss et al 1968; West 1962, 1977). The goal is to reduce closing volume and optimize FRC (Manning et al 1999). The intrapleural pressure becomes less negative down the upright lung. Thus the apices have a greater initial volume and reduced compliance compared with the bases. Because the bases are more compliant in this position, they exhibit greater volume changes during ventilation. In addition to these gravity-dependent inter-regional differences in lung volume, ventilation is influenced by intraregional differences, which are dependent on regional mechanical differences in the compliance of the lung parenchyma and the resistance to airflow in the airways. Perfusion increases down the upright lung such that the V̇/Q̇ ratio in the apices is disproportionately high compared with that in the bases. Ventilation and perfusion matching is optimal in the mid-lung region. Manipulating body position alters both inter-regional and intra-regional determinants of ventilation and perfusion and their matching.

Although the negative effects of the supine position have been well documented for several decades (Dean & Ross 1992b, Dripps & Waters 1941), supine or recumbent positions are frequently assumed by patients in hospital. These positions are associated with significant reductions in lung volumes and flow rates and increased work of breathing (Craig et al 1971, Hsu & Hickey 1976). The decrease in FRC contributes to closure of the dependent airways and reduced arterial oxygenation (Ray et al 1974). This effect has long been known to be accentuated in older persons (Leblanc et al 1970), patients with cardiopulmonary disease (Fowler 1949), patients with abdominal pathology, smokers and individuals who are obese.

The haemodynamic consequences of the supine position are also remarkable. The gravity-dependent increase in central blood volume may precipitate vascular congestion, reduced compliance and pulmonary oedema (Blomqvist & Stone 1983, Sjostrand 1951). The commensurate increase in stroke volume increases the work of the heart (Levine & Lown 1952). Within 6 hours, a compensatory diuresis can lead to a loss of circulating blood volume and orthostatic intolerance, i.e. haemodynamic intolerance to the upright position. Bed rest deconditioning has been attributed to this reduction in blood volume and the impairment of the volume-regulating mechanisms rather than physical deconditioning per se (Hahn-Winslow 1985). Thus the upright position is essential to maximize lung volumes and flow rates and this position is the only means of optimizing fluid shifts such that the circulating blood volume and the volume-regulating mechanisms are maintained. The upright position coupled with movement is necessary to promote normal fluid regulation and balance (Lamb et al 1964). The upright position is a potent stimulus to the sympathetic nervous system. This is an important clinical effect, which offsets impaired blood volume and pressure-regulating mechanisms secondary to recumbency (Hahn-Winslow 1985).

Side-to-side positioning is frequently used in the clinical setting. Adult patients with unilateral lung disease may derive greater benefit when the affected lung is uppermost (Remolina et al 1981). Markedly improved gas exchange without deleterious haemodynamic effects has been reported for patients with severe hypoxaemia secondary to pneumonia (Dreyfuss et al 1992). Arterial oxygen tension is increased secondary to improved ventilation of the unaffected lung when this lung is dependent, in the adult patient. Patients with uniformly distributed bilateral lung disease may derive greater benefit when the right lung is lowermost (Zack et al 1974). In this case, arterial oxygen tension is increased secondary to improved ventilation of the right lung, which may reflect the increased size of the right lung compared with the left and that, in this position, the heart and adjacent lung tissue are subjected to less compression.

The prone position has long been known to have considerable physiological justification in patients with cardiopulmonary compromise (Douglas et al 1977), even those who are critically ill with acute respiratory failure (Bittner et al 1996, Chatte et al 1997, Mure et al 1997), those with acute respiratory distress syndrome (Vollman 2004), and patients with trauma-induced adult respiratory distress syndrome (Fridrich et al 1996). The beneficial effects of the prone position on arterial oxygenation may reflect improved lung compliance secondary to stabilization of the anterior chest wall, tidal ventilation, diaphragmatic excursion, FRC and reduced airway closure (Dean 1985, Pelosi et al 1998).

The response to prone positioning may differ; for example, in early adult respiratory distress syndrome the effect of prone positioning may depend on whether the primary insult is of a pulmonary or non-pulmonary nature (Lim et al 2001). The benefits of the prone position in respiratory distress syndrome have been reported to be additive to invasive medical interventions (Jolliet et al 1997).

Mobilization

Physiological and Scientific Rationale. The negative effects of recumbency during critical illness, combined with the patient's life-threatening pathology, are compounded by progressive deconditioning (Allen et al 1999, Chuley et al 1982). Thus a whole-body rehabilitation approach warrants being considered from the start (Martin et al 2005) to prevent as well as address recumbency and deconditioning effects and their compounded effects on the patient's other problems.

The acute response to mobilization/exercise reflects a commensurate increase in oxygen transport to provide oxygen to the working muscles and other organs. The increase is dependent on the intensity of the mobilization/exercise stimulus. The demand for oxygen and oxygen consumption increases as exercise continues, with commensurate increases in minute ventilation ($\dot{V}_E$), that is, the amount of air inhaled per minute, CO and oxygen extraction at the tissue level. Relatively low intensities of mobilization can have a direct and profound effect on oxygen transport in patients with acute cardiopulmonary dysfunction (Dean 2006a, Dull & Dull 1983, Lewis 1980) and need to be instituted early after the initial pathological insult or surgery (Orlava 1959, Wenger 1982). The resulting exercise hyperpnoea, the increase in $\dot{V}_E$, is effected by an increase in tidal volume and breathing frequency (Zafiropoulos et al 2004). In addition, ventilation and perfusion matching is augmented by the distension and recruitment of lung zones with low ventilation and low perfusion. Spontaneous exercise-induced deep breaths are associated with improved flow rates and mobilization of pulmonary secretions (Wolff et al 1977). When mobilization is performed in the upright position, the anteroposterior diameter of the chest wall assumes a normal configuration compared with the recumbent position in which the anteroposterior diameter is reduced and the transverse diameter is increased. In addition, diaphragmatic excursion is favoured, flow rates are augmented and coughing is mechanically facilitated. The work of breathing may be reduced with caudal displacement of the diaphragm and the work of the heart is minimized by the displacement of fluid away from the central circulation to the legs.

With respect to cardiovascular effects, acute mobilization/exercise increases CO by increasing stroke volume and heart rate. This is associated with increased blood pressure and increased coronary and peripheral muscle perfusion. Despite their energetic demands, mobilization and exercise may augment outcomes even in acute respiratory failure (Wong 2000, 2004), and in patients requiring left ventricular assist devices (Perme 2006).

Passive movement of the limbs may stimulate deep breaths and heart function; however, this effect is considered minimal compared with active movement (West & Luks 2015). In addition, there is little scientific evidence to support any additional benefit from various facilitation techniques (Bethune 1975).

To promote adaptation of the steps in the oxygen transport pathway to the stimulation of mobilization in patients who are acutely ill, the stimulus is administered in a comparable manner to that in an exercise programme prescribed for patients with chronic cardiopulmonary dysfunction and who are medically stable. The components include a pre-exercise period, a warm-up period, a steady-state period, a cool-down period and a recovery period (Blair et al 2005). These components optimize the response to exercise by preparing the cardiopulmonary and cardiovascular systems for steady-state exercise and by permitting these systems to reestablish resting conditions following exercise. The cool-down period, in conjunction with the recovery period, ensures that exercise does not stop abruptly, and allows for biochemical degradation and removal of the by-products of metabolism.

Ongoing monitoring is essential given that subjecting patients to mobilization/exercise stimulation is inherently risky, particularly for patients with cardiopulmonary dysfunction. Indices of overall oxygen transport in addition to indices of the function of the individual steps in the oxygen transport pathway provide a detailed profile of the patient's cardiopulmonary status. Minimally, in the general ward setting, measures of breathing frequency, ABGs, arterial saturation, heart rate, blood pressure and clinical observation provide the basis for ongoing assessment, mobilization/exercise and progression.

A fundamental requirement in defining the parameters for mobilization is that the patient's oxygen transport system is capable of increasing the oxygen supply to meet an increasing metabolic demand. If not, mobilization is absolutely contraindicated and the treatment of choice to optimize oxygen transport is body positioning. However, in the case of a patient being severely haemodynamically unstable or at risk of being so, for example hypotensive or on a high FiO_2, even the stress of positioning may be excessive. Fluctuations in blood gases should correct with appropriate treatment pacing and the provision of supplemental oxygen during treatment. However, if the PaO_2/FiO_2 remains below 250, or the alveolar–arterial (A–a) gradient remains widened, these signs may portend deterioration including acute renal failure (Chawla et al 2005). Acute renal failure is associated with a high mortality rate (Ympa et al 2005). There are some instances where a patient cannot be moved, for example with an open chest, with intra-aortic balloon pumps, on neuromuscular blockade, or hypotensive.

Mechanically adjustable bedside chairs and stretcher chairs constitute an important advance. These chairs adjust to a flat horizontal surface that can be matched to bed height and positioned beneath the patient lying on the bed. Although these beds have potential cardio-pulmonary benefit (Powers & Daniels 2004), they do not replace active positioning and movement.

Kinetic beds have a place in the management of some patients. Patients who are immobile because of induced coma or marked haemodynamic instability may benefit. Patients with multiple injuries have also been shown to benefit substantially from the continual movement of kinetic beds (Stiletto et al 2000).

To Improve Oxygen Transport in Post-Acute and Chronic Cardiopulmonary Dysfunction

Physiological and Scientific Rationale

Although the physiological responses to long-term exercise in patients with chronic cardiopulmonary disease may differ from those in healthy persons, patients can significantly improve their functional work capacity (Table 7-4). In healthy people, an improvement in aerobic capacity reflects improved efficiency of the steps in the oxygen transport pathway to adapt to the increased oxygen demands imposed by exercise stress. This adaptation is effected by both central (cardiopulmonary) and peripheral (at the tissue level) changes (Dean 2006b, Wasserman & Whipp 1975). Such aerobic conditioning is charac-terized by a training-induced bradycardia secondary to an increased stroke volume and increased oxygen extraction capacity of the working muscle. These adaptation or training responses result in an increased maximal oxygen uptake and maximal voluntary ven-tilation and reduced submaximal $\dot{V}_E$, CO, heart rate, blood pressure and perceived exertion. However, patients with chronic lung disease are often unable to exercise at the intensity required to elicit an aerobic training response. Their functional work capacity may be improved by other mechanisms, for example

TABLE 7-4	
Chronic Effects of Mobilization/Exercise on Oxygen Transport	
Systemic Response	**Effect**
Cardiopulmonary	↑ Capacity for gas exchange
	↑ Cardiopulmonary efficiency
	↓ Submaximal minute ventilation
	↓ Work of breathing
Cardiovascular	Exercise-induced bradycardia
	↑ Maximum $\dot{V}O_2$
	↓ Submaximal heart rate, blood pressure, myocardial oxygen demand, stroke volume, cardiac output
	↓ Work of the heart
	↓ Perceived exertion
	↑ Plasma volume
	Cardiac hypertrophy
	↑ Vascularity of the myocardium
Tissue level	↑ Vascularity of working muscle
	↑ Myoglobin content and oxidative enzymes in muscle
	↑ Oxygen extraction capacity

↓, Decreases; ↑, increases; $\dot{V}O_2$, oxygen consumption.

desensitization to breathlessness, improved motiva-tion, improved biomechanical efficiency, increased ventilatory muscle strength and endurance or some combination (Belman & Wasserman 1981, Bernard et al 1999). Aerobic capacity can be increased through peripheral adaptations (Gosselin et al 2003), but peripheral myopathies in patients with primary lung and heart disease have been reported (Storer 2001).

Patients with chronic heart disease, such as those with severe infarcts, may be able to train aerobically; however, training adaptation primarily results from peripheral rather than central factors commensurate with the level of impairment (Bydgman & Wahren 1974; Larsen et al 2001, 2002).

Planning an Exercise Programme

The exercise programme is based on the principle that oxygen delivery and uptake are enhanced in response to an exercise stimulus which is precisely defined for an individual in terms of the type of exercise, its inten-sity, duration, frequency and the course of the training programme. These parameters are based on an exercise test in conjunction with assessment findings. Exercise tests are performed on a cycle ergometer, treadmill or with a walk test (Noonan & Dean 2000). The general procedures and protocols are standardized to maximize the validity and reliability of the results (Blair et al 2005, Dean et al 1989). The principles of, and guidelines for, exercise testing and training patients with chronic lung and heart disease have been well documented (Dean 2006d). The training-sensitive zone is defined by objective and subjective measures of oxygen transport determined from the exercise test. The components of each exercise training session include baseline, warm-up, steady-state portion, cool-down and recovery period (Blair et al 2005, Dean 1993). The cardiopulmonary and cardiovascular systems are gradually primed for sustaining a given level of exercise stress, while in addition the musculoskeletal system adapts correspondingly. Following the steady-state portion of the training session, the cool-down period permits a return to the resting physiological state. Cool-down and recovery periods are essential for the biochemical degradation and elimination of the metabolic by-products of exercise.

Progression. Progression of the exercise programme is based on a repeated exercise test. This is indicated when the exercise prescription no longer elicits the desired physiological responses – specifically when the steady-state work rate consistently elicits responses at the low end or below the lower limit of the training-sensitive zone for the given indices of oxygen transport. This reflects maximal adaptation of the steps in the oxygen transport pathway to the given exercise stimulus. Further details of exercise, physical activity and both Cardiac and Pulmonary rehabilitation are provided in Chapter 12

Summary

'Cardiopulmonary dysfunction' refers to impairment of one or more steps in the oxygen transport pathway that can impair oxygen transport overall. Factors that can impair the transport of oxygen from the atmosphere to the tissues include cardiopulmonary pathology, bed rest, recumbency and restricted mobility, extrinsic factors related to the patient's medical care, intrinsic factors related to the patient or a

combination of these. Positioning and mobilization are two interventions that have potent and direct effects on several of the steps in the oxygen transport pathway. These interventions have a role in improving oxygen transport in acute and chronic cardiopulmonary dysfunction and in averting the negative effects of restricted mobility and recumbency, particularly those related to cardiopulmonary and cardiovascular function.

OXYGEN THERAPY

Introduction

All mammals are dependent upon oxygen for function and survival. Oxygen therapy refers to the therapeutic administration of oxygen at a concentration greater than that of air at sea level (20.94% or FiO_2 0.2094) to increase alveolar oxygen concentration. Oxygen therapy is used to correct or prevent hypoxaemia (abnormally low oxygenation of arterial blood) and tissue hypoxia (insufficient oxygen available to the tissues to meet metabolic needs). It must be delivered using the minimal concentration required to maintain adequate tissue oxygenation, thereby minimizing cardiopulmonary workload. Oxygen therapy is not a treatment for breathlessness or increased work of breathing unless occurring in association with hypoxaemia.

Hypoxaemia is generally defined as PaO_2 <60 mmHg (<8 kPa) or arterial oxygen saturation (SaO_2) <90%, (O'Driscoll et al 2008) and in the absence of hypercapnia is known as type 1 respiratory failure. Type 2 respiratory failure is defined as hypercapnia ($PaCO_2$ >46 mmHg, 6.1 kPa), with or without hypoxaemia. (O'Driscoll et al 2008) In broad terms, hypoxaemia may be caused by hypoventilation, diffusion abnormalities, venous admixture (shunt) or a combination of these factors. (Hypoxaemia may also be caused by reduced FiO_2, for example at high altitude and with haemoglobin deficiency.) When primarily due to hypoventilation or diffusion abnormalities, hypoxaemia may be alleviated or reversed by elevation of FiO_2. However, when hypoxaemia is primarily due to venous admixture, PaO_2 may be restored if the shunt is no greater than 30% of CO, and by administering a high FiO_2 (Lumb 2010).

Oxygen is carried in the blood in two forms, mostly in chemical combination with haemoglobin and to a smaller extent in physical solution in plasma and red blood cells. It is estimated that 100 mL of blood normally carries 20 mL of oxygen bound to haemoglobin and 0.3 mL in physical solution (Lumb 2010). The presence of hypoxaemia is determined by ABG analysis (PaO_2, SaO_2) and may be indicated by pulse oximetry (arterial oxygen saturation as measured by pulse oximetry (SpO_2)). Oximetry (SaO_2, SpO_2) is the measurement of oxyhaemoglobin saturation, which refers to the proportion of available haemoglobin which is carrying oxygen. Reference ranges for these and other ABG parameters in young healthy adults are summarized in (Table 7-5). With the exception of PaO_2, which decreases over time, these measures are not influenced by age. PaO_2 is estimated to decrease from mean (95% CIs) 94 (84–104) mmHg or 12.5 (11.2–13.8) kPa at 20 to 29 years of age, to 74 (64–84) mmHg or 9.9 (8.5–11.2) kPa at 80 to 89 years of age (Lumb 2010).

This section will describe the provision and prescription of oxygen therapy to self-ventilating patients in acute care and domiciliary settings, and the interfaces commonly used for its administration. More comprehensive information and illustrations of the systems described may be found in the British Thoracic Society guidelines for emergency oxygen use and for home oxygen use.

Oxygen Therapy in the Acute Setting

General Principles

Oxygen therapy is used in the acute setting for the treatment of any patient with documented or suspected hypoxaemia (as defined previously) or for rapidly deteriorating patients until aetiology is determined and adequately treated. Indications include any acute illness, following severe trauma and myocardial infarction and short-term use after procedures or surgery (Heuer 2013a, O'Driscoll et al 2008, Wagstaff 2009). Titration, regular monitoring and documentation of the patient's response is essential, using ABG analysis and/or pulse oximetry, with the aim of achieving and maintaining a target PaO_2 or SpO_2. ABG analysis should be performed for all critically ill patients and any previously stable patient who exhibits a sudden or unexpected fall in oxygen saturation or who requires an increased FiO_2 to maintain oxygenation, even if within the target range. This is recommended because SpO_2 may remain normal in patients with significant abnormalities, for example, alterations in $PaCO_2$, acid-base status (pH) and in patients with low blood oxygen content due to anaemia (O'Driscoll et al 2008). ABG analysis will also provide additional, clinically important information regarding other metabolic parameters.

The target oxygen saturation range is typically 94–98%, (O'Driscoll et al 2008) or 92–96% (Beasley et al 2015) that is, normal or near normal levels. However, for patients who have or are at risk of having type 2 respiratory failure or receiving terminal palliative care, the target may be lower (typically 88–92%) (O'Driscoll et al 2008). Type 2 respiratory failure may occur in patients with moderate to severe COPD, previously unrecognized COPD, other chronic pulmonary disease such as bronchiectasis and CF, severe chest wall or spinal deformity, neuromuscular disease and severe obesity (O'Driscoll et al 2008). In such patients, oxygen-induced hypercapnia may occur as a result of reduced hypoxic drive for ventilation and/or reduced hypoxic pulmonary vasoconstriction which may contribute to ventilation–perfusion mismatch (Lumb 2010). Although supplementary oxygen will not improve hypercapnia and may worsen it, the treatment of hypoxaemia is the priority for patients

---

TABLE 7-5		
Reference Ranges for Arterial Blood in Young Healthy Adults		
	Reference Range	
PaO_2	90–110 mmHg, 12.0–14.7 kPa	
$PaCO_2$	34–46 mmHg, 4.6–6.1 kPa	
pH	7.35–7.45 units	
HCO_3^-	22–26 mEq/L	
SaO_2, SpO_2	96–98%	

Beachey, 2013; O'Driscoll et al 2008.

HCO_3^-, Bicarbonate concentration; $PaCO_2$, partial pressure of carbon dioxide; PaO_2, partial pressure of oxygen; SaO_2, arterial oxygen saturation; SpO_2, arterial oxygen saturation by pulse oximeter.

with type 2 respiratory failure, with appropriate monitoring of response, particularly $PaCO_2$ (Heuer 2013a, Lumb 2010, O'Driscoll et al 2008). Hypercapnia may be reduced by improving alveolar ventilation, using strategies to manage its underlying cause or by providing measures such as non-invasive or invasive ventilatory support (Lumb 2010).

Despite maintaining a target SpO_2, supplemental oxygen may mask progressive respiratory failure or other deterioration (Downs 2003). Regular review is required to assess the response to treatment and to monitor for symptoms of deterioration, for example increased breathlessness or work of breathing, drowsiness, confusion and fatigue. It is recommended that oxygen therapy prescription (delivery system and flow rate), and target and measured oxygen saturation be formally and regularly recorded (Heuer 2013a, O'Driscoll et al 2008).

Delivery Systems

In the acute setting, oxygen is usually supplied at high pressure from a centralized bulk storage system via a pipe network throughout the facility. In-built valves reduce the gas pressure to a level suitable for use with devices such as ventilators. For the oxygen therapy devices described in this section, a flow metre is also required (when using a compressed gas cylinder, a regulator is required in addition to a flow metre).

Oxygen delivery systems for the spontaneously breathing patient are broadly categorized according clinical performance and design, into fixed and variable performance systems and enclosure systems (Table 7-6). Fixed-performance devices incorporate wide bore, corrugated tubing (approximately 2-cm diameter), allowing the delivery of humidification with supplemental oxygen. High-flow devices are used in critically ill patients as described in Chapter 9. Variable performance devices use narrow bore oxygen tubing to provide supplemental oxygen only.

The FiO_2 provided by a system depends primarily upon the extent to which the gas flow it delivers meets the patient's peak inspiratory flow (PIF). If PIF exceeds the gas flow delivered, the remainder is drawn from the surrounding air, thus diluting the

TABLE 7-6	
Commonly Used Systems and Interfaces for Delivery of Oxygen Therapy in the Acute Setting	
Systems	**Devices/Interfaces**
Variable performance	Nasal cannula
	Nasal catheter
	Transtracheal catheter
	Reservoir cannulae:
	Nasal reservoir cannula
	Pendant reservoir cannula
	Simple face mask
	Reservoir masks:
	Partial rebreathing mask
	Non-rebreathing mask
Fixed performance	Air entrainment (Venturi) system
	Air entrainment nebulizer system
	Heated humidification systems
	Interfaces:
	Face mask, large holes
	Tracheostomy mask
	Trough mask (face tent)
	T-piece
	High-flow humidified nasal prongs
Enclosure systems	Oxygen tents
	Oxygen hoods
	Incubators

gas delivered and lowering FiO_2. PIF may vary from approximately 25 L/min normally to 60 L/min in a tachypnoeic patient, but in rare circumstances may reach ≥ 100 L/min. A total gas flow of 60 L/min is considered to be adequate to meet PIF in most cases (Heuer 2013a).

Variable Performance Systems.
Variable performance systems deliver oxygen at relatively low flow rates, typically 2–15 L/min (Wagstaff 2009). These systems incorporate small reservoirs and are very sensitive to the patient's ventilatory pattern (PIF, respiratory rate and I:E ratio). While it is not possible to accurately predict the FiO_2 delivered by these devices, for patients with an average respiratory rate and tidal volume it is

estimated that FiO_2 increases by approximately 4% for every 1 L/min increase in oxygen flow (Heuer 2013a). Low-flow metres (0.25 to 2.5 L/min) are available for use when oxygen flows of ≤2 L/min are required.

NASAL CANNULA. The nasal cannula consists of two soft prongs, approximately 1 cm long, which are inserted into the anterior nares and are connected to an oxygen outlet (and flow metre) via narrow bore tubing. The patient's nasopharynx acts as an anatomic reservoir, making this system particularly sensitive to changes in PIF and respiratory rate. However, mouth breathing does not decrease FiO_2 (O'Driscoll et al 2008). The nasal cannula may be used with oxygen flows of 0.25 to 6 L/min, but it is recommended that it not be used at >4 L/min due to excessive nasal dryness and discomfort (O'Driscoll et al 2008).

RESERVOIR CANNULAE. There are two types of reservoir cannulae. These devices incorporate an oxygen reservoir within the cannula tubing, serving as an oxygen conservation system.

The nasal reservoir cannula stores approximately 20 mL of oxygen in a reservoir which is 10 to 15 mm long and sits directly below the nasal prongs across the face. Oxygen is stored during expiration and is inhaled early in inspiration. Disadvantages include discomfort and a bulky appearance.

The pendant reservoir cannula has a reservoir of approximately 7 cm in diameter which sits over the anterior chest wall at mid-sternal level and may be hidden under the patient's clothing. While less visible than the reservoir cannula, disadvantages are that the device is heavier, which may cause ear and facial discomfort.

Both types of reservoir cannula may be used at oxygen flows of 0.25 to 4 L/min. These devices are estimated to reduce oxygen flow requirements by 50–75% in comparison with standard nasal cannulae, particularly at low flow rates (Heuer 2013a). A limitation of these devices is that they contain a reservoir membrane which must be reopened or reset during expiration. This requires expiration to occur through the nose, especially when used with low oxygen flows, which may be particularly difficult during exercise.

NASAL CATHETER. The nasal catheter is a single, soft, narrow tube with several holes at its distal end,

connected to an oxygen outlet via narrow bore tubing. It is inserted into the nasopharynx to a depth equivalent to that of the distance between the nose and ear lobe, or under direct visualization to rest just above the uvula, and is secured to the patient's face with tape (AARC Clinical Practice Guideline 2002b, Heuer 2013a). Oxygen flows (0.24–6 L/min) are delivered to the oropharynx which acts as an anatomical reservoir (AARC Clinical Practice Guideline 2002b). This device is generally used for short-term oxygen delivery during specialized procedures, for example, bronchoscopy, but seldom elsewhere. Disadvantages include difficulty of insertion, gagging or swallowing of gas. It is recommended that the nasal catheter is not used in patients with maxillofacial trauma, basal skull fracture and coagulation disorders (AARC Clinical Practice Guideline 2002b, Heuer 2013a).

TRANSTRACHEAL CATHETER. The transtracheal catheter is inserted into the trachea between the second and third tracheal rings using a guide wire and is secured by a neck chain. Oxygen flows of 0.25–4 L/min are used (Heuer 2013a). Due to the position of the catheter, oxygen builds up in the trachea and upper airway during expiration, extending the patient's anatomic reservoir in comparison with other variable performance devices. In comparison with the standard nasal cannula, the transtracheal catheter provides a higher FiO_2 for a given oxygen flow rate, and is estimated to reduce oxygen flow requirements by 50% to achieve a given PaO_2 (Heuer 2013a). While of considerable economic and practical benefit for patients requiring long-term continuous oxygen therapy (COT), this device has not gained wide acceptance. Disadvantages include its high cost, the possibility of infection around the insertion site and mucus plugging and the rigorous patient education and ongoing professional evaluation required for its maintenance (Heuer 2013a).

SIMPLE OXYGEN MASK. The simple oxygen mask is a semi-rigid plastic device which covers the mouth and nose and has exhalation ports (a number of small holes) in both sides. It has an air inlet at its base which is connected via narrow bore tubing to an oxygen source. Room air is entrained through the inlet into the mask as source oxygen enters, increasing the total flow delivered and flushing exhaled CO_2 from the mask. Additional room air may be drawn through the exhalation ports and around the mask edge. The body of the mask acts as an oxygen reservoir between patient breaths. The simple oxygen mask is used with oxygen flows of 5–10 L/min, to deliver oxygen concentrations of approximately 35–60%. If used with an oxygen flow of <5 L/min, increased resistance to inspiration may occur and the mask gas volume may act as dead space, leading to rebreathing of CO_2 (Heuer 2013a, O'Driscoll et al 2008).

RESERVOIR MASKS. Reservoir masks come in two forms, partial rebreathing and non-rebreathing masks. These masks are similar in design to the simple oxygen mask, with the addition of a 1-L reservoir bag and in the case of the non-rebreathing mask, a series of one-way valves. The reservoir bag increases reservoir volume, providing higher FiO_2 capabilities than the simple mask (Heuer 2013a).

The partial rebreathing mask allows source oxygen to flow to the patient during inspiration, and during expiration source oxygen and approximately the first third of the patient's expired gas enter the bag. As the latter is mostly from the patient's anatomic dead space, early in expiration it contains a relatively high oxygen concentration and low CO_2 concentration. As the bag fills, the last two-thirds of expired gas (higher in CO_2) passes out of the mask exhalation ports (Heuer 2013a). It is recommended that oxygen flow be sufficient to prevent bag deflation (during inspiration) of more than one-third volume to minimize CO_2 rebreathing (Heuer 2013a). With flows of ≥10 L/min, this device may provide oxygen concentrations of 40–70% (AARC Clinical Practice Guideline 2002a, Heuer 2013a).

The non-rebreathing mask incorporates one-way valves at the base of the mask (between it and the reservoir bag) to prevent exhaled gas entering the bag, and over the two exhalation ports in the body of the mask (AARC Clinical Practice Guideline 2002a, Heuer 2013a). During inspiration, negative mask pressure closes the valves over the expiratory ports, preventing air entrainment, and opens the valve over the top of the bag allowing delivery of oxygen from the bag. The reverse occurs during expiration. With flows of ≥10 L/min, this device may provide oxygen concentrations of 60–90% (AARC Clinical Practice Guideline 2002a, Heuer 2013a, O'Driscoll et al 2008).

British guidelines recommend a minimum flow of 15 L/min be used with reservoir masks (British Thoracic Society 2009).

Fixed Performance Systems. Fixed performance systems deliver relatively gas high flows, aimed to equal or exceed the patient's PIF, thereby delivering a known or fixed FiO_2. Commonly used fixed performance systems are the air entrainment mask and air entrainment nebulizer. High-flow heated systems are also available. If these devices are unable to provide sufficient FiO_2 to meet the required target, the use of gas blending systems may be considered. Gas blending systems are connected to air and oxygen outlets and are designed to provide precise control over the mix of the two gases, typically providing flows of >60 L/min (Heuer 2013a).

AIR ENTRAINMENT ('VENTURI') MASK. The body of the air entrainment mask is similar to that of the simple oxygen mask described, but has one larger exhalation port in each side. A short piece of wide bore corrugated tubing (approximately 10 cm long) is attached to its base. This is connected to an adaptor containing a narrow jet orifice surrounded by an air entrainment port or cage. Source oxygen is delivered to the jet via narrow bore tubing and flows through it at high velocity. Air is entrained via the entrainment port due to shearing forces at the boundary of the jet flow, thus diluting the gas delivered to the mask. The total flow delivered by the system depends upon the diameter of the jet orifice, the flow of gas into it and the cross sectional area of the entrainment port.

A range of differently sized adaptors is provided with the air entrainment mask, designed to deliver oxygen concentrations of 24–40% or 60% (AARC Clinical Practice Guideline 2002a, Heuer 2013a, O'Driscoll et al 2008). The required oxygen flow rate is indicated on each adaptor. Those providing a lower FiO_2 have a smaller jet orifice resulting in a higher flow of source oxygen through it, higher entrainment of room air and greater total flow. Conversely, a larger jet orifice provides the highest oxygen delivery to the system, but entrains the least air into the system delivering a lower total flow to the patient. FiO_2 may therefore become variable at higher oxygen settings, particularly >35% (AARC Clinical Practice

Guideline 2002a, Heuer 2013a) and if a patient has a respiratory rate >30 breaths/minute (O'Driscoll et al 2008).

A collar may be attached over the adaptor of the air entrainment mask system to allow humidified gas to be entrained. Humidification (see *Heated Humidifier Systems*) is recommended if oxygen therapy is required at higher concentrations for prolonged periods (more than 24 hours), for patients reporting discomfort due to upper airway dryness and for all patients with a tracheostomy or previous laryngectomy who require oxygen therapy in the acute setting (O'Driscoll et al 2008).

Air entrainment mask systems are recommended for use with patients who need a precise, low FiO_2, but have the disadvantages of being noisy, more claustrophobic and less comfortable than nasal cannulae, and the need to be removed for eating and to enhance communication.

AIR ENTRAINMENT NEBULIZER. Air entrainment nebulizers are large volume, gas-powered jet nebulizers, incorporating an adjustable air-entrainment port. They are designed to deliver low to moderate oxygen concentrations and humidification, and may have temperature control capabilities. A small jet orifice is required to produce aerosol, typically requiring an oxygen flow of 12–15 L/min. The ratio of entrained room air to oxygen delivered by these systems is adjusted by varying the entrainment port size. As for air entrainment mask systems, these devices will deliver a known, fixed oxygen concentration only at lower oxygen settings (≤35 percent) (Heuer 2013a). To increase the total flow delivered, two devices may be connected in parallel using a Y-adaptor, thus doubling the total flow delivered.

HEATED HUMIDIFIER SYSTEMS. Heated humidifier systems incorporate an electric heating element. The heater power may be adjusted to achieve the desired airway temperature.

Air entrainment nebulizers and heated humidifiers are sensitive to down-stream flow resistance, which may be affected by the length of tubing used (typically 1.5 to 1.8 metres), excess condensate within the tubing, or if the entrainment ports of the mask become obstructed. Back pressure may decrease the volume of air entrained, reducing total flow delivered and possibly varying FiO_2 (Heuer 2013a).

INTERFACE DEVICES FOR FIXED PERFORMANCE SYSTEMS. Fixed performance systems may be used with a face mask (as described for air entrainment masks, with large entrainment ports on both sides), a trough mask, a T-tube or tracheostomy mask (shield) (AARC Clinical Practice Guideline 2002a, Heuer 2013a). Humidified nasal prong systems are also available.

A trough mask covers the mouth but is open below the nose, and may be suitable for patients who are unable to tolerate a face mask. A T-tube is used for patients who are orally or nasally intubated or who have a tracheostomy tube (Fink and Ari 2013). The tracheostomy mask is a semi-rigid plastic mask which fits over a tracheostomy, allowing supplemental oxygen to be delivered and secretions and condensate to escape from the airway, thus minimizing resistance to airflow (Fink and Ari 2013). FiO_2 may be fixed or variable with a tracheostomy mask, depending upon whether or not a tracheostomy tube is present, and the status of its cuff. Patients who do not have a tracheostomy tube will inhale air from the nasopharynx, thereby reducing FiO_2 (Heuer 2013a).

Enclosure Systems. Enclosure systems are usually only used for infants and small children. These include oxygen tents and hoods and incubators which provide a temperature-controlled environment. Hoods are designed to provide a fixed FiO_2 but oxygen tents and incubators tend to provide unstable FiO_2, as they have a tendency to leak (AARC Clinical Practice Guideline 2002b, Heuer 2013a).

Domiciliary Oxygen Therapy

Oxygen therapy is provided in domiciliary settings in many countries for continuous, nocturnal or intermittent use, or for patients with documented hypoxaemia (Table 7-7) (AARC Clinical Practice Guideline 2007, Hardinge et al 2015, McDonald et al 2005). The prescription of domiciliary oxygen therapy is based upon the survival and quality of life benefits demonstrated in patients with COPD and severe hypoxaemia (Medical Research Council Working Party 1981, Nocturnal Oxygen Therapy Trial Group 1980).

| | | | | **TABLE 7-7** | |
| | | | | **Domiciliary Oxygen Therapy Delivery and Prescription Guidelines** | |

Classification	Subcategories	Apparatus commonly used	Australasia (McDonald et al 2005)	United States (AARC Clinical Practice Guideline, 2007)	United Kingdom (Hardinge et al 2015)
Continuous oxygen therapy (COT)	Long-term oxygen therapy (LTOT) Short-term oxygen therapy (STOT)	Concentrator (stationary)	PaO_2 ≤55 (kPa ≤7.3) or PaO_2 56–59 (kPa 7.4–7.8) + hypoxic organ damage Stable: ≥4 weeks. Goal: PaO_2 >60 mmHg (8 kPa)	PaO_2 ≤55 (kPa ≤7.3) or PaO_2 56–59 (kPa 7.4–7.8), SpO_2 ≤89% + hypoxic organ damage or SpO_2 ≤88%	PaO_2 ≤55 (kPa ≤7.3) or PaO_2 55–59 (kPa 7.3–7.8) + hypoxic organ damage Stable: ≥5 weeks + 2 × ABG, ≥3 weeks apart
Nocturnal oxygen therapy (NOT)	During sleep	Concentrator (stationary)	PaO_2 <55 mmHg or SpO_2 <88% >⅓ of night	Lung disease + sleep apnoea + nocturnal desaturation PaO_2 ≤55 mmHg	Nocturnal hypoxaemia + fulfill criteria for COT
Intermittent oxygen therapy	Domiciliary ambulatory oxygen (long term)	Transportable apparatus: Compressed gas cylinder Liquid oxygen canister Portable concentrator	SpO_2 ≤88% on air + improvement in exercise capacity or dyspnoea on O_2	PaO_2 ≤55 mmHg (≤7.3 kPa), SpO_2 ≤88% on air	Two of: – SpO_2 corrected to ≥90% – ≥10% ↑ walking distance – ≥1 unit ↑ Borg score
	Palliative	Concentrator (stationary)	Dyspnoea, life expectancy <3 months	Dyspnoea ± hypoxaemia in terminal illness	Intractable breathlessness + no treatment response
	With COT Training oxygen Short burst oxygen therapy (SBOT) Emergency/stand-by Air-travel	Transportable apparatus: Compressed gas cylinder Liquid oxygen canister Portable concentrator			

ABG, Arterial blood gas; *PaO₂,* partial pressure of oxygen; *SpO₂,* arterial oxygen saturation by pulse oximeter.

Domiciliary oxygen therapy is delivered using a variety of systems, depending upon clinical requirements, practicality and expense.

Delivery Systems and Devices. Domiciliary oxygen is supplied using three main delivery systems: oxygen concentrators, compressed gas cylinders and in some centres liquid oxygen systems. The interface most commonly used in the domiciliary setting is the nasal cannula. Occasionally, a transtracheal catheter may be used.

OXYGEN CONCENTRATORS. Oxygen concentrators are electrically powered devices which usually use a molecular sieve to separate oxygen from nitrogen in room air. At low flows (1–2 L/min) concentrators typically deliver oxygen concentrations of 92–95%, but at 5 L/min oxygen concentration may be 85–93%. Stationary oxygen concentrators (connected to mains electricity) are the most cost-efficient delivery system for patients requiring COT at low flows. Portable, battery driven concentrators are also available, but are expensive and battery life may be limiting (Heuer 2013b).

COMPRESSED GAS CYLINDERS. The most commonly used device for supplying portable or ambulatory oxygen is the compressed gas cylinder, transported in a trolley (stroller) or, less commonly, carried in a shoulder bag. Disadvantages include difficulty with portability due to weight, with changeover of the regulator and the requirement of regular deliveries (Heuer 2013b).

LIQUID OXYGEN SYSTEMS. Liquid oxygen systems consist of a large stationary unit from which small, portable canisters may be transfilled. Their use is limited by cost and the requirement of regular deliveries (Heuer 2013b).

CONSERVATION DEVICES. In the domiciliary setting, portable apparatus is commonly used with a demand-flow or pulsed-dose conservation device. This device is placed between the supply device and delivery interface and uses a flow sensor to provide a flow of oxygen on demand at the initiation of inspiration. It may be used with stationary liquid oxygen reservoirs, liquid portable canisters and compressed gas oxygen cylinders, and may be incorporated in some portable concentrator devices (Heuer 2013b).

Domiciliary Oxygen Therapy Prescription. Prescription guidelines for domiciliary oxygen therapy have been published by a number of groups globally, including groups from Australasia (McDonald et al 2005), Britain (Hardinge et al 2015) and North America (AARC Clinical Practice Guideline 2007) (see Table 7-7). Criteria for qualification for COT are essentially consistent internationally, but a number of differences exist regarding the domiciliary provision of intermittent oxygen therapy and assessment procedures.

Oxygen therapy has a major role in the management of patients with COPD, both in the acute and domiciliary settings. With advancing disease severity, chronic respiratory failure is common, both type 1 and type 2, complicated by episodes of acute-on-chronic respiratory failure during exacerbations. Besides ceasing smoking, continuous, long-term, supplemental domiciliary oxygen is the only therapy which has been shown to reduce mortality in patients with COPD (Medical Research Council Working Party 1981, Nocturnal Oxygen Therapy Trial Group 1980). The principles and guidelines for the use of oxygen therapy in this patient group are described in Chapter 12.

Continuous Oxygen Therapy. COT is domiciliary oxygen therapy prescribed for long-term use on a daily basis for ≥15 hours per day, for the treatment of severe, chronic hypoxaemia (PaO_2 ≤55 mmHg, ≤7.3 kPa). (AARC Clinical Practice Guideline 2007, Hardinge et al 2015, McDonald et al 2005) Also known as 'long-term oxygen therapy (LTOT)' (AARC Clinical Practice Guideline, 2007), the term 'COT' is proposed to avoid confusion with oxygen prescribed for long-term nocturnal or intermittent use. COT may also be provided for patients with PaO_2 56–59 (7.4–7.8) in the presence of hypoxic organ damage, defined as secondary polycythaemia (AARC Clinical Practice Guideline 2007, Hardinge et al 2015, McDonald et al 2005), pulmonary hypertension (Hardinge et al 2015, McDonald et al 2005) or right heart failure, cor pulmonale or congestive heart failure (AARC Clinical Practice Guideline 2007, McDonald et al 2005).

COT is most commonly prescribed at low flows, using an oxygen concentrator and nasal cannula. Evidence to support the guidelines for prescription of COT was provided by the combined results of two RCTs which included a total of 290 patients with COPD and severe resting hypoxaemia (Medical Research Council Working Party 1981, Nocturnal Oxygen Therapy Trial Group 1980). The results of these studies have been extrapolated to include the prescription for COT to children and infants older than 28 days (AARC Clinical Practice Guideline 2007), and patients with cyanotic congenital heart disease, congestive heart failure, pulmonary vascular disease, primary pulmonary hypertension and other chronic lung diseases, including interstitial lung disease, advanced lung cancer, bronchiectasis, CF and severe asthma (Hardinge et al 2015, McDonald et al 2005).

Short-Term Oxygen Therapy. Short-term oxygen therapy (STOT) refers to the prescription of COT for patients who are hypoxaemic upon discharge from hospital (Eaton et al 2001). It is recommended that ABGs be re-tested once clinical stability has been reached, as many patients who previously did not qualify for COT will return to their prior status. The suggested time for retesting varies from 1 to 3 months (Hardinge et al 2015, Eaton et al 2001, Heuer 2013b, McDonald et al 2005).

NOCTURNAL OXYGEN. Nocturnal oxygen is recommended for patients with lung disease who do not qualify for COT according to the previously mentioned criteria, but exhibit episodes of hypoxaemia during sleep (McDonald et al 2005). The use of nocturnal oxygen is based upon a double-blinded RCT of 38 patients with COPD, a daytime saturation of ≥90% and nocturnal desaturation (<90% for ≥5 minutes), which demonstrated a reduction in pulmonary artery pressure (Fletcher et al 1992). However, the clinical importance of nocturnal hypoxaemia is unclear and other studies investigating the effects of nocturnal oxygen have had conflicting findings (McDonald et al 2005). Australasian guidelines specifically define nocturnal desaturation in contrast to others (see Table 7-7).

Intermittent Oxygen Therapy

DOMICILIARY AMBULATORY OXYGEN. Domiciliary ambulatory oxygen therapy refers to the provision of oxygen, for use during exertional activities, to patients who demonstrate exertional desaturation but have a resting PaO_2 which precludes them from receiving COT. Prescription is usually also dependent upon demonstration of an acute response to supplemental oxygen during an exercise test, commonly the 6-minute walk test (6MWT) or incremental shuttle walk test (ISWT) (Hardinge et al 2015; McDonald et al 2005). Guidelines for the provision of domiciliary ambulatory oxygen have been set arbitrarily by extrapolation from those for COT, and vary between centres (see Table 7-5). The British guidelines recommend reassessment after 2 months including an interview, review of a diary card of oxygen usage and withdrawal if deemed unhelpful (Hardinge et al 2015). Although not yet evidence-based, domiciliary ambulatory oxygen is widely prescribed for patients who do not

have severe resting hypoxaemia (Moore et al 2011, Ram and Wedzicha 2002).

AMBULATORY OXYGEN IN CONJUNCTION WITH COT. In some centres, transportable oxygen is provided for use conjunction with COT, to encourage maintenance of activity while adhering to the recommendation for COT of ≥15 hours per day. While anticipated to provide the same benefits as COT, this hypothesis has not been confirmed by a double-blinded, randomized, crossover trial designed to test it (Lacasse et al 2005).

TRAINING OXYGEN. Training oxygen refers to the use of supplemental oxygen during specific exercise, for example pulmonary rehabilitation programs. Supplemental oxygen has been shown to improve exertional dyspnoea and exercise performance acutely in some patients with COPD, including those without exertional desaturation (Moore & Berlowitz 2011). The reasons for these acute benefits are believed to be multifactorial and not solely dependent upon the relief of hypoxaemia. Despite a lack of evidence of long-term benefit (Nonoyama et al 2009), these demonstrated acute benefits have prompted the use of training oxygen in some centres (McDonald et al 2005).

SHORT BURST OXYGEN THERAPY. Mainly prescribed in the United Kingdom, short burst oxygen therapy (SBOT) is used for short periods of approximately 10 to 20 minutes, for pre-oxygenation before exertion and to relieve dyspnoea during recovery after exertion or at rest. However, there is no evidence support the use of SBOT (Hardinge et al 2015).

OTHER USES OF INTERMITTENT OXYGEN THERAPY. Supplemental oxygen may also be recommended during air-travel for patients who become severely hypoxic in this circumstance, although assessment methods and prescription vary (Ahmedzai et al 2011, McDonald et al 2005). Palliative oxygen is commonly prescribed for terminally ill patients with the aim of relieving intractable dyspnoea (McDonald et al., 2005), although no evidence of benefit has been demonstrated other than a possible placebo effect (Abernathy et al 2009). Oxygen is occasionally provided for 'stand-by' emergency use for patients who live in isolated areas and suffer life-threatening hypoxaemic episodes, for example during acute asthma (McDonald et al 2005).

Hazards of Oxygen Therapy

Physiological Hazards. High levels of supplemental oxygen and prolonged exposure may result in oxygen toxicity, which may affect the lungs and the central nervous system. Pulmonary manifestations include damage to the capillary endothelium, causing increased capillary permeability, interstitial and alveolar oedema and worsening hypoxaemia (Heuer 2013a, Lumb 2010). Central nervous system effects tend to occur when breathing oxygen at pressures of >1 atmosphere (hyperbaric pressures) and include tremors, twitching and convulsions. It is recommended that exposure to 100% oxygen should be of <24 hours duration where possible, and that oxygen concentration be decreased to 70% within 2 days and 50% or less within 5 days. However, the priority of treatment is to maintain an adequate PaO_2 using the required FiO_2 (Heuer 2013a).

A further physiological hazard is oxygen-induced depression of ventilation which may occur in some patients with chronic hypercapnia (for example, patients with advanced COPD). This may result in further elevation of $PaCO_2$ and progressive deterioration in conscious state. However, for such patients, the primary concern is appropriate management of hypoxaemia, with careful monitoring of response (Heuer 2013a). Other hazards include the risk of absorption atelectasis, which is more significant with FiO_2 >0.50 in patients breathing at low tidal volumes, for example after sedation, or with surgical pain or CNS dysfunction (Heuer 2013a). More rarely, supplemental oxygen given to some premature infants may result in retinopathy (AARC Clinical Practice Guideline 2002b).

Combustion. While oxygen does not explode, it supports combustion. Therefore oxygen therapy should not be used in the presence of open flames, combustible materials such as petroleum based oils, lotions and sprays or equipment capable of creating a spark, such as electrical appliances. Smoking while using supplemental oxygen has resulted in facial burns, inhalation injuries and death.

Inhalation Therapy

Many pharmacological agents are used to treat respiratory disease. Often these medications are administered by inhalation because this increases the proportion of the dose received by the lungs, allowing a smaller total dose and reducing systemic side effects. Many inhaled medications have mechanisms of action that are similar or complementary to the mechanisms of action of some physiotherapy interventions for respiratory disease, particularly when these interventions are targeted towards airway clearance. Because this creates potential for interactions (both beneficial and detrimental) between the two types of therapies, physiotherapists should be aware of the medications that have been prescribed for each of their patients.

Physiotherapists may find it difficult to maintain a comprehensive understanding of all inhaled respiratory medications because the range of medications that is commercially available varies between countries and changes frequently. It can be helpful to think of medications in classes defined by the primary mode of action: bronchodilators, mucoactives, antibiotics, anti-inflammatories, and so on. Within each of these main classes of medication, there are subclasses. For example, the class of mucoactive medications has the subclasses: expectorants, which add water to the airway; mucolytics, which break down the mucus structure; mucoregulators, which change the volume or content of secretions and mucokinetics, which improve cough-mediated clearance by increasing airflow or reducing sputum adhesivity, as presented in Table 7-8. Some medications have multiple mechanisms and so could belong in multiple classes or subclasses. Despite these complexities, thinking about medications by their mechanism(s) of action is valuable because it guides clinical reasoning about how they should be coordinated with respiratory physiotherapy interventions.

TABLE 7-8

Medications in the Mucoactive Class, Arranged by Subclass with Detailed Mechanisms of Action

Subclass

Agent	Detailed Mechanism(s)
Expectorants	
Hypertonic saline	Airway hydration, cough, disrupts biofilms, improves mucus rheology, inhibits bacterial motility
Mannitol	Airway hydration, cough, improves mucus rheology
Mucolytics	
N-acetylcysteine	Disrupts ionic bonds within mucus structure, anti-inflammatory, antioxidant
Nacystelyn	Disrupts ionic bonds within mucus structure, chloride secretion
Dornase alpha	Cleaves DNA polymers in mucus
Mucoregulators	
Carbocysteine	Modulates mucus content, anti-inflammatory, antioxidant
Glucocorticoids	Reduces airway inflammation and mucin secretion
Anticholinergics	Decreases volume of secretions
Mucokinetics	
β_2 agonists	Increase ciliary action, improved cough clearance via expiratory flow
Surfactant	Decreases mucus adherence to epithelium

Modified from Bye et al 2011.

This section of the chapter will review the evidence about hypertonic saline, mannitol, and dornase alpha primarily, although issues related to some other inhaled therapies will also be discussed. For each medication, the mechanisms of action will be discussed in detail, the evidence about clinical efficacy will be summarized and potential interactions with physiotherapy interventions will also be considered. Strategies for maximizing the benefits from these interactions will be discussed, including the order and timing of inhaled therapies in relation to physiotherapy interventions.

In addition however, simple measures of systemic and targeted hydration of the airways can also optimize airway clearance in patients with difficulty clearing mucus. Mucosal function is reported to require optimal conditions of 37°C and 100% relative humidity (Williams et al 1996). The effects of a cold-water jet nebulizer humidification system in combination with PD in adults with non-CF bronchiectasis increased sputum wet weight yield by a median of 6 g when compared with PD alone (Conway et al 1992). In addition, tracheobronchial humidification via a nasal interface at a flow rate between 20 and 25 L/min (warm air fully saturated at 37°C), in 10 adults with non-CF bronchiectasis, resulted in a significant enhancement of MCC and this was sustained over a 6-hour monitoring period. Acute (3 hours) and short-term (3 hours per day for 6 days) clearance effects were assessed using a tracheobronchial radio aerosol retention technique (Hasani et al 2008).

Mouse models have suggested that airway surface dehydration leads to persistent neutrophilic airway inflammation with increased mucus production and resultant emphysema (Mall et al 2008). In a prospective single-centre open-labelled placebo controlled study, 108 patients with moderate to severe COPD and bronchiectasis were either randomized to daily humidification via the Optiflow nasal cannula system (Fisher & Paykel Healthcare Limited, Berkshire, United Kingdom) for 2 or more hours per day (humidified air, fully saturated at 37°C at a flow rate of 20–25 L/min) or to usual care. Patients on long-term humidification had significantly fewer exacerbations (18.2 vs 33.5 days, $p < 0.05$), increased time to first exacerbation (median 52 vs 27 days, $p < 0.05$) and a nonsignificant reduction in exacerbation frequency (2.97 per patient per year vs 3.63 per patient per year, $p > 0.05$) (Rea et al 2010).

There have been no studies investigating the effects of humidification alone in CF. This is possibly due to differences in the pathophysiology of CF compared non-CF bronchiectasis, such that humidification alone would be insufficient to alleviate and restore the depleted airway surface liquid (ASL) height, which is a key factor in secretion retention in CF. Appropriate humidification is a potentially useful adjunctive component in the management of individuals with bronchiectasis and should be considered as part of the airway clearance management.

HYPERTONIC SALINE

Saline concentrations of 3% or higher are called 'hypertonic' because they have a higher salt concentration than the liquid that lines the inner surface of the airways. Typically, concentrations between 3% and 7% are nebulized and inhaled. Once deposited on the airway surface, hypertonic saline generates greater osmotic pressure than the isotonic ASL and draws water into the airway to increase hydration of the airway surface. Although airway hydration appears to be the main mechanism of action, hypertonic saline has several other mechanisms that may be beneficial in a variety of respiratory conditions.

Mechanisms of Action

The osmotic action of hypertonic saline is particularly relevant to CF, where depletion of the ASL causes disruption of normal MCC. This is because enough ASL to cover the cilia is necessary to prevent the mucus from adhering to the cilia and the airway wall, and to allow the cilia to perform their normal action of propelling the overlying mucus towards the mouth (Boucher 2002, 2007). This may seem to suggest that the osmotic action may be unhelpful in other diseases of mucus retention where ASL is preserved, possibly augmenting the ASL so much that the cilia cannot reach the mucus layer. However, excess ASL is absorbed by the mucus layer once the cilia are adequately covered (Button et al 2012). This is also beneficial because the extra water of mucus allows it to flow more readily. This explains why hypertonic saline accelerates MCC not only in people with CF, but also in people with other respiratory tract diseases and even in healthy people (Daviskas et al 1996; Donaldson et al 2006; Robinson et al 1996, 1997; Ural et al 2009).

Commonly, coughing occurs during and immediately after inhalation of hypertonic saline. When a bronchodilator is given as a premedication, excessive coughing prevents use of hypertonic saline by only about 3% of people with CF (Elkins & Bye, 2006) and even fewer with non-CF bronchiectasis (Kellett & Robert 2011, Kellett et al 2005, Nicolson et al 2012). Supervision of the first dose with spirometry and oxyhaemoglobin saturation monitoring before and after the dose are recommended to ensure that sufficient bronchoprotection is provided by the premedication (Elkins & Bye, 2006). For most people, cough is probably a key beneficial mechanism – creating high shear stresses likely to detach mucus that is adhered to the airway wall and thus allowing it be cleared by the mucociliary system. This is evident on radio aerosol scans of osmotic agents where coughing causes an increase in mucus clearance beyond that occurring by MCC alone (Robinson and Bye, 2002).

Adding saline (or even salt alone) to mucus causes significant reductions in viscosity, elasticity and spinnability (King et al 1997, Scheffner et al 1964). This may be due to the sodium and chloride ions allowing a change in the ionic bonding between the macromolecules in the mucus, thereby untangling the mucus structure (Dasgupta & King 1996). These rheological changes allow the mucus to flow more readily along the mucosal surface (Wills et al 1997). These rheological changes become even more favourable with increasing amounts of salt added to the mucus.

Hypertonic saline also reduces the viability and motility of *Pseudomonas aeruginosa* (Behrends et al 2010, Havasi et al 2008) as well as disrupting its bacterial biofilms and inhibiting formation of new ones (Anderson & O'Toole 2008). Hypertonic saline also improves the bactericidal efficiency of some antimicrobial peptides (Bergsson et al., 2009) and increases two CFTR-dependent thiols that are protective against oxidative lung injury (Gould et al., 2010).

Evidence About Efficacy

Hypertonic saline has been shown to be effective in adults and older children (≥6 yr) with CF, with regular inhalation improving lung function within 2 weeks (Donaldson et al 2006, Eng et al 1996). This benefit is maintained while inhalations are continued, at least to 48 weeks (Elkins et al 2006c). The risk of pulmonary exacerbations also decreases significantly, whether defined according to intravenous antibiotic therapy for symptoms, or according to symptoms alone. These benefits are accompanied by a reduction in absenteeism from school and regular sporting fixtures and fewer courses of antibiotics prescribed for exacerbations (Elkins et al 2006c). The quality of life measures also identified significant improvements in mental and emotional health, completion of usual role and perceived health. In a trial in younger children (<6 yr) and infants, hypertonic saline did not reduce the frequency of exacerbations (Rosenfeld et al 2012). However, in the subgroup who underwent infant lung function testing, the forced expiratory volume in 0.5 seconds was improved significantly by hypertonic saline. Further studies in infants are planned.

In adults with non-CF bronchiectasis, regular inhalation of hypertonic saline for 3 months was also associated with significant improvements in lung function and quality of life, as well as significant reductions in annual antibiotic use and emergency healthcare utilization (Kellett & Robert 2011). A subsequent 12-month trial did not identify these benefits (Nicolson et al 2012), but it was substantially underpowered compared to the original trial. As clinically worthwhile benefits were not excluded by the confidence intervals in that trial, an adequately powered long-term trial of hypertonic saline in people with bronchiectasis is in progress (Australian New Zealand Clinical Trials Registry: ACTRN12611001199909).

A Cochrane review of hypertonic saline for infants with bronchiolitis identified 11 trials (Zhang et al 2013). Inpatients treated with nebulized 3% saline had a significantly shorter hospital stay. Hypertonic saline also significantly improved clinical scores in the first 3 days in both inpatients and outpatients. However, when administered in the emergency department, hypertonic saline did not show any significant short-term effects (up to 2 hr) on clinical score and oxygen saturation. No significant adverse events related to hypertonic saline inhalation were reported.

Although hypertonic saline has been considered in other respiratory conditions that can feature secretion retention, the available research does not support its use. In COPD, acute airway narrowing is common after administration of the lowest concentration of hypertonic saline (3%), even with premedication with a bronchodilator (Taube et al 2001). Although additional agents such as montelukast can attenuate the airway narrowing (Zuhlke et al 2003), hypertonic saline does not appear to be helpful among those who can tolerate it (Valderramas & Atallah 2009). In people with asthma, hypertonic saline increases mucus clearance (Daviskas et al 1996) but it is not recommended because the airway narrowing (which can be exacerbated by hypertonic saline) is usually a greater problem than secretion retention.

Interaction with Physiotherapy

Another benefit of a dose of hypertonic saline is that the subjective ease of clearing sputum improves significantly (Elkins et al 2005, Eng et al 1996, Kellett & Robert 2011, Robinson et al 1997). Therefore physiotherapy interventions for airway clearance should be carefully timed with hypertonic saline administration to capitalize on the peak effect. In vitro studies indicate that equalization of the osmotic stimulus of hypertonic saline by movement of water into the airway is rapid and although the ASL may remain augmented for hours, the peak effect lasts only minutes (Donaldson et al 2006, Goralski et al 2010). Several approaches are advocated to capitalize on the peak effect during airway clearance sessions. One approach is to deliver hypertonic saline immediately before physical ACTs are performed, so that the airways are hydrated and mucus rheology is improved before the techniques are commenced. However, it is also possible to deliver hypertonic saline during ACTs, either intermittently (i.e. interspersed with short period of ACTs) or continuously if the techniques being used allow concurrent inhalation of the nebulized hypertonic saline (which may also save time). Delivery of hypertonic saline before or during ACTs appear to be similarly tolerable and effective, and preferable to delivery of hypertonic saline after ACTs (Dentice et al 2012).

Poor tolerability of hypertonic saline may occur – typically due to cough, chest tightness or pharyngitis – due to accumulation of saline in the mouth and throat. Anecdotally, rinsing and gargling with water may be effective in reducing these symptoms (Bye & Elkins 2007), even intermittently during the nebulization period if desired. These symptoms usually reduce in intensity with subsequent doses.

MANNITOL

Mannitol is a naturally occurring non-ionic sugar alcohol. When inhaled, it osmotically draws water into the airway – similar to hypertonic saline. Unlike hypertonic saline, however, mannitol is inhaled as a dry powder. The standard dose is 400 mg, but this is not tolerable in a single inhalation. Therefore each dose is divided into 10 individual capsules, each with 40 mg of mannitol (Teper et al 2011). One capsule is loaded into a handheld inhaler and pierced. The patient then exhales away from the inhaler, seals their lips on the inhaler, inhales through it with a close to full inspiration and inspiratory flow moderately above normal (at least 45–60 L/min and enough to make the capsule rattle), followed by a breath hold of 5 seconds and exhalation. The empty capsule is then ejected from the inhaler and the procedure is repeated for each of the 10 capsules to take one standard dose of 400 mg. Therefore although dry-powder mannitol does not require nebulizer cleaning, this is somewhat offset by the complex inhalation procedures.

Mechanisms of Action

Unlike hypertonic saline, in vitro studies have not been performed to show the osmotic movement of water across the airway epithelium, so the duration of the effect is unknown. However, the osmotic effect of mannitol is well established by its uses elsewhere in the body. Osmotic restoration of airway hydration is therefore the most likely explanation as to why mannitol accelerates MCC in healthy people and in people with various respiratory tract diseases (Daviskas et al 1997, 2008; Robinson et al 1999).

Coughing is common after each capsule of mannitol is inhaled and airway narrowing occurs frequently, so a bronchodilator is recommended as premedication before every dose (Daviskas & Anderson 2006). Despite premedication, 7–16% of people with CF get too much airway narrowing on a test dose of mannitol to safely continue its use (Aitken et al 2012, Bilton et al 2011). The first dose (i.e. 10 capsules) should therefore be supervised to ensure there is sufficient bronchoprotection by assessing oxyhaemoglobin saturation and change in FEV_1 after the dose (Pharmaxis 2011). Once established on mannitol, a further 14% of people with CF discontinue it by choice or due to adverse events (Aitken et al 2012, Bilton et al 2011). Similarly, 16% of people with bronchiectasis do not pass their initial test dose and 14% discontinue it by choice or due to an adverse event (Bilton et al 2013b). The proportions of people with other respiratory diseases who do not pass their initial test dose and who discontinue use are not clearly established (Daviskas et al 2010a). For those who can tolerate mannitol, cough is part of the beneficial mechanism, with clear evidence of acceleration of clearance with coughing on radio aerosol scans above that achieved with mannitol alone (Daviskas et al 2001).

Mannitol reduces both the solids content and the surface tension of sputum from people with CF, bronchiectasis and asthma (Daviskas et al 2007, 2010b, 2010c). While significant changes in viscoelasticity were observed in sputum from people with bronchiectasis when inhaled mannitol was followed by repetitive voluntary coughing, no change in sputum viscoelasticity after 2 weeks of treatment with mannitol was demonstrated in people with CF (Daviskas et al 2010b). No antibacterial or antioxidative mechanisms have been established for mannitol.

Evidence about Efficacy

In people with CF, mannitol improves lung function significantly after 2 weeks and this is maintained with long-term use (Aitken et al 2012, Bilton et al 2011, Jaques et al 2008). The risk of pulmonary exacerbations did not decrease significantly in either of the long-term trials (Aitken et al 2012, Bilton et al 2011). Pooling the data from both trials did not show a decrease in the time to first exacerbation with mannitol (Bilton et al 2013a). The relative risk of an exacerbation did reach statistical significance on the pooled analysis, but the 95% confidence interval did not confirm that the effect is clinically worthwhile. Quality of life did not improve significantly with mannitol.

In people with bronchiectasis, the effect of mannitol has been studied in a 12-week trial (Bilton et al 2013b). One primary outcome was quality of life, which showed no significant effect of mannitol. The other primary outcome was the weight of expectorated sputum collected over 24 hours. This is very difficult to interpret for two reasons. First, it is unclear which should be considered favourable: greater sputum production (i.e. mannitol is still effecting more clearance after 12 weeks) or less sputum production (i.e. mannitol has caused a reduction in the volume of secretions being produced by the lungs after 12 weeks). Second, the significant difference that occurred was due to a decrease in sputum production in the control group while the mannitol group remained unchanged. On high-resolution imaging, there was a statistically significant reduction in mucus plugging due to mannitol, but the effect may be too small to be clinically worthwhile. The remaining outcomes in this study also showed no significant benefits of mannitol for people with bronchiectasis: antibiotic use, pulmonary exacerbations, lung function, diffusion capacity, bacterial density, or exercise capacity (Bilton et al 2013b).

A single dose of mannitol improves MCC in adults with asthma (Daviskas et al 2010a), but the effects of regular use on clinical outcomes have not been examined. The effect of mannitol in other respiratory diseases has not been investigated.

Interaction with Physiotherapy

In all clinical studies to date, mannitol has been delivered before any ACTs or voluntary coughing. The effect of different timing of mannitol delivery in relation to physiotherapy is therefore unknown. However, clinical reasoning suggests that mannitol should be delivered after bronchodilator to reduce airway narrowing and immediately before ACTs to capitalize on the temporary augmentation of ASL. Coughing accelerates clearance on radio aerosol scans above that achieved with mannitol alone (Daviskas et al 2001), suggesting that all patients who use mannitol should be encouraged to follow it with physical ACTs to maximize the effect.

Due to the high rates of discontinuation of regular mannitol inhalations, physiotherapists should offer support in the early stages of regular mannitol use. This support should include coaching patients in the correct inhalation technique. Tilting the head up is reported to minimize cough and maximize delivery. The mouthpiece of the inhaler device should be tilted down so that the capsule drops forwards into the inhaler. The shoulders should remain relaxed during the near maximal inhalation of each capsule. If coughing is triggered, recovery time should be incorporated so that the next inspiratory capacity manoeuvre can be correctly performed. Each capsule should be checked when it is ejected from the inhaler device to ensure that it is empty. Non-empty capsules should be reloaded and emptying re-attempted with repeat inhalation (Pharmaxis 2011). However, the capsule should not be pierced a second time due to risk of creating small fragments of capsule that could be inhaled.

The dry powder inhaler utilizes energy from the patient's inspiration for aerosolization. Thus delivery and dispersion of mannitol is affected by the individual's ability to inhale at a suitably high flow rate. People with severe lung disease may have inadequate pulmonary function to achieve adequate mannitol delivery (Hirsh 2002), although inspiratory flows through the device have been shown to be adequate in ≈92% of adults and children with CF (Elkins et al 2014a) and ≈100% of adults with bronchiectasis (Elkins et al 2014b).

DORNASE ALPHA

Mechanisms of Action

Neutrophilic inflammation is a feature of both CF and bronchiectasis. Degenerating neutrophils release large amounts of DNA into airway mucus, so purulent secretions have an abundance of highly polymerized DNA and poor rheological properties for mucociliary and cough clearance (Voynow & Rubin 2009). Dornase alpha (deoxyribonuclease I (DNase I) (Pulmozyme)) is a highly purified solution of a bioengineered copy of a human proteolytic enzyme that cleaves DNA polymers (Rubin 2002). This cleaving action improves viscosity of sputum as demonstrated by increased 'pourability' 30 minutes after the application of dornase alpha (Shak et al 1990). It was hypothesized that the reduced sputum viscosity would reverse mucus stasis in people with CF, but radio aerosol studies did not demonstrate any immediate or cumulative effect of dornase alpha on MCC (Laube et al 1996, Robinson et al 2000).

Evidence about Efficacy

Despite the absence of evidence of an effect on MCC, clinical trials have demonstrated benefits from regular inhalation of dornase alpha by people with CF. A recent Cochrane review identified 12 trials of dornase alpha versus control in people with CF (Jones & Wallis 2010). The duration of the studies varied from 6 days (Laube et al 1996) to 3 years (Paul et al 2004). Statistically significant and clinically worthwhile benefits were observed in pooled FEV_1 data by 1 month, with the significant benefit maintained through 2 years of regular use (Quan et al 2001). The benefit in FVC was also significant between 1 and 6 months. Dornase alpha also reduced the age-adjusted risk of a pulmonary exacerbation with 6 months of use (Fuchs et al 1994) but not at 2 years (Quan et al 2001). The clinical benefits were accompanied by significant improvements in quality of life in some of the studies. Voice alteration and rash were more common on treatment.

In contrast, clinical studies in non-CF bronchiectasis have shown that dornase alpha is of no benefit, and may even be harmful. In a short-term study, dornase alpha was not associated with any improvement in lung function and quality of life measures in adults with bronchiectasis (Wills et al 1996). In vitro sputum transportability actually fell following the addition of dornase alpha to their sputum. A subsequent international multicentre study randomised 349 patients with stable bronchiectasis to either dornase alpha or placebo over a 24-week period (O'Donnell et al 1998). Pulmonary exacerbations were more frequent and FEV_1 decline was greater in patients who received dornase alpha. The reasons for this difference in response between patients with CF and bronchiectasis remain unclear. This unexpected detrimental finding highlights the importance of performing well-designed studies that address the therapeutic options for bronchiectasis, rather than extrapolating the results of trials involving patients with CF.

People with asthma often have mucus hypersecretion and retention at some times during the course of their disease (Rogers 2004). Three weeks of therapy with dornase alpha was ineffective at improving FEV_1 in adults with acute asthma that was refractory to bronchodilators (Silverman et al 2012). Three weeks of therapy with dornase alpha also did not improve FVC, FEV_1 or forced expiratory flow at 25–75% of FVC (FEF_{25-75}) in children with clinically stable asthma (Bakker et al 2013).

Interaction with Physiotherapy

Traditionally, people with CF have been advised to nebulize dornase alpha 30 minutes prior to ACTs because it makes in vitro sputum pourable within 30 minutes (Shak et al 1990). Alternatively, dornase alpha nebulization after ACTs may improve deposition to peripheral airways due to reduced mucus obstruction. Time of day may also be important. Spontaneous MCC is faster during waking hours than sleep (Bateman et al 1978), so morning nebulization of dornase alpha may capitalize on faster daytime MCC and on the clearance effects of daytime activities such as exercise (Dwyer et al 2011b). Conversely, evening inhalation may be more convenient or may ease expectoration the following morning due to increased dwell time in the airways. However, evening inhalation could theoretically induce cough and impair sleep quality.

A recent Cochrane review identified 4 trials of dornase alpha administration before versus after physiotherapy techniques for airway clearance in people with CF (Dentice & Elkins 2013). The duration of the studies varied from 2 weeks (Bishop et al 2011, Fitzgerald et al 2005) to 8 weeks (Anderson & Morton 2009). Inhalation after instead of before airway clearance did not significantly change FEV_1. Similarly, FVC, FEF_{25-75} and quality of life were not significantly affected. Another small airways measure, FEF_{25}, was significantly worse with dornase alfa inhalation after airway clearance, with a mean difference of 0.17 L (95% CI 0.05 to 0.28), based on the pooled data from two small studies in children (7–19 years) with well-preserved lung function. However, this result relied on a measure with high variability, the studies had variable follow up, and the effect was not reflected in the FEF_{25-75} measure of small airway function. All other secondary outcomes were statistically non-significant. In one additional trial, morning versus evening inhalation had no impact on lung function or symptoms (van der Giessen et al 2007).

For most people with CF, the majority of evidence indicates that the effectiveness of dornase alpha is not influenced by when it is administered with respect to airway clearance or time of day. Therefore the timing of dornase alpha inhalation can be largely based on pragmatic reasons (such as fitting around other medications in the airway clearance regimen) or individual preference. However, for children with well-preserved lung function who are unlikely to be on other medications, inhalation before airway clearance could be recommended, as it may be more beneficial for small airway function.

BRONCHODILATORS

Many inhaled bronchodilators are available commercially and it is beyond the scope of this chapter to review them all. However, the primary mechanism common to all of them (i.e. bronchodilatation) can be used in several ways to improve the efficacy of other interventions.

Improving the regional deposition of inhaled drugs can improve the clinical response obtained (Pritchard 2001). Bronchodilators can be used to improve airway patency and on this basis bronchodilator premedication is recommended to achieve better deposition (and effect) of other inhaled medications, although direct evidence for this is somewhat limited (Harrison & Laube 1994, Heijerman et al 2009). Bronchodilators can also be used prior to ACTs that rely on expiratory airflow, in order to improve airway patency and thereby achieve more effective secretion clearance (Kellett et al 2005, Sutton et al 1988).

Bronchodilators can also provide protection against airway narrowing from subsequent inhaled medications such as antibiotic or osmotic agents (Delvaux et al 2004, Fontana et al 1988). Theoretically bronchodilators may also prevent airway narrowing due to a physiotherapy technique for airway clearance (e.g. if the technique triggers excessive coughing), although it may be more appropriate to choose a less aggravating technique.

Exercise is another physiotherapy intervention that has a range of benefits in patients with respiratory disease (Dwyer et al 2011b, Carson et al 2013, Cindy Ng et al 2012). However, one possible adverse effect of exercise is its potential to cause airway narrowing, which can occur in people with or without chronic asthma (Parsons 2013). A short bout of warm-up exercise can prevent this exercise-induced bronchoconstriction in many patients (Elkins & Brannan, 2012). If necessary, bronchodilator premedication is another effective prevention strategy (Parsons 2013). In people with asthma who develop exercise-induced bronchoconstriction, bronchodilatation occurs in the first 1–2 minutes of exercise, with the onset of bronchoconstriction at 6–8 minutes in adults and a little earlier in children (Hallstrand et al 2013, Weiler et al 2010). Therefore the deposition and effect of the bronchodilator can be improved by administering it 1–2 minutes after the start of exercise (Joseph et al 1976).

STRUCTURING AN AIRWAY CLEARANCE SESSION

Order of Interventions

Combining the information from empirical research presented in the preceding sections of this chapter with clinical reasoning suggests that inhaled medications should be ordered as follows. Bronchodilators should be given first to improve deposition of other medications, to minimize bronchoconstriction from irritant medications, and to maximize airflow during physiotherapy techniques. If an osmotic expectorant such as hypertonic saline or mannitol is used, it should be given after the bronchodilator and before ACTs. Hypertonic saline could also be given during ACTs, either simultaneously or intermittently, although some caveats about combining interventions are discussed in the next section. For most people with CF, if dornase alpha is used, it can be given before or after ACT. However, young children with well-preserved lung function may benefit from taking it before the ACTs. Inhaled antibiotic and anti-inflammatory medications should be administered last so that uniform deposition throughout the lungs is promoted by removing as much mucus obstruction as possible. If airway narrowing is induced by any of the interventions, it would be appropriate to ensure resolution of this before progressing on to the next intervention because it is likely to impair the efficacy of inhaled medications and ACTs.

Combining Interventions

Some people with respiratory disease are interested in combining therapies, such as inhaling a medication during ACTs. Before recommending such procedures, physiotherapists should consider what is known about whether the ACT affects deposition of the inhaled medication and whether the medication affects the efficacy of the ACT. Unfortunately, very few combinations that have been investigated are promising. PEP can be applied via a mask or mouthpiece as an ACT (McIlwaine et al 2015). Nebulizer attachments are available commercially to allow nebulization of medications simultaneously. Although this has mild benefits on the pattern of distribution of the medication within the lungs, the total dose received by the patient is substantially reduced (Laube et al 2005). HFCWO is a physical ACT applied via a pneumatic vest. It does not impair the deposition of inhaled medications (Stites et al 2006). Unfortunately, HFCWO is not as effective as simpler, cheaper methods of airway clearance (McIlwaine et al 2013), so it would not be recommended for use in clinical practice. Physiotherapists should consider the advantages and disadvantages of these combinations carefully before recommending them in clinical practice.

Techniques for Improving Dyspnoea

Dyspnoea is the perceptual experience of distress with breathing. The terms 'dyspnoea' and 'shortness of breath' are often used interchangeably to infer distress with breathing in clinical contexts. While all individuals will have experienced breathlessness at some point in their lives, unless an individual has experienced distress with breathing, the degree of unpleasantness and consequent impact on all aspects of everyday life that this sensation evokes is difficult to appreciate. This may explain why these two terms are often erroneously used as synonyms and why dyspnoea as a symptom is underappreciated and in many cases, inadequately assessed and managed by health professionals.

Dyspnoea is not:

- a single, generic sensation
- simply an intense form of shortness of breath
- something people should endure
- inevitable due to ageing of the cardiovascular, respiratory or musculoskeletal systems.

DIFFERENCES BETWEEN SHORTNESS OF BREATH AND DYSPNOEA

Symptoms can only be described by those experiencing them. Signs are described by people observing the person either as a subjective impression or measured objectively (Fig. 7-51). Dyspnoea is a symptom, whereas shortness of breath can be both a symptom ('I feel short of breath') and a sign described by health professionals observing a person displaying a constellation of signs reflecting an increased work of breathing (see Fig. 7-51). Dyspnoea is always unpleasant and distressing, whereas shortness of breath may be pleasant or unpleasant depending on the individual's expectation, current situation and past experiences. The state of being breathless may range from a pleasant, enjoyable experience welcomed by ultra-athletes, to breathing discomfort with exertion experienced in people with chronic medical conditions, through to the unremitting distress of refractory dyspnoea which persists despite medical management such as experienced by many people with end-stage life-limiting illnesses (see Fig. 7-51).

In acute clinical situations (e.g. acute respiratory failure, infections, bronchospasm, uncompensated heart failure), the degree of dyspnoea may have a predictable relationship with degree of physiological disturbance of cardiovascular and respiratory systems. However, in situations where dyspnoea is a common daily symptom such as in chronic respiratory, cardiovascular, neurological and musculoskeletal conditions,

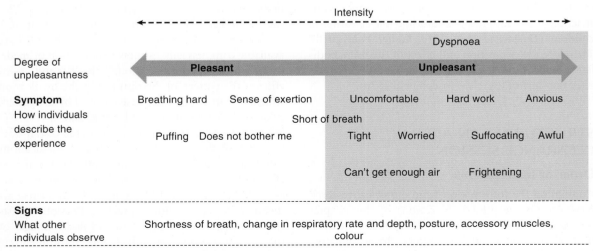

FIGURE 7-51 ■ The landscape of breathlessness.

dyspnoea has a more tenuous relationship with the degree of physiological impairment. For example, in people with COPD, two individuals may have the same degree of impairment in ABGs profiles or airways obstruction yet differ markedly with respect to the degree of dyspnoea experienced at rest or on exertion.

MECHANISMS UNDERPINNING DYSPNOEA

Dyspnoea is the perceptual experience of a sensation. Sensation drives behaviour. Where an activity or context results in a pleasurable sensation, we seek to repeat the activity. Where an activity or context results in an unpleasant sensation especially if associated with a fearful or anxious emotional response, we avoid the activity or context (Williams et al 2012b). From an evolutionary perspective, dyspnoea is a sensation necessary for survival (O'Donnell et al 2007). Similar to other survival sensations (pain, thirst and hunger), where these sensations are sufficiently unpleasant or fear inducing, they motivate the individual to change behaviours. In acute situations, these sensations prompt behaviours to ensure survival of the individual. However, where the individual is repeatedly exposed to these sensations, long-term behaviours are learned in order to avoid the sensation, potentially leading to secondary health consequences (Lansing et al 2009).

Dyspnoea is a multidimensional sensation currently thought to comprise distinct sensory qualities (work/effort, air hunger/unsatisfied inspiration and tightness), that vary in intensity, degree of unpleasantness and subsequent emotional and behavioural impact (Parshall et al 2012). While there may be further sensory qualities, three distinct sensory qualities have been identified, each of which is proposed to result from discrete mechanisms (Parshall et al 2012). The sensation of tightness is thought to arise from afferent output from airways receptors. The sensation of work/effort is likely to derive from a combination of respiratory muscle afferents and the sensory cortex assessing the magnitude of motor drive from the motor cortex. The sensation of air hunger/unsatisfied inspiration is proposed to result from the discrepancy between the motor drive to breathe (sensed by corol-

lary discharge to sensory cortex) and afferent feedback from sources within the respiratory system (Parshall et al 2012). Notably, the sensation of air hunger/unsatisfied inspiration has been reported to be more unpleasant than the sensation of work/effort (Banzett et al 2015).

Lansing et al (2009) proposed a staged model for the perceptual processes underpinning the sensation of breathlessness in which afferent input is initially evaluated for intensity and sensory quality. Subsequently, an assessment of the degree of unpleasantness is made which culminates in immediate and longer-term emotional responses (fear, frustration, anxiety) and behavioural consequences (immediate cessation of activity or life style changes) (Lansing et al 2009).

In order to consciously appreciate and describe the sensation, complex integration is therefore required between afferent information arising from systems within the body and cortical areas associated with respiratory motor drive, attention, memory, expectation and affective state (Parshall et al 2012). Respiratory motor control is an automatic process involving the brainstem respiratory centre which, under normal circumstances, does not require or result in conscious awareness of breathing by the individual (O'Donnell et al 2007). Respiratory motor control can also be voluntarily altered as a result of input from cortical structures (Parshall et al 2012). A respiratory gating model has been proposed in order to explain the connections between systems permitting a conscious appreciation of breathing (Davenport in O'Donnell et al 2007).

A simple schematic derived from O'Donnell et al (2007) and Parshall et al (2012) is presented in Figure 7-52. Unlike pain, there are no specialized receptors for dyspnoea. Parshall et al (2012) comprehensively summarize the variety of sources which may contribute afferent input from systems within the body (chemoreceptors, stretch, irritant, airway, muscle, joint, vascular, skin receptors) and cortical structures (motor cortex, sensory cortex, association cortex and limbic system (see Fig. 7-52A). Many of the respiratory afferents within the body have projections to the respiratory network in the brainstem and projections to higher cortical centres (O'Donnell et al 2007). Between the primary motor cortex, sensory cortex and limbic system, there are inter-connecting neurons which permit information (corollary discharge) to be shared

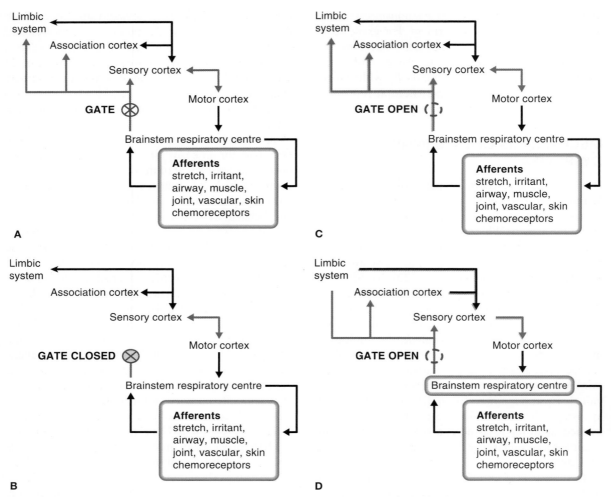

FIGURE 7-52 ■ Simplified version of the respiratory gating model. **(A)** Simplified schematic of the relationships between areas involved in the conscious awareness of breathing. **(B)** At rest and health, gate closed, breathing is automatic and there is no conscious awareness of breathing. **(C)** Where afferent input is increased from body systems, gate opens and individual has the ability to be consciously aware of breathing (bottom-up modulation). **(D)** Where attention is directed to breathing or limbic/association/sensory cortex corollary discharge, gate opens and individual has the ability to be consciously aware of breathing (top-down modulation).

between structures (Gigliotti 2010). These corollary discharges to the sensory cortex provide an avenue for the brain to monitor the state of respiratory activity (Gigliotti 2010).

At rest and in health, respiratory motor control is automatic, and the individual does not have a conscious awareness of the sensation of breathing (see Fig. 7-52B). When afferent information from the body exceeds a threshold (increased work of breathing;

'bottom-up' modulation (see Fig. 7-52C) or where attention is directed to breathing or breathing changes as a result of an emotional/affective event ('top-down' modulation in Figure 7-52D), the gate is opened and there is the potential for conscious appreciation of the sensation of breathing.

O'Donnell et al (2007), proposed that the sensation of breathing is state dependent, where 'state' refers to both the existing background physiological state and the cognitive/behavioural/affective state' (p. 147). It is possible that ineffective respiratory gating or perceptual processing of the sensation of dyspnoea may explain situations where individuals have an increased or decreased awareness of the sensation of dyspnoea leading to increased or delayed medical care seeking behaviours. Recent research suggests that impaired respiratory gating exists in anxious individuals leading to increased perceptions of respiratory sensations (Chan et al 2012, von Leupoldt et al 2011), whereas inaccurate or blunted perceptions of dyspnoea may result in delays in seeking medical assistance resulting in greater costs of medical care and increased mortality in elderly people (Ebihara et al 2012).

ASSESSMENT OF DYSPNOEA

There are a diverse range of instruments available to assess various aspects of breathlessness. In general, these instruments fall into two categories: instruments that assess the sensation of breathlessness (intensity, unpleasantness and sensory quality) and instruments that assess the impact of sensation (respiratory-related quality of life and respiratory-related impairment). The majority of instruments assess the impairment, impact or burden that breathlessness imposes on behaviour or quality of everyday life. In many cases, these instruments have been developed for specific chronic conditions and assess dyspnoea as a subscale within a broader

questionnaire (e.g. Chronic Respiratory Disease Questionnaire (Guyatt et al 1987), Motor Neurone Disease Dyspnoea Rating Scale (Dougan et al 2000)). There are comparatively few instruments which specifically assess the sensation of breathlessness. The instruments which assess the sensation of breathlessness may either assess a single dimension of sensation (such as visual analogue scales (Aitken 1969, von Leupoldt & Dahme 2005) or numeric rating scales for intensity or unpleasantness) or assess multiple dimensions (such as the Dyspnoea–12 (Yorke et al 2010) or Multidimensional Dyspnoea scale (Banzett et al 2015)). The evolution and examples of instruments used to assess dyspnoea are presented in Figure 7-53.

There is no universally accepted instrument for assessing dyspnoea. A number of review or consensus papers have been published concerning assessment of breathlessness or dyspnoea in advanced cardiovascular and pulmonary disease (Bausewein et al 2007, Mahler et al 2010), COPD (Glaab et al 2010), acute and chronic heart failure (Johnson et al 2010, West, R.L. et al 2010), palliative care (Dorman et al 2007, Mularski et al 2010) and obesity (Gerlach et al 2013). In both clinical and research settings, it is recommended that dyspnoea assessment include measures of intensity and sensory quality (Johnson et al 2010, Mahler et al 2010, Mularski et al 2010, Parshall et al 2012, West, R.L. et al 2010), distress or unpleasantness (Mahler et al 2010, Mularski et al 2010) and impact of

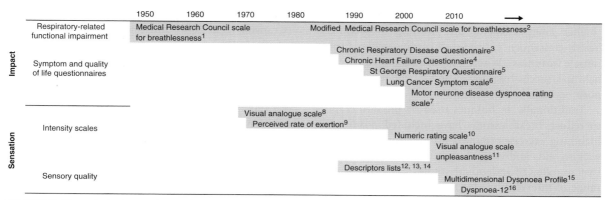

FIGURE 7-53 ■ Evolution and examples of instruments. *(1, Fletcher 1952; 2, Brooks 1982; 3, Guyatt et al 1987; 4, Guyatt et al 1989; 5, Jones et al 1992; 6, Hollen et al 1993; 7, Dougan et al 2000; 8, Aitken 1969; 9, Borg 1970; 10, Gift and Narsavage 1998; 11, Von Leupoldt and Dahme 2005; 12, Simon et al 1989; 13, Simon et al 1990; 14, Mahler et al 1996; 15, Banzett et al 2015; 16, Yorke et al 2010.)*

breathlessness on quality of life (Johnson et al 2010, Parshall et al 2012, West, R.L. et al 2010).

MANAGEMENT STRATEGIES FOR DYSPNOEA

Simplistically, any intervention which alters afferent input from systems within the body or cortical areas associated with respiratory motor drive, attention, memory, expectation and affective state has the potential to alter the sensation of breathlessness. In life-threatening acute situations where respiratory distress results from cardiac or respiratory failure, interventions such as supplemental oxygen, supported ventilation, resuscitation, antibiotics and anti-inflammatories aim to address the physiological disruption (support and reduce work of breathing, improve ventilation/perfusion, CO, reduce inflammation, etc).

In chronic medical conditions where dyspnoea is a common symptom, the initial focus of management is to optimize treatment of underlying medical conditions (Parshall et al 2012). Even when an individual is receiving optimal medical and pharmacological management for the underlying chronic condition, dyspnoea is likely to persist as a daily experience usually, but not always, related to physical exertion. Where physical exertion is associated with dyspnoea, individuals learn to modify their behaviour (and environment) to avoid or reduce the likelihood of experiencing the sensation. As a result, daily activity profiles are likely to shift towards prolonged periods of sedentary behaviours (low energy expenditure) and less frequent periods of moderate to vigorous physical activity (higher energy expenditure) leading to secondary health consequences (reduced cardiovascular fitness, muscle weakness). Where adaptive behaviours become habitual, successful intervention for the relief of dyspnoea becomes more difficult.

Traditionally, techniques used by physiotherapists to reduce breathlessness have included positioning, breathing exercises (pursed lip breathing, BC, IMT), walking aids and exercise training. While there are a vast number of individual studies exploring a wide range of interventions for the relief of dyspnoea, systematic reviews with or without meta-analysis allow synthesis of similar interventions. Table 7-9 presents a summary of systematic reviews of higher level research designs concerning interventions for management of dyspnoea in adults.

For long-term relief of dyspnoea, compelling evidence exists to recommend the use of exercise training and pulmonary rehabilitation (see Chapter 12). The potential mechanisms by which exercise training of sufficient duration and intensity may reduce the sensation of dyspnoea include system efficiency ($\downarrow$ ventilatory effort for same workload), reduced or delayed onset of dynamic hyperinflation during exercise and reduced sensitivity to dyspnoea (Williams et al 2012a).

For short-term relief of dyspnoea, high-level evidence supports the use of chest wall vibration (mediated by muscle spindles) and walking aids (mediated through forwards lean postures, bracing and recruitment of accessory muscles) (Bausewein et al 2008). Training programs of sufficient duration and intensity for both IMT and neuroelectric muscle stimulation of peripheral muscles (mediated through increased strength and endurance of muscles) have been demonstrated to have beneficial effects on dyspnoea (Bausewein et al 2008, Gosselink et al 2011) and may be useful in people who cannot participate in standard exercise programmes.

The evidence to support the efficacy of breathing exercises (e.g. pursed lip breathing, BC) to reduce sensations of dyspnoea is inconsistent. While breathing training/exercises may provide a short-term beneficial effect for some individuals, diaphragmatic breathing (BC) for relief of dyspnoea is not be recommended for people with moderate to severe COPD (Gosselink et al 1995). Supplemental oxygen during end-stage disease provides no further benefit compared to medical air (Cranston et al 2008) but may be beneficial for the relief of dyspnoea in people with COPD who are mildly hypoxemic or who desaturate during exercise (Langer et al 2009, Uronis et al 2011).

While insufficient evidence or low-level support was reported for the use of relaxation exercises, hand-held fans, psychotherapy/counselling, music as a distraction or acupuncture/acupressure for the relief of dyspnoea, this should not be inferred to mean that these interventions have been proven to be ineffective.

It is worth noting, that the development of instruments which assess the multidimensional nature of dyspnoea is relatively recent and consequently the

1992). As inspiratory muscle dysfunction contributes to dyspnoea in COPD, it is evident that specifically targeting the inspiratory muscles may lead to further reductions in dyspnoea (Hill et al 2004).

The inspiratory muscles, like other skeletal muscles, undergo physiological adaptations in response to training. Despite this, the early literature on the use of IMT in patients with COPD presents a mixed picture. In part this is due to the paucity of controlled clinical trials, but more importantly due to the nature of the training adopted. In general the trials were confounded by the training regimens, in which the frequency, duration and intensity of training were less than that required to achieve a true training response, as highlighted in an early meta-analysis (Smith et al 1992). A decade later, Lotters et al (2002) published a second meta-analysis, which included only studies in which the intensity of IMT was controlled and fixed in order to achieve a training response. This review concluded that IMT improved respiratory muscle strength and endurance, although the effects of IMT on exercise capacity remained to be determined. More recently, Geddes et al (2005) published a systematic review in which IMT was shown to be effective not only in terms of increasing inspiratory muscle strength and endurance but also in improving exercise capacity in adults with COPD. However, this review emphasized that the method of IMT employed is important if clinical benefits are to be obtained and that training of the ventilatory muscles must follow the basic principles of training for any striated muscle with regard to the intensity and duration of the stimulus, the specificity of training and the reversibility of training.

The principle of specificity of training is that the effects of training are very specific to the neural and muscular elements of overload. The overload principle asserts that overload must be applied to a muscle for a training response to occur (ACSM's Guidelines for Exercise Testing and Prescription 2014). Overload may be applied by increasing the frequency or duration of training or the intensity of the loading, or a combination of these factors. Generally, training theory suggests that inspiratory muscle strength gains can be achieved at intensities of 80–90% of maximal inspiratory pressure. Strength-endurance gains (maximal effective force that can be maintained) can be achieved at 60–80%, and endurance (the ability to continue a dynamic task for a prolonged period) at approximately 60% of peak, which equates with high-intensity training regimens used in systemic exercise (Kraemer et al 2002).

Overload may also include the concept of incremental loading. This involves decreasing the rest periods between muscle contractions (Komi & Hakkinen 1991), which has been shown to recruit a larger proportion of muscle fibres and, hence, a larger pool of fibres are trained for subsequent lower but potentially fatiguing loads (Reid & Samrai 1995, Reid et al 1994). In studies that used the principle of high-intensity incremental IMT, improvements in lung volumes, diaphragm thickness and exercise capacity were obtained in healthy individuals and in patients with CF (Enright et al 2004, 2006).

In previous investigations, training methodologies varied between flow, pressure or volume loads imposed on the respiratory muscles (McCool 1992). A low-pressure high-flow load was first described in 1976 by Leith & Bradley which involved training the respiratory muscles by voluntarily ventilating at high levels for a prolonged period (usually 15 minutes). This was analogous to the high ventilatory demands imposed on the inspiratory muscles during high-intensity exercise (Belman 1993). The load imposed on the inspiratory muscles required a high flow rate at low pressure, now considered impractical, as it requires the assembly of complex breathing circuits in order to ensure that the individual remains normocapnic. In addition, breathless patients find this method of IMT uncomfortable to maintain and hence this method of IMT tends to be reserved for laboratory-based investigations rather than being used in a clinical setting (Scherer et al 2000).

In contrast to a flow load, a high-pressure low-flow load occurs with any process that increases the transpulmonary pressure required to breathe in. These loads can be experimentally imposed by inhaling from a rigid chamber or by breathing through an external resistance. Such loads can be achieved by either resistive or threshold devices. Resistive training devices incorporate a range of apertures, which vary in size in order to apply the prescribed resistive load. Threshold devices impose a threshold or a critical inspiratory opening pressure that the individual is required to overcome before the start of an inspiratory flow. The efficacy of both these modes of IMT have been the subject of some debate, although it has been shown that targeted resistive IMT is as effective as threshold IMT for adults with COPD (Hsiao et al 2003). On a practical level, some issues require consideration; for example, targeted resistive devices provide visual feedback which enhances motivation, although ensuring that the patient is maintaining the required training intensity can be problematic. Conversely, threshold trainers provide a more constant resistance, although the loss of visual feedback may result in loss of motivation.

In addition to the mode of training adopted, the frequency of training in IMT interventions, the duration of the training intervention and the issue of reversibility of training requires consideration. Standard guidelines of the American College of Sports Medicine (ACSM's Guidelines for Exercise Testing and Prescription 2014) suggest a training frequency of one to two times per day for a total duration of 20–30 minutes, three to five times per week for 6 weeks. However, functional improvements and adaptive cellular changes in the inspiratory muscles have been shown to occur following 5 weeks of training (Ramirez-Sarmiento et al 2002), although training must be maintained for the cellular training effects to be sustained (McArdle et al 2014). In summary, the optimal frequency of training is thought to be three times weekly, to continue beyond 4 weeks and with maintenance achieved by continuing training at one or two times weekly (Fleck 1994).

In conclusion, although there is much conflicting evidence in the literature, which has cast doubt on the place of IMT in patients with respiratory muscle dysfunction, more recent data that have incorporated the appropriate physiological training principles during IMT look promising (Geddes et al 2005). The use of targeted inspiratory resistive or threshold modes of IMT as opposed to non-targeted inspiratory resistive modes ensures that the training intensity is achieved and maintained. Thus with effective IMT regimens, exercise intolerance, dyspnoea and hypercapnic ventilatory failure may be prevented or alleviated. In addition, another indication for IMT is that weakness of the inspiratory muscles may lead to an inability to generate an adequate flow to assure lung deposition when using dry powder inhalers. Hence strengthening the inspiratory muscles may improve the efficacy of inhaled drug therapy (Weiner & Weiner 2006). These considerations are vital if IMT is to find a proven place in pulmonary rehabilitation programmes (Hill & Eastwood 2005).

BREATHING CONTROL

Breathing techniques can be considered in two categories; normal breathing, known as 'breathing control (BC)', where the pattern of breathing is maximally efficient for the individual with minimal effort expended, and 'breathing exercises', where either inspiration is emphasized (as in TEEs and IMT) or expiration is emphasized (as in the huff of the FET).

BC is normal tidal breathing using the lower chest and encouraging relaxation of the upper chest and shoulders. This was also known historically as 'diaphragmatic breathing', but the term is a misnomer, as during normal tidal breathing there is activity not only in the diaphragm but also in the internal and external intercostal muscles, the abdominal and scalene muscles (Green & Moxham 1985). This pattern of breathing is not appropriate for everyone. Dyspnoea has been shown to increase in some people with COPD using 'diaphragmatic breathing' owing to an increase in asynchronous and paradoxical breathing movements (Gosselink 2004, Gosselink et al 1995).

To be taught BC, the patient should be in a comfortable, well-supported position either sitting (Fig. 7-54) or in high side lying (Fig. 7-55). The patient is encouraged to relax the upper chest, shoulders and arms. One hand, which may be either the patient's or the physiotherapist's or one hand of each, can be positioned lightly on the upper abdomen. As the patient breathes in, the hand should be felt to rise up and out; as the patient breathes out, the hand sinks down and in. Inspiration using the lower chest in this way is the active phase. Expiration should be relaxed and passive, and both inspiration and expiration should be barely audible. Inspiration through the nose allows the air to be warmed, humidified and filtered before it reaches the upper airways. If the nose is blocked, breathing through the mouth will reduce the resistance to the flow of air and reduce the work of breathing. If the patient is very breathless, breathing through the mouth will reduce the anatomical dead space.

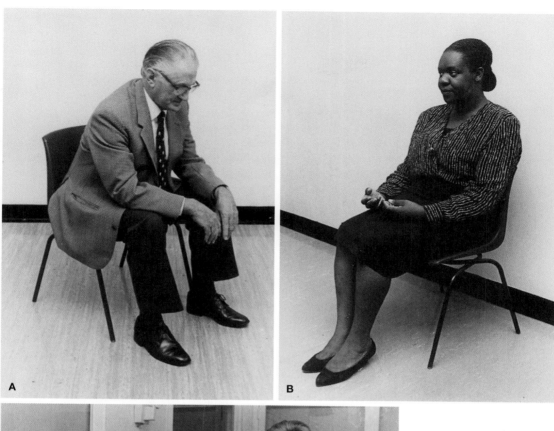

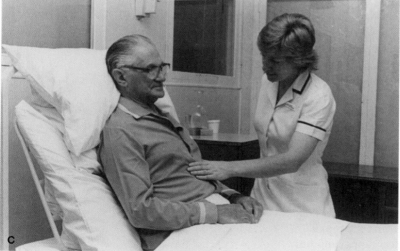

FIGURE 7-54 ▪ (A, B and C) Breathing control in sitting.

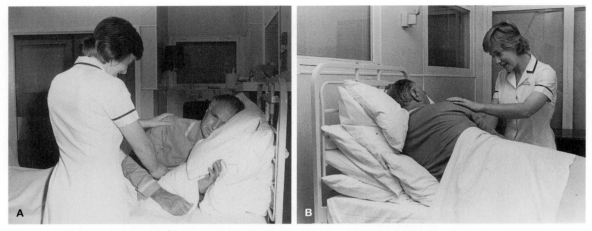

FIGURE 7-55 ■ **(A** and **B)** Breathing control in high side lying.

Many breathless patients, for example those with emphysema, asthma, pulmonary fibrosis or lung cancer, may benefit from using BC in positions that encourage relaxation of the upper chest and shoulders and allow movement of the lower chest and abdomen. These positions also optimize, by lengthening, the length tension status of the diaphragm (Dean 1985, O'Neill & McCarthy 1983, Parshall et al 2012, Sharp et al 1980). When the patient is sitting or standing leaning forwards, the abdominal contents raise the anterior part of the diaphragm, probably facilitating its contraction during inspiration. A similar effect can be seen in the side lying and high side lying positions where the curvature of the dependent part of the diaphragm is increased. This effect, combined with relaxation of the head, neck and shoulders, promotes the pattern of BC.

Useful positions are:

■ Relaxed sitting (see Fig. 7-54)
■ High side lying (see Fig. 7-55): for maximal relaxation of the head, neck and upper chest, the neck should be slightly flexed and the top pillow should be above the shoulder, supporting only the head and neck
■ Forwards lean standing (Fig. 7-56)
■ Relaxed standing (Fig. 7-57)
■ Kneeling position (Fig. 7-58): this may be preferred by children.

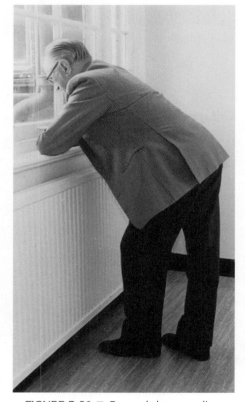

FIGURE 7-56 ■ Forwards lean standing.

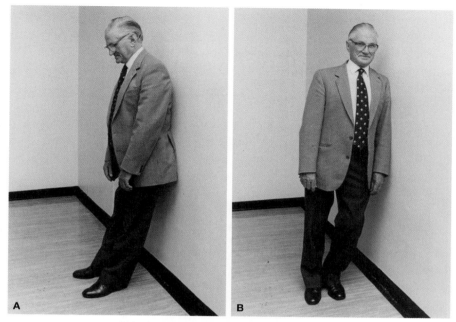

FIGURE 7-57 ■ **(A** and **B)** Relaxed standing.

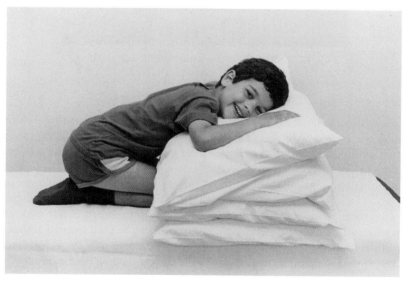

FIGURE 7-58 ■ Forwards kneeling.

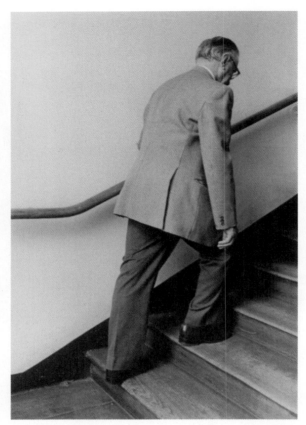

FIGURE 7-59 ■ Breathing control while stair climbing.

These positions discourage the tendency of breathless patients to push down or grip with their hands, which causes elevation of the shoulders and overuse of the accessory muscles of breathing, and may result in a more effective length tension status of the diaphragm.

BC may also be used to improve exercise capacity in breathless patients when walking up slopes, hills and stairs (Fig. 7-59). Breathless patients tend to hold their breath on exertion and rush, for example, up a flight of stairs, arriving at the top extremely breathless and unable to speak. The simple technique of relaxing the arms and shoulders, reducing the walking speed a little and using the pattern of breathing in on climbing up one step and breathing out on climbing up the next step may lead to a marked reduction in breathlessness

(Webber 1991). When this technique has been mastered, some patients, on days when they are less breathless, may find breathing in for one step and out for two steps more comfortable. The severely breathless patient may also find the combination of BC with walking helpful when walking on level ground. A respiratory walking frame (Fig. 7-60) with or without portable oxygen can be used to assist ambulation in the severely breathless patient.

BC can also be used to control a bout or paroxysm of coughing. Some people with chronic respiratory disease automatically use pursed-lip breathing. Breathing through pursed lips has the effect of generating a small positive pressure during expiration, which may to some extent reduce the collapse of unstable airways.

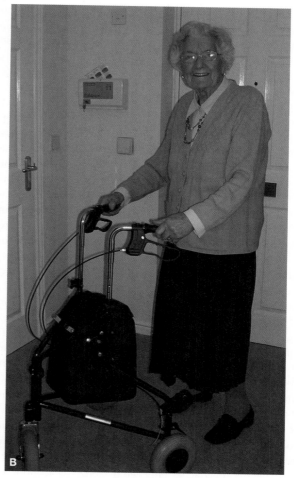

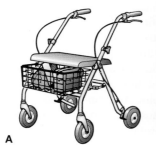

A **B**

FIGURE 7-60 ■ **(A)** Diagrammatic representation of a four-wheeled rollator. **(B)** Using a three-wheeled walker.

Techniques for Improving Dysfunctional Breathing

The reader is directed to the section on Hyperventilation Syndrome in Chapter 5 for an overview of dysfunction breathing in relation to that respiratory disorder.

MANUAL THERAPY TECHNIQUES FOR MUSCULOSKELETAL DYSFUNCTION

Musculoskeletal dysfunction is common in people with respiratory disease. People with chronic cardiorespiratory disease may often demonstrate skeletal, musculoskeletal and nervous systems adaptations over time, related to the severity and management of their disease. As age increases, the incidence of musculoskeletal deterioration will also increase (Parasa & Maffulli 1999). Any postural or degenerative changes are likely to have implications for physical function and quality of life as well as influencing the cardiorespiratory system.

Postural and skeletal changes occurring over time relate to the overuse of upper chest breathing patterns, lack of lower rib expansion and reduction in the more efficient pattern of diaphragmatic breathing. Chronic hyperinflation typically leads to the development of a barrel-shaped chest with an increase in the antero-posterior diameter of the chest. Pain may limit rib expansion and abdominal breathing, particularly in patients following abdominal surgery.

Secondary malalignment of the scapulae is associated with prolonged coughing using trunk flexion and the increased outward pressure on the chest wall. More sputum may mean more pain and less efficient airway clearance (Massery 2005).

In a study of 143 young adults with CF, Henderson and Specter (1994) found 77% of females and 36% of males over 15 years of age had a kyphosis of more than 40° (the upper limit of normal). Kyphosis tends to worsen with age and disease severity (Massie et al 1998).

The neck and shoulder girdle structures adapt to counterbalance the flexed-trunk sitting position. Neutral neck and head position is compromised as the neck and head are drawn forwards by the large superficial muscle groups and hyperactivity of the suboccipital extensors. The greater the thoracic kyphosis, the more likely it is that the middle and upper cervical regions will become lordotic, as the upper cervical spine hyperextends and tilts the head upward to maintain a vertical orientation of the face.

This upper cervical spine hyperextension and forwards head posture combine with a loss of endurance of the deep cervical flexor muscles to increase the likelihood of cervicogenic headache (Jull et al 2002, Watson & Trott 1993). Chronic headaches may also be associated with medical causes in patients with cardiorespiratory disease (Festini et al 2004, Ravilly et al 1996).

The incidence of musculoskeletal chest pain in people with CF tends to increase as the disease progresses. Painful stiffness in the chest may inhibit airway clearance and increase the work of breathing (Massery 2005). A decrease in muscle strength and mobility in the trunk, chest and shoulders has been demonstrated in people with CF (Ross et al 1987).

In the presence of an inefficient, upper chest breathing pattern, the overactive scalene muscles elevate the first and second ribs while the levator scapulae depress and rotate the lateral shoulder girdle (Fig. 7-61). Shortening of upper trapezius and tightness of pecto-ralis minor and major elevate and anteriorly tilt the scapulae, respectively. At the same time the antagonist and stabilizing muscles, serratus anterior and the middle and lower fibres of trapezius lengthen and weaken, causing winging and inferior rotation of the scapulae (Sahrmann 2005). Over time, the long thoracic extensors and multifidus lose their segmental stabilizing capacity and endurance, and become less able to sustain the upright sitting neutral posture.

The sternocleidomastoids are used excessively during coughing. Muscle fatigue related to the excess work of breathing may further accentuate poor posture in people with moderate to severe chronic lung disease. The existing kyphosis of the thoracic spine is increased due to prolonged bed rest and reductions in general exercise tolerance. Habitual slouching due to dyspnoea and feeling unwell will place more kyphotic strain on the thoracic and lumbar spines, and the lumbopelvic angle will be flexed instead of lordotic.

Vertebral intersegmental motion will be gradually lost as the chest becomes fixed in elevation and flexion. Reduced range of thoracic extension will contribute to loss of the final 30° of shoulder flexion and abduction; while tightness in anterior deltoid, teres major and latissimus dorsi muscles and disturbance of normal scapulothoracic rhythm will decrease the free range of external rotation and flexion available at the glenohumeral joint. As a consequence, the overstretching of infraspinatus and teres minor, associated with the internally rotated position of the humerus, may lead to poor stability of the humerus in the glenoid fossa (Fig. 7-62).

These muscular and skeletal aberrations are likely to have consequences on the range and quality of pelvic position in sitting, neck and shoulder motion, and both general and specific trunk and shoulder movement and function. In particular they cause a physical limit to the end range of shoulder elevation and an alteration in muscle recruitment likely to increase the risk of shoulder tendon impingement and wear.

Individuals with respiratory disease may complain of acute or chronic cervical, thoracic or rib joint pain, which may decrease chest expansion as measured by a reduction in VC. Joint manifestations (mainly hypertrophic osteoarthropathy) are common in children with CF, affecting 2–8.5% of patients (Botton et al

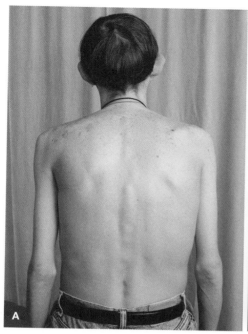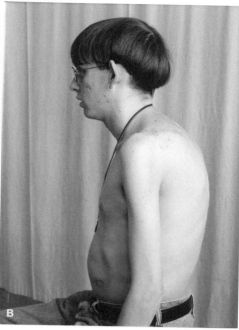

FIGURE 7-61 ■ CJ, aged 16, cystic fibrosis. **(A)** Relaxed sitting posture (posterior view). Note forwards head position, tight suboccipital and mid-cervical extensors, tight upper and middle fibres of trapezius, asymmetry and abducted and protracted position of the scapulae, increased thoracic kyphosis, reduced upper lumbar lordosis and posterior rotation of pelvis. **(B)** Relaxed sitting posture (side view). Note forwards head position, increased sternocleidomastoid activity, increased low cervical lordosis and thoracic kyphosis, abducted and protracted scapulae, anterior position of humerus in glenoid fossa, internal rotation of humerus and lax abdominal muscles.

2003, Parasa & Maffulli 1999). Back pain may be due to CF-related arthropy, and arthritis due to coexistent conditions or drug reactions, as well as the more obvious mechanical reasons. Mechanical back pain in people with CF has been described in the literature, but the incidence and prevalence have not been reliably established for the different age groups.

With increasing longevity in people with CF, musculoskeletal changes will become more important. Decreased bone mineral density is common at all ages but further reduction tends to occur with time, increasing illness and adverse effects of medication. With an increased emphasis on encouraging general exercise to improve respiratory and general health and bone density, musculoskeletal problems may become more prevalent, requiring careful monitoring (Buntain et al 2004).

With chronic respiratory disease, fracture rates are reported to be approximately twice as high in women

aged 16 to 32 years and the same increase is observed at a slightly later stage in men (Parasa & Maffulli 1999). Low bone mineral density is related to poor nutrition, reduced weight bearing, resistive muscle activity and the use of corticosteroids (Aris et al 1998, Bachrach et al 1994, Henderson & Madsen 1996). The combination of vertebral wedging, soft tissue contractures, poor posture and coughing may also cause persistent back pain in these patients (Fok et al 2002).

There is a high prevalence of acute episodes of pain in adults with CF (Festini et al 2004). As children with chest pain and CF are more likely to have a lower FEV_1 percentage predicted and poorer quality of life, the assessment of musculoskeletal pain in this client group should be routine (Koh et al 2005).

Pain may restrict the ability to attain an upright posture and to use an efficient muscle pattern. Tensioning or compression of the neural tissues, as they exit from the cervical spine and proceed through the

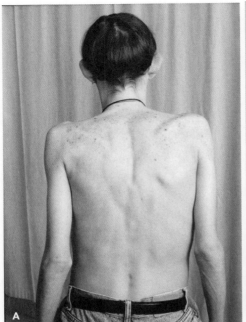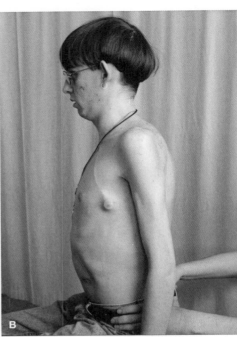

FIGURE 7-62 ■ **(A)** Sitting posture (posterior view) following active assisted anterior rotation of pelvis. Note decreased mid-cervical lordosis, improved position of scapulae, reduced thoracic kyphosis, neutral rotation of pelvis and improved lumbar lordosis. **(B)** Sitting posture (side view) following active assisted anterior rotation of pelvis. Note less forwards head position, activation of deep cervical flexors, reduced sternocleidomastoid activity, improved scapulae and humeral position and thoracic kyphosis.

axilla, may also occur in some individuals (Butler 1991) and is associated with chronic overuse of the accessory muscles of respiration, elevated first rib and a depressed lateral shoulder girdle.

Subjective Assessment

Assessment of those with chronic respiratory disease or following heart or chest surgery should include questioning regarding headache, neck, thoracic or lumbar pain and any upper limb pain or distal arm paraesthesia. The use of valid and reliable outcome measures improves evaluation of the effect of treatment. The area of pain can be recorded on a body chart and the intensity quantified using an absolute visual analogue scale (AVAS). The impact of any pain or movement restriction on activities of daily living may be assessed using a functional disability scale (e.g. Neck Disability Index (Vernon & Mior 1991), Shoulder, Arm and Hand Disability Index (Institute for

Work & Health 1996) or headache questionnaire (Niere & Jerak 2004)). Individual involvement in the identification of treatment goals and expectations will enable clearer planning and prioritization. In those with dyspnoea, it will be helpful to quantify dyspnoea intensity using an AVAS or Borg scale (Pfeiffer et al 2002) before any postural correction or treatment. Questioning about the behaviour of musculoskeletal pain during the night and in the morning will help to clarify the degree of inflammation involved. Headache may be multifactorial in origin and may be related to upper cervical spine dysfunction or to various other physiological and biochemical changes.

Activities that aggravate the problem may include sustained end-range postures of the neck or thoracic spine, trunk movements which require a reversal of the thoracic kyphosis or activities involving shoulder elevation. Repetitive coughing will load the costotransverse joints and may result in localized pain.

Additionally, the increased abdominal pressure related to persistent cough may result in increased lumbar disc pressure and rupture, while the repetitive flexion and extension of the spine during coughing may aggravate existing cervical pathology or dysfunction.

Physical Assessment: Posture

Musculoskeletal assessment should proceed in a systematic manner from evaluation of posture to assessment of joint mobility, muscle recruitment patterns, muscle length, strength and endurance, keeping in mind the specific function loss or pain area and type reported. Any change in symptoms during assessment should be noted. In particular any improvement in pain when posture is modified may assist motivation to change.

In the presence of chronic respiratory disease, the physiotherapist will need to keep in mind the possibility of reduced bone density and fragile skin tissue related to age or the long-term use of systemic steroids. Pain, dyspnoea and fatigue will also need to be monitored concurrently and the assessment adjusted as necessary. The presence of wound and drain sites in the postsurgical patient may require modified assessment positions. While the assessment is ideally performed in sitting, supine and prone, examination of those with dyspnoea may need to be conducted in semi-supine, sitting or high side lying.

With the individual in relaxed sitting, the following should be noted:

1. The relaxed posture of the pelvis, lumbar, thoracic and cervical spines
2. The point of maximal curve of each of these segments
3. Whether the spinal posture is fixed or able to be corrected
4. The position of the scapulae and the location of the humeral head within the glenoid
5. The posture of the neck and head and alignment with the trunk and pelvis.

If it is possible to assist the pelvis to roll anteriorly to move the body weight on to the ischial tuberosities, note whether the thoracic kyphosis, cervical lordosis and head forwards positions all automatically improve (see Fig. 7-62). Is the lumbosacral flexed position able to be reversed as the pelvis is assisted to roll forwards?

The cervical spine and the head may need to be guided to move the centre of gravity of the body over the pelvis and the head placed in a less protracted position to assess the reversibility of the resting posture. The inability to maintain this corrected position will indicate the extent of loss of endurance of the postural muscles.

Observe where the scapulae are resting and how the arms are hanging in standing and then in sitting. Usually if the position of the pelvis and spine is faulty, the scapulae will be elevated or dropped, protracted and winging with either upward or downward rotation. This 'weak' position of the scapulae means that stress will be transferred to the shoulder and neck joint structures during overhead activities. Arm elevation will also be weak. If the arms rest in an internally rotated position, this will interfere with smooth coordinated arm elevation and increase the risk of shoulder tendon impingement.

Physical Assessment: Range of Motion

Total range of thoracic motion is dependent on the mobility of the apophyseal, costovertebral, costotransverse joints and ribs and in particular the extensibility of the intercostal, pectoralis and latissimus dorsi muscles. Stiffness in the upper thoracic spine may be indicated by an inability to reverse the kyphosis on request or during cervical extension and shoulder abduction. A flattened or lordotic area in the mid-thoracic region usually indicates hypomobility (Boyling & Palastanga 1994). People with chronic respiratory disease and breathlessness are often unable to lie flat during the night due to difficulty breathing and/or persistent coughing, and the spine is not rested in extension.

The major portion of thoracic rotation is expected to be in the middle thoracic spine (T6–T8) (Gregersen & Lucas 1967) with lateral flexion occurring as a conjunct movement (White & Panjabi 1990). During lateral flexion, the ribs should flare and spread on the contralateral side and approximate on the ipsilateral side (Boyling & Palastanga 1994). The end-feel of normal thoracic rotation is springy due to limitation by ligamentous tissue and joint capsules. Age or postural changes at the costovertebral joints may restrict rib motion and lead to a harder end-feel (Nathan 1962). Gentle overpressure applied at end-range will assist determination of the quality of restriction, but overpressure should be used with caution if the risk of osteoporosis or existing fracture is suspected.

During spinal flexion, the inferior facets of the apophyseal joint of the superior vertebra normally glide superoanteriorly on the facets of the inferior vertebra. In extension the reverse movement occurs. Although the initial limitation to extension is from the anterior ligaments, the anterior annulus and the posterior longitudinal ligament, the normal end-feel is one of bony impingement as the inferior articular facets contact the lamina of the caudad vertebrae (White & Panjabi 1990). The mobility of the upper and middle ribs may be assessed by palpating bilaterally anteriorly and posteriorly during a deep inspiration; the lower ribs are assessed by palpating laterally during a full cycle of inspiration and expiration (Lee 2003).

The range of glenohumeral rotation will depend on the resting position of the humerus and tightness of the anterior and posterior shoulder capsule and muscles. During normal bilateral shoulder flexion and abduction the thoracic spine extends (particularly in the younger age group). Any restriction in the range of thoracic lateral flexion and rotation will limit the range of unilateral shoulder elevation (Boyling & Palastanga 1994). Shortened or overactive latissimus dorsi and teres major will add further limitation.

Observing posteriorly during shoulder elevation should enable assessment of any abnormal patterns of muscle recruitment. The upper trapezius and levator scapulae muscles, sternocleidomastoid and the scalenes tend to be overactive in people with respiratory disease, while the deep upper cervical and scapular stabilizers will be underactive (Fig. 7-63). Abnormal scapulohumeral rhythm is usually most obvious as shoulder movement is initiated and then again towards the end of range. Assessing passive shoulder motion in supine (or half sitting in those with dyspnoea) will enable better differentiation between scapulohumeral and scapulothoracic motions. The excursion, strength and endurance of specific muscle groups identified as overactive or underactive need to be examined individually in order to determine the relationship of movement impairment to pain and disability. Neural tissue provocation tests (Butler 1991) and tests for reflexes, power and sensation should be performed if

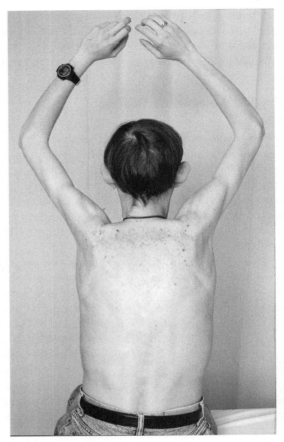

FIGURE 7-63 ■ Shoulder abduction. Note overactivity of upper trapezius, poor reversal of thoracic kyphosis, abducted, protracted and rotated scapulae, shortened teres major and latissimus dorsi and absence of lower trapezius activity.

any arm or hand pain or paraesthesia is reported. Thoracic outlet disorder may develop in the chronic respiratory disease due to the fixed and limited posture of the neck and upper body structures.

Physiotherapy Management

Prioritization of the main problems is important before treatment is started; the severity of musculoskeletal and cardiorespiratory dysfunction and the chronicity of the pain and disability need to be assessed. The time available and ability to perform home treatment techniques need to be considered in the choice of technique and in estimated prognosis.

Postural Correction and Motor Control Training

Postural correction may change the breathing pattern and the intensity of dyspnoea. These factors need to be monitored carefully during treatment. As the individual becomes familiar with the gentle effort required to activate the correct muscles, oxygen consumption may be reduced. Adherence to a home exercise programme will be improved if a direct link can be demonstrated between improvement in posture and relief of pain or shortness of breath. The 'ideal' posture is one where the body is positioned so that the spine, pelvis and shoulder girdle are in their neutral zone, allowing the muscles to work in the most efficient manner. In the ideal posture the deep neck flexors, lower trapezius, transversus abdominus, gluteus medius and the pelvic floor will be softly activated milliseconds before the movement is begun.

Posture may be improved by educating awareness of positioning of the pelvis in sitting and the use of more efficient movement patterns using visual, auditory and sensory feedback. Postural correction utilizes motor learning with training of the holding ability of the postural stabilizers, while avoiding substitution by the stronger prime movers (White & Sahrmann 1994). The principles of motor control require frequent gentle repetition of the corrected movement or position. The initial focus should be on correcting any posterior pelvic rotation in sitting and on reducing the lumbar and thoracic kyphosis to bring the head back over the trunk. A small pillow or lumbar roll may then be used to maintain this position. If necessary, postural correction can be started in semi-supine or high side lying and then incorporated into maintenance of corrected posture during specific activities. The use of the diaphragm, abdominal and neck shoulder muscles will need to be monitored and changed if inappropriate.

Mobilization Techniques

Physiotherapy management of joint restriction and pain may include passive mobilizations of cervical and thoracic apophyseal, costotransverse, costochondral and sternochondral joints and the glenohumeral joint (Bray 1994, Vibekk 1991). Manipulation is usually contraindicated. The focus of treatment will most commonly be on improving the range and quality of

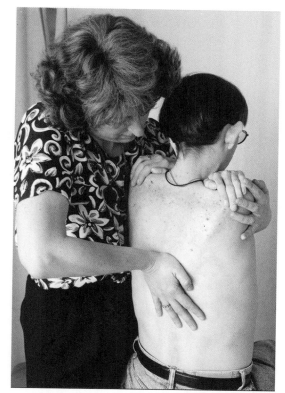

FIGURE 7-64 ■ Mobilization of thoracic extension. Passive or active assisted, with fulcrum at T8.

thoracic extension and rotation and on increasing the mobility of the ribs. Positioning during treatment will need to be carefully selected to minimize dyspnoea or pain. Specific joint restrictions may be treated with passive mobilization techniques in static positions or functional movements, and then optimally followed by active assisted or active exercises. General techniques to the upper, mid or lower regions of the spine or localized techniques to a specific vertebral level or rib can be performed in sitting, forwards lean sitting or in high side lying (Lee 2003) (Figs 7-64 and 7-65). Mobilization of the ribs may be performed in side lying, with the upper arm elevated to stretch the intercostal muscles or in sitting, using active shoulder abduction combined with lateral flexion. In forwards lean sitting with the head and arms supported on pillows, the ribcage will be free to move during mobilization techniques.

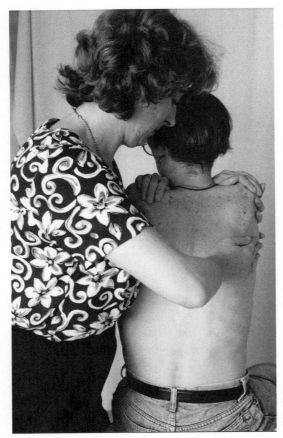

FIGURE 7-65 ■ Mobilization of thoracic rotation. Passive or active assisted, with postero-anterior pressure on ribs 7 and 8.

Active or passive bilateral arm flexion and spine extension may be combined with deep inspiration and expiration to improve rib mobility. In sitting, the active extension or rotation can be performed while the therapist assists the movement to encourage an increase in range. Self-mobilizations can be performed over the back of a chair, in four-point kneel or leaning against a wall using a rolled towel for localization (Fig. 7-66). Home mobilization exercises will be necessary if the respiratory condition is chronic and the musculoskeletal dysfunction long term. A mirror, or training a family member, will assist self-treatment and provide helpful feedback.

Following surgery via sternotomy or thoracotomy, specific gentle passive mobilizations of the sternocostal joints or costotransverse joints may be required, if localized painful limitation of shoulder or thoracic movement or pain on breathing are present. Following thoracotomy, patients may tend to immobilize the arm on the side of the incision and need to be encouraged to move within pain limits as early as possible to reduce the risk of frozen shoulder. The scapula may be taken through its range of protraction, retraction, elevation and depression while the patient is in side lying. Bilateral arm movements are preferred in the early stage following surgery, initially avoiding abduction and external rotation to reduce stress on the scar.

The long-term ventilated patient may also develop musculoskeletal problems. Routine passive mobilization of the shoulder through its full range of flexion, external rotation and abduction should be mandatory. Lateral flexion and extension of the thoracic spine can be performed via arm elevation when in side lying. Gentle passive rotation of the thoracic spine can also be performed in this position with the upper arm resting on the lateral chest wall.

Muscle-Lengthening Techniques

Stretching of tight muscle groups may precede or accompany endurance training of the lengthened muscle groups (Janda 1994). Stretching of the anterior deltoid and pectoralis major muscles, using a proprioceptive neuromuscular facilitation hold–relax technique, has been shown to increase VC and shoulder range of movement (Putt & Paratz 1996). Other muscles that may require careful stretching are: sternocleidomastoid, the scalenes, upper and middle fibres of trapezius, levator scapulae, pectoralis minor, teres major, latissimus dorsi, subscapularis and the suboccipital extensors (Table 7-10). Sustained stretches may be facilitated by conscious or reflex relaxation of the muscle during exhalation. Hold–relax techniques using the agonist or contract–relax techniques using the antagonist of the shortened muscle (White & Sahrmann 1994) may augment sustained stretches and myofascial release massage along the line of the muscle fibres. Where possible, individuals should be taught to perform their own stretches and mobilizations as part of long-term maintenance.

Taping

Taping of the scapula in a more neutral position, or of the thoracic spine in a reduced kyphosis, may

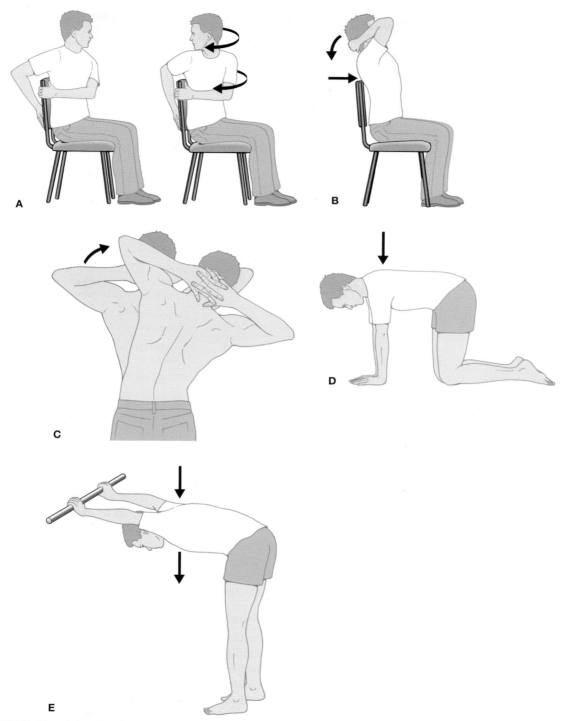

FIGURE 7-66 ■ **(A)** Assisted active exercise for rotation of cervical and thoracic spine. **(B)** Active assisted exercise for thoracic spine extension. **(C)** Active exercise for thoracic spine lateral flexion and stretching of the intercostal muscles. **(D)** Active mobilization exercise for mid-thoracic extension. **(E)** Passive stretch of anterior shoulder muscles and mobilization of thoracic extension.

TABLE 7-10		
Assessment of Muscle Length		
Muscle	Observation if Muscle Tight	Length Testing Position
Pectoralis major	Internal rotation and anterior translation of the humerus	Horizontal extension and abduction to 140°
Pectoralis minor	Anterior and inferior position of coracoid process and elevation of ribs 3–5	Retraction and depression of scapula
Upper cervical extensors	Forwards position of head on neck, increased upper cervical lordosis	Flexion of the head on the upper cervical spine
Upper trapezius	Elevation of scapula, palpable anterior border of trapezius (occiput to distal clavicle)	Cervical flexion with contralateral lateral flexion and ipsilateral rotation
Levator scapula	Increased muscle bulk anterior to upper trapezius and posterior to sternocleidomastoid from C2–C4 to superior angle of scapula	Cervical flexion, contralateral lateral flexion and contralateral rotation, keeping the medial superior scapula border depressed
Sternocleidomastoid	Forwards position of head on neck, elevated first rib and prominence at the clavicular insertion of sternocleidomastoid	Upper cervical flexion with lower cervical extension
Anterior scalenes	Elevation of ribs 1–3, ipsilateral lateral flexion of head on neck	Exhalation with depression of ribs 1–3 and upper cervical flexion
Latissimus dorsi	Internal rotation of humerus	Elevation of shoulder in external rotation with posterior pelvic tilt
Teres major	Medial rotation of humerus, protracted and upward rotation of scapula	Flex shoulder while sustaining scapular retraction and depression
Diaphragm	Flexed thorax and localized lordosis at the thoracolumbar junction	Relaxed diaphragmatic breathing

temporarily unload the affected tissue to gain pain relief and facilitate healing. It will also provide a feeling as to which posture will assist pain reduction of the thoracic kyphosis and what may need to be assisted until the holding capacity of the thoracic extensors and lower fibres of trapezius has been improved. Strapping tape (over anti-allergy tape) applied in the corrected sitting may give proprioceptive feedback in the early stages of retraining. It is important to ensure comfort and that cervical motion is freer following taping. Appropriate warnings and instructions regarding removal of the tape should be given.

There are many different approaches to taping. A long piece of tape starting anteriorly above the clavicle and crossing the mid-fibres of trapezius may inhibit overactivity of this muscle. The tape is then crossed over at the peak of the thoracic kyphosis and extended down to the lumbar spine if necessary. It should not be so firm that pain is produced or neural symptoms provoked. A horizontal tape to lift the lateral edge of

the acromion and a tape around the inferior border of the scapula to facilitate serratus anterior action may both help. Tape under the axilla to lift the scapula and relieve neural tension may also assist pain reduction, but care needs to be taken with the sensitive skin of the axilla. All taping should be designed and applied related to the individual's specific and individual needs. Retesting range of motion and pain on aggravating movements will allow direct appraisal of the effectiveness of taping. Warnings regarding possible skin reaction and pain provocation should be given.

Muscle Retraining (Strength and Endurance)

Training of scapular retraction and depression using middle and lower fibres of trapezius is important to complement any gain in range of thoracic extension and to improve scapular stability (Fig. 7-67). The holding capacity of the deep upper cervical flexors and cervicothoracic extensors will need to be trained to reduce the degree of forwards head posture and to

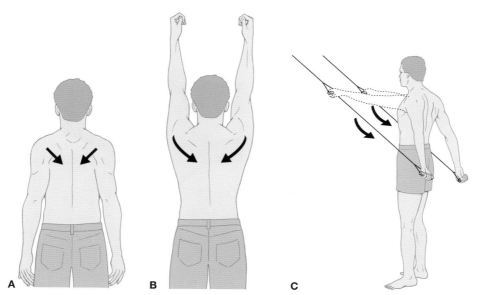

FIGURE 7-67 ■ **(A)** Active scapulae retraction/depression (rhomboids, middle and lower trapezius). **(B)** Active scapulae retraction/depression in shoulder elevation. **(C)** Active scapulae retraction/depression in shoulder extension.

TABLE 7-11	
Assessment of Holding Capacity of Lengthened Muscles	
Muscle	**Test Position**
Deep upper cervical flexors	Half supine, nodding of head on neck; test holding ability.
Middle and lower trapezius	With patient prone (or sitting if short of breath), test holding ability by placing scapula in retraction and depression and asking patient to hold.
Serratus anterior	Note ability to maintain scapula against chest wall during a partial push-up against a wall.
Infraspinatus	Test strength of external rotation.

assist relaxation of sternocleidomastoid and the scalene muscles (Table 7-11). The longus colli and rectus capitus anterior major may be trained initially in high sitting, then progressed to supine if shortness of breath allows (Fig. 7-68). Alternatively, gentle nodding of the head on the neck against slight self-applied resistance using the thumb can be taught in sitting. The serratus anterior action of holding the scapula against the chest wall will be improved with training using a half push-up action against a wall (taking care that upper trapezius is not overactive) (O'Leary et al 2007).

A gym ball may be useful for encouraging a more upright sitting posture in younger clients. Prone positions over the ball may be used to stimulate the antigravity muscles. Side lying over the ball will assist with rib mobility and stretching of the intercostal muscles if mobility and shortness of breath allow. Thera-Band can be used to apply resistance to weak motion and to give more specific directional feedback.

Neural Tissue Techniques

When neural tissue provocation tests reveal irritation or restriction, the primary aim of treatment will be to mobilize the tight adjacent structures and improve posture to reduce load on the sensitive tissues. The effect on the neural system should be monitored during and after treatment. If progress is inadequate, gentle mobilization (not stretching) of the neural tissues at the site of restriction may be required.

Summary

People with chronic respiratory disease may have postural dysfunction and musculoskeletal pathology in

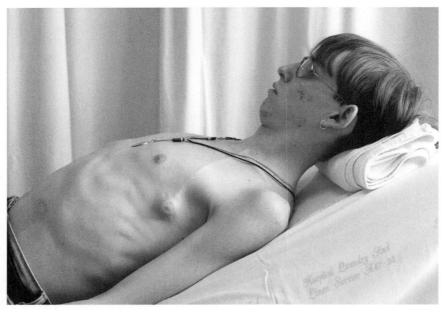

FIGURE 7-68 ■ Position for training activation of deep upper cervical flexors and lower trapezius and for stretching of upper cervical extensors and pectoralis minor and major.

addition to their cardiothoracic disease. Early identification of disability and musculoskeletal limitations will provide the physiotherapist with the opportunity to teach preventative strategies and enable early, more effective intervention. Postural awareness and education with a home mobilizing and strengthening programme may be usefully included in a holistic home programme.

Clinical research is required to evaluate whether the musculoskeletal complications described in this section can be prevented or minimized by an early intervention programme, and whether improving the function of the musculoskeletal system has a positive effect on respiratory function.

NEUROPHYSIOLOGICAL FACILITATION OF RESPIRATION

The respiration of mammals involves a ventilatory system in which the essential part, the lung, effects exchange between the surrounding air and the blood. Even though this organ is richly supplied with nerves, it does not have an autonomous function. It under-

takes this task by the conjoint action of two elements, the ribcage and the diaphragm, which form the chamber enclosing it (Duron & Rose 1997).

Breathing is a complex behaviour. It is governed by a variety of regulating mechanisms under the control of large parts of the central nervous system. Ongoing research into the respiratory ventilatory system (ribcage and diaphragm) has dramatically altered traditional understanding of the respiratory muscles and their neural control. The motor synergy of respiration includes the major and accessory respiratory muscles and motor neuron pools from the level of the fifth cranial nerve down to the upper lumbar segments (von Euler 1986).

Respiratory rhythmicity, as with other rhythmical repetitive motor actions (i.e. locomotion and mastication), is supported in the central nervous system by a central pattern generator (CPG). CPGs are neuronal networks capable of generating the characteristic rhythmic patterns in the complete absence of extrinsic reflexes and feedback loops (Atwood & MacKay 1989, Gordon 1991, von Euler 1986). However, in order to adapt the ventilatory system to prevailing and anticipated needs and to achieve coordination with the cardiovascular system, breathing is regulated by a multitude of reflexes, negative feedback circuits and feedforward mechanisms (Ainsworth l997, Koepchen et al 1986, von Euler 1986).

Neurophysiological facilitation of respiration is the use of selective external proprioceptive and tactile stimuli that produce reflexive movement responses in the ventilatory apparatus to assist respiration. The responses they elicit appear to alter the rate and depth of breathing and can be demonstrated to occur in other mammals (dogs) as well as in humans (Bethune 1975, 1976). These procedures are particularly useful in the chest care of the unconscious patient and of the conscious postsurgical patient who frequently find that the reflexive nature of the respiratory movements reduces the perception of pain (Bethune 1991). The present models of the neural control of respiration, with their emphasis on the roles of spinal neurons and on the importance of afferent (sensory) input, provide further biological support for neurophysiological facilitation procedures, i.e. clinical use of selective afferent input in respiratory care.

Neural Control

Research on ventilatory muscle control presently places considerable emphasis on spinal respiratory motor neurons and their controlling or modifying influence on central respiratory programmes. One of the theoretical models of the functional organization of the neural control of breathing identifies three major central nervous system levels: suprabulbar mechanisms, bulbar mechanisms and spinal motor neuron pools and integrating mechanisms (von Euler 1986) (Fig. 7-69).

Based on a similar model, Miller et al (1997) have considered the many neural structures that can potentially modify the final output of the ventilatory muscles. Input from peripheral sensory structures (proprioceptive, cutaneous, vagal and chemoceptive) and from a variety of brain regions (cerebral cortex, pons, cerebellum and others) is all integrated in the premotor bulbospinal respiratory neurons. Adjustments to the respiratory control of these multifunctional muscles occurs in order to support their many non-respiratory behaviours including speech, swallowing, coughing, vomiting. The motor neuron pools that drive these

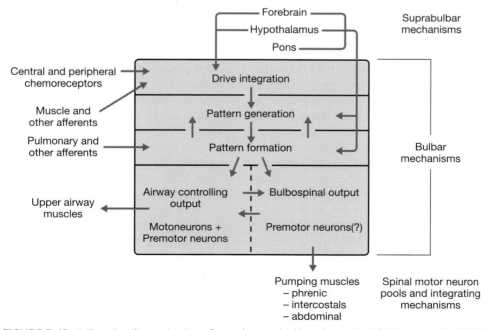

FIGURE 7-69 ■ Functional organization of neural control of breathing. *(Modified from von Euler 1986).*

multifunctional ventilatory muscles are subjected to changes in activity pattern due to their control by the neuronal networks, recruited on the basis of the different incoming stimuli. The spinal respiratory motor neurons are the final common pathway. They determine the output of the major respiratory muscles including their 'rhythmic breath-by-breath respiratory drive'. The actions of the ventilatory apparatus only during eupneic respiration (normal easy breathing) will be discussed.

Breathing in all mammalian species depends on a bilateral neuronal respiratory network within the lower brainstem, which generates three neural phases: inspiration, post-inspiration and expiration. Inspiration involves augmenting activity in the inspiratory nerves and muscles. The post-inspiratory phase represents declining activity in the inspiratory nerves (early expiration). During late or active expiration the expiratory nerves and muscles exhibit augmenting activity which ends abruptly at the next inspiration. All phase activities are generated without the need for peripheral feedback. Although classical research proposed a hierarchical organization of various 'centres' in the pons and medulla, studies have revealed that supramedullary structures are not essential for the maintenance of respiratory rhythm. Respiratory neurons in the rostral pons, previously known as the 'pneumotaxic centre,' controlling respiratory rhythm, are not necessary for rhythm generation. These pontine neurons are now thought to stabilize the respiratory pattern, slow the rhythm and influence timing. Efferent axons from the medullary neurons project to the inspiratory neurons in the spinal cord (Atwood & MacKay 1989, Bianchi & Pasaro 1997, Richler et al 1997).

The origin of the respiratory rhythm remains unclear as precise knowledge of all possible interactions among neurons in the respiratory network is incomplete. 'Respiratory drive is regulated by information from sensory receptors within the airway, lungs and respiratory muscles, as well as central and peripheral chemoceptors' (Frazier et al 1997).

Proprioceptive information arising from respiratory muscles may regulate the motor activity through long loop reflexes that include the medullary respiratory centres. Proprioceptive information through segmental and intersegmental loops at the spinal level may also influence the motor activity. Although complex spinal circuitry exists for modulating diaphragmatic activity through large and small phrenic afferents, proprioceptive regulation of phrenic motor neurons seems weak or absent. Afferent information from the lower intercostals and the abdominal muscles (T9–T10) may facilitate phrenic motor neurons by a spinal reflex. Emerging evidence suggests that phrenic afferents are more involved in respiratory regulation during stressed breathing (Frazier et al 1997, Hilaire & Monteau 1997). There are apparent differences between the neural mechanisms controlling the diaphragm and those controlling the thoracic muscles. While phrenic motor neurons appear mainly under medullary control and seem insensitive to proprioception, thoracic respiratory neurons seem to receive respiratory drive mainly via a network of thoracic interneurons.

Respiratory Muscles

The Diaphragm

The diaphragm is the major inspiratory muscle in humans. Current understanding of its action suggests that it does not expand the entire chest wall, as previously proposed. Actions of the diaphragm are being investigated with more attention being paid to the direction of the muscle fibres that compose it and the insertional and 'appositional' forces that are generated. The insertional forces are the result of muscular attachments. The appositional force is the pleural pressure that develops on the inner aspect of the lower ribs between the ribs and the diaphragm where the diaphragmatic fibres, that are directed cranially, are in direct contact with the ribcage (De Troyer 1997).

Diaphragmatic muscle fibres originate from three major sites: the xiphisternal junction, the costal margin of the lower ribcage and the transverse processes of the lumbar vertebrae (see Chapter 1). All fibres insert into the central tendon. Thus the orientation of these fibres differs. For example, midcostal diaphragmatic muscle fibres are perpendicular to midsternal and midcrural fibres. In humans, diaphragmatic muscle fibres have tendinous insertions within the muscle and do not traverse the full length of the muscle from origin to insertion, as in some smaller animals. Therefore the mechanical action of these fibres is complex, depending on relationships imposed by the specific attachments and the loads imposed by the ribcage and abdominal wall.

Older literature raised the possibility that there might be motor innervation of some parts of the diaphragm from intercostal nerves. It is now clear that the only innervation is the phrenic nerve via the phrenic motor neurons originating in the third, fourth and fifth segments of the cervical cord in humans. Animal studies have demonstrated that the diaphragm is somatotopically innervated. In the cat, C5 innervates the ventral portions of both costal and crural diaphragmatic fibres, while their dorsal portions are innervated by C6. Studies in other animals have produced similar data. The compartmentalization related to these innervation patterns and the further sub-compartmentalization of motor unit territories within these areas 'provide the potential for differential control' of different regions of diaphragmatic muscle. The differences between the diaphragmatic fibres from the three sites of origin have prompted some investigators to suggest that the crural portion is a separate muscle, under separate neuromotor control (Sieck & Prakash 1997). The crural portion has no costal attachment. Crural fibres surrounding the oesophagus may be under separate neural control in order to act as a sphincter. Detailed histochemical studies have demonstrated other differences between fibres from the three originating sites. A recognized uniqueness of the diaphragm is that it has few muscle spindles. When they are present, they are found primarily in the crural portion (Agostoni & Sant' Ambrogio 1970, Sieck & Prakash 1997).

Studies of isolated diaphragmatic contractions, examined by electrical stimulation of the phrenic nerve in dogs, demonstrated that while the lower ribs moved cranially and the cross-sectional area of the lower ribcage increased, the upper ribs moved caudally and the cross-sectional area of the upper ribcage decreased. Similar results have been obtained in human subjects with phrenic nerve pacing following traumatic transaction of the upper cord and during spontaneous breathing in subjects with transaction of the lower cord, who use the diaphragm exclusively. In seated humans (as in the dog) the diaphragm has both an expiratory action on the upper ribcage and an inspiratory action on the lower ribcage, which increases in its transverse diameter.

It has been established that the inspiratory action of the diaphragm on the ribcage is due in part to the insertional force of its attachment to the lower ribs. During inspiration the muscle fibres of the diaphragm shorten and the dome descends relative to the costal insertions of the muscle. The descent of the dome, which remains relatively constant in size and shape during breathing, expands the thorax vertically, resulting in a fall in pleural pressure. The descent also displaces abdominal viscera caudally, increasing abdominal pressure, which pushes the abdominal wall outwards. The diaphragmatic fibres inserting on the upper borders of the lower six ribs also apply a force on these ribs when they contract. This force equals the force exerted on the central tendon. If the abdominal viscera effectively oppose the diaphragmatic descent, the lower ribs are lifted and rotated outwards.

The inspiratory force of the diaphragm is also related to its apposition to the ribcage. This is best explained in the words of De Troyer (1997):

The zone of apposition makes the lower rib cage in effect part of the abdominal container and measurements in dogs have established that during breathing the changes in pressure in the pleural recess between the apposed diaphragm and the rib cage are almost equal to the changes in abdominal pressure. Pressure in the pleural recess rises, rather than falls during inspiration, thus indicating that the rise in abdominal pressure is truly transmitted through the apposed diaphragm to expand the lower rib cage.

The inspiratory efficiency of the insertional and appositional forces is largely dependent on the resistance the abdominal viscera provide to diaphragmatic descent. If the resistance of the abdominal contents was eliminated, the zone of apposition would disappear during inspiration and the contracting diaphragmatic muscle would become orientated transversely at their attachments onto the ribs. In this case, the insertional force would have an expiratory action on the lower ribs. These studies reinforce the view of Goldman (1974) that abdominal muscle contraction, commonly associated only with an expiratory action, appears to have an important role in defending diaphragmatic length during inspiration.

The Intercostal Muscles

The place of the intercostal muscles has been more difficult to establish. Conventional wisdom regards the external intercostals as inspiratory in function, elevating the ribs, and the internal intercostals as expiratory in function, depressing the ribs. This theory was based on geometric considerations proposed in 1848 (the Hamberger theory) and it has been challenged since 1867, when electrical stimulation of the intercostal muscles was undertaken for the first time. These latter studies suggested that the external and internal intercostal muscles were synergistic in action. The Hamberger theory is regarded as being incomplete. Its theoretical model is planar but real ribs are curved. Therefore the changes in length of the intercostal muscles (i.e. their mechanical advantage) vary with respect to the position of the muscle fibres along the rib. Also, the Hamberger theory assumed that all ribs rotate by equal amounts around parallel axes. The radii of curvature of the different ribs are different (Duron & Rose 1997).

Histological and electrophysiological studies have disclosed that the ribcage is non-homogeneous. It has motor components that vary with their location in the upper or lower thorax. In addition, each intercostal can be functionally different depending on its position in the same intercostal space (Gray 1973). It is now generally accepted that most of the external intercostal muscles do not participate in the ventilatory process during quiet breathing (De Troyer 1997, Duron & Rose 1997). Unlike the diaphragm, the intercostal muscles also have a postural function. Detailed studies of the respiratory and postural actions of the intercostal muscles have revealed functional differences from segment to segment and between external and internal intercostal muscles within the same segment. The major place of each intercostal muscle in postural activity and/or respiratory cycles has yet to be established. Nevertheless, Duron & Rose (1997) reviewed extensive studies in animal and human subjects and report precise distributions of inspiratory and expiratory activity. A summary of their findings follows:

1. In addition to the diaphragm, the inspiratory muscles active during normal breathing are the ventral intercartilaginous part of the intercostal muscles and the dorsal levator costae muscle.
2. The lateral part of the external and internal intercostal muscles of the upper rib spaces are synergistic muscles. They often have a postural type of activity. Their motor neurons may be activated by the central inspiratory drive; thus they may participate in respiration.
3. In the four lowest intercostal spaces, the lateral parts of the external and internal intercostal muscles are also synergistic. The lateral part of the internal intercostal is active in expiration during quiet breathing. The lateral part of the external intercostal is also expiratory but only during dyspnoea, similar to abdominal expiratory action.
4. The lateral part of the intercostal muscles are antagonistic in the fifth through eighth intercostal spaces. The external intercostals are inspiratory and the internal intercostals are expiratory.
5. In every intercostal space the dorsal part of the external (inspiratory) and the dorsal part of the internal (expiratory) muscles are antagonistic during quiet breathing.
6. All intercostal muscles of the lateral part of the ribcage participate in posture. There appears to be a clear distinction between the dorsal and ventral part of each intercostal space from which phasic respiratory activities are always recorded and the lateral part of each intercostal space where tonic postural activities are observed.

The insertions of both the external and internal intercostal muscles suggest that their orientation would assist rotation of the thorax. Indeed, electromyography (EMG) studies on normal human subjects have demonstrated that external intercostals on the right were activated when the torso was rotated to the left, but silent when the torso was rotated to the right. On the other hand, the internal intercostals on the right were only active when the torso was rotated to the right. The abundance of muscle spindles and the preponderance of type I (slow) muscle fibres in intercostal muscles are consistent with postural activity. Eighty-five percent of external intercostal muscle fibres in dogs are type 1, a percentage that is higher than that of antigravity limb muscles.

Accessory Muscles of Inspiration

The scalene muscles in humans have traditionally been considered as accessory inspiratory muscles. However, EMG studies have established that scalene muscles invariably contract with the diaphragm and parasternal intercostals during inspiration. No clinical situation exists in which paralysis of all inspiratory muscles occurs without also affecting the scalene muscles, so it is impossible to accurately define the isolated action of these muscles on the human ribcage. Observations on quadriplegic patients have demonstrated that persistent inspiratory action in scalene muscles is observed in those individuals with a spinal transection at C7 or lower that preserves scalene innervation. In these situations the antero-posterior diameter of the ribcage remains constant or increases, as opposed to the inward displacement of the upper ribcage when the level of transection interferes with scalene innervation (De Troyer 1997). Accessory muscles of the neck assist thoracic respiration by stabilizing the upper ribcage. This is a minor function in normal persons at rest. These muscles become more active during exercise and in the presence of diseases such as asthma and COPD. Generally, neck and upper airway muscles have a higher proportion of fast muscle fibres, faster isometric contraction times and lower fatigue resistance than the diaphragm (Lunteren & Dick 1997).

Many other muscles can elevate the ribs when they contract and are therefore truly 'accessory' muscles of inspiration. These are muscles running between the head and the ribcage, shoulder girdle and ribcage, spine and shoulder girdle. Such muscles as the sternocleidomastoid, pectoralis minor, trapezius, serrati and erector spinae are primarily postural in function. They are active in respiration in healthy humans only during increased respiratory effort. Of these accessory muscles, only the sternocleidomastoids have been extensively studied. In patients with transection of the upper cord causing paralysis of the diaphragm, intercostals, scalene and abdominal muscles, the sternocleidomastoids (innervation from cranial nerve 11) contract forcefully during unassisted inspiration, causing a large increase in the expansion of the upper ribcage but an inspiratory decrease in the transverse diameter of the lower ribcage (De Troyer 1997).

The Abdominal Muscles

The four muscles of the ventrolateral wall of the abdomen, the rectus abdominis, the external oblique, the internal oblique and the transversus abdominis, have significant respiratory function in humans. The fibres in each of these muscles assume a direction different from each other; consequently, the mechanical action of an abdominal muscle contraction depends on fibre direction and the concurrent action of the other abdominal muscles. Added to this complexity is the fact that the force generated by the abdominal wall is applied to a load that is determined by viscous and non-linear elastic resistances. The capacity of the abdominal wall to function adequately varies markedly among individuals and correlates well with an individual's activity level, gender, corpulence and age.

Abdominal muscle fibres are similar to those of other skeletal muscle. Differences in fibre composition between them are minor. Generally speaking, type 1 (slow) muscle fibres predominate. Bishop (1997) reports that although details of the morphology of abdominal motor units are not known and information on the number and distribution of muscle proprioceptors (muscle spindles and tendon organs) in abdominal muscle is scarce, proprioceptive feedback is recognized as an important modulator of abdominal motor neuron excitability. Electrically evoked reflexes studied in cats under the conditions of bilateral rhizotomy of the lumbar segments or C6 spinal cord transection demonstrated that both segmental feedback and supraspinal signals control abdominal motor neurons. Furthermore, studies on the phasic and tonic abdominal stretch reflexes suggest a special functional significance for the γ-spindle loop. Normal individuals, when standing, develop tonic abdominal muscle activity unrelated to respiratory phases.

Many brain regions can modify abdominal motor neuron output via multiple descending pathways. Spinal abdominal motor neurons receive strong projections from the brainstem. However, brainstem and spinal abdominal motor neurons receive direct and indirect projections from the premotor cortex, the motor cortex, the cerebellum, the hypothalamus, the pons and many other regions of the brain. The voluntary control over the abdominal muscles via the motor cortex is very similar to control by the cortex over muscles of the limbs and digits.

The respiratory action of the abdominal muscles is first to contract and pull the abdominal wall inward and so increase abdominal pressure. This pressure causes the diaphragm to move upwards into the thoracic cavity, which in turn results in an increase in pleural pressure and a decrease in lung volume. The abdominal muscles also displace the ribcage. By virtue of their insertions on the ribs, it would appear that the action of the abdominal muscles is to pull the lower ribs caudally and thus deflate the ribcage in another expiratory action. However, experiments in dogs have shown that these muscles also have an inspiratory action. Because of the large zone where the diaphragm is directly apposed to the ribcage, the rise in abdominal pressure due to abdominal muscle contraction is transmitted to the lower ribcage. In addition, the rise in abdominal pressure forcing the diaphragm cranially and the consecutive increase in passive diaphragmatic tension also tend to raise the lower ribs and expand the lower ribcage (insertional force of the diaphragm). Regardless of their actions on the ribs, the abdominal muscles are primarily expiratory muscles through their actions on the diaphragm and the lung.

Neurophysiological Facilitatory Stimuli

The proprioceptive and tactile stimuli selected below produce remarkably consistent reflexive responses in the ventilatory muscles. Inspiratory expansion of the ribs, increased epigastric excursion, visibly increased and often palpably increased tone in the abdominal muscles and change in the respiratory rate (usually slower) are among the responses observed. In the clinical setting, these responses are often accompanied by involuntary coughing, changes in breath sounds on auscultation, rapid return of mechanical chest wall stability, less necessity for suctioning, a more normal respiratory pattern and retention of the improved breathing pattern for some time after the treatment period. In some unconscious patients there is an apparent increase in the level of consciousness (more reaction to other stimuli). These effects appear to be cumulative. Successive application of the stimuli elicits faster responses and longer retention of the altered pattern. The changes noted during treatment application are frequently dramatic. The responses are most pronounced in the most deeply unconscious. The facilitatory stimuli are:

- Intercostal stretch
- Vertebral pressure to the upper thoracic spine
- Vertebral pressure to the lower thoracic spine
- Anterior-stretch lift of the posterior basal area
- Moderate manual pressure
- Perioral pressure
- Abdominal co-contraction.

The foregoing discussion of neural control models, with the emphasis on the importance of afferent input and the place of spinal motor neurons, indicates that the majority of the responses to these stimuli are mediated by muscle stretch receptors via dorsal roots and intersegmental reflexes (Table 7-12).

Intercostal Stretch

Intercostal stretch (Fig 7-70A) is provided by applying pressure to the upper border of a rib in a direction that will widen the intercostal space above it. The pressure should be applied in a downward direction, not pushing inward into the patient. The application of the stretch is timed with an exhalation and the stretched position is then maintained as the patient continues to breathe in his usual manner. As the stretch is maintained, a gradual increase in inspiratory movements in and around the area being stretched occurs. This may be done as a unilateral or bilateral procedure. It should not be performed on fractured or floating ribs. Care must be exercised around sensitive mammary tissue in females. When performed over areas of instability, as in the presence of paradoxical movement of the upper ribcage or over areas of decreased mobility, this procedure is effective in restoring normal breathing patterns. Epigastric excursions can be observed if intercostal stretch is performed over the lower ribs, but above the floating ribs. This may represent the reflexive activation of the diaphragm by the intercostal afferents that innervate its margins.

Vertebral Pressure

Firm pressure applied directly over the vertebrae of the upper and lower thoracic cage (Fig. 7-70B) activates the dorsal intercostal muscles. Pressure should be applied with an open hand for comfort and must

TABLE 7-12

Neurophysiological Facilitation for the Chest

Procedure	Method	Observations	Suggested Mechanism
Perioral stimulation	Pressure is applied to the patient's top lip by the therapist's finger and maintained	■ Increased epigastric excursion ■ 'Deep breathing' ■ Sighing ■ Mouth closure ■ Swallowing ■ 'Snout phenomena'	Primitive reflex response related to sucking
Vertebral pressure T2–T5	Manual pressure to thoracic vertebrae in region of T2–T5	■ Increased epigastric excursions ■ 'Deep breathing'	Dorsal root-mediated intersegmental reflex
Vertebral pressure T7–T10	Manual pressure to thoracic vertebrae in region of T7–T10	Increased respiratory movements of apical thorax	
Anterior stretch – lifting posterior basal area	■ Patient supine ■ Hands under lower ribs ■ Ribs lifted upward	■ Expansion of posterior basal area ■ Increased epigastric movements	■ Dorsal root as for vertebral pressure high ■ Stretch receptors in intercostals, back muscles
Co-contraction – abdomen	■ Pressure laterally over lower ribs and pelvis ■ Alternate right and left sides	■ Increased epigastric movements ■ Increased muscle contraction (rectus abdominus) ■ Decreased girth in obese ■ Increased firmness to palpation ■ Depression of umbilicus	Stretch receptors in abdominal muscles? Intercostal to phrenic reflex
Intercostal stretch	Stretch on expiratory phase maintained	Increased movement of area being stretched	Intercostal stretch receptors
Moderate manual pressure	Moderate pressure open palm	Gradually increased excursion of area under contact	Cutaneous afferents

be firm enough to provide some (intrafusal) stretch. For this reason it is easier to apply when the patient is supine, as in the supine position it is not necessary to stabilize the body and one may also observe the patient's reactions. Afferent input that activates the dorsal intercostal muscles is consistent with the observations of Duron & Rose (1997) that in every intercostal space the dorsal part of the external (inspiratory) and the dorsal part of the internal (expiratory) intercostal muscles are antagonistic during quiet breathing.

Firm pressure over the uppermost thoracic vertebrae results in increased epigastric excursions in the presence of a relaxed abdominal wall. Pressure over the lower thoracic vertebrae results in increased inspiratory movements of the apical thorax. These responses correlate with the observations of Helen Coombs

(1918) who demonstrated that section of the thoracic roots diminished costal respiration. She stated:

If the spinal roots are cut in the thoracic region alone there is diminution of costal respiration although abdominal respiration remains unaltered and the rate is very little changed: if the cervical dorsal roots are also involved, independent costal respiration disappears.

In 1930, in research with kittens, Coombs and Pike said:

… when dorsal roots of spinal nerves are divided in the thoracic region, costal respiration in kittens from birth to ten days old almost ceases … when dorsal roots of cervical nerves are sectioned, the thoracic

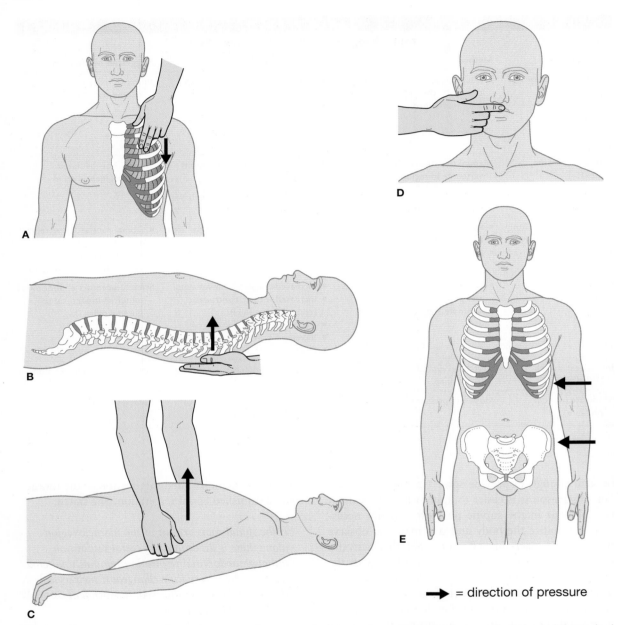

= direction of pressure

FIGURE 7-70 ▪ **(A)** Intercostal stretch: pressure down towards the next rib, not 'in' towards the patient's back. **(B)** Vertebral pressure over T2, 3, 4, 5. **(C)** Lifting posterior basal area. **(D)** Perioral stimulation: moderate pressure on top lip (the airway should not be occluded). **(E)** Co-contraction of abdominal muscles: pressure over lower ribs and pelvic bone.

nerves being intact, the movements of the diaphragm are much cut down and the respiratory rate is slower at no matter what age.

There is little to be found in the literature defining intersegmental respiratory reflexes. Sieck & Prakash (1997) noted that phrenic motor neurons do not receive a major excitatory input from muscle spindle afferents. However, they recognize that there are extrasegmental reflexes that affect phrenic motor neuron activation. Group I and II afferents from intercostal nerves have been shown to exert both inhibitory and facilitatory influences on phrenic nerve activity.

Anterior-Stretch Basal Lift

This procedure is performed by placing the hands under the ribs of the supine patient and lifting gently upwards (Fig. 7-70C). The lift is maintained and provides a maintained stretch and pressure posteriorly and an anterior stretch as well. This may be done bilaterally if the patient is small enough. If this is not possible or necessary, it should also be effective when performed unilaterally. As the lift is sustained, stretch is maintained and increasing movement of the ribs in a lateral and posterior direction can be seen and felt. Increased epigastric movements also often become obvious. The lift to the back places some stretch on the dorsal intercostal area and should also stretch the spaces between some of the mid-thoracic ribs (5–8). These are both areas where the intercostal muscles are considered to be antagonistic in action. The epigastric movements suggest that the diaphragm is being activated by intercostal afferents.

Maintained Manual Pressure

When firm contact of the open hand(s) is maintained over an area in which expansion is desired, gradual increasing excursion of the ribs under the contact will be felt. This is a useful procedure to obtain expansion in any situation where pain is present; for instance, when there are chest tubes or after cardiac surgery which may have required splitting of the sternum. Manual contact over the posterior chest wall is also useful and comfortable for persons with COPD. The inspiratory response is thought to be due to cutaneous tactile receptors. The contact should be firm so that it does not tickle.

In 1963 Sumi studied hair, tactile receptors and pressure receptors in the cat and reported thoracic cutaneous fields for both inspiratory and expiratory motor neurons. He proposed that since the excitatory skin fields for inspiratory motor neurons were more extensive than those for expiratory motor neurons, more inspiratory motor neurons could be excited by a single skin stimulus. Local cutaneous stimulation of the thoracic region would then tend to reflexively produce an inspiratory position of the ribcage. Duron & Bars (1986) also studied thoracic cutaneous stimulation in the cat. They directly electrically stimulated desheathed lateral cutaneous nerves in anaesthetized decerebrate cats and cats that were both decerebrate and spinal. Among their findings was widespread inhibition on both inspiratory and expiratory activity after stimulation of the cutaneous nerve. Their observations also suggested that responses from the upper and lower thoracic areas were different. They acknowledge that the place of each of the different cutaneous afferent components needs to be identified.

Perioral Pressure

Perioral stimulation is provided by applying firm maintained pressure to the patient's top lip (Fig. 7-70D), being careful not to occlude the nasal passage. (The use of surgical gloves is advised to avoid contamination.) The response to this stimulus is a brief (approximately 5-second) period of apnoea followed by increased epigastric excursions. The initial response may frequently be observed as a large maintained epigastric swell. Pressure is maintained for the length of time the therapist wishes the patient to breathe in the activated pattern. As the stimulus is maintained the epigastric excursions may increase so that movement is transmitted to the upper chest and the patient appears to be deep breathing. Respiratory rate is usually slower. The patient may sigh on initiation of the procedure or sometime after the response has become established.

The paucity of muscle spindles in the diaphragm determines that phrenic motor neurons, which provide its motor activation, do not receive any significant excitatory input from muscle spindle afferents and there are few, if any, γ motor neurons in the phrenic motor nucleus (Sieck & Prakash 1997). Information regarding afferent facilitation of phrenic motor neurons and/or other reflex interactions influencing their excitability is sparse. The responses that are observed on application of this stimulus correlate very well with the work of Peiper (1963).

When this perioral stimulus is applied to the unconscious patient if the mouth is open, it will close. Swallowing is noted and sucking movements are often evident even in the presence of oral airways. Swallowing and sucking may not be evident initially, but may appear in the more deeply unconscious after repeated stimulation. Occasionally such a patient has been observed to push pursed lips forwards in a 'mouth phenomenon' or 'lip phenomenon' or 'snout phenomenon'. These observations are similar to observations made by Peiper (1963) while studying the neurology of respiration and the neurology of food intake and the relationship between sucking, swallowing and breathing in infants. The 'mouth', 'lip' or 'snout phenomenon' has been reported by Peiper and other investigators as a reflex response to gentle tapping on the upper lip noted in young normal infants and in adults with severe cerebral disorders. Movement of the lips, sucking, swallowing and chewing motions have been reported on stroking the lips of comatose adults and are thought to be related to infantile rooting reflexes.

Peiper observed that three centrally directed rhythmic movements arise during an infant's food intake: sucking, breathing and swallowing. Earlier experiments on young animals had established that there was a sucking centre located bilaterally in the medulla. Peiper established the dominance of the sucking centre over respiration. Infants can breathe while they nurse, partly due to the high position of the larynx. The initiation of sucking was observed to immediately disturb respiration. There was initial lowering of the diaphragm for 5 seconds or more before respirations began at a new rhythm led by the sucking centre. When the sucking movements ceased, the respiratory movements continued in the new pattern for a period (in this instance, faster rhythm). The similarity between the observations recorded by Peiper and those observed in response to the perioral stimulus suggests that these phenomena are related. The stimulus on the top lip is thought to imitate, in part, the pressure of the mother's breast against the lips of a nursing infant. The lack of recent recorded material would seem to indicate that the investigation into sucking centres per se has not been pursued much further. The related activity of swallowing has been investigated, especially with respect to its interactions with respiration.

Swallowing is a complex behaviour. Although it is one of the most elaborate of motor functions in humans, swallowing is a primitive reflex with implications of a stereotyped and fixed behaviour (Jean et al 1997). In most mammals, including humans, all the muscles concerned with swallowing are striated. Similar to respiration, swallowing is considered an autonomic function, but is governed by the same neural principles as those serving some somatic functions, such as locomotion. Great differences among species are observed concerning swallowing during the respiratory cycle. Most of the significant data were obtained from sheep. The oropharynx serves both deglutition and respiration. Several muscles in the mouth, pharynx and larynx are active to ensure the patency of the upper airways and to regulate the airflow during the respiratory cycle. In humans, swallows occur mainly during expiration. When the swallowing rhythm is regular, one swallow occurs for every one or few breaths. A brief minor inspiration called a 'swallow breath' ('Schluckatmung' by pioneer investigators) occurs at the onset of swallowing. The functional significance of this brief inspiration is not known.

The CPG for swallowing is located in the medulla in two main groups of neurons in two regions that also contain respiratory neurons. The mechanisms that generate its rhythms are not understood. The factors regulating the functional interactions between swallowing and respiration have yet to be determined. Margaret Rood (1973) taught the use of perioral stimulation to reduce spastic muscle tone. She believed that it induced a parasympathetic bias (as opposed to a sympathetic bias) and that it promoted general relaxation. It was a prerequisite for her light, moving touch facilitation procedure to activate limb muscles. Rood's treatment focus and patient population probably accounts for her lack of awareness of the respiratory responses to this stimulus.

Co-Contraction of the Abdomen

Rood (1973) taught co-contraction of the abdomen (Fig. 7-70E) as a procedure to facilitate respiration. Pressure is applied simultaneously over the patient's lower lateral ribs and over the ilium in a direction at right angles to the patient. Moderate force is applied and maintained. Rood believed that this procedure increased tone in the abdominal muscles and also activated the diaphragm. She proposed that the pressure directed across the abdomen produced intrafusal stretch, thus activating the muscle spindles (mainly in the rectus). She thought that the side contralateral to the pressure reacted first. As those muscles responded to the stretch and shortened, they would stretch the intrafusal fibres of the opposite muscles, which in turn would activate their homonymous extrafusal muscles, which would contract, shorten and stretch the first set again and so the cycle would be repeated. A series of alternating contractions was thought to occur as long as the pressure was maintained. Co-contraction of the abdomen should be performed bilaterally with pressure applied alternately and maintained for some seconds on either side. The maintained pressure is repeated as necessary to obtain and maintain the response for the desired period.

In practice, activation of the abdominal muscles does not always occur in the contralateral side first. There can be considerable variation in individual responses. Preexisting muscle tone, corpulence, postoperative status and the integrity of the abdominal wall are some of the influencing factors. Lax abdominal muscles (for any reason) appear to respond more slowly. If activation is slow, it is often helpful to observe the umbilicus, which may exhibit changes in its movement pattern, becoming more depressed on exhalations before changes in the muscles can be detected.

This is an effective procedure. As pressure is maintained, increasing abdominal tone can be both seen and palpated. In the presence of retained secretions, abdominal co-contractions may produce coughing more readily than the other procedures. As ventilation increases with any procedure, coughing may occur. In obese patients, abdominal co-contraction has frequently resulted in decreased abdominal girth.

Clinical Application

In the clinical setting auscultation and standard chest assessment should be undertaken before, during and after treatment. Ventilatory movement patterns should be noted. Is chest expansion simultaneous and equal? Are there paradoxical movements or any areas of indrawing on inspiration? The therapist must be aware of the patterns of ventilation and how they are changing. Since the patient's response determines the duration of treatment, assessment is critical. The procedure of choice is continued until the desired treatment effect has been achieved, whether increased breath sounds, cough or stabilized respiratory pattern. Many patients raise secretions and cough. (Advice given to therapists was frequently 'co-contract and duck'.) Unconscious patients need assistance to get rid of their secretions, but suctioning may not be required as often or as deeply. Some unconscious patients appear to become less obtunded. Eyelids may flutter, eyes may open or there may be spontaneous movements. Sometimes, such a patient will initially turn the head away or push the therapist's hand away. These are positive signs as these patients are often thought to be unresponsive.

Responses to the facilitatory procedures are individual reactions and therefore every patient will not demonstrate the same level of responsiveness to each procedure. It is not necessary to do each procedure with every patient, but it is imperative to observe the individual response and modify treatment accordingly. Treatment should not be continued in the presence of an undesirable response. Anecdotally, a dramatic example of an undesirable response was observed in a decerebrate patient who was so hypertonic that abdominal co-contractions applied in the supine position began to elevate him into a sitting position. Such a response necessitates the use of other procedures. Conscious medical patients often appreciate the sense of relaxation and the lack of a sense of effort when facilitation procedures are used in their care. Many perform their own perioral stimulation. Acute and chronic neurological conditions such as amyotrophic lateral sclerosis, Guillain–Barré syndrome, cerebral vascular accidents and others may also be treated with these procedures and derive benefit.

REFERENCES

AARC Clinical Practice Guideline, 2002a. Oxygen therapy for adults in the acute care facility: 2002 update. Respir. Care 47, 717–720.

AARC Clinical Practice Guideline, 2002b. Selection of an oxygen delivery device for neonatal and pediatric patients: 2002 revision and update. Respir. Care 47, 707–716.

AARC Clinical Practice Guideline, 2007. Oxygen therapy in the home or alternate site health care facility. Respir. Care 52, 1063–1068.

Abernathy, A., McDonald, C., Frith, P., et al., 2009. Palliative oxygen versus medical air for relief of dyspnea: results of an international, multi-site randomised controlled trial. Respirology 14, A29.

Adler, D., Perrig, S., Takahashi, H., et al., 2012. Polysomnography in stable COPD under non-invasive ventilation to reduce patient-ventilator asynchrony and morning breathlessness. Sleep Breath. 16, 1081–1090.

Agarwal, R., Reddy, C., Aggarwal, A., et al., 2006. Is there a role for noninvasive ventilation in acute respiratory distress syndrome? A meta-analysis. Respir. Med. 100, 2235–2238.

Agostini, P., Knowles, N., 2007. Autogenic drainage: the technique, physiological basis and evidence. Physiotherapy 93, 157–163.

Agostoni, E., Sant'Ambrogio, G., 1970. The diaphragm. In: Campbell, E.J.M., Agostoni, E., Newsom Davies, J. (Eds.), The Respiratory Muscles, Mechanics and Neural Control. WB Saunders, Philadelphia.

Ahmedzai, S., Balfour-Lynn, I., Bewick, T., et al., 2011. Managing passengers with stable respiratory disease planning air travel: British Thoracic Society recommendations. Thorax 66, i1–i30.

Aitken, R.C., 1969. Measurement of feelings using visual analogue scales. Proc. R. Soc. Med. 62, 989–993.

Aitken, M.L., Bellon, G., De Boeck, K., 2012. Long-term inhaled dry powder mannitol in cystic fibrosis: an international randomized study. Am. J. Respir. Crit. Care Med. 185, 645–652.

Aldridge, A., 2005. Glossopharyngeal breathing in multiple sclerosis. Personal communication. (Lymington New Forest Hospital, Hampshire).

Allan, J.S., Garrity, J.M., Donahue, D.M., 2003. The utility of high-frequency chest wall oscillation therapy in the post-operative management of thoracic surgical patients. Chest 124, 235s.

Allen, C., Glasziou, P., Delman, C., 1999. Bedrest: a potentially harmful treatment needing more careful evaluation. Lancet 354, 1229–1233.

Almeida, C.C., Ribeiro, J.D., Almeida-Junior, A.A., Zeferino, A.M., 2005. Effect of expiratory flow increase technique on pulmonary function of infants on mechanical ventilation. Physiother. Res. Int. 10 (4), 213–221.

Altaus, P., 2009. Oscillating PEP. In: Physiotherapy for the Treatment of Cystic Fibrosis (CF), 4th ed. International Physiotherapy Group for Cystic Fibrosis (IPG/CF) ed, pp 18–22 <www.cfww.org/docs/ipg-cf/bluebook/bluebooklet2009webseversion.pdf> (accessed 12 October 2013.).

Alvarez, S.E., Peterson, M., Lunsford, B.R., 1981. Respiratory treatment of the adult patient with spinal cord injury. Phys. Ther. 6 (12), 1737–1745.

Ambrosino, N., Callegari, G., Galloni, C., et al., 1995. Clinical evaluation of oscillating positive expiratory pressure for enhancing expectoration in diseases other than cystic fibrosis. Monaldi Arch. Chest Dis. 50, 269–275.

American Association for Respiratory Care, 2003. AARC clinical practice guideline: intermittent positive pressure breathing. Respir. Care 48 (5), 540–546.

American Association for Respiratory Care, 2004. AARC clinical practice guideline: nasotracheal suctioning. Respir. Care 49 (9), 1080–1084.

ACSM's Guidelines for Exercise Testing and Prescription, ninth ed. 2014. Linda S Pescatello, Ross Arena, Deborah Riebe, Paul D Thompson Wolters Kluwer/Lippincott Williams & Wilkins, Philadelphia, PA.

Anderson, A., Alexanders, J., Sinani, C., et al., 2015. Effects of ventilator vs manual hyperinflation in adults receiving mechanical ventilation: a systematic review of randomised clinical trial. Physiotherapy 101, 103–110.

Anderson, P., Morton, J., 2009. Evaluation of two different timings of Pulmozyme nebulisation in relation to chest physiotherapy in children with cystic fibrosis [abstract]. J. Cyst. Fibros. 9, S74.

Anderson, G.G., O'Toole, G.A., 2008. Innate and induced resistance mechanisms of bacterial biofilms. In: Romeo, T. (Ed.), Bacterial Biofilms. Springer, Heidelberg.

Antonaglia, V., Ferluga, M., Molino, R., et al., 2011. Comparison of noninvasive ventilation by sequential use of mask and helmet versus mask in acute exacerbation of chronic obstructive pulmonary disease: a preliminary study. Respiration 82, 148–154.

Antonaglia, V., Lucangelo, U., Zin, W.A., et al., 2006. Intrapulmonary percussive ventilation improves the outcome of patients with acute exacerbation of chronic obstructive pulmonary disease using a helmet. Crit. Care Med. 34, 2940–2945.

Antonelli, M., Conti, G., Bufi, M., et al., 2000. Noninvasive ventilation for treatment of acute respiratory failure in patients undergoing solid organ transplantation: a randomized trial. J. Am. Med. Assoc. 283, 235–241.

App, E., Kieselmann, R., Reinhardt, D., et al., 1998. Sputum rheology changes in cystic fibrosis lung disease following two different types of physiotherapy: flutter vs autogenic drainage. Chest 114, 171–177.

Arens, R., Gozal, D., Omlin, K., et al., 1994. Comparison of high frequency chest compression and conventional chest physiotherapy in hospitalized patients with cystic fibrosis. Am. J. Respir. Crit. Care Med. 150, 1154–1157.

Aris, R.M., Renner, J.B., Winders, A.D., et al., 1998. Increased rate of fractures and severe kyphosis: sequelae of living into adulthood with cystic fibrosis. Ann. Intern. Med. 128, 186–193.

Armstrong, D.S., Grimwood, K., Carzino, R., et al., 1995. Lower respiratory infection and inflammation in infants with newly diagnosed cystic fibrosis. BMJ 310, 1571–1572.

Arnulf, I., Similowski, T., Salachas, F., et al., 2000. Sleep disorders and diaphragmatic function in patients with amyotrophic lateral sclerosis. Am. J. Respir. Crit. Care Med. 161, 849–856.

Atwood, H.L., MacKay, W.A., 1989. Essentials of Neurophysiology. Decker, Toronto.

Auriant, I., Jallot, A., Herve, P., et al., 2001. Noninvasive ventilation reduces mortality in acute respiratory failure following lung resection. Am. J. Respir. Crit. Care Med. 164, 1231–1235.

Ayres, S.M., Kozam, R.L., Lukas, D.S., 1963. The effects of intermittent positive pressure breathing on intrathoracic pressure, pulmonary mechanics and the work of breathing. Am. Rev. Respir. Dis. 87, 370–379.

Bach, J.R., 1993. Mechanical insufflation-exsufflation: a comparison of peak expiratory flows with manually assisted coughing techniques. Chest 104, 1553–1562.

Bach, J.R., 1994. Update and perspective on noninvasive respiratory muscle aids. Part 2. The expiratory aids. Chest 105, 1538–1544.

Bach, J.R., 1992. Airway secretion management and general pulmonary rehabilitation considerations for patients with neuromuscular ventilatory failure. J. Neurol. Rehabil. 6, 75–80.

Bach, J.R., 1995. Respiratory muscle aids for the prevention of pulmonary morbidity and mortality. Semin. Neurol. 15 (1), 72–83.

Bach, J.R., 2003. Mechanical insufflation/exsufflation: has it come of age? A commentary. Eur. Respir. J. 21, 385–386.

Bach, J.R., 2012. Noninvasive respiratory management of high level spinal cord injury. J. Spinal Cord Med. 35 (2), 72–80.

Bach, J.R., Alba, A.S., 1990. Noninvasive options for ventilatory support of the traumatic high level quadriplegic patient. Chest 98 (3), 613–619.

Bach, J.R., Alba, A.S., Bodofsky, E., et al., 1987. Glossopharyngeal breathing and noninvasive aids in the management of post-polio respiratory insufficiency. Birth Defects 23, 99–113.

Bach, J.R., Baird, J.S., Plosky, D., et al., 2002. Spinal muscular atrophy type 1: management and outcomes. Pediatr. Pulmonol. 34, 16–22.

Bach, J.R., Bianchi, C., Vidigal-Lopes, M., et al., 2007. Lung inflation by glossopharyngeal breathing and 'air stacking' in Duchenne muscular dystrophy. Am. J. Phys. Med. Rehabil. 86 (4), 295–300.

Bach, J.R., Goncalves, M.R., Hamdani, I., Winck, J.C., 2010. Extubation of patients with neuromuscular weakness: a new management paradigm. Chest 137, 1033–1039.

Bach, J.R., Ishikawa, Y., Kim, H., 1997. Prevention of pulmonary morbidity for patients with Duchenne muscular dystrophy. Chest 112, 1024–1028.

Bach, J.R., Smith, W.H., Michaels, J., et al., 1993. Airway secretion clearance by mechanical exsufflation for post-poliomyelitis ventilator assisted individuals. Arch. Phys. Med. Rehabil. 74, 170–177.

Bach, J.R., Vis, N., Weaver, B., 2000. Spinal muscular atrophy type 1, a non-invasive management approach. Chest 117, 1100–1105.

Bachrach, L.K., Loutit, C.W., Moss, R.B., Marcus, R., 1994. Osteopenia in adults with cystic fibrosis. Am. J. Med. 96, 27–34.

Badr, C., Elkins, M., Ellis, E., 2002. The effect of body position on maximal expiratory pressure and flow. Aust J. Physiother. 48, 95–102.

Bakker, E.M., van der Wiel-Kooij, E.C., Mullinger, B., et al., 2013. Small-airways deposition of dornase alfa in children with asthma and persistent airway obstruction. J. Allergy Clin. Immunol. 132, 482–485.

Banerjee, S.K., Davies, M., Sharples, L., et al., 2013. The role of facemask spirometry in motor neurone disease. Thorax 68, 385–386.

Banzett, R., O'Donnell, C.R., Guilfoyle, T.E., et al., 2015. Multidimensional dyspnoea profile (MDP): an instrument for laboratory and clinical research. Eur. Resp. J. 45 (6), 1681–1691.

Barach, A.L., Beck, G.J., 1954. Ventilatory effect of head-down position in pulmonary emphysema. Am. J. Med. 16, 55–60.

Baratz, D.M., Westbrook, P.R., Shah, P.K., et al., 1992. Effect of nasal continuous positive airway pressure on cardiac output and oxygen delivery in patients with congestive heart failure. Chest 102, 1397–1401.

Barbato, A., Frischer, T., Kuehni, C.E., et al., 2009. Primary ciliary dyskinesia: a consensus statement on diagnostic and treatment approaches in children. Eur. Respir. J. 34, 1264–1276.

Bateman, J.R., Pavia, D., Clark, S.W., 1978. The retention of lung secretions during the night in normal subjects. Clin. Sci. Mol. Med. 55 (6), 523–527.

Bauer, M., McDougal, J., Schoumacher, R., 1994. Comparison of manual and mechanical chest percussion in hospitalized patients with cystic fibrosis. J. Pediatr. 124, 250–254.

Bausewein, C., Booth, S., Gysels, M., et al., 2008. Non-pharmacological interventions for breathlessness in advanced stages of malignant and non-malignant diseases. Cochrane Database Syst. Rev. 16 (2), Art. No.: CD005623, doi:10.1002/14651858.CD005623.pub2.

Bausewein, C., Farguhar, M., Booth, S., et al., 2007. Measurement of breathlessness in advanced disease. Respir. Med. 101, 399–410.

Baydur, A., Adkins, R.H., Milic-Emili, J., 2001. Lung mechanics in individuals with spinal cord injury: effects of injury level and posture. J. Appl. Physiol. 90 (2), 405–411.

Baydur, A., Gilgoff, I., Prentice, W., et al., 1990. Decline in respiratory function and experience with long-term assisted ventilation in advanced Duchenne's muscular dystrophy. Chest 97, 884–889.

Beachey, W., 2013. Acid-base balance. In: Kacmarek, R., Stoller, J., Heuer, A. (Eds.), Egan's Fundamentals of Respiratory Care, 10th ed. Elsevier Mosby, St. Louis.

Beasley, R., Chien, J., Douglas, J., et al., 2015. TSANZ Oxygen guidelines for acute oxygen use in adults; swimming between the flags. Respirology 20 (8), 1182–1191.

Beck, L.A., 1998. Morbid obesity and spinal cord injury: a case study. SCI Nurs. 15, 3–5.

Beck, G., Barach, A., 1954. Value of mechanical aids in the management of a patient with poliomyelitis. Ann. Intern. Med. 40, 1081–1094.

Beck, G.J., Scarrone, L.A., 1956. Physiological effects of exsufflation with negative pressure (EWNP). Dis. Chest 29, 80–95.

Becker, H.F., Piper, A.J., Flynn, W.E., et al., 1999. Breathing during sleep in patients with nocturnal desaturation. Am. J. Respir. Crit. Care Med. 159, 112–118.

Behrends, V., Ryall, B., Wang, X., et al., 2010. Metabolic profiling of *Pseudomonas aeruginosa* demonstrates that the anti-sigma factor MucA modulates osmotic stress tolerance. Mol. Biosyst. 6 (3), 562–569.

Bellone, A., Lascioli, R., Raschi, S., et al., 2000. Chest physical therapy in patients with acute exacerbation of chronic bronchitis: effectiveness of three methods. Arch. Phys. Med. Rehabil. 81, 558–560.

Bellone, A., Spagnolatti, L., Massobrio, M., 2002. Short-term effects of expiration under positive expiratory pressure in patients with acute exacerbation of chronic obstructive pulmonary disease and mild acidosis requiring non-invasive positive pressure ventilation. Intensive Care Med. 28, 581–585.

Belman, M.J., 1993. Exercise in patients with chronic obstructive pulmonary disease. Thorax 48, 936–946.

Belman, M.J., Wasserman, K., 1981. Exercise training and testing in patients with chronic obstructive pulmonary disease. Basics Respirat. Dis. 10, 1–6.

Ben-Dov, I., Zlobinski, R., Segel, M.J., et al., 2009. Ventilatory response to hypercapnia in C(5–8) chronic tetraplegia: the effect of posture. Arch. Phys. Med. Rehabil. 90 (8), 1414–1417.

Bennett, W.D., Chapman, W.F., Gerrity, T.R., 1992. Ineffectiveness of cough for enhancing mucus clearance in asymptomatic smokers. Chest 102, 412–416.

Bennett, W.D., Foster, W.M., Chapman, W.F., 1990. Cough-enhanced mucus clearance in the normal lung. J. Appl. Physiol. 69, 1670–1675.

Bereiter, M., 2001. Glossopharyngeal breathing in motor neurone disease. Personal communication. Schweizer Paraplegiker Zentrum, Switzerland.

Bergsson, G., Reeves, E.P., McNally, P., et al., 2009. LL-37 complexation with glycosaminoglycans in cystic fibrosis lungs inhibits antimicrobial activity, which can be restored by hypertonic saline. J. Immunol. 183, 543–551.

Bernard, S., Whittom, F., Leblanc, P., et al., 1999. Aerobic and strength training in patients with chronic obstructive lung disease. Am. J. Respir. Crit. Care Med. 159, 896–901.

Berney, S., Denehy, L., 2002. A comparison of the effects of manual and ventilator hyperinflation on static lung compliance and sputum production in intubated and ventilated intensive care patients. Physiother. Res. Int. 7 (2), 100–108.

Berney, S., Denehy, L., Pretto, J., 2004. Head-down tilt and manual hyperinflation enhances sputum clearance in patients who are intubated and ventilated. Aust J. Physiother. 50 (1), 9–14.

Berry, R., Chediak, A., Brown, L., et al., 2010. Best clinical practices for the sleep center adjustment of noninvasive positive pressure ventilation (NPPV) in stable chronic alveolar hypoventilation syndromes. J. Clin. Sleep Med. 6, 491–509.

Bethune, D.D., 1975. Neurophysiological facilitation of respiration in the unconscious patient. Physiother. Can. 27, 241–245.

Bethune, D., 1976. Facilitation of respiration in unconscious adult patients. Respiratory Technology 12 (4), 18–21.

Bethune, D., 1991. Neurophysiological facilitation of respiration. In: Pryor, J.A. (Ed.), Respiratory Care. Churchill Livingstone, Edinburgh.

Bianchi, L., Foglio, K., Porta, R., et al., 2002. Lack of additional effect of adjunct of assisted ventilation to pulmonary rehabilitation in mild COPD patients. Respir. Med. 96, 359–367.

Bianchi, R., Gigliotti, F., Romagnoli, I., et al., 2011. Impact of a rehabilitation program on dyspnea intensity and quality in patients with chronic obstructive pulmonary disease. Respiration 81, 186–195.

Bianchi, C., Grandi, M., Felisari, G., 2004. Efficacy of glossopharyngeal breathing for a ventilator-dependent, high-level tetraplegic patient after cervical cord tumor resection and tracheotomy. Am. J. Phys. Med. Rehabil. 83 (3), 216–219.

Bianchi, A.L., Pasaro, R., 1997. Organization of central respiratory neurons. In: Miller, A.D., Bianchi, A.L., Bishop, B.P. (Eds.), Neural Control of the Respiratory Muscles. CRC Press, New York.

Bickerman, H., 1954. Exsufflation with negative pressure (EWNP); elimination of radiopaque material and foreign bodies from bronchi of anesthetized dogs. AMA Arch. Intern. Med. 93, 698–704.

Bihari, S., Bersten, A., 2012. Chronic heart failure modifies the response to positive end-expiratory pressure in patients with chronic obstructive pulmonary disease. J. Crit. Care 27, 639–646.

Bilton, D., Bellon, G., Charlton, B., et al., 2013a. Pooled analysis of two large randomised phase III inhaled mannitol studies in cystic fibrosis. J. Cyst. Fibros. 12, 367–376.

Bilton, D., Daviskas, E., Anderson, S.D., et al., 2013b. Phase 3 randomized study of the efficacy and safety of inhaled dry powder mannitol for the symptomatic treatment of non-cystic fibrosis bronchiectasis. Chest 144, 215–225.

Bilton, D., Dodd, M.E., Abbot, J.V., Webb, A.K., 1992. The benefits of exercise combined with physiotherapy in the treatment of adults with cystic fibrosis. Respir. Med. 86, 507–511.

Bilton, D., Robinson, P., Cooper, P., et al., 2011. Inhaled dry powder mannitol in cystic fibrosis: an efficacy and safety study. Eur. Respir. J. 38, 1071–1080.

Bishop, B.P., 1997. The abdominal muscles. In: Miller, A.D., Bianchi, A., Bishop, B.P. (Eds.), Neural Control of the Respiratory Muscles. CRC Press, New York.

Bishop, J.R., Erskine, O.J., Middleton, P.G., 2011. Timing of dornase alpha inhalation does not affect the efficacy of the airway clearance regimen in adults with cystic fibrosis: a randomised crossover trial. J. Physiother. 57, 223–229.

Bittner, E., Chendrasekhar, A., Pillai, S., 1996. Changes in oxygenation and compliance as related to body position in acute lung injury. Am. J. Surg. 62, 1038–1041.

Blair, S.N., Painter, P., Pate, R.R., et al., 2005. Resource Manual for Guidelines for Exercise Testing and Prescription, 5th ed. Lea and Febiger, Philadelphia.

Blazey, S., Jenkins, S., Smith, R., 1998. Rate and force of application of manual chest percussion by physiotherapists. Aust. J. Physiother. 44, 257–264.

Blomqvist, C.G., Stone, H.L., 1983. Cardiovascular adjustments to gravitational stress. In: Shepherd, J.T., Abboud, F.M. (Eds.), Handbook of Physiology. Section 2: Circulation, vol. 2. American Physiological Society, Bethesda, pp. 1025–1063.

Blumenthal, I., Lealman, G.T., 1982. Effects of posture on gastro-oesophageal reflux in the newborn. Arch. Dis. Child. 57, 555–556.

Borel, J.C., Wuyam, B., Chouri-Pontarollo, N., et al., 2008. During exercise non-invasive ventilation in chronic restrictive respiratory failure. Respir. Med. 102, 711–719.

Borg, G., 1970. Perceived exertion as an indicator of somatic stress. Scand. J. Rehabil. Med. 2, 92–98.

Borghi-Silva, A., Di Thommazo, L., Pantoni, C.B., et al., 2009. Non-invasive ventilation improves peripheral oxygen saturation and reduces fatigability of quadriceps in patients with COPD. Respirology 14, 537–544.

Borghi-Silva, A., Mendes, R.G., Toledo, A.C., et al., 2010. Adjuncts to physical training of patients with severe COPD: oxygen or noninvasive ventilation? Respir. Care 55, 885–894.

Bott, J., Keilty, S.E.J., Noone, L., 1992. Intermittent positive pressure breathing – a dying art? Physiotherapy 78, 656–660.

Bott, J., Blumenthal, S., Buxton, M., et al., 2009. Guidelines for the physiotherapy management of the adult, medical, spontaneously breathing patient. Thorax 64 (Suppl. 1), i1–i51.

Botton, E., Saraux, A., Laselve, H., et al., 2003. Musculoskeletal manifestations in cystic fibrosis. Joint Bone Spine 70 (5), 327–335.

Boucher, R.C., 2002. An overview of the pathogenesis of cystic fibrosis lung disease. Adv. Drug Deliv. Rev. 54, 1359–1371.

Boucher, R.C., 2007. Evidence for airway surface dehydration as the initiating event in CF airway disease. J. Intern. Med. 261, 5–16.

Boyling, J.D., Palastanga, N., 1994. In: Grieve, G.P. (Ed.), Modern Manual Therapy of the Vertebral Column, second ed. Churchill Livingstone, Edinburgh.

Brackbill, Y., Douthitt, T.C., West, H., 1973. Psychophysiological effects in the neonate of prone versus supine placement. J. Pediatr. 82, 82–83.

Bradley, J., Moran, F., 2008. Physical training for cystic fibrosis. Cochrane Database Syst. Rev. (1), CD002768.

Bradley, J., Moran, F., Greenstone, M., 2002. Physical training for bronchiectasis. Cochrane Database Syst. Rev. (3), CD002166.

Braggion, C., Cappelletti, L.M., Cornacchia, M., et al., 1995. Short-term effects of three chest physiotherapy regimens in patients hospitalized for pulmonary exacerbations of cystic fibrosis: a cross-over randomized study. Pediatr. Pulmonol. 19, 16–22.

Brasher, P.A., McClelland, K.H., Denehy, L., Story, I., 2003. Does removal of deep breathing exercises from a physiotherapy program including pre-operative education and early mobilisation after cardiac surgery alter patient outcomes? Aust. J. Physiother. 49, 165–173.

Bray, C., 1994. Thoracic mobilisation in the management of respiratory and cardiac problems. In: The Forgotten Thoracic Spine. Manipulative Physiotherapists Association of Australia Symposium, University of Sydney, Australia.

Brazier, D., 1999. Endotracheal suction technique: putting research into practice. J. Association Chart. Physiother. Respir. Care 32, 13–17.

Brewin, C.R., Bradley, C., 1989. Patient preferences and randomised clinical trials. BMJ 299, 313–315.

British Thoracic Society, 2009. Emergency oxygen use in adults patients: updates <https://www.brit-thoracic.org.uk/document-library/clinical-information/oxygen/emergency-oxygen-use-in-adult-patients-guideline/emergency-oxygen-use-in-adult-patients-guideline/>.

British Thoracic Society/Association of Chartered Physiotherapists in Respiratory Care, 2009. Guidelines for the physiotherapy management of the adult, medical, spontaneously breathing patient: glossopharyngeal breathing in section 6c neuromuscular disease. Thorax 64 (Suppl. 1), 39.

Brooks, S.M. (Chairman), 1982. Task group on surveillance for respiratory hazards in the occupational setting. Surveillance for respiratory hazards. ATS News 126, 952–956.

Brooks, D., Anderson, C., Carter, M., et al., 2001. Clinical practice guidelines for suctioning the airway of the intubated and nonintubated patient. Can. Respir. J. 8, 163–181.

Browne, W.J., Wood, C.J., Desai, M., Weller, P.H., 2009. Urinary incontinence in 9–16 year olds with cystic fibrosis compared to other respiratory conditions and a normal group. J. Cyst. Fibros. 8, 50–57.

Buntain, H.M., Greer, R.M., Schluter, P.J., et al., 2004. Bone mineral density in Australian children, adolescents and adults with cystic fibrosis: a controlled cross sectional study. Thorax 59, 149–155.

Burns, K.E., Adhikari, N.K., Keenan, S.P., et al., 2010. Noninvasive positive pressure ventilation as a weaning strategy for intubated adults with respiratory failure. Cochrane Database Syst. Rev. CD004127, doi:10.1002/14651858.CD004127.pub2CD004127.

Burns, J.R., Jones, F.L., 1975. Early ambulation of patients requiring ventilatory assistance. Chest 68, 608.

Butler, D.S., 1991. Mobilisation of the Nervous System. Churchill Livingstone, Melbourne.

Button, B., Cai, L.H., Ehre, C., et al., 2012. A periciliary brush promotes lung health by separating the mucus layer from airway epithelia. Science 337, 937–941.

Button, B.M., Heine, R.G., Catto-Smith, A.G., et al., 2004. Chest physiotherapy, gastro-oesophageal reflux, and arousal in infants with cystic fibrosis. Arch. Dis. Child. 89, 435–439.

Bydgman, S., Wahren, J., 1974. Influence of body position on the anginal threshold during leg exercise. Eur. J. Clin. Invest. 4, 201–206.

Bye, P.T., Ellis, E.R., Issa, F.G., et al., 1990. Respiratory failure and sleep in neuromuscular disease. Thorax 45, 241–247.

Bye, P.T.P., Elkins, M.R., 2007. Other mucoactive agents for cystic fibrosis. Paediatr. Respir. Rev. 8, 30–39.

Bye, P.T., Lau, E.M.T., Elkins, M.R., 2011. Pharmacological airway clearance strategies in bronchiectasis. Eur. Respir. Monogr. 52, 1–9.

Cameron, M.H., Monroe, L., 2011. Physical Rehabilitation for the Physical Therapist Assistant, Saunders.

Campbell, T., Ferguson, N., McKinlay, R., 1986. The use of a simple self-administered method of positive expiratory pressure (PEP) in chest physiotherapy after abdominal surgery. Physiotherapy 72, 498–500.

Campbell, A., O'Connell, J., Wilson, F., 1975. The effect of chest physiotherapy upon the FEV_1 in chronic bronchitis. Med. J. Aust. 1, 33–35.

Carlucci, A., Richard, J., Wysocki, M., et al., 2001. Noninvasive versus conventional mechanical ventilation: an epidemiologic survey. Am. J. Respir. Crit. Care Med. 163, 874–880.

Carrillo, A., Ferrer, M., Gonzalez-Diaz, G., et al., 2012b. Noninvasive ventilation in acute hypercapnic respiratory failure caused by obesity hypoventilation syndrome and chronic obstructive pulmonary disease. Am. J. Respir. Crit. Care Med. 186, 1279–1285.

Carrillo, A., Gonzalez-Diaz, G., Ferrer, M., et al., 2012a. Non-invasive ventilation in community-acquired pneumonia and severe acute respiratory failure. Intensive Care Med. 38, 458–466.

Carron, M., Freo, U., BaHammam, A.S., et al., 2013. Complications of non-invasive ventilation techniques: a comprehensive qualitative review of randomized trials. Br. J. Anaesth. 110, 896–914.

Carson, K.V., Chandratilleke, M.G., Picot, J., et al., 2013. Physical training for asthma. Cochrane Database Syst. Rev. Art. No.: CD001116, doi:10.1002/14651858.CD001116.pub4.

Casaburi, R., Patessio, A., Loli, F., et al., 1991. Reductions in exercise lactic acidosis and ventilation as a result of exercise training in patients with obstructive pulmonary disease. Am. Rev. Respir. Dis. 143, 9–18.

Casadro-Flores, J., Martinez de Azagra, A., Ruiz-Lopez, M.J., et al., 2002. Pediatric ARDS: effect of supine-prone postural changes on oxygenation. Intensive Care Med. 28, 1792–1796.

Cecins, N.M., Jenkins, S.C., Pengelley, J., Ryan, G., 1999. The active cycle of breathing techniques: to tip or not to tip? Respir. Med. 93, 660–665.

Cegla, U., Bautz, M., Fröde, G., Werner, T., 1997. Physical therapy in patients with COPD and tracheobronchial instability: comparison of 2 oscillating PEP systems (RC-Cornet, VRP1 Desitin). Results of a randomized prospective study of 90 patients. Pneumologie 51, 129–136.

Cegla, U., Jost, H., Harten, A., et al., 2002. Course of severe COPD with and without physiotherapy with the RC-Cornet. Pneumologie 56, 418–424.

Chaboyer, W., Gass, E., Foster, M., 2004. Patterns of chest physiotherapy in Australian intensive care units. J. Crit. Care 19, 145–151.

Chan, P., von Leupoldt, A., Bradley, M., et al., 2012. The effect of anxiety on respiratory sensory gating measured by respiratory-related evoked potentials. Biol. Psychol. 91, 185–189.

Chandra, D., Stamm, J.A., Taylor, B., et al., 2012. Outcomes of noninvasive ventilation for acute exacerbations of chronic obstructive pulmonary disease in the United States, 1998–2008. Am. J. Respir. Crit. Care Med. 185, 152–159.

Chang, H., Weber, M., King, M., 1988. Mucus transport by high-frequency nonsymmetrical oscillatory airflow. J. Appl. Physiol. 65, 1203–1209.

Chatham, K., Marshall, C., Campbell, I., Prescott, R., 1993. The Flutter VRP1 device in post-thoracotomy patients. Physiotherapy 79, 95–98.

Chatte, G., Sab, J.-M., Dubois, J.-M., 1997. Prone position in mechanically ventilated patients with severe acute respiratory failure. Am. J. Critical Care Med. 155, 473–478.

Chatwin, M., Bush, A., Simonds, A.K., 2011. Outcome of goal-directed non-invasive ventilation and mechanical insufflation/exsufflation in spinal muscular atrophy type I. Arch. Dis. Child. 96, 426–432.

Chatwin, M., Bush, A., Macrae, D.J., et al., 2013. Risk management protocol for gastrostomy and jejunostomy insertion in ventilator dependent infants. Neuromuscul. Disord. 23, 289–297.

Chatwin, M., O'Driscoll, D., Corfield, D., et al., 2004. Controlled trial of intrapulmonary percussion in adults and children with stable severe neuromuscular disease. Am. J. Crit. Care Med. 169, A438.

Chatwin, M., Ross, E., Hart, N., et al., 2003. Cough augmentation with mechanical insufflation/exsufflation in patients with neuromuscular weakness. Eur. Respir. J. 21, 502–508.

Chatwin, M., Simonds, A., 2009. The addition of mechanical insufflation/exsufflation shortens airway-clearance sessions in neuromuscular patients with chest infection. Respir. Care 24, 1473–1479.

Chawla, L.S., Abell, L., Mazhari, R., et al., 2005. Identifying critically ill patients at high risk for developing acute renal failure: a pilot study. Kidney Int. 68, 2274–2280.

Chevaillier, J., 1984. Autogenic drainage (AD). In: Lawson, D. (Ed.), Cystic Fibrosis: Horizons. John Wiley, Chichester, p. 235.

Chevaillier, J., 2009. Autogenic drainage (AD). In: Physiotherapy for the Treatment of Cystic Fibrosis (CF), 4th ed. International Physiotherapy Group for Cystic Fibrosis (IPG/CF) ed, pp 8–9 <www.cfww.org/docs/ipg-cf/bluebook/bluebooklet2009website version.pdf> (accessed 12 October 2013).

Chiappetta, A., Beckerman, R., 1995. High frequency chest wall oscillation in spinal muscular atrophy (SMA). RT J. Respir. Care Pract. 8 (4), 112–114.

Choi, J.S., Jones, A.Y., 2005. Effects of manual hyperinflation and suctioning on respiratory mechanics in mechanically ventilated patients with ventilator-associated pneumonia. Aust J. Physiother. 51, 25–30.

Christensen, E., Nedergaard, T., Dahl, R., 1990. Long-term treatment of chronic bronchitis with positive expiratory pressure mask and chest physiotherapy. Chest 97, 645–650.

Chuley, M., Brown, J., Summer, W., 1982. Effect of postoperative immobilization after coronary artery bypass surgery. Crit. Care Med. 10, 176–178.

Cindy Ng, L.W., Mackney, J., Jenkins, S., Hill, K., 2012. Does exercise training change physical activity in people with COPD? A systematic review and meta-analysis. Chron. Respir. Dis. 9 (1), 17–26.

Clark, A.P., Winslow, E.H., Tyler, D.O., White, K.M., 1990. Effects of endotracheal suctioning on mixed venous oxygen saturation and heart rate in critically ill adults. Heart Lung 19, 552–557.

Clarke, R.C., Kelly, B.E., Convery, P.N., Fee, J.P., 1999. Ventilatory characteristics in mechanically ventilated patients during manual hyperventilation for chest physiotherapy. Anaesthesia 54, 936–940.

Clauss, R.H., Scalabrini, B.Y., Ray, R.F., Reed, G.E., 1968. Effects of changing body position upon improved ventilation– perfusion relationships. Circulation 37 (Suppl. 2), 214–217.

Clement, A.J., Hübsch, S.K., 1968. Chest physiotherapy by the 'bag squeezing' method: a guide to technique. Physiotherapy 54, 355–359.

Clini, E., Antoni, F., Vitacca, M., et al., 2006. Intrapulmonary percussive ventilation in tracheostomized patients: a randomized controlled trial. Intensive Care Med. 32, 1994–2001.

Confalonieri, M., Garuti, G., Cattaruzza, M.S., et al., 2005. A chart of failure risk for noninvasive ventilation in patients with COPD exacerbation. Eur. Respir. J. 25, 348–355.

Confalonieri, M., Potena, A., Carbone, G., et al., 1999. Acute respiratory failure in patients with severe community-acquired pneumonia: a prospective randomized evaluation of noninvasive ventilation. Am. J. Respir. Crit. Care Med. 160, 1585–1591.

Connors, A.J., Hammon, W., Martin, R., Rogers, R., 1980. Chest physical therapy: the immediate effect on oxygenation in acutely ill patients. Chest 78, 559–564.

Consensus Conference Report, 1999. Clinical indications for noninvasive positive pressure ventilation in chronic respiratory failure due to restrictive lung disease, COPD, and nocturnal hypoventilation: a consensus Conference report. Chest 116, 521–534.

Contal, O., Vignaux, L., Combescure, C., et al., 2012. Monitoring of noninvasive ventilation by built-in software of home bilevel ventilators: a bench study. Chest 141, 469–476.

Conway, J.H., Fleming, J.S., Perring, S., Holgate, S.T., 1992. Humidification as an adjunct to chest physiotherapy in aiding tracheo-bronchial clearance in patients with bronchiectasis. Respir. Med. 86 (2), 109–114.

Coombs, H.C., 1918. The relation of the dorsal roots of the spinal nerves and the mesencephalon to the control of respiratory movements. Am. J. Physiol. 46, 459–471.

Cornacchia, M., Zenorini, A., Perobelli, S., et al., 2001. Prevalence of urinary incontinence in women with cystic fibrosis. BJU Int. 88, 44–48.

Costantini, D., Brivio, A., Brusa, D., et al., 2001. PEP mask versus postural drainage in CF infants a long-term comparative trial. Pediatr. Pulmonol. (Suppl. 22), 308.

Craig, D.B., Wahba, W.M., Don, H.F., 1971. 'Closing volume' and its relationship to gas exchange in seated and supine positions. J. Appl. Physiol. 31, 717–721.

Cranston, J.M., Crockett, A., Currow, D., 2008. Oxygen therapy for dyspnoea in adults. Cochrane Database Syst. Rev. (3), Art. No.: CD004769, doi:10.1002/14651858.CD004769.pub2.

Crescimanno, G., Marrone, O., Vianello, A., 2011. Efficacy and comfort of volume-guaranteed pressure support in patients with chronic ventilatory failure of neuromuscular origin. Respirology 16, 672–679.

Crimi, C., Noto, A., Princi, P., et al., 2010. A European survey of noninvasive ventilation practices. Eur. Respir. J. 36, 362–369.

Cross, J., Elender, F., Barton, G., et al., 2012. Evaluation of the effectiveness of manual chest physiotherapy techniques on quality of life at six months post exacerbation of COPD (MATREX): a randomized controlled equivalence trial. BMC Pulm. Med. 12, 1–9.

Currie, D.C., Munro, C., Gaskell, D., Cole, P.J., 1986. Practice, problems and compliance with postural drainage: a survey of chronic sputum producers. Br. J. Dis. Chest 80, 249–253.

Cuvelier, A., Pujol, W., Pramil, S., et al., 2009. Cephalic versus oronasal mask for noninvasive ventilation in acute hypercapnic respiratory failure. Intensive Care Med. 35, 519–526.

Czarnik, R.E., Stone, K.S., Everhart, C.C. Jr., Preusser, B.A., 1991. Differential effects of continuous versus intermittent suction on tracheal tissue. Heart Lung 20, 144–151.

Dab, I., Alexander, F., 1979. The mechanism of autogenic drainage studied with flow volume curves. Monogr. Paediatr. 10, 50–53.

Dai, B., Kang, J., Yu, N., et al., 2013. Oxygen injection site affects FiO_2 during noninvasive ventilation. Respir. Care 58, 1630–1636.

Dail, C.W., 1951. 'Glossopharyngeal breathing' by paralyzed patients. Calif. Med. 75, 217–218.

Dail, C.W., Affeldt, J.E., Collier, C.R., 1955. Clinical aspects of glossopharyngeal breathing. J. Am. Med. Assoc. 158, 445–449.

Dantzker, D.R., 1983. The influence of cardiovascular function on gas exchange. Clin. Chest Med. 4, 149–159.

Darbee, J.C., Kanga, J.F., Ohtake, P.J., 2005. Physiologic evidence for high-frequency chest wall oscillation and positive expiratory pressure breathing in hospitalized subjects with cystic fibrosis. Phys. Ther. 85, 1278–1289.

Darbee, J., Ohtake, P., Grant, B., Cerny, F., 2004. Physiological evidence for the efficacy of positive expiratory pressure as an airway clearance technique in patients with cystic fibrosis. Phys. Ther. 84, 524–537.

Dasgupta, B., King, M., 1996. Reduction in viscoelasticity in cystic fibrosis sputum in vitro using combined treatment with nacystelyn and rhDNase. Pediatr. Pulmonol. 22, 161–166.

David, A., 1991. Autogenic drainage: the German approach. In: Pryor, J. (Ed.), Respiratory Care, 1st ed. Churchill Livingstone, Edinburgh, pp. 65–78.

Davies, H., Kitchman, R., Gordon, G., Helms, P., 1985. Regional ventilation in infancy. Reversal of the adult pattern. NEJM 313, 1627–1628.

Daviskas, E., Anderson, S.D., 2006. Hyperosmolar agents and clearance of mucus in the diseased airway. J. Aerosol Med. 19, 100–109.

Daviskas, E., Anderson, S.D., Brannan, J.D., et al., 1997. Inhalation of dry-powder mannitol increases mucociliary clearance. Eur. Respir. J. 10, 2449–2454.

Daviskas, E., Anderson, S.D., Young, I.H., 2007. Inhaled mannitol changes the sputum properties in asthmatics with mucus hypersecretion. Respirology 12, 683–691.

Daviskas, E., Anderson, S.D., Young, I.H., 2010c. Effect of mannitol and repetitive coughing on the sputum properties in bronchiectasis. Respir. Med. 104, 371–377.

Daviskas, E., Anderson, S.D., Eberl, S., et al., 2001. The 24-h effect of mannitol on the clearance of mucus in patients with bronchiectasis. Chest 119, 414–421.

Daviskas, E., Anderson, S.D., Eberl, S., Young, I.H., 2008. Effect of increasing doses of mannitol on mucus clearance in patients with bronchiectasis. Eur. Respir. J. 31, 765–772.

Daviskas, E., Anderson, S.D., Eberl, S., Young, I.H., 2010a. Beneficial effect of inhaled mannitol and cough in asthmatics with mucociliary dysfunction. Respir. Med. 104, 1645–1653.

Daviskas, E., Anderson, S.D., Gonda, I., et al., 1995. Changes in mucociliary clearance during and after isocapnic hyperventilation in asthmatic and healthy subjects. Eur. Respir. J. 8, 742–751.

Daviskas, E., Anderson, S.D., Gonda, I., et al., 1996. Inhalation of hypertonic saline aerosol enhances mucociliary clearance in asthmatic and healthy subjects. Eur. Respir. J. 9, 725–732.

Daviskas, E., Anderson, S.D., Jaques, A., Charlton, B., 2010b. Inhaled mannitol improves the hydration and surface properties of sputum in patients with cystic fibrosis. Chest 137, 861–868.

Dean, E., 1985. Effect of body position on pulmonary function. Phys. Ther. 65, 613–618.

Dean, E., 1993. Bedrest and deconditioning. Neurol. Report 17, 6–9.

Dean, E., 1994a. Oxygen transport: a physiologically-based conceptual framework for the practice of cardiopulmonary physiotherapy. Physiotherapy 80, 347–359.

Dean, E., 2006a. Optimizing outcomes: relating interventions to an individual's needs. In: Frownfelter, D., Dean, E. (Eds.), Cardiovascular and Pulmonary Physical Therapy: Evidence and Practice, 4th ed. Mosby, St Louis.

Dean, E., 2006b. Mobilization and exercise. In: Frownfelter, D., Dean, E. (Eds.), Cardiovascular and Pulmonary Physical Therapy: Evidence and Practice, 4th ed. Mosby, St Louis.

Dean, E., 2006c. Body positioning. In: Frownfelter, D., Dean, E. (Eds.), Cardiovascular and Pulmonary Physical Therapy: Evidence and Practice, 4th ed. Mosby, St Louis.

Dean, E., 2006d. Exercise testing and training for individuals with primary cardiopulmonary dysfunction. In: Frownfelter, D., Dean, E. (Eds.), Cardiovascular and Pulmonary Physical Therapy: Evidence and Practice, 4th ed. Mosby, St Louis.

Dean, E., Ross, J., 1992a. Oxygen transport: the basis for contemporary cardiopulmonary physical therapy and its optimization with body positioning and mobilization. Phys. Ther. Pract. 1, 34–44.

Dean, E., Ross, J., 1992b. Discordance between cardiopulmonary physiology and physical therapy: toward a rational basis for practice. Chest 101, 1694–1698.

Dean, E., Ross, J., Bartz, J., Purves, S., 1989. Improving the validity of exercise testing: the effect of practice on performance. Arch. Phys. Med. Rehabil. 70, 599–604.

Delvaux, M., Henket, M., Lau, L., et al., 2004. Nebulised salbutamol administered during sputum induction improves bronchoprotection in patients with asthma. Thorax 59, 111–115.

Denehy, L., Berney, S., 2001. The use of positive pressure devices by physiotherapists. Eur. Respir. J. 17, 821–829.

Denehy, L., Berney, S., 2006. Physiotherapy in the intensive care unit. Phys. Ther. Rev. 11, 49–56.

Dentice, R., Elkins, M., 2013. Timing of dornase alfa inhalation for cystic fibrosis. Cochrane Database Syst. Rev. (6), CD007923, doi:10.1002/14651858.CD007923.pub3.

Dentice, R.L., Elkins, M.R., Bye, P.T.P., 2012. Adults with cystic fibrosis prefer hypertonic saline before or during airway clearance techniques: a randomised crossover trial. J. Physiother. 58, 33–40.

De Troyer, A., 1997. Mechanics of the chest wall muscles. In: Miller, A.D., Bianchi, A.L., Bishop, B.P. (Eds.), Neural Control of the Respiratory Muscles. CRC Press, New York.

Di Marco, F., Centanni, S., Bellone, A., et al., 2011. Optimization of ventilator setting by flow and pressure waveforms analysis during noninvasive ventilation for acute exacerbations of COPD: a multicentric randomized controlled trial. Critical Care 15, R283.

Diaz, O., Begin, P., Torrealba, B., et al., 2002. Effects of noninvasive ventilation on lung hyperinflation in stable hypercapnic COPD. Eur. Respir. J. 20, 1490–1498. distributed by J. B. Lippincott.

Donaldson, S.H., Bennett, W.D., Zeman, K.L., et al., 2006. Mucus clearance and lung function in cystic fibrosis with hypertonic saline. NEJM 354, 241–250.

do Nascimento Junior, P., Módolo, N.S.P., Andrade, S., et al., 2014. Incentive spirometry for prevention of postoperative pulmonary complications in upper abdominal surgery. Cochrane Database Syst. Rev. (2), CD006058.

Dorman, S., Byrne, A., Edwards, A., 2007. Which measurement scales should be used to assess breathlessness in palliative care? A systematic review. Palliat. Med. 21, 177–191.

Dougan, C.F., Connell, C.O., Thornton, E., et al., 2000. Development of a patient-specific dyspnoea questionnaire in motor neurone disease (MND): the MND dyspnoea rating scale (MDRS). J. Neurol. Sci. 180, 86–93.

Douglas, W.W., Rehder, K., Froukje, B.M., 1977. Improved oxygenation in patients with acute respiratory failure: the prone position. Am. Rev. Respir. Dis. 115, 559–566.

Downs, J., 2003. Has oxygen administration delayed appropriate respiratory care? Fallacies regarding oxygen therapy. Respir. Care 48, 611–620.

Dreher, M., Storre, J.H., Windisch, W., 2007. Noninvasive ventilation during walking in patients with severe COPD: a randomised cross-over trial. Eur. Respir. J. 29, 930–936.

Dreyfuss, D., Djedaini, K., Lanore, J.-J., et al., 1992. A comparative study of the effects of almitrine bismesylate and lateral position during unilateral bacterial pneumonia with severe hypoxemia. Am. Rev. Respir. Dis. 148, 295–299.

Dripps, R.D., Waters, R.M., 1941. Nursing care of surgical patients. I. The 'stir-up'. Am. J. Nurs. 41, 530–534.

Duggal, A., Perez, P., Golan, E., et al., 2013. Safety and efficacy of noninvasive ventilation in patients with blunt chest trauma: a systematic review. Critical Care 17, R142.

Duiverman, M., Wempe, J., Bladder, G., et al., 2011. Two-year home-based nocturnal noninvasive ventilation added to rehabilitation in chronic obstructive pulmonary disease patients: a randomized controlled trial. Respir. Res. 12, 112.

Duiverman, M.L., Wempe, J.B., Bladder, G., et al., 2008. Nocturnal noninvasive ventilation in addition to rehabilitation in hypercapnic COPD patients. Thorax 63, 1052–1057.

Duron, B., Bars, P., 1986. Effect of thoracic cutaneous nerve stimulations on the activity of the intercostal muscles and motoneurons of the cat. In: Euler, C., Lagercrantz, A. (Eds.), Neurobiology of the Control of Breathing (Nobel Conference Series). Raven Press, New York.

Duron, B., Rose, D., 1997. The intercostal muscles. In: Miller, A.D., Bianchi, A.L., Bishop, B.P. (Eds.), Neural Control of the Respiratory Muscles. CRC Press, New York.

Dull, J.L., Dull, W.L., 1983. Are maximal inspiratory breathing exercises or incentive spirometry better than early mobilization after cardiopulmonary bypass? Phys. Ther. 63, 655–659.

Dwyer, T.J., Alison, J.A., McKeough, Z.J., et al., 2011a. Effects of exercise on respiratory flow and sputum properties in patients with cystic fibrosis. Chest 139, 870–877.

Dwyer, T.J., Elkins, M.R., Bye, P.T., 2011b. The role of exercise in maintaining health in cystic fibrosis. Curr. Opin. Pulm. Med. 6, 455–460.

Eaton, T.E., Grey, C., Garrett, J.E., 2001. An evaluation of short-term oxygen therapy: the prescription of oxygen to patients with chronic lung disease hypoxic at discharge from hospital. Respir. Med. 95, 582–587.

Eaton, T., Young, P., Zeng, I., et al., 2007. A randomized evaluation of the acute efficacy, acceptability and tolerability of flutter and active cycle of breathing with and without postural drainage in noncystic fibrosis bronchiectasis. Chron. Respir. Dis. 4, 23–30.

Ebihara, S., Niu, K., Ebihara, T., et al., 2012. Impact of blunted perception of dyspnea on medical care use and expenditure, and mortality in elderly people. Frontiers Physio. 3, 238 Published online 2012 July 4. doi:10.3389/fphys.2012.00238.

Elkins, M., Alison, J., Bye, P., 2005. Effect of body position on maximal expiratory pressure and flow. Pediatr. Pulmonol. 2005, 385–391.

Elkins, M.R., Anderson, S.D., Perry, C.P., et al., 2014b. Inspiratory flows and volumes in subjects with non-CF bronchiectasis using a new dry powder inhaler device. Open Respir. Med. J. 7, 95–100.

Elkins, M.R., Brannan, J.D., 2012. Warm-up exercise can reduce exercise-induced bronchoconstriction. Br. J. Sports Med. 46, 657–658.

Elkins, M.R., Bye, P.T.P., 2006b. Inhaled hypertonic saline as a therapy for cystic fibrosis. Curr. Opin. Pulm. Med. 12, 445–452.

Elkins, M., Jones, A., van der Schans, C.P., 2006a. Positive expiratory pressure physiotherapy for airway clearance in people with cystic fibrosis. Cochrane Database Syst. Rev. (2), Art. No.: CD003147, doi:10.1002/14651858.CD003147.pub3.

Elkins, M.R., Robinson, M., Rose, B.R., et al., 2006c. A controlled trial of long-term inhaled hypertonic saline in patients with cystic fibrosis. NEJM 354 (3), 229–240.

Elkins, M.R., Robinson, P., Anderson, S.D., et al., 2014a. Inspiratory flows and volumes in subjects with Cystic Fibrosis using a new dry powder inhaler device. Open Respir. Med. J. 7, 88–94.

Eng, P.A., Morton, J., Douglass, J.A., et al., 1996. Short-term efficacy of ultrasonically nebulized hypertonic saline in cystic fibrosis. Pediatr. Pulmonol. 21, 77–83.

Enright, S., Chatham, K., Ionescu, A.A., et al., 2004. Inspiratory muscle training improves lung function and exercise capacity in adults with cystic fibrosis. Chest 126, 406–411.

Enright, S.J., Unnithan, V.B., Heward, C., et al., 2006. Effect of high-intensity inspiratory muscle training on lung volumes, diaphragm thickness, and exercise capacity in subjects who are healthy. Phys. Ther. 86 (3), 345–354.

Esquinas Rodriguez, A.M., Scala, R., Soroksky, A., et al., 2011. Clinical review. Humidifiers during non-invasive ventilation: key topics and practical implications. Critical Care 16, 203.

Esteban, A., Frutos-Vivar, F., Ferguson, N.D., et al., 2004. Noninvasive positive-pressure ventilation for respiratory failure after extubation. NEJM 350, 2452–2460.

Ewart, W., 1901. The treatment of bronchiectasis and of chronic bronchial affections by posture and by respiratory exercises. Lancet 2, 70–72.

Falk, M., Andersen, J., 1991. Positive expiratory pressure (PEP) mask. In: Pryor, J. (Ed.), Respiratory Care, first ed. Churchill Livingstone, Edinburgh, pp. 51–63.

Falk, M., Kelstrup, M., Andersen, J.B., et al., 1984. Improving the ketchup bottle method with positive expiratory pressure, PEP, in cystic fibrosis. Eur. J. Respir. Dis. 65 (6), 423–432.

Fanfulla, F., Taurino, A.E., Lupo, N.D., et al., 2007. Effect of sleep on patient/ventilator asynchrony in patients undergoing chronic non-invasive mechanical ventilation. Respir. Med. 101, 1702–1707.

Fauroux, B., Boule, M., Lofaso, F., et al., 1999. Chest physiotherapy in cystic fibrosis: improved tolerance with nasal pressure support ventilation. Pediatrics 103, E32.

Fauroux, B., Guillemot, N., Aubertin, G., et al., 2008. Physiologic benefits of mechanical insufflation-exsufflation in children with neuromuscular diseases. Chest 133, 161–168.

Fauroux, B., Lavis, J.F., Nicot, F., et al., 2005. Facial side effects during noninvasive positive pressure ventilation in children. Intensive Care Med. 31, 965–969.

Ferrer, M., Esquinas, A., Leon, M., et al., 2003. Noninvasive ventilation in severe hypoxemic respiratory failure: a randomized clinical trial. Am. J. Respir. Crit. Care Med. 168, 1438–1444.

Ferrer, M., Sellares, J., Valencia, M., et al., 2009. Non-invasive ventilation after extubation in hypercapnic patients with chronic respiratory disorders: randomised controlled trial. Lancet 374, 1082–1088.

Ferrer, M., Valencia, M., Nicolas, J.M., et al., 2006. Early noninvasive ventilation averts extubation failure in patients at risk: a randomized trial. Am. J. Respir. Crit. Care Med. 173, 164–170.

Festini, F., Ballarin, S., Codamo, T., et al., 2004. Prevalence of pain in adults with cystic fibrosis. J. Cyst. Fibros. 3 (1), 51–57.

Figueiredo, P., Zin, W., Guimarães, F., 2012. Flutter valve improves respiratory mechanics and sputum production in patients with bronchiectasis. Physiother. Res. Int. 17, 12–20.

Fink, J.B., 2007. Forced expiratory technique, directed cough, and autogenic drainage. Respir. Care 52 (9), 1210–1221, discussion 1221–1223.

Fink, J., Ari, A., 2013. Humidity and bland aerosol therapy. In: Kacmarek, R., Stoller, J., Heuer, A. (Eds.), Egan's Fundamentals of Respiratory Care, tenth ed. Elsevier Mosby, St. Louis.

Fink, J.B., Mahlmeister, M.J., 2002. High-frequency oscillation of the airway and chest wall. Respir. Care 47, 797–807.

Fitzgerald, D.A., Hilton, J., Jepson, B., Smith, L., 2005. A crossover, randomized, controlled trial of dornase alfa before versus after physiotherapy in cystic fibrosis. Pediatrics 116 (4), 549–554.

Flandreau, G., Bourdin, G., Leray, V., et al., 2011. Management and long-term outcome of patients with chronic neuromuscular disease admitted to the intensive care unit for acute respiratory failure: a single-center retrospective study. Respir. Care 56, 953–960.

Fleck, S., 1994. Detraining: its effects on endurance and strength. Strength Cond. J. 2, 22–28.

Fletcher, C.M., 1952. The clinical diagnosis of pulmonary emphysema: an experimental study. Proc. R. Soc. Med. 45 (9), 577–584. PMID: 13003946.

Fletcher, E., Luckett, R., Goodnight-White, S., et al., 1992. A double-blind trial of nocturnal supplemental oxygen for sleep desaturation in patients with chronic obstructive pulmonary disease and a daytime PaO_2 above 60 mmHg. Am. Rev. Respir. Dis. 145, 1070–1076.

Flight, W.G., Shaw, J., Johnson, S., et al., 2012. Long-term non-invasive ventilation in cystic fibrosis: experience over two decades. J. Cyst. Fibros. 11, 187–192.

Flude, L.J., Agent, P., Bilton, D., 2012. Chest physiotherapy techniques in bronchiectasis. Clin. Chest Med. 33 (2), 351–361.

Fok, J., Brown, N.E., Zuberbuhler, P., et al., 2002. Low bone mineral density in cystic fibrosis patients. Can. J. Diet. Pract. Res. 63, 192–197.

Fontana, G.A., Hanson, P.J.V., Cardellicchio, S., et al., 1988. Effect of aminophylline aerosol on the bronchial response to ultrasonic mist of distilled water in asthmatic patients. Respiration 54, 241–246.

Fowler, W.S., 1949. Lung function studies. III. Uneven pulmonary ventilation in normal subjects and patients with pulmonary disease. J. Appl. Physiol. 2, 283–299.

Frazier, D.T., Xu, F., Lee, L.-Y., 1997. Respiratory-related reflexes and the cerebellum. In: Miller, A.D., Bianchi, A.L., Bishop, B.P. (Eds.), Neural Control of the Respiratory Muscles. CRC Press, New York.

Freitag, L., Bremme, J., Schroer, M., 1989. High-frequency oscillation for respiratory physiotherapy. Br. J. Anaesth. 63, S44–S46.

Freitas, E.R.F.S., Soares, B.G.O., Cardoso, J.R., Atallah, A.N., 2012. Incentive spirometry for preventing pulmonary complications after coronary artery bypass graft. Cochrane Database Syst. Rev. (9), CD004466.

Fridrich, P., Krafft, P., Hochleuthner, H., 1996. The effects of long-term prone positioning in patients with trauma-induced adult respiratory distress syndrome. Anesth. Analg. 83, 1206–1211.

Frownfelter, D.L., Dean, E.W., 2006. Cardiovascular and Pulmonary Physical Therapy: Evidence and Practice. Mosby Elsevier, St. Louis, Missouri USA.

Fuchs, H.J., Borowitz, D.S., Christiansen, D.H., et al., 1994. Effect of aerosolized recombinant human DNase on exacerbations of respiratory symptoms and on pulmonary function in patients with cystic fibrosis. The Pulmozyme Study Group. NEJM 331, 637–642.

Fuschillo, S., De Felice, A., Gaudiosi, C., et al., 2003. Nocturnal mechanical ventilation improves exercise capacity in kyphoscoliotic patients with respiratory impairment. Monaldi Arch. Chest Dis. 59, 281–286.

Gallon, A., 1991. Evaluation of chest percussion in the treatment of patients with copious sputum production. Respir. Med. 85, 45–51.

Gallon, A., 1992. The use of percussion. Physiotherapy 78, 85–89.

Garner, D.J., Berlowitz, D.J., Douglas, J., et al., 2013. Home mechanical ventilation in Australia and New Zealand. Eur. Respir. J. 41, 39–45.

Garrard, C., A'Court, C., 1995. The diagnosis of pneumonia in the critically-ill. Chest 108, S17–S25.

Garrod, R., Mikelsons, C., Paul, E.A., et al., 2000. Randomized controlled trial of domiciliary noninvasive positive pressure ventilation and physical training in severe chronic obstructive pulmonary disease. Am. J. Respir. Crit. Care Med. 162, 1335–1341.

Geddes, E.L., Reid, D.W., Crowe, J., et al., 2005. Inspiratory muscle training in adults with chronic obstructive pulmonary disease: a systematic review. Respir. Med. 99, 1440–1458.

Gerlach, Y., Coates, A., Williams, M.T., 2013. Weighing up the evidence: a systematic review of measures used for the sensation of breathlessness in obesity. Int. J. Obes. 27, 341–349.

Gift, A.G., Narsavage, G., 1998. Validity of the numeric rating scale as a measure of dyspnea. Am. J. Crit. Care 7, 200–204.

Gigliotti, F., 2010. Mechanisms of dyspnoea in health subjects. Multidisciplinary Respir. Med. 5, 195–201.

Giles, D., Wagener, J., Accurso, F., Butler-Simon, N., 1995. Short-term effects of postural drainage with clapping vs autogenic drainage on oxygen saturation and sputum recovery in patients with cystic fibrosis. Chest 108, 952–954.

Girault, C., Richard, J.C., Chevron, V., et al., 1997. Comparative physiologic effects of noninvasive assist-control and pressure support ventilation in acute hypercapnic respiratory failure. Chest 111, 1639–1648.

Glaab, T., Vogelmeier, C., Buhl, R., 2010. Outcome measures in chronic obstructive pulmonary disease (COPD): strengths and limitations. Respir. Res. 11 (79), 1–11.

Glossop, A., Shepherd, N., Bryden, D., et al., 2012. Non-invasive ventilation for weaning, avoiding reintubation after extubation and in the postoperative period: a meta-analysis. Br. J. Anaesth. 109, 305–314.

Gokdemir, Y., Karadag-Saygi, E., Erdem, E., et al., 2014. Comparison of conventional pulmonary rehabilitation and high-frequency chest wall oscillation in primary ciliary dyskinesia. Pediatr. Pulmonol. 49, 611–616.

Goldman, M., 1974. Mechanical coupling of the diaphragm and the rib cage. In: Pengelly, L.D., Rebuck, A.S., Campbell, E.J.M. (Eds.), Loaded Breathing. Proceedings of an international symposium, 'The effects of mechanical loads on breathing'. Longman Canada, Don Mills, Ontario.

Gomez-Merino, E., Bach, J.R., 2002. Duchenne muscular dystrophy: prolongation of life by noninvasive ventilation and mechanically assisted coughing. Am. J. Phys. Med. Rehabil. 81, 411–415.

Goncalves, M.R., Honrado, T., Winck, J.C., Paiva, J.A., 2012. Effects of mechanical insufflation-exsufflation in preventing respiratory failure after extubation: a randomized controlled trial. Crit. Care 16, R48.

Gordon, J., 1991. Spinal mechanisms of motor coordination. In: Kandel, E.R., Schwartz, J.H., Jessel, J.M. (Eds.), Principles of Neural Science. Appleton & Lange, Connecticut.

Gondor, M., Nixon, P., Mutich, R., et al., 1999. Comparison of Flutter device and chest physical therapy in the treatment of cystic fibrosis pulmonary exacerbation. Pediatr. Pulmonol. 28, 255–260.

Goralski, J.L., Boucher, R.C., Button, B., 2010. Osmolytes and ion transport modulator: new strategies for airway surface rehydration. Curr. Opin. Pharmacol. 10, 294–299.

Gormezano, J., Branthwaite, M.A., 1972. Pulmonary physiotherapy with assisted ventilation. Anaesthesia 27, 249–257.

Gosselin, N., Lambert, K., Poulain, M., et al., 2003. Endurance training improves skeletal muscle electrical activity in active COPD patients. Muscle Nerve 28, 744–753.

Gosselink, R., 2004. Breathing techniques in patients with chronic obstructive pulmonary disease (COPD). Chron. Respir. Dis. 1, 163–172.

Gosselink, R., De Vos, J., van den Heuvel, S.P., et al., 2011. Impact of inspiratory muscle training in patients with COPD: what is the evidence? Eur. Respir. J. 37, 416–425.

Gosselink, R., Schrever, K., Cops, P., et al., 2000. Incentive spirometry does not enhance recovery after thoracic surgery. Crit. Care Med. 28 (3), 679–683.

Gosselink, R.A., Wagenaar, R.C., Rijswijk, H., et al., 1995. Diaphragmatic breathing reduces efficiency of breathing in patients with chronic obstructive pulmonary disease. Am. J. Respir. Crit. Care Med. 151, 1136–1142.

Gould, N.S., Gauthier, S., Kariya, C.T., et al., 2010. Hypertonic saline increases lung epithelial lining fluid glutathione and thiocyanate: two protective CFTR-dependent thiols against oxidative injury. Respir. Res. 11, 119.

Gozal, D., 1997. Nocturnal ventilatory support in patients with cystic fibrosis: comparison with supplemental oxygen. Eur. Respir. J. 10, 1999–2003.

Gray's Anatomy, 1973. Longman, Edinburgh

Green, M., Moxham, J., 1985. The respiratory muscles. Clin. Sci. 68, 1–10.

Gregersen, G.G., Lucas, D.L., 1967. An in vivo study of the axial rotation of the human thoraco-lumbar spine. J. Bone Joint Surg. 49A, 247–262.

Gregson, R.K., Shannon, H., Stocks, J., et al., 2012. The unique contribution of manual chest compression-vibrations to airflow during physiotherapy in sedated, fully ventilated children. Pediatr. Crit. Care Med. 13, e97–e102.

Gregson, R.K., Stocks, J., Petley, G.W., et al., 2007. Simultaneous measurement of force and respiratory profiles during chest physiotherapy in ventilated children. Physiol. Meas. 28, 1017–1028.

Gross, D., Zidulka, A., O'Brien, C., et al., 1985. Peripheral mucociliary clearance with high-frequency chest wall compression. J. Appl. Physiol. (1985) 58, 1157–1163.

Guideline, A.C.P., 1992. Nasotracheal suctioning. American Association for Respiratory Care. Respir. Care 37, 898–901.

Guimarães, F.S., Moço, V.J., Menezes, S.L., et al., 2012. Effects of ELTGOL and Flutter VRP1® on the dynamic and static pulmonary volumes and on the secretion clearance of patients with bronchiectasis. Rev. Bras Fisioter 16, 108–113.

Guimarães, F., Lopes, A., Constantino, S., et al., 2013. Expiratory rib cage compression, secretion clearance and respiratory mechanics in mechanically ventilated patients: a randomized crossover trial. Respir. Care, [Epub ahead of print].

Gumery, L., Lee, J., Whitehouse, J., Honeybourne, D., 2005. The prevalence of urinary incontinence in adult cystic fibrosis males. J. Cyst. Fibros. 4 (Suppl. 1), S97.

Guo, Y.F., Sforza, E., Janssens, J.P., 2007. Respiratory patterns during sleep in obesity-hypoventilation patients treated with nocturnal pressure support: a preliminary report. Chest 131, 1090–1099.

Gursel, G., Aydogdu, M., Gulbas, G., et al., 2011. The influence of severe obesity on non-invasive ventilation (NIV) strategies and responses in patients with acute hypercapnic respiratory failure attacks in the ICU. Minerva Anestesiol. 77, 17–25.

Guyatt, G.H., Berman, L.B., Townsend, M., et al., 1987. A measure of quality of life for clinical trials in chronic lung disease. Thorax 42, 773–778.

Guyatt, G.H., Nogradi, S., Halcrow, S., et al., 1989. Development and testing of a new measure of health status for clinical trials in heart failure. J. Gen. Intern. Med. 4, 101–107.

Haeffener, M.P., Ferreira, G.M., Barreto, S.S.M., et al., 2008. Incentive spirometry with expiratory positive airway pressure reduces pulmonary complications, improves pulmonary function and 6-minute walk distance in patients undergoing coronary artery bypass graft surgery. Am. Heart J. 156 (5), 900.e2–900.e7. [DOI: 101016].

Hahn-Winslow, E., 1985. Cardiovascular consequences of bed rest. Heart Lung 14, 236–246.

Hallstrand, T.S., Kippelen, P., Larsson, J., et al., 2013. Where to from here for exercise-induced bronchoconstriction. Immunol. Allergy Clin. North Am. 33 (3), 3.

Hansen, L., Warwick, W., 1990. High-frequency chest compression system to aid in clearance of mucus from the lung. Biomed. Instrum. Technol. 24, 289–294.

Hansen, L., Warwick, W., Hansen, K., 1994. Mucus transport mechanisms in relation to the effect of high frequency chest compression (HFCC) on mucus clearance. Pediatr. Pulmonol. 17, 113–118.

Hardinge, M., Annandale, J., Bourne, S., 2015. British Thoracic Society guidelines for home oxygen use in adults. Thorax 70 (Suppl. 1), i1–i43.

Harrison, K.S., Laube, B.L., 1994. Bronchodilator pretreatment improves aerosol deposition uniformity in HIV-positive patients who cough while inhaling aerosolized pentamidine. Chest 106 (2), 421–426.

Hasani, A., Chapman, T.H., McCool, D., et al., 2008. Domiciliary humidification improves lung mucociliary clearance in patients with bronchiectasis. Chron. Respir. Dis. 5 (2), 81–86.

Hasani, A., Pavia, D., Agnew, J.E., et al., 1994a. Regional clearance during cough and forced expiration technique (FET): effects of flow and viscoelasticity. Thorax 49, 557–561.

Hasani, A., Pavia, D., Agnew, J.E., et al., 1994b. Regional mucus transport following unproductive cough and forced expiration technique in patients with airway obstruction. Chest 105, 1420–1425.

Hasani, A., Pavia, D., Agnew, J.E., Clarke, S.W., 1991. The effect of unproductive coughing/FET on regional mucus movement in the human lungs. Respir. Med. 85 (Suppl. A), 23–26.

Havasi, V., Hurst, C.O., Briles, T.C., et al., 2008. Inhibitory effects of hypertonic saline on P. aeruginosa motility. J. Cyst. Fibros. 7 (4), 267–269.

Hebestreit, A., Kersting, U., Basler, B., et al., 2001. Exercise inhibits epithelial sodium channels in patients with cystic fibrosis. Am. J. Respir. Crit. Care Med. 164, 443–446.

Heijerman, H., Westerman, E., Conway, S., et al., 2009. Inhaled medication and inhalation devices for lung disease in patients with cystic fibrosis: a European consensus. J. Cyst. Fibros. 8 (5), 295–315.

Heine, R.G., Button, B.M., Olinsky, A., et al., 1998. Gastro-oesophageal reflux in infants under 6 months with cystic fibrosis. Arch. Dis. Child. 78, 44–48.

Henderson, R.C., Madsen, C.D., 1996. Bone density in children and adolescents with cystic fibrosis. J. Pediatr. 128, 28–34.

Henderson, R.C., Specter, B.B., 1994. Kyphosis and fractures in children and young adults with cystic fibrosis. J. Pediatr. 125, 208–212.

Heuer, A., 2013a. Medical gas therapy. In: Kacmarek, R., Stoller, J., Heuer, A. (Eds.), Egan's Fundamentals of Respiratory Care, tenth ed. Elsevier Mosby, St. Louis.

Heuer, A., 2013b. Respiratory care in alternative settings. In: Kacmarek, R., Stoller, J., Heuer, A. (Eds.), Egan's Fundamentals of Respiratory Care, tenth ed. Elsevier Mosby, St. Louis.

Hilaire, G., Monteau, R., 1997. Brainstem and spinal control of respiratory muscles during breathing. In: Miller, A.D., Bianchi, A.L., Bishop, B.P. (Eds.), Neural Control of the Respiratory Muscles. CRC Press, New York.

Hilbert, G., Gruson, D., Vargas, F., et al., 2001. Noninvasive ventilation in immunosuppressed patients with pulmonary infiltrates, fever, and acute respiratory failure. NEJM 344, 481–487.

Hill, K., Jenkins, S.C., Hillman Eastwood, P.R., 2004. Dyspnoea in COPD: can inspiratory muscle training help? Aust. J. Physiother. 50, 169–180.

Hill, K., Eastwood, P.R., 2005. Respiratory muscle training: the con argument. Chron. Respir. Dis. 2 (4), 223–224.

Hill, K., Patman, S., Brooks, D., 2010. Effect of airway clearance techniques in patients experiencing an acute exacerbation of chronic obstructive pulmonary disease: a systematic review. Chron. Respir. Dis. 7, 9–17.

Hirsh, A.J., 2002. Altering airway surface liquid volume: inhalation therapy with amiloride and hyperosmotic agents. Adv. Drug Deliv. Rev. 54, 1445–1462.

Hsiao, S.F., Wu, Y.T., Wu, H.D., Wang, T.G., 2003. Comparison of the effectivness of pressure threshold and targeted resistive muscle training in patients with chronic obstructive pulmonary disease. J. Formos. Med. Assoc. 102, 204–205.

Hodgson, C., Carroll, S., Denehy, L., 1999. A survey of manual hyperinflation in Australian hospitals. Aust J. Physiother. 45, 185–193.

Hodgson, C., Denehy, L., Ntoumenopoulos, G., et al., 2000. An investigation of the early effects of manual lung hyperinflation in critically ill patients. Anaesth. Intensive Care 28, 255–261.

Holland, A., Button, B., 2006. Is there a role for airway clearance techniques in chronic obstructive pulmonary disease? Chron. Respir. Dis. 3, 83–91.

Holland, A.E., Denehy, L., Buchan, C.A., et al., 2007. Efficacy of a heated passover humidifier during noninvasive ventilation: a bench study. Respir. Care 52, 38–44.

Holland, A.E., Denehy, L., Ntoumenopoulos, G., et al., 2003. Non-invasive ventilation assists chest physiotherapy in adults with acute exacerbations of cystic fibrosis. Thorax 58, 880–884.

Holland, A.E., Hill, C., 2008. Physical training for interstitial lung disease. Cochrane Database Syst. Rev. (4), Art. No.: CD006322, doi:10.1002/14651858.CD006322.pub2.

Holland, A.E., Hill, C.J., Jones, A.Y., McDonald, C.F., 2012. Breathing exercises for chronic obstructive pulmonary disease. Cochrane Database Syst. Rev. (10), Art. No.: CD008250, doi:10.1002/14651858.CD008250.pub2.

Hollen, P.J., Gralla, R.J., Kris, M.G., et al., 1993. Quality of life assessment in individuals with lung cancer: testing the Lung Cancer Symptom Scale (LCSS). Eur. J. Cancer 29A (Suppl. 1), S51–S58.

Homnick, D., Anderson, K., Marks, J., 1998. Comparison of the Flutter device to standard chest physiotherapy in hospitalized patients with cystic fibrosis: a pilot study. Chest 114, 993–997.

Horiuchi, K., Jordan, D., Cohen, D., et al., 1997. Insights into the increased oxygen demand during chest physiotherapy. Crit. Care Med. 25, 1347–1351.

Hsu, H.O., Hickey, R.F., 1976. Effect of posture on functional residual capacity postoperatively. Anesthesiology 44, 520–521.

Imle, P.C., Klemic, N., 1989. Changes with immobility and methods of mobilization. In: Mackenzie, C.F. (Ed.), Chest Physiotherapy in the Intensive Care Unit, second ed. Williams and Wilkins, Baltimore, pp. 188–214.

Inal-Ince, D., Savci, S., Topeli, A., et al., 2004. Active cycle of breathing techniques in non-invasive ventilation for acute hypercapnic respiratory failure. Aust J. Physiother. 50, 67–73.

Ingwersen, U., Larsen, K., Bertelsen, M., et al., 1993. Three different mask physiotherapy regimens for prevention of post-operative pulmonary complications after heart and pulmonary surgery. Intensive Care Med. 19, 294–298.

Institute for Work & Health, 1996. DASH Index. The American Academy of Orthopaedic Surgeons (AAOS). <www.iwh.on.ca> (accessed 5 July 2007).

Jaber, S., Chanques, G., Matecki, S., et al., 2002. Comparison of the effects of heat and moisture exchangers and heated humidifiers on ventilation and gas exchange during non-invasive ventilation. Intensive Care Med. 28, 1590–1594.

Jacob, W., 1990. Physiotherapy in the ICU. In: Oh, T.E. (Ed.), Intensive Care Manual, third ed. Butterworths, Sydney, p. 24. (Chapter 4).

Janda, V., 1994. Muscles and motor control in cervicogenic disorders: assessment and management physical therapy for the cervical and thoracic spine. In: Grant, R. (Ed.), Clinics in Physical Therapy, second ed. Churchill Livingstone, New York.

Jaques, A., Daviskas, E., Turton, J.A., et al., 2008. Inhaled mannitol improves lung function in cystic fibrosis. Chest 133, 1388–1396.

Jean, A., Car, A., Kessler, J.P., 1997. Brainstem organization of swallowing and its interaction with respiration. In: Miller, A.D., Bianchi, A.L., Bishop, B.P. (Eds.), Neural Control of the Respiratory Muscles. CRC Press, New York.

Jiang, J.S., Kao, S.J., Wang, S.N., 1999. Effect of early application of biphasic positive airway pressure on the outcome of extubation in ventilator weaning. Respirology 4, 161–165.

Johansson, K.M., Nygren-Bonnier, M., Schalling, E., 2012. Effects of glossopharyngeal breathing on speech and respiration in multiple sclerosis: a case report. Mult. Scler. 18 (6), 905–908.

Johnson, J.E., Gavin, D.J., Adams-Dramiga, S., 2002. Effects of training with heliox and noninvasive positive pressure ventilation on exercise ability in patients with severe COPD. Chest 122, 464–472.

Johnson, M.J., Oxberry, S.G., Cleland, J.G.F., et al., 2010. Measurement of breathlessness in clinical trials in patients with chronic heart failure; the need for a standardised approach: a systemic review. Eur J. Heart Fail. 12, 137–147.

Jolliet, P., Bulpa, P., Ritz, M., et al., 1997. Additive beneficial effects of the prone position, nitric oxide, and almitrine bismesylate on gas exchange and oxygen transport in acute respiratory distress syndrome. Crit. Care Med. 25, 786–794.

Jones, A.P., Wallis, C., 2010. Dornase alfa for cystic fibrosis. Cochrane Database Syst. Rev. 17 (3), CD001127.

Jones, A.Y.M., Hutchinson, R.C., Oh, T.E., 1992. Chest physiotherapy in intensive care units in Australia, the UK and Hong Kong. Physiother. Theory Pract. 8, 39–47.

Jones, P.W., Quirk, F.H., Baveystock, C.M., et al., 1992. A self-complete measure for chronic airflow limitation: the St George's Respiratory Questionnaire. Am. Rev. Respir. Dis. 145, 1321–1327.

Joris, J.L., Sottiaux, T.M., Chiche, J.D., et al., 1997. Effect of bi-level positive airway pressure (BiPAP) nasal ventilation on the postoperative pulmonary restrictive syndrome in obese patients undergoing gastroplasty. Chest 111, 665–670.

Joseph, J., Bandler, L., Anderson, S.D., 1976. Exercise as a bronchodilator. Aust J. Physiother. 22, 47–50.

Jull, G., Trott, P., Potter, H., et al., 2002. A randomized controlled trial of exercise and manipulative therapy for cervicogenic headache. Spine 27 (17), 1835–1843.

Kamishima, K., Yamamoto, H., Shida, A., et al., 1983. Effect of voluntary coughing on bronchial mucociliary clearance in smokers and patients with chronic obstructive pulmonary disease. Am Rev. Respir. Dis. 127 (Suppl.), 165.

Kang, S.W., Bach, J.R., 2000. Maximum insufflation capacity. Chest 118, 61–65.

Keenan, S.P., Powers, C., McCormack, D.G., et al., 2002. Noninvasive positive-pressure ventilation for postextubation respiratory distress: a randomized controlled trial. J. Am. Med. Assoc. 287, 3238–3244.

Keenan, S.P., Sinuff, T., Burns, K.E., et al., 2011. Clinical practice guidelines for the use of noninvasive positive-pressure ventilation and noninvasive continuous positive airway pressure in the acute care setting. Can. Med. Assoc. J. 183, E195–E214.

Keenan, S.P., Sinuff, T., Cook, D.J., et al., 2003. Which patients with acute exacerbation of chronic obstructive pulmonary disease benefit from noninvasive positive-pressure ventilation? A systematic review of the literature. Ann. Intern. Med. 138, 861–870.

Kelleher, W.H., Parida, R.K., 1957. Glossopharyngeal breathing. Br. Med. J. 2, 740–743.

Kellett, F., Redfern, J., Niven, R.M., 2005. Evaluation of nebulised hypertonic saline (7 percent) as an adjunct to physiotherapy in patients with stable bronchiectasis. Respir. Med. 99, 27–31.

Kellett, F., Robert, N.M., 2011. Nebulised 7 percent hypertonic saline improves lung function and quality of life in bronchiectasis. Respir. Med. 105, 1831–1835.

Kerem, E., Yatsiv, I., Goitein, K.J., 1990. Effect of endotracheal suctioning on arterial blood gases in children. Intensive Care Med. 16, 95–99.

Khamiees, M., Raju, P., DeGirolamo, A., et al., 2001. Predictors of extubation outcome in patients who have successfully completed a spontaneous breathing trial. Chest 120, 1262–1270.

Khan, T.Z., Wagener, J.S., Bost, T., et al., 1995. Early pulmonary inflammation in infants with cystic fibrosis. Am. J. Respir. Crit. Care Med. 151, 1075–1082.

Kim, C.S., Greene, M.A., Sankaran, S., Sackner, M.A., 1986a. Mucus transport in the airways by two-phase gas-liquid flow mechanism: continuous flow model. J. Appl. Physiol. (1985) 60, 908–917.

Kim, C.S., Iglesias, A.J., Sackner, M.A., 1987. Mucus clearance by two-phase gas–liquid flow mechanism: asymmetric periodic flow model. J. Appl. Physiol. 62, 959–971.

Kim, C.S., Rodriguez, C.R., Eldridge, M.A., Sackner, M.A., 1986b. Criteria for mucus transport in the airways by two-phase gas-liquid flow mechanism. J. Appl. Physiol. (1985) 60, 901–907.

King, M., 1998. Experimental models for studying mucociliary clearance. Eur. Respir. J. 11, 222–228.

King, M., Brock, G., Lundell, C., 1985. Clearance of mucus by simulated cough. J. Appl. Physiol. (1985) 58, 1776–1782.

King, M., Dasgupta, B., Tomkiewicz, R.P., Brown, N.E., 1997. Rheology of cystic fibrosis sputum after in vitro treatment with hypertonic saline alone and in combination with recombinant human deoxyribonuclease I. Am. J. Respir. Crit. Care Med. 156, 173–177.

King, D., Morrell, A., 1992. A survey on manual hyperinflation as a physiotherapy technique in intensive care units. Physiotherapy 78, 747–750.

King, M., Phillips, D.M., Gross, D., et al., 1983. Enhanced tracheal mucus clearance with high frequency chest wall compression. Am. Rev. Respir. Dis. 128, 511–515.

King, M., Phillips, D.M., Zidulka, A., Chang, H.K., 1984. Tracheal mucus clearance in high-frequency oscillation. II. Chest wall versus mouth oscillation. Am. Rev. Respir. Dis. 130, 703–706.

King, M., Zidulka, A., Phillips, D.M., et al., 1990. Tracheal mucus clearance in high-frequency oscillation: effect of peak flow rate bias. Eur. Respir. J. 3, 6–13.

Kluft, J., Beker, L., Castagnino, M., et al., 1996. A comparison of bronchial drainage treatments in cystic fibrosis. Pediatr. Pulmonol. 22, 271–274.

Knudson, R.J., Mead, J., Knudson, D.E., 1974. Contribution of airway collapse to supramaximal expiratory flows. J. Appl. Physiol. 36, 653–667.

Koepchen, H.P., Abel, H.-H., Klussendorf, D., Lazar, H., 1986. Respiratory and cardiovascular rhythmicity. In: Euler, C., Lagercrantz, A. (Eds.), Neurobiology of the Control of Breathing (Nobel Conference Series). Raven Press, New York.

Koh, J.L., Harrison, D., Palermo, T.M., et al., 2005. Assessment of acute and chronic pain symptoms in children with cystic fibrosis. Pediatr. Pulmonol. 40 (4), 330–335.

Kohlenberg, A., Schwab, F., Behnke, M., et al., 2010. Pneumonia associated with invasive and noninvasive ventilation: an analysis of the German nosocomial infection surveillance system database. Intensive Care Med. 36, 971–978.

Komi, P.V., Hakkinen, K., 1991. Strength and power. In: Dirix, A., Knuttgen, H.G., Tittel, K. (Eds.), The Olympic Book of Sports Medicine. Blackwell, Oxford, pp. 181–193.

Konstan, M., Stern, R., Doershuk, C., 1994. Efficacy of the Flutter device for airway mucus clearance in patients with cystic fibrosis. Journal of Pediatrics 124, 689–693.

Koomans, H.A., Boer, W.H., 1997. Causes of edema in the intensive care unit. Kidney Int. Suppl. 59, S105–S110.

Kraemer, W., Adams, K., Cararelli, E., et al., 2002. American College of Sports Medicine position stand. Progressive models in resistance training for healthy adults. Med. Sci. Sports Exerc. 34, 364–380.

Krause, M.F., Hoehn, T., 2000. Chest physiotherapy in mechanically ventilated children: a review. Crit. Care Med. 28, 1648–1651.

Kwok, H., McCormack, J., Cece, R., et al., 2003. Controlled trial of oronasal versus nasal mask ventilation in the treatment of acute respiratory failure. Crit. Care Med. 31, 468–473.

Kyroussis, D., Polkey, M.I., Hamnegard, C.H., et al., 2000. Respiratory muscle activity in patients with COPD walking to exhaustion with and without pressure support. Eur. Respir. J. 15, 649–655.

Lacasse, Y., Goldstein, R., Lasserson, T.J., Martin, S., 2006. Pulmonary rehabilitation for chronic obstructive pulmonary disease. Cochrane Database Syst. Rev. (4), Art. No.: CD003793, doi:10.1002/14651858.CD003793.pub2.

Lacasse, Y., Lecours, R., Pelletier, C., et al., 2005. Randomised trial of ambulatory oxygen in oxygen-dependent COPD. Eur. Respir. J. 25, 1032–1038.

Laghi, F., Tobin, M.J., 2003. Disorders of the respiratory muscles. Am. J. Respir. Crit. Care Med. 168, 10–48.

Lamb, L.E., Johnson, R.L., Stevens, P.M., 1964. Cardiovascular deconditioning during chair rest. Aerosp. Med. 23, 646–649.

Langenderfer, B., 1998. Alternatives to percussion and postural drainage. A review of mucus clearance therapies: percussion and postural drainage, autogenic drainage, positive expiratory pressure, flutter valve, intrapulmonary percussive ventilation, and high-frequency chest compression with the ThAIRapy Vest. J. Cardiopulm. Rehabil. 18, 283–289.

Langer, D., Hendriks, E., Burtin, C., et al., 2009. A clinical practice guideline for physiotherapists treating patients with chronic obstructive pulmonary disease based on a systematic review of available evidence. Clin. Rehabil. 23, 445–462.

Langlands, J., 1967. The dynamics of cough in health and in chronic bronchitis. Thorax 22, 88–96.

Lannefors, L., Button, B.M., McIlwaine, M., 2004. Physiotherapy in infants and young children with cystic fibrosis: current practice and future developments. J. R. Soc. Med. 97 (Suppl. 44), 8–25.

Lannefors, L., Wollmer, P., 1992. Mucus clearance with three chest physiotherapy regimes in cystic fibrosis: a comparison between postural drainage, PEP and physical exercise. Eur. Respir. J. 5, 748–753.

Lansing, R., Gracely, R., Banzett, R., 2009. The multiple dimensions of dyspnoea: review and hypothesis. Respir. Physiol. Neurobiol. 167, 53–60.

Lapin, C., 2000. Mixing and matching airway clearance techniques to patients. Pediatr. Pulmonol. 30 (Suppl. 21), 144–146.

Lapin, C., 2002. Airway physiology, autogenic drainage and active cycle of breathing. Respir. Care 47, 778–785.

Larsen, A.I., Aarsland, T., Kristiansen, M., et al., 2001. Assessing the effect of exercise training in men with heart failure: comparison of maximal, submaximal and endurance exercise protocols. Eur. Heart J. 22, 684–692.

Larsen, A.I., Lindal, S., Aukrust, P., et al., 2002. Effect of exercise training on skeletal muscle fibre characteristics in men with chronic heart failure: correlation between muscle alterations, cytokines, and exercise capacity. Int. J. Cardiol. 83, 25–32.

Laube, B.L., Auci, R.M., Shields, D.E., et al., 1996. Effect of rhDNase on airflow obstruction and mucociliary clearance in cystic fibrosis. Am. J. Respir. Crit. Care Med. 153, 752–760.

Laube, B.L., Geller, D.E., Lin, T.C., et al., 2005. Positive expiratory pressure changes aerosol distribution in patients with cystic fibrosis. Respir. Care 50 (11), 1438–1444.

Laurin, L.P., Jobin, V., Bellemare, F., 2012. Sternum length and rib cage dimensions compared with bodily proportions in adults with cystic fibrosis. Can. Respir. J. 19, 196–200.

Lawrence, V.A., Cornell, J.E., Smetana, G.W., 2006. Strategies to reduce postoperative pulmonary complications after noncardiothoracic surgery: systematic review for the American College of Physicians. Ann. Intern. Med. 144 (8), 596–608.

Leblanc, P., Ruff, F., Milic-Emili, J., 1970. Effects of age and body position on airway closure in man. J. Appl. Physiol. 28, 448–451.

Lee, D., 2003. The Thorax: An Integrated Approach, second ed. Orthopaedic Physical Therapy, Minneapolis.

Lee, A.L., Burge, A.T., Holland, A.E., 2013. Airway clearance techniques for bronchiectasis. Cochrane Database Syst. Rev. (5), Art. No.: CD008351.

Lee, A.L., Williamson, H.C., Lorensini, S., Spencer, L.M., 2015. The effects of oscillating positive expiratory pressure therapy in adults with stable non-cystic fibrosis bronchiectasis: a systematic review. Chron. Respir. Dis. 12 (1), 36–46.

Leith, D.E., 1968. Cough. Phys. Ther. 48, 439–447.

Leith, D.E., 1977. Cough. In: Brain, J.D., Proctor, D.F., Reid, L.M. (Eds.), Respiratory Defence Mechanisms Part II. Marcel Dekker Inc, New York, pp. 545–591.

Leith, D.E., Bradley, M., 1976. Ventilatory muscle strength and endurance training. J. Appl. Physiol. 41, 508–516.

Leith, D.E., 1985. The development of cough. Am. Rev. Respir. Dis. 131, S39–S42.

Lellouche, F., Maggiore, S., Deye, N., et al., 2002. Effect of the humidification device on the work of breathing during noninvasive ventilation. Intensive Care Med. 28, 1582–1589.

Lenique, F., Habis, M., Lofaso, F., et al., 1997. Ventilatory and hemodynamic effects of continuous positive airway pressure in left heart failure. Am. J. Respir. Crit. Care Med. 155, 500–505.

Levine, S.A., Lown, B., 1952. Armchair' treatment of acute coronary thrombosis. J. Am. Med. Assoc. 148, 1365–1369.

Levy, M., Tanios, M., Nelson, D., et al., 2004. Outcomes of patients with do-not-intubate orders treated with noninvasive ventilation. Crit. Care Med. 32, 2002–2007.

Lewis, F.R., 1980. Management of atelectasis and pneumonia. Surg. Clin. North Am. 60, 1391–1401.

Lewis, L., Williams, M., Olds, T., 2012. The active cycle of breathing technique: a systematic review and meta-analysis. Respir. Med. 106, 155–172.

Lewis, L.K., Williams, M.T., Olds, T., 2007. Short-term effects on the mechanism of intervention and physiological outcomes but insufficient evidence of clinical benefits for breathing control: a systematic review. Aust J. Physiother. 53, 219–227.

Lightowler, J.V., Wedzicha, J.A., Elliott, M.W., et al., 2003. Noninvasive positive pressure ventilation to treat respiratory failure resulting from exacerbations of chronic obstructive pulmonary disease: Cochrane systematic review and meta-analysis. Br. Med. J. 326, 185.

Lim, C.M., Kim, E.K., Lee, J.S., et al., 2001. Comparison of the response to the prone position between pulmonary and extrapulmonary acute respiratory distress syndrome. Intensive Care Med. 27, 477–485.

Lim, W.J., Mohammed, A.R., Carson, K.V., et al., 2012. Non-invasive positive pressure ventilation for treatment of respiratory failure due to severe acute exacerbations of asthma. Cochrane Database Syst. Rev. Art. No.: CD004360, doi:10.1002/14651858.CD004360. pub4.

Lima, C.A., De Andrade Ade, F., Campos, S.L., et al., 2014. Effects of noninvasive ventilation on treadmill 6-min walk distance and regional chest wall volumes in cystic fibrosis: randomized controlled trial. Respir. Med. 108, 1460–1468.

Lindemann, H., 1992. Zum Stellenwert der Physiotherapie mit dem VRP 1-Desitin ('Flutter'). Pneumologie 46, 626–630.

Lindemann, H., Boldt, A., Kieselmann, R., 1990. Autogenic drainage: efficacy of a simplified method. Acta Univ. Carol. [Med.] (Praha) 36, 210–212.

Lindholm, P., Nyren, S., 2005. Studies on inspiratory and expiratory glossopharyngeal breathing in breath-hold divers employing magnetic resonance imaging and spirometry. Eur. J. Appl. Physiol. 94 (5–6), 646–651.

Lobato, S.D., Rodriguez, E.P., Alises, S.M., 2011. Portable pulse-dose oxygen concentrators should not be used with noninvasive ventilation. Respir. Care 56, 1950–1952.

Lopez-Vidriero, M.T., Reid, L., 1978. Bronchial mucus in health and disease. Br. Med. Bull. 34, 63–74.

Lotters, F., van Tol, B., Kwakkel, G., Gosselink, R., 2002. Effect of controlled inspiratory muscle training in patients with COPD: a meta-analysis. Eur. Respir. J. 20, 570–576.

Lumb, A., 2010. Nunn's Applied Respiratory Physiology, seventh ed. Churchill Livingstone Elsevier, Edinburgh.

Lunteren, E., Dick, T.E., 1997. Muscles of the upper airway and accessory respiratory muscles. In: Miller, A.D., Bianchi, A.L., Bishop, B.P. (Eds.), Neural Control of the Respiratory Muscles. CRC Press, New York.

Maa, S.H., Hung, T.J., Hsu, K.H., et al., 2005. Manual hyperinflation improves alveolar recruitment in difficult-to-wean patients. Chest 128, 2714–2721.

MacDonnell, T., McNicholas, W.T., FitzGerald, M.X., 1986. Hypoxaemia during chest physiotherapy in patients with cystic fibrosis. Int. J. Med. S 155 (10), 345–348.

Macklem, P.T., 1974. Physiology of cough. Ann. Otology Rhinol. Laryngol. 83, 761–768.

Mahajan, A.K., Diette, G.B., Hatipoglu, U., et al., 2011. High frequency chest wall oscillation for asthma and chronic obstructive pulmonary disease exacerbations: a randomized sham-controlled clinical trial. Respir. Res. 12, 120.

Mahler, D.A., Harver, A., Lenine, T., et al., 1996. Descriptors of breathlessness in cardiorespiratory disease. Am. J. Respir. Crit. Care Med. 154, 1357–1363.

Mahler, D.A., Slecky, P.A., Harrod, C.G., et al., 2010. American College of Chest Physicians consensus statement on the management of dyspnea in patients with advanced lung disease. Chest 137, 674–691.

Main, E., 2013. What is the best airway clearance technique in cystic fibrosis? Paediatr. Respir. Rev. 14 (Suppl. 1), 10–12.

Main, E., Grillo, L., Rand, S., 2015. Airway clearance strategies in cystic fibrosis and non-cystic fibrosis bronchiectasis. Semin. Respir. Crit. Care Med. 36 (2), 251–266. doi:10.1055/s-0035-1546820.

Main, E., Prasad, A., van der Schans, C.P., 2005. Conventional chest physiotherapy compared to other airway clearance techniques for cystic fibrosis. Cochrane Database Syst. Rev. (1), Art. No.:CD002011, doi:10.1002/14651858.CD002011.pub2.

Main, E., Tannenbaum, E., Stanojevic, S., et al., 2006. The effects of positive expiratory pressure (PEP) or oscillatory positive pressure (RC Cornet) on FEV_1 and lung clearance index over a twelve month period in children with CF. Pediatr. Pulmonol. 41 (Suppl. 29), 351.

Make, B.J., Hill, N.S., Goldberg, A.L., et al., 1998. Mechanical ventilation beyond the intensive care unit: report of a consensus conference of the American College of Chest Physicians. Chest 113 (Suppl. 5), 289S–344S.

Mall, M.A., Harkema, J.R., Trojanek, J.B., et al., 2008. Development of chronic bronchitis and emphysema in beta-epithelial Na^+ channel-overexpressing mice. Am. J. Respir Crit. Care Med. 177 (7), 730–742.

Maltais, F., Le Blanc, P., Jobin, J., Caraburi, R., 2000. Peripheral muscle dysfunction in chronic obstructive pulmonary disease. Clin. Chest Med. 21, 665–677.

Manning, F., Dean, E., Ross, J., Abboud, R.A.T., 1999. Lung function in side lying positions compared with supine in older healthy individuals. Phys. Ther. 79, 456–466.

Marks, J.H., 2007. Airway clearance devices in cystic fibrosis. Paediatr. Respir. Rev. 8 (1), 17–23.

Marti, J., Li Bassi, G., Rigol, M., et al., 2013. Effects of manual rib cage compressions on expiratory flow and mucus clearance during mechanical ventilation. Crit. Care Med. 41, 850–856.

Martin, V., Hincapie, L., Nimbuck, M., et al., 2005. Impact of whole-body rehabilitation in patients receiving chronic mechanical ventilation. Crit. Care Med. 33, 2255–2265.

Massery, M., 2005. Musculoskeletal and neuromuscular interventions: a physical approach to cystic fibrosis. J. R. Soc. Med. 98 (Suppl. 45), 55–66.

Massie, J., Clements, B., 2005. Diagnosis of cystic fibrosis after newborn screening. The Australasian experience: twenty years and five million babies later – a consensus statement from the Australasian Paediatric Respiratory Group. Pediatr. Pulmonol. 39, 440–446.

Massie, R.J., Towns, S.J., Bernard, E., et al., 1998. The musculoskeletal complications of cystic fibrosis. J. Paediatr. Child Health 34 (5), 467–470.

Maxwell, L.J., Ellis, E.R., 2003. The effect of circuit type, volume delivered and 'rapid release' on flow rates during manual hyperinflation. Aust J. Physiother. 49, 31–38.

Mazzocco, M., Owens, G., Kirilloff, L., Rogers, R., 1985. Chest percussion and postural drainage in patients with bronchiectasis. Chest 88, 360–363.

McArdle, W.D., Katch, F.I., Katch, V.L., 2014. Exercise Physiology, Energy, Nutrition and Human Performance, eighth ed. Wolters Kluwer, Lippincott Williams & Wilkins.

McCarren, B., Alison, J.A., 2006. Physiological effects of vibration in subjects with cystic fibrosis. Eur. Respir. J. 27, 1204–1209.

McCarren, B., Alison, J.A., Herbert, R.D., 2006a. Manual vibration increases expiratory flow rate via increased intrapleural pressure in healthy adults: an experimental study. Aust. J. Physiother. 52, 267–271.

McCarren, B., Alison, J.A., Herbert, R.D., 2006b. Vibration and its effect on the respiratory system. Aust. J. Physiother. 52, 39–43.

McCarren, B., Alison, J., Lansbury, G., 2003. The use of vibration in public hospitals in Australia. Physiother. Theory Pract. 19, 87–98.

McCarren, B., Chow, M.C., 1996. Manual hyperinflation: a description of the technique. Aust J. Physiother. 42, 203–208.

McCool, F.D., 1992. Inspiratory muscle weakness and fatigue. RT: The Journal for Respiratory Care Practitioners 5 (6), 32–41.

McDonald, C., Crockett, A., Young, I., 2005. Adult domiciliary oxygen therapy: position statement of the Thoracic Society of Australia and New Zealand. Med. J. Aust. 182, 621–626.

McIlwaine, M.P., Alarie, N., Davidson, G.F., et al., 2013. Long-term multicentre randomised controlled study of high frequency chest wall oscillation versus positive expiratory pressure mask in cystic fibrosis. Thorax 68, 746–751.

McIlwaine, M., Button, B., Dwan, K., 2015. Positive expiratory pressure physiotherapy for airway clearance in people with cystic fibrosis. Cochrane Database Syst. Rev. (6), Art. No.: CD003147, doi:10.1002/14651858.CD003147.pub4.

McIlwaine, M., Wong, L., Chilvers, M., Davidson, G., 2010. Long-term comparative trial of two different physiotherapy techniques; postural drainage with percussion and autogenic drainage, in the treatment of cystic fibrosis. Pediatr. Pulmonol. 45, 1064–1069.

McIlwaine, P.M., Wong, L.T., Peacock, D., Davidson, A.G., 1997. Long-term comparative trial of conventional postural drainage and percussion versus positive expiratory pressure physiotherapy in the treatment of cystic fibrosis. J. Pediatr. 131, 570–574.

McIlwaine, P.M., Wong, L.T., Peacock, D., Davidson, A.G., 2001. Long-term comparative trial of positive expiratory pressure versus oscillating positive expiratory pressure (flutter) physiotherapy in the treatment of cystic fibrosis. J. Pediatr. 138, 845–850.

McKim, D.A., Road, J., Avendano, M., et al., 2011. Home mechanical ventilation: a Canadian Thoracic Society clinical practice guideline. Can. Respir. J. 18, 197–215.

McKoy, N., Saldanha, I., Odelola, O., Robinson, K., 2012. Active cycle of breathing technique for cystic fibrosis. Cochrane Database Syst. Rev. (12), Art.No.:CD007862, doi:10.1002/14651858.CD007862.pub3.

Mead, J., Takishima, T., Leith, D., 1970. Stress distribution in lungs: a model of pulmonary elasticity. J. Appl. Physiol. 28, 596–608.

Medical Research Council Working Party, 1981. Long term domiciliary oxygen therapy in chronic hypoxic cor pulmonale complicating chronic bronchitis and emphysema. Lancet 1, 681–686.

Menadue, C., Alison, J.A., Piper, A.J., et al., 2009. Non-invasive ventilation during arm exercise and ground walking in patients with chronic hypercapnic respiratory failure. Respirology 14, 251–259.

Menadue, C., Alison, J.A., Piper, A.J., et al., 2010a. Bilevel ventilation during exercise in acute on chronic respiratory failure: a preliminary study. Respir. Med. 104, 219–227.

Menadue, C., Alison, J.A., Piper, A.J., et al., 2010b. High and low level pressure support during walking in people with severe kyphoscoliosis. Eur. Respir. J. 36, 370–378.

Menkes, H., Traystman, R., 1977. Collateral ventilation. Am. Rev. Respir. Dis. 116, 287–309.

Mestriner, R.G., Fernandes, R.O., Steffen, L.C., Donadio, M.V., 2009. Optimum design parameters for a therapist-constructed positive-expiratory-pressure therapy bottle device. Respir. Care 54, 504–508.

Milla, C.E., Hansen, L.G., Warwick, W.J., 2006. Different frequencies should be prescribed for different high frequency chest compression machines. Biomed. Instrum. Technol. 40, 319–324.

Miller, J.M., Ashton-Miller, J.A., DeLancey, J.O., 1998. A pelvic muscle precontraction can reduce cough-related urine loss in selected women with mild SUI. J. Am. Geriatr. Soc. 46 (7), 870–874.

Miller, A.D., Bianchi, A.L., Bishop, B.P., 1997. Overview of the neural control of the respiratory muscles. In: Miller, A.D., Bianchi, A.L., Bishop, B.P. (Eds.), Neural Control of the Respiratory Muscles. CRC Press, New York.

Miller, S., Hall, D., Clayton, C., Nelson, R., 1995. Chest physiotherapy in cystic fibrosis: a comparative study of autogenic drainage and the active cycle of breathing techniques with postural drainage. Thorax 50, 165–169.

Miske, L.J., Hickey, E.M., Kolb, S.M., et al., 2004. Use of the mechanical in-exsufflator in pediatric patients with neuromuscular disease and impaired cough. Chest 125, 1406–1412.

Mohsenifar, Z., Rosenberg, N., Goldberg, H., Koerner, S., 1985. Mechanical vibration and conventional chest physiotherapy in outpatients with stable chronic obstructive pulmonary disease. Chest 87, 483–485.

Moore, R., Berlowitz, D., 2011. Dyspnoea and oxygen therapy in chronic obstructive pulmonary disease. Phys. Ther. Rev. 16, 10–18.

Moore, R., Berlowitz, D., Denehy, L., et al., 2011. A randomised trial of domiciliary, ambulatory oxygen in patients with COPD and dyspnoea but without resting hypoxaemia. Thorax 66, 32–37.

Moraes, T., Carpenter, S., Taylor, L., 2002. Cystic fibrosis incontinence in children. Pediatr. Pulmonol. Suppl. 24, 315.

Moran, F., Bradley, J., Elborn, J., et al., 2005. Physiotherapy involvement in non-invasive ventilation hospital services: a British Isles survey. Int. J. Clin. Pract. 59, 453–456.

Moran, F., Bradley, J.M., Piper, A.J., 2009. Non-invasive ventilation for cystic fibrosis. Cochrane Database Syst. Rev. CD002769.

Morgan, R.K., McNally, S., Alexander, M., et al., 2005. Use of sniff nasal-inspiratory force to predict survival in amyotrophic lateral sclerosis. Am. J. Respir. Crit. Care Med. 171, 269–274.

Morgan, M.D.L., Silver, J.R., Williams, S.J., 1986. The respiratory system of the spinal cord patient. In: Bloch, R.F., Basbaum, M. (Eds.), Management of Spinal Cord Injuries. Williams and Wilkins, Baltimore, pp. 78–115.

Morrison, L., Agnew, J., 2009. Oscillating devices for airway clearance in people with cystic fibrosis. Cochrane Database Syst. Rev. (1), Art. No.: CD006842.

Mortensen, J., Falk, M., Groth, S., Jensen, C., 1991. The effects of postural drainage and positive expiratory pressure physiotherapy on tracheobronchial clearance in cystic fibrosis. Chest 100, 1350–1357.

Mularski, R.A., Campbell, M.L., Asch, S.M., et al., 2010. A review of quality of care evaluation for the palliation of dyspnea. Am. J. Respir. Crit. Care Med. 181, 534–538.

Mure, M., Martling, C.-R., Lindahl, S.G.E., 1997. Dramatic effect on oxygenation in patients with severe acute lung insufficiency treated in the prone position. Crit. Care Med. 25, 1539–1544.

Murphy, P.B., Davidson, C., Hind, M.D., et al., 2012. Volume targeted versus pressure support non-invasive ventilation in patients with super obesity and chronic respiratory failure: a randomised controlled trial. Thorax 67, 727–734.

Murray, M., Pentland, J., Hill, A., 2009. A randomized crossover trial of chest physiotherapy in non-cystic fibrosis bronchiectasis. Eur. Respir. J. 34, 1086–1092.

Mustfa, N., Aiello, M., Lyall, R.A., et al., 2003. Cough augmentation in amyotrophic lateral sclerosis. Neurology 61, 1285–1287.

Myers, L.B., 2009. An exploratory study investigating factors associated with adherence to chest physiotherapy and exercise in adults with cystic fibrosis. J. Cyst. Fibros. 8, 425–427.

Nankivell, G., Caldwell, P., Follett, J., 2010. Urinary incontinence in adolescent females with cystic fibrosis. Paediatr. Respir. Rev. 11, 95–99.

Naraparaju, S., Vaishali, K., Venkatesan, P., Acharya, V., 2010. A comparison of the Acapella and a threshold inspiratory muscle trainer for sputum clearance in bronchiectasis – a pilot study. Physiother. Theory Pract. 26, 353–357.

Nathan, H., 1962. Osteophytes of the vertebral column. An anatomical study of their development according to age, race and sex with considerations as to their aetiology and significance. Journal of Bone and Joint Surgery 44, A243.

National Institute for Cardiovascular Outcomes Research (NICOR), 2011. <https://data.gov.uk/dataset/national-adult-cardiac-surgery-audit-report-data-2010-11>.

National Institute for Health and Clinical Excellence Urinary incontinence in women: management. <https://www.nice.org.uk/guidance/cg171/chapter/1-recommendations>.

Naughton, M.T., Rahman, M.A., Hara, K., et al., 1995. Effect of continuous positive airway pressure on intrathoracic and left ventricular transmural pressures in patients with congestive heart failure. Circulation 91, 1725–1731.

Nava, S., Barbarito, N., Piaggi, G., et al., 2006. Physiological response to intrapulmonary percussive ventilation in stable COPD patients. Respir. Med. 100, 1526–1533.

Nava, S., Carbone, G., DiBattista, N., et al., 2003. Noninvasive ventilation in cardiogenic pulmonary edema: a multicenter randomized trial. Am. J. Respir. Crit. Care Med. 168, 1432–1437.

Nava, S., Cirio, S., Fanfulla, F., et al., 2008. Comparison of two humidification systems for long-term noninvasive mechanical ventilation. Eur. Respir. J. 32, 460–464.

Nava, S., Ferrer, M., Esquinas, A., et al., 2013. Palliative use of non-invasive ventilation in end-of-life patients with solid tumours: a randomised feasibility trial. Lancet Oncol. 14, 219–227.

Navalesi, P., Costa, R., Ceriana, P., et al., 2007. Non-invasive ventilation in chronic obstructive pulmonary disease patients: helmet versus facial mask. Intensive Care Med. 33, 74–81.

Navalesi, P., Fanfulla, F., Frigerio, P., et al., 2000. Physiologic evaluation of noninvasive mechanical ventilation delivered with three types of masks in patients with chronic hypercapnic respiratory failure. Crit. Care Med. 28, 1785–1790.

Nelson, H.P., 1934. Postural drainage of the lungs. Br. Med. J. 2, 251–255.

Nevins, M.L., Epstein, S.K., 2001. Weaning from prolonged mechanical ventilation. Clin. Chest Med. 22, 13–33.

Newall, C., Stockley, R.A., Hill, S.L., 2005. Exercise training and inspiratory muscle training in patients with bronchiectasis. Thorax 60, 943–948.

Newbold, M.E., Tullis, E., Corey, M., et al., 2005. The Flutter Device versus the PEP Mask in the Treatment of Adults with Cystic Fibrosis. Physiotherapy Canada 57, 199–207.

Newhouse, P.A., White, F., Marks, J.H., Homnick, D.N., 1998. The intrapulmonary percussive ventilator and flutter device compared to standard chest physiotherapy in patients with cystic fibrosis. Clin. Pediatr. (Phila) 37, 427–432.

Nguyen, T.T., Thia, L.P., Hoo, A.F., et al., 2014. Evolution of lung function during the first year of life in newborn screened cystic fibrosis infants. Thorax 69, 910–917.

Nicolini, A., Cardini, F., Landucci, N., et al., 2013. Effectiveness of treatment with high-frequency chest wall oscillation in patients with bronchiectasis. BMC Pulm. Med. 13, 21.

Nicolson, C.H.H., Stirling, R.G., Borg, B.M., et al., 2012. The long term effect of inhaled hypertonic saline 6 percent in non-cystic fibrosis bronchiectasis. Respir. Med. 106, 661–667.

Niere, K., Jerak, A., 2004. Measurement of headache frequency, intensity and duration: comparison of patient report by questionnaire and headache diary. Physiother. Res. Int. 9 (4), 149–156.

Nocturnal Oxygen Therapy Trial Group, 1980. Continuous or nocturnal oxygen therapy in hypoxemic chronic obstructive lung disease: a clinical trial. Ann. Intern. Med. 93, 391–398.

Nonoyama, M., Brooks, D., Lacasse, Y., et al., 2009. Oxygen therapy during exercise training in chronic obstructive pulmonary disease (review). Cochrane Database Syst. Rev. (2), Art. No. CD005372.

Noonan, V., Dean, E., 2000. Submaximal exercise testing: clinical application and interpretation. Phys. Ther. 80, 782–807.

Ntoumenopoulos, G., 2005. Indications for manual lung hyperinflation (MHI) in the mechanically ventilated patient with chronic obstructive pulmonary disease. Chron. Respir. Dis. 2, 199–207.

Nygren-Bonnier, M., Markstrom, A., Lindholm, P., et al., 2009a. Glossopharyngeal pistoning for lung insufflation in children with spinal muscular atrophy type II. Acta Paediatr. 98 (8), 1324–1328.

Nygren-Bonnier, M., Wahman, K., Lindholm, P., et al., 2009b. Glossopharyngeal pistoning for lung insufflation in patients with cervical spinal cord injury. Spinal Cord 47 (5), 418–422.

Oberwaldner, B., Evans, J., Zach, M., 1986. Forced expirations against a variable resistance: a new chest physiotherapy method in cystic fibrosis. Pediatr. Pulmonol. 2, 358–367.

Oberwaldner, B., Theissl, B., Rucker, A., Zach, M., 1991. Chest physiotherapy in hospitalized patients with cystic fibrosis: a study of lung function effects and sputum production. Eur. Respir. J. 4, 152–158.

O'Connor, C., Bridge, P., 2005. Can the interrupter technique be used as an outcome measure for autogenic drainage in bronchiectatic patients? A pilot study. Journal of the Association of Chartered Physiotherapists in Respiratory Care 37, 29–34.

O'Donnell, A.E., Barker, A.F., Ilowite, J.S., Fick, R.B., 1998. Treatment of idiopathic bronchiectasis with aerosolized recombinant human DNase I. rhDNase Study Group. Chest 113, 1329–1334.

O'Donnell, D.E., Banzett, B.B., Carrieri-Kohlman, V., et al., 2007. Pathophysiology of dyspnea in chronic obstructive pulmonary disease: a roundtable. Proc. Am. Thorac. Soc. 4, 145–168.

O'Donnell, D.E., McGuire, M., Samis, L., Webb, K.A., 1995. The impact of exercise reconditioning on breathlessness in severe chronic airflow limitation. Am. J. Respir. Crit. Care Med. 152, 2005–2013.

O'Donohoe, R., Fullen, B.M., 2014. Adherence of subjects with cystic fibrosis to their home program: a systematic review. Respir. Care 59, 1731–1746.

O'Driscoll, B., Howard, L., Davison, A., 2008. BTS guideline for emergency oxygen use in adult patients. Thorax 63 (Suppl. VI), vi1–vi68.

O'Leary, S., Jull, G., Kim, M., Vicenzino, B., 2007. Cranio-cervical flexor muscle impairment at maximal, moderate, and low loads is a feature of neck pain. Man. Ther. 12 (1), 34–39.

O'Neill, S.O., McCarthy, D.S., 1983. Postural relief of dyspnoea in severe chronic airflow limitation: relationship to respiratory muscle strength. Thorax 38, 595–600.

Oermann, C.M., Sockrider, M.M., Giles, D., et al., 2001. Comparison of high-frequency chest wall oscillation and oscillating positive expiratory pressure in the home management of cystic fibrosis: a pilot study. Pediatr. Pulmonol. 32, 372–377.

Oh, T.E., 1990. Intensive Care Manual, Sydney. Butterworths, Boston.

Olsen, M., Lonroth, H., Bake, B., 1999. Effects of breathing exercises on breathing patterns in obese and non-obese subjects. Clin. Physiol. 19, 251–257.

Orlava, O.E., 1959. Therapeutic physical culture in the complex treatment of pneumonia. Phys. Ther. Rev. 39, 153–160.

Orman, J., Westerdahl, E., 2010. Chest physiotherapy with positive expiratory pressure breathing after abdominal and thoracic surgery: a systematic review. Acta Anaesthesiol. Scand. 54, 261–267.

Orr, A., McVean, R.J., Web, A.K., Dodd, M.E., 2001. Questionnaire survey of urinary incontinence in women with cystic fibrosis. Br. Med. J. 322, 1521.

Osadnik, C.R., McDonald, C.F., Jones, A.P., Holland, A.E., 2012. Airway clearance techniques for chronic obstructive pulmonary disease. Cochrane Database Syst. Rev. (3), CD008328.

Osadnik, C.R., McDonald, C.F., Miller, B.R., et al., 2014. The effect of positive expiratory pressure (PEP) therapy on symptoms, quality of life and incidence of re-exacerbation in patients with acute exacerbations of chronic obstructive pulmonary disease: a multicentre, randomised controlled trial. Thorax 69, 137–143.

Oscroft, N.S., Ali, M., Gulati, A., et al., 2010. A randomised crossover trial comparing volume assured and pressure pre-set noninvasive ventilation in stable hypercapnic COPD. COPD 7, 398–403.

Osman, L.P., Roughton, M., Hodson, M.E., Pryor, J.A., 2010. Short-term comparative study of high frequency chest wall oscillation and European airway clearance techniques in patients with cystic fibrosis. Thorax 65, 196–200.

Overend, T.J., Anderson, C.M., Lucy, S.D., et al., 2001. The effect of incentive spirometry on postoperative pulmonary complications. Chest 120, 971–978.

Ozsancak, A., Sidhom, S.S., Liesching, T.N., et al., 2011. Evaluation of the total face mask for noninvasive ventilation to treat acute respiratory failure. Chest 139, 1034–1041.

Padman, R., Geouque, D.M., Engelhardt, M.T., 1999. Effects of the Flutter device on pulmonary function studies among pediatric cystic fibrosis patients. Del. Med. J. 71, 13–18.

Paneroni, M., Clini, E., Simonelli, C., et al., 2011. Safety and efficacy of short-term intrapulmonary percussive ventilation in patients with bronchiectasis. Respir. Care 56 (7), 984–988.

Parasa, R.B., Maffulli, N., 1999. Musculoskeletal involvement in cystic fibrosis. Bull. Hosp. Joint Dis. 58 (1), 37–44.

Paratz, J., Lipman, J., McAuliffe, M., 2002. Effects of manual hyperinflation on haemodynamics, gas exchange, and respiratory mechanics in ventilated patients. J. Intensive Care Med. 17, 317–324.

Parshall, M.B., Schwartzstein, R.M., Adams, L., et al., 2012. An official American thoracic society statement: update on the mechanisms, assessment, and management of dyspnea. Am. J. Respir. Crit. Care Med. 185, 435–452.

Parsons, J.P., 2013. Exercise-induced bronchoconstriction. Otolaryngol. Clin. North Am. 47 (1), 119–126.

Pasquina, P., Tramers, M.R., Walder, B., 2003. Prophylactic respiratory physiotherapy after cardiac surgery: systematic review. BMJ 327 (7428), 1379–1381.

Pasquina, P., Merlani, P., Granier, J.M., et al., 2004. Continuous positive airway pressure versus noninvasive pressure support ventilation to treat atelectasis after cardiac surgery. Anesth. Analg. 99, 1001–1008.

Pasteur, M.C., Bilton, D., Hill, A.T., 2010. British Thoracic Society guideline for non-CF bronchiectasis. Thorax 65 (Suppl. 1), i1–i58.

Patman, S., Jenkins, S., Stiller, K., 2000. Manual hyperinflation: effects on respiratory parameters. Physiother. Res. Int. 5, 157–171.

Patterson, J.E., Bradley, J.M., Hewitt, O., et al., 2005. Airway clearance in bronchiectasis: a randomized crossover trial of active cycle of breathing techniques versus Acapella. Respiration 72, 239–242.

Patterson, J.E., Hewitt, O., Kent, L., et al., 2007. Acapella versus 'usual airway clearance' during acute exacerbation in bronchiectasis: a randomized crossover trial. Chron. Respir. Dis. 4, 67–74.

Paul, K., Rietschel, E., Ballmann, M., et al., 2004. Effect of treatment with dornase alpha on airway inflammation in patients with cystic fibrosis. Am. J. Respir. Crit. Care Med. 169 (6), 719–725.

Paulus, F., Binnekade, J.M., Schultz, M.J., 2008. Bagging: an (early) harmful or (late) beneficial maneuver? Crit. Care Med. 36 (12), 3278–3279.

Pavia, D., Webber, B., Agnew, J.E., et al., 1988. The role of intermittent positive pressure breathing (IPPB) in bronchial toilet. Eur. Respir. J. 1 (Suppl. 2), 250S.

Peiper, A., 1963. Cerebral Function in Infancy and Childhood. Consultants Bureau, New York.

Pelosi, P., Tubiolo, D., Mascheroni, D., 1998. Effects of the prone position on respiratory mechanics and gas exchange during acute lung injury. Am. J. Critical Care Med. 157, 387–393.

Perme, C., 2006. Early mobilization of LVAD recipients who require prolonged mechanical ventilation. Tex. Heart Inst. J. 33, 130–134.

Perrin, C., Jullien, V., Venissac, N., et al., 2007. Prophylactic use of noninvasive ventilation in patients undergoing lung resectional surgery. Respir. Med. 101, 1572–1578.

Perry, R.J., Man, G.C., Jones, R.L., 1998. Effects of positive end-expiratory pressure on oscillated flow rate during high-frequency chest compression. Chest 113, 1028–1033.

Pfeiffer, K.A., Pivarnik, J.M., Womack, C.J., et al., 2002. Reliability and validity of the Borg and OMNI rating of perceived exertion scales in adolescent girls. Med. Sci. Sports Exerc. 34 (12), 2057–2061.

Pfleger, A., Theissl, B., Oberwaldner, B., Zach, M., 1992. Self-administered chest physiotherapy in cystic fibrosis: a comparative study of high-pressure PEP and autogenic drainage. Lung 170, 323–330.

Phang, P.T., Russell, J.A., 1993. When does $\dot{V}O2$ depend on $\dot{V}O2$? Respir. Care 38, 618–630.

Pharmaxis, 2011. Bronchitol Product Information. Blackwell Scientific Publications, Philadelphia. Pharmaxis, Sydney.

Piper, A., 2010. Discharge planning and management for patients with chronic respiratory failure using home mechanical ventilation. Breathe 6, 322–333.

Piper, A.J., Menadue, C., 2009. Noninvasive ventilation as an adjunct to exercise training in patients with chronic respiratory disease. Breathe 5, 334–345.

Piper, A.J., Moran, F.M., 2006. Non-invasive ventilation and the physiotherapist: current state and future trends. Phys. Ther. Rev. 11, 37–43.

Piper, A.J., Parker, S., Torzillo, P.J., et al., 1992. Nocturnal nasal IPPV stabilizes patients with cystic fibrosis and hypercapnic respiratory failure. Chest 102, 846–850.

Plant, P.K., Owen, J.L., Elliott, M.W., 2000. Early use of non-invasive ventilation for acute exacerbations of chronic obstructive pulmonary disease on general respiratory wards: a multicentre randomised controlled trial. Lancet 355, 1931–1935.

Powers, J., Daniels, D., 2004. Turning points: implementing kinetic therapy in the ICU. Nurs. Manage. 35 (Suppl.), 1–7.

Prasad, S.A., Balfour-Lynn, I.M., Carr, S.B., Madge, S.L., 2006. A comparison of the prevalence of urinary incontinence in girls with cystic fibrosis, asthma, and healthy controls. Pediatr. Pulmonol. 41 (11), 1065–1068.

Prasad, S.A., Main, E., Dodd, M.E., 2008. Finding consensus on the physiotherapy management of asymptomatic infants with cystic fibrosis. Pediatr. Pulmonol. 43, 236–244.

Principi, T., Pantanetti, S., Catani, F., et al., 2004. Noninvasive continuous positive airway pressure delivered by helmet in hematological malignancy patients with hypoxemic acute respiratory failure. Intensive Care Med. 30, 147–150.

Pritchard, J.N., 2001. The influence of lung deposition on clinical response. J. Aerosol Med. 14, 19–26.

Pryor, J., Tannenbaum, E., Scott, S., et al., 2010a. Beyond postural drainage and percussion: airway clearance in people with cystic fibrosis. J. Cyst. Fibros. 9, 187–192.

Pryor, J., Webber, B., 1979. An evaluation of the forced expiration technique as adjunct to postural drainage. Physiotherapy 65, 304–307.

Pryor, J., Webber, B., Hodson, M., Batten, J., 1979. Evaluation of the forced expiration technique as an adjunct to postural drainage in treatment of cystic fibrosis. Br. Med. J. 2, 417–418.

Pryor, J.A., 1991. The forced expiration technique. In: Pryor, J.A. (Ed.), Respiratory Care. Churchill Livingstone, Edinburgh, pp. 79–100.

Pryor, J.A., Tannenbaum, E., Scott, S.F., et al., 2010b. Beyond postural drainage and percussion: airway clearance in people with cystic fibrosis. J. Cyst. Fibros. 9, 187–192.

Pryor, J.A., Webber, B.A., Hodson, M.E., 1990. Effect of chest physiotherapy on oxygen saturation in patients with cystic fibrosis. Thorax 45, 77.

Putensen, C., Zech, S., Wrigge, H., et al., 2001. Long-term effects of spontaneous breathing during ventilatory support in patients with acute lung injury. Am. J. Respir. Care Med. 164, 43–49.

Putt, M.T., Paratz, J.D., 1996. The effect of stretching pectoralis major and anterior deltoid muscles on the restrictive component of chronic airflow limitation. In: Proceedings of the National Physiotherapy Conference, Brisbane, Queensland. Australian Physiotherapy Association, Brisbane, Queensland.

Quan, J.M., Tiddens, H.A., Sy, J.P., et al., 2001. A two-year randomized, placebo-controlled trial of dornase alfa in young patients with cystic fibrosis with mild lung function abnormalities. J. Pediatr. 139, 813–820.

Rabec, C., Georges, M., Kabeya, N.K., et al., 2009. Evaluating noninvasive ventilation using a monitoring system coupled to a ventilator: a bench-to-bedside study. Eur. Respir. J. 34, 902–913.

Racca, F., Appendini, L., Berta, G., et al., 2009. Helmet ventilation for acute respiratory failure and nasal skin breakdown in neuromuscular disorders. Anesth. Analg. 109, 164–167.

Ragette, R., Mellies, U., Schwake, C., et al., 2002. Patterns and predictors of sleep disordered breathing in primary myopathies. Thorax 57, 724–728.

Ram, F., Wedzicha, J., 2002. Ambulatory oxygen for chronic obstructive pulmonary disease. Cochrane Database Syst. Rev. (1), Art No.: CD000238.

Ram, F.S., Picot, J., Lightowler, J., et al., 2004. Non-invasive positive pressure ventilation for treatment of respiratory failure due to exacerbations of chronic obstructive pulmonary disease. Cochrane Database Syst. Rev. Art. No.:CD004104, doi:10.1002/14651858.CD004104.pub3.

Ramirez, A., Delord, V., Khirani, S., et al., 2012. Interfaces for long-term noninvasive positive pressure ventilation in children. Intensive Care Med. 38, 655–662.

Ramirez-Sarmiento, A., Orozco-Levi, M., Guell, R., et al., 2002. Inspiratory muscle training in patients with chronic obstructive pulmonary disease: structural adaptations and physiological outcomes. Am. J. Respir. Crit. Care Med. 166, 1491–1797.

Ramos, E., Ramos, D., Iyomasa, D., et al., 2009. Influence that oscillating positive expiratory pressure using predetermined expiratory pressures has on the viscosity and transportability of sputum in patients with bronchiectasis. J. Bas. Pneumologie 35, 1190–1197.

Rand, S., Hill, L., Prasad, S.A., 2013. Physiotherapy in cystic fibrosis: optimising techniques to improve outcomes. Paediatr. Respir. Rev. 14, 263–269.

Ravilly, S., Robinson, W., Suresh, S., et al., 1996. Chronic pain in cystic fibrosis. Pediatrics 98 (4 Pt 1), 741–747.

Ray, J.F., Yost, L., Moallem, S., et al., 1974. Immobility, hypoxemia and pulmonary arteriovenous shunting. Arch. Surg. 109, 537–541.

Rea, H., McAuley, S., Jayaram, L., et al., 2010. The clinical utility of long-term humidification therapy in chronic airway disease. Respir. Med. 104 (4), 525–533.

Rees, J., Tedd, H., Soyza, A.D., 2013. Managing urinary incontinence in adults with bronchiectasis. Br. J. Nurs. 22, S15–S16, S18.

Reeve, J., Ewan, S., 2005. The physiotherapy management of the coronary artery bypass graft patient: a survey of current practice throughout the United Kingdom. ACPRC 37, 35–45.

Reid, W.D., Huang, J., Bryson, S., 1994. Diaphragm injury and myofibrillar structure induced by resistive loading. J. Appl. Physiol. 76, 176–184.

Reid, W.D., Samrai, B., 1995. Respiratory muscle training for patients with chronic obstructive pulmonary disease. Phys. Ther. 75 (11), 996–1005.

Remolina, C., Khan, A.V., Santiago, T.V., Edelman, N.H., 1981. Positional hypoxemia in unilateral lung disease. NEJM 304, 523–525.

Restrepo, R.D., Wettstein, R., Wittnebel, L., Tracy, M., 2011. AARC (American Association for Respiratory Care) clinical practice guideline. Incentive spirometry: 2011. Respir. Care 56, 1600–1604.

Richards, G., Cistulli, P., Ungar, R., et al., 1996. Mouth leak with nasal continuous positive airway pressure increases nasal airway resistance. Am. J. Respir. Crit. Care Med. 154, 182–186.

Richler, D.W., Ballanyi, K., Ramirez, J.-M., 1997. Respiratory rhythm generation. In: Miller, A.D., Bianchi, A.L., Bishop, B.P. (Eds.), Neural Control of the Respiratory Muscles. CRC Press, New York.

Ries, A.L., Bauldoff, G.S., Carlin, B.W., et al., 2007. Pulmonary rehabilitation: joint ACCP/AACVPR evidence-based clinical practice guidelines. Chest 131, 4S–42S.

Roberts, C., Brown, J., Reinhardt, A., et al., 2008. Non-invasive ventilation in chronic obstructive pulmonary disease: management of acute type 2 respiratory failure. Clin. Med. (Northfield Il) 8, 517–521.

Robinson, K.A., McKoy, N., Saldanha, I., Odelola, O.A., 2010. Active cycle of breathing technique for cystic fibrosis. Cochrane Database Syst. Rev. (11), CD007862, doi:10.1002/14651858.CD007862 .pub2.

Robinson, M., Bye, P.T., 2002. Mucociliary clearance in cystic fibrosis. Pediatr. Pulmonol. 33, 293–306.

Robinson, M., Daviskas, E., Eberl, S., et al., 1999. The effect of inhaled mannitol on bronchial mucus clearance in cystic fibrosis patients: a pilot study. Eur. Respir. J. 14, 678–685.

Robinson, M., Hemming, A.L., Moriarty, C., et al., 2000. Effect of a short course of rhDNase on cough and mucociliary clearance in patients with cystic fibrosis. Pediatr. Pulmonol. 30, 16–24.

Robinson, M., Hemming, A.L., Regnis, J.A., et al., 1997. Effect of increasing doses of hypertonic saline on mucociliary clearance in patients with cystic fibrosis. Thorax 52, 900–903.

Robinson, M., Regnis, J.A., Bailey, D.L., et al., 1996. Effect of hypertonic saline, amiloride, and cough on mucociliary clearance in patients with cystic fibrosis. Am. J. Respir. Crit. Care Med. 153, 1503–1509.

Rogers, D.F., 2004. Airway mucus hypersecretion in asthma: an undervalued pathology? Curr. Opin. Pharmacol. 4 (3), 241–250.

Rood, M., 1973. Unpublished lectures given at the University of Western Ontario, London, Ontario.

Rosenfeld, M., Gibson, R.L., McNamara, S., et al., 2001. Early pulmonary infection, inflammation, and clinical outcomes in infants with cystic fibrosis. Pediatr. Pulmonol. 32, 356–366.

Rosenfeld, M., Ratjen, F., Brumback, L., et al., 2012. Inhaled hypertonic saline in infants and children less than six years of age with cystic fibrosis: the ISIS randomized trial. JAMA 307, 2269.

Ross, J., Dean, E., 1992. Body positioning. In: Zadai, C. (Ed.), Pulmonary Management in Physical Therapy. Churchill Livingstone, New York.

Ross, J., Gamble, J., Schultz, A., Lewiston, N., 1987. Back pain and spinal deformity in cystic fibrosis. Am. J. Dis. Child. 141 (12), 1313–1316.

Rossi, A., Ganassini, A., Tantucci, C., Grassi, V., 1996. Aging and the respiratory system. Aging (Milano) 8, 143–161. (English abstract).

Rothen, H., Sporre, B., Engberg, G., et al., 1993. Re-expansion of atelectasis during general anaesthesia: a computed tomography study. Br. J. Anaesth. 71, 788–795.

Rubin, B.K., 2002. The pharmacologic approach to airway clearance: mucoactive agents. Respir. Care 47 (7), 818–822.

Sackner, M.A., Kim, C.S., 1987. Phasic flow mechanisms of mucus clearance. Eur. J. Respir. Dis. Suppl. 153, 159–164.

Salh, W., Bilton, D., Dodd, M., Webb, A.K., 1989. Effect of exercise and physiotherapy in aiding sputum expectoration in adults with cystic fibrosis. Thorax 44, 1006–1008.

Samuels, S., Samuels, M., Dinwiddie, R., Prasad, A., 1995. A survey of physiotherapy techniques used in specialist clinics for cystic fibrosis in the United Kingdom. Physiotherapy 81, 279–283.

Sancho, J., Servera, E., Diaz, J., Marin, J., 2004. Efficacy of mechanical insufflation-exsufflation in medically stable patients with amyotrophic lateral sclerosis. Chest 125, 1400–1405.

Sanderson, M.J., Charles, A.C., Dirksen, E.R., 1990. Mechanical stimulation and intercellular communication increases intracellular Ca^+ in epithelial cells. Cell Regul. 1, 585–596.

Sanderson, M.J., Chow, I., Dirksen, E.R., 1988. Intercellular communication between ciliated cells in culture. Am. J. Physiol. 254, C63–C74.

Savian, C., Paratz, J., Davis, A., 2006. Comparison of the effectiveness of manual and ventilator hyperinflation at different levels of positive end-expiratory pressure in artificially ventilated and intubated intensive care patients. Heart Lung 35 (3), 334–341.

Savci, S., Ince, D., Arikan, H., 2000. A comparison of autogenic drainage and the active cycle of breathing techniques in patients with chronic obstructive pulmonary diseases. J. Cardiopulm. Rehabil. 20, 37–43.

Schechter, M.S., 2007. Airway clearance applications in infants and children. Respir. Care 52, 1382–1390, discussion 1390-1.

Scheffner, A.L., Medler, E.M., Jacobs, L.W., Sarett, H.P., 1964. The in vitro reduction in viscosity of human tracheobronchial secretions by acetylcysteine. Am. Rev. Respir. Dis. 90, 721–729.

Scherer, T.A., Barandun, J., Martinez, E., et al., 1998. Effect of high-frequency oral airway and chest wall oscillation and conventional chest physical therapy on expectoration in patients with stable cystic fibrosis. Chest 113, 1019–1027.

Scherer, T.A., Spengler, C.M., Owassapian, D., et al., 2000. Respiratory muscle endurance training in chronic obstructive lung disease. Am. J. Respir. Crit. Care Med. 162, 1709–1714.

Schettino, G.P., Chatmongkolchart, S., Hess, D.R., et al., 2003. Position of exhalation port and mask design affect CO_2 rebreathing during noninvasive positive pressure ventilation. Crit. Care Med. 31, 2178–2182.

Schneiderman-Walker, J., Pollock, S., Corey, M., et al., 2000. A randomized controlled trial of a 3-year home exercise program in cystic fibrosis. J. Pediatr. 136, 304–310.

Schonhofer, B., Dellweg, D., Suchi, S., et al., 2008. Exercise endurance before and after long-term noninvasive ventilation in patients with chronic respiratory failure. Respiration 75, 296–303.

Schöni, M., 1989. Autogenic drainage: a modern approach to physiotherapy in cystic fibrosis. J. R. Soc. Med. 82 (Suppl. 16), 32–37.

Scottish Intercollegiate Guidelines Network, 2004. Management of urinary incontinence in primary care. <http://www.sign.ac.uk/pdf/qrg79.pdf> (accessed 2016).

Selsby, D., Jones, J.G., 1990. Some physiological and clinical aspects of chest physiotherapy. Br. J. Anaesth. 64, 621–631.

Sevransky, J.F., Haponik, E.F., 2003. Respiratory failure in elderly patients. Clin. Geriatr. Med. 19, 205–224.

Seymour, C.W., Martinez, A., Christie, J.D., Fuchs, B.D., 2004. The outcome of extubation failure in a community hospital intensive care unit: a cohort study. Critical Care 8, R322–R327.

Shabari, Prem, V., Alaparthi, G.K., et al., 2011. Comparison of Acapella and RC-Cornet for airway clearance in bronchiectasis: a pilot study. Int. J. Curr. Res. Rev. 3, 138.

Shah, A.R., Kurth, C.D., Gwiazdowski, S.G., et al., 1992. Fluctuations in cerebral oxygenation and blood volume during endotracheal suctioning in premature infants. J. Pediatr. 120, 769–774.

Shak, S., Capon, D.J., Hellmiss, R., et al., 1990. Recombinant human DNase I reduces the viscosity of cystic fibrosis sputum. Proc. Natl. Acad. Sci. U.S.A. 87, 9188–9192.

Shannon, H., Gregson, R., Stocks, J., et al., 2009. Repeatability of physiotherapy chest wall vibrations applied to spontaneously breathing adults. Physiotherapy 95, 36–42.

Shannon, H., Stocks, J., Gregson, R.K., et al., 2015. Clinical effects of specialist and on-call respiratory physiotherapy treatments in mechanically ventilated children: a randomised crossover trial. Physiotherapy 101, 349–356.

Sahrmann, S.A., 2005. Diagnosis and Treatment of Movement Impairment Syndromes. Mosby, St Louis.

Sharp, J.T., Drutz, W.S., Moisan, T., et al., 1980. Postural relief of dyspnea in severe chronic obstructive pulmonary disease. Am. Rev. Respir. Dis. 122, 201–211.

Sieck, G.C., Prakash, Y.S., 1997. The diaphragm muscle. In: Miller, A.D., Bianchi, A.L., Bishop, B.P. (Eds.), Neural Control of the Respiratory Muscles. CRC Press, New York.

Silverman, R.A., Foley, F., Dalipi, R., et al., 2012. The use of rhDNAse in severely ill, non-intubated adult asthmatics refractory to bronchodilators: a pilot study. Respir. Med. 106, 1096–1102.

Simon, P.M., Schwartzstein, R.M., Woodrow Weiss, J., 1989. Distinguishable sensations of breathlessness in normal volunteers. Am. Rev. Respir. Dis. 148, 1021–1027.

Simon, P.M., Schwartzstein, R.M., Woodrow Weiss, J., et al., 1990. Distinguishable types of dyspnoea in patients with shortness of breath. Am. Rev. Respir. Dis. 142, 1009–1014.

Simonds, A.K., 2004. Pneumothorax: an important complication of non-invasive ventilation in neuromuscular disease. Neuromuscul. Disord. 14, 351–352.

Simonelli, C., Paneroni, M., Vitacca, M., 2013. An implementation protocol for noninvasive ventilation prescription: the physiotherapist's role in an Italian hospital. Respir. Care 58, 662–668.

Singer, M., Vermaat, J., Hall, G., et al., 1994. Haemodynamic effects of manual hyperinflation in critically ill mechanically ventilated patients. Chest 106, 1182–1187.

Sinha, R., Bergofsky, E., 1972. Prolonged alteration of lung mechanics in kyphoscoliosis by positive pressure hyperinflation. Am. Rev. Respir. Dis. 106, 47–57.

Sivasothy, P., Brown, L., Smith, I.E., Shneerson, J.M., 2001. Effect of manually assisted cough and mechanical insufflation on cough flow of normal subjects, patients with chronic obstructive pulmonary disease (COPD), and patients with respiratory muscle weakness. Thorax 56, 438–444.

Sjostrand, T., 1951. Determination of changes in the intrathoracic blood volume in man. Acta Physiol. Scand. 22, 116–128.

Smith, K., Cook, D., Guyatt, G.H., et al., 1992. Respiratory muscle training in chronic airflow limitation: a meta-analysis. Am. Rev. Respir. Dis. 145, 533–539.

Solcher, J., Dechman, G., 1998. Inspiratory muscle function in chronic obstructive pulmonary disease (COPD). Phys. Ther. Rev. 3, 31–39.

Sole, M.L., Byers, J.F., Ludy, J.E., et al., 2003. A multisite survey of suctioning techniques and airway management practices. Am. J. Crit. Care 12, 220–230, quiz 231-2.

Sontag, M.K., Quittner, A.L., Modi, A.C., et al., 2010. Lessons learned from a randomized trial of airway secretion clearance techniques in cystic fibrosis. Pediatr. Pulmonol. 45, 291–300.

Southall, D.P., Samuels, M.P., 1992. Reducing risks in the sudden infant death syndrome. Br. Med. J. 304, 260–265.

Southern, K.W., Munck, A., Pollitt, R., et al., 2007. A survey of newborn screening for cystic fibrosis in Europe. J. Cyst. Fibros. 6, 57–65.

Squadrone, V., Coha, M., Cerutti, E., et al., 2005. Continuous positive airway pressure for treatment of postoperative hypoxemia: a randomized controlled trial. J. Am. Med. Assoc. 293, 589–595.

Starke, I.D., Webber, B.A., Branthwaite, M.A., 1979. IPPB and hypercapnia in respiratory failure: the effect of different concentrations of inspired oxygen on arterial blood gas tensions. Anaesthesia 34, 283–287.

Stiletto, R., Gotzen, L., Goubeaud, S., 2000. Kinetic therapy for therapy and prevention of post-traumatic lung failure: results of a prospective study of 111 polytrauma patients. Unfallchirurgie 103, 1057–1064. (English abstract).

Stiller, K., 2000. Physiotherapy in intensive care: towards an evidence-based practice. Chest 118, 1801–1813.

Stiller, K., Geake, T., Taylor, R., Hall, B., 1990. Acute lobar atelectasis: a comparison of two chest physiotherapy regimens. Chest 98, 1336–1340.

Stiller, K., Simionato, R., Rice, K., Hall, B., 1992. The effect of intermittent positive pressure breathing on lung volumes in acute quadriparesis. Paraplegia 30 (2), 121–126.

Stites, S.W., Perry, G.V., Peddicord, T., et al., 2006. Effect of high-frequency chest wall oscillation on the central and peripheral distribution of aerosolized diethylene triamine penta-acetic acid as compared to standard chest physiotherapy in cystic fibrosis. Chest 129, 712–717.

Stone, K.S., Turner, B., 1989. Endotracheal suctioning. Annu. Rev. Nurs. Res. 7, 27–49.

Storer, T.W., 2001. Exercise in chronic pulmonary disease: resistance exercise prescription. Med. Sci. Sport Exer. 33 (Suppl. 7), S680–S692.

Storre, J.H., Huttmann, S.E., Ekkernkamp, E., et al., 2014. Oxygen supplementation in noninvasive home mechanical ventilation: the crucial roles of CO_2 exhalation systems and leakages. Respir. Care 59, 113–120.

Storre, J.H., Seuthe, B., Fiechter, R., et al., 2006. Average volume-assured pressure support in obesity hypoventilation: a randomized crossover trial. Chest 130, 815–821.

Sukumalchantra, Y., Park, S.S., Williams, M.H., 1965. The effect of intermittent positive pressure breathing (IPPB) in acute ventilatory failure. Am. Rev. Respir. Dis. 92, 885–889.

Suri, P., Burns, S., Bach, J., 2008. Pneumothorax associated with mechanical insufflation-exsufflation and related factors. Am. J. Phys. Med. Rehabil. 87, 951–955.

Sutton, P., Lopez-Vidriero, M., Pavia, D., et al., 1985. Assessment of percussion, vibratory-shaking and breathing exercises in chest physiotherapy. Eur. J. Respir. Dis. 66, 147–152.

Sutton, P.P., Gemmell, H.G., Innes, N., et al., 1988. Use of nebulised saline and nebulised terbutaline as an adjunct to chest physiotherapy. Thorax 43, 57–60.

Sutton, P.P., Parker, R.A., Webber, B.A., et al., 1983. Assessment of the forced expiration technique, postural drainage and directed coughing in chest physiotherapy. Eur. J. Respir. Dis. 64, 62–68.

Svanberg, L., 1957. Influence of position on the lung volumes, ventilation and circulation in normals. Scand. J. Lab. Invest. 25 (Suppl.), 7–175.

Syed, N., Maiya, A., Kumar, S., 2009. Active cycle of breathing technique (ACBT) versus conventional chest physical therapy on airway clearance in bronchiectasis: a crossover trial. Adv Physiother 11, 193–198.

Sykes, M.K., McNicol, M.W., Campbell, E.J.M., 1976. Respiratory Failure, second ed. Blackwell Science, Oxford, p. 153.

Szeinberg, A., Tabachnik, E., Rashed, N., et al., 1988. Cough capacity in patients with muscular dystrophy. Chest 94, 1232–1235.

Tambascio, J., De Souza, L., Lisboa, R., et al., 2011. The influence of Flutter VRP1 components on mucus transport of patients with bronchiectasis. Respir. Med. 105, 1316–1321.

Tang, C.Y., Taylor, N.F., Blackstock, F.C., 2010. Chest physiotherapy for patients admitted to hospital with an acute exacerbation of chronic obstructive pulmonary disease (COPD): a systematic review. Physiotherapy 96, 1–13.

Taube, C., Holz, O., Mucke, M., et al., 2001. Airway response to inhaled hypertonic saline in patients with moderate to severe chronic obstructive pulmonary disease. Am. J. Respir. Crit. Care Med. 164, 1810–1815.

Teper, A., Jaques, A., Charlton, B., 2011. Inhaled mannitol in patients with cystic fibrosis: a randomised open-label dose response trial. J. Cyst. Fibros. 10, 1–8.

Thompson, C.S., Harrison, S., Ashley, J., et al., 2002. Randomised crossover study of the Flutter device and the active cycle of breathing technique in non-cystic fibrosis bronchiectasis. Thorax 57, 446–448.

Thoracic Society, 1950. The nomenclature of bronchopulmonary anatomy. Thorax 5, 222–228.

Thoresen, M., Cavan, F., Whitelaw, A., 1988. Effect of tilting on oxygenation in newborn infants. Arch. Dis. Child. 63, 315–317.

Toledo, A., Borghi-Silva, A., Sampaio, L.M., et al., 2007. The impact of noninvasive ventilation during the physical training in patients with moderate-to-severe chronic obstructive pulmonary disease (COPD). Clinics 62, 113–120.

Tomashefski, J.F., Jr., Bruce, M., Goldberg, H.I., Dearborn, D.G., 1986. Regional distribution of macroscopic lung disease in cystic fibrosis. Am. Rev. Respir. Dis. 133, 535–540.

Tomkiewicz, R., Biviji, A., King, M., 1994. Effects of oscillating air flow on the rheological properties and clearability of mucous gel simulants. Biorheology 31, 511–520.

Toussaint, M., De Win, H., Steens, M., Soudon, P., 2003. Effect of intrapulmonary percussive ventilation on mucus clearance in Duchenne muscular dystrophy patients: a preliminary report. Respir. Care 48, 940–947.

Toussaint, M., Guillet, M.-C., Paternotte, S., et al., 2012. Intrapulmonary effects of setting parameters in portable intrapulmonary percussive ventilation devices. Respir. Care 57, 735–742.

Tucker, B., Jenkins, S., Cheong, D., Robinson, P., 1999. Effect of unilateral breathing exercises on regional lung ventilation. Nucl. Med. Commun. 20, 815–821.

Tudehope, D.I., Bagley, C., 1980. Techniques of physiotherapy in intubated babies with the respiratory distress syndrome. Aust. Paediatr. J. 16, 226–228.

Tuggey, J., Elliott, M., 2005. Randomised crossover study of pressure and volume non-invasive ventilation in chest wall deformity. Thorax 60, 859–864.

Tzeng, A.C., Bach, J.R., 2000. Prevention of pulmonary morbidity for patients with neuromuscular disease. Chest 118, 1390–1396.

Ural, A., Oktemer, T.K., Kizil, Y., et al., 2009. Impact of isotonic and hypertonic saline solutions on mucociliary activity in various nasal pathologies: clinical study. J. Laryngol. Otol. 123, 517–521.

Urell, C., Emtner, M., Hedenstrom, H., et al., 2011. Deep breathing exercises with positive expiratory pressure at a higher rate improve oxygenation in the early period after cardiac surgery: a randomised controlled trial. Eur. J. Cardiothorac Surg. 40, 162–167.

Uronis, H., McCrory, D.C., Samsa, G., et al., 2011. Symptomatic oxygen for non-hypoxaemic chronic obstructive pulmonary disease. Cochrane Database Syst. Rev. (6), Art. No.: CD006429, doi:10.1002/14651858.CD006429.pub2.

Valderramas, S.R., Atallah, A.N., 2009. Effectiveness and safety of hypertonic saline inhalation combined with exercise training in patients with chronic obstructive pulmonary disease: a randomized trial. Respir. Care 54, 327–333.

van der Giessen, L.J., Gosselink, R., Hop, W.C., Tiddens, H.A., 2007. Recombinant human DNase nebulisation in children with cystic fibrosis: before bedtime or after waking up? Eur. Respir. J. 30, 763–768.

van der Schans, C., 1997. Forced expiratory manoeuvres to increase transport of bronchial mucus: a mechanistic approach. Monaldi Arch. Chest Dis. 52, 367–370.

van der Schans, C., Piers, D., Beekhuis, H., et al., 1990. Effect of forced expirations on mucus clearance in patients with chronic airflow obstruction: effect of lung recoil pressure. Thorax 45, 623–627.

van der Schans, C., Piers, D., Postma, D., 1986. Effect of manual percussion on tracheobronchial clearance in patients with chronic airflow obstruction and excessive tracheobronchial secretion. Thorax 41, 448–452.

van der Schans, C.P., Postma, D.S., Koeter, G.H., Rubin, B.K., 1999. Physiotherapy and bronchial mucus transport. Eur. Respir. J. 13, 1477–1486.

van der Schans, C., Van Der Mark, T., De Vries, G., et al., 1991. Effect of positive expiratory pressure breathing in patients with cystic fibrosis. Thorax 46, 252–256.

van Ginderdeuren, F., Malfroot, A., Verdonck, J., 2003. Influence of assisted autogenic drainage (AAD) and AAD combined with bouncing on gastro-oesophageal reflux (GOR) in infants under the age of 5 months. J. Cyst. Fibrosis 2, A251.

van Ginderdeuren, F., Verbanck, S., Van Cauwelaert, K., et al., 2008. Chest physiotherapy in cystic fibrosis: short-term effects of autogenic drainage preceded by wet inhalation of saline versus autogenic drainage preceded by intrapulmonary percussive ventilation with saline. Respiration 76, 175–180.

van 't Hul, A., Gosselink, R., Hollander, P., et al., 2004. Acute effects of inspiratory pressure support during exercise in patients with COPD. Eur. Respir. J. 23, 34–40.

Van 't Hul, A., Gosselink, R., Hollander, P., et al., 2006. Training with inspiratory pressure support in patients with severe COPD. Eur. Respir. J. 27, 65–72.

van Winden, C.M., Visser, A., Hop, W., et al., 1998. Effects of flutter and PEP mask physiotherapy on symptoms and lung function in children with cystic fibrosis. Eur. Respir. J. 12, 143–147.

Varekojis, S.M., Douce, F.H., Flucke, R.L., et al., 2003. A comparison of the therapeutic effectiveness of and preference for postural drainage and percussion, intrapulmonary percussive ventilation, and high-frequency chest wall compression in hospitalized cystic fibrosis patients. Respir. Care 48, 24–28.

Vargas, F., Bui, H., Boyer, A., et al., 2005. Intrapulmonary percussive ventilation in acute exacerbations of COPD patients with mild respiratory acidosis: a randomized controlled trial [ISRCTN17802078]. Critical Care 9, R382–R389.

Vernon, H., Mior, S., 1991. The Neck Disability Index: a study of reliability and validity. J. Manipulative Physiol. Ther. 14, 409–415.

Vianello, A., Bevilacqua, M., Arcaro, G., et al., 2000. Non-invasive ventilatory approach to treatment of acute respiratory failure in neuromuscular disorders: a comparison with endotracheal intubation. Intensive Care Med. 26, 384–390.

Vianello, A., Corrado, A., Arcaro, G., et al., 2005. Mechanical insufflation-exsufflation improves outcomes for neuromuscular disease patients with respiratory tract infections. Am. J. Phys. Med. Rehabil. 84, 83–88.

Vibekk, P., 1991. Chest mobilisation and respiratory function. In: Pryor, J.A. (Ed.), Respiratory Care. Churchill Livingstone, Edinburgh, pp. 103–119.

Vignaux, L., Vargas, F., Roeseler, J., et al., 2009. Patient-ventilator asynchrony during non-invasive ventilation for acute respiratory failure: a multicenter study. Intensive Care Med. 35, 840–846.

Villa, M.P., Pagani, J., Ambrosio, R., et al., 2002. Mid-face hypoplasia after long-term nasal ventilation. Am. J. Respir Crit. Care Med. 166, 1142–1143.

Vital, F., Ladeira, M., Atallah, Á., 2013. Non-invasive positive pressure ventilation (CPAP or bilevel NPPV) for cardiogenic pulmonary oedema. Cochrane Database Syst. Rev. Art. No.: CD005351, doi:10.1002/14651858.CD005351.pub3.

Vollman, K.M., 2004. Prone positioning in the patient who has acute respiratory distress syndrome: the art and science. Crit. Care Nurs. Clin. North Am. 16, 319–336.

Volsko, T.A., Difiore, J., Chatburn, R.L., 2003. Performance comparison of two oscillating positive expiratory pressure devices: Acapella versus Flutter. Respir. Care 48, 124–130.

von Euler, C., 1986. Breathing behavior. In: von Euler, C., Lagercrantz, A. (Eds.), Neurobiology of the Control of Breathing (Nobel Conference Series). Raven Press, New York.

von Leupoldt, A., Balewski, S., Petersen, S., et al., 2007. Verbal descriptors of dyspnea in patients with COPD at different intensity levels of dyspnea. Chest 132, 141–147.

von Leupoldt, A., Chan, P., Bradley, M., et al., 2011. The impact of anxiety of neural processing of respiratory sensations. Neuroimage 55, 247–252.

von Leupoldt, A., Dahme, B., 2005. Differentiation between the sensory and affective dimension of dyspnea during resistive load breathing in normal subjects. Chest 128, 3345–3349.

Voynow, J.A., Rubin, B.K., 2009. Mucins, mucus, and sputum. Chest 135, 505–512.

Wadell, K., Webb, K.A., Preston, M.E., et al., 2013. Impact of pulmonary rehabilitation on the major dimensions of dyspnea in COPD. COPD 10 (4), 425–435. doi:10.3109/15412555.2012.758696; [Epub 2013 Mar 28].

Wagstaff, A., 2009. Oxygen therapy. In: Bersten, A.D., Soni, N. (Eds.), Oh's Intensive Care Manual, sixth Edition. Butterworth Heinemann Elsevier, Philadelphia, pp. 315–326.

Walkey, A.J., Wiener, R.S., 2013. Use of noninvasive ventilation in patients with acute respiratory failure, 2000–2009: a population-based study. Ann. Am. Thorac. Soc. 10, 10–17.

Wallgren-Pettersson, C., Bushby, K., Mellies, U., et al., 2004. 117th ENMC Workshop. Ventilatory support in congenital neuromuscular disorders: congenital myopathies, congenital muscular dystrophies, congenital myotonic dystrophy and SMA (II). Neuromuscul. Disord. 14, 56–69.

Walterspacher, S., Scholz, T., Tetzlaff, K., Sorichter, S., 2011. Breath-hold diving: respiratory function on the longer term. Med. Sci. Sports Exerc. 43 (7), 1214–1219.

Wanner, A., 1984. Does chest physical therapy move airway secretions? Am. Rev. Respir. Dis. 130, 701–702.

Ward, K., Horobin, H., 2012. Does the application of an algorithm for non-invasive ventilation in chronic obstructive pulmonary disease improve the initiation process and patient outcomes? Physiotherapy 98, 151–159.

Ward, S., Chatwin, M., Heather, S., et al., 2005. Randomised controlled trial of non-invasive ventilation (NIV) for nocturnal hypoventilation in neuromuscular and chest wall disease patients with daytime normocapnia. Thorax 60, 1019–1024.

Warnock, L., Gates, A., Van Der Schans, C.P., 2013. Chest physiotherapy compared to no chest physiotherapy for cystic fibrosis. Cochrane Database Syst. Rev. (9), CD001401.

Warwick, W.J., Hansen, L.G., 1991. The long-term effect of high-frequency chest compression therapy on pulmonary complications of cystic fibrosis. Pediatr. Pulmonol. 11, 265–271.

Warwick, W.J., Wielinski, C.L., Hansen, L.G., 2004. Comparison of expectorated sputum after manual chest physical therapy and high-frequency chest compression. Biomed. Instrum. Technol. 38, 470–475.

Wasserman, K., Hansen, J.E., Sue, D.Y., Whipp, B.J., 1987. Principles of Exercise Testing and Interpretation. Lea and Febiger, Philadelphia.

Wasserman, K., Whipp, B.J., 1975. Exercise physiology in health and disease. Am. Rev. Respir. Dis. 112, 219–249.

Watson, D., Trott, P., 1993. Cervical headache – an investigation of natural head posture and upper cervical flexor muscle performance. Cephalalgia 13, 272–284.

Webber, B.A., Hofmeyr, J.L., Morgan, M.D., Hodson, M.E., 1986. Effects of postural drainage, incorporating the forced expiration technique, on pulmonary function in cystic fibrosis. Br. J. Dis. Chest 80, 353–359.

Webber, B., Parker, R., Hofmeyr, J., Hodson, M., 1985. Evaluation of self percussion during postural drainage using the forced expiration technique. Physiother. Pract. 1, 42–45.

Webber, B.A., 1991. The role of the physiotherapist in medical chest problems. Respiratory Disease in Practice Feb/Mar, 12–15.

Webber, B.A., Higgens, J.M., 1999. Glossopharyngeal ('frog') breathing: what, when and how? DVD available from ACPRC: email <secretary@acprc.org.uk>.

Weber, K.T., Janicki, J.S., Shroff, S.G., Likoff, M.J., 1983. The cardiopulmonary unit: the body's gas transport system. Clin. Chest Med. 4, 101–110.

Webber, B.A., Shenfield, G.M., Paterson, J.W., 1974. A comparison of three different techniques for giving nebulized albuterol to asthmatic patients. Am. Rev. Respir. Dis. 109, 293–295.

Weiler, J.M., Anderson, S.D., Randolph, C., et al., 2010. Pathogenesis, prevalence, diagnosis, and management of exercise-induced bronchoconstriction: a practice parameter. Ann. Allergy Asthma Immunol. 105, S1–S47.

Weindler, J., Kiefer, R.T., 2001. The efficacy of postoperative incentive spirometry is influenced by the device-specific imposed work of breathing. Chest 119, 1858–1864.

Weiner, P., Azgad, Y., Garnam, R., 1992. Inspiratory muscle training combined with general exercise training in COPD. Chest 102, 1351–1356.

Weiner, P., Weiner, M., 2006. Inspiratory muscle training may increase peak inspiratory flow in chronic obstructive pulmonary disease. Respiration 73, 151–156.

Wen, A.S., Woo, M.S., Keens, T.G., 1996. Safety of chest physiotherapy in asthma. Am. J. Respir. Crit. Care Med. 153, A77.

Wenger, N.K., 1982. Early ambulation: the physiologic basis revisited. Adv. Cardiol. 31, 138–141.

West, J.B., 1962. Regional differences in gas exchange in the lung of erect man. J. Appl. Physiol. 17, 893–898.

West, J.B., 1977. Ventilation and perfusion relationships. Am. Rev. Respir. Dis. 116, 919–943.

West, R.L., Hernandez, A.F., O'Connor, C.M., et al., 2010. A review of dyspnoea in acute heart failure syndromes. Am. Heart J. 160, 209–214.

West, J., Luks, A., 2015. West's Respiratory Physiology: The Essentials. Lippincott Williams and Wilkins, Baltimore.

West, K., Wallen, M., Follett, J., 2010. Acapella vs. PEP mask therapy: a randomized trial in children with cystic fibrosis during respiratory exacerbation. Physiother. Theory Pract. 26, 143–149.

Westerdahl, E., Lindmark, B., Almgren, S.-O., Tenling, A., 2001. Chest physiotherapy after coronary artery bypass graft surgery: a comparison of three different deep breathing techniques. J. Rehabil. Med. 33, 79–86.

White, A.A., Panjabi, M.M., 1990. Clinical Biomechanics of the Spine, second ed. Lippincott, Philadelphia.

White, S., Sahrmann, S., 1994. Physical therapy for the cervical and thoracic spine. In: Grant, R. (Ed.), Clinics in Physical Therapy, second ed. Churchill Livingstone, New York.

White, D., Stiller, K., Roney, F., 2000. The prevalence and severity of symptoms of incontinence in adult cystic fibrosis patients. Physiother. Theory Pract. 16, 35–42.

Whitman, J., Van Beusekom, R., Olson, S., et al., 1993. Preliminary evaluation of high-frequency chest compression for secretion clearance in mechanically ventilated patients. Respir. Care 38, 1081–1087.

Williams, C., 1995. Haemoglobin: is more better? Nephrol. Dial. Transplant 2 (Suppl.), 48–55.

Williams, M.T., 2011. Applicability and generalizability of palliative interventions for dyspnoea: one size fits all, some or none? Curr. Opin. Suppor. Palliat. Care 5, 92–100.

Williams, M.T., Gerlach, Y., Moseley, L., 2012b. The 'survival perceptions': time to put some bacon on our plates? J. Physiother. 58, 73–75.

Williams, M.T., Petkov, J., Olds, T., et al., 2012a. A reduction in the use of volunteered descriptors of air hunger is associated with increased walking distance in people with COPD. Respir. Care 57, 1431–1441.

Williams, R., Rankin, N., Smith, T., et al., 1996. Relationship between the humidity and temperature of inspired gas and the function of the airway mucosa. Crit. Care Med. 24 (11), 1920–1929.

Wills, P.J., Hall, R.L., Chan, W.M., Cole, P.J., 1997. Sodium chloride increases the ciliary transportability of cystic fibrosis and bronchiectasis sputum on the mucus-depleted bovine trachea. J. Clin. Invest. 99, 9–13.

Wills, P.J., Wodehouse, T., Corkery, K., et al., 1996. Short-term recombinant human DNase in bronchiectasis: effect on clinical state and in vitro sputum transportability. Am. J. Respir. Crit. Care Med. 154, 413–417.

Wilson, G., Baldwin, A., Walshaw, M., 1985. A comparison of traditional chest physiotherapy with the active cycle of breathing in patients with chronic suppurative lung disease. Eur. Respir. J. 8 (Suppl. 19), S171.

Willson, G., Piper, A., Norman, M., et al., 2004. Nasal versus full face mask for noninvasive ventilation in chronic respiratory failure. Eur. Respir. J. 23, 605–609.

Winck, J.C., Goncalves, M.R., Lourenco, C., et al., 2004. Effects of mechanical insufflation-exsufflation on respiratory parameters for patients with chronic airway secretion encumbrance. Chest 126, 774–780.

Windisch, W., Storre, J.H., 2012. Target volume settings for home mechanical ventilation: great progress or just a gadget? Thorax 67, 663–665.

Wolff, R.K., Dolovich, M.B., Obminski, G., Newhouse, M.T., 1977. Effects of exercise and eucapnic hyperventilation on bronchial clearance in man. J. Appl. Physiol. 43, 46–50.

Wollmer, P., Ursing, K., Midgren, B., Eriksson, L., 1985. Inefficiency of chest percussion in the physical therapy of chronic bronchitis. Eur. J. Respir. Dis. 66, 233–239.

Wong, W., Paratz, J., Wilson, K., Burns, Y., 2003. Hemodynamic and ventilatory effects of manual respiratory physiotherapy techniques of chest clapping, vibration, and shaking in an animal model. J. Appl. Physiol. 95, 991–998.

Wong, W.P., 2000. Physical therapy for a patient in acute respiratory failure. Phys. Ther. 80, 662–670.

Wong, W.P., 2004. Use of body positioning in the mechanically ventilated patient with acute respiratory failure: application of the Sackett's rules of evidence. Physiother. Theory Pract. 15, 25–41.

Wood, C.J., 1998. Endotracheal suctioning: a literature review. Intensive Crit. Care Nurs. 14, 124–136.

Wood, K.E., Flaten, A.L., Backes, W.J., 2000. Inspissated secretions: a life-threatening complication of prolonged noninvasive ventilation. Respir. Care 45, 491–493.

Wood, K.A., Lewis, L., Von Harz, B., et al., 1998. The use of noninvasive positive pressure ventilation in the emergency department: results of a randomized clinical trial. Chest 113, 1339–1346.

Wynne, R., Botti, M., 2004. Postoperative pulmonary dysfunction in adults after cardiac surgery with cardiopulmonary bypass: Clinical significance and implications for practice. Am. J. Crit. Care 13, 384–393.

Yamauchi, L.Y., Travaglia, T.C., Bernardes, S.R., et al., 2012. Noninvasive positive-pressure ventilation in clinical practice at a large university-affiliated Brazilian hospital. Clinics 67, 767–772.

Yánez-Brage, I., Pita-Fernández, S., Juffé-Stein, A., et al., 2009. Respiratory physiotherapy and incidence of pulmonary complications in off-pump coronary artery bypass graft surgery: an observational follow-up study. BMC Pulm. Med. 9, 36. doi:10.1186/1471-2466-9-36.

Ympa, Y.P., Sakr, Y., Reinhart, K., Vincent, J.L., 2005. Has mortality from acute renal failure decreased? A systematic review of the literature. Am. J. Med. 118, 827–832.

Yorke, J., Moosavi, S.H., Shuldham, C., 2010. Quantification of dyspnoea using descriptors: development and initial testing of the dyspnoea-12. Thorax 65, 21–26.

Young, A.C., Wilson, J.W., Kotsimbos, T.C., Naughton, M.T., 2008. Randomised placebo controlled trial of non-invasive ventilation for hypercapnia in cystic fibrosis. Thorax 63, 72–77.

Zach, M.S., Oberwaldner, B., 1987. Chest physiotherapy: the mechanical approach to antiinfective therapy in cystic fibrosis. Infection 15, 381–384.

Zack, M.B., Pontoppidan, H., Kazemi, H., 1974. The effect of lateral positions on gas exchange in pulmonary disease. Am. Rev. Respir. Dis. 110, 49–55.

Zafiropoulos, B., Alison, J., McCarren, B., 2004. Physiological responses to the early mobilization of the intubated, ventilated abdominal surgery patient. Aust J. Physiother. 50, 95–100.

Zarbock, A., Mueller, E., Netzer, S., et al., 2009. Prophylactic nasal continuous positive airway pressure following cardiac surgery protects from postoperative pulmonary complications: a prospective, randomized, controlled trial in 500 patients. Chest 135, 1252–1259.

Zhang, L., Mendoza-Sassi, R.A., Wainwright, C., Klassen, T.P., 2013. Nebulised hypertonic saline solution for acute bronchiolitis in infants. The Cochrane Database Syst. Rev. 7, Art. No.: CD006458.

Zhao, Y., Markides, C.N., Matar, O.K., Hewitt, G.F., 2013. Disturbance wave development in two-phase gas-liquid upwards vertical annular flow. Int. J. Multiphase Flow 55, 111–129.

Zuffo, S., Gambazza, S., Capra, A., 2012. Noninvasive ventilation in cystic fibrosis: the Italian physiotherapists' point of view. Eur. Respir. J. 39, 1539–1540.

Zuhlke, I.E., Kanniess, F., Richter, K., et al., 2003. Montelukast attenuates the airway response to hypertonic saline in moderate-to-severe COPD. Eur. Respir. J. 22, 926–930.

ZuWallack, R., Hedges, H., 2008. Primary care of the patient with chronic obstructive pulmonary disease. Part 3. Pulmonary rehabilitation and comprehensive care for the patient with chronic obstructive pulmonary disease. Am. J. Med. 121, S25–S32.

OPTIMIZING ENGAGEMENT AND ADHERENCE WITH THERAPEUTIC INTERVENTIONS

MANDY BRYON

CHAPTER OUTLINE

INTRODUCTION 402

IMPACT OF DIAGNOSIS 402
Diagnosis in Childhood 402
Impact of Diagnosis in Adulthood 403
Following Diagnosis 404

LIVING WITH CARDIORESPIRATORY
ILLNESS 405
Managing Treatment Regimens 405
Peer and Social Relationships 407
Emotional Impact of a Medical Illness 407

ENGAGEMENT WITH MEDICAL TEAMS 410
Adolescence 410
Team Work and Technology 411

CONCLUSION 412

REFERENCES 412

INTRODUCTION

One of the most common causes of morbidity and mortality in people with a chronic health condition is poor adherence to prescribed treatment. In the case of cardiorespiratory conditions, this refers not only to medication but also lifestyle recommendations such as diet and exercise (Quittner et al 2014). Healthcare professionals (HCPs) recognize that adherence to treatment is a problem and therefore seek solutions. Unfortunately the approach is often conceptually misguided; it follows the tenet that 'the patient is not doing as we suggest so how can I make them do more treatment or follow my advice regarding lifestyle?' In doing so, the response to improving adherence is to burden the patient further. A psychosocial model would be to consider the patient and the HCP as part of the problem and both need to be incorporated into the solution; i.e. how can the HCP modify prescribed treatment to ensure the patient is engaged with a treatment package that suits them personally? This chapter considers the impact of diagnosis of a chronic cardiorespiratory condition on the adult patient and the parents of children similarly diagnosed. Attention is paid to living with the medical condition and engaging with medical teams to optimize treatment adherence.

IMPACT OF DIAGNOSIS

Diagnosis in Childhood

Diagnoses of cardiorespiratory conditions made within the first few months of life have a particular impact, as they come at a time when parents are feeling intense emotions towards their newborn infant, and they are asked to assimilate the information that their baby has a potentially life-limiting illness such as cystic fibrosis (CF) or heart problems. Parents who had been prepared for acquiring child-rearing skills now must learn nursing and medical skills and incorporate a group of uninvited strangers comprising the medical team into their lives. Clearly, this time will be one of stress and sorrow for parents and a frequently asked question is: 'Does a diagnosis of a medical condition given early in the child's life carry with it a risk for damage to the parent–child bond?'

There is very little research investigating the impact of a diagnosis of a chronic life-threatening illness on the parent–child bond. The studies published suggest the majority demonstrate a secure attachment with the mother, with some showing an insecure–avoidant pattern where the child shows little distress on separation and actively avoids the mother on reunion. There are no significant differences reported in rates of insecure attachments found from the healthy controls, but the implications are that those children with insecure attachments to a primary care-giver will be vulnerable at times of stress as a result of the illness (Simmons and Goldberg 2001).

This suggests that the parent–child instinctive drives to form a bond are not affected by the diagnosis of CF and the same could be said to be true for other cardiorespiratory conditions. Concerns have been raised that the infant diagnosed with CF via newborn screening techniques may harm the parent–child attachment by disrupting the relationship with the disclosure of a life-threatening illness in an infant that had not displayed any symptoms of disease (Grob 2008). It has been reported, however, that mothers of children diagnosed by newborn screening have higher frequencies of 'at-risk' scores for parenting stress than mothers of traditionally diagnosed children (Baroni et al 1997), though these authors suggest that the significant variables influencing maternal well-being are the way in which the diagnosis is communicated and subsequent parental support and engagement with the medical team.

Parents of children with a medical condition are at risk for overprotection of their children. A fear of infection can result in parents restricting the physical movements and toys of their young children. Attendance at playschools and nurseries may be denied; possibly even contact with other healthy children may be limited. Studies of the play interactions of parents of preschool children with CF indicate that mothers are much more interfering and less supportive of their children and the child correspondingly shows less persistence and compliance in play activities (Goldberg et al 1995). The child-rearing practices of parents of children with CF may be affected by the overwhelming need to protect the child. All daily interactions from dressing to feeding to bedtimes may be indirectly altered by the diagnosis.

Children with chronic illness are capable of more a sophisticated understanding of their illness than previously thought. However, there is a barrier to effective communication with children. On interview about their condition, children with CF tend to give consistently similar responses to questions irrespective of age; they know that CF affects the respiratory (85%) and digestive (80%) systems, though they don't know why or how and the majority don't know the importance of nutrition (70%) (Angst 2001). This suggests that they are repeating received information without assimilating true understanding. Children tend to hold a glossary of CF terms which is separate from how it affects them personally. Though they are quite capable of a decent knowledge of their own health and engage in patient–clinician discussions about treatment, the tendency is to avoid this. Children with CF define themselves as 'healthy' irrespective of actual health status and this phenomenon is also found in other chronic health conditions: asthma (Frey 1996) and heart disease (Veldtman et al 2001). This is fundamental to engaging with children in discussion about their treatment. Particularly when treatment in many cardiorespiratory conditions is preventative, the child is well and must implement daily therapies to stay well. When a child perceives themselves to be well and has limited conceptual understanding of the medical condition and how it impacts, there is little motivation to comply with time-consuming treatments.

This dual comprehension of CF – a knowledge of the physical components of the disease but an unwillingness to apply them to the self – may come about in part from a parental desire to protect the child from the potentially distressing aspects of CF, what Bluebond-Langner (1991) terms a 'conspiracy of silence', and in part from the reluctance of CF health professionals to include the child in consultations. Parents are used by children as envoys and information brokers; they act as buffers from unpleasant information (Young et al 2003).

Impact of Diagnosis in Adulthood

There will have been a degree of preparation done by an adult patient prior to receiving a diagnosis. The adult will often come to the consultation with thoughts and beliefs about the symptoms that have led to the diagnosis appointment. How the individual's thoughts match the information that is presented may determine whether the diagnosis is received with acceptance, distress or, in some situations, relief.

Considerable research exploring patients' thoughts about physical health problems suggests that for any condition an individual will have a 'common sense' understanding about the condition which has been termed an 'illness representation' (Leventhal et al 1984). This is a set of beliefs which revolves around five key themes. These include:

- *identity,* which describes the symptoms and label that the individual associates with an illness
- *timeline,* which is related to how long the condition is thought to last, i.e. whether it is acute, chronic or cyclical
- *consequences,* which incorporates thoughts about how serious the condition is and the effect that it will have on the lives of both themselves and individuals close to them
- *control,* including thoughts about the extent that they as an individual can control their illness and thoughts about whether treatment can control the illness
- *cause,* which are beliefs relating to what the person attributes the cause of their condition to.

These thoughts are a way for individuals to make sense of any symptoms they experience and will influence the behavioural response; they may be present even before diagnosis. For example if an individual has chest pain and identifies it as due to indigestion, they may be unlikely to visit a doctor. However, if the same pain was interpreted as a heart attack, a very different response might be expected. Such beliefs are important at all stages of illness from diagnosis to the end stages of a condition and are related to outcomes both physical and psychological. For example the more chronic in nature the condition is perceived to be, the poorer the psychological reaction to the condition. In contrast if the individual perceives that the condition will be controllable or is caused by factors which may be amenable to change, e.g. by changing lifestyle factors such as diet or exercise, their reaction to the condition is generally more positive (Hagger and Orbell 2003).

Illness beliefs come from a range of sources including general lay information about health, such as might be gained through the media or increasingly the Internet, information from the social environment including authoritative advice such as from medical personnel and also knowledge of other individuals with similar symptoms, and finally personal experience which relates to the individual's own previous experience of such symptoms. The range of sources which feed illness beliefs may explain the variability in reaction to diagnosis of physical health problems and differences in management. Such beliefs must therefore be taken into account at all stages of managing physical illness.

One particularly difficult form of diagnosis in adulthood is that which would normally have been made during childhood, such as late diagnosis of CF. Patients diagnosed with CF as adults can be left feeling confused as often there is uncertainty around diagnosis, with perhaps multiple tests before diagnosis is confirmed (Widerman 2002). For the HCP working with adults diagnosed with CF over the age of 18, it is important to recognize the significant effect of such a diagnosis and to acknowledge that informational needs may be different from that of a patient diagnosed as a child. Providing time for questions and being alert to the meaning of this for both the patient and their plans for the future, e.g. reproductive health, will be important. The patient and HCP will be engaging in a long-term relationship and the first impressions created at the time of the diagnosis will have prolonged consequences.

Following Diagnosis

Fundamental to the patient–HCP relationship is good communication. Nowadays there is an accepted shift from prescription to collaboration (Kinmonth et al 1998). Such a patient-centred approach sees the HCP and patient as the meeting of two experts: the patient an expert on the impact of the illness on their individual lives and the HCP expert on the clinical management of the condition. Evidence of the benefits of a collaborative or patient-centred approach is demonstrated on a range of outcomes including satisfaction, treatment adherence, quality of life and physical health outcomes (Michie et al 2003). Accurate understanding of one's own medical condition correlates with less distress, less confusion, improved relationships with the medical team, better adherence to medication and an improved emotional well-being (Veldtman et al 2001).

Collaboration may be more straightforward with the adult patient than the child. How to involve the child in such a collaborative relationship is therefore often something the HCP may need to guide the parents on. This process can be complex and requires ongoing support. Practical guidelines have been recommended (Towle and Godolphin 1999):

- Develop a collaboration with the parents for ongoing information-sharing with the child.
- Establish the parents' preferences for managing communication.
- Inform parents of the advantages of including the child as collaborator in their medical treatment.
- Ensure parents have accurate knowledge.
- Avoid jargon and technical explanations.
- Expect that information will be forgotten – ensure repetition at consultations.
- When speaking to a child ask them what they know about a subject first, expand that knowledge using their own words.

Although targeted at involving children in care, these principles apply equally well when the patient is an adult.

LIVING WITH CARDIORESPIRATORY ILLNESS

Following diagnosis with a cardiac or respiratory condition the adult patient, parent or child will be faced with a number of demands in managing their condition. The challenges inherent in living with a physical illness include having to manage persistent symptoms without cure, continuous medication use, adapting to behavioural changes, e.g. diet/exercise, undergoing changes to social and work circumstances, managing emotional distress and participating in decisions about medical treatment. Given these significant effects, it is perhaps not surprising that individuals with cardiac or respiratory conditions typically experience reduced quality of life compared with individuals without health conditions (Poon et al 2014). A key objective in working with people with respiratory or cardiac conditions should therefore be helping to improve quality of life while managing these demands.

Managing Treatment Regimens

The life expectancy of children and adults diagnosed with a cardiorespiratory condition has improved greatly. Even people with conditions such as CF, which a few years ago would have resulted in childhood death, can now live to their 40th and 50th decade. Improved surgical techniques and more aggressive medical treatments account for this improvement, including management by a multidisciplinary team. People with cardiorespiratory chronic conditions can, these days, expect to engage in and aspire to those aspects of life which occupy their healthy peers. This engagement, however, is only possible if patients can find a way to accommodate hefty treatment regimens and lifestyle demands such as exercise and nutritional programmes into their daily routine. Poor adherence to treatment regimen is perhaps the most well documented area of difficulty in managing chronic cardiorespiratory health conditions no matter what age the patient (Quittner et al 2014).

Generally there is good evidence that in adults, like children, adherence is less than optimal. For example adherence to physiotherapy in CF on a daily basis has been reported to be only 29.5% (Myers and Horn 2006). Other studies (Abbott et al 1994, Conway et al 1996, Shepherd et al 1990) have reported adherence to oral antibiotics to be 68–93% and exercise to be 69–75%.

The level of poor adherence to CF treatment, especially with physiotherapy and diet and to a lesser extent with nebulized therapy, indicates that patients are making decisions about treatment management based on factors other than purely clinician advice (Ketler et al 2002). Patients or parents may deliberately alter treatment regimens according to their own beliefs and personal quality of life assessment, which may not match the aims of treatment held by health professionals (Horne and Weinman 1999). Importantly there is little evidence to suggest that adherence is associated with either the seriousness of the condition or sociodemographic variables such as education levels (Abbott et al 1994).

The prescribers of treatment must therefore accept that a degree of poor adherence will be normal. A traditional prescriptive approach will fail to uncover any incompatibility between medical criteria and the patients' criteria for treatment success. Recent recommendations have suggested that a more fruitful approach, in line with collaborative care, is to understand the patient's illness behaviours in terms of self-management (Bodenheimer et al 2002). This encompasses the idea that people manage their condition, including its treatments, in a social and emotional world, and good quality of life is achieved by balancing all of these aspects.

Improving Self-Management and Collaborative Care

Given individuals make decisions about the management of their illness based on their priorities within their broader day-to-day life, the role of the HCP is to support the individual to make informed decisions and address the patient's identified priorities. Understanding patients' or parents' treatment beliefs is key to this. Studies suggest that thoughts about the *necessity* of the medication or treatment and secondly *concerns* about the medication or treatment, e.g. worries about side effects, are particularly important in predicting adherence. In both asthma and cardiac conditions, patients' greater belief in necessity and lower concerns about medication have been shown to be related to greater adherence (Horne et al 2013). Where concerns outweigh beliefs in necessity then adherence will be lower.

In addition, the meaning associated with treatment is important particularly as an illness progresses and treatments become more demanding. For example, the requirement of an individual to use oxygen is often associated with an adverse reaction by the patient. Frequently this is less to do with the practicalities of oxygen use, but more significantly the representation of this as an indicator that health is deteriorating. At this point, understanding what the treatment represents and aiding adjustment to deterioration in health may be an important factor in facilitating use of the treatment.

The implications of these findings for practice are that in working with patients or parents to improve self-management, their beliefs about the behaviour including worries, concerns and self-efficacy must be elicited. This should supplement traditional approaches of general education and advice giving, which although

important are often insufficient for behaviour change (Kolbe et al 1996). Psychological interventions that target beliefs include cognitive behavioural interventions such as motivational interviewing as a strategy to improve adherence (Duff and Latchford 2013). Motivational interviewing is a person-centred intervention which views motivation as a fluctuating state which can be targeted through trained HCPs facilitating individuals to understand and resolve their ambivalence about behaviour change. It also draws on the concept that individuals may vary in their readiness to change a behaviour and has been shown to have use in a range of healthcare settings (Duff and Latchford 2013).

The Role of Parenting in Managing Medical Treatments

Levels of parental stress have been found to positively correlate with reported child behaviour difficulties but not to correlate with severity of illness, number of hospitalizations or time taken for treatment (Simmons and Goldberg 2001). The daily demands of child rearing for any parent become a major strain especially around two years of age when the child begins to assert autonomy. Oppositional behaviour around treatment can be a major difficulty. When parents face daily challenges to their authority they lose confidence and become coerced into withdrawing their commands for compliance to any instruction whether or not connected with delivering treatment (Patterson 2002).

In delivering paediatric care, the HCP is not always dealing directly with the patient; most medical consultations are with the parent, acting as the patient's advocate. There is often an accepted belief by HCPs that the parents will implement treatment exactly as prescribed. Unfortunately, the HCP rarely asks the parent if they will be able to get their child to do as they are told. Treatment refusal in young children is not necessarily directed at the treatment per se, but part of normal non-compliance to parental instruction. There is little difference between a child refusing to clean their teeth and refusing to take their medicine; the behavioural opposition is technically the same. What makes this often a more entrenched problem is that the parental emotional response to treatment refusal is greater than it would be for more benign behaviours. Inadvertently, parents' frantic attempts to gain compliance make the problem worse. Behaviour therapy, such as behavioural contracting, parent management training and modelling, has been found to be empirically supported as an effective intervention for use with children and parents (Kendall and Chambless 1998). Parent management training, in particular, is advantageous for the medical team as it can be standardized and implemented from a manual by non-psychologists (Kendall et al 1998). HCPs often overlook simple parenting strategies as they too become entrenched in the belief that compliance to parental instruction to take medicine somehow requires a more specialist intervention. In short, if a parent knows how to teach their child to clean their teeth every day, they can apply the same techniques to performing treatment routinely.

Peer and Social Relationships

It may be a key priority for HCPs that patients should adhere to treatments, but for the child or adult this treatment must occur within their social world. Qualitative research indicates that one of the most pervasive emotional difficulties facing the school age child with a chronic medical condition is a feeling of difference compared with peers (Angst 2001). Children will go to great lengths to minimize observable differences between themselves and their peers, and this puts them at risk from failing to conduct necessary treatments.

For all children and adolescents, peer relationships provide the arena for the development of social skills and a positive self-concept. Children and adolescents with a long-term medical condition may avoid discussion of their illness with peers due to anxiety that shared knowledge of the condition might make them less acceptable as a friend or make them vulnerable to bullying. In medical conditions like many in cardiorespiratory illnesses where there are no or few visible differences, it is easier to hide the diagnosis. Psychologically, the burden of withholding information can be more damaging than the potential support available from a peer group. Again this is a question of managing the balance between accepting the imposition of a chronic illness while trying to make life as normal and routine as possible. School age children can be helped to include their friends in knowledge about their condition and this is more likely to sustain

and strengthen a relationship than, as is often feared, result in rejection. Friends can help the school age child with CF to incorporate CF into their self-image and learn to live with a chronic illness (Gallant 2003). There is caution around the artificial creation of peer support groups and mentoring schemes developed with the intention of providing age-contemporaneous support. These schemes have been found to be potentially detrimental when a power imbalance is formed. These schemes should be used with sensitive support (Embuldeniva et al 2013). The importance of school attendance is obvious and the multidisciplinary team needs to enquire about absence rates and ensure that parents are promoting school attendance. Including childhood peer relationships in medical consultations as a means to improve engagement is not evaluated, the ethical questions in designing such studies are perhaps prohibitive.

For adults social relationships are key, and there is now considerable evidence to suggest that an individual's social context and particularly the support the patient or parent receives from their social network can significantly affect adjustment to chronic illness. In general the important factor is not necessarily how large the social network is, but how satisfied the individual is with their relationships (DiMatteo 2004). This may reflect the fact that although a social network may be present, if interactions are negative or unhelpful then support will not be received from the network; for example conflict within a relationship has been shown to be associated with poorer health outcomes (Smith and Ruiz 2002).

Emotional Impact of a Medical Illness

Given the areas of life that can be affected by illness, it is perhaps not surprising that cardiac and respiratory conditions have an impact on psychological well-being in both adults and children. The illness can also put considerable strain on relationships or act as barriers to developing relationships. For example, adolescents with chronic illness must undergo the same developmental tasks as their healthy peers: physical and sexual growth, personal individuation, intimate relationships, finding a comfortable social group, educational goals and preparation for an occupation. Adult patients with CF may have worries about entering into friendships or sexual relationships because of concern that others may not be able to cope with their illness. The possibility of not being able to have children may also be of concern within a relationship. Evidence suggests that although rates of marriage may be lower than in individuals without CF it is still common with up to 45% of adults reported to be, or have been, married (Yankaskas and Fernald 1999).

Living with a cardiac or respiratory condition can also have significant implications for employment. As illness progresses the individual may become too physically unwell to work full time and may need to work fewer hours, change their line of work or ultimately give up work. The implications of this can be both financial and social. From a financial perspective loss of earnings can place significant burden on a family. Although welfare benefits may be available, these may not equate with previous earnings. In addition some individuals may associate the receipt of benefits with stigma. Helping individuals overcome the psychological barrier to receiving benefits is important to help individuals maintain as good a quality of life as possible.

A major emotional impact of long-term illness is the affect it has on an individual's self-image and self-respect. Diagnosis of a cardiac or respiratory condition, or a major exacerbation of a long-term condition can impact on maintenance of image-defining roles, e.g. as parent, child, spouse or financial provider. HCPs must be aware of and sensitive to the challenges an illness can have not just in terms of changes to treatment management, an inpatient admission or on prognosis, but on changes to defining roles. For example, adults who worked to provide an income for their family but can no longer remain in full time employment may feel they have lost their significant role in the family and as perceived by society. Changes in roles can lead to major loss of self-respect and can result in negative emotions and possibly depression if not managed well. It is therefore important to understand the different roles that are challenged by the individual's illness and not just focus on treatment management. Although role changes are often thought of in terms of those undergone by the patient, significant role changes may also be experienced by those close to the patient. For example, the partner or spouse of an ill individual may have to take up employment to support the family or conversely may feel they are

unquestioningly forced into a caring role. Although for many people this is done without resentment, in some instances it may cause difficulties and it is important that these individuals are provided with sufficient support.

The term 'coping' has often been used to refer to how well individuals manage both the physical and emotional impact of their health condition. Lazarus and Folkman (1984) developed a simple model to explain stress: people make an assessment of the demands a situation presents (primary appraisal) and then the resources they have to meet these demands (secondary appraisal). Where demand outstrips resources, the situation is said to be perceived as stressful and actions are then needed to manage the situation. Coping refers to those actions taken to manage the stress. In cardiorespiratory illness people have many demands placed on them and hence it is not surprising people find the situation stressful. For example, parents of recently diagnosed children and preschoolers report higher levels of parenting stress and depressive symptoms than normal controls (Quittner et al 1992, Simmons et al 1993). Parent stress levels have been found to have a negative effect on the physical health of a child. Problems with family, friends, school and finances correlated with lower pulmonary function and lower height/weight indices over a 15-month prospective study (Finkelstein et al 1992).

In coping with the stress of illness people use a wide range of strategies. Research in a range of cardiac and respiratory conditions tends to suggest that more problem-focused coping is associated with better psychological adjustment, while avoidant strategies are less helpful. For example, Abbott et al (2001) reported avoidant strategies to be associated with poorer adherence to physiotherapy and enzyme regimens; Barton et al (2003) report emotion-focused coping to be associated with poorer adherence, more hospital admissions and more frequent asthma attacks in patients with asthma and Hesselink et al (2004) found emotional coping style to be associated with poorer health-related quality of life in both asthma and COPD. These studies must be treated with caution, however, as the usefulness of a coping strategy will very often be dependent on the particular situation.

Anxiety

Anxiety and panic are common in both respiratory and cardiac conditions, with prevalence typically higher than in individuals without physical health problems (Goodwin et al 2004). The causal relationship between anxiety and particularly respiratory conditions is often not clear, in some instances the experience of breathlessness may precipitate anxiety, in other instances anxiety precipitates breathlessness. Correct diagnosis of anxiety is important for treatment; however, the similarity of the symptoms of anxiety, such as increased breathing and heart rate, sweating, etc., with physiological characteristics of disease can complicate this. In diagnosing anxiety it is therefore important to also focus on the thoughts and feelings associated with anxiety such as feelings of dread, powerlessness or predictions of catastrophe.

Although anxiety can be related to a range of factors in respiratory and cardiac conditions it is commonly precipitated by increased exertion and the fear that activity will cause breathlessness. If individuals fear that they can not manage breathlessness they may then avoid activity; however, this can engender a vicious cycle whereby through lack of activity the person becomes physically deconditioned and hence more easily breathless on exertion, which reinforces the sense of panic and anxiety (Fig. 8-1).

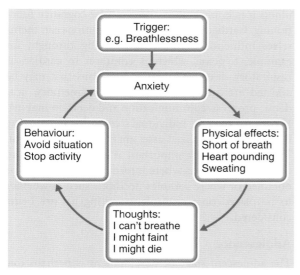

FIGURE 8-1 ■ Cycle of anxious responding.

In managing anxiety a range of interventions may be useful. Explanation of the cycle of anxiety and reduced functioning can be beneficial to help individuals differentiate symptoms due to anxiety versus those caused by their physical illness. Attendance at cardiac or pulmonary rehabilitation programmes where individuals have the opportunity to build confidence in exercising can also be helpful. Where anxiety is chronic or interfering with daily functioning, it may be necessary to refer the individual for specialist psychological input where techniques such as cognitive behaviour therapy have been shown to be of benefit (National Collaborating Centre for Primary Care 2004).

Depression

Like anxiety, depression is common in individuals with chronic illness. In heart failure prevalence rates have been estimated to range from 13% to 77% depending on how depression is assessed (Thomas et al 2003). In a major study looking at long-term risk for depressive symptoms following diagnosis from a range of medical conditions, individuals diagnosed with respiratory and cardiac disease were at higher risk 2 years after initial diagnosis than a number of other conditions including diabetes, hypertension, stroke or arthritis (Polsky et al 2005). A recent study of over 2000 adolescents and adults with CF from 39 centres in the UK urges caution in reporting depressive symptomatology, as rates were not found to be elevated above the general population (Duff et al 2014). There are further studies that throw more light on the importance of diagnostic screening measures used (Quittner et al 2014).

Depression has been shown to be associated with significantly poorer physical outcomes than in individuals without depression. For example in patients with coronary heart disease, depression is associated with poorer adherence with higher mortality and reduced prognosis (Gehi et al 2005).

Unfortunately the physical limitations that cardiac and respiratory conditions place on individuals can trigger a vicious cycle of withdrawal from activity, negative evaluations of life, deepening depression and further withdrawal. Where depression is mild, rehabilitation programmes which incorporate mood and adjustment have been shown to reduce emotional distress and subsequent morbidity and mortality. This is true for both cardiac (Denollet and Brutsaert 2001) and pulmonary rehabilitation programmes (Alexopoulos et al 2006). Alternatively if depression is more severe, referral to a psychologist may be beneficial. Work may then focus on recognizing the association between limitations from the illness and mood state, managing changes in activity levels, scheduling pleasurable events, addressing negative thoughts and focussing on coping strategies to aid adjustment to the current physical state. For individuals where depression is severe and a more cognitive approach is not appropriate, antidepressant medication may be beneficial, although interaction with any current medications for the cardiac or respiratory condition should be taken into account. Importantly, all HCP teams should ensure that annual screening for emotional well-being is conducted (Quittner et al 2014).

End Stage of Life

One of the final challenges for any individual with cardiac or respiratory disease is managing the terminal phase of illness and impending death. It has been theorized that when faced with the certain knowledge of one's end of life, the individual goes through a sequence of reactions (Kubler-Ross 1969); these have also been applied to those grieving following a bereavement. It is now known that this is not an exact series of steps, although many patients find the description of the feelings reassuring. These were described as:

- denial – represented by a lack of acknowledgement of the prognosis
- anger – this may be directed at a range of people or situations or may be turned inwards towards oneself and occurs once the reality of the situation begins to be accepted
- bargaining – often with relation to God
- depression – once bargaining is unsuccessful the patient is said to experience a period of sadness, sometimes to the level of depression
- acceptance – this final stage is said to be where the person accepts the reality and can become at peace with the situation.

In working with people at the end stage of their lives it is important that the HCP gives the patient, whether adult or child, the space to ask questions and also gives permission to discuss this stage of their illness (see von Gunten et al (2000) for discussion of communication techniques at end of life). In discussing dying with patients it is important to elicit specific fears the individual has; for example these may be related to how they may die, whether they will experience pain or more existential issues. Only by identifying the individual's unique worries will appropriate intervention be possible.

A common challenge when working with people who are dying is when family members request that the patient is not told of what is happening. This request may be particularly common with relatives of child patients but can occur with adults as well. Evidence suggests, however, that individuals want information about their health status and that this can help both the patient and family avoid uncertainty, maximize control, bring order to chaos and make sense of the illness (Fallowfield et al 2002). In working with families who request the patient is not told it is important to help the family member understand the advantages of telling the patient, such as allowing open communication about worries and concerns, and the risks of not discussing information with the patient: for example not providing an opportunity to say goodbye.

ENGAGEMENT WITH MEDICAL TEAMS

In managing an individual with cardiac or respiratory illness it is important to also consider cognitive functioning. Cardiac and respiratory conditions can themselves influence cognitive functioning through, for example, hypoxia, which is common in cardiac or respiratory disease. Cognitive functions that may be affected are attention, concentration, memory, academic progress, communication and decision making. If concern over an individual's cognitive functioning is apparent, specialized assessment should be sought. This is particularly important if an individual is to undergo procedures where informed consent must be obtained or where complex decisions such as whether to be placed on a transplant waiting list are being considered.

Adolescence

The adolescent stage of development is perhaps one of the most challenging for children and parents to negotiate; when the teenager also has a life-threatening chronic illness the potential for even greater problems is enormous. It has been termed 'the health paradox of adolescence': on almost every measure adolescence is the healthiest and most resilient stage of childhood development. Adolescents show improvements in speed, strength, reaction time, intelligence, immune function and resistance to cold, heat, dehydration and hunger, and yet overall non-medically related morbidity and mortality rates increase by a great extent compared with that of earlier stages of childhood (Blum and Qureshi 2011). The primary causes of death and injury in the healthy adolescent years are related to problems with poor behavioural and emotional control. The phase is marked by risk-taking and erratic behaviour and the major restructuring of the brain in the adolescent to early adulthood years could be a big clue as to why.

Improvements in neurophysiological assessment show that the adolescent brain undergoes large changes of white to grey matter in the prefrontal cortex, an area responsible for decision making and impulse control. Additionally, the brain embarks on a process of thinning and pruning any unused neural pathways, as well as an increase in myelination. Both these neurological changes result in improved connections between parts of the brain which produces increased speed and enhanced information processing and leads to higher level control of behaviour (Geidd et al 1999).

During this stage of neurological restructuring the underdeveloped prefrontal cortex functions in ways that means the teenager/young adult has difficulty in interpreting emotional expression, displays uninhibited and impulsive behaviours lacking in reasoning, has difficulty modulating negative emotions and fails to consider long-term consequences of actions. So it can be postulated that the teenager and young adult with a chronic health condition does not intend to cause themselves harm by failing to manage their health and treatment but is open to such risky behaviour. By the mid-twenties, most young people have acquired a more mature adult brain which is marked by the development of executive cognitive functioning. This produces the adult-like abilities to plan, organize, assess cost-benefits before acting, act reasonably and allocate attention where it is required. Prior to that stage the adolescent 'brain in development' is more

likely to have a high sensitivity to rewards and a low sensitivity to risk (Lopez et al 2008). It is not surprising therefore that parents find it too risky to hand over control for medical treatment management to their teenage children. The HCP must be fully aware of the neurological and neuropsychological changes that are occurring in the adolescent brain in order to gear engagement effectively and negotiate treatment requirements and goals. There should be avoidance of any suggestion to push the adolescent into independent treatment management too soon. At the same time, the young person should be enabled to take responsibility with controlled risk, being given feedback about the consequences of their treatment choices on their health, not nagged to do it the adult way.

Team Work and Technology

One of the difficulties healthcare teams have is that in many cases there is no clear evidence or sensitive change in measures of the impact of specific treatment on individual health. People with cardiorespiratory conditions show deterioration despite high quality treatment interventions and optimum adherence to those regimens. Adherence to treatment is difficult to measure. Self-report is notoriously unreliable and there is even variance in the estimates of different HCPs in the adherence behaviour of their patient, with physiotherapists being most likely to make a correct assessment (Daniels et al 2011).

There is nowadays the technology to 'chip' drug delivery devices in order to measure rates of adherence in asthma pumps, nebulizers and potentially airway clearance devices commonly used in cardiorespiratory conditions. The initial value of electronic devices was in research to show rates of adherence of drug use in clinical trials and interestingly, rates of adherence appear to be much higher in those patients enrolled in a clinical trial than those on normal treatment regimens (Van Onzenoort et al 2011).

There has been concern that monitoring adherence rates with electronic devices is overly controlling by the medical teams, but in fact quite the opposite can be the case. Studies of adults with CF using a chipped nebulizer provided the healthcare teams with valuable information about ease of use (Daniels et al 2011). People with CF found the timing of the morning dose was almost impossible to maintain over time. Even people with CF who thought they were adherent were surprised by the evidence of their own usage. The outcome was that consultations between patient and HCP became naturally more collaborative. It is possible to download drug usage and compare this to other assessed health parameters such as lung function (Wildman and Hoo 2014). Therefore more accurate and tailored treatment is possible.

The potential to include microchip technology in a range of treatment delivery systems producing downloadable medical and health information that is both physical and psychological is exciting. The advent of smart medicine where test results, adherence rates and lifestyle choices can be available to the patient on mobile phones as well as transmitted to healthcare teams enables a new phase of interactive medicine where collaboration is a normal component in medical review (McDonald, 2013).

CONCLUSION

Cardiorespiratory health conditions require frequently non-negotiable complex daily treatment management, adherence to a nutritional plan and changes in lifestyles. It is not surprising that rates of adherence to daily treatment regimens are low. Engagement with the HCP is essential for collaborative and acceptable treatment management. From the moment of diagnosis the relationship with the HCP is key, whether supporting parents in managing their children or with adults in recognizing the impact of social and emotional factors in living with a chronic medical condition. Physical health status can be affected by the individual's emotional well-being, directly via anxiety or depressive reactions and indirectly in terms of coping styles and perceptions of health status. Health beliefs affect attitudes to treatment adherence and the changes occurring in an adolescent brain give clear direction to the HCP in assessing levels of adherence. Medical teams need to embrace future technological developments to increase the monitoring, feedback and collaborative opportunities for working with patients.

REFERENCES

Abbott, J., Baumann, U., Conway, S., et al., 2001. Cross-cultural differences in health related quality of life in adolescents with cystic fibrosis. Disabil. Rehabil. 23, 837–844.

Abbott, J., Dodd, M., Bilton, D., Webb, A.K., 1994. Treatment compliance in adults with cystic fibrosis. Thorax 49, 115–120.

Alexopoulos, G.S., Sirey, J.A., Raue, P.J., et al., 2006. Outcomes of depressed patients undergoing inpatient pulmonary rehabilitation. Am. J. Geriatr. Psychiatry 14, 466.

Angst, D.B., 2001. School-age children. In: Bluebond-Langner, M., Lask, B., Angst, D.B. (Eds.), Psychosocial Aspects of Cystic Fibrosis. Arnold, London, pp. 125–138.

Baroni, M.A., Anderson, Y.E., Mischler, E., 1997. Cystic fibrosis newborn screening: impact of early screening on parental stress. Pediatr. Nurs. 23, 143–151.

Barton, C., Clarke, D., Sulaiman, N., Abramson, M., 2003. Coping as a mediator of psychosocial impediments to optimal management and control of asthma. Respir. Med. 97, 747–761.

Bluebond-Langner, M., 1991. Living with cystic fibrosis: a family affair. In: Morgan, J. (Ed.), Young people and death. Charles Press, Philadelphia, pp. 46–62.

Blum, R.W., Qureshi, F., 2011. Morbidity and mortality among adolescents and young adults in the United States. <www.jhsph.org>.

Bodenheimer, T., Lorig, K., Holman, H., Grumbach, K., 2002. Patient self-management of chronic disease in primary care. JAMA 288 (19), 2469–2475.

Conway, S., Pond, M.N., Hamnett, T., Watson, A., 1996. Compliance with treatment in adult patients with cystic fibrosis. Thorax 51, 29–33.

Daniels, T., Goodacre, L., Sutton, C., et al., 2011. Accurate assessment of adherence: self-report and clinician report vs electronic monitoring of nebulisers. Chest 140 (2), 425–432.

Denollet, J., Brutsaert, D.L., 2001. Reducing emotional distress improves prognosis in coronary heart disease: 9-year mortality in a clinical trial of rehabilitation. Circulation 104, 2018–2023.

DiMatteo, M.R., 2004. Social support and patient adherence to medical treatment: a meta-analysis. Health Psychol. 2, 207–218.

Duff, A.J.A., Abbott, J., Cowperthwaite, C., et al., 2014. Depression and anxiety in adolescents with cystic fibrosis in the UK: a cross-sectional study. J. Cyst. Fibros. 13 (6), 745–753. in press.

Duff, A.J.A., Latchford, G.J., 2013. Motivational interviewing for adherence problems in cystic fibrosis: evaluation of training healthcare professionals. J Clin Med Res. 5 (6), 475–480.

Embuldeniva, G., Veinot, P., Bell, E., et al., 2013. The experience and impact of chronic disease peer support interventions: a qualitative synthesis. Patient Educ. Couns. 92 (1), 3–12.

Fallowfield, L., Jenkins, V., Beveridge, H., 2002. Truth may hurt but deceit hurts more: communication in palliative care. Palliat. Med. 16, 297–303.

Finkelstein, S., Petzel, J., Budd, S., et al., 1992. Comparative study of physical and behavioral status in cystic fibrosis. Pediatr. Pulmonol. (Suppl. 8), 221.

Frey, M., 1996. Behavioural correlates of health and illness in youths with chronic illness. Appl. Nurs. Res. 9, 167–176.

Gallant, M.P., 2003. The influence of social support on chronic illness self-management: a review and directions for research. Health Educ. Behav. 30, 170–195.

Gehi, A., Haas, D., Pipkin, S., Whooley, M.A., 2005. Depression and medication adherence in outpatients with coronary heart disease:

findings from the Heart and Soul study. Archives Internal Medicine 165, 2508–2513.

Geidd, J.N., Blumenthal, J., Jeffries, N.O., et al., 1999. Brain development during childhood and adolescence: a longitudinal MRI study. Nat Neurosci. 2, 861–863.

Goldberg, S., Gotowiec, A., Simmons, R.J., 1995. Behaviour problems in chronically ill children. J Dev Psychopathology 7, 267–282.

Goodwin, R.D., Fergusson, D.M., Horwood, C.J., 2004. Asthma and depressive and anxiety disorders among young people in the community. Psychol. Med. 34, 1465–1474.

Grob, R., 2008. Is my sick child healthy? Is my healthy child sick? Changing parental experiences of cystic fibrosis in the age of expanded newborn screening. Soc. Sci. Med. 67 (7), 1056–1064.

Hagger, M.S., Orbell, S., 2003. A meta-analytic review of the common-sense model of illness representations. Psychol. Health 18 (2), 141–184.

Hesselink, A.E., Penninx, B.W.J.H., Schlosser, M.A.G., et al., 2004. The role of coping resources and coping style in quality of life of patients with asthma and COPD. Qual. Life Res. 13, 509–518.

Horne, R., Chapman, S.C.E., Forbes, A., et al., 2013. Understanding patients' adherence-related beliefs about prescribed medications: a meta-analytic review of the necessity-concerns framework. PloS ONE 8 (12), e80633. <plosone.org>.

Horne, R., Weinman, J., 1999. Patients' beliefs about prescribed medicines and their role in adherence to treatment in chronic physical illness. J. Psychosom. Res. 47, 555–567.

Kendall, P.C., Chambless, D.L. (Eds.), 1998. Empirically supported psychological therapies. J. Consult. Clin. Psychol. 66, 3–167. (special edition).

Kendall, P.C., Chu, B., Gifford, A., et al., 1998. Breathing life into a manual: flexibility and creativity with manual-based treatments. Cogn. Behav. Pract. 5, 177–198.

Ketler L.J., Sawyer S.M., Winefield H.R., Greville H.W., 2002. Determinants of adherence in adults with cystic fibrosis. Thorax 57, 459–464

Kinmonth, A.L., Woodcock, A., Griffin, S., et al., 1998. Randomised controlled trial of patient centred care of diabetes in general practice: impact on current wellbeing and future disease risk. BMJ 317 (7167), 1202–1208. Oct 31.

Kolbe, J., Vamos, M., Fergusson, W., et al., 1996. Differential influences on asthma self-management knowledge and self-management behavior in acute severe asthma. Chest 110, 1463–1468.

Kubler-Ross, E., 1969. On death and dying. Tavistock/Routledge, London.

Lazarus, R.S., Folkman, S., 1984. Stress appraisal and coping. Springer, New York.

Leventhal, H., Nerenz, D.R., Steele, D.F., 1984. Illness representations and coping with health threats. In: Baum, A., Singer, J. (Eds.), A Handbook of Psychology and Health. Erlbaum, Hillsdale, NJ, pp. 219–252.

Lopez, B., Schwarz, S.J., Prado, G., et al., 2008. Adolescent neurological development and its implications for adolescent substance use prevention. J. Prim. Prev. 29 (1), 5–35.

McDonald, K., 2013. Cystic fibrosis project to trial web real-time communications and shared electronic health record. <Pulseitmagazine.com>.au, April.

Michie, S., Miles, J., Weinman, J., 2003. Patient-centredness in chronic illness: what is it and does it matter? Patient Educ. Couns. 51, 197–206.

Myers, L.B., Horn, S.A., 2006. Adherence to chest physiotherapy in adults with cystic fibrosis. J. Health Psychol. 11 (6), 915–926. 2: 207–218.

National Collaborating Centre for Primary Care, 2004. Anxiety: management of anxiety (panic disorder, with or without agoraphobia & generalized anxiety disorder) in adults in primary, secondary & community care. National Institute of Clinical Excellence, London.

Patterson, G.R., 2002. The early development of coercive family process. In: Reid, J.B., Patterson, G.R., Snyder, J. (Eds.), Antisocial behaviour in children and adolescents: a developmental analysis and model for intervention. American Psychological Association, Washington DC, USA, pp. 25–44.

Polsky, D., Doshi, J.A., Marcus, S., et al., 2005. Long-term risk for depressive symptoms after a medical diagnosis. Arch. Intern. Med. 165, 1260–1266.

Poon, J.L., Doctor, J.N., Nichol, M.B., 2014. Longitudinal changes in health-related quality of life for chronic diseases: an example in haemophilia A. J. Gen. Intern. Med. 29(3) S760–S766.

Quittner, Al, Goldbeck, L., Abbott, J., et al., 2014. Prevalence of depression and anxiety in patients with cystic fibrosis and their caregivers: results of the International Depression Epidemiological Study (TIDES) across nine countries. Thorax 69 (12), 1090–1097. in press.

Quittner, A.L., DiGirolamo, A.M., Michel, A., Eigen, H., 1992. Parental response to cystic fibrosis: a contextual analysis of the diagnostic phase. J. Pediatr. Psychol. 17, 683–704.

Quittner, A.L., Zhang, J., Marychenko, M., et al., 2014. Medication adherence in healthcare use in cystic fibrosis. Chest. 46 (1), 142–151.

Shepherd, S.L., Hover, M.F., Harwood, I.R., et al., 1990. A comparative study of the psychosocial assets of adults with cystic fibrosis and their healthy peers. Chest 97, 1310–1316.

Simmons, R.J., Goldberg, S., 2001. Infants and pre-school children. In: Lask, B., Bluebond-Langner, M., Angst, D. (Eds.), Psychosocial aspects of cystic fibrosis. Arnold Publishers, London, pp. 110–124.

Simmons, R.J., Goldberg, S., Washington, J., 1993. Parenting stress and chronic illness in children. Paper presentation. Society of Behavioural Pediatrics, Providence, Rhode Island.

Smith, T.W., Ruiz, J.M., 2002. Psychosocial influences on the development and course of coronary heart disease: current status and implications for research and practice. J Cons and Clin Psychol. 70, 548–568.

Thomas, S.A., Friedmann, E., Khatta, M., et al., 2003. Depression in patients with heart failure: physiologic effects, incidence, and relation to mortality. AACN Clinical Issues. 14, 3–12.

Towle, A., Godolphin, W., 1999. Framework for teaching and learning informed shared decision-making. BMJ 319, 766–771.

Van Onzenoort, H.A.W., Menger, F.E., Neef, C., et al., 2011. Participation in a clinical trial enhances adherence and persistence to treatment. Hypertension 58, 573–578.

Veldtman, G.R., Matley, S.L., Kendall, L., et al., 2001. Illness understanding in children and adolescents with heart disease. Western J. Med. 174, 171–174.

von Gunten, C.F., Ferris, F.D., Emanuel, L.L., 2000. Ensuring competency in end of life care: communication and relational skills. J. Am. Med. Assoc. 284, 3051–3057.

Widerman, E., 2002. Communicating a diagnosis of cystic fibrosis to an adult: what physicians need to know. Behav. Med. 28, 45–52.

Wildman, M.J., Hoo, Z.H., 2014. Moving cystic fibrosis care from rescue to prevention by embedding adherence measurement in routine care. Paediatr. Respir. Rev. 13 (15), 16–18.

Yankaskas, J.R., Fernald, G.W., 1999. Adult social issues. In: Yankaskas, J.R., Knowles, M.R. (Eds.), Cystic Fibrosis in Adults. Lippincott-Raven, Philadelphia.

Young, B., Dixon-Woods, M., Windridge, K.C., Heney, D., 2003. Managing communication with young people who have a potentially life-threatening chronic illness: qualitative study of patients and parents. Br. Med. J. 326, 305–314.

9

ADULT INTENSIVE CARE

JENNIFER PARATZ ■ GEORGE NTOUMENOPOULOS ■
ALICE Y M JONES ■ CLAIRE FITZGERALD

CHAPTER OUTLINE

INTRODUCTION 415

MONITORING AND MECHANICAL
SUPPORT 416
Mechanical Ventilation 416
Monitoring of the Body Systems 419

PROBLEM IDENTIFICATION AND
PHYSIOTHERAPEUTIC INTERVENTIONS
IN ICU 423
Broad Problems 424
Interventions 426
Specific Conditions in ICU 430

PHYSIOTHERAPY MANAGEMENT OF WORK OF
BREATHING AND CONCEPTS OF WEANING
FROM MECHANICAL VENTILATION 435

Work of Breathing 436
Waveform Analysis – Assessment of Patient–
Ventilator Synchrony 436
Lung/Thoracoabdominal Compliance and Airway
Resistance 440
Respiratory Muscle Strength and Weaning 440
Weaning from Mechanical Ventilation 441

CONCLUSION 447

REFERENCES 449

INTRODUCTION

Management of the intensive care patient involves both respiratory management and early intervention to prevent and improve muscle and joint function. The major role of the physiotherapist in the intensive care unit (ICU) is to maintain lung volume, improve oxygenation and ventilation, optimize secretion clearance as well as maximize musculoskeletal function and facilitate return of independent function upon ICU discharge. In some centres, our role may also lead to advanced or extended scope of practice that includes extubation/decannulation, ventilator weaning, lung recruitment and troubleshooting mechanical ventilation problems. Physiotherapists should not only acquire competency in techniques necessary for treatment intervention but must also demonstrate the ability to manage complications that might arise as a consequence of their actions.

Furthermore, a greater understanding by the physiotherapist of the relationship between other organ systems, haemodynamics and ventilatory management will optimize the quality of patient care and lead to an extension of the physiotherapist's scope of practice, in liaison with a multidisciplinary team.

This chapter will discuss methods of monitoring and supporting the major organ systems of the body and the implications for physiotherapy intervention. The second section of the chapter adopts a problem-based approach and will focus on the place of physiotherapy in the ICU.

MONITORING AND MECHANICAL SUPPORT

Mechanical Ventilation

Mechanical ventilation is used for patients with respiratory failure or to support other organ systems. Traditional (and most common) modes of ventilation include **volume-controlled ventilation** (ventilator rate and fixed volume), **pressure-controlled ventilation** (ventilator rate and fixed pressure) and **pressure-supported ventilation** (spontaneous mode with pressure support and positive end expiratory pressure as adjuncts) (Fig. 9-1). *The general move towards less use of sedation and 'sedation breaks' (Kress et al 2012) promotes the use of spontaneous ventilation modes and reduces time on ventilation and delirium.*

In general, 'open lung/protective ventilation' is the preferable ventilation strategy for patients post major insult and at risk of ventilator induced lung injury (VILI), wet lungs and acute respiratory distress syndrome (ARDS). Open lung/protective ventilation refers to ventilation with small tidal volumes (6–8 mL/kg) and plateau pressures (<30 cmH$_2$0) (Serpa et al 2012). The partial pressure of carbon dioxide in arterial blood (PaCO$_2$) may be allowed to rise and the alveoli remain inflated with optimal positive end-expiratory pressure (PEEP) (Levitt and Matthay 2006). There is level 1 evidence for low tidal volumes compared to larger tidal volumes, leading to a decrease in mortality (Petrucci and Iacovelli 2007).

With the aim of limiting lung damage and preserving spontaneous breathing, methods of ventilation such as bi-level ventilation are more commonly used. Biphasic positive airway pressure (BiPAP)/bi-level is pressure-controlled ventilation with two levels of continuous positive airway pressure (CPAP) (P$_{high}$ and P$_{low}$), with a set mandatory breathing rate. The inspiratory to expiratory (I:E) ratio can be adjusted. The mandatory breaths are pressure-controlled and the spontaneous breaths can occur throughout the respiratory cycle and can also be pressure supported (often only at P$_{low}$). Thus bi-level ventilation can be used as pressure-controlled ventilation initially in sedated or paralyzed patients, with progression to spontaneous breathing in this mode to optimize gas exchange. Weaning to CPAP and pressure-supported mode (to allow spontaneous breathing) and then to CPAP alone is the commonly used process to liberate the patient from mechanical ventilation. Figure 9-2 shows the biphasic waveform on a ventilator monitor screen.

Less conventional methods of ventilation still aiming to limit lung damage and preserve spontaneous breathing are also utilized; these include:

- pressure control–inverse ratio ventilation (PC–IRV)
- airway pressure release ventilation (APRV)
- high-frequency ventilation (oscillatory or jet or percussive ventilation).

The following descriptions are summarized from the review by Hess (2002).

Pressure Control–Inverse Ratio Ventilation (PC–IRV)

This mode of ventilation aims to maintain a constant pressure during inspiration. The physiological basis for adopting this mode of ventilation is that the 'prolonged' inspiration promotes alveolar expansion through alveolar recruitment with increased mean airway pressures. The I:E ratio is higher (e.g. 1:1 or 2:1) compared with the traditional 1:2. Thus complete exhalation from the alveoli with slower time constants is prevented by the short expiratory time; expansion of the alveoli is maintained by auto-PEEP (generated by the longer inspiratory time). The combination of decelerating flow and maintenance of airway pressure over time results in the inflation of stiff (non-compliant) lung units with long time constants, for example, in patients with ARDS.

Airway Pressure Release Ventilation (APRV)

This mode of ventilation maintains CPAP with intermittent release of the pressure (essentially an inverse ratio form of bi-level ventilation). The duration of release is rather short and similar to PC–IRV, and results in an inverse I:E ratio mode of ventilation. Patients who are able to breathe spontaneously with a relatively low work of breathing can utilize APRV, thereby minimizing barotrauma and circulatory compromise and optimizing gas exchange. This mode of ventilation may not be suitable for patients with asthma or severe chronic obstructive pulmonary disease (COPD), as expiratory flow is not optimal with the short expiratory time.

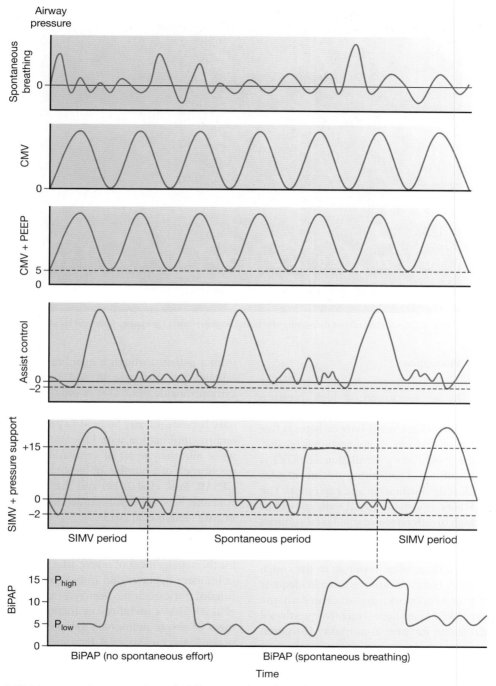

FIGURE 9-1 ■ Diagrammatic presentation of different modes of ventilation. BiPAP, Biphasic positive airway pressure; CMV, controlled mandatory ventilation; PEEP, positive end-expiratory pressure; SIMV, synchronized intermittent mandatory ventilation.

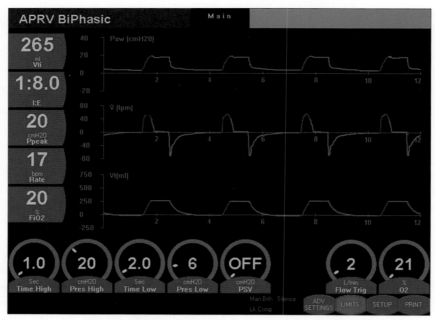

FIGURE 9-2 ■ A monitor screen displaying the biphasic waveforms (pressure, flow and tidal volume).

High-Frequency Ventilation

High-frequency ventilation can be jet ventilation or oscillation. In jet ventilation, a high pressure (30–300 kPa) of air with supplementary oxygen is delivered to the airway via a small-bore catheter at frequencies between 60 and 300 Hz. Expiration is passive.

High-frequency oscillatory ventilation (HFOV) is oscillation of a continuous distending pressure at rates of 3–15 Hz with active inspiration and expiration. The advantage of HFOV is a stable CPAP, with control of ventilation at high breath rates and small tidal volumes (50–100 mL). The patient needs to be very heavily sedated and/or paralyzed to minimize or prevent spontaneous respiration, often resulting in the cough reflex being abated. Humidification is often inadequate with this form of ventilatory support. The early use of HFOV for ARDS has been recently questioned with potential for an increase in mortality (Ferguson et al 2013).

Other Forms of Ventilation and Adjuncts

Extracorporeal membrane oxygenation (ECMO) and *extracorporeal carbon dioxide (CO₂) removal (ECCO₂R)* are processes whereby blood is continuously pumped from a patient through a membrane oxygenator that imitates gas exchange to add oxygen and remove carbon dioxide (*ECCO₂R* is only for CO_2 removal). These devices are not too dissimilar to cardiopulmonary bypass and may be used to provide gas exchange and in combination with lung rest, and may be used when all other forms of ventilation have failed. The publication of a number of recent trials (most notably CESAR, Peek et al 2010) and the 'swine-flu' (H1N1) epidemic have led to substantial increases in the use of ECMO (Pham et al 2013).

Inhaled *nitric oxide* can be used as a selective pulmonary vasodilator. It has been used for many decades for the management of severe arterial hypoxaemia and pulmonary hypertension in both adults and children. Inhaled nitric oxide has been recommended (Germann et al 2005) as a useful rescue therapy for the management of severe pulmonary arterial hypertension and severe refractory arterial hypoxaemia, but does not confer any survival benefits in adults.

Monitoring of Patients on Mechanical Ventilation

Careful observation of the patient data from the mechanical ventilator including pressure, flow and volume waveforms will assist the physiotherapist in identifying the level of synchrony between the patient and the mechanical ventilator, including any potential causes of increased work of breathing or changes in lung/thorax compliance (e.g. lung collapse) or airway resistance (e.g. bronchospasm, airway secretions) in a mechanically ventilated patient.

Monitoring Respiratory Muscle Function. Respiratory muscle weakness can be associated with prolonged mechanical ventilation and weaning delay or failure. Maximal static inspiratory and expiratory efforts, electromyography of respiratory muscles, respiratory rate, carbon dioxide level, pressure–time product, vital capacity and maximum voluntary ventilation are all variables which reflect respiratory muscle function. Respiratory rate and tidal volume presently remain the most convenient and frequently used indices of respiratory muscle function (e.g. respiratory rate/tidal volume provides a rapid shallow breathing index (Bissett et al 2012). These measures may be used to assess the readiness of the patient to breathe spontaneously and to be weaned from ventilatory support.

Lung Mechanics. Improvement in lung volume is associated with improvement in the elastic properties of the lung. The relationship between changes in lung volume and transpulmonary pressure is referred to as 'static lung compliance (l/cmH_2O)'. Static lung compliance should be measured during 'cessation of air flow', when elastic recoil is independent of airway resistance. Dynamic lung compliance can be measured during 'uninterrupted' respiration.

The change in lung volume and pressure are measured at end-inspiration (compliance) and end-expiration (auto-PEEP); this is when airflow 'momentarily' ceases during the 'normal' respiratory cycle. Most mechanical ventilators in ICU display/calculate dynamic lung compliance, and auto-PEEP as well as airway resistance.

Monitoring of the Body Systems

Rapid, potentially lethal physiological and pathological changes can occur in an acutely ill patient; hence essential bodily function must be adequately monitored and supported to optimize patient care. While monitors and equipment are essential for primary measurement and support, the interpretation of the data in concert with astute patient observation ensures that patients will be safely and effectively managed.

Respiratory System

Respiratory function is best assessed by analysis of measures of oxygenation and ventilation, such as oxygen saturation and arterial blood gases. An understanding of the mechanics of breathing is essential to determine the work of breathing required to achieve a certain level of gas exchange. Emerging modalities in assessment for physiotherapists also include electrical impedance tomography (Caruana et al 2011) and ultrasound (Via et al 2012). Lung ultrasound is a real-time imaging modality that is radiation free, non-invasive and has increasing popularity within critical care. Lung ultrasound has proven to be more accurate that the bedside portable chest radiograph for the detection of consolidation, pneumonia, pneumothorax, pleural effusion and pulmonary oedema (Xirouchaki et al 2011). However, it has yet to be adopted by physiotherapists within critical care. Lung ultrasound may prove to be an ideal modality to enhance our understanding of the conditions managed within critical care and the responses to physiotherapy intervention. Further information on lung ultrasound can be found in Chapter 7.

Oxygenation

ARTERIAL BLOOD GASES. Arterial blood gases (partial pressure of oxygen, carbon dioxide, and pH) provide essential information about a patient's metabolic and respiratory status. Interpretation of arterial blood gases, the oxygenation ratio and alveolar–arterial oxygen (A–a) gradient are discussed in Chapter 2.

Pulse oximetry and inline capnography are essential monitoring for the intensive care patient. Mechanisms and interpretation are described in detail in Chapter 2. Detailed 'indications' for capnography can be found in the American Association for Respiratory Care (AARC) Clinical Practice Guidelines on Capnography/Capnometry during Mechanical Ventilation (AARC 2011).

Cardiovascular System

Arterial Blood Pressure. Intra-arterial measurement (commonly radial or femoral artery) should normally be considered accurate, but the systolic pressure may be overestimated due to systolic 'overshoot' (a property of the fluid–pressure transducer monitoring system). The 'area' under the arterial tracing can provide a rough estimate of the cardiac output (Michard 2005). If the arterial trace dips on inspiration (arterial swing), this is an indication that the patient is hypovolaemic and may require fluid. Positive pressure techniques such as manual or ventilator hyperinflation should be avoided or modified until fluid balance is adjusted. The use of automated non-invasive blood pressure (NIBP) devices is common. The **mean arterial pressure (MAP)** ((systolic − diastolic)/3 + diastolic blood pressure) most closely approximates capillary perfusion pressure and is thus a useful measurement.

Central Venous Pressure. Central venous pressure (CVP) reflects systemic blood volume, venous return and right heart filling pressures. This is sufficient to guide fluid therapy in the majority of patients. It is usually monitored by a catheter inserted via the internal jugular or subclavian vein, and less frequently via the femoral vein. Normal values are 8–10 mmHg in the non-ventilated patient, and 12–16 mmHg if the patient is on positive pressure ventilation; however, as the right ventricular preload is determined by the volume and not the pressure, the absolute value of CVP is less meaningful. The response to a fluid load is more useful information. A high CVP value, however, may be associated with conditions that cause a rise in the right atrial pressure (for example right heart failure, reduced right ventricular diastolic compliance, hypervolaemia and pulmonary hypertension) (Gray et al 2002), whereas a low CVP value may suggest hypovolaemia.

Urine Output. Urine output is an index of renal perfusion and is a guide to adequacy of cardiac output. With normal renal perfusion, the urine output should be at least 0.5 mL/kg hour^{-1}.

Electrocardiogram. The electrocardiogram provides information on the rate and rhythm of the heart; it also assists in the diagnosis and identification of the possible site of myocardial infarction. Interpretation of the electrocardiogram is discussed in detail in Chapter 4.

As critically ill patients are more complex and potentially more unstable, a higher level of monitoring is often required, providing information on cardiac output, vasodilatory state, venous saturation, right heart function and fluid responsiveness. A number of monitors both invasive and non-invasive are utilized. The parameters provided by each monitor and clinical implications are described in Table 9-1. It is important to note that in some conditions there is a 'pattern of response' (Table 9-2), and a normal value in this case would represent lack of compensation; for example systemic vascular resistance is increased above normal in hypovolaemic or cardiac shock. A number of monitors can be utilized for these measures, including the highly invasive but accurate pulmonary artery thermodilution catheter ranging to less invasive methods utilizing Doppler technology. The most commonly used in ICUs today are pulse pressure methods, which measure the pressure in an artery over time to derive a waveform, such as PiCCO (Fig. 9-3) and LiDCO-*plus*. Echocardiography, both transthoracic and transoesophageal, is also increasingly used within the ICU.

Neurological System

Level of Consciousness. The Glasgow Coma Scale (GCS) (Bordini et al 2010) is the most common way to measure the level of consciousness. GCS scores range from 3 to 15. A score of 8 or less suggests severe head injury, 9–12 moderate injury and 13–15 mild injury. Pupil size and level of reactivity to light provide an index of neurological integrity (pupils equal and reactive to light (PERL)). A fixed dilated unilateral pupil indicates pressure on the oculomotor nerve and urgent investigation is necessary. Fixed dilated pupils indicate severe neurological impairment (often indicating sustained severe increase in intracranial pressure (ICP)), which may be made worse by hypoxia or biochemical abnormalities and are often a sign of brainstem death. A number of scoring systems are used in intensive care to asses the level of sedation, with the most commonly used being Richmond Agitation Sedation Scale (RASS), Riker scale and the Comfort scale (De Jonghe et al 2000). These can be a useful guide to the level of cooperation available from the patient. Importantly the majority of these scales also assess agitation and can be safety measures in treatment planning.

TABLE 9-1
Haemodynamic Variables, Normal Values and Implications for Management

Variable	Definition	Normal Values	Explanation	Implications for Management
Cardiac output (CO)	Stroke volume × heart rate, volume of blood pumped by heart in one minute	4–8 L/min	<4 L/min heart is not pumping adequately, often poor prognosis	Abnormal values may be due to a number of conditions, need to look at other variables
Cardiac function index (CFI)	Inotrophic state of heart	4.5–6.5 L/min	<4.5 L/min indicates poor myocardial contractility	If less than 4.5 L/min may not tolerate techniques which require an increased demand from myocardium
Pulmonary artery occlusion pressure or 'wedge pressure' (PAOP)	Indicator of left ventricular filling pressures	6–12 mmHg	Response to a fluid load is important, <6 mmHg with no response to fluid indicates hypovolaemia, >15 mmHg indicates overload	If low, may not be able to tolerate positive pressure techniques, e.g. MHI, VHI or upright positioning
Intrathoracic blood volume index (ITBVI)	Indicator of circulating blood volume and cardiac preload	850–1050 mL/m^2	<850 = underfilled, >1050 = adequate to overfilled	If low may not be able to tolerate positive pressure techniques, e.g. MHI, VHI or upright positioning
Extra vascular lung water index (EVLWI)	Water content in lungs	3.0–7.0 mL/kg	>7.0 mL/kg leakiness, ↑ in left heart failure, ARDS, pneumonia, sepsis, burns	Can discriminate and predict acute lung injury. If increased take precautions for potential ventilator induced lung injury, i.e. low inspiratory pressures, low tidal volumes and maintenance of PEEP
Systemic venous resistance (SVR)	Measure of vasoconstriction/ dilatation of peripheral blood vessels, i.e. afterload, 80 × (mean arterial pressure − mean pulmonary capillary wedge pressure)/cardiac output	700–1600 dyn/s cm^{-5}	<700 dyn/s cm^{-5} vasodilated	If less than 700 may not be able to tolerate positive pressure techniques, e.g. MHI, VHI or upright positioning
Pulmonary vascular resistance (PVR)	Resistance offered by vasculature in lungs, 80 × (mean pulmonary arterial pressure − mean pulmonary capillary wedge pressure)/cardiac output	20–130 dyn/s cm^{-5}	>130 dyn/s cm^{-5} vasoconstricted, increases due to hypoxaemia, right heart failure, obstruction	Important to identify cause, relieving hypoxaemia will decrease PVR

Continued on following page

TABLE 9-1				
Haemodynamic Variables, Normal Values and Implications for Management *(Continued)*				
Variable	Definition	Normal Values	Explanation	Implications for Management
Stroke volume variation (SVV)	Difference in SV over 30 seconds	10–15% normal	15% underfilled SVV <10% overloaded	If greater than 15%, is hypovolaemic and may be unable to tolerate positive pressure techniques, e.g. MHI, VHI or upright positioning
Mixed venous oxygen saturation (SvO_2)	Tissue oxygenation	60–80%	Balance between oxygen supply and demand	If SvO_2 low, O_2 supply insufficient or O_2 demand ↑, metabolic stress If SvO_2 high, then O_2 demand has ↓ or O_2 supply has ↑

ARDS, acute respiratory distress syndrome; *MHI,* manual hyperinflation; *PEEP,* positive end-expiratory pressure; *SV,* stroke volume; *VHI,* ventilator hyperinflation.

TABLE 9-2							
Clinical Patterns in Various Shock States							
	Cardiac Output	Systemic Venous Resistance	Pulmonary Vascular Resistance	Arterial Blood Pressure	Heart Rate	Central Venous Pressure/PCWP	Peripheries
Hypovolaemic shock	Low	High	Normal	Low	High	Low	Cold
Cardiogenic shock	Low	High	High	Low	High	High	Cold, clammy
Distributive, e.g. sepsis, shock	High	Low	Normal → High	Low	High	Normal	Warm, dry
Pulmonary embolus	Low	High	High	Low	High	Normal → High	Cold
Cardiac tamponade	Low	High	High	Low	High	High	Cold
Spinal shock	Low	Low	Normal	Low	Low	Low	Warm, dry

PCWP, pulmonary capillary wedge pressure.
NB: Note that these patterns can vary according to whether the patient is compensated or decompensated and patients may have more than one clinical problem.

Cranial Computed Tomography Scan. Computed tomography (CT) of the head provides information about the brain and skull. A plain skull radiograph may identify fractures of the skull and CT with contrast is used for investigation of intracranial space-occupying lesions (haemorrhage, tumour or abscess). Magnetic resonance imaging (MRI) is now more commonly used when scanning neurological patients.

Intracranial Pressure. ICP is measured by insertion of a catheter through the skull into the lateral ventricle or by means of an extradural or subarachnoid bolt (Feyen et al 2012). ICP is often monitored in patients with head injuries, post brain surgery and for patients with intracranial and subarachnoid haemorrhage. The intraventricular catheter has the advantage of allowing drainage of cerebrospinal fluid (CSF) when the ICP is

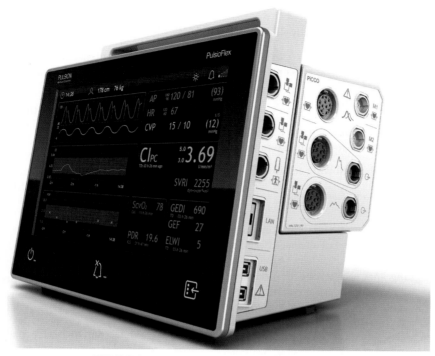

FIGURE 9-3 ■ PiCCO. *(©Pulsion Medical Systems AG)*

BOX 9-1
CALCULATION OF CEREBRAL
PERFUSION PRESSURE (CPP)

CPP = MAP − ICP

CPP, Cerebral perfusion pressure; *ICP*, intracranial pressure; *MAP*, mean arterial pressure.
Ulatowski (1997)

high but because it penetrates the dura, there is a greater accompanying risk of intracranial infection. Any change in the ICP is dependent upon the relative amounts of blood, brain and CSF within the adult skull. ICP allows determination of global cerebral perfusion pressure (CPP), which relates closely to cerebral blood flow (CBF) (Box 9-1).

Raised $PaCO_2$ results in an increase in CBF, which will cause a rise in ICP and a lowering of CPP. Controlled hyperventilation may lower the $PaCO_2$, thus reducing cerebral vasodilatation and CBF, thereby lowering the ICP. **Normal ICP is 10–15 mmHg**, but baseline levels are often higher in neurosurgical patients. In order to provide adequate perfusion to the brain, it is generally recommended that **CPP should be maintained at a level greater than 60 mmHg** (Huang et al 2006).

PROBLEM IDENTIFICATION AND PHYSIOTHERAPEUTIC INTERVENTIONS IN ICU

Quality of patient care depends on appropriate patient assessment and identification of problems associated with presenting symptoms. Appropriate intervention involves complex decision-making processes. This section discusses broad problems encountered by patients in the ICU and the rationale for interventions to be undertaken. Case studies or common patient scenarios are presented to illustrate the principles of intervention.

Broad Problems

Problems particularly relevant to critically ill patients include:

- decreased lung volumes/lung compliance
- decreased gas exchange
- decreased mucociliary clearance
- increased work of breathing
- weakness of peripheral and respiratory muscles
- development of intensive care acquired weakness.

These are discussed in the following section.

Decreased Lung Volumes, Lung Compliance and Gas Exchange

Intubation, mechanical ventilation and the accompanying sedation can result in a number of adverse effects on the respiratory and cardiovascular system. Ventilation/perfusion mismatching may occur due to preferential ventilation of the non-dependent areas (increased dead space) of the lung, while the poorly ventilated dependent areas still receive preferential perfusion (increased shunt), especially in the supine position. The monotonous pattern of positive pressure ventilation without spontaneous respiration may impair gas exchange (Hedenstierna et al 1985) and the absence of sighs during mechanical ventilation leads to decreased surfactant release, decreased lung compliance and progressive pulmonary atelectasis (Antonaglia et al 2006). Decreased functional residual capacity (FRC) also occurs because of cephalad displacement of the diaphragm and loss of lung volumes, both of which occur predominantly in the dependent zones. Alveoli may develop different levels of resistance, those with high resistance taking a longer time to inflate. The different mechanical properties of alveoli may be interpreted as having varying *time constants* (the product of alveolar *compliance* × *resistance*). A long time constant indicates an alveolus that opens slowly during tidal inflation.

In the immobilized ventilated patient, progressive atelectasis will result in a further decrease in lung compliance and gas exchange. The patient may also have a diffusion defect due to factors such as pneumonia, alveolar thickening or ARDS.

Decreased Mucociliary/Secretion Clearance

Normal mucociliary clearance depends on a complex interaction between ciliated columnar cells in the tracheobronchial tree and special viscoelastic properties of the bronchial secretions. As well as the presence of an invasive airway, immobility and decreased conscious level, the intensive care patient may have a number of factors that specifically impair mucociliary clearance, which include:

- ciliary denudation by the endotracheal or nasotracheal tube
- pharmacological agents, including barbiturates
- activation of the inflammatory mediator system
- high levels of inspired oxygen
- high inspiratory pressures/PEEP
- low tidal volume
- trauma from suctioning
- volatile anaesthetic agents
- impaired cough
- sub-optimal humidification
- inspiratory flow bias during mechanical ventilation and gravity (causing the retrograde flow of mucus) (Li Bassi et al 2012).

Premorbid factors such as a history of smoking, chronic respiratory disease and/or severe neuromuscular disorders other than impaired respiratory muscle strength may also further impair mucociliary/secretion clearance.

Intubation and mechanical ventilation can inhibit normal mucociliary clearance and be associated with secretion retention and pneumonia (Konrad et al 1994). Current ventilator strategies predispose towards an inspiratory flow bias (Ntoumenopoulos et al 2011), which may predispose towards secretion retention. Remaining intubated and ventilated for longer than 48 hours is reported to cause heavy colonization with anaerobic bacteria (Agvald-Ohman et al 2003). The colonization of bacteria may be partly due to suction-induced lesions of mucous membranes. These bacteria are then capable of synthesizing and releasing toxins capable of further impairing ciliary mobility and causing a loss in epithelial integrity. It is important that the physiotherapist understands the mechanisms of impaired mucociliary clearance in the intubated ventilated patient and appreciates which methods of intervention are most effective.

Mucociliary clearance in healthy, non-intubated patients includes the cough mechanism. In the intubated patient, mucociliary clearance may be facilitated by the mechanism of annular two-phase gas liquid transport (Chapter 7) In brief, this is a non-ciliary dependent phasic flow with energy transmitted from moving air to static liquid, resulting in shearing of the secretions (for example forced expiratory manoeuvres, manual lung hyperinflation). The detection of secretion retention is often based on clinical examination; however, we have yet to develop a gold standard for its diagnosis. Novel outcome tools have been explored such as vibration response imaging, essentially a computerized lung sound monitoring device (Ntoumenopoulos and Glickman 2012). Other devices such as TBA Care are connected in circuit to the endotracheal tube (ETT) and detect the presence of airway crackles, and may be useful as an indicator of the need for airway suctioning (Lucchini et al 2011).

Weakness of Respiratory and Peripheral Muscles

Mechanical ventilation for as little as 48 hours has been demonstrated to decrease diaphragm strength (Sassoon et al 2002) and endurance of respiratory muscles (Chang et al 2005, Picard et al 2012) and is associated with mitochondrial dysfunction and lipid accumulation. Respiratory and peripheral muscle weakness due both to immobilization and muscle degradation and myocyte degeneration result in hospital acquired infections, increased time on mechanical ventilation, longer hospital stay and reductions in quality of life with significant functional limitations.

Increased Work of Breathing

There are many means of assessing the lung/thorax mechanics, work of breathing and metabolic cost of breathing in an intubated and mechanically ventilated patient (Table 9-3).

Work of breathing in the mechanically ventilated patient will increase if there is asynchrony between the patient and the ventilator: that is, the ability of the mechanical ventilator to respond promptly to patient demand for flow during inspiration, to cycle from inspiration to expiration and to allow an unimpeded expiration.

TABLE 9-3		
Measures of Work of Breathing, Lung Thorax/Mechanics and Metabolic Consumption		
■ $P_{0.1}$	Amount of negative pressure generated (effort) in first 100 msec of inspiration	Most modern ventilators can measure this value automatically, with normal values of 2–5 cmH_2O. Increased $P_{0.1}$ indicates excessive work of breathing to trigger inspiration and hence may require increased inspiratory support and/or reduced ventilator trigger sensitivity or increased sedation.
■ NIF/MIP	Maximal inspiratory force generated – effort dependent, normal values 70–100 cmH_2O	
■ Intrinsic PEEP/gas trapping	Amount of PEEP generated at the end of a normal passive expiration estimating the amount of gas trapped in the lung	normal = 0 cmH_2O
■ Oesophageal balloon monitoring	Oesophageal balloon catheter placed to measure negative oesophageal pressures as an estimation of pleural pressure	
■ Direct/indirect calorimetry	Expired ventilator gas measure of oxygen consumption and carbon dioxide production as a measure of metabolic consumption of the patient	
■ Weaning indices – f/V_T	Breath frequency in bpm divided by tidal volume as fraction of 1 L with value of <105 being potentially predictive of weaning success	For example, for a patient with respiratory rate 50 bpm and tidal volume 400 mL, the weaning index will be 50/0.4 = 125, and thus not suitable for weaning.

bpm, breaths per minute; *f/Vt*, rapid shallow breathing index; *MIP*, maximal inspiratory pressure; *NIF*, negative inspiratory force; $P_{0.1}$, effort in first 100 msec in inspiration; *PEEP*, positive end-expiratory pressure.

An understanding of the basic waveform of ventilatory pattern allows the physiotherapist to obtain much information associated with the patient's work of breathing during mechanical ventilation.

Interventions

The chapter on physiotherapy interventions (Chapter 7) contains several techniques that are also used in the ICU; these include hyperinflation and manual techniques. Only details specific to ICU patients are discussed in this chapter and more detailed information regarding the techniques can be found in Chapter 7. In addition, while the evidence for physiotherapy intervention in critically ill patients is at times conflicting, the algorithm developed by Hanekom et al (a) (2011) (Fig. 9-4) summarizes the best evidence and combined this with expert opinion through the Delphi process.

Hyperinflation Techniques

The ventilated, critically ill patient often has an underlying problem associated with progressive atelectasis due to low tidal volume and/or monotonous breathing patterns, immobility with recumbency in bed and loss of lung compliance combined with impaired mucociliary clearance. Manual hyperinflation (MHI) and ventilator hyperinflation (VHI) have been introduced in an effort to improve ventilation and secretion mobilization through enhanced expiratory flow bias. Recruitment manoeuvres, i.e. a sustained increase in airway pressure with the goal to recruit atelectatic lung tissue, are increasingly in use in ICUs. These techniques are described in Chapter 7.

Manual Techniques

Percussion and Vibration. Evidence for manual techniques such as percussion of the chest wall and vibration during the expiratory phase is discussed in Chapter 7. Precautions applied to manual techniques have been discussed. In intensive care patients, precautions also include decreased platelet levels, skin wounds and chest trauma.

Secretion Removal Techniques

Suction – Open/Closed. As critically ill patients are usually intubated, regular pulmonary toilet must be applied to maintain airway patency. Formerly this was always via the open suction technique: that is disconnection from mechanical ventilation, instillation of a sterile catheter into the ETT to trigger a cough and application of a negative pressure to aspirate secretions. As the patient did not receive ventilation during this period, an efficient technique in less than 15 seconds was always deemed necessary from a safety perspective. Most ICUs now utilize the 'in-line' suction technique (closed-suctioning), whereby a sealed catheter is connected to the ETT and suction is possible without disconnection from the ventilator. The AARC provides evidence-based guidelines on the practice of airway suctioning in intubated and mechanically ventilated patients (2010). This technique has been associated with less risk of desaturation and reduction in lung volume (Cereda et al 2001), fewer arrhythmias, less cardiovascular changes and less reduction of PEEP (Maggiore et al 2003). However, in pressure-controlled modes of mechanical ventilation, the negative pressure from the suction catheter may trigger ventilator breaths, and the inspiratory flow from the ventilator may force the secretions away from the catheter tip, resulting in fewer secretions being aspirated (Lasocki et al 2006). After suctioning, a lung recruitment technique such as MHI or VHI may be required to minimize the risk of atelectasis induced by the negative pressure suctioning generated by either the open or closed system, but this should be judged on patient need.

Nasopharyngeal/Oropharyngeal Suction and Mini-Tracheotomy. Nasopharyngeal and oropharyngeal suction have been discussed in detail in Chapter 7. These techniques are often necessary before and during extubation, as well as in attempt to prevent intubation in patients with ineffective coughing efforts or increased secretions.

Minitracheotomy is often utilized in intensive care and is invaluable for patients with secretion retention, weak cough and contraindications to or intolerance of oral/nasopharyngeal airways. This is also discussed in Chapter 7.

Increased Moisture to Airways

Humidification. Humidification has been discussed in Chapter 7. Humidification is mandatory for patients on mechanical ventilation to reverse some of the

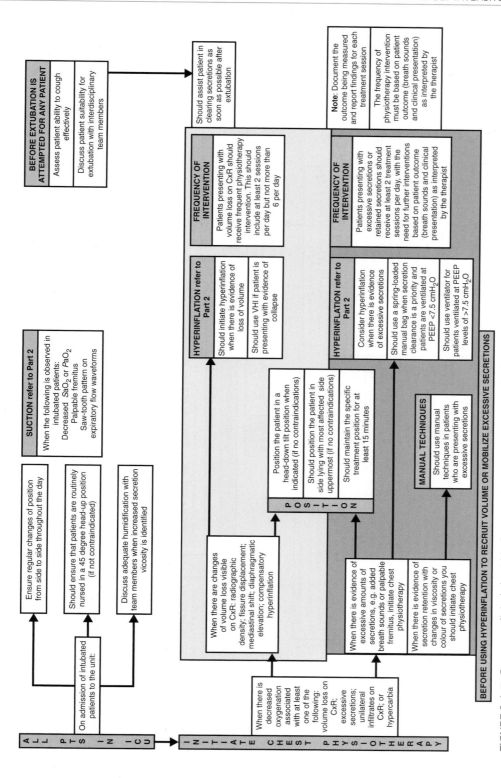

FIGURE 9-4 ■ Consensus clinical algorithm for prevention and management of pulmonary dysfunction in intubated patients. ARDS, Acute respiratory distress syndrome; CPAP, continuous positive airway pressure; CxR, chest radiograph; ICU, intensive care unit; PaO_2, partial pressure of carbon dioxide in arterial blood; PEEP, positive end-expiratory pressure; PTS, patients; SaO_2, oxyhaemoglobin saturation by arterial blood gas VHI, ventilator hyperinflation. (*Reproduced from Hanekom S, Berney S, Morrow B et al (2011) with the permission of John Wiley & Sons.*)

Continued on following page

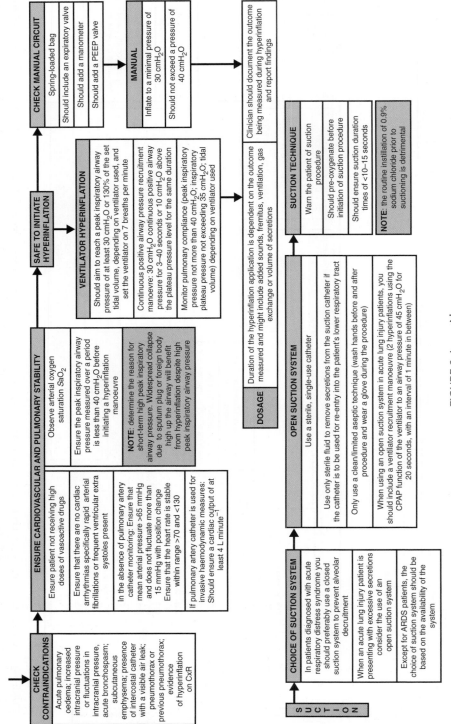

CHECK CONTRAINDICATIONS

Acute pulmonary oedema; increased intracranial pressure or fluctuations in intracranial pressure; acute bronchospasm; subcutaneous emphysema; presence of intercostal catheter with a visible air leak; pneumothorax or previous pneumothorax; evidence of hyperinflation on CxR

ENSURE CARDIOVASCULAR AND PULMONARY STABILITY

Ensure patient not receiving high doses of vasoactive drugs

Observe arterial oxygen saturation SaO₂

Ensure that there are no cardiac arrhythmias specifically rapid arterial fibrillations or frequent ventricular extra systoles present

Ensure the peak inspiratory airway pressure measured over a period is less than 40 cmH₂O before initiating a hyperinflation manoeuvre

In the absence of pulmonary artery catheter monitoring: Ensure that mean arterial pressure >65 mmHg and does not fluctuate more than 15 mmHg with position change Ensure that the heart rate is stable within range >70 and <130

NOTE: determine the reason for short-term high peak inspiratory airway pressure. Widespread collapse due to sputum plug or foreign body high up the airway will benefit from hyperinflation despite high peak inspiratory airway pressure

If pulmonary artery catheter is used for invasive haemodynamic measures: Should ensure a cardiac output of at least 4 L minute⁻¹

SAFE TO INITIATE HYPERINFLATION

CHECK MANUAL CIRCUIT

Spring-loaded bag

Should include an expiratory valve

Should add a manometer

Should add a PEEP valve

MANUAL

Inflate to a minimal pressure of 30 cmH₂O

Should not exceed a pressure of 40 cmH₂O

VENTILATOR HYPERINFLATION

Should aim to reach a peak inspiratory airway pressure of at least 30 cmH₂O or 130% of the set tidal volume, depending on ventilator used, and set the ventilator on 7 breaths per minute

Continuous positive airway pressure recruitment manoeuvre: 30 cmH₂O continuous positive airway pressure for 3–40 seconds or 10 cmH₂O above the plateau pressure level for the same duration

Monitor pulmonary compliance (peak inspiratory pressure not more than 40 cmH₂O; inspiratory plateau pressure not exceeding 35 cmH₂O; tidal volume) depending on ventilator used

Clinician should document the outcome being measured during hyperinflation and report findings

DOSAGE

Duration of the hyperinflation application is dependent on the outcome measured and might include added sounds, fremitus, ventilation, gas exchange or volume of secretions

SUCTION

CHOICE OF SUCTION SYSTEM

In patients diagnosed with acute respiratory distress syndrome you should preferably use a closed suction system to prevent alveolar decruitment

When an acute lung injury patient is presenting with excessive secretions consider the use of an open suction system

Except for ARDS patients, the choice of suction system should be based on the availability of the system

OPEN SUCTION SYSTEM

Use a sterile, single-use catheter

Use only sterile fluid to remove secretions from the suction catheter if the catheter is to be used for re-entry into the patient's lower respiratory tract

Only use a clean/limited aseptic technique (wash hands before and after procedure and wear a glove during the procedure)

When using an open suction system in acute lung injury patients, you should include a ventilator recruitment manoeuvre (2 hyperinflations using the CPAP function of the ventilator to an airway pressure of 45 cmH₂O for 20 seconds, with an interval of 1 minute in between)

SUCTION TECHNIQUE

Warn the patient of suction procedure

Should pre-oxygenate before initiation of suction procedure

Should ensure suction duration times of <10–15 seconds

NOTE: the routine instillation of 0.9% sodium chloride prior to suctioning is detrimental

FIGURE 9-4, cont'd

adverse effects of intubation such as reduced tracheal mucus velocity and cilial impairment.

A critically ill patient on high concentration of inspired oxygen will also benefit from heated humidification. However, a heat and moisture exchanger (HME) can be used as an alternative but has been associated with increased circuit dead space and resistance to airflow and may also increase the viscosity of secretions and lead to increased artificial airway occlusions with increased days of use. It may also be associated with an increased work of breathing in spontaneously breathing patients who are on low levels of respiratory support (Boots et al 2006). The use of HMEs may increase $PaCO_2$ in patients with acute lung injury (ALI)/ARDS (Moran et al 2006) due to increases in dead space. Nebulization with normal saline via the ventilator circuit has been reported to increase the yield of airway secretions (O'Riordan et al 2006).

Saline Instillation. Direct instillation of normal saline into the endotracheal or tracheostomy tube during or prior to suction in an attempt to decrease viscosity of secretions is a frequently used yet sometimes controversial technique. While a number of studies have found that this practice results in temporary decreased oxyhaemoglobin saturation measured by arterial blood gas (SaO_2) and/or mixed venous saturation, no increase in secretion yield and possible dislodgement/dispersion of microorganisms into the lower respiratory tract, there were methodological limitations in these studies (Paratz and Stockton 2009). A recent single-centre trial reported that use of saline instillation during suctioning resulted in lower rates of ventilator-associated pneumonia (VAP) (Caruso et al 2009). This technique requires further investigation.

Positioning

The physiological effects and rationale of positioning have been covered in detail in Chapter 7. Altering the position of a critically ill patient is a powerful tool and may result in both beneficial and adverse effects. Cardiovascular changes associated with positional changes, especially in critically ill patients, should be closely monitored during physiotherapy. An adequate understanding of the pathophysiology of positioning and its predicted effects is essential.

Gravity-Assisted Positioning. Traditional gravity-assisted positions (Chapter 7) are often not utilized in intensive care patients as full positioning may be hindered by cardiovascular instability, equipment and lack of patient cooperation. However, evidence suggests that specifically positioning the patient for the affected lobe results in increased expiratory flow rate, better oxygenation, increased sputum clearance and faster resolution of lobar collapse without adverse effects on haemodynamic stability (Berney et al 2004, Li Bassi et al 2011). Head-down positioning (lateral Trendelenburg) may also assist to prevent VAP and is currently the subject of a large multicentre trial (Zanella et al 2012).

Prone Positioning. Prone positioning for extended periods of time has been advocated as a method to improve oxygenation and lung mechanics in patients with ACI and ARDS. There is strong evidence that this method results in improved lung mechanics and oxygenation due to expansion of the collapsed dorsal regions of the lung (Messerole et al 2002) with reductions in alveolar instability and lung hyperinflation. This technique is most useful if used early in the disease process and may also result in increased secretion clearance due to drainage of the collapsed dorsal regions of the lung. The recent PROSEVA trial (Guérin et al 2013), reported that in the intervention arm nursed prone for 16 hours per day, there was a halving of 28- and 90-day mortality.

Lateral Positioning. The effects of lateral positioning will depend on pathology of the lung, whether unilateral or bilateral and mode of ventilation. To maximize alveolar expansion, lung segments to be expanded are often placed in the uppermost (non-dependent) lateral position for facilitation of aeration, especially with positive pressure ventilation. However, blood flow will preferentially move to the dependent lung (even more so during positive pressure ventilation); hence there may be potent effects on gas exchange dependent upon the extent of pulmonary disease (unilateral or bilateral).

In patients with unilateral lung disease, lying the patient on the non-diseased lung may improve gas exchange and facilitate secretion drainage (Ibanez et al 1981). However, a small trial failed to demonstrate any consistent benefits with lateral positioning (Thomas et al 2007). In adopting lateral positioning to optimize gas exchange, the physiotherapist should be aware of the mode of ventilation, monitored variables (tidal volume, airway pressures), inotropic and vasoactive requirements and cardiovascular status (blood pressure, heart rate). For example re-positioning a heavily sedated intubated patient who is receiving a pressure-controlled mode of ventilation (such as pressure support) and who has copious secretions and a poor cough may lead to severe reductions in tidal volume (and hence minute ventilation) due to the movement of secretions in the major airways, which may alter airway resistance.

Continuous Lateral Rotation Therapy or Kinetic Therapy. Continuous lateral rotation therapy or kinetic therapy consists of continually changing the position of the patient (to extreme lateral position) in specially designed hydraulic beds. The beds are costly but have been proposed to increase the clearance of airway secretions (Davis et al 2001), reduce the rate of development of VAP (Dodek et al 2004, Kirschenbaum et al 2002), resolve atelectasis if combined with percussion (Raoof et al 1999) and improve inflammatory mediators after trauma (Bein et al 2012). There is some preliminary evidence of improvements in major patient outcomes in specific patients groups such as cardiogenic shock (Simonis et al 2012) and post-traumatic ALI (Bein et al 2012); however, there are also reports of impairment in respiratory mechanics and ventilation with prolonged steep lateral positions (Schellongowski et al 2007), and reports of high rates of patient intolerance of the beds. Further research is warranted for this technique.

Non-Invasive Ventilation (NIV)

BiPAP, CPAP and intermittent positive pressure breathing (IPPB) have been covered earlier in Chapter 7. These modes of ventilation are of particular use in the critically ill patient in attempting to prevent intubation in respiratory failure or in weaning and extubation. Patients with chronic obstructive airways disease, chronic heart failure, obesity and renal failure are often at risk of reintubation and ventilation following extubation. These patients may benefit from some form of NIV post extubation.

High Flow Oxygen

Humidified high flow nasal prong (cannula) (HFNP) oxygen therapy is a method for providing oxygen and enables flows exceeding a patient's peak inspiratory flow. HFNP may act as a bridge between low flow oxygen and ventilation, reduce the need for nasal CPAP/intubation or provide support post extubation. At high flow of 2 L/kg min^{-1}, using appropriate nasal prongs, a positive distending pressure of 4–8 cmH$_2$O is achieved. This improves FRC, thereby reducing work of breathing. Because flows used are high, heated water humidification is necessary to avoid drying of respiratory secretions and for maintaining nasal cilia function (Ricard 2012).

Mobilization in Critical Care

Greater numbers of patients are surviving intensive care but a new syndrome of 'post–intensive-care syndrome' has appeared with residual physical (30–50%), cognitive and psychosocial problems (30–60%) lasting from 5 to 15 years (Oeyen et al 2010). A combination of the catabolic effects of the major illness, stress response, hospital-acquired infections and certain pharmacological agents can result in the loss of large amounts of muscle mass attributed to a proteolytic or protein degradation process or specific critical care weakness syndromes (Griffiths et al 2010) All of these factors have a major impact on the health and productivity of survivors and carers. Rehabilitation for these patients is discussed in detail in Chapter 13.

Specific Conditions in ICU

This section describes the management of some conditions commonly encountered in the ICU. Common problems associated with the conditions are illustrated as case studies.

Acute Respiratory Distress Syndrome

ARDS and ALI refer to a clinical syndrome potentially caused by a wide variety of insults to the body and characterized by acute onset, refractory hypoxaemia, decreased compliance and bilateral diffuse infiltrates on chest radiograph. The criteria for diagnosis for ARDS has been recently updated and is now termed the 'Berlin definition' (Ranieri et al 2012):

■ timing – within 1 week of a known clinical insult or new or worsening respiratory symptoms

- diffuse bilateral infiltrates seen on chest radiographs, not explained by effusions, lobar/lung collapse, or nodules
- no clinical evidence of congestive heart failure – with the use of echocardiography to rule out hydrostatic oedema if there are no risk factors for ARDS
- mild – 200 mmHg $<PaO_2$/fraction of inspired oxygen (FiO$_2$) $\leq$300 mm Hg with PEEP or CPAP $\geq$5 cmH$_2$O
- moderate – 100 mmHg $<PaO_2$/FiO$_2$ $\leq$200 mmHg with PEEP $\leq$5 cmH$_2$O
- severe – PaO_2/FiO$_2$ <100 mmHg with PEEP $\geq$5 cmH$_2$O
- thoracic imaging (both plain radiographs and CT) is one of the essential components in diagnosis and assessment of ARDS.

Pathogenesis of Acute Respiratory Distress Syndrome. ARDS once carried a mortality rate of 50–80% (Metnitz et al 1999) but this has decreased over time (Sigurdsson et al 2013). The exact mechanisms involved in the pathogenesis of ARDS are unknown, although infiltrating leukocytes and widespread endothelial injury are typical. Alveolar and pulmonary microcirculatory endothelial injury leads to normal inflammatory responses characterized by the release of cytokines and recruitment of neutrophils to the area of inflammation (Boyle et al 2014). This initiates a number of reactions in the lungs, which lead to hypoxaemia.

These conditions cause a general inflammatory response with damage to the alveolar–capillary interface, leading to leakage of fluid into the interstitial space/alveoli and resulting in reduced lung compliance and shunting. Patients are dyspnoeic, tachypnoeic and severely hypoxaemic. Management revolves around 'protective ventilation'; that is low tidal volumes and the maintenance of optimal PEEP (Silversides & Ferguson 2013). If high tidal volumes are given and the ventilator is frequently disconnected, barotrauma, volutrauma and and/or atelectrauma may result. These syndromes are the result of damage from high pressure, high volume and repeated deflation and inflation of alveoli. Biotrauma may also result, where high pressure, volume or shearing of alveoli may result in leaking of inflammatory substances from the lung that

circulate to effect other organs causing multi–organ system failure.

Prone positioning may be beneficial in patients with more severe ARDS (Gattinoni et al 2010, Guérin et al 2013). In the past, physiotherapists were advised that any intervention should occur when the patient was in the subacute stage of ARDS. However, it is reported that certain interventions such as recruitment of the lung and prone positioning may be more successful if introduced early in the disease (Pelosi et al 2002).

Ventilator-Associated Events (VAEs) and Ventilator-Associated Pneumonia (VAP)

VAEs include a number of conditions that can cause worsening of oxygenation in the ventilated patient. If there is additional evidence of infection, this is termed 'ventilator-associated pneumonia' (Raoof et al 2014).

Specific Criteria for the Diagnosis of VAP

- Hypoxaemia in a ventilated patient for more than than 2 days requiring greater than 20% increase in FiO$_2$ or greater than 3 cmH$_2$O increase in PEEP
- Hypoxaemia in the setting of generalized infection or inflammation and antibiotics instituted for a minimum of 4 days
- Laboratory evidence of white blood cells on Gram stain of material from a respiratory infection secretion OR possible/probable presence of respiratory pathogens on quantitative cultures.

Treatment of VAP. The mortality attributable to VAP is significant, and therefore prompt administration of appropriate empiric antibiotic therapy directed at the most prevalent and virulent pathogens is essential. As the most common pathogens are *Pseudomonas, Enterobacter, Acinetobacter,* as well as Gram-positive organisms, multi-drug therapy is often required, although the use of monotherapy versus combination therapy remains controversial (Wilke and Grube 2013).

There is strong evidence (Li Bassi and Torres 2011, Minei et al 2006) that measures such as semi-recumbent positioning, continuous turning, handwashing, aspiration of subglottic secretions, selective digestive contamination and early tracheotomy all result in a decreased incidence of VAP. Physiotherapists may have a role in the prevention of VAP. Some small trials have demonstrated improvements in outcome associated with respiratory physiotherapy including Ntoumenopoulos et al (2002), who found a decreased incidence of VAP (39% vs 8%) as a consequence of respiratory physiotherapy, and Pattanshetty et al (2010, 2011), who also reported improvements in time on ventilation and mortality.

Sepsis and Systemic Inflammatory Response Syndrome (SIRS)

Patients admitted with or acquiring an infection in ICU often develop **sepsis**, that is a systemic response to infection. The diagnosis (Levy et al 2003) involves:

- proven or highly probable infection
- heart rate (HR) ≥90 beats per minute
- respiratory rate (RR) ≥20 breaths per minute
- temperature ≥38.0°C or ≤36.0°C
- white blood cell (WBC) count ≥12 000/mm^3 or ≤4000/mm^3 or >10% immature neutrophils.

If this condition worsens, **sepsis syndrome**, that is sepsis with evidence of organ dysfunction, for example hypotension or renal failure, may develop.

Septic shock is the most extreme manifestation of this condition and refers to sepsis syndrome with hypotension despite adequate fluid resuscitation. There is widespread fluid leakage, peripheral vasodilatation and often an inadequate circulating volume. Patients require vasoactive and/or inotropic support to maintain an adequate blood pressure and cardiac output, and are often monitored with a PiCCO device to enable monitoring of haemodynamic function.

An inflammatory reaction may also develop to a non-infectious insult such as pancreatitis, burns or post organ transplantation. This is termed '**systemic inflammatory response syndrome (SIRS)**'. Criteria for the diagnosis of SIRS include the values listed (HR, RR, temperature, WBC count) without infection present (Klouwenberg et al 2012). Patients with SIRS are generally more haemodynamically stable than patients with sepsis and can tolerate most physiotherapy interventions.

In 2002, at the European Society of Intensive Care Annual Congress, the 'Surviving Sepsis Campaign' was launched, leading to publication of a document for critical care providers and health agencies to reduce the sepsis mortality rate by 25% in 5 years (Schorr and

Dellinger 2014). The recommendations include a 'sepsis care bundle' to optimize patient care. Some of the measures in the 'bundle' are the early provision of antimicrobial therapy, early fluid resuscitation and 'source control' and protective lung ventilatory strategy (to minimize airway pressures/tidal volumes). It is demonstrated that lack of adherence to 'sepsis care bundles' in the first 24 hours of sepsis, results in worse patient outcome (Gao et al 2005).

The scenarios in Case Study 9-1 are common in patients with SIRS and/or sepsis.

Chest Trauma

Chest trauma can range from a single rib fracture to multiple rib fractures with a 'flail' segment and underlying contusions. Accompanying injuries may also include haemothoraxes, pneumothoraxes and solid organ injury (for example to the liver). Patients are admitted to intensive care based on whether they can effectively maintain ventilation, but other criteria depend on whether there are other injuries such as head trauma or laceration to organs such as the liver or spleen. Further risk factors for deterioration following chest trauma include age greater than 65 years old and pre-existing respiratory disease. Elderly patients with three or more rib fractures have been shown to have a five times greater increase in mortality and a four times greater increase in the incidence of pneumonia (Stawicki et al 2004).

The current management of chest trauma is directed towards effective pain relief, avoidance of fluid overloading, early mobilization and avoidance of invasive ventilation if possible. If a flail segment is present, an adequate end-expiratory pressure is required to 'splint' the flail segment in order for the patient to ventilate effectively, which may be successfully managed through NIV.

Figures 9-5A and 9-5B describe the pathophysiological changes present in a severe chest trauma with a lung contusion and the physiological consequences.

These consequences often do not occur until day 2 or 3, leading to a late deterioration. Management of the chest trauma patient must therefore be proactive and aimed at restoring effective ventilation, reversing atelectasis and mobilizing secretions, using a combination of management techniques. Transcutaneous electrical stimulation (TENS) can be an effective adjunct for pain relief even with an epidural in situ.

CASE STUDY 9-1

Synopsis

A 46-year-old female is admitted in respiratory failure following diagnosis of severe community-acquired pneumonia, and ventilated on synchronized intermittent mandatory ventilation (SIMV) 12 breaths × 600 mL, PEEP 7.5 cmH$_2$O, FiO$_2$ 0.4 and pressure support 10 cmH$_2$O. Her chest radiograph demonstrates right middle lobe consolidation and she has purulent secretions on suction. Three hours later, her blood pressure decreases to 85/60 mmHg and heart rate increases to 110/minute. A PiCCO monitor demonstrates the values of cardiac index 5.5 L/min (normal 3.0–5.0 L/min), systemic vascular resistance index (SVRI 800 dyn/s cm^{-5} m^{-2} (normal *1250–1750* dyn/s cm^{-5} m^{-2}), extra vascular lung water index (EVLWI) 7.0 mL/kg (normal 3.0–7.0 mL/kg), intrathoracic blood volume index (ITBVI) 800 mL/m^3 (normal *850–1050 mL/m³*) and cardiac function index (CFI) 6.0 L/min (normal 4.5–6.5 L/min). She is given a large volume of fluid resuscitation and her blood pressure increases to 95/60 mmHg. Noradrenaline 5 µg/min increasing to 9 µg/min over 2 hours is administered.

CLINICAL DECISION MAKING

This patient has developed septic shock and she is in a 'hyperdynamic state.' The low SVRI indicates that the peripheral circulation is widely vasodilated. If an intervention of either increased positive pressure (MHI or VHI) or mobility against gravity was given at this stage, there would be inadequate compensatory reflexes and the circulation would fail. The physiotherapist needs **to delay these procedures until fluid resuscitation is complete; inotrope/vasopressor levels are decreasing;** *and blood pressure and SVRI values are in the normal range* (Paratz and Lipman 2006). However, directed positioning and manual techniques could be used in order to provide 'source control', i.e. removal of the infected organism. Intervention can be well tolerated in critically ill patients (Berney and Denehy 2003). It has been shown that the infectious agent together with inflammatory substances cause direct myopathy due to both decreased protein synthesis and an increased proteolysis within 3 days of the infectious insult. Early physical intervention such as passive movements and functional electrical stimulation should be started, progressing to more upright and active measures (sitting over edge of bed) as she becomes more cardiovascularly stable.

Haematological Problems

Patients with haematological conditions (e.g. leukaemia) commonly develop secondary respiratory problems following bone marrow or peripheral stem cell transplantation and require admission to intensive care as well as mechanical ventilation. This is more likely in patients with decreased lung volumes due to pulmonary fibrosis caused by pre-transplant irradiation (Shankar and Cohen 2001). It is reported that NIV applied proactively in haematological patients with lung infiltrates and hypoxaemia results in decreased mortality (Hilbert et al 2001, Wemke et al 2012).

It is essential for the platelet count of these patients to be checked before invasive interventions (e.g. nasopharyngeal suctioning). Patients with a low platelet count (<20 × 10^9/L) may bleed spontaneously and techniques such as percussion, vibration, resisted exercise and insertion of a nasopharyngeal airway should be avoided. Soft-tipped catheters should be used for airway suction in patients with low platelet counts. Alternative methods of secretion removal such as the active cycle of breathing techniques, mechanical inexsufflation, positive expiratory pressure (PEP), oscillatory PEP and autogenic drainage should be considered if the patient is able to cooperate.

Brain Injury

Injury to the brain may occur due to trauma (local haematoma or diffuse brain injury) or subarachnoid haemorrhage. It is important to remember that while primary damage is irreversible, the outcome can also be affected by indirect or secondary damage to the

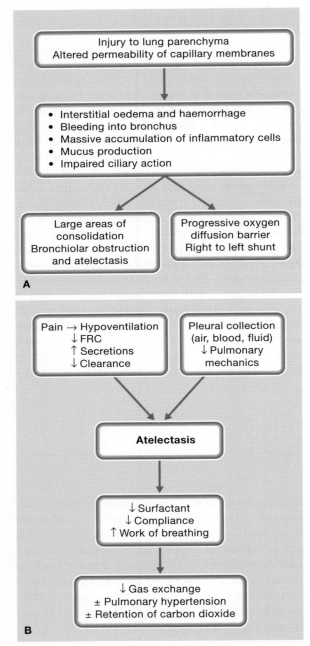

A

B

FIGURE 9-5 ■ **(A)** Pathophysiological changes following chest trauma with lung contusion. **(B)** Physiological consequences of severe chest trauma. FRC, Functional residual capacity.

brain due to such events as hypoxaemia, hypercarbia, cerebral oedema or hypotension. The patient with a brain injury therefore needs to be expertly managed. Normal management of the head-injured patient involves the following principles (Dutton and McCunn 2003):

- control of intracranial volume
- ensuring adequate oxygenation and perfusion of brain
- minimizing metabolism of the brain.

This is achieved by the following management strategies, which may address either one or all three of the above aims:

- maintaining 30 degrees head-up positioning
- monitoring ICP
- drainage of CSF via the external ventricular drain, if indicated
- maintaining the patient in a hypernatraemic state (less water content in brain cells)
- sedation and paralysis in the early stage (days 1–3) in order to limit increases in ICP from coughing and struggling and also to decrease brain metabolism
- prevention of seizures
- hypothermia
- ensuring optimal arterial blood gases
- hyperventilation to maintain $PaCO_2$ 30–35 mmHg
- ensuring CPP ≥60 mmHg using noradrenaline
- barbiturates*
- decompression craniotomy.*

Factors such as ICP, CPP, brain CT scan, changes on chest radiograph and arterial blood gases need to be noted in order to balance the significance of injury of one system over the other. For example a patient with chest radiograph changes, borderline arterial blood gases and low to medium ICP may receive active physiotherapy intervention but a patient with a clear chest radiograph, normal arterial blood gases and high ICP may be treated with position changes only.

---

*These last two methods of management are only used in cases of uncontrollable ICP, and of note a large multicentre trial reported an increase in unfavourable neurological outcomes in patients with decompressive craniectomy (Cooper et al 2011).

When planning intervention in a patient with acute severe head injury, consideration should be given to the following.

- Patient should be treated in a maximally sedated state.
- Treat when ICP is low, <20 mmHg if possible.
- Keep neck strictly in midline – rotation will block CSF and venous blood and increase ICP. Nurse with head up 30 degrees.
- Suction will increase ICP; severe increases in ICP following suction may be prevented by intravenous or topical lidocaine (lignocaine) (Brucia et al 1992).
- ICP is likely to increase during a combined physiotherapy intervention (MHI, suction, manual techniques). Short treatment sessions (<8 minutes) are preferable to a long session (Paratz and Burns 1993, Rudy et al 1991).
- Percussion or vibration if indicated, as sole techniques, do not increase ICP (Paratz and Burns 1993).
- Coordinate management – try to avoid too many interventions e.g. chest radiography, turning, physiotherapy in quick succession. This is more likely to cause increased ICP.
- During MHI an end tidal CO_2 monitor should be used in order to control the $PaCO_2$ between 30 and 35 mmHg or baseline value.
- Head-down postural drainage or prone positions are likely to increase ICP. Research has shown that prone positioning may be well tolerated (in terms of ICP) in head-injured patients (Neklu-dov et al 2006, Thelandersson et al 2006).

Severe Neuromuscular Disease

Acute chest infection with an increase in respiratory secretions may precipitate an acute or chronic episode of respiratory failure in patients with chest wall and/or neuromuscular disease (i.e. motor neuron disease, Duchenne muscular dystrophy, amyotrophic lateral sclerosis). Intubation and mechanical ventilation further impair secretion clearance and increases the risk of VAP (Konrad et al 1994) and patients with neuromuscular disease often require prolonged weaning from mechanical ventilation (Bach 1993). Improved secretion clearance may be important in the recovery process, but is yet to be proven effective. Boitano (2006) provides a comprehensive review of the factors necessary for, and optimal means of, enhancing secretion clearance in the neuromuscular diseased patient.

Patients with severe neuromuscular dysfunction often have a combination of problems, including reduced inspiratory and expiratory muscle strength, increased volume and tenacity of airway secretions, bulbar dysfunction (non-intubated), increased airway resistance and reduced lung/thorax compliance (Boitano 2006). For these patients, conventional chest physiotherapy techniques may be less effective (Ntoumenopoulos and Shipsides 2007). Hence, newer mechanical devices such as the mechanical In-Exsufflator (JH Emerson Co, Mass, USA) have been introduced (Chapter 7). The technique has been poorly investigated to date in intubated patients (Pillastrini et al 2006, Sancho et al 2003). Manual-assisted cough (abdominal compression during the expiration phase following a maximal inspiration) (Chapter 7) is another effective means of enhancing expiratory flow and hence secretion clearance (Boitano 2006).

PHYSIOTHERAPY MANAGEMENT OF WORK OF BREATHING AND CONCEPTS OF WEANING FROM MECHANICAL VENTILATION

While increased sedative and narcotic use can achieve greater patient–ventilator synchrony, in the short term (Richman et al 2006) these agents, as well as neuromuscular blocking agents, have been shown to be associated with an increased duration of mechanical ventilation, weaning time and time in the ICU (Arroliga et al 2005). During activities when the patient's demand for ventilation may increase (e.g. physiotherapy or situations such as anxiety and sepsis) a simple manoeuvre such as increasing the inspiratory flow rate or a change over to a pressure-controlled mode may increase patient comfort and assist in the reduction of sedative requirement. A better understanding of the interaction between the ventilator and the patient will thus facilitate the role of the physiotherapist in the management of patients receiving mechanical ventilation. This section will discuss the concepts of work of breathing in patients receiving mechanical ventilation and issues that facilitate the weaning of patients from mechanical ventilation.

Work of Breathing

Work of breathing may include the work undertaken by the patient as well as the work by the ventilator. While minimizing the patient's work of breathing is the main interest for most clinicians, the optimal balance between the level of work from the patient and the level of support from the ventilator is still unknown. For example, too much respiratory rest as may be achieved with mandatory modes or high levels of pressure support may lead to diaphragm atrophy (Grosu et al 2012). The patient's work of breathing is dependent on the type of pulmonary disease, respiratory muscle strength, airway (and/or tracheal tube) diameter, airway secretions, anxiety, sedatives, narcotics, neuromuscular blocking agents, the mode of mechanical ventilation/settings and the level of synchrony between the patient and the mechanical ventilator.

A patient's work of breathing may be described as the amount of muscle activity required to overcome the elastic (lung tissue, chest wall and abdominal compartments) and resistive (airways, flow rate) elements of the respiratory system.

The waveform of the patient's ventilatory pattern can provide much information about the lung/thoracic compliance and airway resistance. Figure 9-6 illustrates a typical volume-delivered breath with an inspiratory pause (generated by closure of the ventilator valves at the end of inspiration).

The main cause of high peak airway pressure (in volume-controlled mode) or low tidal volume (in pressure-controlled mode) in an intubated patient may be related to problems with airways resistance: for example, a small ETT, high flow rates, secretions, bronchospasm, patient biting the ETT or the patient 'fighting' the ventilator. In patients with volume-controlled or dual-mode ventilation, if both the peak and plateau pressures (see Fig. 9-6) are high relative to the tidal volume delivered (5–6 mL/kg), this may indicate stiff or poorly compliant lung, e.g. diffuse parenchymal disease such as ARDS or pneumonia.

A more accurate measure of static lung/thorax compliance requires the delivery of a volume-controlled breath with a known plateau/pause pressure with the patient deeply sedated not making any respiratory effort, using the formula:

Tidal volume/(Plateau pressure − PEEP).

An accurate plateau pressure exists only if a long enough inspiratory pause (with zero flow) of 1–3 seconds is incorporated in the ventilator pattern (Barberis et al 2003). In order to optimize the interaction between the patient and the mechanical ventilation, it is important to ensure patient–ventilator synchrony (ability of the mechanical ventilator to promptly respond to patient demand for flow during inspiration and to allow an unimpeded expiration), which may increase patient comfort and reduce energy expenditure and the requirements for sedation.

Waveform Analysis – Assessment of Patient–Ventilator Synchrony

Considering that most mechanical ventilators now display real-time ventilator waveforms such as pressure, flow and volume across time or as loops (pressure/volume, flow/volume), it is important that

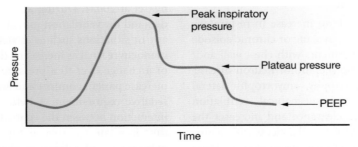

FIGURE 9-6 ■ The waveform of a typical volume-controlled breath, illustrating a reliable plateau pressure that allows measurement of dynamic lung/thorax compliance (= TV / [PIP − PEEP]) and static lung/thorax compliance (= TV / [Plateau pressure − PEEP]).

physiotherapists familiarize themselves with basic waveform analysis and the expected changes with therapy or alterations to mechanical ventilatory support.

Specific patient interventions, such as patient re-positioning and secretion movement, may adversely affect ventilation (reduced tidal volume, minute volume), particularly in pressure-controlled modes such as PCV or BiPAP. The early detection of untoward changes in waveforms allows the clinician to optimize the ventilator settings (by altering the PEEP or pressure settings), modify treatment (increase the head up tilt) and provide intervention (airway suctioning) to minimize any disruptions to the ventilation delivered or suggest the need for emergency manual lung ventilation when insufficient mechanical ventilation occurs (e.g. due to airway occlusion).

Bedside waveform analysis (Tables 9-4 and 9-5) can be used to determine the presence of specific clinical problems such as excessive patient trigger, missed breath attempts, inadequate inspiratory flow, prolonged inspiration, gas trapping and airway secretions.

For this section it will be assumed that the patient is able to breathe in an assisted mode of ventilation (e.g. SIMV with pressure support). The normal pressure waveform is shown in Figure 9-6.

The three variables that determine the patient interaction with a mechanical ventilator are:

- initiation of inspiratory flow (flow or pressure trigger) – the 'trigger' variable
- the volume or pressure to be delivered – the 'set inspiratory' variable, and
- the transition from inspiration to expiration phase – the 'cycling off' variable (Georgopoulos et al 2006).

Troubleshooting for Ventilator Triggering. See Table 9-4 Curve A and Curve B.

Troubleshooting for Inadequate Inspiratory Flow Rate (Volume Modes). See Table 9-4 Curve C.

Troubleshooting – Cycling from Inspiration to Expiration. See Table 9-4 Curve D.

Troubleshooting – Gas Trapping/Intrinsic–Peep. See Table 9-5 Curve A.

Intrinsic PEEP

Gas trapping due to intrinsic PEEP may lead to ventilator asynchrony (Murias et al 2013). Patients with intrinsic PEEP who are triggering breaths have to generate a larger negative intrapleural pressure that is at least equal to the level of intrinsic PEEP plus the trigger sensitivity level of the ventilator before a breath can be triggered and delivered. Thus if the PEEP is set at 5 cmH$_2$O, and intrinsic PEEP is 5 cmH$_2$O, the total PEEP is in fact 10 cmH$_2$O; i.e. although the set inspiratory trigger is –1 cmH$_2$O (below PEEP), the patient has to generate a negative intrapleural pressure of at least 6 cmH$_2$O to trigger a breath. This may result in ineffective or wasted patient effort to trigger a ventilator breath, resulting in patient–ventilator asynchrony (see Table 9-4 Curve B). The expiratory flow waveforms should also be checked to ensure complete exhalation before the next breath delivery (see Table 9-5 Curve A). Adequate exhalation before the next inspiration should occur, not only during mandatory breath delivery but also during spontaneous ventilation modes such as CPAP and pressure support. Incomplete exhalation (to zero flow or baseline) puts the patient at risk of attempting to trigger inspiratory gas flow before expiration is complete (see Table 9-5 Curves A and B). This may also potentially lead to ineffective triggering efforts and patient–ventilator asynchrony (see Table 9-5 Curve B), with missed breath attempts.

Airway Secretions. Airway secretions in the mechanically ventilated patient may be difficult to detect through conventional means (auscultation, chest palpation) for the following reasons:

- inability to position the patient properly for examination
- inadequate inspiratory and expiratory flow rates to create turbulent flow (e.g. due to low levels of CPAP and pressure support).

Ventilator flow waveform analysis can assist in the detection of airway secretions, as it could induce a 'saw-tooth' pattern or jagged waveform during the expiratory flow (see Table 9-5 Curve C). The removal of the condensate from the ventilator circuit is necessary as it may cause the artefact of sawtoothing, and lead to the false impression of secretion retention.

TABLE 9-4

Pressure Waveforms of Common Clinical Problems, Causes and Clinical Signs (Volume-Controlled)

Abnormal Ventilator Waveform Appearance	Description and Potential Causes
A Pressure Curve (Triggering) *Excessive trigger* 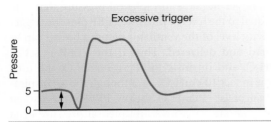	**Pressure Curve** At the start of pressure curve there is a negative deflexion greater than 1–2 cmH$_2$O, followed by positive pressure breath delivery Potential causes: ■ excessive trigger settings (e.g. pressure trigger set at −4 cmH$_2$O) ■ patient distress/agitation/ETT intolerance ■ inadequate inspiratory support ■ respiratory muscle weakness Clinical signs: ■ accessory muscle use at start of breath ■ increased work of breathing/patient distress.
B Pressure Curve (Breath Attempts) *Missed breath attempts* 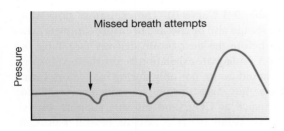	**Pressure Curve** Negative deflexion(s) in the pressure curve *(arrows)*, below PEEP level without inspiratory flow or positive pressure being delivered Potential causes: ■ excessive trigger setting (pressure or flow setting) ■ intrinsic PEEP ■ ineffective patient effort Clinical signs: ■ respiratory distress/accessory muscle use ■ paradoxical respiratory attempts ■ mismatch between respiratory rate on ventilator and actual patient respiratory rate/attempts at breathing (e.g. total ventilator respiratory rate 12, but calculated rate on basis of observation 22 bpm).
C Pressure Curve (Flow Rate) *Inadequate flow rate* 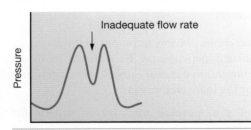	**Pressure Curve** Negative inflexion in the pressure curve during inspiratory phase *(arrow)*, due to patient inspiratory effort exceeding set ventilator flow rate, often coined 'bunny ears' in appearance with no change in inspiratory flow rate Potential causes: ■ volume-controlled mode with inadequate fixed inspiratory flow rate. Clinical signs: ■ patient appears to be triggering an additional breath during ventilator breath ■ paradoxical respiratory attempts during ventilator.
D Pressure Curve (Inspiratory Time) *Prolonged inspiration* 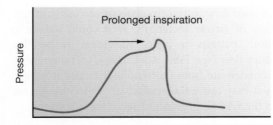	**Pressure Curve** A positive inflexion at the end of inspiration on the pressure/time curve *(arrow)*, indicating the patient is attempting to exhale while the ventilator is still delivering inspiratory flow Potential causes: ■ prolonged inspiratory time or excessive inspiratory pressure/tidal volume. Clinical signs ■ expiratory muscle activation at end of inspiratory phase of respiration of ventilator.

bpm, Breaths per minute; *ETT*, endotracheal tube; *PEEP*, positive end-expiratory pressure.

TABLE 9-5
Flow Waveforms of Common Clinical Problems, Causes and Clinical Signs (Volume-Controlled)

Abnormal Ventilator Waveform Appearance	Description and Potential Causes
A Flow Curve (Expiratory Flow) *Gas trapping* 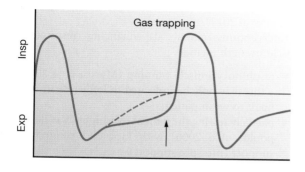	**Expiratory Flow Curve (End Curve)** Expiratory gas trapping (*arrow* indicates that expiratory flow is still occurring before next positive pressure breath is delivered). Normal exhalation Potential causes: ■ bronchospasm ■ COPD ■ ARDS/ALI ■ high set respiratory rate, long inspiratory time, with insufficient expiratory time ■ insufficient PEEP. Clinical signs: ■ expiratory muscle use during expiration ■ hyperinflated appearance. May result in reduced blood pressure due to raised intrathoracic pressure *(Note: some intensivists disconnect the patient from mechanical ventilator at end of expiration to assess a rebound increase in blood pressure)*
B Flow Curve (Expiratory Flow) *Missed breath attempts* 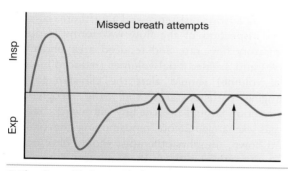	**Expiratory Flow Curve** Missed breath attempts *(arrows)* – patient attempts to trigger inspiratory flow Potential causes: ■ bronchospasm ■ COPD ■ ALI/ARDS ■ insufficient PEEP. Clinical signs: ■ respiratory distress/accessory muscle use ■ paradoxical respiratory attempts ■ mismatch between respiratory rate on ventilator and actual patient respiratory rate/attempts at breathing (e.g. total ventilator respiratory rate 12 mismatches, patients' actual breath attempts of 22 bpm).
C Flow Curve (Expiratory Flow) Saw-tooth pattern 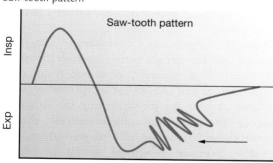	**Expiratory Flow Curve** Saw-tooth pattern *(arrow)* on expiration Potential causes: ■ indicative of secretions in major airways ■ condensate in ventilator tubing. Clinical signs ■ palpable fremitus (chest wall or ventilator tubing) ■ auscultatory signs of airway secretions (crackles, wheezes).

ALI, Acute lung injury; *ARDS*, acute respiratory distress syndrome; *bpm*, breaths per minute; *COPD*, chronic obstructive pulmonary disease; *PEEP*, positive end-expiratory pressure.

Lung/Thoracoabdominal Compliance and Airway Resistance

Reduced lung/thoracoabdominal compliance or increased airway resistance are common causes of increased work of breathing. The mode of ventilation (volume-controlled vs pressure-controlled) may have an impact on the physiological effects of physiotherapy treatment.

Case Study 9-2 examines some issues on ventilation and positioning.

Respiratory Muscle Strength and Weaning

The critically ill patient is predisposed to develop muscle dysfunction/wasting due mainly to inactivity and sepsis, with the consequence of poor activity tolerance, reduced strength and prolonged time on mechanical ventilation in intensive care (Winkelman 2004). The evidence supporting inspiratory muscle training to date has focused on the long-term, difficult-to-wean patient (Aldrich et al 1989, Martin et al 2002). However, inspiratory muscle training may improve respiratory muscle strength or shorten weaning time (Bissett et al 2012).

Interventions aimed at enhancing respiratory muscle strength include:

- respiratory muscle training (Martin et al 2002) – this may only be indicated in longer-term, difficult to wean patients
- partially resting the patient overnight (Vassilakopoulos et al 2006) with increased respiratory support (pressure support)

CASE STUDY 9-2

A 70-year-old female patient has had abdominal surgery complicated by sepsis and ALI due to an infected peritoneum. This patient was ventilated in BiPAP mode, set rate 20 bpm, P_{high} 30 cmH$_2$O, P_{low} 10 cmH$_2$O, FiO$_2$ 0.8, with exhaled tidal volume of 400 mL. The morning chest radiograph demonstrated bilateral diffuse pulmonary infiltrates (alveolar shadowing). The physiotherapist examined the patient and reported bilateral crackles on auscultation with palpable fremitus throughout the left hemithorax. The physiotherapist repositioned the patient into right side lying with the head of the bed flat. The tidal volume reduced from 400 mL to 250 mL, with the respiratory rate unchanged.

What are the implications of the treatment decisions of this physiotherapist?

ANALYSIS

The reductions in tidal volume may relate to the reduced FRC as a result of altered head-down posturing (from head up to head flat) in combination with a pressure-controlled mode of ventilation. In addition, as the patient had palpable fremitus unilaterally, this is indicative of airway secretions, and repositioning into side lying may have caused the movement of secretions to the more central airways or caused direct aspiration of secretions into the dependent lung. The set inspiratory pressure in a pressure-controlled mode (such as bi-level ventilation) does not ensure constant tidal volume with changing airways resistance and lung/thorax compliance. Inspection of the flow waveforms (reduced inspiratory flow rate and reduced area under the curve) and exhaled tidal volumes (reduced exhaled tidal volume) should alert the clinician to the changing patient status and early recognition/intervention should prevent any untoward changes in gas exchange. Before repositioning the patient head down, the physiotherapist should have noted the saw-tooth pattern on the expiratory flow waveform (see Table 9-5 Curve C) and suctioned the airway to clear secretions from central airways to minimize the risk of airway occlusion during patient re-positioning.

Reduced lung/thorax compliance may be improved with the upright sitting position (Behrakis et al 1983). This, however, does not mean that patients cannot and should not be turned for pressure area care or for physiotherapy for secretion clearance (however, the physiotherapist should monitor the tidal volume in pressure modes and inspiratory pressure in volume modes to ensure sufficient minute ventilation is maintained during interventions).

■ general exercise training including activities of daily living such as sitting over the edge of the bed, standing and ambulation (Chiang et al 2006, Zafiropoulos et al 2004).

Weaning from Mechanical Ventilation

Although mechanical ventilation may be lifesaving, it is associated with numerous complications such as VAP, cardiovascular compromise, barotrauma and VILI (Haas and Loik 2012). Mechanical ventilation may be associated with diaphragmatic dysfunction (Jubran 2006) and reduced inspiratory muscle endurance (Chang et al 2005). Once clinical improvement has occurred, emphasis is placed on weaning or liberating the patient from mechanical ventilation (Haas and Loik 2012). However, the value of weaning the patient from the ventilator as soon as possible must be balanced against the risks of premature withdrawal, which may be associated with reintubation, in turn associated with increased mortality (MacIntyre 2004). The imbalance between increased respiratory workload, decreased respiratory muscle strength and endurance may be important factors associated with ventilator dependence (Caruso et al 2005). Shock on admission, increased APACHE II score, ARDS and multiple organ dysfunction are variables significantly associated with prolonged time (>21 days) on mechanical ventilation. These patients also suffer from a high rate of failed extubations, unsuccessful weaning, malnutrition and infection (Estenssoro et al 2006).

Key issues in the management of the ventilated patient are outlined in Box 9-2. Suggested guidelines for extubation are given in Box 9-3.

Weaning Strategies

When the patient's medical condition has been stabilized, weaning off mechanical ventilation is often started. Kuo et al (2006) demonstrated improved predictive accuracy of the measurement of the rapid shallow breathing index at the end of a 2-hour period of spontaneous breathing compared with the traditional method when the measurement is taken at the beginning of the trial. The optimal means to assess appropriateness for weaning and extubation is still evolving.

Controversy exists regarding the most appropriate weaning strategy, the indicators used to assess readiness for weaning/extubation and the use of weaning protocols. Early work (Kollef et al 1997) demonstrated a significantly lower weaning time, when weaning was protocol-led by nurse and therapist compared with physician-led. Weaning protocols may have minimal impact in an intensive care environment where there is a high number of qualified nurses, high physician input, good collaboration between the team members and autonomous nursing decision making in relation to weaning practices (Rose and Nelson 2006). Other weaning strategies include daily T-piece trials, pressure support and extubation to NIV to facilitate the process (Girault et al 1999).

The Physiotherapist's Role in Weaning from Mechanical Ventilation

Non-physician and nurse-led weaning may significantly improve weaning outcomes, but the impact may depend on the medical staffing levels (Krishnan et al

---

BOX 9-2
KEY ISSUES THAT MUST BE ADDRESSED IN THE OVERALL MANAGEMENT OF THE MECHANICALLY VENTILATED PATIENT

When it has been determined that the disease process or processes have begun to stabilize or reverse, clinicians should:

1. understand the reasons why the patient may still require mechanical ventilation (e.g. respiratory system mechanics, resistance, gas exchange, neuromuscular dysfunction, cardiac failure) and their treatment (e.g. secretions, bronchospasm, pleural effusion, cardiac function)
2. use assessment techniques to identify whether the patient can tolerate withdrawal of ventilation (e.g. spontaneous breathing trials, wean off pressure support, rapid shallow breathing index)
3. determine whether the patient requires continued ventilation, and develop an appropriate ventilator management strategy (daily spontaneous breathing trials, mobilization, weaning sedation)
4. provide an extended management plan for the patient who is likely to remain ventilator-dependent.

(MacIntyre 2004)

2004). The physiotherapist's role in weaning could be directed towards:

- early assessment of patient rehabilitation potential (strength, endurance, bed mobility, transfer training)
- assistance with secretion clearance
- respiratory muscle training
- ambulatory ventilation where appropriate
- identification of readiness for extubation (e.g. minimal secretions, effective cough, airway reflexes present, neurological status)
- facilitation of early appropriate endotracheal extubation to institute NIV where appropriate
- assistance with tracheostomy weaning (e.g. periods of spontaneous breathing interspersed with periods of respiratory muscle rest on mechanical ventilation)
- recognizing patients at risk of difficulties in weaning: e.g. COPD, heart failure, obesity,

chronic renal failure, flail chest and being proactive in applying NIV
- appropriate respiratory management including titration of PEEP and pressure support settings to facilitate 'leak speech' or the use of speaking valves.

Tracheostomy

A tracheostomy is often performed in an intensive care patient when long-term ventilation (≥7–10 days) is anticipated. Tracheostomy is also performed if there is concurrent upper airway obstruction, e.g. tumour, trauma, or if equipment dead space poses an unacceptable hindrance to weaning. A tracheostomy may be instituted either percutaneously or surgically, depending on the urgency and physical features of the patient, such as body mass index, condition and head/neck anatomy. Percutaneous tracheostomy is performed at the bedside and uses a Seldinger dilation technique, which usually leaves only a small residual scar. Surgical tracheostomy requires patient transfer to the operating room, a surgical incision and dissection through to the trachea. In some cases, removal of the cricoid cartilage is necessary but the cosmetic result is less acceptable (Friedman 2006). Tracheostomy assists weaning from mechanical ventilation by reducing dead space, decreasing airway resistance, improving secretion clearance and decreasing the need for sedation (Pierson 2005).

Physiotherapists are usually required to optimize lung function in tracheostomized patients and therefore it is important that they understand the functional characteristics of the tracheostomy tube design and the implications for patient care. Tracheostomy tubes are available in different sizes and styles (Hess 2005). They can be of different dimensions, cuffed or uncuffed, single or dual cannula, and fenestrated or non-fenestrated.

Cuffed tubes possess a cuff or balloon that directs all airflow via the tracheostomy tube when inflated, bypassing the native upper airway. This enables the effective delivery of positive pressure ventilation. It also provides some airway protection from subglottic secretions, which is advantageous given that aspiration of oropharyngeal organisms is a major cause of VAP (Safdar et al 2005). This protection is not absolute, although fluid leakage can be minimised with the use of low-volume, low-pressure cuffs (Young et al 2006).

A cuff pressure of 15–25 mmHg is advisable to safeguard an adequate seal for positive pressure ventilation and minimise aspiration whilst maintaining tracheal perfusion (Heffner and Hess 2001). Over-inflation of the tracheostomy cuff has the potential to result in numerous complications such as fistulae, tracheal stenosis and tracheomalacia (Bourjeily et al 2002). If higher cuff pressures are required due to the presence of cuff leak this may indicate a tube too small in diameter, tracheal dilation or malposition of the tube (Morris 2010a).

Cuff deflation restores some of a patient's breathing to the upper airway, allowing potential to regain vocalisation and functional swallow (Bach and Alba 1990). This is conditional in-part on sufficient airflow around the tracheostomy tube. The presence of the floppy deflated cuff provides significantly more resistance to airflow than observed in cuff absence (Beard and Monaco 1993; Hussey and Bishop 1996). Use of an uncuffed tube may therefore be suitable in the patient requiring long-term tracheostomy, even in the presence of an ongoing requirement for mechanical ventilation. However, patients require adequate oropharyngeal muscle strength and pulmonary compliance to effectively use an uncuffed tube (Hess 2005), and their risk of aspiration should be considered low.

Dual-cannula tracheostomy tubes have an inner cannula that is disposable or reusable.

Removal of the inner cannula allows the quick restoration of a patent airway should the tube become occluded, avoiding the risks associated with having to change the entire tracheostomy tube. This makes this tube type particularly desirable in patients with a high sputum load. The negative aspect of using an inner cannula is the reduction in the internal diameter (ID) of the tracheostomy tube imposed by its presence. This can significantly affect work of breathing in a spontaneously breathing individual (Cowan et al 2001). A single cannula tube may be preferred in a patient unable to tolerate such respiratory effort, perhaps in the presence of airway pathology or ventilator dependency.

Regular cleaning of the inner cannula is considered good practice (Mitchell et al 2013), although the frequency for this is variable in the literature. A starting point of four-hourly is reasonable (St George's Healthcare NHS trust 2013), with adjustments to this depending on the tenacity and quantity of a patient's sputum. This may avoid a build-up of secretions that would increase a patient's work of breathing and lead to potential tube obstruction. It may also prevent biofilm formation on the inside of the tube (Bjorling et al 2007), which has been associated with the development of VAP. Cleaning brushes/swabs if used must be soft and non-abrasive to avoid damaging the inner surface of the cannula and promoting biofilm formation.

Fenestrated tracheostomy tubes have a single large or multiple small openings in the posterior wall of the outer tracheostomy cannula. Insertion of a non-fenestrated inner cannula in a dual cannula fenestrated tube allows the tube to function as an ordinary tracheostomy tube. However, there is a risk of surgical emphysema when using positive pressure ventilation with this tube type even when a non-fenestrated inner cannula is in place (Intensive Care Society 2008). The majority of ICUs in the UK therefore use non-fenestrated tracheostomy tubes initially (78%) (Powell et al 2011). It should be noted that suction should not be performed with a fenestrated inner cannula in situ, as this may cause tracheal damage.

Fenestrated tubes allow additional airflow through the native airway and over the vocal cords, and are typically reserved for the patient desiring speech or undergoing weaning from tracheostomy. In the absence of cuff inflation, substantial resistance to inspiratory airflow across the non-fenestrated tracheostomy tube was determined when using a tracheostomy occlusion cap in a tracheal model (Hussey & Bishop 1996). This was significantly reduced with a fenestrated tracheostomy, allowing airflow both through as well as around the tube. The reduction in work of breathing presented by a fenestrated tube should theoretically improve tolerance of tube capping.

In practice, the misalignment of fenestrations is common, and they may become blocked by secretions. An increased risk of granulation tissue formation within fenestrations is also described when they are not properly centred in the airway (Conlan and Kopec 2000). If considering a fenestrated tube it is advisable to regularly check the position and patency of the fenestrations. Another option would be to downsize or change to an uncuffed tube, since this can achieve similar benefits to changes in airflow (Intensive Care Society 2008).

Tracheostomy tubes with subglottic suction capability are also available (e.g. Portex® Blue Line Ultra Suctionaid). Such tubes have a suction port situated above the cuff, allowing intermittent or continuous drainage of secretions to minimise their aspiration into the tracheobronchial tree (Coffman et al 2008). Endotracheal tubes with the capacity for subglottic suctioning have been associated with reduced incidence of VAP (Frost et al 2013), although the clinical efficacy of tracheostomy tubes with this capability has not yet been reported. It should also be considered that a wider outer diameter of the tracheostomy tube is necessitated to accommodate the suction port (Hess 2005).

Dimensions of a tracheostomy tube refer to the length, internal and external diameter, and curvature of the tube. Standard length tubes have been criticised as too short for the average patient in critical care (Mallick et al 2008). Extended length tubes are available with a fixed or adjustable flange. Extended proximal tracheostomy tube length (horizontally) is necessary in patients with an increased pre-tracheal space due to such reasons as obesity, oedema, or distorted anatomy. Increased distal tracheostomy tube length (vertically) may be needed to bypass an area of tracheomalacia or obstruction.

A wider tube provides less resistance to airflow, and is appropriate for the patient expected to breathe entirely through the tube for more comfortable breathing (Mullins et al 1993). However, wider tubes are associated with more difficult speech, swallow and ability to tolerate a tube cap or speaking valve (Beard & Monaco 1993; Hussey & Bishop 1996). Too wide a tube can also lead to damage to the tracheal wall. It is recommended that the outer diameter of the tracheostomy tube should be no larger than two-thirds of the tracheal diameter (Russell 2004).

A narrower tube is preferable for the patient expected to breathe at least partially around the tube, reducing the obstruction to airflow. Caution should be taken when selecting a tube with smaller diameter if continuous cuff inflation is ongoing since this will increase respiratory effort, and high cuff pressures may be required to create an airway seal.

Two different tracheostomy tube sizing systems are in existence; the International Standards Organisation (ISO) sizing system and the Jackson sizing system. The ISO system relates to the ID of the tube, although for dual cannula tubes there is disparity in how manufacturers translate this. For Portex® tubes the sizing refers to the ID of the outer cannula, whereas for Tracoe® it refers to the ID of the inner tube. The inner cannula ID can vary by 1–2 mm between the purportedly same sized Portex® and Tracoe® tubes, which would have a significant impact upon the patient's imposed work of breathing (St John and Malen 2004). The Jackson sizing system as used by Shiley® does not relate directly to tube ID.

Tube Changes. Most manufacturers guide that a tracheostomy tube should be in place no longer than 30 days (Regan and Hunt 2008). Single cannula tubes should be changed every 7–14 days to prevent tube blockage from an excess of secretions (St George's Healthcare NHS trust 2013). The first tracheostomy tube change is recommended to take place at least 5–7 days after initial tube insertion (Kost 2008). This allows time for maturation of the stomal tissue tract, reducing the risk of airway loss or creation of a false passage into the pre-tracheal space. This change ideally should be performed by a practitioner with advanced airway management skills, with subsequent changes performed by individuals with appropriate training (Intensive Care Society 2008).

Routine Tracheostomy Care. The aims of tracheostomy care are to prevent tube dislodgement, maintain skin integrity and airway patency, and ensure patient comfort (Poovathor et al 2011). Correct cuff inflation, inner cannula care, suctioning, humidification and stoma care are key principles in tracheostomy management.

The normal heating, humidification and filtering system of the upper airways is bypassed in breathing via a tracheostomy tube. Supplementary humidification is hence essential in all tracheostomy patients. Humidification systems include heated and cold water systems, and heat and moisture exchangers (HME). A HME retains heat and moisture in a patient's expired air and exploits this to humidify subsequent breaths.

Examples of this include the Thermovent® T (Swedish nose) and Buchanan® protector. A HME can become blocked by secretions and so should be inspected regularly. For the patient requiring oxygen therapy it is preferable to use a heated humidification system (Regan & Hunt 2008). It should be noted that saline nebulisation only complements the different humidification systems (Billau 2004).

Although suctioning may maintain tube patency and reduce the risk of respiratory compromise, routine tracheostomy suctioning is generally not recommended (Barnett 2012). Suctioning should instead be undertaken when secretions are evident visually or audibly in the airway, airway obstruction is suspected, or when tube changes and cuff deflation are performed (Mitchell et al 2013). It is suggested to assess patients for signs of airway secretions every 1 to 2 hours (St John & Malen 2004).

Essential equipment should be kept at the bedside of tracheostomy patients regardless of their location to facilitate emergency care (Intensive Care Society 2008). Continuous waveform capnography monitoring is also advised in all mechanically ventilated tracheostomy patients to enable prompt diagnosis of tube displacement (McGrath et al 2012). However, this may restrict movement of more active patients, and the weight this adds to the tube potentially contributes to displacement.

In the UK specialist multidisciplinary tracheostomy teams are becoming increasingly prevalent (Mace et al 2006), aiming to drive standards in tracheostomy care (Cetto et al 2011). Key team members may include a specialist physician (e.g. ENT or intensivist), head and neck or critical care nurse, a physiotherapist and speech and language therapist. Most teams report meeting a minimum of once-weekly. Such specialist teams have been associated with reduced time to decannulation, adverse events and hospital or ICU length of stay (Garrubba et al 2009; Speed and Harding 2013).

Swallow. Aspiration frequency is high in tracheostomy patients, Ding and Logemann (2005) reporting this in the range of 50–87%, with almost half of aspirators doing so silently. This asymptomatic aspiration was greater in the cuff inflated state. In anchoring the larynx and hindering expiratory airflow, the cuff can impede laryngeal elevation and desensitise the larynx, and may also cause compression of the oesophagus (Morris 2010b).

The modified Evans blue dye has a low sensitivity for detecting clinical aspiration, and is no longer advocated over more formal swallow testing, such as fibreoptic endoscopic evaluation of swallow (FEES) (Regan & Hunt 2008). Compared to FEES, clinical examination of swallow has also been associated with inaccurate estimation of aspiration (Hales et al 2008; Warnecke et al 2013). Radionuclide salivagram may be a more sensitive test of aspiration yet, and frequent suctioning need has also been found to correlate with salivary aspiration in both FEES and salivagram (Kang et al 2013). In the absence of formal testing capability, suctioning requirements alone may hence provide indication of a patient's aspiration status.

Speech. Speech is interrupted in the cuff inflated condition since air bypasses the vocal cords. When cuff deflation is tolerable, speech is still only enabled with the development of sufficient tracheal pressure to drive airflow via the upper airway (Morris 2010c). This can be facilitated by tube occlusion or with the application of positive pressure.

Tube occlusion can be by simple digital occlusion or by the application of a cap or one-way speaking valve (in the absence of cuff inflation). A speaking valve allows inspiratory airflow via the tracheostomy tube, closing on expiration to promote airflow through the upper airway and over the vocal cords. Speaking valves have been associated with restored smell and taste (Regan & Hunt 2008), and reduced incidence of aspiration (Suiter et al 2003). Speech will be augmented when airflow around the tube is maximised, such as with the use of uncuffed and fenestrated tubes, and those with smaller diameters.

Although certain speaking valves can be applied in ventilator circuits, ventilated patients undertaking at least partial cuff deflation may not require this to achieve 'leak speech'. This is enhanced in using PEEP. Low-level PEEP was concluded to be as effective as the Passy-Muir ventilator speaking valve in establishing good patient speech quality (Prigent et al 2010), and speech is further improved in using higher levels of PEEP (Garguilo et al 2013).

Weaning. The presence of a tracheostomy tube is associated with numerous potential complications and impairment of vocalisation, swallow and cough. Unless an irreversible requirement for tracheostomy is present, the minimisation of tracheostomy cannulation time should be sought. Tracheostomy tube removal, or decannulation, may also facilitate discharge from a more acute care setting (O'Connor and White 2010).

Numerous approaches to tracheostomy weaning have been described, including variable durations of cuff deflation, tube downsizing or exchange to a fenestrated tracheostomy tube, and periods of tube occlusion via a cap (Choate et al 2009). There is no consensus as yet of the optimal weaning strategy (Regan & Hunt 2008), and studies comparing tracheostomy weaning processes are limited.

In an international survey of physicians and respiratory therapists, toleration of tube capping was one of the most important decannulation determinants (Stelfox et al 2008). It is believed that the adequacy of the native airway and sufficiency of the patient's ventilatory reserve can be confirmed in the patient successfully breathing around the capped tracheostomy tube (Heffner & Hess 2001). Duration of capping varies in studies from 12 hours (Hunt and McGowan 2005) to up to 96 hours (Ceriana et al 2003). The inability to endure capping potentially requires change to a smaller or fenestrated tracheostomy tube.

Yet capping of the tracheostomy tube does not simulate normal breathing. The remaining tube in the airway imposes a significant obstruction to airflow, and some patients unable to tolerate this extra load on their breathing may still be ready for decannulation (Gao et al 2008; Intensive Care Society 2008). One study has retrospectively compared an older routine of tube downsizing and capping to a newer protocol without the requirement for downsizing or capping (Thompson-Ward et al 1999). Only ability to tolerate cuff deflation for 24–48 hour without need for suctioning was required before decannulation. The newer protocol resulted in a significant decrease in time to weaning of five days ($p < 0.01$) without a significant increase in weaning failure.

A one-step method to planned tube removal has also been proposed (Lewarski 2005; St John & Malen 2004). When the patient meets certain criteria for decannulation, including verification of airflow through the upper airway on cuff deflation, the tracheostomy tube is immediately removed without a period of cuff deflation or tube capping. This has been successfully applied to patients with temporary tracheostomy following oral or oropharyngeal tumour resections (Wasserzug et al 2010), and in a large cohort of ICU patients (Choate et al 2009). In the latter study decannulations occurred in both ICU and ward environments. A low decannulation failure rate was reported (4.8%) and there was no mortality related to decannulation failure.

Clearance of oropharyngeal secretions is advisable prior to cuff deflation, and in the process of cuff deflation simultaneous suctioning below the cuff can be employed. There should be close monitoring of respiratory rate, respiratory muscle work, oxygen saturation and cardiovascular parameters. Respiratory distress, desaturation ($\geq$5%), cardiovascular instability or failure to protect the airway would indicate the need for cuff re-inflation. Assessing the patency of the upper airway can be undertaken by simple finger occlusion of the tracheostomy tube for 60 seconds once cuff deflation is successful, and the absence of desaturation, respiratory distress or stridor may guide readiness for decannulation.

Decannulation. Several studies have explored objective measures to predict successful decannulation, such as upper airway resistance (Gao et al 2008), maximal expiratory pressure (Lima et al 2011) and peak cough flow either through the mouth or via the tracheostomy tube (Chan et al 2010; Fitzgerald et al 2013; McKim et al 2012). These studies have had various limitations, including small patient numbers, and patient groups studied have been heterogeneous making conclusions and recommendations difficult.

In all cases decannulation should be a multidisciplinary decision. Recommended decannulation criteria are listed in Box 9-4. Given sputum retention is a main cause of decannulation failure, attributed to 52.5% of failures in a large observational study of ICU patients (Choate et al 2009), consideration of cough efficacy is particularly important. Consensus opinion also suggests the use of fibreoptic laryngoscopy as a prerequisite to confirm airway patency (Mitchell, et al 2013). A FEES protocol during cuff deflation has

BOX 9-4
CRITERIA FOR DECANNULATION

- Resolution or significant improvement in the original indication for tracheostomy
- Self-ventilating off mechanical ventilation, and considered to have sufficient ventilatory reserve
- $FiO_2 \leq 0.35$
- Effective cough
- Minimal secretions with, suctioning needs < 2 hourly
- No signs of bronchopulmonary infection
- Able to manage their oral secretions (by swallow, expectoration or Yankauer suction)
- Consistent and adequate consciousness level for airway protection
- Cardiovascularly stable
- No significant gastro-oesophageal reflux
- Absent or minimal head and neck oedema
- Airway is maintained with cuff deflation, and airflow via the upper airway is demonstrated without stridor
- No general anaesthesia requirement in the near future

additionally been shown to be highly effective in identifying readiness for decannulation in the critically unwell neurologic patient population (Warnecke, Suntrup, Teismann, Hamacher, Oelenberg, & Dziewas 2013). Patients demonstrating management of their secretions during this protocol could be decannulated immediately without interim weaning steps, with a decannulation failure rate of only 1.9%.

Following tube removal close monitoring should take place for signs of decannulation failure, particularly in the first 24 hours. Emergency equipment should be kept at the patient's bedside during this period. The stoma dressing should be changed once to twice daily, and more frequently if it is becoming soiled, until such time that the site has healed. In most cases this takes around 10 days (De Leyn et al 2007), although rarely surgical closure is required.

A mini-tracheostomy (cuffless tracheal tube) may be appropriate following decannulation if the patient requires assistance with secretion clearance. However, since they are limited to using size 10 French gauge suction catheters they are not useful in the patient with thick, tenacious secretions. As an adjunct to optimise sputum clearance in adults with an acute condition, the evidence for mini-tracheostomies is inconclusive (Beach et al 2013).

Criteria employed to assess each aspect and stage of weaning are controversial. The 'blue dye' test used to assess swallowing is cited in the major international guidelines (Heffner and Hess 2001) but has been shown to have low sensitivity and may give a false-negative result, especially when compared with video fluoroscopy (Ceriana et al 2003). Actual cough strength and ability to clear secretions can be subjective; therefore maximal expiratory pressure (MEP) and/or peak flow measurements have been used to predict the likelihood of being weaned from tracheotomy. A peak cough rate of at least 29 L/min as measured by a Piko-I peak flow metre was suggested to be necessary for successful decannulation in a cohort of neurosurgical patients (Chan et al 2010). During mechanical ventilation, in a stable patient, cuff deflation can be used to facilitate verbal communication (termed 'leak speech' without the use of a speaking valve). Troubleshooting for the management of patients receiving mechanical ventilation is summarized in Table 9-6.

CONCLUSION

The extended role of the physiotherapist in intensive care is topical (McPherson et al 2006). While the role and responsibilities of the physiotherapist vary from country to country and even hospital to hospital in the same city, over recent years physiotherapists have successfully gained greater autonomy and their role within the ICU in weaning, extubation, ventilator and tracheostomy management, fibre-optic bronchoscopy, ICU outreach, post ICU clinics and bedside thoracic ultrasound. Rehabilitation for ICU patients has also emerged as an important treatment and role for physiotherapists in ICU.

This chapter has described various means of monitoring and supporting the major organ systems of the body and the implications for physiotherapy intervention, and adopted a problem-based discussion of various physiotherapeutic interventions in the ICU. The inclusion of waveform analysis associated with mechanical ventilation, concepts of weaning from the ventilator and the role of the physiotherapist in optimization of work of breathing, all aim to encourage a greater awareness of the extended scope of their role in intensive care. Tables 9-4 and 9-5 provide a quick reference table for ventilator troubleshooting and

TABLE 9-6

Troubleshooting – Management of Patients Receiving Mechanical Ventilation

Events	Possible Causes	Possible Action
High-pressure alarm signals (volume- or dual-controlled modes)	Patient is restless and/or with asynchronous breathing	■ Calm the patient ■ Auscultate breath sounds – right and left side equal? ■ Check tidal volume ■ Check with nurse/doctor for sedation ■ If the patient has adequate respiratory drive, check with doctor to consider pressure-controlled/CPAP/pressure support modes which might be more comfortable for the patient
	Increased airway resistance ■ Position of ETT ■ Secretions ■ Bronchospasm	■ Check ETT ■ Auscultate – coarse crackles/wheezes? ■ Suction airway ■ Discuss with medical team – bronchodilators
	Obstruction in airway ■ Secretions ■ Patient biting the tube	■ Suction airway ■ Insert Guedel airway or bite block to stop biting of ETT ■ MHI and saline lavage
	Poor compliance (stiff lung) ■ Pulmonary oedema ■ Pleural effusion ■ Pneumothorax	■ Auscultate breath sounds – right and left side equal? ■ Check chest radiograph and appropriate management of condition ■ Consider reducing set inspiratory flow rate in volume-controlled or change over to pressure- or dual-controlled ventilation
Low-pressure alarm signals	■ Disconnection of circuit ■ Cuff leak ■ Large negative pressure patient effort ■ Malfunction of the ventilator	■ Check tidal volume/expired minute volume ■ Manually ventilate the patient while checking and reconnecting the circuit ■ Check cuff pressure ■ Check function of ventilator
Slight drop (1 to 2 cmH₂O) in airway pressure in volume-controlled mode is normal after physiotherapy (no alarm signal)	The patient's lung compliance and/or airway resistance has improved (e.g. after secretion clearance)	■ No action required
Hypoxaemia	Incorrect settings	■ Increase FiO₂ ■ Check settings (tidal volume, rate, PEEP) and alter settings if necessary
	Circuit/airway disconnection	■ Check tidal volume/expired minute volume ■ Auscultate breath sounds ■ Manually ventilate the patient while checking and reconnecting the circuit
	Secretions	■ Auscultate breath sounds ■ Suction airway (if secretions are tenacious and/or poor cough, saline and/or MHI may be required)
	Malposition of the tracheal tube (e.g. down right main bronchus)	■ Auscultate breath sounds ■ Check position of ETT at lip level, check ETT ties ■ Check chest radiograph
	Pneumothorax/pleural effusion	■ Auscultate breath sounds – right and left side equal ■ Check chest radiograph
	Onset of new medical problem (e.g. sputum plugging, atelectasis, pulmonary oedema)	■ Check chest radiograph ■ Auscultate/palpate chest ■ Bronchoscopy
	Medications (vasodilators)	■ Increase FiO₂

CPAP, continuous positive airway pressure; ETT, endotracheal tube; FiO₂, fractional inspired oxygen concentration; MHI, manual hyperinflation; PEEP, positive end-expiratory pressure.

management. The adoption of newer non-invasive technologies such as electrical impedance tomography and lung ultrasound will assist to advance our understanding of the conditions we can more easily detect and use to monitor therapy effectiveness.

In addition to clinical research, it is essential that documentary evidence of the cost-effectiveness of physiotherapy in intensive care is explored, to provide outcomes and to direct clinical practice in the future. Opportunities include engagement in collaborative approaches, multi-centre trials and large observational databases.

REFERENCES

Agvald-Ohman, C., Wernerman, J., Nord, C.E., Edlund, C., 2003. Anaerobic bacteria commonly colonize the lower airways of intubated ICU patients. Clin. Microbiol. Infect. 9 (5), 397–405.

Aldrich, T.K., Karpel, J.P., Uhrlass, R.M., et al., 1989. Weaning from mechanical ventilation: adjunctive use of inspiratory muscle resistive training. Crit. Care Med. 17 (2), 143–147.

American Association for Respiratory Care (AARC), 2010. Clinical Practice Guidelines: endotracheal suctioning of mechanically ventilated patients with artificial airways 2010. Respir. Care 55 (6), 758–764.

American Association for Respiratory Care (AARC), 2011. Clinical practice guidelines: capnography/capnometry during mechanical ventilation. Respir. Care 56 (4), 503–509.

Antonaglia, V., Pascotto, S., Simoni, L.D., Zin, W.A., 2006. Effects of a sigh on the respiratory mechanical properties in ALI patients. J. Clin. Monit. Comput. 20 (4), 243–249.

Arroliga, A., Frutos-Vivar, F., Hall, J., et al., 2005. Use of sedatives and neuromuscular blockers in a cohort of patients receiving mechanical ventilation. Chest 128 (2), 496–506.

Bach, J.R., 1993. Mechanical insufflation-exsufflation: comparison of peak expiratory flows with manually assisted and unassisted coughing techniques. Chest 104 (5), 1553–1562.

Bach, J.R., Alba, A.S., 1990. Tracheostomy ventilation. A study of efficacy with deflated cuffs and cuffless tubes. Chest 97 (3), 679–683.

Barberis, L., Manno, E., Guérin, C., 2003. Effect of end-inspiratory pause duration on plateau pressure in mechanically ventilated patients. Intensive Care Med. 29 (1), 130–134.

Barnett, M., 2012. Back to basics: caring for people with a tracheostomy. Nurs. Res. Care 14 (8), 390–394.

Beach, L., Denehy, L., Lee, A., 2013. The efficacy of minitracheostomy for the management of sputum retention: a systematic review. Physiotherapy 99 (4), 271–277.

Beard, B., Monaco, F.J., 1993. Tracheostomy discontinuation: impact of tube selection on resistance during tube occlusion. Respir. Care 38, 267–270.

Behrakis, P.K., Baydur, A., Jaeger, M.J., Milic-Emili, J., 1983. Lung mechanics in sitting and horizontal body positions. Chest 83 (4), 643–646.

Bein, T., Zimmerman, M., Scwiewe-Langgartner, F., et al., 2012. Continuous lateral rotational therapy and systemic inflammatory response in posttraumatic acute lung injury: results from a prospective randomised study. Injury 43 (11), 1982–1987.

Berney, S., Denehy, L., 2003. The effect of physiotherapy treatment on oxygen consumption and haemodynamics in patients who are critically ill. Aust J Physiother 49 (2), 99–105.

Berney, S., Denehy, L., Pretto, J., 2004. Head-down tilt and manual hyperinflation enhance sputum clearance in patients who are intubated and ventilated. Aust J Physiother 50 (1), 9–14.

Billau, C., 2004. Humidification. In: Russell, C., Matta, B. (Eds.), Tracheostomy: A Multi-Professional Handbook. Cambridge University Press, Cambridge, pp. 143–156.

Bissett, B., Leditschke, I.A., Paratz, J., Boots, R., 2012. Respiratory dysfunction in ventilated patients: can inspiratory muscle training help? Anaesth. Intensive Care 40 (2), 236–246.

Bjorling, G., Belin, A.L., Hellstrom, C., et al., 2007. Tracheostomy inner cannula care: a randomized crossover study of two decontamination procedures. Am. J. Infect. Control 35 (9), 600–605.

Boitano, L.J., 2006. Management of airway clearance in neuromuscular disease. Respir. Care 51 (8), 913–922.

Boots, R.J., George, N., Faoagali, J.L., et al., 2006. Double-heater-wire circuits and heat-and-moisture exchangers and the risk of ventilator-associated pneumonia. Crit. Care Med. 34 (3), 687–693.

Bordini, A.L., Luiz, T.F., Fernandes, M., et al., 2010. Coma scales: a historical review. Arq. Neuropsiquiatr 68 (6), 930–937.

Bourjeily, G., Habr, F., Supinski, G., 2002. Review of tracheostomy usage: complications and decannulation procedures. Part II. Clin. Pulm. Med. 9 (5), 273–278.

Boyle, A.J., McNamee, J.J., McAuley, D.F., 2014. Biological therapies in the acute respiratory distress syndrome. Expert Opin. Biol. Ther. 14 (7), 969–981.

Brucia, J.J., Owen, D.C., Rudy, E.B., 1992. The effects of lidocaine on intracranial hypertension. J Neurosci Nurs 24 (4), 205–214.

Caruana, L., Paratz, J., Chang, A., Fraser, J.F., 2011. Electrical impedance tomography in the clinical assessment of lung volumes following recruitment manoeuvres. Phys. Ther. Rev. 16 (9), 66–73.

Caruso, P., Denari, S.D., Ruiz, S.A., et al., 2005. Inspiratory muscle training is ineffective in mechanically ventilated critically ill patients. Clinics 60 (6), 479–484.

Caruso, P., Denari, S., Ruiz, S.A., et al., 2009. Saline instillation before tracheal suctioning decreases the incidence of ventilator-associated pneumonia. Crit. Care Med. 37 (1), 32–38.

Cereda, M., Villa, F., Colombo, E., et al., 2001. Closed system endotracheal suctioning maintains lung volume during volume-controlled mechanical ventilation. Intensive Care Med. 27 (4), 648–654.

Ceriana, P., Carlucci, A., Navalesi, P., et al., 2003. Weaning from tracheotomy in long-term mechanically ventilated patients: feasibility of a decisional flowchart and clinical outcome. Intensive Care Med. 29 (5), 845–848.

Cetto, R., Arora, A., Hettige, R., et al., 2011. Improving tracheostomy care: a prospective study of the multidisciplinary approach. Clin. Otolaryngol. 36 (5), 482–488.

Chan, L.Y.Y., Jones, A.Y.M., Chung, R.C.K., Hung, K.N., 2010. Peak flow rate during induced cough: a predictor of successful decannulation of a tracheotomy tube in neurosurgical patients. Am. J. Crit. Care 19 (3), 278–284.

Chang, A.T., Boots, R.J., Brown, M.G., et al., 2005. Reduced inspiratory muscle endurance following successful weaning from prolonged mechanical ventilation. Chest 128 (2), 553–559.

Chiang, L.L., Wang, L.Y., Wu, C.P., et al., 2006. Effects of physical training on functional status in patients with prolonged mechanical ventilation. Phys. Ther. 86 (9), 1271–1281.

Choate, K., Barbetti, J., Currey, J., 2009. Tracheostomy decannulation failure rate following critical illness: a prospective descriptive study. Aust. Crit. Care 22 (1), 8–15.

Coffman, H.M., Rees, C.J., Sievers, A.E., Belafsky, P.C., 2008. Proximal suction tracheotomy tube reduces aspiration volume. Otolaryngol. Head Neck Surg. 138 (4), 441–445.

Conlan, A.A., Kopec, S.E., 2000. Tracheostomy in the ICU. J. Intensive Care Med. 15 (1), 1–13.

Cooper, D.J., Rosenfeld, J.V., Murray, L., et al., 2011. Decompressive craniectomy in diffuse traumatic brain injury. N. Engl. J. Med. 364 (16), 1493–1502.

Cowan, T., Op't Holt, T.B., Gegenheimer, C., et al., 2001. Effect of inner cannula removal on the work of breathing imposed by tracheostomy tubes: a bench study. Respir. Care 46 (5), 460–465.

Davis, K., Johannigman, J.A., Campbell, R.S., et al., 2001. The acute effects of body position strategies and respiratory therapy in paralyzed patients with acute lung injury. Crit. Care 5 (2), 81–87.

De Jonghe, B., Cook, D., Appere-De-Vecchi, C., et al., 2000. Using and understanding sedation scoring systems: a systematic review. Intensive Care Med. 26, 275–285.

De Leyn, P., Bedert, L., Delcroix, M., et al., 2007. Tracheotomy: clinical review and guidelines. Eur. J. Cardiothorac. Surg. 32 (3), 412–421.

Ding, R., Logemann, J.A., 2005. Swallow physiology in patients with trach cuff inflated or deflated: a retrospective study. Head Neck 27 (9), 809–813.

Dodek, P., Keenan, S., Cook, D., et al., 2004. Evidence-based clinical practice guideline for the prevention of ventilator-associated pneumonia. Ann. Intern. Med. 141 (4), 305–313.

Dutton, R.P., McCunn, M., 2003. Traumatic brain injury. Curr. Opin. Crit. Care 9 (6), 503–509.

Estenssoro, E., Reina, R., Canales, H.S., et al., 2006. The distinct clinical profile of chronically critically ill patients: a cohort study. Crit. Care 10 (3), R89.

Ferguson, N.D., Cook, D.J., Guyatt, G.H., et al., 2013. High-frequency oscillation in early acute respiratory distress syndrome. N. Engl. J. Med. 368 (9), 795–805.

Feyen, B.F., Sener, S., Jorens, P.G., et al., 2012. Neuromonitoring in traumatic brain injury. Minerva Anestesiol. 78 (8), 949–958.

Fitzgerald, C., Main, E., Brown, C., 2013. Peak cough flow via tracheostomy – a useful assessment tool before decannulation? J. Assoc. Chart. Physiother. Respir. Care 45, 43.

Friedman, Y., 2006. Percutaneous versus surgical tracheostomy: the continuing saga. Crit. Care Med. 34 (8), 2250–2251.

Frost, S.A., Azeem, A., Alexandrou, E., et al., 2013. Subglottic secretion drainage for preventing ventilator associated pneumonia: a meta-analysis. Aust. Crit. Care 26 (4), 180–188.

Gao, F., Melody, T., Daniels, D.F., et al., 2005. The impact of compliance with 6-hour and 24-hour sepsis bundles on hospital mortality in patients with severe sepsis: a prospective observational study. Crit. Care 9 (6), R764–R770.

Gao, C., Zhou, L., Wei, C., et al., 2008. The evaluation of physiologic decannulation readiness according to upper airway resistance measurement. Otolaryngol. Head Neck Surg. 139 (4), 535–540.

Garguilo, M., Leroux, K., Lejaille, M., et al., 2013. Patient-controlled positive end-expiratory pressure with neuromuscular disease: effect on speech in patients with tracheostomy and mechanical ventilation support. Chest 143 (5), 1243–1251.

Garrubba, M., Turner, T., Grieveson, C., 2009. Multidisciplinary care for tracheostomy patients: a systematic review. Crit. Care 13 (6), R177.

Gattinoni, L., Carlesso, E., Taccone, P., et al., 2010. Prone positioning improves survival in severe ARDS: a pathophysiological review and individual patient meta-analysis. Minerva Anestiol 76 (6), 448–454.

Georgopoulos, D., Prinianakis, G., Kondili, E., 2006. Bedside waveforms interpretation as a tool to identify patient-ventilator asynchronies. Intensive Care Med. 32 (1), 34–47.

Germann, P., Braschi, A., Della Rocca, G., et al., 2005. Inhaled nitric oxide therapy in adults: European expert recommendations. Intensive Care Med. 31 (8), 1029–1041.

Girault, C., Daudenthun, I., Chevron, V., et al., 1999. Non-invasive ventilation as a systematic extubation and weaning technique in acute-on-chronic respiratory failure: a prospective, randomized controlled study. Am. J. Respir. Crit. Care Med. 160 (1), 86–92.

Gray, H.H., Dawkins, K.D., Morgan, J.M., Simpson, I.A., 2002. Examination of the cardiovascular system. In: Lecture Notes on Cardiology, fourth ed. Blackwell Publishing, Denmark, p. 12.

Griffiths, R.D., Hall, J.B., 2010. Intensive care unit-acquired weakness. Crit. Care Med. 38, 779–787.

Grosu, H.B., Lee, Y.I., Lee, J., et al., 2012. Diaphragm muscle thinning in patients who are mechanically ventilated. Chest 142 (6), 1455–1460.

Guérin, C., Reignier, J., Richard, J.C., PROSEVA Study Group, 2013. Prone positioning in severe acute respiratory distress syndrome. N. Engl. J. Med. 368 (23), 2159–2168.

Haas, C.F., Loik, P.S., 2012. Ventilator discontinuation protocols. Respir. Care 57 (10), 1649–1662.

Hales, P.A., Drinnan, M.J., Wilson, J.A., 2008. The added value of fibreoptic endoscopic evaluation of swallowing in tracheostomy weaning. Clin. Otolaryngol. 33 (4), 319–324.

Hanekom, S., Berney, S., Morrow, B (a), et al., 2011. The validation of a clinical algorithm for the prevention and management of pulmonary dysfunction in intubated adults: a synthesis of evidence and expert opinion. J. Eval. Clin. Pract. 17 (4), 801–810.

Hedenstierna, G., Brismar, B., Strandberg, A., et al., 1985. New aspects on atelectasis during anaesthesia. Clin Physiol 5 (Suppl. 3), 127–131.

Heffner, J.E., 2005. Management of the chronically ventilated patient with a tracheostomy. Chron. Respir. Dis. 2 (3), 151–161.

Heffner, J.E., Hess, D., 2001. Tracheostomy management in the chronically ventilated patient. Clin Chest Med 22 (1), 55–69.

Hess, D.R., 2002. Mechanical ventilation strategies: what's new and what's worth keeping? Respir. Care 47 (9), 1007–1017. Review.

Hess, D.R., 2005. Tracheostomy tubes and related appliances. Respir. Care 50 (4), 497–510.

Hilbert, G., Gruson, D., Vargas, F., et al., 2001. Noninvasive ventilation in immunosuppressed patients with pulmonary infiltrates, fever, and acute respiratory failure. NEJM 344 (7), 481–487.

Huang, S.J., Hong, W.C., Han, Y.Y., et al., 2006. Clinical outcome of severe head injury using three different ICP and CPP protocol-driven therapies. J. Clin. Neurosci. 13 (8), 818–822.

Hunt, K., McGowan, S., 2005. Tracheostomy management in the neurosciences: a systematic multidisciplinary approach. Br. J. Neurosci. Nurs.

Hussey, J.D., Bishop, M.J., 1996. Pressures required to move gas through the native airway in the presence of a fenestrated vs a nonfenestrated tracheostomy tube. Chest 110 (2), 494–497.

Ibanez, J., Raurich, J.M., Abizanda, R., et al., 1981. The effect of lateral positions on gas exchange in patients with unilateral lung disease during mechanical ventilation. Intensive Care Med. 7 (5), 231–234.

Intensive Care Society. Standards for the care of adult patients with a temporary tracheostomy. http://www.ics.ac.uk/intensive_care_professional/standards__safety_and_quality. 2008. 6-12-2011.

Jubran, A., 2006. Critical illness and mechanical ventilation: effects on the diaphragm. Respir. Care 51 (9), 1054–1061.

Kang, Y., Chun, M.H., Lee, S.J., 2013. Evaluation of salivary aspiration in brain-injured patients with tracheostomy. Ann. Rehabil. Med. 37 (1), 96–102.

Kirschenbaum, L., Azzi, E., Sfeir, T., et al., 2002. Effect of continuous lateral rotational therapy on the prevalence of ventilator-associated pneumonia in patients requiring long-term ventilatory care. Crit. Care Med. 30 (9), 1983–1986.

Klouwenberg, K., Ong, D.S., Bonten, M.J., et al., 2012. Classification of sepsis, severe sepsis and septic shock: the impact of minor variations in data capture and definition of SIRS criteria. Intensive Care Med. 38 (5), 811–819.

Kollef, M.H., Shapiro, S.D., Silver, P., et al., 1997. A randomized, controlled trial of protocol-directed versus physician-directed weaning from mechanical ventilation. Crit. Care Med. 25 (4), 567–574.

Konrad, F., Schreiber, T., Brecht-Kraus, D., Georgieff, M., 1994. Mucociliary transport in ICU patients. Chest 105 (1), 237–241.

Kost, K.M., 2008. Tracheostomy in the intensive care unit setting. In: Myers, E.N., Johnson, J.T. (Eds.), Tracheotomy: Airway Management, Communication, and Swallowing, second ed. Singular Pub. Group, San Diego, pp. 83–116.

Kress, J.P., Hall, J.B., 2012. The changing landscape of ICU sedation. JAMA 308 (19), 2030–2031.

Krishnan, J.A., Moore, D., Robeson, C., et al., 2004. A prospective, controlled trial of a protocol-based strategy to discontinue mechanical ventilation. Am. J. Respir. Crit. Care Med. 169 (6), 673–678.

Kuo, P.H., Wu, H.D., Lu, B.Y., et al., 2006. Predictive value of rapid shallow breathing index measured at initiation and termination of a 2-hour spontaneous breathing trial for weaning outcome in ICU patients. J. Formos. Med. Assoc. 105 (5), 390–398.

Ladyshewsky, A., Gousseau, A., 1996. Successful tracheal weaning. Can. Nurse 92 (2), 35–38.

Lasocki, S., Lu, Q., Sartorius, A., et al., 2006. Open and closed-circuit endotracheal suctioning in acute lung injury: efficiency and effects on gas exchange. Anesthesiology 104 (1), 39–47.

Levitt, J.E., Matthay, M.A., 2006. Treatment of acute lung injury: historical perspective and potential future therapies. Semin Respiratory. Crit. Care Med. 27 (4), 426–437.

Levy, M.M., Fink, M.P., Marshall, J.C., et al., 2003. SCCM/ESICM/ACCP/ATS/SIS International Sepsis Definitions Conference. Intensive Care Med. 29 (4), 530–538.

Lewarski, J.S., 2005. Long-term care of the patient with a tracheostomy. Respir. Care 50 (4), 534–537.

Li Bassi, G., Saucedo, L., Marti, J.D., et al., 2012. Effects of duty cycle and positive end-expiratory pressure on mucus clearance during mechanical ventilation. Crit. Care Med. 40 (3), 895–902.

Li Bassi, G., Torres, A., 2011. Ventilator-associated pneumonia: role of positioning. Curr. Opin. Crit. Care 17 (1), 57–63.

Lima, C.A., Siqueira, T.B., Travassos, E.F., et al., 2011. Influence of peripheral muscle strength on the decannulation success rate. Rev. Bras. Ter. Intensiva 23 (1), 56–61.

Lucchini, A., Zanella, A., Bellani, G., et al., 2011. Tracheal secretion management in the mechanically ventilated patient: comparison of standard assessment and an acoustic secretion detector. Respir. Care 56 (5), 596–603.

Mace, A.D., Patel, N.N., Mainwaring, F., 2006. Current standards of tracheostomy care in the UK. Otolaryngol. 1 (1), 37–39.

MacIntyre, N.R., 2004. Evidence-based ventilator weaning and discontinuation. Respir. Care 49 (7), 830–836.

Maggiore, S.M., Lellouche, F., Pigeot, J., et al., 2003. Prevention of endotracheal suctioning-induced alveolar derecruitment in acute lung injury. Am. J. Respir. Crit. Care Med. 167 (9), 1215–1224.

Mallick, A., Bodenham, A., Elliot, S., Oram, J., 2008. An investigation into the length of standard tracheostomy tubes in critical care patients. Anaesthesia 63 (3), 302–306.

Martin, A.D., Davenport, P.D., Franceschi, A.C., Harman, E., 2002. Use of inspiratory muscle strength training to facilitate ventilator weaning: a series of 10 consecutive patients. Chest 122 (1), 192–196.

McGrath, B.A., Bates, L., Atkinson, D., Moore, J.A., 2012. Multidisciplinary guidelines for the management of tracheostomy and laryngectomy airway emergencies. Anaesthesia 67 (9), 1025–1041.

McKim, D.A., Hendin, A., Leblanc, C., et al., 2012. Tracheostomy decannulation and cough peak flows in patients with neuromuscular weakness. Am. J. Phys. Med. Rehabil. 91 (8), 666–670.

McPherson, K., Kersten, P., George, S., et al., 2006. A systematic review of evidence about extended roles for allied health professionals. J. Health Serv. Res. Policy 11 (4), 240–247.

Messerole, E., Peine, P., Wittkopp, S., et al., 2002. The pragmatics of prone positioning. Am. J. Respir. Crit. Care Med. 165 (10), 1359–1363.

Metnitz, P.G., Bartens, C., Fischer, M., et al., 1999. Antioxidant status in patients with acute respiratory distress syndrome. Intensive Care Med. 25 (2), 180–185.

Michard, F., 2005. Changes in arterial pressure during mechanical ventilation. Anesthesiology 103 (2), 419–428.

Minei, J.P., Nathens, A.B., West, M., et al., 2006. Inflammation and the host response to injury, a large-scale collaborative project: patient-oriented research core-standard operating procedures for clinical care. II. Guidelines for prevention, diagnosis and treatment of ventilator-associated pneumonia (VAP) in the trauma patient. J Trauma 60 (5), 1106–1113.

Mitchell, R.B., Hussey, H.M., Setzen, G., et al., 2013. Clinical consensus statement: tracheostomy care. Otolaryngol. Head Neck Surg. 148 (1), 6–20.

Moran, T., Bellapart, J., Vari, A., Mancebo, J., 2006. Heat and moisture exchangers and heated humidifiers in acute lung injury/acute respiratory distress syndrome patients: effects on respiratory mechanics and gas exchange. Intensive Care Med. 32 (4), 524–531.

Morris, L., 2010a. Care of the tracheostomy patient. In: Morris, L., Afifi, M.S. (Eds.), Tracheostomies: The Complete Guide. Springer Publishing Company, LLC, New York, pp. 211–241.

Morris, L., 2010b. Downsizing and decannulation. In: Morris, L., Afifi, M.S. (Eds.), Tracheostomies: The Complete Guide. Springer Publishing Company, LLC, New York, pp. 303–322.

Morris, L., 2010c. Phonation with a tracheostomy. In: Morris, L., Afifi, M.S. (Eds.), Tracheostomies: The Complete Guide. Springer Publishing Company, LLC, New York, pp. 181–209.

Mullins, J.B., Templer, J.W., Kong, J., et al., 1993. Airway resistance and work of breathing in tracheostomy tubes. Laryngoscope 103 (12), 1367–1372.

Murias, G., Villagra, A., Blanch, L., 2013. Patient-ventilator dyssynchrony during assisted invasive mechanical ventilation. Minerva Anestesiol. 79 (4), 434–444.

Nekludov, M., Bellander, B., Mure, M., 2006. Oxygenation and cerebral perfusion pressure improved in prone position. Acta Anaesthesiol. Scand. 50 (8), 932–936.

Ntoumenopoulos, G., Glickman, Y., 2012. Computerised lung sound monitoring to assess effectiveness of chest physiotherapy and secretion removal: a feasibility study. Physiotherapy 98 (3), 250–255.

Ntoumenopoulos, G., Presneill, J.J., McElholum, M., Cade, J.F., 2002. Chest physiotherapy for the prevention of ventilator-associated pneumonia. Intensive Care Med. 28 (7), 850–856.

Ntoumenopoulos, G., Shannon, H., Main, E., 2011. Do commonly used ventilator settings for mechanically ventilated adults have the potential to embed secretions or promote clearance? Respir. Care 56 (12), 1887–1892.

Ntoumenopoulos, G., Shipsides, T., 2007. Proposal for a more effective chest physiotherapy treatment in the neuromuscular patient with copious secretions, bulbar dysfunction and poor cough: a case report. Physiotherapy 93 (2), 164–167.

O'Connor, H.H., White, A.C., 2010. Tracheostomy decannulation. Respir. Care 55 (8), 1076–1081.

O'Riordan, T.G., Mao, W., Palmer, L.B., Chen, J.J., 2006. Assessing the effects of racemic and single-enantiomer albuterol on airway secretions in long-term intubated patients. Chest 129 (1), 124–132.

Oeyen, S.G., Vandijck, D.M., Benoit, D.B., et al., 2010. Quality of life after intensive care: a systematic review of the literature. Crit. Care Med. 38 (12), 2386–2400.

Paratz, J., Burns, Y., 1993. The effect of respiratory physiotherapy on intracranial pressure, mean arterial pressure, cerebral perfusion pressure, and end tidal carbon dioxide in ventilated neurosurgical patients. Physiother. Theory Pract. 9 (1), 3–11.

Paratz, J., Lipman, J., 2006. Manual hyperinflation causes norepinephrine release. Heart Lung 35 (4), 262–268.

Paratz, J., Stockton, K., 2009. Efficacy and safety of normal saline instillation: a systematic review. Physiotherapy 95 (4), 241–250.

Pattanshetty, R.B., Gaude, G.S., 2010. Effect of multimodality chest physiotherapy in prevention of ventilator-associated pneumonia: a randomized clinical trial. Indian J Crit Care Med 14 (2), 70–76.

Pattanshetty, R.B., Gaude, G.S., 2011. Effect of multimodality chest physiotherapy on the rate of recovery and prevention of complications in patients with mechanical ventilation: a prospective study in medical and surgical intensive care units. Indian J. Med. Sci. 65 (5), 175–185.

Peek, G.J., Elbourne, D., Mugford, M., et al., 2010. Randomised controlled trial and parallel economic evaluation of conventional ventilatory support versus extracorporeal membrane oxygenation for severe adult respiratory failure (CESAR). Health Technol. Assess. 14 (35), 1–46.

Pelosi, P., Brazzi, L., Gattinoni, L., 2002. Prone position in acute respiratory distress syndrome. Eur Respir J 20 (4), 1017–1028.

Petrucci, N., Iacovelli, W., 2007. Lung protective strategy for the acute respiratory distress syndrome. Cochrane Database Syst. Rev. 18 (3), CD003844.

Pham, T., Combes, A., Rozé, H., et al., 2013. Extracorporeal membrane oxygenation for pandemic influenza A(H1N1)-induced acute respiratory distress syndrome: a cohort study and propensity-matched analysis. Am. J. Respir. Crit. Care Med. 187 (3), 276–285.

Picard, M., Jung, B., Liang, F., et al., 2012. Mitochondrial dysfunction and lipid accumulation in the human diaphragm during mechanical ventilation. Am. J. Respir. Crit. Care Med. 186 (11), 1140–1149.

Pierson, D.J., 2005. Tracheostomy and weaning. Respir. Care 50 (4), 526–533.

Pillastrini, P., Bordini, S., Bazzocchi, G., et al., 2006. Study of the effectiveness of bronchial clearance in subjects with upper spinal cord injuries: examination of a rehabilitation programme involving mechanical insufflation and exsufflation. Spinal Cord 44 (10), 614–616.

Poovathor, S., Posner, E., Vosswinkel, J., Seidman, P.A., 2011. Intensive care unit tracheostomy care. In: Seidman, P.A., Goldenberg, D., Sinz, E. (Eds.), Tracheotomy Management: A Multidisciplinary Approach. Cambridge University Press, Cambridge, UK, pp. 117–125.

Powell, H.R.F., Hanna-Jumma, S., Philpott, J.M., Higgins, D., 2011. National survey of fenestrated versus non-fenestrated tracheostomy tube use and the incidence of surgical emphysema in UK adult intensive care units. J. Intensive Care Soc. 12 (1), 25–28.

Prigent, H., Garguilo, M., Pascal, S., et al., 2010. Speech effects of a speaking valve versus external PEEP in tracheostomized ventilator-dependent neuromuscular patients. Intensive Care Med. 36 (10), 1681–1687.

PULSION Medical Systems AG: PiCCO technology. <http://www.pulsion.com/index.php?id=6334> (accessed 15 May 2013).

Ranieri, V., Rubenfield, G., the ARDS Definition Task Force, 2012. Acute respiratory distress syndrome: the Berlin definition. JAMA 307 (23), 2526–2533.

Raoof, S., Baumann, M.H., the Critical Care Societies Collaboration, 2014. An official multi-society statement: ventilator-associated events: the new definition. Crit. Care Med. 42 (1), 228–229.

Raoof, S., Chowdhrey, N., Raoof, S., et al., 1999. Effect of combined kinetic therapy and percussion therapy on the resolution of atelectasis in critically ill patients. Chest 115 (6), 1658–1666.

Regan, K., Hunt, K., 2008. Tracheostomy management. Contin. Educ. Anaesth. Crit. Care Pain 8 (1), 31–35.

Ricard, J.D., 2012. High flow nasal oxygen in acute respiratory failure. Minerva Anestesiol. 78 (7), 836–841.

Richman, P.S., et al., 2006. Sedation during mechanical ventilation: a trial of benzodiazepine and opiate in combination. Crit. Care Med. 34 (5), 1395–1401.

Rose, L., Nelson, S., 2006. Issues in weaning from mechanical ventilation: literature review. J. Adv. Nurs. 54 (1), 73–85.

Rudy, E.B., Turner, B.S., Baun, M., et al., 1991. Endotracheal suctioning in adults with head injury. Heart Lung 20 (6), 667–674.

Russell, C., 2004. Tracheostomy tubes. In: Russell, C., Matta, B. (Eds.), Tracheostomy: A Multi-Professional Handbook. Cambridge University Press, Cambridge, pp. 97–114.

Safdar, N., Crnich, C.J., Maki, D.G., 2005. The pathogenesis of ventilator-associated pneumonia: its relevance to developing effective strategies for prevention. Respir. Care 50 (6), 725–739.

Sancho, J., Servera, E., Vergara, P., Marin, J., 2003. Mechanical insufflation-exsufflation vs. tracheal suctioning via tracheostomy tubes for patients with amyotrophic lateral sclerosis: a pilot study. Am J Phys Med and Rehabil 82 (10), 750–753.

Sassoon, C.S., Caiozzo, V.J., Manka, A., Sieck, G.C., 2002. Altered diaphragm contractile properties with controlled mechanical ventilation. J. Appl. Physiol. 92 (6), 2585–2595.

Schellongowski, P., Losert, H., Locker, G.J., et al., 2007. Prolonged lateral steep position impairs respiratory mechanics during continuous lateral rotation therapy in respiratory failure. Intensive Care Med. 33 (4), 625–631.

Schorr, C.A., Dellinger, R.P., 2014. The Surviving Sepsis Campaign: past, present and future. Trends Mol. Med. 20 (4), 192–194.

Serpa Neto, A., Cardoso, S.O., Manetta, J.A., et al., 2012. Association between use of lung-protective ventilation with lower tidal volumes and clinical outcomes among patients without acute respiratory distress syndrome: a meta-analysis. JAMA 308 (16), 1651–1659.

Shankar, G., Cohen, D.A., 2001. Idiopathic pneumonia syndrome after bone marrow transplantation: the role of pre-transplant radiation conditioning and local cytokine dysregulation in promoting inflammation and fibrosis. Int. J. Exp. Pathol. 82 (2), 101–113.

Sigurdsson, M.I., Sigvaldason, K., Gunnarsson, T.S., et al., 2013. Acute respiratory distress syndrome: nationwide changes in incidence, treatment and mortality over 23 years. Acta Anaesthesiol. Scand. 57 (1), 37–45.

Silversides, J.A., Ferguson, N.D., 2013. Clinical review: acute respiratory distress syndrome: clinical ventilator management and adjunct therapy. Crit. Care 17 (2), 225.

Simonis, G., Steiding, K., Schaefer, K., et al., 2012. A prospective, randomized trial of continuous lateral rotation ('kinetic therapy') in patients with cardiogenic shock. Clin. Res. Cardiol. 101 (12), 955–962.

Speed, L., Harding, K.E., 2013. Tracheostomy teams reduce total tracheostomy time and increase speaking valve use: a systematic review and meta-analysis. J. Crit. Care 28 (2), 216.e1–216.e10.

Stawicki, S.P., Grossman, M.D., Hoey, B.A., et al., 2004. Rib fractures in the elderly: a marker of injury severity. J. Am. Geriatr. Soc. 52 (5), 805–808.

Stelfox, H.T., Crimi, C., Berra, L., et al., 2008. Determinants of tracheostomy decannulation: an international survey. Crit. Care 12 (1), R26.

St George's Healthcare NHS trust. Tracheostomy Guidelines. http://www.stgeorges.nhs.uk/trachindex.asp. 2013. 22-9-0013.

St John, R.E., Malen, J.F., 2004. Contemporary issues in adult tracheostomy management. Crit. Care Nurs. Clin. North Am. 16 (3), 413–430.

Suiter, D.M., McCullough, G.H., Powell, P.W., 2003. Effects of cuff deflation and one-way tracheostomy speaking valve placement on swallow physiology. Dysphagia 18 (4), 284–292.

Thelandersson, A., Cider, A., Nellgard, B., 2006. Prone position in mechanically ventilated patients with reduced intracranial compliance. Acta Anaesthesiol. Scand. 50 (8), 937–941.

Thomas, P.J., Paratz, J.D., Lipman, J., Stanton, W.R., 2007. Lateral positioning of ventilated intensive care patients: a study of oxygenation, respiratory mechanics hemodynamics and adverse events. Heart Lung 36 (4), L277–L288.

Thompson-Ward, E., Boots, R., Frisby, J., et al., 1999. Evaluating suitability for tracheostomy decannulation: a critical evaluation of two management protocols. J. Med. Speech Lang. Pathol. 7 (4), 273–281.

Tonnelier, J.M., Prat, G., Le Gal, G., et al., 2005. Impact of a nurses' protocol-directed weaning procedure on outcomes in patients undergoing mechanical ventilation for longer than 48 hours: a prospective cohort study with a matched historical control group. Crit Care 9 (2), R83–R89.

Ulatowski, J., 1997. Cerebral protection. In: Oh, T.E. (Ed.), Intensive Care Manual, fourth ed. Butterworth-Heinemann, Oxford, pp. 403–411.

Vassilakopoulos, T., Zakynthinos, S., Roussos, C., 2006. Bench-to-bedside review: weaning failure – should we rest the respiratory muscles with controlled mechanical ventilation? Crit Care 10 (1), 204.

Via, G., Storti, E., Gulati, G., et al., 2012. Lung ultrasound in the ICU: from diagnostic instrument to respiratory monitoring tool. Minerva Anestesiol. 78 (11), 1282–1296.

Warnecke, T., Suntrup, S., Teismann, I.K., et al., 2013. Standardized endoscopic swallowing evaluation for tracheostomy decannulation in critically ill neurologic patients. Crit. Care Med. 41 (7), 1728–1732.

Wasserzug, O., Adi, N., Cavel, O., et al., 2010. One-stage decannulation procedure for patients undergoing oral and oropharyngeal oncological surgeries and prophylactic tracheotomy. Open Otorhinolaryngol. J. 4, 73–76.

Wemke, M., Schiemanck, S., Hoffken, G., et al., 2012. Respiratory failure in patients undergoing allogeneic hematopoietic SCT: a randomized trial on early non-invasive ventilation based on standard care hematology wards. Bone Marrow Transplant. 47 (4), 574–580.

Wilke, M., Grube, R., 2013. Update on management options in the treatment of nosocomial and ventilator associated pneumonia: review of actual guidelines and economic aspects of therapy. Infect Drug Resist 18 (7), 1–7.

Winkelman, C., 2004. Inactivity and inflammation: selected cytokines as biologic mediators in muscle dysfunction during critical illness. Review. AACN Clin. Issues 15 (1), 74–82.

Xirouchaki, N., Magkanas, E., Vaporidi, K., 2011. Lung ultrasound in critically ill patients: comparison with bedside chest radiography. Intensive Care Med. 37 (9), 1488–1493.

Young, P.J., Pakeerathan, S., Blunt, M.C., Subramanya, S., 2006. A low-volume, low-pressure tracheal tube cuff reduces pulmonary aspiration. Crit. Care Med. 34 (3), 632–639.

Zafiropoulos, B., Alison, J.A., McCarren, B., 2004. Physiological responses to the early mobilisation of the intubated, ventilated abdominal surgery patient. Aust. J. Physiother. 50 (2), 95–100.

Zanella, A., Cressoni, M., Epp, M., et al., 2012. Effects of tracheal orientation on development of ventilator-associated pneumonia. Intensive Care Med. 38 (4), 677–685.

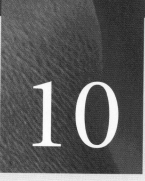

PAEDIATRIC INTENSIVE CARE

Paediatric Mechanical Support

STEWART REID ■ MARK J PETERS

Physiotherapy Management of Ventilated Infants and Children

ELEANOR MAIN ■ ALICIA J SPITTLE

■ ■ ■ ■ ■ ■ ■ ■ ■ ■ ■ ■ ■ ■ ■ ■ ■ ■ ■ ■

CHAPTER OUTLINE

INTRODUCTION 456

PAEDIATRIC MECHANICAL SUPPORT 456
Epidemiology of Acute Respiratory Failure in Children 456
  Pattern and Time Course of Disease 457
  Acute Hypoxaemic Respiratory Failure 458
Indications for Supportive Respiratory Therapy 458
  Hypoxia 458
  Hypercarbia 459
  Endotracheal Intubation 460
Mechanical Ventilation 461
  General Ventilatory Care 461
  Acute Deterioration and 'Troubleshooting' 464
  Commonly Used Modes of Mechanical Ventilation in Children 464
Newer Ventilatory Support Techniques 466
  High-Frequency Oscillatory Ventilation 466
  Extracorporeal Membrane Oxygenation 466
Ventilation Strategies for Specific Disease 467
  Acute Bronchiolitis 467
  Acute Hypoxaemic Respiratory Failure 469
  Recruitment Manoeuvres 469
Other Considerations During Mechanical Ventilation 470
  Monitoring During Mechanical Ventilation 470
  Weaning From Mechanical Ventilation 471
  Non-Invasive Support 472

PHYSIOTHERAPY MANAGEMENT OF VENTILATED INFANTS AND CHILDREN 473
  Chest Percussion and Vibration 477
  Manual Lung Inflation 479
  Endotracheal and Nasopharyngeal Airway Suction 480
  Saline Instillation 481
  Positioning 481

NEONATAL INTENSIVE CARE AND SPECIAL CARE NURSERIES 482
  Level of Perinatal Care 482
  Reasons for Admission to NICU 482
  Congenital Diaphragmatic Hernia 483
  Oesophageal Atresia and Tracheo-Oesophageal Fistula 483
  Gastroschisis and Exomphalos (Omphalocoele) 483
Pulmonary Conditions 484
  Respiratory Distress Syndrome 484
  Bronchopulmonary Dysplasia 484
  Meconium Aspiration 485
  Pulmonary Haemorrhage 485
  Periventricular Haemorrhage and Periventricular Leucomalacia 485
  Patent Ductus Arteriosus 485
  Physiological Jaundice 486
Treatments Available for Respiratory Conditions in the NICU 486
  Pharmaceutical Interventions 486
  Mechanical Support 487

Physiotherapy Interventions in the NICU 488
Manual Techniques 488
Special Considerations in the NICU 489
General Paediatric Intensive Care 490
Common Reasons for PICU Admission 490
Asthma 491
Bronchiolitis 493
Pertussis 493
Pneumonia 493
Pleural Infection 494
Acute Laryngotracheobronchitis (Croup) 494
Acute Epiglottitis 494
Bronchopulmonary Dysplasia 494
Inhaled Foreign Body 496
Children with Neurological and Neuromuscular
    Impairment 496
Need for High-Frequency Oscillatory Ventilation 496
Management of Surgical Patients 497

Pulmonary Problems Following Liver
    Transplantation 497
Paediatric Cardiac Intensive Care 498
Common Paediatric Cardiac Surgery Procedures 498
Palliative Procedures 498
Corrective Surgery: Closed Procedures 498
Corrective Surgery: Open Procedures 499
Cardiac Valve Abnormalities 502
Transplantation Surgery in Children 503
Need for Extracorporeal Membrane Oxygenation 503
Tracheal Repair: Tracheal Stenosis and Slide
    Tracheoplasty 504
Clinical Problems Encountered in the CICU 504
Pulmonary Hypertensive Crisis 504
Delayed Sternal Closure 505
Phrenic Nerve Damage 505
REFERENCES 505

INTRODUCTION

Babies and children with a wide variety of medical and surgical problems are admitted to neonatal, general paediatric or cardiac intensive care units (ICUs). Respiratory failure in acutely ill infants and children may have various origins, and respiratory support in children needs to be informed by an understanding of age-specific pathophysiology. The most common causes of respiratory failure in children vary with age and are distinct from adult causes. In the newborn infant, asphyxia, transient tachypnoea of the newborn, respiratory distress syndrome (RDS), meconium aspiration syndrome (MAS), pneumothorax, persistent pulmonary hypertension, hypoxic-ischaemic encephalopathy and congenital malformations (cardiac, pulmonary or gastro-intestinal) are the most common causes of respiratory distress.

Under 2 years of age, bronchopneumonia, bronchiolitis, croup, status asthmaticus, foreign body inhalation and congenital heart and airway anomalies are important. Among older children, asthma, accidental poisoning and central nervous system infection (e.g. meningitis), trauma and cerebral hypoxia/ischaemia are common causes of a new episode of respiratory failure. Increasingly, however, respiratory support is required in the context of acute-on-chronic respiratory failure from chronic respiratory or underlying neurological diseases.

Paediatric Mechanical Support

Although the principles of when and how mechanical support should be undertaken in paediatric patients are, broadly speaking, similar to those applied in adults, there are differences in epidemiology, pathophysiology and management that warrant consideration. The emphasis, therefore, of this section will be on a paediatric perspective of respiratory supportive therapy.

EPIDEMIOLOGY OF ACUTE RESPIRATORY FAILURE IN CHILDREN

Respiratory failure develops when the rate of gas exchange between the alveolar air and the blood fails to match the body's metabolic demands. The patient therefore loses the ability to provide sufficient oxygen to the blood and develops hypoxaemia, or the patient is unable to ventilate adequately and develops hypercarbia. Epidemiologically, there is little information in children about the incidence of acute respiratory failure. Adult definitions using blood gas parameters may be appropriate for certain age groups but in others, they may not be useful. For example, in infants with acute bronchiolitis, acute respiratory failure is usually defined as:

$PaCO_2$ ≥8 kPa (60 mmHg) with PaO_2 ≤8 kPa (60 mmHg) when using FiO_2 = 0.6 (where $PaCO_2$ = partial pressure of carbon dioxide in arterial blood, PaO_2 = partial pressure of oxygen in arterial blood and FiO_2 = fraction of inspired oxygen concentration) or, in the case of patients with respiratory arrest, a preceding history of severe respiratory distress accompanied by cyanosis.

However, when trying to look at large populations, in the absence of blood gases, a more pragmatic definition for acute respiratory failure is needed. For example, when using the definition of 'acute airway management necessitating endotracheal (ET) tube intubation' (Tasker 2000), it is possible to explore issues such as the pattern and time course of paediatric disease that have some bearing on how mechanical support should be undertaken.

Pattern and Time Course of Disease

Table 10-1 summarizes a retrospective analysis of 1000 infants and children (aged older than 28 days and younger than 17 years) who required ET intubation for acute respiratory failure complicating acutely acquired medical, rather than surgical, disease (Tasker 2000). The three major categories relate to the system or problem underlying respiratory failure (respiratory tract disorder, central nervous system disorder or systemic disorder) and the subcategories relate to the clinical diagnostic entities commonly encountered in intensive care. Respiratory tract problems due to infection are, not surprisingly, the most common problems seen. The time course of recovery in survivors is

TABLE 10-1

Diagnostic Distribution of 1000 Children Requiring Endotracheal Tube Intubation During Acute Medical Illness Ordered by Number (n), Age and Length of Stay on the Intensive Care Unit in Survivors

System Disorder	n	Age in Months Median (IQR)	Length of Stay in Survivors Median (IQR) Days m:f
Respiratory tract	**521**	**13 (4–40)**	
Upper airway infection	80	21 (12–35)	4 (3–5):3 (3–5)
Bronchiolitis	89	3 (2–6)	5 (4–9):6 (3–9)
Asthma	25	37 (21–86)	4 (3–5):4 (3–5)
Pneumonia	90	10 (4–40)	8 (5–12):9 (4–14)
Pneumonia and immunodeficiency	120	16 (5–51)	9 (5–16):9 (7–14)
Neuromuscular disease	66	22 (7–88)	10 (5–19):8 (5–20)
Non-infective LRTD	51	16 (7–69)	5 (3–8):6 (4–10)
Central nervous	**342**	**18 (6–62)**	
Infection	117	22 (8–65)	4 (2–6):4 (3–7)
Hypoxia-ischaemia	78	14 (4–34)	5 (2–10):3 (1–8)
Other encephalopathy	147	17 (6–70)	5 (3–8):5 (2–8)
Systemic	**137**	**19 (6–52)**	
Septicaemia	90	19 (4–69)	6 (4–10):6 (4–12)
Inflammatory syndromes	47	19 (6–32)	4 (3–9):5 (3–8)

IQR, Interquartile range; *LRTD*, lower respiratory tract disease; m:f, males to females.

influenced by the site within the airways that infection has reached. This is reflected by an increase in the length of stay in the ICU with more distally affected tissues (i.e. upper airway compared with lower airway). In relating such information to clinical practice, one can use the expected time course to decide on an agenda for treatment or 'care pathway'. For example, given that the expected time course for intensive care recovery in pneumonia necessitating intubation is around 8 days (interquartile range 5–12 days), one can then predict when certain targets should be met. The same applies to the other 11 distinct diagnosis-related entities. This idea will be revisited later in this section where three clinical examples are discussed.

Acute Hypoxaemic Respiratory Failure

Acute hypoxaemic respiratory failure (AHRF) signifies respiratory failure at the more severe end of the pathophysiological spectrum, irrespective of underlying aetiology. Previously for paediatric practice, we identified this state by using diagnostic criteria that were modified from the American-European Consensus Conference diagnostic criteria for acute respiratory distress syndrome (ARDS) (Bernard et al 1994). These criteria include:

- acute onset of respiratory failure over less than 48 hours
- evidence of a severe defect in oxygenation (PaO_2/FiO_2 of less than 26.7 kPa, 200 mmHg) for at least 6 consecutive hours on the day of admission
- no evidence of left atrial hypertension
- four-quadrant interstitial shadowing on chest radiograph.

More recently for ARDS the modified Berlin definitions have been applied effectively to younger populations. The previous two categories of acute lung injury non-ARDS (ALI non-ARDS) and ARDS have been expanded to mild, moderate and severe ARDS with defining ranges of PaO_2/FiO_2 ratios and specifying a positive end-expiratory pressure (PEEP) or continuous positive airway pressure (CPAP) ≥ 5 cmH$_2$O. (Mild = 200–300 mmHg; moderate = 100–200 mmHg; severe <100 mmHg). These new classifications relate closely with the risk of death (De Luca, 2013).

Children meeting all the criteria except the characteristic chest radiographic appearances of ARDS

(last criterion) are described as cases of AHRF. The significance of AHRF is that it implies a certain severity of illness and risk of mortality. These factors are important when it comes to deciding which ventilatory strategy should be adopted, and which adjunctive therapies (see Ventilation Strategies for Specific Disease). For example, in a prospective epidemiological study, Peters and colleagues (1998) found that out of 850 mechanically ventilated infants and children, AHRF occurred in 118 patients (14%, 95% confidence interval (CI) 12–16%). Of these 118 patients, 52 met the criteria for ARDS (44%, 35–53%). Mortality was four times higher in those with AHRF than the mortality seen in those patients without AHRF. In the AHRF patients, mortality was three times higher for those with ARDS (Peters et al 1998). In a study from North America, the Pediatric Acute Lung Injury and Sepsis Investigators (PALISI) network reported a mortality from ARDS of 4.3% (Randolph et al 2003). This coincides with the adoption of protective modes of ventilation for this condition. Therefore identifying these entities (AHRF and ARDS) at an early stage is important so as to institute the most appropriate method of ventilation.

INDICATIONS FOR SUPPORTIVE RESPIRATORY THERAPY

For practical purposes we can consider the treatment of respiratory dysfunction in terms of treating hypoxia and hypercarbia. Appropriate management is aimed first at prevention, second at early diagnosis and third at a clear understanding of the pathophysiology and way in which the proposed treatment works to maintain or restore good lung function.

Hypoxia

Hypoxia must be treated first; give oxygen. At the same time attempts should be made to correct the underlying problem. Local processes in the lung, such as atelectasis and bronchopneumonia, can result in a portion of the pulmonary blood flow perfusing unventilated alveoli (i.e. intrapulmonary shunt), which in some cases may be effectively treated by airway clearance techniques and postural change. With a large shunt fraction – greater than 25% of pulmonary blood flow – PaO_2 is not significantly improved by solely increasing the FiO_2. In these cases a diffuse pulmonary process

TABLE 10-2

Methods of Oxygen Administration

Method	Maximum Achievable FiO$_2$ at 6–10 L/min of Oxygen (%)
Nasopharyngeal catheter	50
Nasal prongs	50
Mask without reservoir bag	50
Mask with reservoir bag (partial rebreathing)	70
Mask with reservoir bag (non-rebreathing)	95
Venturi	24, 28, 35, 40
Incubator	40
Canopy tent	50
Head box	95

FiO$_2$, Fractional inspired oxygen concentration.

is usually present and a form of assisted positive airway pressure is required. Such assistance may also be required for severe impairment of chest wall mechanics (e.g. rib fractures, pain, weakness, etc.) even in the absence of pulmonary parenchymal disease.

In infants and children, there are several methods of administering oxygen (Table 10-2). Young patients do not usually tolerate nasal catheters and cannulae. Face masks with a reservoir and a non-rebreathing valve can be used to increase the FiO$_2$. Alternatively, high-flow oxygen via the appropriate Venturi-valve mask can be used. Oxygen delivered via the oxygen inlet of an incubator rarely exceeds an FiO$_2$ of 0.4. When supplemental oxygen is delivered into a tent, the concentration varies depending on any leaks in the system. Regardless of the technique, it is essential that the administered oxygen is warm and humidified. To avoid damage to the lungs, oxygen administration should be discontinued as soon as possible (as indicated by blood gas measurements). An FiO$_2$ below 0.6 is preferred to minimize the risk of oxygen toxicity. Reduction in the FiO$_2$ should be carried out cautiously in a stepwise manner. To facilitate this process, both the concentration and duration of oxygen therapy must be recorded accurately. A well-calibrated oxygen analyzer is used to check the inspired concentration every 2 hours when using a tent or head box or when adding oxygen into an incubator. The need

for monitoring PaO$_2$ in preterm newborn infants is related to the potential for pulmonary oxygen toxicity and the danger of retrolental fibroplasia. Aside from reasons specific to neonates, there is evidence for avoidance of hyperoxia, as it has been associated with worsening survival and neurological outcomes following cardiac arrest (Elmer et al 2015) and perhaps in other scenarios.

So, in any patient, oxygen should be administered at the lowest concentration sufficient to maintain the PaO$_2$ between 6.7 and 13.3 kPa (50–100 mmHg). Continuous measurement or monitoring of transcutaneous oxygen or pulse oximetry arterial oxygen saturation (SpO$_2$) are essential additions to the direct, and intermittent, measurement of arterial blood gases. In some instances, supplemental oxygen may cause respiratory depression if there has been chronic respiratory failure and the patient has a hypoxic drive to ventilation (as opposed to the normal situation where the PaCO$_2$ is the most important factor in the control of ventilation). This phenomenon is generally uncommon in paediatric practice but has been encountered in children with cystic fibrosis, cerebral palsy and bronchopulmonary dysplasia (BPD).

In addition to oxygen, some type of positive pressure may be useful in the management of hypoxia. Mask and nasal CPAP or bi-level positive airway pressure (BiPAP) increase lung compliance by recruiting additional areas of the lung for ventilation. Also, lung recruitment improves oxygenation by decreasing intrapulmonary shunt. These modes of non-invasive ventilation (NIV) are being used more frequently as the step before invasive mechanical ventilation. When invasive mechanical ventilation is used, the addition of some PEEP is a common practice in maintaining adequate functional residual capacity. However, PEEP may adversely affect the patient lung mechanics if hyperinflation occurs. This problem results in impaired pulmonary perfusion and further accentuates any ventilation–perfusion ($\dot{V}/\dot{Q}$) mismatch. Therefore PEEP above 4 cmH$_2$O should be used judiciously if there is already regional hyperinflation, such as occurs in BPD (Box 10-1). In this context a strategy for treating hypoxia is outlined in Box 10-2.

Hypercarbia

When shallow (or ineffectual) breathing is present, the dead space (i.e. ventilated but non-perfused regions)

BOX 10-1
POSITIVE END-EXPIRATORY PRESSURE

ADVANTAGES

Increased functional residual capacity
Recruits additional lung units, improving compliance
Reduces pulmonary shunt fraction
Allows for a decrease in fractional inspired oxygen · concentration (FiO_2)

DISADVANTAGES

Increases mean airway pressure, leading to reduced venous return
Can increase 'dead space' by impairing perfusion to hyperinflated regions
Can increase pulmonary vascular resistance and right heart dysfunction
Altered renal blood flow with increase in antidiuretic hormone release
Barotrauma caused by increased airway pressure

BOX 10-2
INITIAL TREATMENT OF HYPOXIA

1. Increase FiO_2 to maintain SaO_2 >90% (see Table 10-2)
2. Consider positive pressure and PEEP, if large shunt. Indications:
   hypoxaemia with FiO_2 > 0.5
   diffuse lung disease
   need to maintain lung volume
3. Initiate regular effective airway clearance
4. Eliminate the underlying cause:
   pain
   fluid overload
   atelectasis
   bronchopneumonia
5. Correct systemic abnormalities:
   hypovolaemia
   sepsis
   carbon monoxide poisoning

FiO_2, Fractional inspired oxygen concentration; PEEP, positive end-expiratory pressure;
SaO_2, arterial oxygen saturation.

---

becomes a larger fraction of each breath. This change results in a decrease in alveolar ventilation, even if the lung parenchyma is normal. When hypercarbia has been found and its cause considered, NIV can be tried a step before invasive mechanical ventilation. This may be useful when hypercarbia is secondary to neuromuscular weakness. If the patient needs invasive mechanical ventilation, then increasing tidal volume or respiratory rate can bring about increased alveolar ventilation. However, these changes may increase mean airway pressure that may generate detrimental effects on pulmonary vascular resistance and $\dot{V}/\dot{Q}$ matching.

If the patient is treated with full mechanical ventilation, the first step is to make sure that the patient is receiving an appropriate tidal volume and minute ventilation.

Ventilatory system leaks and loss of a portion of the tidal volume through compressive loss in the tubing, as well as abnormalities in ETT function, are common problems that need rectifying. Previously, uncuffed ETTs were used due to anatomical differences in the paediatric airway and concerns over tracheal injury from high pressures exerted on the mucosa by the cuff. This led to a variable degree of 'leak' around the cuff, which could compromise ventilation. The use of newer, low-pressure high-volume cuffed ETTs is increasingly accepted (Weiss et al 2009).

Having excluded mechanical factors, the other causes of hypercarbia may be related to an increase in CO_2 production or an increase in dead-space ventilation. An increase in dead space may be due to excessive PEEP (particularly when there is already hyperinflation or hypovolaemia) and it may be corrected by intravenous volume to increase preload to the heart.

Endotracheal Intubation

There are four absolute indications for controlling the airway by ET intubation:

- maintain the patency of the airway where problems are present or anticipated (e.g. direct airway trauma, oedema or infection)
- to protect the airway from aspiration in states of altered consciousness, where airway-protective mechanisms may be lost or impaired
- to facilitate airway clearance techniques and avoid airway obstruction when there is marked atelectasis and pulmonary infection – an inadequate cough might necessitate more direct access to the airways for suctioning
- when positive pressure breathing is indicated because of inadequate spontaneous ventilation.

In practice, experienced staff should carry out establishing airway and respiratory support for the acutely ill child, because such patients can deteriorate rapidly, particularly at the time of inducing anaesthesia. Following pre-oxygenation with 100% inspired oxygen, a variety of agents are used to facilitate ET intubation. Intravenous induction is often used in the paediatric (PICU) setting, combining hypnotic drugs such as midazolam or ketamine with opioid analgesics such as fentanyl and muscle relaxants, e.g. suxamethonium or rocuronium. Alternatively, an inhalational induction with the volatile agent sevoflurane may be used. Table 10-3 provides a guide to the appropriate ETT size, length and suction catheter used in the paediatric age range and Figure 10-1 illustrates a commonly used method of ETT fixation.

MECHANICAL VENTILATION

Many of the ventilatory techniques are similar for children and adults. However, there are some differences between these two groups that are highlighted in the following section.

General Ventilatory Care

A variety of ventilators can be used in paediatric mechanical ventilation (Fig. 10-2). There are specific ventilators designed for neonates and small infants that are used mainly in neonatal units to ventilate premature babies. Fortunately, most modern ventilators can be used across the whole age spectrum and they can deliver different modes of pressure control ventilation (PCV) and volume control ventilation (VCV) (Donn & Sinha 2003).

One of the main goals during mechanical ventilation is to minimize dyssynchrony and optimize patient–ventilator interaction. Adequate patient comfort will potentially decrease the need for pharmacological sedation and may help to minimize the duration of mechanical ventilation. The addition of PEEP at 3–5 cmH$_2$O above atmospheric pressure is routinely

TABLE 10-3
Endotracheal Tube Size and Suction Catheters

Age	Weight (kg)	Endotracheal Tube (ID mm)	Length at Lip (cm)	Length at Nose (cm)	Suction Catheter (ED French Gauge)
Newborn	<0.7	2.0	5.0	6.0	5.0
	<1	2.5	5.5	7.0	5.0
	1	3.0	6.0	7.5	6.0
	2	3.0	7.0	9.0	6.0
	3	3.0	8.5	10.5	6.0
	3.5	3.5	9.0	11	7.0
3 months	6.0	3.5	10	12	7.0
1 year	10	4.0	11	14	8.0
2 years	12	4.5	12	15	8.0
3 years	14	4.5	13	16	8.0
4 years	16	5.0	14	17	10
6 years	20	5.5	15	19	10
8 years	24	6.0	16	20	12
10 years	30	6.5	17	21	12
12 years	38	7.0	18	22	12–14
14 years	50	7.5	19	23	14

ID: internal diameter, ED: external diameter, 3 French Gauge = 1 mm

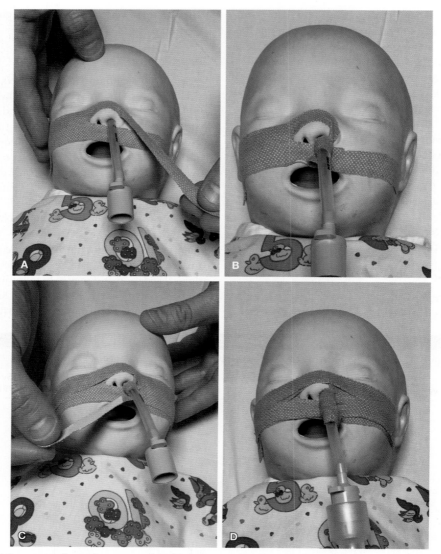

FIGURE 10-1 ■ Sequence of securing an nasal endotracheal tube in an infant. **(A)** First 'trouser-leg' tape with lower part secured below nose and upper part wrapping around tube. **(B)** First tape in place. **(C)** Second tape with upper part secured across nose, lower part wrapping around tube. **(D)** Taping complete.

used unless there is a contraindication. This helps to avoid alveolar collapse during mechanical ventilation. The amount of PEEP may need to be increased in conditions associated with low lung volume, such as neonatal RDS, atelectasis, severe pneumonia (e.g. viral, *Pneumocystis carinii*) or ARDS. One recent study in respiratory syncytial virus (RSV) bronchiolitis suggested that a PEEP around 7 cmH$_2$O is most often

associated with optimal lung volumes but that each child should be assessed individually (Essouri et al 2011).

Complications of ventilator therapy occur frequently, and all intensive care staff should be continually aware of the potential hazards (Box 10-3). Aseptic technique is important for tracheal airway care because nosocomial infection constitutes a large and

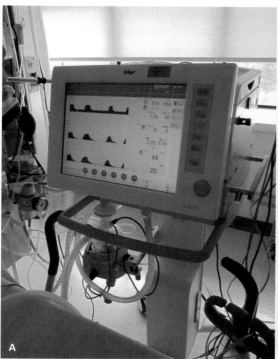
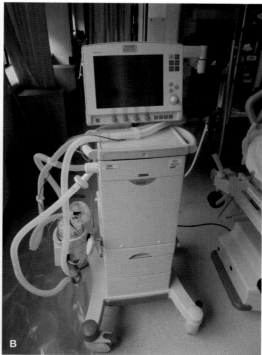

FIGURE 10-2 ■ Examples of ventilators used in paediatric intensive care unit for conventional ventilation. **(A)** Drager Evita XL (Drägerwerk AG & Co. KGaA, Germany). **(B)** Maquet Servo-I (MAQUET Holding B.V. & Co. KG, Germany).

BOX 10-3
COMPLICATIONS ASSOCIATED WITH MECHANICAL VENTILATION

RESPIRATORY

Tracheal lesions, e.g. erosions, oedema, stenosis, granuloma, obstruction

Accidental endotracheal tube displacement into bronchus, oesophagus or hypopharynx

Infection

Air leaks, e.g. pneumothorax, pneumomediastinum, interstitial emphysema

Air trapping causing hyperinflation

Excessive secretions resulting in atelectasis

Oxygen hazards, e.g. depression of ventilation, bronchopulmonary dysplasia

Pulmonary haemorrhage

CIRCULATORY

Impaired venous return resulting in decreased cardiac output and systemic hypotension

Oxygen hazards, e.g. retrolental fibroplasia, cerebral vasoconstriction

Septicaemia

Intracranial haemorrhage, e.g. intraventricular, subarachnoid

Hyperventilation leading to decreased cerebral blood flow

METABOLIC

Increased work of breathing because of 'fighting' the ventilator

Alkalosis due to potassium depletion or excessive bicarbonate therapy

RENAL AND FLUID BALANCE

Antidiuresis

Excess water in the inspired gas

EQUIPMENT MALFUNCTION (MECHANICAL)

Ventilator leaks or valve dysfunction

Overheating of inspired gases

Kinked or disconnected tubes

preventable problem. The application of PEEP, increased tidal volumes and increased airway pressure can also produce complications. Potential disruption of normal $\dot{V}/\dot{Q}$ matching seen with spontaneous breathing can occur with lung overexpansion and leads to regional hypoperfusion. A decrease in venous return, an increase in pulmonary vascular resistance and a decrease in left ventricular output can impair cardiac output and oxygen delivery. The more compliant the lung or the less compliant the chest wall, the greater the transmission of positive airway pressure to the mediastinum and the greater the negative effect on cardiac function. Volume loading or inotropic support can overcome the concomitant decrease in cardiac output, in large part.

The significance of ventilator-induced lung injury (VILI) has been appreciated more during the last few years. It now seems clear that the pathogenesis of respiratory failure is greatly influenced by the way the lungs are ventilated. Barotrauma and volutrauma have been used to describe VILI. However, there is some controversy as to which of these is the more damaging. Both can produce overdistension, and it is this problem that appears to cause the injury. To complicate matters, another factor appears to be 'atelectrauma', i.e. where the repeated collapse and re-expansion of areas of the lung produce shearing injury that contributes to inflammation and lung damage (Slutsky 2013). The best ventilator strategy should therefore aim to keep tidal volume to a minimum with optimum PEEP and, sometimes, neuromuscular blockade. Theoretically, these manoeuvres should reduce atelectasis and patient–ventilator interactions.

In regard to other problems, pulmonary interstitial emphysema, pneumomediastinum, pneumoperitoneum and subcutaneous emphysema do not require specific treatment unless there is significant haemodynamic impairment. Poor renal function, as exhibited by decreased glomerular filtration rate, urine production and sodium excretion, can be a consequence of hypoxia and hypercarbia. This may be further compounded by the effects of mechanical ventilation with PEEP on producing an antidiuretic hormone-mediated salt and water-retaining effect (probably secondary to decreased cardiac output), an increased renal vein pressure and a neural reflex from the pressure-distorted atrial wall.

Acute Deterioration and 'Troubleshooting'

In mechanically ventilated patients, the adequacy of gas exchange and ventilation should be assessed frequently. Changes in therapy should then be titrated against expected parameters or targets (see Table 10-5). When there is an acute deterioration during mechanical ventilation, problem solving or 'troubleshooting' should begin with making the patient safe. In the first instance this means disconnecting the patient from the ventilator and support breathing with bag ventilation using FiO_2 of 1.0. Easy ventilation and patient stabilization with the bag suggests a ventilator problem that should be systematically addressed (e.g. check the circuit for leaks, check ventilator function, check gas flow). However, it should be remembered that 'hand-bagging' might result in increased tidal volume, which can also be responsible for the patient's improvement. Patients with stiff lungs are frequently dyspnoeic despite adequate gas exchange. Increasing the tidal volume will correct this subjective feeling and may also account for patient improvement.

Difficult bagging at the time of disconnecting the ventilator strongly suggests a problem with the ETT or the lung–to–chest-wall complex. A suction catheter (see Table 10-3) should be passed down the ETT to check for narrowing or blockage. Chest examination, blood gases and chest radiography should be ordered. A blocked ETT should be replaced urgently by an appropriately experienced physician, or an alternative technique used to oxygenate in the interim, e.g. face mask ventilation or laryngeal mask airway. A pneumothorax requires chest tube placement. If neither of these is the cause for deterioration, then the possibilities may include new problems, such as an increased oxygen demand due to sepsis, impaired oxygen delivery due to heart failure or acute pulmonary injury due to gastric aspiration. These and other causes need to be sought and treated appropriately.

Commonly Used Modes of Mechanical Ventilation in Children

Pressure Versus Volume Control

In VCV a set tidal volume is delivered and the peak inspiratory pressure (PIP) will depend on lung compliance, inspiratory flow and airway resistance. The plateau pressure, which occurs when there is zero flow

TABLE 10-4

Advantages and Disadvantages of Pressure-Limited and Volume-Limited Ventilation

	Pressure-Limited	Volume-Limited
Advantages	Avoids excessive inflating pressures Decreased risk of barotrauma	Constant volume delivered High inflating pressures reflect changes in mechanics
Disadvantages	Variable volume delivered No signs of altered mechanics	Capable of generating very high inflating pressures Increased risk of barotrauma

in the airways during the inspiratory pause, is a more accurate measurement of actual alveolar pressure and it will be mainly influenced by lung compliance. The ventilator rate and inspiratory time are set by the clinician. This mode has the advantage of guaranteeing minute ventilation, especially in conditions when optimum minute ventilation is required (e.g. head injury). However, a decrease in compliance can lead to excessively high pressures with risk of lung injury (Table 10-4).

In PCV the delivered breath is limited by pressure. The tidal volume is determined by preset pressure limit, inspiratory time and lung compliance; it may also vary with the condition of the lung. The flow is decelerating, meaning that it slows down progressively after reaching the set inspiratory pressure. As in VCV, the ventilator rate and inspiratory time are set by the clinician. PCV has the advantage of decelerating flow and it has been considered to be less injurious because lower pressures are usually achieved, compared with volume control. However, a decrease in lung compliance, such as that caused by accumulation of secretions, may be associated with a decrease in tidal volume. This situation may go unrecognized because the ventilator will continue to cycle at the preset pressure (see Table 10-4). Use of continuous end tidal CO_2 monitoring can detect this occurrence earlier, as can careful setting of modern ventilator alarm limits for minute volume or tidal volume.

There are few controlled studies in children comparing these various modes of ventilation. Usually the final choice of ventilator mode depends on personal experience, the availability of technology and the underlying disease. Whatever mode is chosen it is essential to ensure that the expected tidal volume, minute ventilation and pressures are achieved.

Low Tidal Volume Ventilation

In patients with AHRF or ARDS, ventilation using low tidal volumes has been widely accepted. In 2000, the ARDS network reported a decreased mortality in adults when using tidal volumes of 6 mL/kg as compared to 12 mL/kg (Acute Respiratory Distress Syndrome Network 2000). These results are probably applicable to children. The risk of using smaller tidal volumes for mechanical ventilation is that it can lead to insufficient minute ventilation and hypercarbia. Therefore the strategy commonly adopted when using low tidal volume ventilation is to accept a higher $PaCO_2$, provided the arterial pH is 7.25 or above. In practice, the ventilator is set so that PIPs are limited below 30 cmH_2O (30 cmH_2O of plateau pressure when using volume control) while employing high mean airway pressures to ensure maximum lung volume recruitment via the use of PEEP. Avoidance of VILI and optimizing ventilation settings has remained an area of intense research. A recent meta-analysis of nine ARDS ventilation studies suggested that the driving pressure (dP) of ventilation is the most strongly associated variable with survival in ARDS (Amato 2015). In practice this is the plateau pressure minus the applied PEEP, and relates to the restriction of lung volume by reduced compliance in this condition. The study excluded patients receiving pressure control ventilation strategies and those not making spontaneous efforts so its application to paediatric critical care practice is unclear.

Pressure-Regulated Volume Control (PRVC) Ventilation

This mode of ventilation is available in newer ventilators. This mode delivers a preset tidal volume in a pressure-limited manner using the lowest possible pressure with a decelerating flow. To guarantee the set tidal volume, the gas flow and pressure change constantly in each delivered breath, depending on lung compliance and airway resistance. This method has the advantage of guaranteeing tidal volume and using decelerating flow. As lung compliance improves during the course of pulmonary disease, the ventilator will automatically wean inspiratory pressures. Even though PRVC seems to have advantages over other modes, clinical controlled trials to evaluate its benefits are few in children with those carried out showing no benefit (D'Angio 2005).

NEWER VENTILATORY SUPPORT TECHNIQUES

High-Frequency Oscillatory Ventilation

High-frequency ventilation techniques, including high-frequency positive pressure ventilation, high-frequency jet ventilation and high-frequency oscillatory ventilation (HFOV), achieve adequate ventilation by employing tidal volumes that are often less than actual dead space and respiratory rates of 60–3000 cycles/min (Fig. 10-3). The most widely used of these

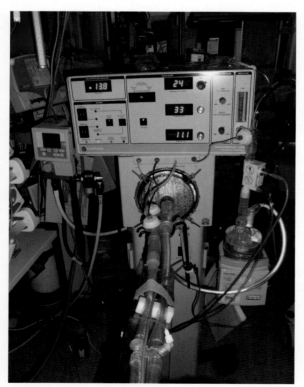

FIGURE 10-3 ■ CareFusion Sensormedics 3000 (CareFusion, USA) used for high-frequency oscillation ventilation (HFOV).

modes in children is the HFOV. The theoretical advantage of HFOV is that it keeps the lungs open by using a relatively high mean airway pressure and it delivers very low tidal volumes, thereby minimizing lung damage caused by high volumes and high inspiratory pressures. The high mean airway pressure allows lung-volume recruitment and improves oxygenation.

The most common indication for this form of ventilation is refractory hypoxaemia. However, HFOV has been used in bronchopleural fistula and some types of obstructive disease and bronchiolitis (Kneyber et al 2005, Scottish Intercollegiate Guidelines Network, 2006, Slee-Wijffels et al 2005). Unfortunately, there is a paucity of published clinical trials on the use of HFOV in the paediatric population and its benefits have not been clearly established as compared with conventional mechanical ventilation. Despite this lack of evidence, HFOV is frequently used in the treatment of hypoxaemic respiratory disease. When used, early institution of this therapy seems to be more beneficial in this group of patients (Arnold et al 1994). The experience reported by Watkins and colleagues (2000) in 100 courses of such ventilation would suggest that, in the presence of AHRF or ARDS, a threshold mean airway pressure of 16 cmH$_2$O is an appropriate indication. As an established part of neonatal critical care for many years, there is evidence that in extremely premature infants, those ventilated by HFOV had similar functional outcomes but measurably better lung function results later in life (Zivanovic 2014). Unfortunately, in adult critical care practice, recent studies have shown no improvement and potentially an increase in mortality using HFOV in ARDS patients (Ferguson et al 2013). Further study will be required in the paediatric population to clarify the use of this modality.

Extracorporeal Membrane Oxygenation

Extracorporeal membrane oxygenation (ECMO) is designed to provide a variable degree of cardiopulmonary support for a predetermined period of time over which the underlying pulmonary disorder is expected to recover. Potentially, ECMO allows recovery without subjecting the lungs to the risks of VILI or oxygen toxicity. Venoarterial systems may be used to completely take over the child's own heart and lung function (Fig. 10-4), although in practice, extracorporeal flows may be limited by venous drainage (usually from

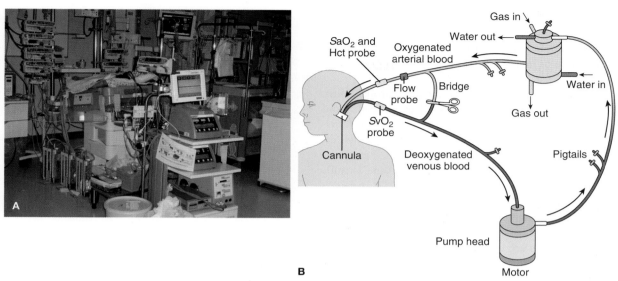

FIGURE 10-4 ■ **(A)** Extracorporeal membrane oxygenation (ECMO) support system. **(B)** ECMO circuit. SaO_2, Arterial oxygen saturation; SvO_2, venous oxygen saturation. (*B reproduced courtesy of ECMO Service/Medical Illustration, Great Ormond Street Hospital.*)

the right internal jugular vein). Venovenous systems have been used for CO_2 removal, although a retrospective study concluded that venovenous ECMO could effectively provide adequate oxygenation for children with severe acute respiratory failure (Pettignano et al 2003). In the complete absence of pulmonary function, venovenous ECMO will provide SpO_2 of 80%. Using extracorporeal support, success has been achieved in some children with acute lung injury (Pearson et al 1993). However, appropriate patient selection is a critical and contentious issue. One method, proposed by Bartlett (1982, 1990), is to identify neonates at high risk for failing to respond to conventional therapy by applying an index of oxygenation, which is related to the mean airway pressure and the FiO_2 during mechanical ventilation, and the achieved PaO_2:

$$\text{Oxygenation index (OI)} = (\text{mean airway pressure} \times FiO_2 \times 100)/PaO_2 \ (\text{mmHg})$$

In Bartlett's proposal (1990), OI greater than 25 predicted 50% mortality and OI greater than 40 predicted 80% mortality. Anecdotally, in children, Goldman and colleagues (1997) have found in meningococcal sepsis that ARDS that fails to respond to HFOV may be reasonably treated with ECMO. As a result of recent pandemics of severe respiratory infections e.g. H1N1 influenza, use of ECMO for respiratory support has increased significantly. As a specialized, equipment- and labour-intensive treatment, it remains confined to a small number of paediatric intensive care units. The CESAR study (conventional ventilatory support versus extracorporeal membrane oxygenation for severe adult respiratory failure) (Peek et al., 2009) assessed the clinical efficacy and also financial viability of transferring adults with severe reversible respiratory failure to ECMO centres for specialist management. This was found to significantly increase survival and decrease long-term disability. It is likely that the situation will be the same for the paediatric population.

VENTILATION STRATEGIES FOR SPECIFIC DISEASE

In paediatric practice, there are some specific diseases or problems that do require a specific ventilatory strategy. These issues are illustrated by the examples that follow.

Acute Bronchiolitis

The typical features of bronchiolitis are:

■ acute generalized peripheral airway obstruction ('air trapping') with tachypnoea, decreased breath sounds and low hemidiaphragms on chest radiography

- infant less than 2 years of age
- little or no evidence of past similar episodes.

RSV is the most frequent cause of bronchiolitis. Other viral causes include adenovirus, influenza and parainfluenza viruses and rhinovirus. Cytomegalovirus can produce a bronchiolitis or pneumonitis-like illness in immunocompromised children. Rare nonviral causes of the bronchiolitis syndrome include *Mycoplasma pneumoniae* and *Bordetella pertussis* infection.

Sixteen percent of infants hospitalized for RSV have apnoea and its course is usually short-lived. Clinically these episodes are diaphragmatic or non-obstructive with complete absence of respiratory effort. In these cases, ET intubation with minimal support is required until the problem resolves. In patients with worsening respiratory distress due to pulmonary parenchymal changes, mechanical support does not necessarily require ET intubation. In some instances, nasopharyngeal prong CPAP, which maintains positive transpulmonary pressure during spontaneous breathing, can be used to avoid mechanical ventilation. Other forms of non-invasive ventilator support are being used to similar effect, such as high-flow nasal cannula (HFNC) systems. When infants with RSV infection require mechanical ventilation, there are many similarities with mechanical ventilation of adults with status asthmaticus (Box 10-4). Clinical observation of inspiratory and expiratory chest excursion, as well as regular auscultation, is important if overventilation with associated hyperinflation and barotrauma is to be avoided. The aim is to maintain or achieve adequate arterial oxygenation and control of respiratory acidosis. This may even necessitate ventilating at slow rates with prolonged expiratory times to permit adequate CO_2 clearance. Low levels of PEEP are used to decrease airway resistance and improve gas exchange, although in studies of lung mechanics, this has not been verified. The presence of inadvertent or auto-PEEP requires that extrinsic PEEP be applied to the same level in order to maintain expiratory flow.

In patients with hyperinflation, the ventilator strategy should aim to limit ventilator-associated dynamic hyperinflation and impaired minute ventilation. The

ventilator should be set at a slow rate (10–15 breaths/min) and with a prolonged expiratory time. Time-cycled PCV is used in this instance while aiming for an arterial pH >7.25 and an SpO_2 of 88–92%. When indicated, neuromuscular blockade and antibiotics will need to be prescribed. All patients should receive adequate analgesia and sedation during mechanical ventilation. Bronchodilators can be administered if patients demonstrate a therapeutic response to an initial trial dose. In the acute phase of illness, fluids, electrolytes and hydration must be closely monitored while generally restricting fluid to 67–75% of

---

BOX 10-4
VENTILATION OF ACUTE BRONCHIOLITIS

OXYGENATION

Aim: PaO_2 9–10 kPa, using PEEP and supplemental oxygen

If: FiO_2 ≥0.6, increase PEEP

If: PaO_2 ≥11.3 kPa, decrease FiO_2 to 0.6:
- then decrease PEEP to 4 cmH_2O
- then decrease FiO_2

CARBON DIOXIDE

Aim: $PaCO_2$ 5.3–6.5 kPa, using rate 10–15/min, tidal volume 15 mL/kg or whatever PIP to achieve adequate chest movement

If PIP ≥30 cmH_2O or if agitated, then paralyze

If: $PaCO_2$ ≥7 kPa, pressure-limited ventilation:
- increase PIP before rate if chest excursion inadequate

Volume ventilation:
- increase minute ventilation with rate up to 20/min

If: $PaCO_2$ ≤4.7 kPa, lower tidal volume to 7 mL/kg:
- PIP to 25 cmH_2O
- then rate

EXTUBATION CRITERIA

PaO_2 ≥9.3 kPa	PEEP/CPAP ≥4 cmH_2O
FiO_2 ≤0.4	
$PaCO_2$ ≤6 kPa	Rate ≤6/min

Continue with supplemental oxygen until SpO_2 ≥0.95 in room air

CPAP, Continuous positive airway pressure; FiO_2, fractional inspired oxygen concentration; $PaCO_2$, partial pressure of carbon dioxide in arterial blood; PaO_2, partial pressure of oxygen in arterial blood; *PEEP*, positive end-expiratory pressure; *PIP*, peak inspirator pressure; SpO_2, pulse oximetry arterial oxygen saturation.

maintenance requirements. In the weaning phase, patients can be removed from ventilator support when safe to do so. In regard to blood gas parameters this means, in general, adequate oxygenation with an FiO_2 <0.4 and normal pH, with good respiratory drive, in the absence of hypercarbia. Discharge from the ICU can then be considered once the patient has managed at least 12–24 hours without any respiratory assistance. Overall these patients will, on average, spend about 7 days (interquartile range 4–8 days) on the ICU (Tasker et al 2000).

In about one-fifth of mechanically ventilated patients with RSV more severe disease is seen (Tasker et al 2000). In this instance, more extensive pulmonary pathology results in a picture of pneumonitis with diffuse alveolar consolidation rather than bronchiolitis with lung hyperinflation. These infants have the clinical features of ARDS, as they exhibit four-quadrant consolidation on chest radiograph. The aim of mechanical support should be to recruit lung volume with the addition of PEEP.

Sometimes HFOV or ECMO is required if lung injury becomes more extensive with likely development of interstitial emphysema and pneumothorax. The time course of this problem is very different to the usual course of bronchiolitis and, on average, patients spend at least 2 weeks on the ICU (Tasker et al 2000).

Acute Hypoxaemic Respiratory Failure

In patients with AHRF or ARDS the low tidal volume strategy in addition to PEEP helps to minimize VILI. The level of PEEP should be adjusted so as ensure maximum lung volume recruitment. Adequate recruitment improves oxygenation and avoids repeated alveolar collapse and reopening that lead to shear injuries. If oxygenation continues being inadequate with a mean airway pressure of 16 cmH_2O or greater, then HFOV should be considered, particularly if the problem is one of diffuse parenchymal changes or consolidation. A series of adjunctive therapies have been proposed for this condition.

Prone Positioning

Prone positioning has been shown to improve oxygenation during hypoxaemic respiratory disease in a number of adult and paediatric studies (Curley et al 2005, Pelosi et al 2002). These observations together with the simplicity of the procedure have justified the inclusion of this technique as standard practice. The incidence of serious adverse effects has not been reported to increase during prone position and only mild complications (e.g. facial oedema and pressure ulcers) have been described. During ventilation in the supine position the dorsal areas of the lung become preferentially consolidated or collapsed. The change to prone position allows recruitment of the dorsal areas of the lung and generates a more even distribution of ventilation and improved $\dot{V}/\dot{Q}$ matching. Previous studies have not shown any impact on outcome despite improved oxygenation with proning (Curley et al 2005). However, a recent multicentre prospective study of early prone positioning for more prolonged periods in ARDS suggested a significant survival benefit (Guerin 2013).

Recruitment Manoeuvres

Recruitment manoeuvres are aimed at recovering collapsed areas of the lung during ALI, especially after specific manipulations such a suctioning and disconnection of the ventilator. A variety of manoeuvres have been described, including increases in the level of PEEP while maintaining constant inspiratory pressures, prolonged increases in pressure (i.e. 40 mmHg for 40 sec) as a single manoeuvre or using stepwise increases and the use of high tidal volumes. There is a risk of VILI as well as cardiovascular instability as a result of these techniques, however. Gattinoni et al (2006) used computed tomography (CT) imaging with recruitment manoeuvers in ARDS patients to assess the percentage of recruitable lung, which they found to be extremely variable and closely correlated to baseline aeration with PEEP applied. Also, they noted that higher percentages of recruitable lung were associated with more severe disease and poorer outcome. There are no controlled studies and there is no consensus regarding these manoeuvres and their safety in children.

Nitric Oxide

Nitric oxide (NO) is an endogenous, endothelium-derived vasodilator. Inhaled NO has the theoretical advantage of producing selective reduction in pulmonary vascular resistance. The fact that inhaled NO acts on the vessels of the aerated areas of the lung during

ARDS suggests that it should improve $\dot{V}/\dot{Q}$ mismatch and therefore should be helpful during the management of this condition. Unfortunately, even though NO has been shown to transiently improve oxygenation in ARDS, it does not seem to improve outcome (Afshari et al 2010) and may even have an increased risk of renal impairment.

Surfactant

The use of exogenous surfactant in adults with ARDS has been shown to be feasible and safe; however, it has not proven to be effective in adult ALI (Stevens et al 2004). A recent multicentre, randomized, blinded trial of calfactant (extract of natural surfactant from calf lungs) compared with placebo in 153 infants with ALI showed improvement in oxygenation and a decrease in mortality in the patients that had received surfactant (Willson et al 2005).

OTHER CONSIDERATIONS DURING MECHANICAL VENTILATION

Position During Mechanical Ventilation

Changes in position during mechanical ventilation can be used to improve lung volumes, $\dot{V}/\dot{Q}$ matching and the clearance of airway secretions, or to improve comfort and work of breathing. Changes in position can also be used to avoid or treat pressure lesions. Elevation of the bed head may also help to reduce gastro-oesophageal reflux and pulmonary aspiration (Torres et al 1992). This has been adopted as a standard part of ventilator-associated infection prevention care bundles.

Humidification

During mechanical ventilation most of the upper airway is bypassed by the ETT or tracheostomy tube, and the rest of the airway may not be able to supply enough heat and moisture to the delivered gases that are dry and colder than body temperature. Humidification and heating is therefore essential to avoid complications such as hypothermia, inspissation of airway secretions, destruction of airway epithelium and atelectasis. In adults, humidifying filters (which operate passively by storing heat and moisture from the patient's exhaled gas) are frequently used for this purpose; however, in children, active heating of humidified air is necessary. In order to achieve this, a humidifier that operates to increase the heat and water vapour content of the gases is interposed in the inspiratory limb of the ventilator circuit and the temperature is usually set to deliver approximately 37°C to the distal area of the circuit.

Suctioning

Suctioning of the airway to remove secretions is part of the routine care of patients receiving artificial ventilation. However, suctioning can lead to side effects including hypoxaemia, haemodynamic instability, mucosal damage, increase in intracranial pressure (ICP) and patient discomfort. The use of adequate sedation, reassurance, preoxygenation and a good technique may help to minimize these complications.

Physiotherapy

Physiotherapy is frequently used as an integral part of the management of children receiving mechanical ventilation. However, the place, frequency and techniques of physiotherapy vary widely among units. Frequent techniques used in mechanically ventilated patients are manual hyperinflation, percussion, vibration and positioning, all of which are believed to increase the clearance of secretions. These are covered later in this chapter.

Monitoring During Mechanical Ventilation

Adequate monitoring of the parameters affected by mechanical ventilation is essential. The information helps to characterize the pathophysiology of the underlying condition, to improve ventilation, to enhance patient comfort, and to guide weaning. Blood gas measurement is the gold standard for assessing pulmonary gas exchange, but this technique is limited by the fact that measurements are not continuous because they require invasive techniques. The use of pulse oximeters and end-tidal carbon dioxide concentration helps to minimize the number of blood gas samples. Transcutaneous carbon dioxide measurement is another way of continuously monitoring the CO_2 status.

Monitoring of the respiratory mechanics and analysis of the patient–ventilator interaction should be part of the routine care during mechanical ventilation. Most modern mechanical ventilators provide a graphical display of gas flow, airway pressures and tidal and minute volumes. In small infants and neonates, the information obtained with a pneumotachometer positioned at the end of the ETT instead of inside the mechanical ventilator can be more reliable. These data, together with measurements of pulmonary gas exchange, help to assess the adequacy of ventilation.

A new technique, electroimpedance tomography, analyzes the distribution of ventilation and can be used at the bedside. This technique uses 16 electrodes placed around the chest. Injection of an alternating electrical current between sequential pairs of adjacent electrodes and the repeated measurement of the differences in voltage through the array of electrodes permits the detection of changes in impedance. Since air is a poor conductor of electricity compared with other tissues, computer-assisted use of a mathematical algorithm then allows the reconstruction of a spatial image of a section of the chest. This method has the advantage of being non-invasive, radiation free, portable and dynamic. Different studies have shown its usefulness to assess regional lung ventilation (Bikker et al. 2011, Victorino et al 2004) but it has yet to be adopted widely.

Weaning from Mechanical Ventilation

Stopping mechanical ventilation as soon as the child is ready to be weaned from support is essential to avoid complications. Prolonged mechanical ventilation has been associated with higher risk of nosocomial pneumonia, progressive ventilator-associated lung injury, airway injury, physiological dependence on sedative and narcotic drugs and even higher mortality. In children who need mechanical ventilation for respiratory failure, the usual approach is to wean the ventilator settings gradually until the patient is considered to be ready for extubation. However, this gradual weaning process is now being questioned. A randomized controlled trial (RCT) comparing weaning protocols versus standard physician-guided weaning in children did not show any impact on the duration of mechanical ventilation. This study also showed that gradual weaning may not be indicated for the majority of children receiving mechanical ventilation due to respiratory failure, and that a large group of children were ready to be extubated when the physicians determined that they were ready to begin a weaning process

---

BOX 10-5

ELIGIBILITY CRITERIA FOR READINESS FOR EXTUBATION TESTING

1. Spontaneous respiratory effort
2. Gag or cough reflexes with suctioning
3. Presence of air leak around the ET tube
4. pH of 7.32–7.47 on blood gas
5. PEEP of 7 or lower
6. FiO_2 of 0.6 or less
7. Acceptable level of consciousness
8. Improvement of the underlying process that led to intubation
9. No need of increased ventilation during the last 24 hours
10. No planned administration of heavy sedation during the next 12 hours

ET, Endotracheal; FiO_2, fractional inspired oxygen concentration; PEEP, positive end-expiratory pressure.

(Randolph et al 2002). Readiness for extubation can be evaluated using a daily test as soon as the patient meets the criteria for testing (Box 10-5). Different tests for extubation readiness have been proposed. In one paediatric study, patients were extubated if they passed a trial of spontaneous breathing with either pressure support of 10 cmH$_2$O or T-piece for up to 2 hours. Mechanical ventilation was reinstituted if any of the following signs appeared:

1. respiratory rate higher than the 90th centile for the age
2. signs of increased respiratory work
3. diaphoresis and anxiety
4. heart rate higher than the 90th centile for the age
5. change in mental status
6. blood pressure lower than the third centile for the age
7. oxygen saturation lower than 90%
8. PaCO$_2$ more than 50 mmHg or an increase of more than 10 mmHg
9. arterial pH lower than 7.30 (Farias et al 2002).

Use of sedation has an impact on the duration of mechanical ventilation. Improved management of sedatives, including the use of objective sedation scores, should be part of the standard care for children receiving mechanical ventilation.

Non-Invasive Support

NIV is the delivery of supportive ventilation without the use of an ET airway. NIV is usually delivered as positive pressure ventilation using CPAP or BiPAP; however, negative pressure ventilation by mean of a cuirass is still useful for some conditions. Initially the use of NIV was mostly used in children with neuromuscular disease. Now it is used in most types of respiratory failure.

In neonates and small infants the most frequent way of delivering non-invasive positive pressure ventilation (NPPV) is by means of nasal CPAP, although modern technology also incorporates the possibility of delivering BiPAP. The most frequent indication is bronchiolitis and other infections with apnoea. In bigger children NPPV is frequently delivered as BiPAP (Fig. 10-5), although CPAP can also be used. In this age it is used for different forms of acute hypoxaemic or hypercarbic respiratory failure including asthma

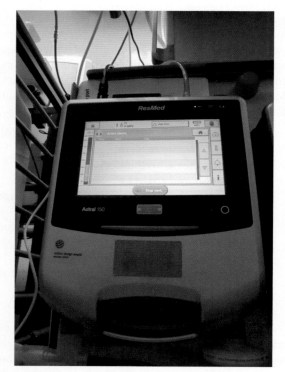

FIGURE 10-5 ▪ ResMed Astral 150 (ResMed, USA) suitable for long-term non-invasive ventilation.

and neuromuscular disease, or after extubation in children who have received long periods of mechanical ventilation. The usual way of applying this form of support is via a nasal mask or a face mask. Nasal masks are better tolerated, but many patients with respiratory distress are mouth breathers and therefore a face mask might be necessary (Fig. 10-6).

In order to tolerate NPPV some sedation is needed in the young infant. In older children, explanation, reassurance and familiarity with the therapy should suffice.

To increase the tolerance, NPPV can be started at low pressure settings that are then increased progressively until the target pressures are obtained. Nasogastric tubes can be used when the accumulation of air in the stomach is a concern, especially in children with face masks. However, many clinicians prefer not to use nasogastric tubes, as their placement with tapes can reduce the tightness of the seal between the mask and the face.

A review of clinical studies using NPPV has shown that improvement usually occurs after the first 3 hours of therapy (Akingbola & Hopkins 2001). NPPV is not recommended in ARDS (Essouri et al 2006). The contraindications for NPPV include respiratory arrest, inability to use the mask because of trauma or surgery, difficult secretion management, haemodynamic instability, altered mental state, risk of aspiration, intolerance to the therapy and life-threatening refractory hypoxaemia or hypercarbia.

A recent alternative method of non-invasive support is through the use of humidified high-flow nasal cannula systems, which have become increasingly widespread. The mechanism of ventilation assistance is multifactorial with a degree of distending pressure (PEEP) applied from the higher flows and gas exchange assisted by greater than minute ventilation flows in the airway. These systems are well tolerated by patients without the need for sedation/anxiolysis. A recent study comparing high-flow oxygen systems with normal low-flow oxygen and non-invasive mask ventilation in patients with hypoxic respiratory failure showed similar rates of intubation but a decrease in 90-day mortality and greater number of ventilator-free days in the high-flow groups (Frat et al 2015).

Finally, one technique that has historically been used effectively in children with neuromuscular disease

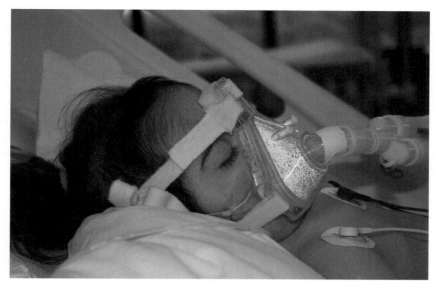

FIGURE 10-6 ■ Face mask for non-invasive ventilation.

since the poliomyelitis epidemics in the 1950s is extrathoracic negative pressure ventilation with a cuirass (Lassen 1953). There has been renewed interest in this form of ventilation (Meessen et al 1994). There are many physiological reasons why negative pressure support should be beneficial, such as its ability to increase tonic activity in the diaphragm and intercostal muscles. In children with neuromuscular disease who are on positive pressure mechanical support, analgesia and sedation can be discontinued quite quickly when negative pressure support is introduced after weaning and extubation (Chisakuta & Tasker 1998). This approach should limit the unavoidable iatrogenic worsening of respiratory drive that results from the

coadministration of analgesia and sedation (which is invariably necessary for children in order that they may tolerate the ETT). In myasthenic patients, the time course of mechanical ventilatory support can be more than halved using this technique. A retrospective analysis comparing two centres, one using negative pressure ventilation and the other using conventional therapies for bronchiolitis-related apnoeas, concluded that the use of negative pressure ventilation was associated with a reduced rate of ET intubation, and shorter PICU stay (Al-balkhi et al 2005). As more portable and easier-to-use ventilators become available, this form of respiratory support may be used more frequently.

Acknowledgement: Tomas Iolster, Robert C Tasker

Physiotherapy Management of Ventilated Infants and Children

Paediatric ICUs are stressful and demanding environments and ventilated children must be thoroughly assessed before any physiotherapy intervention is considered. A report from the nurse caring for the baby will provide important information about the

current haemodynamic status and stability of the child. A recent chest radiograph will be helpful in identifying any focal areas of respiratory compromise and should be examined in conjunction with careful auscultation in order to decide on the appropriateness of intervention. Evaluation of fluid status, urine output, heart rate and rhythm, blood pressure, platelets, bleeding, inotropic support and level of sedation will all contribute to a decision on how and if any treatment should be performed.

When children are critically ill, intubated and ventilated, therapists often have to use complex clinical reasoning to make difficult decisions. A careful risk–benefit analysis should always precede an intervention and this should include an overview of haemodynamic instability and orthopaedic or neurological contraindications to treatment that might supersede physiotherapy requirements at that time. Classic contraindications to certain treatment techniques may sometimes be superseded by more compelling clinical needs, for example a small pneumothorax may be considered less important than acute lobar atelectasis. This is not always an easy decision to make, and timely effective treatment can often prevent a critically ill infant from significant acute deterioration. Treatments should never be performed routinely, as they are never without risk of potentially detrimental effects (Horiuchi et al 1997, Krause & Hoehn 2000, Stiller 2000).

The effects of surgery, anaesthesia and immobility are the same for infants and children as for adults (see Chapter 11). However, anatomical and physiological differences between these populations make children more vulnerable to these respiratory complications (Chapter 1). Infants and children who have undergone major surgery therefore require regular accurate assessment by a physiotherapist, and successful treatments depend on thorough and continuous evaluation of clinical data during treatment from a multitude of different sources, including haemodynamic and respiratory information, observation and auscultation. Experience and competence are essential in the management of the most critically ill babies, as is a complete knowledge of underlying anatomical and physiological processes likely to influence the outcome of treatment. For example, treating a child with a univentricular pulmonary and systemic circulation with high bagging pressures or high oxygen concentration would dramatically influence the flow of blood to the lungs with potentially life-threatening consequences. Similarly, treating a child with head injury without appreciating the relationship between ICP, mean arterial pressure and cerebral perfusion pressure (CPP)

could have serious immediate and long-term consequences for their recovery. Treatments should also be timed carefully to avoid problems associated with vomiting and aspiration after feeds.

Physiotherapists working in an ICU should be familiar with the equipment used (Fig. 10-7). They should be able to respond when a problem is indicated by the monitors and be able to ascertain whether the problem is patient- or equipment-related. Children may be intubated with either nasal or oral ETTs (see Fig. 10-1). The narrowest part of the upper airways in babies and small children is the circular cricoid ring. Thus perfectly sized uncuffed tubes can be passed nasally and form a good seal in the cricoid ring, reducing the risk of damage to the tracheal mucosa from larger cuffed tubes (Deakers et al 1994, Khine et al 1997). Another advantage to nasal intubation is that the mouth is free to suck a sponge or pacifier during ventilation, so that normal feeding can be started as soon after extubation as possible. An important disadvantage to ill-fitting uncuffed tubes is the potential risk of ETT leak, in terms of both inconsistent delivery of ventilation and inaccurate monitoring of respiratory function (Kuo et al 1996, Main et al 2001a).

Details of oxygen delivery and paediatric mechanical support are described earlier in this chapter. However, modern ventilators incorporate pressure and flow sensors which allow continuous monitoring and calculation of tidal breathing parameters or respiratory mechanics from which an assessment of respiratory function can be made (MacNaughton & Evans 1999). It is essential that physiotherapists familiarize themselves with these devices, the interpretation of data generated from them and their limitations in the clinical environment (Castle et al 2002). There is great potential for such equipment to provide objective feedback about efficacy and tolerance of treatments in individual patients and to provide excellent tools for systematic evaluation of physiotherapy treatment in mechanically ventilated infants. Standard monitoring equipment is often similar to those used on adult ICUs (see Chapter 9), although normal physiological values vary according to age (Table 10-5).

Physiotherapy for infants receiving intensive care is an area of specialist practice. Evidence suggests that the level of staff expertise may be important to patient outcomes, and poor clinical decision making and a

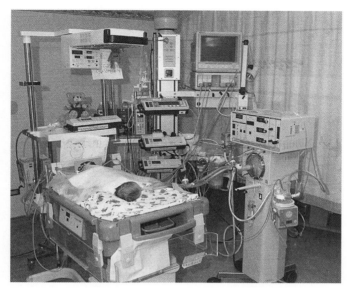

FIGURE 10-7 ■ Equipment used in a paediatric intensive care unit. Figure shows an infant undergoing high-frequency oscillatory ventilation.

TABLE 10-5
Normal Values

Age Group	Heart Rate Mean (Range) (Beats/Min)	Respiratory Rate (Range) (Breaths/Min)	Blood Pressure Systolic/Diastolic (mmHg)	Arterial Blood pH	$PaCO_2$ mmHg	PaO_2 mmHg
Preterm	150 (100–200) 120–170	40–60 at rest	39–59/16–36	7.25–7.40	40–50 (4–4.7 kPa)	50–70 (6.7–9.3 kPa)
Newborn–1 year	140 (80–180) (80–90 if asleep, 160+ distressed)	30–60	50–90/25–60	7.30–7.40	30–35 (4–4.7 kPa)	60–90 (8–12 kPa)
1–3 years	95 (70–140)	20–40	80–110/34–67	7.30–7.40	30–35 (4–4.7 kPa)	80–100 (10.7–13.3 kPa)
3–6 years	85 (65–110)	20–30	86–116/44–74	7.35–7.45	35–45 (4.7–6 kPa)	80–100 (10.7–13.3 kPa)
>6 years	75 (60–90)	15–20	91–125/53–82	7.35–7.45	35–45 (4.7–6 kPa)	80–100 (10.7–13.3 kPa)
>12 years	70 (55–85)	12–18	101–136/59–84	7.35–7.45	35–45 (4.7–6 kPa)	80–100 (10.7–13.3 kPa)

$PaCO_2$, Partial pressure of carbon dioxide in arterial blood; PaO_2, partial pressure of oxygen in arterial blood.

lack of input from senior staff may contribute to poor outcomes (Shannon 2015a, Shannon 2015b). Independent research has shown that physiotherapy competence is vital if adverse events are to be avoided and benefits optimized. A careful review of the material in Chapter 2 of this book, relating to comprehensive assessment of patients, in conjunction with consideration of the differences in the cardiorespiratory system between adults and children in Chapter 1, would provide a helpful basis for assessment of paediatric patients in the ICU. It is important to conclude examination of the child with a list of prioritized clinical

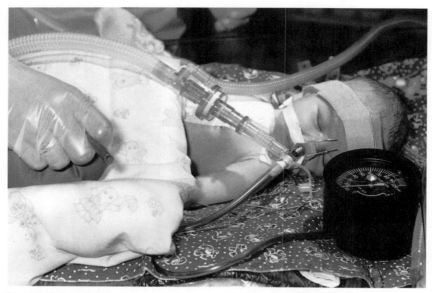

FIGURE 10-8 ■ Manual hyperinflation in a small child, showing pressure gauge in circuit.

problems and a clear idea of which important problems would be likely to respond to physiotherapy interventions, as well as a plan for treatment selection. As anticipated, clinical problems that may typically benefit would include mucus plugging, loss of lung volume due to atelectasis, a weak or absent cough, and a deterioration of effective gas exchange for any reason.

Physiotherapy treatment cycles for ventilated children in the United Kingdom commonly consist of combinations of saline instillation, manual lung inflations, chest wall vibrations and ETT suction. Treatments sometimes involve simultaneous application of chest wall vibrations during ETT suction in patients who are not sufficiently conscious to cough spontaneously during suction. This comprises insertion of the suction catheter and application of manual chest wall vibrations while applying negative pressure to the suction catheter and withdrawing it from the open tracheal tube (this dual activity being performed by a single physiotherapist, not as the two-person treatment often seen in adult practice). Full assessment appears to take between 12 and 19 minutes on average for experienced and novice practitioners respectively. Treatments take between 7 and 9 minutes for experienced and novice practitioners, and include on average three cycles of treatment (Shannon 2015b). They are therefore generally short interventions in this critically ill population.

At the end of treatments, experienced practitioners almost routinely apply a series of slow, pressure limited manual inflation recruitment breaths with an inspiratory hold before returning the patients to the ventilator at the end of a treatment (Fig. 10-8). Although a vital part of airway hygiene, ETT suction is associated with a rapid reduction in functional residual capacity and has been cited as a cause of atelectasis, which is likely to be exacerbated further when applying additional external chest wall compression to the compliant paediatric chest wall (Fig. 10-9). In isolation, physiotherapy treatment components such as those involving saline instillation, suction and chest wall vibrations may cause further acute de-recruitment of the small airways. Lung recruitment breaths may therefore play an important role in increasing alveolar ventilation and oxygenating the lung following physiotherapy treatments which include these components (Shannon 2015b).

Physiotherapy interventions for different clinical problems are covered in some detail in Chapter 7. However, a number of points related to the care of paediatric patients in intensive care are considered in the following sections.

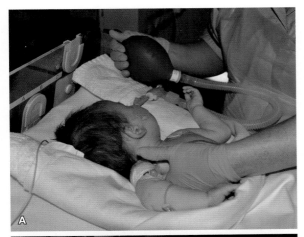

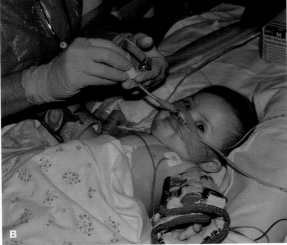

FIGURE 10-9 ■ **(A)** Manual lung inflation with chest wall vibrations. **(B)** Endotracheal tube suction.

Chest Percussion and Vibration

Chest percussion (sometimes referred to as 'chest clapping', see Fig. 7-16) can be modified in children by using a single hand, fingers or a face mask. It is generally well tolerated and widely used in children. In neonates and preterm infants 'tenting' (using the first three or four fingers of one hand with slight elevation of the middle finger) or the use of a soft, plastic, cup-shaped object such as a face mask may be more appropriate (see Figs 10-12 and 7-17) (Tudehope & Bagley 1980).

Chest wall vibrations involve the application of a rapid extrathoracic compressive force at the beginning of expiration, followed by oscillatory compressions until expiration is complete. The compressions and oscillations applied during chest wall vibrations are believed to aid secretion clearance via a number of physiological mechanisms, including increasing peak expiratory flow to move secretions towards the large airways for removal by suction or cough (Kim et al 1987, King 1998, McCarren et al 2006, Ntoumenopoulos 2005, van der Schans et al 1999, Wanner 1984).

Chest wall vibrations remain objectively undefined and may vary considerably between practitioners and units. The terms 'chest vibrations', 'compressions', 'shaking' and 'expiratory flow increase techniques' have been used variously in the literature (Almeida et al 2005, Sutton et al 1985, Wong et al 2003). Chest wall vibrations appear to be used more frequently in ventilated children than percussion, probably because the glottis is held open by the ETT, facilitating rapid expiratory flow during vibrations that improve mucus clearance. There is a strong linear relationship between the maximum force applied during chest wall vibrations and the age of the child, most likely reflecting modification of techniques to accommodate changes in chest wall compliance (Gregson et al 2007a). Maximum force applied during physiotherapy can vary substantially between physiotherapists. Similarly there is marked variability in the pattern of force–time profiles between physiotherapists with respect to the duration of vibration, and amplitude, number and frequency of oscillations. Figure 10-10 illustrates the style of force profiles delivered to four infants, all aged between 5 and 14 months by four different physiotherapists. However, there is remarkable consistency within and between each physiotherapist's treatment sessions (Gregson et al 2007b, 2012). The clinical consequences for such variation in treatment profiles remain unclear.

In children who are not intubated, vibrations can be applied effectively when reflex glottic closure does not occur and when the respiratory rate is normal or near normal (30–40 breaths/min). If infants are breathing very rapidly, the expiratory phase is so short that vibrations are more difficult to perform. Chest wall vibrations in ventilated children are effective, possibly because the combination of compliant chest wall and open glottic splinting by the ETT, facilitate rapid expiratory flow during vibrations that improve mucus clearance (Main et al 2004, Shannon 2015a, 2015b).

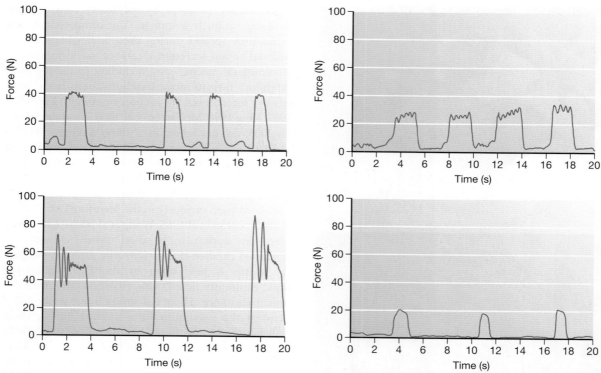

FIGURE 10-10 ■ Force–time profiles of chest wall vibrations delivered by four different physiotherapists to four infants (5–14 months). The patterns are repeatable within each treatment but vary considerably between therapists with respect to magnitude and duration of vibration, and amplitude, number and frequency of oscillations.

However, it is then important to consider incorporating effective re-recruitment manoeuvres into the treatment cycle, to counteract any treatment related atelectasis that may accrue during the chest compressions.

Physiotherapy treatments for ventilated children involving manual techniques have been shown to have an advantage over routine suction in reducing respiratory resistance, which may be of substantial benefit in patients with evidence of acute atelectasis (Main et al 2004). Within individuals, physiotherapy treatments are also more likely to produce improvements in tidal volume, respiratory compliance and resistance than suction alone, but both physiotherapy and suction procedures can produce short-term deterioration in a significant minority of children. Sensitive tools still need to be identified for selection of patients most likely to benefit from physiotherapy (Main et al 2004).

Research has also shown significant disparities in treatment outcomes when paediatric ICU respiratory physiotherapy was delivered by non-respiratory on-call physiotherapists, compared with specialist respiratory physiotherapists (Shannon et al 2015a, Shannon et al 2015b). While there were significant improvements in respiratory compliance following both on-call and respiratory physiotherapists' treatments (mean increase, 0.07 and 0.08 mL/cmH$_2$O kg^{-1} respectively, p < 0.01), on a case-by-case basis, there were fewer clinically important improvements following non–respiratory physiotherapists' treatments compared with the respiratory physiotherapists' (n = 27 (43%) versus n = 40 (63%), p = 0.03). Adverse events were also more frequent and severe following non-respiratory physiotherapists' treatments (11 vs 8). These differences in outcome may have been related to differences in both the selection and application of techniques. Both non-respiratory on-call physiotherapists and specialist respiratory physiotherapists used combinations of saline instillation, manual lung inflations, chest wall vibrations and ETT suction during treatments. However, specialist respiratory physiotherapists used simultaneous chest wall vibrations with suction and recruitment manoeuvres significantly more frequently than non-respiratory on-call physiotherapists (92% versus 52%, and 87% versus 46% of treatments, respectively, p < 0.001). Chest wall vibrations delivered by non-respiratory on-call physiotherapists were 15% less effective at increasing peak expiratory flow. This suggests an important training need for non-respiratory on-call physiotherapists, particularly in the effective delivery of physiotherapy techniques (Shannon 2015a, Shannon 2015b).

In children with dietary deficiencies, liver disease, bone mineral deficiency (e.g. rickets) or coagulopathies, manual techniques should be applied with caution. Manual techniques may not be appropriate in extremely premature infants and specific issues related to this group of patients are discussed later.

Manual Lung Inflation

Manual lung inflation involves disconnection of the patient from mechanical ventilation to provide temporary manual ventilation. The same contraindications apply for children and adults (see Chapters 7 and 9). However, special consideration should be applied in preterm infants whose lung tissue is easily damaged by high inflation pressures and in children with hyperinflated lungs (e.g. asthma and bronchiolitis) in whom there is a greater risk of pneumothorax. For infants, 500-mL bags are recommended, and 1-L bags for older children. They may be valved or open-ended, so that expulsion of excess pressure is controlled by the operator's fingers, but self-inflating bags are used in some units. A manometer should be placed in the circuit to monitor the inflation pressures (see Fig. 10-8). As a general guideline, manual ventilation pressures during physiotherapy should not exceed 30 cmH_2O or 10 cmH_2O above peak ventilator pressure. In order to prevent airway collapse, some positive end-expiratory pressure (PEEP) can be maintained in the bag. The flow rate of gas is adjusted according to the size of the child: 4 l/min for infants, increasing to 8 l/min for children.

In paediatric patients, manual ventilation is used to achieve hyperinflation, hyperoxygenation, and hyperventilation, as discussed in the following sections.

Hyperinflation

Hyperinflation is a long, slow inspiration with an inspiratory pause followed by rapid release of the bag. The aim of this technique is to recruit lung units by improving collateral ventilation and increasing lung volume. However, in acute respiratory distress, the proportion of recruitable lung may be extremely variable (Gattinoni et al 2006). Following hyperinflation, a high expiratory flow may assist in mobilizing secretions towards central airways. Some studies support the use of hyperinflation for improving respiratory mechanics (Choi & Jones 2005, Marcus et al 2002). However, there remains some controversy over the safety and effectiveness of manual lung hyperinflation as the volumes, pressures and FiO_2 are not always controlled and there are inherent dangers of barotrauma (Berney & Denehy 2002, Gattinoni et al 1993, Savian et al 2006). In addition, collateral ventilation channels are poorly developed in small infants (Menkes & Traystman 1977). In children with compromised cardiac output, the long inspiratory phase with pause may be contraindicated.

Hyperoxygenation

Hyperoxygenation may be used before suction in order to reduce suction-induced hypoxia or pulmonary hypertension. A review of the efficacy of ventilator versus manual hyperinflation in delivering hyperoxygenation or hyperinflation breaths before, during and/or after ETT suctioning found that hyperoxygenation or hyperinflation breaths at 100% oxygen delivered via the ventilator were either superior or equivalent to manually delivered breaths in preventing suction-induced hypoxaemia. However, delivery of manual hyperinflation breaths resulted in increased airway pressure and increased haemodynamic consequences (Stone 1990, Stone & Turner 1989). In the presence of pulmonary hypertension, it is generally not advisable to use an FiO_2 of 1.0 during manual hyperinflation, as this may further increase blood flow to the lungs.

Hyperventilation

Hyperventilation is a known method of rapidly lowering ICP in patients with head injury. Cerebral blood flow is dependent on $PaCO_2$, which decreases during hyperventilation, leading to arterial vasoconstriction and lower ICP. So that physiotherapy can be safely undertaken, hyperventilation should be used only for short periods and only to normocapnia ($PaCO_2$ 4.0 kPa). In those patients with a large cardiac shunt, hyperventilation may be contraindicated.

Endotracheal and Nasopharyngeal Airway Suction

Airway suction is discussed further in Chapters 7 and 9. Suction techniques may be either nasopharyngeal, oropharyngeal or endotracheal, depending on whether there is an artificial airway in situ. Adverse effects have frequently been reported and include hypoxaemia, mechanical trauma, apnoea, bronchospasm, pneumothorax, atelectasis, cardiac arrhythmias and even death on rare occasions (Clark et al 1990, Clarke et al 1999, Czarnik et al 1991, Kerem et al 1990, Shah et al 1992, Singer et al 1994, Stone & Turner 1989, Wood 1998). Practice varies widely among centres and where available local guidelines should be taken in to consideration (Sole et al 2003).

Complications associated with suction may be reduced by:

- Pre-oxygenation before suction using ventilator or manually delivered breaths with a higher FiO_2 (Chulay & Graeber 1988, Goodnough 1985). Pre-oxygenation with ventilator breaths has been recommended in preference to disconnection and manual hyperinflation because of the reduced risk of barotrauma, loss of PEEP and FiO_2 (Glass et al 1993, McCabe & Smeltzer 1993, Stone et al 1991). Particular care should be taken in preterm infants to avoid hyperoxia, as this is associated with retinopathy of prematurity (Roberton 1996).
- Suctioning via a port adaptor or closed suction systems in patients who require maintenance of PEEP and/or positive pressure ventilation during suction (Harshbarger et al 1992).
- Avoiding cross-infection, particularly in vulnerable infants, by meticulous hand washing and adherence to local infection control policies.
- Keeping suction pressures as low as possible, without compromising the efficacy of secretion

clearance. High negative pressures have been associated with mechanical trauma of the tracheal mucous membranes (Kleiber et al 1988).
- Selecting a suction catheter with an external diameter which does not exceed 50% of the internal diameter of the airway (Imle & Klemic 1989). Most commonly used catheters are 6 and 8 French gauge (FG). Size 5 FG and below are usually ineffective in removing thick secretions. Size 10 FG and above should be reserved for use with older children.
- Using graduated catheters with centimetre markings to gauge how far the catheter has been passed. Pneumothorax due to direct perforation of a segmental bronchus by a suction catheter has been reported in intubated preterm infants (Vaughan et al 1978).
- Positioning in side lying and restraining the nonintubated child who requires nasopharyngeal suction, to avoid potential aspiration of gastric contents (Fig. 10-11). Constant reassurance should be given throughout the procedure. Supplemental oxygenation and resuscitation equipment should be available. Nasopharyngeal suction of neonates may cause reflex bradycardia and apnoea.
- Avoiding nasopharyngeal suction if the child has stridor or has recently been extubated, as this may precipitate laryngospasm.

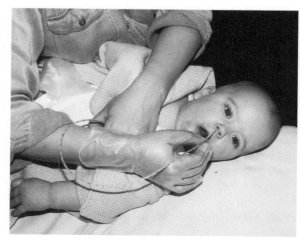

FIGURE 10-11 ■ Nasopharyngeal suction.

Saline Instillation

Saline instillation into the tracheal tube of ventilated patients aims to loosen thick or sticky secretions to facilitate easy removal with suction (Schreuder & Jones 2004). Evidence for the practice is variable and therefore saline should be used only where there is a clear indication. Some suggest that saline instillation at best is not effective and at worst is harmful (Blackwood 1999, Hagler & Traver 1994, Kinloch 1999, McKelvie 1998, Ridling et al 2003), while others suggest it is well tolerated even in infants and may be helpful in removing secretions adherent to the chest wall (Shorten et al 1991). Other mucolytics (*N*-acetylcysteine) in aliquots of 0.5–5 mL may be used to enhance secretion clearance. Larger quantities of saline are sometimes used as part of bronchoalveolar lavage procedures.

Positioning

When appropriate, modified gravity-assisted positions can be used in children to assist with clearance of bronchial secretions. The upper lobes, particularly the right side, are more frequently affected by respiratory problems and appropriate positioning may be helpful. A few studies have specifically examined the efficacy of gravity-assisted positioning in infants and children. Although it remains a useful technique in the presence of copious secretions, the possible risks of gastro-oesophageal reflux and aspiration must be considered (Button et al 1997, Button et al 2003, Button et al 2004).

A head-down tip should be avoided in children with raised ICP or in preterm infants because of the risk of periventricular haemorrhage (PVH). Abdominal distension places the diaphragm at a mechanical disadvantage and a head-down tilt is likely to exacerbate this further. In some cases, modified postural drainage may be prudent and equally effective (Fig. 10-12).

Positioning may be used to optimize respiratory function. The supine position has been shown to be the least beneficial, while prone positioning has been shown to improve respiratory function (see Chapter 7), decrease gastro-oesophageal reflux (Blumenthal & Lealman 1982) and reduce energy expenditure (Brackbill et al 1973). It is often used in closely monitored infants with respiratory problems in a hospital setting, but parents should be cautious of using this position when babies are sleeping unattended because of its association with sudden infant death (Southall & Samuels 1992).

Patterns of regional ventilation in infants differ significantly from adults (Bhuyan et al 1989, Davies et al 1985, Heaf et al 1983), with ventilation in infants and small children being preferentially distributed to the uppermost regions of the lungs. In acutely ill children with unilateral lung disease, care should be taken if positioning the child with the affected lung uppermost as this may cause rapid deterioration of respiratory status. Spontaneously breathing newborn infants are better oxygenated when tilted slightly head up (Thoresen et al 1988) and show a drop in PaO_2 if placed flat or tilted head down.

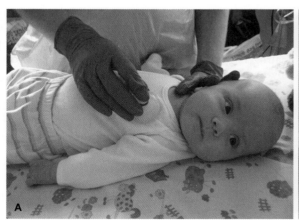 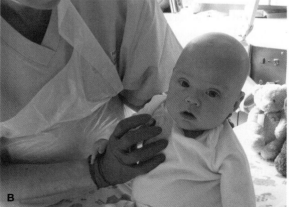

FIGURE 10-12 ■ Modified postural drainage in an infant, using a face mask for percussion **(A)** in supine and **(B)** in sitting for the upper lobes.

Neonatal Intensive Care and Special Care Nurseries

A neonatal ICU (NICU) and special care nursery specializes in the care of critically ill or premature newborn infants who have specific and differing needs to those of the broader paediatric population. Newborns in the NICU are among the most fragile patients that physiotherapists treat, and detrimental effects can occur as a result of care procedures and inappropriate handling. Therefore advanced knowledge of fetal and infant development, physiological assessment and monitoring, newborn pathologies and treatments and outcomes are needed (Sweeney et al 2009). Breathing difficulties, which are associated with preterm birth, low birth weight, congenital abnormalities and other perinatal complications, such as meconium aspiration, are the main reason for admission to the NICU or special care nursery.

Level of Perinatal Care

There are four levels of perinatal hospital care classified by the American Academy of Pediatrics (American Academy of Pediatrics Committee on Fetus Newborn, 2012):

- Level I (nursery): able to provide neonatal resuscitation, postnatal care of healthy newborn and physiologically stable infants born >35 weeks' gestational age (GA) and stabilize ill newborn infants or infants born at <35 weeks' GA until transfer to appropriate level of care.
- Level II (special care nursery): able to provide care to infants born >32 weeks' GA and/or weighing >1500 g at birth, and moderately ill infants that are not anticipated to need subspecialty services on an urgent basis. CPAP can be provided, with mechanical ventilation only available for brief durations (less than 24 hours).
- Level III (NICU): able to provide continuous life support and comprehensive care for extremely high-risk newborn infants and those with critical illness, including infants born weighing <1500 g or at <32 weeks' GA. These units routinely provide assisted ventilation and have ready access to a full range of paediatric medical subspecialists.
- Level IV (NICU): able to provide the same services as a level III NICU and are located within institutions that can provide on-site surgical repair of serious congenital or acquired malformations.

Reasons for Admission to NICU

Preterm Birth

Preterm birth, defined as any birth occurring at <37 weeks' GA, accounts for 11% (range: 5–18%) of all births worldwide (Blencowe et al 2012). The rates of preterm birth are increasing throughout the world and due to advances in obstetric and neonatal care, survival rates are also rising (Saigal and Doyle 2008). The reasons for the increase in the preterm birth rate include increasing maternal age, artificial reproductive technologies, multiple births and pregnancy complications (Cheong and Doyle 2012). Children born preterm are divided into three categories depending on their GA at birth: late preterm (32–36 weeks' GA), very preterm (<32 weeks' GA) and extremely preterm (<28 weeks' GA). Some infants are born as early as 23 weeks' gestation and are considered at the edge of viability. The degree of neonatal care, health problems and long-term neurodevelopmental outcomes are related to GA, with those born earliest most at risk (Saigal and Doyle 2008). The lungs and the brain are the most vulnerable organs to the consequences of preterm birth, with prematurity the main reason for admission to a NICU (American Academy of Pediatrics Committee on Fetus Newborn 2012, Saigal and Doyle 2008). Neonatal care, while essential, causes a number of iatrogenic problems; the preterm lung is easily injured by mechanical ventilation, oxygen, infection and nutritional deficits, and the brain is vulnerable to hypotension, hypoxia and prolonged stress (Jobe 2013, Sweeney et al 2009). The preterm infant is also particularly vulnerable to infection. Early-onset sepsis can occur during the first days of life.

Low Birth Weight

Low birth weight is often associated with being born preterm; however, more mature infants can be classified as low birth weight if there is poor intrauterine growth. 'Intrauterine growth restriction' (IUGR) refers to a condition where the infant is unable to achieve its genetically determined potential size due to underlying pathology. Small for gestational age (SGA), defined as birth weight at less than 10th centile or less than two standard deviations on population specific growth charts for GA, is not synonymous with IUGR, as some infants may be constitutionally small. Causes of low birth weight include placental dysfunction, smoking during pregnancy, infection, poor maternal nutrition and chromosomal abnormalities (Jansson and Powell 2007).

Congenital Abnormalities

Congenital abnormalities seen in the NICU may include congenital diaphragmatic hernia (CDH), oesophageal atresia, tracheo-oesophageal fistula, abdominal wall defects and congenital heart disease.

Congenital Diaphragmatic Hernia

CDH occurs when abnormal fetal development weakens the muscular diaphragmatic barrier between the abdomen and thoracic cavity. The abdominal contents (usually stomach or small bowel) are displaced into the thoracic cavity, posteriorly and most commonly on the left side. CDH occurs roughly once per 3000 births and is associated with pulmonary hypoplasia on the affected side, as the abdominal viscera occupy the space normally available for the growing lung (Schultz et al 2007, Smith et al 2005). Survival rates range between 50% and 90% for infants with CDH, with degree of pulmonary hypoplasia being the main determinant of survival (Wenstrom et al 1991). Commonly associated anomalies such as persistent fetal circulation and abnormalities of the pulmonary vasculature can complicate outcome, and the contralateral lung is often smaller than expected because of compression by mediastinal shift during fetal development. The adoption of lung-preserving strategies, including high-frequency oscillatory ventilation and ECMO have improved survival (Chiu & Hedrick 2008, Morini et al 2006). The infant with CDH is often very unwell and surgical correction is needed via a laparotomy to carefully return the abdominal viscera into the abdominal cavity and close the defect in the diaphragm. Physiotherapy may be indicated if there is retention of secretions. Manual hyperinflation techniques should avoid generating excessive pressures, which can damage hypoplastic lungs. Children with CDH have an increased risk of long-term respiratory, gastro-intestinal, neurological and musculoskeletal problems and therefore follow-up is required following hospital discharge (Chiu and Hedrick 2008).

Oesophageal Atresia and Tracheo-Oesophageal Fistula

There are five recognized types of this anomaly. In the most common variant of this congenital abnormality (approximately 86% of cases) the upper oesophageal segment ends in a blind pouch (atresia) with a fistula connecting the distal oesophageal segment to the trachea. The incidence is approximately 1 in 4000 births (Depaepe et al 1993, Nassar et al 2012). The condition may be suspected antenatally if there is polyhydramnios (excess amniotic fluid) or failure to detect the stomach on ultrasound.

The infant presents postnatally with episodes of choking, coughing and respiratory distress due to an inability to swallow saliva or feeds and consequent aspiration into the larynx or trachea. It is often difficult to pass a nasogastric tube, which on chest radiograph appears curled in the upper oesophagus. Surgical correction is usually attempted as soon as possible and involves division of the fistula and anastomosis of the ends of the oesophagus. If recurrent or continuous aspiration occurs before corrective surgery, physiotherapy (in the head-up position) may be indicated to clear excess secretions or treat lung collapse due to aspiration of gastric contents.

Postoperatively, head-down postural drainage is contraindicated and patients are often nursed in the head-up position for the first few days, to reduce the risk of aspiration. Care must be taken not to extend the neck, especially in patients with a tight oesophageal anastomosis. Nasopharyngeal or oropharyngeal suction should not in general exceed the external distance between the nasal cavity and the ear. This distance is effective at producing cough and inadvertent damage to the oesophageal anastomosis is avoided.

Gastroschisis and Exomphalos (Omphalocoele)

Gastroschisis and exomphalos are relatively rare abdominal wall defects, occurring about once in 5000 births (Baird & MacDonald 1982). Gastroschisis refers to a full-thickness abdominal wall defect next to the umbilical opening, through which the small and large bowel herniate, not usually covered by a membrane. Exomphalos occurs when the anterior abdominal wall fails to close at the base of the umbilical cord, allowing the abdominal contents and sometimes the liver to herniate through the umbilical ring and develop externally in utero. A translucent membranous sac encloses the hernial contents. The defect is usually diagnosed antenatally by ultrasound and is classified as major or minor depending on whether the defect is bigger or smaller than 5 cm. Affected infants often have other major associated anomalies.

Immediately after birth, the abdominal contents are covered to prevent heat and fluid loss until corrective surgery can be undertaken. In most cases primary repair is possible but where the defect is large, a staged procedure is required, with gradual reduction of the bowels into the abdominal cavity. Postoperatively the infant may require ventilation as the tightly packed, rigid abdomen causes respiratory embarrassment and compromises venous return. Where a staged procedure is necessary, prolonged ventilation may be required. Some infants have impaired antenatal lung growth and some continue to have abnormal lung function during infancy.

These infants are particularly at risk from retention of secretions and lobar collapse due to the distended abdomen and predominantly supine nursing position (with the abdominal contents suspended above the abdomen). If treatment is required, techniques that increase intrathoracic pressure and consequently intra-abdominal pressure, such as vibrations or manual hyperinflation, should be used very cautiously. Postoperative respiratory compromise, if related to increased abdominal pressure, is unlikely to respond to physiotherapy. A slightly head-up position may relieve the thorax of some of the weight of the abdominal contents and reduce the work of breathing.

PULMONARY CONDITIONS

Respiratory Distress Syndrome

RDS occurs in very preterm infants due to structural and biochemical immaturity of the lung (including lack of surfactant) and cardiovascular system, and a very distensible chest wall (Rojas-Reyes et al., 2012). The incidence of RDS increases with decreasing gestational age and symptoms can develop within 4 hours of delivery with sternal and costal recession, nasal flaring, grunting and tachypnoea. Survival rates for infants with RDS have improved with surfactant therapy, with both prophylactic and early surfactant replacement therapy shown to reduce mortality and pulmonary complications in ventilated infants with RDS. Children who have RDS and require mechanical ventilation are at risk of BPD in the neonatal period and respiratory abnormalities later in infancy, including recurrent wheezing, asthma, respiratory infection and pulmonary-function test abnormalities. As lung collapse in RDS is primarily caused by lack of surfactant, physiotherapy is not required for this condition. Secretions may become a problem after the infant has been intubated for more than 48 hours, owing to irritation of the tracheal mucosa by the ETT. These secretions may be cleared easily by suction alone.

Respiratory distress in the preterm infant can also be caused by perinatal pneumonia, which may be bacterial, viral or fungal in origin. The presenting features of serious bacterial group B *Streptococcus pneumoniae* are similar to RDS with an indistinguishable chest radiograph. Group B streptococcal pneumonia can be rapidly fatal unless antibiotic therapy is started early.

Bronchopulmonary Dysplasia

BPD may develop in neonates being treated with oxygen and positive pressure ventilation for respiratory failure, often, but not always due to RDS. BPD, also known as 'chronic lung disease (CLD)', involves abnormal development of hyaline membranes in the alveoli in the lung tissue as a result of inflammation and scarring of the lungs. BPD is defined by the continued need for supplemental oxygen at 36 weeks' postmenstrual age for very preterm infants, or >28 days for children born at older gestations (Jobe and Bancalari 2001). A cut-off of 36 weeks' GA has been shown to have the best sensitivity and specificity for predicting long-term respiratory problems in preterm children and is likely associated with the alveolar stage of lung development occurring from 36 weeks' GA. While the incidence of lung damage has decreased with developments such as antenatal corticosteroids, postnatal surfactant and more gentle approaches to mechanical ventilation, the incidence of BPD remains between 30% and 40% for infants born extremely preterm (Jobe 2013). It also occurs in a variety of other conditions including oesophageal atresia, aspiration pneumonia, congenital heart disease and meconium aspiration (Gardner et al 2011). The incidence of BPD differs between hospitals due to variations in respiratory management, barotrauma and volutrauma. Clinical signs and symptoms can include tachypnoea and rib or sternal retraction, and some children may require oxygen and/or ventilation for months or years. Children with BPD have an increased rate of hospitalization during the first few years of life.

Meconium Aspiration

Meconium aspiration syndrome (MAS) usually occurs in full-term infants who become hypoxic due to a prolonged and difficult labour. Hypoxia causes the infant to pass meconium into the amniotic fluid and to make gasping movements, thereby drawing meconium into the pharynx. The irritant properties of meconium can cause a chemical pneumonitis and meconium aspiration can also lead to significant gas trapping and thoracic air leak. It is characterized by early onset respiratory distress, with tachypnoea, cyanosis and variable hyperinflation. Many infants with MAS can be treated effectively with oxygen. Moderate cases will need further respiratory support such as nasal CPAP or intubation and positive pressure ventilation. Severe MAS is treated with high-frequency oscillation and NO, or ECMO.

Physiotherapy can be very helpful in the management of meconium aspiration, in facilitating removal of extremely thick and tenacious green meconium secretions. However, in severe cases where pneumonitis has developed following meconium aspiration, babies may be less able to tolerate treatments, which should be undertaken cautiously.

Pulmonary Haemorrhage

Pulmonary haemorrhage is defined as acute intrapulmonary bleeding. It is relatively uncommon but may be a life-threatening event. Physiotherapy is contraindicated, although regular suctioning may be required to keep the airway clear. When fresh blood is no longer being aspirated, physiotherapy techniques may assist removal of residual blood. Prognosis is often poor.

Periventricular Haemorrhage and Periventricular Leucomalacia

Intraventricular bleeding in preterm infants occurs more frequently and severely in the smallest and least mature infants. Haemorrhage in the capillaries in the floor of the lateral ventricles is common in very low birthweight infants. The bleeding may extend into the ventricles and subarachnoid space. Several factors contribute to the risk of bleeding. These include hypoxia, fluctuations in blood pressure and cerebral blood flow and venous congestion. Cerebral ultrasound scanning is used to diagnose periventricular bleeds and they are graded according to the extent of the bleeding:

- grade I: bleeding into the floor of the ventricle
- grade II: bleeding into the ventricle (intraventricular haemorrhage (IVH))
- grade III–IVH: with dilatation of the ventricle
- grade IV–IVH: and bleeding into the cerebral cortex causing areas of ischaemia.

The smaller bleeds (grades I and II) have a good prognosis. They usually require no treatment and have no long-term sequelae. Neurological development following a grade I or II bleed seems to be similar to that of an infant with a comparable gestation. Larger bleeds may need treatment with shunting and the outcome is dependent on the grade of the bleed. More severe bleeds are associated with ischaemic brain damage and therefore have a high mortality and morbidity.

Periventricular leucomalacia (PVL) may occur on its own or associated with PVH. Ischaemia of cerebral tissue adjacent to the ventricles causes formation of cystic lesions. There is an association with neurological problems, particularly diplegia.

Patent Ductus Arteriosus

Patent ductus arteriosus (PDA) occurs in up to one-third of all preterm infants who weigh less than 1500 g at birth (Zahka & Patel 2002). In the full-term infant the duct, which is a fetal circulatory vessel, closes within the first 24 hours of life. A persistent patent duct in the preterm infant may lead to increased pulmonary blood flow. If symptomatic, a PDA can be treated medically (using indomethacin) or surgically (with ligation), depending on the infant's clinical status.

Physiological Jaundice

Physiological jaundice is common in the normal full-term infant owing to the breakdown of fetal haemoglobin, causing a raised level of unconjugated bilirubin in the blood. It usually begins 2 days after birth and disappears after 1 week to 10 days. High levels of unconjugated bilirubin may diffuse into the basal ganglia and lead to a condition called 'kernicterus', characterized by athetoid cerebral palsy, deafness and mental retardation. Preterm infants are particularly prone to developing jaundice and run an increased risk of subsequent kernicterus, though this condition is now extremely rare. Serum bilirubin levels are closely monitored and phototherapy may be required. Phototherapy units consist of traditional white or blue lamps, which emit light of wavelength 400–500 nm, or newer fibre-optic phototherapy blankets. Phototherapy oxidizes unconjugated bilirubin into harmless derivatives. In severe cases of jaundice an exchange transfusion (where small amounts of blood are replaced by donor blood until twice the infant's blood volume has been exchanged) may be required. Adequate calorie intake and weight gain are important in preterm and low birthweight infants to avoid hypoglycaemia, persistent jaundice and delayed recovery from RDS. Feeding should be started as soon as possible, either enterally in those who can tolerate it, or intravenously. Preterm infants often have poor sucking, gag and cough reflexes, so will be fed nasogastrically until these develop.

TREATMENTS AVAILABLE FOR RESPIRATORY CONDITIONS IN THE NICU

Many of the types of respiratory support available in paediatric and adult ICUs are used in the NICU; however, they are modified due to vulnerability of the developing lung and brain. Further, there are some treatments that are specific to the NICU that have been shown to improve lung development, including the use of antenatal corticosteroids, surfactant and caffeine (Morley et al 2008).

Pharmaceutical Interventions

Caffeine

Methylxanthines reduce the frequency of apnoea of prematurity, incidence of BPD and need for mechanical ventilation (Schmidt et al 2006). It is often administered to promote weaning of extremely preterm infants with RDS from ventilator support (Henderson-Smart & Davis 2003).

Corticosteroids

Antenatal corticosteroids are used to stimulate structural maturation and surfactant synthesis in the fetal lung (Jobe 1993). They are administered to women at risk of preterm birth prior to delivery and have been shown to increase survival, assist in rapid ventilator weaning, and decrease the need for supplemental oxygen when treatment occurs between 25 and 36 weeks' GA, and for infants born 1–7 days after the treatment commences (Roberts & Dalziel, 2006).

Postnatally, steroid use may also reduce lung inflammation and improve pulmonary function in severe RDS. However, it is associated with serious adverse side effects to the central nervous system, including cerebral palsy. Therefore the use of postnatal steroids is reserved for the sickest infants who would otherwise not be able to be weaned from mechanical ventilation (Stark et al 2001).

Surfactant Therapy

Surfactant is essential for normal lung function in infants. Surfactant lines the alveolar surface and is involved in all aspects of the respiratory cycle, with particular importance in preventing atelectasis at end expiration (Rojas-Reyes et al 2012). Surfactant replacement therapy involves the administration of artificial surfactant through an ETT. It can be used to treat RDS or prevent its development when administered in the delivery room. Surfactant therapy reduces the need for ventilator support and decreases the risk of pneumothorax, pulmonary interstitial emphysema, BPD and death (Engle & American Academy of Pediatrics Committee on Fetus and Newborn, 2008). Its use has resulted in significant improvements in the survival rates of very preterm infants and until recently was part of standard care (D'Angio et al 2002, Rojas-Reyes et al 2012). However, surfactant needs to be delivered through an ETT and the process of intubating a fragile infant can itself be destabilizing (O'Donnell et al 2006). Further, recent evidence suggests that not all extremely preterm infants need surfactant if they are stabilized with CPAP at birth (Morley et al 2008). Therefore although initial studies suggested that very preterm infants given prophylactic surfactant had improved outcomes, more recent research suggests that surfactant treatment should only be given to those infants developing lung problems, as prophylactic administration at birth via an ETT does not improve clinical outcome, and is associated with increased risk of BPD or death (Rojas-Reyes et al 2012). Surfactant replacement therapy is also used to treat acute respiratory morbidity in late preterm and term neonates with MAS, pneumonia/sepsis and perhaps pulmonary haemorrhage (Engle & American Academy of Pediatrics Committee on Fetus and Newborn 2008).

Supplemental Oxygen

Supplemental oxygen may be required for newborns with respiratory difficulties to ensure organs are appropriately oxygenated. However, high levels of oxygen can inflame the lining of the lungs, injure the airways and slow lung development in preterm infants (Gardner et al 2011). Historically, use of unrestricted and unmonitored oxygen therapy in neonates was accompanied by potential harm from oxygen free radicals and was associated with increased incidence of BPD, retinopathy of prematurity (leading to permanent visual impairment) and brain damage (Gardner et al 2011). Therefore current target rates for oxygen saturation are lower for very preterm infants prior to term age than those traditionally used for adults in order to minimize harm from supplemental oxygen.

Respiratory Support

Intermittent Positive Pressure Ventilation

Mechanical ventilation via ETT was previously given to all very preterm infants at birth to support their immature respiratory system and to administer surfactant. However, nasal CPAP has been shown to be as effective as intubation at birth and may be associated with reduced rates of BPD, as it causes less trauma (Morley et al 2008). There are some infants who will need more respiratory support and will require

intubation, including positive pressure ventilation, and possibly surfactant. Once an infant has recovered from an acute respiratory problem, it is important that they are weaned from the ventilation to minimize long-term complications of respiratory support. Pressures on ventilators need to be reduced where possible to prevent barotrauma and the use of volume-controlled ventilation settings reduces volutrauma.

Non-Invasive Ventilation

NIV techniques were developed to reduce the adverse effects that are associated with ventilation via ETT in the newborn.

Continuous Positive Airway Pressure

In the neonate, CPAP can be delivered by face mask, nasal pharyngeal tubes, nasal prongs or ETT (Gardner et al 2011). The most common delivery of CPAP in the NICU and special care nursery is via nasal prongs. Compared to mechanical ventilation via an ETT, it is less invasive, results in improved oxygenation and decreased work of breathing, reduces the complications of intubation, decreases the need for surfactant and reduces the incidence of BPD (Davis et al 2009). However, there is risk of pneumothorax and pressures need to be closely monitored. It is important that the appropriate size nasal prongs are used to avoid displacement of the prongs and erosion of the nasal tissue.

High-Flow Nasal Cannulae

High-Flow Nasal Cannulae (HFNC) have been used to provide non-invasive respiratory support by delivering blended air and oxygen with a flow rate >1 L/min (Manley et al 2013). It is becoming more commonly used in the NICU in preference to nasal CPAP, as it is considered to be less invasive and thought to be more comfortable for the baby. Recent RCTs comparing nasal CPAP and HFNC have shown no difference in treatment failure, requirement for reintubation (defined as ETT with 7 days) or pneumothoraces when used to wean preterm infants from ETT (Manley et al 2013, Yoder et al 2013). Importantly, nasal trauma was less with HFNC. It should only be delivered using heated and humidified systems, and the recommended flow rate should be between 2 and 8 L/min, with many recommending 5–7 L/min initially.

Physiotherapy Interventions in the NICU

The role of the physiotherapist in the NICU has changed from providing prophylactic respiratory physiotherapy in the 1980s and 1990s to focusing on the neurodevelopment of the critically ill or preterm infant, and only treating infants for respiratory problems when pathology likely to respond to physiotherapy is clearly present (e.g. atelectasis). This is due to a numbers of reasons, including lack of evidence to support routine post-extubation physiotherapy and advances in respiratory support, particularly the use of CPAP, along with the recognition of potential risks associated with manual physiotherapy techniques such as percussions and vibrations (Gardner et al 2011, Hudson and Box 2003). Preterm and critically ill neonates tolerate handling poorly and should be handled as little as possible. The skin of a preterm baby is very thin and easily damaged. Manual techniques should be applied with care. Physiotherapy and suction should only be carried out when indicated and careful assessment is essential before any intervention.

Manual Techniques

A unique brain injury called 'encephaloclastic porencephaly', similar to brain injury seen in children with 'shaken baby syndrome' was identified in two hospitals (UK and New Zealand) in the 1990s. A possible association between this brain lesion and the chest physiotherapy which was delivered four times hourly (cupping with a face mask) in very preterm infants was postulated (Harding et al 1998, Knight et al 2001). This study involved a retrospective analysis of 454 infants with birth weights less than 1500 g delivered between 24 and 27 weeks' gestation. Affected individuals received more frequent chest physiotherapy treatments, but also had more prolonged and severe episodes of hypotension in the first week than controls and were less likely to have had a cephalic presentation at delivery. Analysis showed that it was not statistically possible to differentiate any contribution of physiotherapy to this cerebral destruction brain injury from other factors, including duration of hypotension, and presentation at delivery.

Since Harding's publication, several authors have disputed the association between encephaloclastic porencephaly and chest physiotherapy (Beby et al 1998, Gray et al 1999, Vincon 1999). The significant methodological errors in the original retrospective trial have been highlighted and it is possible that these lesions occurred only in the sickest infants and the frequency of chest physiotherapy was a reflection of this (Gray et al 1999). No cases of encephaloclastic porencephaly were reported over the same 3-year period in two separate studies, despite similar criteria for initiation of chest physiotherapy (Beby et al 1998, Gray et al 1999). Follow-up data from the centre in New Zealand which first reported this problem later suggested that identification of encephaloclastic porencephaly emerged at a time when the use of chest physiotherapy had already decreased and that the cluster of cases seen between 1992 and 1994, although associated with the number of chest physiotherapy treatments given, may have been due to some other factor (Knight et al 2001). Although an association between chest physiotherapy and encephaloclastic porencephaly seems unlikely, it highlights the need for very careful assessment of preterm infants and a judicious approach to treatment. If chest physiotherapy is indicated and chest percussion thought appropriate, the baby should be kept in a stable position, with the head and shoulders well supported, and vital signs carefully monitored throughout treatment.

An active programme of pre- and post-extubation chest physiotherapy may result in a lower incidence of lobar collapse and reintubation within 24 hours (Flenady & Gray 2002). However, a large single-centre RCT in Australia, testing the effects of a neonatal post-extubation programme on the incidence of post-extubation collapse found no differences between the physiotherapy and control groups in terms of the rate of post-extubation collapse, adverse events (apnoea or bradycardia), duration of requirement of supplemental oxygen or the need for re-intubation within 24 hours (Bagley et al 2005). There is still insufficient evidence for the beneficial effects of routinely performed neonatal chest physiotherapy (Flenady & Gray, 2002). Neonates should therefore only be treated with manual techniques (positioning, percussion and vibration) if there is a clear clinical indication (e.g. atelectasis) and the infant is able to tolerate the procedure (Harding et al 1998, Ramsay 1995). Percussion should only be used when secretions are not cleared by suction alone and the head must be supported. Percussions and vibrations are not recommended for very preterm infants in the first month of life, as the immature brain is vulnerable to the shaking movements (Harding et al 1998). Further, percussions and vibrations need to be administered gently due to the fragility of the ribs of neonates, particularly in preterm infants with BPD who are at risk of osteopenia (Wood 1987).

Developmental Care

Developmental care is defined as a broad range of interventions designed to minimize the stress of the infant and family while in the NICU environment, such as control of external stimuli (vestibular, auditory, visual, tactile), positioning and/or swaddling of the preterm infant (Symington & Pinelli 2009). The focus of developmental care is to promote infant organization as indicated by homoeostasis of both the physiological and behavioural systems.

Positioning

The positioning of infants receiving mechanical ventilation in NICU may have an impact on clinical outcome. The lateral decubitus positions, prone and supine are all used, although there is a tendency to nurse ventilated infants in the prone position. A systematic review of 11 trials involving 206 infants reported that prone positioning did have some advantage in terms of improved oxygenation but that there was no evidence to suggest that any one position during mechanical ventilation was more effective in producing a clinically relevant and sustained improvement (Balaguer et al 2006).

Physiotherapists play an important role in making recommendations on positioning infants in the NICU due to their advanced knowledge of both the musculoskeletal and cardiorespiratory systems (Sweeney et al 2010). Prolonged atypical positioning in the NICU has been associated with long-term musculoskeletal problems including torticollis and lower limb malalignment (Bracewell & Marlow 2002, Sweeney et al 2010). Recent studies suggest ventilation distribution in preterm infants is not gravity-dependent but follows an anatomical pattern in preterm infants on CPAP, or in spontaneously breathing infants in the supine or prone position (Hough et al 2012). The prone position has many physiological benefits compared with supine, including improved oxygen saturation and reduced episodes of desaturation (Wells et al 2005). Clinicians often position preterm infants in prone, especially in the weeks following birth. It is important to encourage regular position changes for infants in the NICU as being nursed in prone or supine for long periods can be associated with positioning plagiocephaly (Nuysink 2009). All infants in the nursery should transition to sleeping in supine prior to discharge to comply with the recommendations to prevent sudden infant death syndrome (Lockridge et al 1999).

Special Considerations in the NICU

Sepsis

Infants are particularly vulnerable to infection and meticulous attention to hygiene by staff and visitors is essential. Sepsis is related to GA and is more common in those born very preterm and those who are post term (>42 weeks' GA). Sepsis in the newborn period is associated with higher rates of mortality in infants born preterm, with 20% of preterm infants dying due to sepsis compared with 1–2% of term-born infants (Weston et al 2011).

Clustering of Care

Infants' care procedures (e.g. feeding, bathing, position changes) are 'clustered' together to promote sleeping and minimize disruption to the infants' sleep/wake cycle (Symington and Pinelli 2009). Physiotherapy assessment and treatment should coincide with care times when feasible, and usually before a feed to minimize the risk of gastro-oesophageal reflux.

Temperature Control

Preterm and low birthweight infants have difficulty maintaining their body temperature, as they have sparse brown fat available for heat production, a small liver with limited glycogen stores for energy and heat production, large surface area to body mass posing huge potential for heat loss and immature response of the central nervous system to cold stress. Cold stress can lead to feeding intolerance, respiratory and metabolic acidosis, hypoglycaemia and hypoxia. Therefore infants who cannot maintain their temperature in an open cot should be kept in a thermoneutral environment (incubators or under radiant warmers). Extremely preterm infants are nursed in a humidified cot until 2 weeks of age or until they weigh more than

1 kg. Heat shields may be used to reduce radiant heat loss and the ambient room temperature is kept high at 27–28°C. A core temperature of less than 36.5°C in preterm infants indicates that non-essential handling should be delayed until the infant's temperature has risen.

Parent-Infant Bonding

Infants who have been resuscitated and require immediate admission to a NICU shortly after birth will not have had the chance for early physical contact with their parents. Incubators and other equipment may be a further barrier to contact. Parents need to be supported by the NICU team throughout this difficult period and should be encouraged to have as close contact as possible with their baby and to help with routine care. This can be enhanced with kangaroo care, where the parent holds their infant skin to skin. Kangaroo care is associated with many benefits including decreased length of stay, lower incidence of sepsis and respiratory tract infection, and greater maternal satisfaction with care (Symington and Pinelli 2009).

GENERAL PAEDIATRIC INTENSIVE CARE

Accidents are the most common cause of child death after the first year of life and 50% are road traffic accidents. Children who have been severely injured may require intensive care and mechanical ventilation in the paediatric intensive care unit (PICU), particularly after head injury.

COMMON REASONS FOR PICU ADMISSION

Trauma, Head Injury and Raised Intracranial Pressure

Raised ICP represents an increase in the volume of the intracranial contents. In addition to trauma, it can be caused by space-occupying lesions or encephalopathy. Normal values for ICP are usually below 15 mmHg. The CPP is the dP for cerebral blood flow and is defined as the difference between mean arterial blood pressure and ICP. It is a crucial parameter which lies within the range of 50–70 mmHg. A variety of methods to monitor ICP can be used including intraventricular catheters, subdural or subarachnoid monitors and cerebral intraparenchymal catheters.

The most common presentation of acute, severe head injury in children is coma. Clinical scores, such as the paediatric modifications of the Glasgow Coma Scale (GCS) (Tasker 2000, Teasdale & Jennett 1974), allow bedside assessment of neurological function and the degree of impairment of consciousness in children. Such scores are designed to allow early identification of pathology when it is still potentially reversible by medical or surgical intervention. Coma in children may present after a longer interval than in adults. Continued extradural bleeding following a relatively minor injury may lead to a deteriorating level of consciousness. Cerebral oedema may be focal or generalized; the latter may result in an increase in ICP and cause a more rapid deterioration.

In the acutely head-injured child, the primary injury refers to the damage sustained during trauma caused by bleeding, contusion or neuronal shearing. Secondary injury is due to the resultant complicating events. These may be intracranial factors such as bleeding, swelling, seizures and raised ICP, or systemic factors such as hypoxia, hypercarbia, hypertension or hypotension, hyperglycaemia or hypoglycaemia and fever. In the United Kingdom, 90–95% of injuries are managed without the need for neurosurgical intervention (Tasker et al 2001, Tasker et al 2006). When required, for example in the presence of an acute subdural bleed, surgical evaluation should be facilitated immediately.

Once the child is stabilized, medical management aims to avoid or minimize secondary brain injury. Factors that may precipitate a rise in ICP, resulting in a potential fall in CPP, should be avoided. Intubation and mechanical hyperventilation have been sometimes been used to reduce ICP. This has been controversial, as hyperventilation (and hypocapnia) may induce cerebral ischaemia. In general, this is still sometimes used for short periods during acute deterioration or when intracranial hypertension is unresponsive to other therapy. The management of children with acute head injury has been reviewed extensively (https://www.nice.org.uk/guidance/cg176/chapter/1 -recommendations). Many of the strategies for management are similar to adults and discussed in Chapters 9 and 13.

Physiotherapy

Immobility, impaired cough, depression of the respiratory centre and pulmonary dysfunction due to anaesthetic and paralyzing agents predispose patients to pulmonary complications. The frequency of pneumonia in severely head-injured patients requiring prolonged mechanical ventilation has been reported to be as high as 70% (Demling & Riessen 1993). Safe and effective treatment should be based on careful assessment and judicious use of appropriate physiotherapy techniques (Prasad & Tasker 1990). The use of bolus doses of analgesics and sedatives or, in more unstable cases, thiopental before an intervention can help reduce acute swings in ICP. Duration of physiotherapy treatments is an important factor, with longer treatment more likely to produce larger elevations of ICP. Sustained increases in ICP during cumulative interventions should be avoided by allowing a return to baseline values between procedures. Careful monitoring of CPP during treatment is essential and treatment should be withheld or abandoned if levels fall below 50 mmHg.

The head-down position is generally contraindicated and any change in position should maintain the head midline in relation to body position. A 30° head-up tilt has been shown to significantly reduce ICP in the majority of patients (Feldman et al 1992). The presence of a bone flap from decompressive craniotomy may limit options for positioning. Chest clapping may be better tolerated than vibrations and manual hyperinflation may be used with careful monitoring (Prasad & Tasker 1995). ETT suctioning may have severe prolonged effects on ICP (Gemma et al 2002) and great care must be taken to avoid hypoxia. A protocol for physiotherapy management is shown in Figure 10-13.

Passive movements to maintain joint mobility may be necessary and it has been shown that these can be undertaken without detrimental effect on ICP in adults, provided that Valsalva-like manoeuvres are avoided (Brimioulle et al 1997).

Asthma

There is considerable global variation in the prevalence of asthma, with the highest rates reported in America, Australasia and the United Kingdom. Much lower rates are reported in prevalence studies from Africa and Asia. Prevalence also varies considerably within countries regionally. In the 1980s to early 1990s, several cross-sectional studies from widely varying regions of the world reported an increase in the prevalence of asthma. Although many of these studies relied on self-reported symptoms, there were also reports of a parallel increase in hospitalizations and mortality rates. However, repeat cross-sectional studies have suggested a levelling off or even a decrease in prevalence (Bauer et al 2007, British Thoracic Society (BTS) 2003, Toelle & Marks 2005). Atopic (allergic) disease in general has increased over the past few decades and possible explanations for this rise include outdoor pollution, social deprivation/socioeconomic status, dietary factors and passive smoking (particularly maternal smoking during pregnancy). In addition, modern westernized homes, which tend to be highly insulated (e.g. double glazing) and have increased humidity, have been recognized to be 'dust mite-friendly' environments. Thick pile carpets, heavily padded furniture and conventional bedding are all potential sites for dust mite activity, a known trigger for allergic reaction.

The main pathophysiological mechanism of asthma in children is inflammation within the airway, resulting in recurrent episodes of wheezing, breathlessness and cough. There is an increased responsiveness of the smooth muscle in the bronchial wall to various stimuli. Hypertrophy of the mucous glands may lead to mucus plugging. These changes cause variable airway obstruction, which may become chronic and severe.

The child with acute asthma may need to be admitted to hospital, and in severe cases may require mechanical ventilation (Inwald et al 2001). Mucus plugging, retained secretions and atelectasis are common sequelae in children who require ventilator support for acute asthma, and chest physiotherapy may be of benefit. It is important that bronchospasm is adequately controlled before physiotherapy techniques are commenced. Treatment should proceed cautiously and be terminated early if bronchospasm is exacerbated. Although there is no routine indication for chest physiotherapy in asthma (Holloway & Ram 2004, Hondras et al 2000), children with persistent areas of lung collapse following an acute attack may respond well to appropriate airway clearance techniques after discharge.

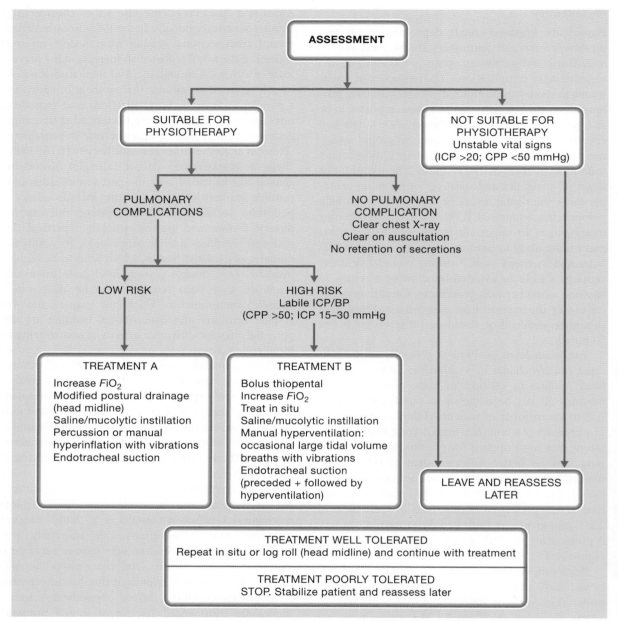

FIGURE 10-13 ■ Flow diagram of an approach to chest physiotherapy in children with raised intracranial pressure. *BP,* Blood pressure; *CPP,* cerebral perfusion pressure; FiO$_2$, fraction of inspired oxygen; *ICP,* intracranial pressure. *(Reproduced with permission from Prasad and Tasker 1990.)*

Bronchiolitis

Bronchiolitis caused by human RSV is the most common severe lower respiratory tract disease in infancy, with RSV being the main agent in more than 70% of cases. It is a seasonal viral disorder, occurring most frequently in the winter months and mainly affecting infants under 2 years of age, with as many as 1–2% of these requiring hospital admission (Hodge & Chetcuti 2000), 90% of whom are under 12 months of age. Bronchiolar inflammation occurs with necrosis and destruction of cilia and epithelial cells, leading to obstruction of the small airways. $\dot{V}/\dot{Q}$ mismatch may cause hypoxia and hypercapnia. Management of this condition is mainly supportive. In those with severe respiratory distress, blood gas monitoring and even ventilatory support may be necessary. Physiotherapy is not indicated in the acute stage of bronchiolitis when the infant has signs of respiratory distress. Studies that have examined the efficacy of physiotherapy intervention compared to no treatment in these patients have not shown any benefit in terms of the course of the disease (Nicholas et al 1999, Webb et al 1985). A systematic review based on the results of three RCTs concluded that chest physiotherapy using vibration and percussion techniques does not reduce length of hospital stay, oxygen requirements, or improve the clinical severity score in infants with acute bronchiolitis who are not under mechanical ventilation and who do not have any other comorbidity (Perrotta et al 2005). The ventilated infant with bronchiolitis needs careful assessment, and physiotherapy techniques should be applied only when sputum retention or mucus plugging is a problem and only if the intervention is tolerated.

Pertussis

Pertussis, commonly called 'whooping cough', is caused by the organism *B. pertussis*. It occurs in epidemics every 3–4 years and is largely preventable by immunization, although immunity may not be lifelong (Raguckas et al 2007), with the highest incidence of pertussis since 1959 being reported in 2004. Pertussis is particularly dangerous in infants less than 6 months of age and in children with underlying cardiopulmonary problems, for example congenital heart disease, asthma, CLD and cystic fibrosis. The cough becomes paroxysmal and can be provoked by crying, feeding or any other disturbance. The spasms of coughing may cause hypoxia and apnoea, especially in infants, and may lead to further problems such as convulsions, intracranial bleeding and encephalopathy.

At the end of the coughing spasm, the inspiratory whoop may occur followed by vomiting, when thick, tenacious sputum can be expectorated. This phase of paroxysmal coughing may last 6–8 weeks and is exhausting for the child and parents. Bronchopneumonia is the most common complication, particularly in infants, and is due to the primary disease itself or to secondary bacterial infection with other organisms such as *Staphylococcus, Haemophilus* or *Pneumococcus*. Infants and children with pneumonia may need admission to hospital. Treatment is supportive. Minimal handling in a quiet environment is essential for the infant with pertussis in order to reduce disturbance, which may precipitate coughing spasms. A small number of cases, particularly infants who have had frequent apnoeic attacks or hypoxic convulsions, will need intensive care and mechanical ventilation. Any physiotherapy manoeuvre during the acute phase can precipitate the paroxysmal cough with its complications. Treatment is therefore contraindicated in children during this stage.

If the child or infant requires ventilation, physiotherapy is important to remove extremely tenacious secretions, which easily block large and small airways and ETTs. The paroxysmal cough is of less concern during treatment when the infant is adequately sedated for mechanical ventilatory support. When the stage of paroxysmal coughing is over, there may occasionally be persistent lobar collapse, which should be responsive to appropriate airway clearance techniques and lung recruitment strategies.

Pneumonia

The most common cause of pneumonia in the neonate is *Staphylococcus aureus;* in the infant, RSV or *M. pneumoniae* and in the child *M. pneumoniae, S. pneumoniae* or *Haemophilus influenzae*. However, in a significant number of cases no pathogen is identified (British Thoracic Society 2002).

In many cases of pneumonia there is consolidation of lung tissue with no excess secretions and there is no evidence that physiotherapy is of benefit (Stiller 2000). Where sputum retention is a problem, an appropriate airway clearance technique may be used. Reassessment of the child is often necessary, as retention of secretions may become a recurrent problem as the pneumonia resolves. If mechanical ventilation is required, physiotherapy is useful in maintaining airway patency, reducing mucus plugging and optimizing ventilation.

Pleural Infection

Pleural infections, although relatively uncommon, have become more prevalent in the United Kingdom and the United States of America in recent years. Empyemas are a significant cause of morbidity in children, but differ from pleural infections in adults in that the final outcome is usually very good (Balfour-Lynn et al 2005). A pleural effusion in a relatively well child is usually a secondary occurrence to an acute bacterial pneumonia. The effusion is usually unilateral. Very occasionally pleural effusions in children represent an underlying malignancy; otherwise, most effusions are associated with an underlying infection. Once the presence of an effusion has been confirmed by chest radiograph or chest ultrasound and other causes ruled out, most children are started on intravenous antibiotics. A loculated effusion is treated either locally, with chest drain insertion and intrapleural fibrinolytics, or surgically with video-assisted thoracic surgery (VATS) or mini-thoracotomy. Although these children do not always have a primary problem with bronchial secretions, immobility and the presence of a chest drain can result in retained secretions and a weak cough. Airway clearance may be necessary, using an appropriate technique. As soon as the clinical condition allows, the child should be encouraged to mobilize as much as possible.

Acute Laryngotracheobronchitis (Croup)

Croup is a common problem occurring between the ages of 6 months and 4 years. The illness is usually viral and produces acute inflammation and oedema of the upper airways, causing fever, a harsh barking cough and a hoarse voice. Stridor, initially inspiratory only, is much worse at night and may become inspiratory and expiratory. The acute stage of respiratory obstruction may only last 1–2 days but the stridor and cough may continue for 7–10 days (Moore & Little 2006, Russell et al 2004). More severely affected infants will be admitted to hospital and given humidified oxygen if hypoxic or distressed. Treatment is supportive but with minimal handling, as any disturbance that upsets the child will increase the laryngeal obstruction.

Very few children with croup who are admitted to hospital go on to require intubation to maintain the airway due to severe respiratory obstruction. A few of these, particularly infants, may also require some additional form of respiratory support, e.g. intermittent positive pressure ventilation or CPAP. Physiotherapy is contraindicated in the non-intubated child with croup. Treatment may be required when the child is intubated, if secretions cannot be cleared by suction alone.

Acute Epiglottitis

Epiglottitis is caused by *H. influenzae* but is now rarely seen due to the introduction of the Hib *(H. influenzae)* vaccine. It is, however, a very dangerous condition, which occurs between the ages of 1 and 7 years. The onset is sudden, with a severe sore throat and high temperature. Stridor and dysphagia develop rapidly; the child drools and is unable to swallow saliva. The neck is held extended in an attempt to open the airway. Acute and possibly fatal obstruction of the airway can develop. The child with suspected epiglottitis should not be disturbed in any way. No attempt should be made to examine the throat, as this may precipitate acute life-threatening obstruction. Usual management is intubation with a nasotracheal tube. In extreme circumstances tracheostomy may be necessary, but should be required only for 3–4 days, following which there is usually complete recovery. Physiotherapy is contraindicated in the non-intubated child with epiglottitis, but airway clearance techniques may be required in the intubated child if secretions cannot be removed by suction alone.

Bronchopulmonary Dysplasia

Infants who remain oxygen-dependent and have abnormal findings on chest radiograph are described as having BPD. BPD covers a broad range of disease and a variety of terminology has been used to describe this disorder, including CLD. Although both CLD and BPD are both still commonly used, it is felt that BPD distinguishes this disorder as a neonatal lung process rather than other chronic respiratory diseases (Jobe & Bancalari 2001, Ryan 2006). The classification of BPD into mild, moderate and severe, depending on oxygen and positive pressure requirement, may offer a better description of underlying pulmonary disease and has been reported to correlate with the infant's maturity, growth and overall severity of illness (Ehrenkranz et al 2005). BPD is seen in extremely low birthweight infants and severity is inversely related to gestational age (Johnson et al 2002). Reported incidence of BPD varies from 15% to 50%, although this is likely to be related to the difference in populations (i.e. number of very premature infants) among the studies.

The pathology of BPD has changed considerably over the past few decades, reflecting the use of newer modalities of mechanical ventilation, introduction of new treatments (such as surfactant) and also improved survival of extremely premature infants. The pathology of BPD used to be associated with fibrosis and airway obstruction but now the problem is one of abnormal lung growth (in particular a marked reduction in alveolar numbers) (Kotecha 2000). This pathological picture is sometimes termed 'new' BPD (Greenough et al 2006).

In addition to prematurity and low birth weight there are several other risk factors for BPD, in particular the requirement of mechanical ventilation and oxygen therapy. High peak pressures in positive pressure ventilation cause barotrauma and high inspired oxygen concentrations cause an acute inflammatory response leading to local tissue damage. Other factors that also influence the pathogenesis of BPD include the presence of a persistent arterial duct–PDA and infection.

Despite several studies, the optimum ventilation mode whereby BPD can be prevented has not been identified. Preventative strategies aim to minimize lung injury. These include using less mechanical ventilatory support, refining the methods of mechanical ventilation and using alternative techniques: permissive hypercapnia, minimal peak pressures, rapid ventilatory rates, early use of CPAP and rapid weaning and extubation (Ambalavanan & Carlo 2006). High-frequency ventilation, in particular high-frequency oscillation, may have a place in preventing BPD but this is as yet unclear (Greenough et al 2006). The infant with BPD shows an increased oxygen requirement and carbon dioxide retention and has decreased lung compliance with increased airway resistance. Tachypnoea and persistent sternal and costal recession are often present. The condition may be progressive, requiring more ventilatory support and eventually leading to respiratory and cardiac failure. Radiographic appearance can vary, but in classic BPD shows interstitial fibrosis and cystic abnormalities. The radiographic appearance in 'new' BPD is often of small lung volumes and hazy lung fields.

Supplementary oxygen is the mainstay of the baby with BPD. The most appropriate target for the oxygen saturation level requires further study (Greenough et al 2006). Good nutrition is essential and the infant may require fluid restriction and diuretics. Some infants respond to bronchodilators and steroids, although the effect of long-term steroids on lung and brain growth is an issue of concern. Antibiotics may be required, as these infants are prone to recurrent chest infections. Babies with a chronic oxygen requirement but who have a reasonable growth rate and do not have frequent episodes of desaturation can be discharged with home oxygen. These families require appropriate community support. The long-term prognosis for those who survive the first 2 years is good, although infants with BPD have significant pulmonary sequelae during childhood and adolescence (Bhandari & Panitch 2006).

Physiotherapy

Infants with CLD are particularly prone to chest infections and have an increased rate of hospital admission in the first 2 years of life. Physiotherapy may be indicated if secretion retention is a problem. However, these infants often wheeze and may have airway collapse. Detailed assessment is important before any intervention and if wheezing is not too severe, careful treatment may be possible. Inhaled β_2-agonists may temporarily improve lung function in these babies (Ng et al 2001) and may be a useful premedication for physiotherapy. Modified gravity-assisted positions with chest percussion may be useful in infants, but nasopharyngeal suction may be required if retained secretions are causing concern. In older children appropriate airway clearance techniques should be used, either during episodes of infection or if retained secretions are a persistent problem. Children, particularly infants in whom supplemental oxygen is delivered via nasal cannulae, often have a problem with thick, dry nasal secretions and may benefit from humidification.

Inhaled Foreign Body

Aspiration of a foreign body into the respiratory tract can occur at all ages, but is most common between the ages of 1 and 3 years. All types of foodstuffs may be aspirated, for example peanuts, pieces of fruit and vegetables, as well as small plastic or metal toys. Objects are most commonly aspirated into the right main bronchus. The left main bronchus and trachea are the next most common, and smaller objects may be inhaled into right middle and lower lobe bronchi or occasionally into the left lower lobe bronchus.

When aspiration has been witnessed by parents or carers, the child should be taken immediately to hospital. On examination there may be wheeze and some signs of respiratory distress. Breath sounds may be reduced over the affected lung. The chest radiograph, taken on expiration, may show gas trapping in the area distal to the blockage.

In some cases, the aspiration is not witnessed and the acute changes just described may be assumed to be the onset of a respiratory infection. The bronchial wall becomes oedematous, especially if the inhaled object is vegetable matter. Total obstruction of the bronchus gradually occurs and secondary pneumonic changes develop in the area distal to the obstruction. After a few days the child may become unwell with a persistent cough. The longer the obstruction remains, the more permanent the lung damage, eventually leading to bronchiectasis (Dinwiddie 1997). An inhaled foreign body should be suspected in any child with a pneumonia that does not respond to conventional treatment.

Management

All children who have aspirated a foreign body into the airway should have an urgent rigid bronchoscopy for removal of the foreign body. If symptoms persist, a repeat bronchoscopy may be necessary to ensure complete removal. Rarely, bronchoscopic removal may fail and thoracotomy may be required.

Physiotherapy

Physiotherapy is not indicated to attempt to remove the object before bronchoscopy. Usually physiotherapy is ineffective, as the object is firmly wedged in the bronchus. However, if the object is dislodged by physiotherapy manoeuvres, it may travel up the bronchial tree and obstruct the trachea, leading to respiratory arrest.

Following bronchoscopy, gravity-assisted positioning and chest clapping may be necessary to clear excess secretions, particularly if the object has been aspirated for some time and secondary bacterial infection has occurred.

Children with Neurological and Neuromuscular Impairment

Impaired cough, as a consequence of weakness from neuromuscular disease such as Duchenne muscular dystrophy and spinal muscular atrophy or neurological impairment, can cause serious respiratory complications including atelectasis, pneumonia, airway obstruction and acidosis (Miske et al 2004). Chronic respiratory insufficiency and respiratory failure will ultimately result from chronic weakness of respiratory muscles, shallow breathing and ineffective cough. For these children, independently performed airway clearance techniques are not usually feasible, but options such as the 'cough assist' (mechanical insufflation/ exsufflation device) and other non-invasive forms of positive pressure ventilation are safe and well tolerated, with growing evidence to support their efficacy (Chatwin et al 2003, Panitch 2006, Vianello et al 2005). They are discussed more comprehensively in Chapter 7. Not all patients with neuromuscular disease are good candidates for the use of non-invasive respiratory aids. Potential contraindications include an inability to manage oropharyngeal secretions, mental status changes or cognitive impairment and cardiovascular instability. For some patients, including those with the most severe spinal muscular atrophy, sole reliance on non-invasive methods of assisted cough and ventilation is inadequate, and they may require repeated episodes of intubation and mechanical ventilation in the ICU to prolong survival (Birnkrant 2002).

Need for High-Frequency Oscillatory Ventilation

HFOV theoretically provides gentle ventilatory support by employing very small tidal volumes and high respiratory rates (1–15 Hz) with high mean airway pressures to achieve adequate ventilation. It has been shown to be safe and effective in the treatment of respiratory failure in paediatric practice (Arnold 1996).

In theory, disconnecting infants from such ventilation for physiotherapy treatments, including manual inflation techniques, would contradict the principles of reducing volume loss, bulk flow of air and the shearing forces associated with such ventilation (Lindgren et al 2007). However, many experienced physiotherapists find that unless children are disconnected for brief and effective treatments, these children are vulnerable to airway obstruction and atelectasis. The loss of volume after disconnection and suction is significant but transient (Tingay et al 2007). The key to successful physiotherapy treatments of children on HFOV lies in adequate preoxygenation, proper assessment and quick, competent and effective treatments, which do not permit de-recruitment within any treatment cycle.

Management of Surgical Patients

In some hospitals, preoperative visits and information leaflets are available to help reduce some of the fear of coming to or being in hospital. Except in emergency admissions, it is helpful for children and their parents to be seen by a physiotherapist before their surgery. Appropriate explanation of postoperative procedures should be given at the level of the child's age and understanding, without overloading the child with information they do not understand and increasing stress and anxiety. If parents understand the need for postoperative physiotherapy intervention, they can play an important role in facilitating postoperative mobility.

Physiotherapy assessment should include cardiorespiratory status and physical and motor development. The assessment of respiratory status provides an opportunity to evaluate postoperative risks and the need for preoperative treatment. If indicated, older children may be taught an airway clearance technique. Techniques for clearing secretions and resolving atelectasis following thoracic and abdominal surgery are discussed further in Chapter 7.

When a child has pre-existing pulmonary disease, for example cystic fibrosis, they may need to be admitted some time before surgery for prophylactic antibiotics and for effective airway clearance. Such children may require physiotherapy and suction in the anaesthetic room following intubation and before surgery (Tannenbaum et al 2007).

Several congenital cardiac anomalies are associated with a broader spectrum of embryological malformations, some of which result in developmental delay. These children may require long-term developmental follow-up. Any preoperative neurological problems or developmental delay should be documented and appropriate management plans formulated.

Physiotherapy

When sedation is stopped and children are able to take a more active role in their treatment, effective pain relief is essential. Pain due to the incision and presence of intercostal drains may cause splinting of the chest wall and reduced excursion. Adequate pain relief can be provided through continuous infusion or patient-controlled systems in older children. It may be difficult to assess the severity of pain in children, although the development of specific paediatric pain scales has made it easier in recent years (Razmus & Wilson 2006). Children in pain can be withdrawn and immobile and infants in pain may be tachycardic and tachypnoeic. Some children who have a fear of needles will deny pain in order to avoid injections.

Treatment is directed towards early extubation and mobilization. When in bed, children should be comfortably positioned in alternate side lying or sitting upright, and the 'slumped posture' should be avoided. As soon as possible, children should be sat out of bed and walking encouraged when appropriate. Drips, drains and catheters can all be carried to allow early ambulation. Attention to posture is important, particularly following thoracotomy when arm and shoulder exercises to the affected side are also essential. If sputum retention is a problem postoperatively, airway clearance techniques may be required. A child may prefer not to have his wound supported or to support his own wound when coughing.

Pulmonary Problems Following Liver Transplantation

Liver transplantation is used for chronic end-stage liver disease and fulminant hepatic failure. Shortage of paediatric donors means that more and more grafts are reductions of adult livers. In some situations one donor liver can be used for two patients. Postoperative complications include bleeding and splinting of the right side of the diaphragm. Patients invariably develop a pleural effusion, which is usually right-sided but may be bilateral. Acute rejection is common 5–7 days post transplant. Some patients develop chronic rejection and require re-transplantation (Salt et al 1992). Physiotherapists may have the opportunity to assess these patients preoperatively, but often patients with fulminant hepatic failure are operated on as an emergency or are too ill to be seen preoperatively.

Postoperatively, the risk of bleeding in some patients means that handling is kept to a minimum. Patients are assessed regularly and treated as appropriate. Following extubation, ambulation is encouraged as soon as possible. Large pleural effusions coupled with ascites mean patients are often very breathless and it is a challenge to assist them to mobilize.

PAEDIATRIC CARDIAC INTENSIVE CARE

Congenital heart problems in infants and children are the primary reasons for admission to the paediatric cardiac ICU (CICU). They are the most common congenital anomaly with the incidence of moderate and severe forms about 6 in 1000 live births, and of all forms about 75 in 1000 live births (Hoffman & Kaplan 2002). Roughly one-third of these will require surgical intervention, and overall mortality has fallen to less than 5% in the best units (Elliott & Hussey 1995, Stark et al 2000). Early complete repair is attempted whenever possible, with the majority of operations being performed in the first year of life. Management of congenital heart defects must involve agreement between cardiologist, surgeon, family and the child, if he or she is old enough. Each aspect of the child's care is an integrated process requiring the skills of a multidisciplinary team before, during and after surgery.

Common Paediatric Cardiac Surgery Procedures

The normal anatomy of the heart is shown in Chapter 1 (see Fig. 1-20).

Palliative Procedures

When a primary repair is not possible, palliative or staging procedures will provide temporary or extended relief of symptoms. They are usually indicated to deal with excessive pulmonary blood flow, inadequate pulmonary blood flow or inadequate mixing between oxygenated and deoxygenated blood in the heart.

Pulmonary Artery Band

The pulmonary artery band is designed to restrict excessive blood flow to the lungs by reducing the diameter of the pulmonary artery with a constricting tape. A child with excessive pulmonary blood flow (ventricular and atrioventricular septal defects or truncus arteriosus) may present with poor feeding, heart failure, tachypnoea and, if uncorrected, pulmonary hypertension. If a corrective procedure is not possible, pulmonary artery banding may be performed via a left thoracotomy, to protect the lungs from the progression of pulmonary vascular disease. The pulmonary artery pressure is reduced to approximately one-third of the systemic pressure.

The Modified Blalock–Taussig Shunt

The modified Blalock–Taussig shunt (MBTS) is the most common palliative procedure used to improve pulmonary blood flow by placing a conduit between the subclavian artery and the pulmonary artery via sternotomy or thoracotomy. Inadequate pulmonary blood flow will result in poorly oxygenated blood and central cyanosis (e.g. tetralogy of Fallot, pulmonary or tricuspid atresia). If primary repair is not possible, the MBTS temporarily improves pulmonary perfusion, thereby significantly improving oxygen saturation (80–85%). The shunt is usually ligated at the time of definitive repair.

Septostomy

In defects such as transposition of the great arteries (TGA), where there is inadequate mixing of oxygenated and deoxygenated blood within the heart, the foramen ovale may be enlarged using either a balloon atrial septostomy in neonates or surgically in older children via a Blalock–Hanlon septectomy.

Corrective Surgery: Closed Procedures
Patent Ductus Arteriosus

The ductus arteriosus is the fetal vascular connection between the main pulmonary trunk and the aorta (usually distal to the origin of the left subclavian artery), which normally closes soon after birth. If it remains open, excessive blood shunts from the aorta to the lungs, causing pulmonary oedema and, in the long term, pulmonary vascular disease. Symptoms may be mild or severe, depending on the magnitude of the left-to-right shunt. This defect occurs very commonly in premature infants and may cause difficulty weaning from ventilation or congestive cardiac failure.

In some circumstances (for instance, neonates with TGA), it is desirable to delay closure of the ductus arteriosus and this may be achieved by the administration of prostaglandin.

It may also be possible to induce closure of the duct in preterm infants with indomethacin. Surgical correction involves a left thoracotomy and ligation. In older infants closure may be achieved via cardiac catheterization using a double umbrella device.

Coarctation of the Aorta

This is a congenital narrowing of the aorta. It usually occurs proximal to the junction of the ductus arteriosus and distal to the left subclavian artery origin. Neonatal presentation with symptoms of congestive heart failure requires early surgical repair. This is usually performed by resection of the stenosis and end-to-end anastomosis. If the aortic arch is extensively hypoplastic, aortic arch angioplasty may be necessary. Repair of simple coarctation carries almost zero mortality. For severe forms of coarctation such as interrupted aortic arch (where upper and lower aortic arches are separated) mortality is higher. Paraplegia is an extremely rare complication specific to correction of this defect (Brewer et al 1972) and may be associated with longer cross-clamping times.

Vascular Ring

This defect is caused when malformations of the aorta or pulmonary artery compress the trachea, oesophagus or both (examples include double aortic arch, abnormally positioned innominate artery or abnormal course of the left pulmonary artery crossing behind the trachea). Symptoms include stridor, respiratory difficulties, repeated chest infections or feeding problems. Surgical decompression of the vascular ring will often improve symptoms, but tracheal stenosis or malacia are frequently associated with vascular rings and further surgery may be required to repair tracheal or bronchial obstruction.

Corrective Surgery: Open Procedures

Open procedures require cardiopulmonary bypass, modified for children in terms of size, flow rate, perfusion, temperature and drugs (Elliott & Hussey 1995).

Atrial Septal Defect (ASD)

ASD is one of the most common congenital cardiac anomalies, characterized by a hole in the septum that separates the left and right atria. Types of ASD include ostium primum defects, also referred to as 'partial atrioventricular septal defects (AVSDs)', discussed in a later section, and ostium secundum defects due to failure of fusion of the two atrial septa and patency of the foramen ovale. Ostium secundum ASD may be associated with one or more of the superior pulmonary veins draining into the superior vena cava.

Children with ASD are generally asymptomatic and diagnosis is usually made after a murmur is detected at routine examination. If undiagnosed, slow development of symptoms may occur with rising pulmonary artery pressure and pulmonary vascular disease. If pulmonary vascular disease becomes severe and pulmonary hypertension is irreversible, then corrective surgery is not possible and heart–lung transplantation is the only palliative option. Because of the severe late consequences of pulmonary hypertension, repair is usually undertaken before the age of 5 years via median sternotomy or right anterior thoracotomy. Late diagnosis and surgical intervention are rare in developed countries. The septal defect is usually closed by direct suture or pericardial or synthetic patch. Umbrella or balloon devices have also been used successfully to close small, round defects via cardiac catheterization.

Ventricular Septal Defect (VSD)

VSDs are the most common congenital cardiac lesions, defined by a hole in the septum that separates left and right ventricles. VSDs are often found in conjunction with other cardiac defects and the clinical presentation will depend on the size of the VSD and the presence or absence of other cardiac anomalies. Infants may present with congestive cardiac failure, recurrent chest infections and failure to thrive. More than half of all VSDs close spontaneously and do not require surgery (Elliott & Hussey 1995). However, as with ASDs, undiagnosed larger defects can lead ultimately to severe irreversible pulmonary hypertension.

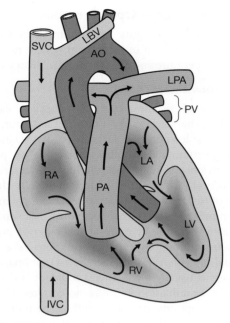

FIGURE 10-14 ■ Ventricular septal defect, showing mixing of blood between the left and right ventricle. *AO,* Aorta; *IVC,* inferior vena cava; *LA,* left atrium; *LBV,* left brachiocephalic vein; *LPA,* left pulmonary artery; *LV,* left ventricle; *PA,* pulmonary artery; *RA,* right atrium; *RV,* right ventricle; *PV,* pulmonary veins; *SVC,* superior vena cava.

VSDs (Fig. 10-14) are defined according to their position in either the perimembranous inlet, the trabecular portion or the muscular outlet of the ventricular septum. Primary repair is usually performed using synthetic or bovine pericardial patches via median sternotomy, with the cardiac approach varying according to the position of the defect. Conduction disturbances are common following surgery.

Although operative mortality approaches zero for isolated septal defects, multiple VSDs or 'Swiss cheese' defects carry a higher risk (De Leval 1994a).

Atrioventricular Septal Defect (AVSD)

Incomplete development of the inferior atrial septum, superior ventricular septum and atrioventricular valves results in a spectrum of anomalies termed 'atrioventricular septal defects' (AVSDs). Symptoms vary in severity according to the magnitude and direction of the shunt and the extent of the ASD, VSD, valve incompetence or combination of these. They may be associated with other cardiac defects (TGA, tetralogy of Fallot) and are also strongly associated with chromosomal abnormalities such as Down syndrome. Some patients may be asymptomatic despite high pulmonary vascular resistance, but a high left-to-right shunt causes dyspnoea, recurrent chest infection and congestive cardiac failure.

Partial AVSD refers to an ostium primum type of ASD above the mitral and tricuspid valves, which are displaced into the ventricles and may be incompetent. The development of pulmonary vascular disease is uncommon.

Complete AVSD is distinguished by a single six-leafed atrioventricular valve between the right and left atrioventricular chambers and continuous with the ASD above and VSD below. Over 50% of infants with this defect will die within the first year of life because of pulmonary vascular disease if left untreated. The remaining children will almost all have died within 5 years.

Both types of AVSD are repaired with patches on cardiopulmonary bypass via a median sternotomy. Hospital mortality is usually less than 10% but may be greater in patients with major associated anomalies. Early complete repair is preferred so that irreversible development of pulmonary vascular disease may be avoided, but conduction problems and valve incompetence are relatively common postoperatively.

Tetralogy of Fallot

The four components of Fallot's tetralogy are classically described as a large VSD, right ventricular (infundibular) outflow or valve obstruction, overriding aorta and right ventricular hypertrophy (Fig. 10-15).

Inadequate blood flow to the pulmonary circulation and preferential flow of deoxygenated blood to the aorta may cause cyanosis, but severity of symptoms will depend on the degree of obstructed pulmonary blood flow. The majority of infants are pink at birth but become progressively cyanosed as they grow. Periodic spasm of the infundibulum prevents blood flow to the lungs and may cause 'spelling' episodes in which infants become irritable. Continued crying leads to increasing cyanosis and eventual loss of consciousness. The spasm then relaxes and the child gradually recovers. These episodes are dangerous and may lead to death or cerebral anoxia. Older undiagnosed children may intuitively squat following exercise,

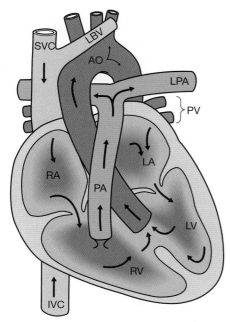

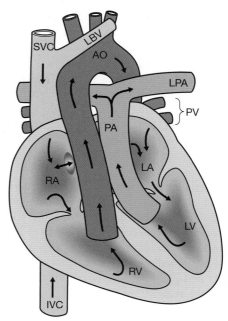

FIGURE 10-15 ▪ Tetralogy of Fallot, showing ventricular septal defect, right ventricular hypertrophy, aorta overriding both ventricles and stenosis of the pulmonary artery. *AO,* Aorta; *IVC,* inferior vena cava; *LA,* left atrium; *LBV,* left brachiocephalic vein; *LPA,* left pulmonary artery; *LV,* left ventricle; *PA,* pulmonary artery; *RA,* right atrium; *RV,* right ventricle; *PV,* pulmonary veins; *SVC,* superior vena cava.

FIGURE 10-16 ▪ Transposition of the great arteries. Shaded area shows either position of a patent foramen ovale or site of balloon septostomy, allowing some mixing of oxygenated and deoxygenated blood between the systemic and pulmonary circulations. *AO,* Aorta; *IVC,* inferior vena cava; *LA,* left atrium; *LBV,* left brachiocephalic vein; *LPA,* left pulmonary artery; *LV,* left ventricle; *PA,* pulmonary artery; *RA,* right atrium; *RV,* right ventricle; *PV,* pulmonary veins; *SVC,* superior vena cava.

which reduces blood flow to and from the lower extremities in an effort to compensate for the large oxygen debt accrued during physical activity. In the presence of cyanosis, this behaviour may suggest diagnosis of this defect.

Some controversy exists about whether it is better to do primary repair or palliative shunt with repair when the child is older. Corrective surgery will involve closure of the VSD, resection of the hypertrophied infundibulum and reconstruction of the pulmonary arteries. Long-term results are good with actuarial survival of 93% at 15 years and good quality of life (Castenda 1994).

Pulmonary Atresia

The infant with pulmonary atresia may be cyanosed at birth and this may become rapidly worse as the ductus arteriosus closes. Palliation in the form of a MBTS is the immediate treatment of choice so that adequate

blood supply to the lungs can be established. Prostaglandins may be used to delay closure of the ductus arteriosus until surgery. In the absence of right ventricular hypoplasia and coronary artery abnormalities, mortality is very low. However, this defect can occur with a VSD, in which case the right ventricle may be hypertrophied or hypoplastic and the pulmonary valve atretic. Sometimes the coronary arteries are supplied with desaturated blood from the right ventricle and major aortopulmonary collateral arteries (MAPCAs) can augment pulmonary blood flow. The technique used for definitive surgical repair is variable depending on the size of the right ventricle.

Transposition of the Great Arteries

This defect is characterized by the aorta originating from the right ventricle and the pulmonary artery from the left (Fig. 10-16). Oxygenated pulmonary blood recirculates through the lungs without reaching the body and deoxygenated blood recirculates through the body without reaching the lungs. The two closed circulations would quickly lead to death but there is usually a degree of mixing through the PDA and, if present, associated anomalies such as ASD or VSD. Babies therefore present soon after birth with cyanosis, and immediate treatment aims include keeping the ductus arteriosus open with prostaglandins until surgery. Before corrective surgery, cardiac catheterization and balloon atrial septostomy may also be necessary.

The arterial switch operation has been performed with good results since 1985 and is the preferred option for simple TGA or for TGA with VSD. It is generally performed in the first 2–3 weeks of life, while the pulmonary vascular resistance is high and the left ventricle is 'trained' to receive the systemic workload. The aorta and pulmonary arteries (above the level of the coronary vessels) are transected and transferred to their correct anatomical positions. The coronary arteries are also transferred to their appropriate positions. Operative mortality is low (<2%) and long-term results appear to be far superior to the earlier Mustard or Senning operations, which redirected blood flow via intra-atrial tunnels (Freed et al 2006).

Interrupted Aortic Arch

This rare condition is characterized by a discontinuous aortic arch and will result in death within the first month of life if left untreated. The most common site for interruption is distal to the left carotid artery. A VSD is almost always present, as is a PDA through which blood flows to the distal aorta. Soon after birth, when the ductus arteriosus begins to close, the pulmonary vascular resistance increases and severe congestive cardiac failure develops. Early surgical repair is the treatment of choice, but is technically difficult and the postoperative course is often prolonged.

Partial or Total Anomalous Pulmonary Venous Connection (PAPVC or TAPVC)

These anomalies are rare and involve some or all four pulmonary veins connecting to the systemic venous circulation. Supracardiac connections (50%) involve blood draining to the innominate vein or the superior vena cava. Cardiac connections (20%) involve blood draining into the coronary sinus or directly into right atrium. Infradiaphragmatic connections (20%) drain into the portal or hepatic veins. The final 10% are mixed connections. The reduced left atrial pressure keeps the foramen ovale open postnatally and mixed arterial and venous blood is transported systemically. Thus symptoms in the first few days of life will include congestive cardiac failure and cyanosis. There are often associated cardiac anomalies and surgical repair will depend on the nature of these, if present.

Truncus Arteriosus

Truncus arteriosus is characterized by a single arterial trunk arising from both ventricles and from which the aorta and pulmonary arteries originate via a single semilunar valve. A VSD permits flow up the common trunk. Congestive cardiac failure and irreversible pulmonary vascular disease rapidly develop in early infancy and untreated infants rarely survive beyond their first year. Surgical treatment involves the closure of the VSD with a patch to divert the left ventricular flow up the aorta. The pulmonary arteries are then detached from the common artery (truncus arteriosus) and connected to the right ventricle using a conduit.

Cardiac Valve Abnormalities

Aortic Stenosis

Obstruction to left ventricular outflow may occur in isolation or in combination with other cardiac defects. They may be found at valvular, subvalvular, supravalvular or combined levels. Critical stenoses present neonatally with congestive cardiac failure and reduced peripheral pulses, and require immediate intervention. Relief of aortic stenosis may be obtained with aortic valvotomy, aortic valve replacement, homograft insertion or balloon dilatation. However, mortality is high (10%) and reoperation common (Elliott & Hussey 1995). Aortic stenosis may not cause problems until adulthood, although by then, a degree of left ventricular hypertrophy may have developed.

Pulmonary Stenosis

The neonate with pulmonary stenosis may become progressively more cyanosed as the PDA closes and this may be reversed or delayed by the use of prostaglandins to keep the PDA patent. Management is similar to that of pulmonary atresia, with surgery dependent on the nature and extent, if any, of associated cardiac anomalies. Homograft valve replacement may be required at a later stage. Less critical pulmonary stenosis may present later in life with breathlessness on exertion and fatigue.

Tricuspid Valve

Tricuspid valve disease is rare in childhood but is seen in Ebstein anomaly. Patients present with severe cardiac failure, cyanosis and dysrhythmia. Neonatal surgery carries a high mortality and a palliative approach with a later Fontan procedure may be preferred (De Leval 1994b). In the older child it is possible to perform a more complex repair of the anomaly.

Mitral Valve

Mitral valve problems present either as stenosis or incompetence, usually associated with other cardiac anomalies. Repair is the preferred option, although replacement may be the only option. Early replacement is associated with a high mortality (20%) (Carpenter 1994).

Hypoplastic Left Heart Syndrome

This defect is defined by aortic valve stenosis or atresia associated with severe left ventricular hypoplasia. Early mortality in untreated patients is high. The systemic blood flow derives almost entirely from the right ventricle through the ductus arteriosus and, depending on the size of it, peripheral pulses may be normal, reduced or absent. Immediate management involves keeping the ductus arteriosus open with prostaglandins. Surgical management options include early heart–lung transplantation or a three-staged surgical procedure that makes the child's circulation function with only two of the heart's four chambers. The first step (Norwood procedure) makes the right ventricle pump blood to the whole body and to the lungs. The second stage (Glenn procedure) allows greater blood flow to the upper body and reduces some of the workload from the right ventricle. The final procedure (Fontan procedure or total cavopulmonary connection) allows blood to return passively to the lungs (rather than being pumped there) and allows the right ventricle to only pump blood out to the body (Norwood & Jacobs 1994). The Norwood procedure is generally performed within a week of birth, the second stage at 3–6 months

of age, and the Fontan at 18 months to 4 years of age. Success of these types of surgery depends on the lungs being free of pulmonary vascular disease and a good balance between pulmonary and systemic circulations.

Transplantation Surgery in Children

The problems of cardiac, lung and heart–lung transplant surgery in children are similar to those in adults, and are discussed in detail in Chapter 13.

Need for Extracorporeal Membrane Oxygenation

ECMO provides complete or partial cardiopulmonary bypass support for the heart and lungs or lungs alone when extremely ill children have severe but potentially reversible cardiac or respiratory failure (Huang et al 2007). It has been reported to be beneficial in both neonates and children with acute lung injury and respiratory failure (Pearson et al 1993, Swaniker et al 2000, UK Collaborative ECMO Trial Group 1996).

In some respects, physiotherapy treatments for children on ECMO may seem relatively less difficult for the physiotherapist. Children on full cardiopulmonary ECMO support are not reliant on mechanical ventilation for adequate oxygenation and it may not be as important to connect ventilation circuits as quickly or complete suction cycles as quickly. However, children on ECMO are heparinized and thus very vulnerable to bleeding, with potentially devastating consequences for survival or long-term outcome. Too much movement or coughing during physiotherapy may raise ICP and cause brain or pulmonary bleeding. If the nursing report suggests active haemorrhage, therapists should consider whether it is appropriate to apply manual techniques or treat at all. Adequate blood flow through the ECMO circuit is often dependent upon body position and the therapist should ensure that turning during treatments does not compromise flow through the cannulae.

Frequently children on ECMO for respiratory failure demonstrate a complete 'whiteout' of the lung fields on chest radiograph within the first day of ECMO support. During this time respiratory compliance is extremely low and little chest movement is seen or achieved during treatments. Children are often on 'resting' ventilation with low respiratory pressures and rates. During this time physiotherapy treatments may only consist of a quick assessment during the day, until it becomes apparent that the chest wall is beginning to move and air bronchograms are beginning to appear on chest radiograph. At this time, it is appropriate to start more regular treatments in order to recruit functional airways and to facilitate early weaning from ECMO.

Tracheal Repair: Tracheal Stenosis and Slide Tracheoplasty

Subglottic stenosis occurs in some infants following prolonged intubation and leads to upper airway obstruction. It could be avoided by attention to tracheal tube placement and fixation and care with suction (Albert 1995). Acquired neonatal tracheobronchial stenosis (particularly in preterm infants) has a poor outcome. Stridor is often present and may respond to adrenaline via a nebulizer. In more severe cases a tracheostomy may be necessary until the airway has increased sufficiently in size to allow adequate ventilation. Some patients will also require surgical laryngotracheoplasty before successful decannulation of the tracheostomy can be achieved. More recently, primary repair of subglottic stenosis with laryngotracheal reconstruction has been successfully developed.

Children born with tracheal stenosis have had a high mortality. Now the development of various surgical tracheal reconstructions, replacements and slide tracheoplasty procedures has provided a new hope for such patients (Beierlein & Elliott 2006). ECMO may be required preoperatively or postoperatively to provide ventilatory support for patients undergoing critical tracheobronchial reconstruction. Manual hyperinflation following tracheal repair may be associated with greater risk of pneumothorax because of the tracheal anastomosis. In addition, the tracheal anastomosis may extend distal to the tracheal tube and suction procedures should avoid traumatizing the site.

Some degree of tracheomalacia is often present and the fact that children are either paralyzed or very well sedated in the early postoperative period means there is often air trapping and impaired airway clearance. It is thus essential that treatments are quick, competent and effective, and include decompression, if necessary, of any trapped air. In the long term, such children may

need follow-up in the community and may continue to have noisy breathing and problems with airway clearance.

Clinical Problems Encountered in the CICU

In addition to the altered pulmonary dynamics and respiratory insufficiency seen after general anaesthesia, open heart surgery with cardiopulmonary bypass leads to further changes in respiratory function. The lungs may be compressed during surgery, contributing to atelectasis, loss of perfusion and diminished surfactant production, all of which contribute to poor respiratory compliance postoperatively. Children and infants should be regularly reviewed and treated as required. Effective pain relief is essential after surgery, as children will find it difficult to cooperate if they feel pain due to the incision or intercostal drains.

Physiotherapy support following cardiac surgery is as anticipated: avoidance of complications related to surgery, airway clearance, resolution of atelectasis if present, optimization of gas exchange and early mobilization. Drips, drains and catheters can all be carried to allow early ambulation. Attention to posture is important, particularly following thoracotomy when arm and shoulder exercises to the affected side are also essential.

The unique difficulties that physiotherapists working in the CICU may encounter are usually related to the ways in which physiotherapy treatments may alter the finely balanced haemodynamic cardiovascular system in vulnerable children. This requires a detailed knowledge of the underlying pathophysiology of the range of congenital cardiac defects. In addition, knowledge of the way in which the cardiac and systemic blood circulations may change following specific surgical corrections, during mechanical ventilation, when NO is entrained into the ventilation and when cardiogenic drugs are administered. Respiratory physiotherapy has the potential to both avert and precipitate critical events in the CICU, and it is the responsibility of professionals to optimize outcomes.

Pulmonary Hypertensive Crisis

Pulmonary hypertensive crisis is described as an acute elevation of the pulmonary artery pressure (owing to contraction of the pulmonary arteriolar musculature), which restricts blood flow through the lungs. It is associated with a fall in left atrial pressure and a dramatic fall in cardiac output. Pulmonary artery pressure may approach or even exceed systemic pressure. It is seen in the presence of hypertrophic reactive arteriolar muscle in the lungs and is therefore common in those patients who have had significant left-to-right shunts (VSD, AVSD, truncus arteriosus). This phenomenon is a critical, life-threatening event and prevention of such an incident is desirable. Airway suction and chest physiotherapy have the potential both for precipitating a hypertensive crisis (by creating an imbalance in the pulmonary/systemic flow ratio) and for correcting an imbalance (caused by excess secretions). The partial pressures of blood oxygen and carbon dioxide relative to each other will determine the ratio of systemic–pulmonary blood flow. Low oxygen and high carbon dioxide will increase pulmonary vascular resistance and reduce pulmonary blood flow. High oxygen and low carbon dioxide cause an increase in pulmonary blood flow.

In children prone to pulmonary hypertensive crisis, treatment should be undertaken with great caution. Inspired oxygen should be increased during chest physiotherapy (but not too much if a child is dependent on a univentricular circulation), and treatment times kept to a minimum. Particular attention should be paid to oxygen saturation and the pulmonary artery pressure in relation to systemic blood pressure. Often children will require a bolus of sedation before treatment and if there is already NO entrained in the ventilator circuit, care should be taken to ensure this supply is maintained during manual ventilation with a bag. NO gas has a potent pulmonary vasodilatory effect and can be delivered directly to the lungs via the ventilator circuit for the effective relief of pulmonary hypertension in infants and children. Very small doses are used to reduce pulmonary arterial pressures, while systemic blood pressure is not affected (doses larger than 80 parts per million can be toxic) (Cheifetz 2000, Haddad et al 2000, Kinsella & Abman 2000).

Delayed Sternal Closure

Occasionally postoperative closure of the sternum is impeded by pulmonary, myocardial or chest wall oedema (due either to prolonged bypass times or particularly complicated intracardiac repairs). If sternal closure is likely to constrict cardiopulmonary function, closure may be delayed for days or even weeks. During this period children are paralyzed or very well sedated and are preferentially nursed in supine. They are therefore at much greater risk of pulmonary complications. However, if stable and if the sternum is stented (to keep its edges separate), the child can, with care, be quarter turned from supine. Manual hyperinflation is usually well tolerated and gentle posterior and posterolateral vibrations may be applied. When the sternum is finally closed, there is often short-term deterioration in respiratory function and it may be useful to suggest an increase in ventilatory support if treatments are to be undertaken soon after sternal closure or to delay physiotherapy treatments until respiratory function has stabilized again (Main et al 2001b).

Phrenic Nerve Damage

Damage to the phrenic nerve is a well-documented complication of paediatric cardiac surgery (Mok et al 1991). It occurs most commonly where dissection is required close to the mediastinal vessels and pericardium, with which its course is closely associated. The result may be difficulty weaning from mechanical ventilation or severe respiratory compromise once extubated. Paradoxical movement during inspiration may compress the ipsilateral lung and cause mediastinal shift to the contralateral side, causing a further loss in lung volume. Physiotherapy intervention will depend on clinical symptoms, but it is important that the patient is positioned head up to relieve the pressure from the abdominal viscera and reduce the work of breathing. It is sometimes necessary to surgically plicate the affected diaphragm.

REFERENCES

Acute Respiratory Distress Syndrome Network, 2000. Ventilation with lower tidal volumes as compared with traditional tidal volumes for acute lung injury and the acute respiratory distress syndrome. NEJM 342 (18), 1301–1308.

Akingbola, O.A., Hopkins, R.L., 2001. Pediatric noninvasive positive pressure ventilation. Pediatr. Crit. Care Med. 2 (2), 164–169.

Al-balkhi, A., Klonin, H., Marinaki, K., et al., 2005. Review of treatment of bronchiolitis related apnoea in two centres. Arch. Dis. Child. 90 (3), 288–291.

Albert, D., 1995. Management of suspected tracheobronchial stenosis in ventilated neonates. Arch. Dis. Child. 72, 1–2.

Almeida, C.C., Ribeiro, J.D., Almeida-Junior, A.A., Zeferino, A.M., 2005. Effect of expiratory flow increase technique on pulmonary function of infants on mechanical ventilation. Physiother. Res. Int. 10 (4), 213–221.

Ambalavanan, N., Carlo, W.A., 2006. Ventilatory strategies in the prevention and management of bronchopulmonary dysplasia. Semin. Perinatol. 30 (4), 192–199.

American Academy of Pediatrics Committee on Fetus Newborn, 2012. Levels of neonatal care. Pediatrics 130 (3), 587–597. doi: 10.1542/peds.2012-1999.

Arnold, J.H., 1996. High frequency oscillatory ventilation: theory and practice in paediatric patients. Paediatr. Anaesth. 6, 437–441.

Arnold, J.H., Hanson, J.H., Toro-Figuero, L.O., et al., 1994. Prospective, randomized comparison of high-frequency oscillatory ventilation and conventional mechanical ventilation in pediatric respiratory failure. Crit. Care Med. 22 (10), 1530–1539.

Bagley, C.E., Gray, P.H., Tudehope, D.I., et al., 2005. Routine neonatal post-extubation chest physiotherapy: a randomized controlled trial. J. Paediatr. Child Health 41 (11), 592–597.

Baird, P.A., MacDonald, E.C., 1982. An epidemiologic study of congenital malformations of the anterior abdominal wall in more than half a million consecutive live births. Am. J. Hum. Genet. 34, 517–521.

Balaguer, A., Escribano, J., Roque, M., 2006. Infant position in neonates receiving mechanical ventilation. Cochrane Database Syst. Rev. (4), Art No: CD003668, doi: 10.1002/14651858. CD003668.pub2.

Balfour-Lynn, I.M., Abrahamson, E., Cohen, G., et al., 2005. BTS Guidelines for the management of pleural infection in children (on behalf of the Paediatric Pleural Diseases Subcommittee of the BTS Standards of Care Committee). Thorax 60, 1–21.

Bartlett, R.H., 1990. Extracorporeal life support for cardiopulmonary failure. Curr. Probl. Surg. 27 (10), 621–705.

Bartlett, R.H., Andrews, A.F., Toomasian, J.M., et al., 1982. Extracorporeal membrane oxygenation for newborn respiratory failure: forty-five cases. Surgery 92 (2), 425–433.

Bauer, M., Hoek, G., Smit, H.A., et al., 2007. Air pollution and development of asthma, allergy and infections in a birth cohort. Eur. Respir. J. 29, 879–888.

Beby, P.J., Henderson-Smart, D.J., Lacey, J.L., Rieger, I., 1998. Short and long term neurological outcomes following neonatal chest physiotherapy. Journal of Paediatric and Child Health 34, 60–62.

Beierlein, W., Elliott, M.J., 2006. Variations in the technique of slide tracheoplasty to repair complex forms of long-segment congenital tracheal stenoses. Ann. Thorac. Surg. 82, 1540–1542.

Bernard, G.R., Artigas, A., Brigham, K.L., et al., 1994. The American-European Consensus Conference on ARDS: definitions, mechanisms, relevant outcomes and clinical trial coordination. Am. J. Respir. Crit. Care Med. 149 (3 Pt 1), 818–824.

Berney, S., Denehy, L., 2002. A comparison of the effects of manual and ventilator hyperinflation on static lung compliance and sputum production in intubated and ventilated intensive care patients. Physiother. Res. Int. 7 (2), 100–108.

Bhandari, A., Panitch, H.B., 2006. Pulmonary outcomes in bronchopulmonary dysplasia. Semin. Perinatol. 30 (4), 219–226.

Bhuyan, U., Peters, A.M., Gordon, I., Helms, P., 1989. Effect of posture on the distribution of pulmonary ventilation and perfusion in children and adults. Thorax 44, 480–484.

Bikker, I.G., et al., 2011. Electrical impedance tomography measured at two thoracic levels can visualize the ventilation distribution changes at the bedside during a decremental positive end-expiratory lung pressure trial. Crit. Care 15 (4), R193.

Birnkrant, D.J., 2002. The assessment and management of the respiratory complications of pediatric neuromuscular diseases. Clin. Pediatr. (Phila.) 41 (5), 301–308.

Blackwood, B., 1999. Normal saline instillation with endotracheal suctioning: *primum non nocere* (first do no harm). J. Adv. Nurs. 29, 928–934.

Blencowe, H., Cousens, S., Oestergaard, M.Z., et al., 2012. National, regional, and worldwide estimates of preterm birth rates in the year 2010 with time trends since 1990 for selected countries: a systematic analysis and implications. Lancet 379 (9832), 2162–2172. doi: 10.1016/S0140-6736(12)60820-4.

Blumenthal, I., Lealman, G.T., 1982. Effects of posture on gastro-oesophageal reflux in the newborn. Arch. Dis. Child. 57, 555–556.

Bracewell, M., Marlow, N., 2002. Patterns of motor disability in very preterm children. Ment. Retard. Dev. Disabil. Res. Rev. 8 (4), 241–248. doi: 10.1002/mrdd.10049.

Brackbill, Y., Douthitt, T.C., West, H., 1973. Psychophysiological effects in the neonate of prone versus supine placement. J. Pediatr. 82, 82–83.

Brewer, L.A., Fosburg, R.G., Mulder, G.A., Verska, J.J., 1972. Spinal cord complications following surgery for coarctation of the aorta: a study of 66 cases. J. Thorac. Cardiovasc. Surg. 64, 368–381.

Brimioulle, S., Moraine, J.J., Norrenberg, K., Kahn, R.J., 1997. Effect of positioning and exercise on intracranial pressure in a neurosurgical intensive care unit. Phys. Ther. 77, 1682–1689.

British Thoracic Society (BTS), Scottish Intercollegiate Guidelines Network (SIGN), 2003. British guideline on the management of asthma. Thorax 58 (Suppl. I), i1–i94.

British Thoracic Society Standards of Care Committee, 2002. Guidelines for the management of community acquired pneumonia in childhood. Thorax 57, 1–24.

Button, B.M., Heine, R.G., Catto-Smith, A.G., et al., 1997. Postural drainage and gastro-oesophageal reflux in infants with cystic fibrosis. Arch. Dis. Child. 76, 148–150.

Button, B.M., Heine, R.G., Catto-Smith, A.G., et al., 2003. Chest physiotherapy in infants with cystic fibrosis: to tip or not? A five-year study. Pediatr. Pulmonol. 35 (3), 208–213.

Button, B.M., Heine, R.G., Catto-Smith, A.G., et al., 2004. Chest physiotherapy, gastro-oesophageal reflux, and arousal in infants with cystic fibrosis. Arch. Dis. Child. 89 (5), 435–439.

Carpenter, A., 1994. Congenital malformation of the mitral valve. In: Stark, J., De Leval, M. (Eds.), Surgery for Congenital Heart Defects, second ed. WB Saunders, Philadelphia, pp. 599–614.

Castenda, A.R., 1994. Tetralogy of Fallot. In: Stark, J., De Leval, M. (Eds.), Surgery for Congenital Heart Defects, second ed. WB Saunders, Philadelphia, pp. 405–416.

Castle, R.A., Dunne, C.J., Mok, Q., et al., 2002. Accuracy of displayed values of tidal volume in the pediatric intensive care unit. Crit. Care Med. 30 (11), 2566–2574.

Chatwin, M., Ross, E., Hart, N., et al., 2003. Cough augmentation with mechanical insufflation/exsufflation in patients with neuromuscular weakness. Eur. Respir. J. 21 (3), 502–508.

Cheifetz, I.M., 2000. Inhaled nitric oxide: plenty of data, no consensus. Crit. Care Med. 28, 902–903.

Cheong, J.L., Doyle, L.W., 2012. Increasing rates of prematurity and epidemiology of late preterm birth. J. Paediatr. Child Health 48 (9), 784–788. doi: 10.1111/j.1440-1754.2012.02536.x.

Chisakuta, A., Tasker, R.C., 1998. Respiratory failure in myasthenia gravis and negative pressure support. Pediatr. Neurol. 19 (3), 225–226.

Chiu, P., Hedrick, H.L., 2008. Postnatal management and long-term outcome for survivors with congenital diaphragmatic hernia. Prenat. Diagn. 28 (7), 592–603. doi: 10.1002/pd.2007.

Choi, J.S., Jones, A.Y., 2005. Effects of manual hyperinflation and suctioning in respiratory mechanics in mechanically ventilated patients with ventilator-associated pneumonia. Aust. J. Physiother. 51, 25–30.

Chulay, M., Graeber, G.M., 1988. Efficacy of a hyperinflation and hyperoxygenation suctioning intervention. Heart and Lung 17, 15–22.

Clark, A.P., Winslow, E.H., Tyler, D.O., White, K.M., 1990. Effects of endotracheal suctioning on mixed venous oxygen saturation and heart rate in critically ill adults. Heart and Lung 19, 552–557.

Clarke, R.C., Kelly, B.E., Convery, P.N., Fee, J.P., 1999. Ventilatory characteristics in mechanically ventilated patients during manual hyperventilation for chest physiotherapy. Anaesthesia 54, 936–940.

Curley, M.A., Hibberd, P.L., Fineman, L.D., et al., 2005. Effect of prone positioning on clinical outcomes in children with acute lung injury: a randomized controlled trial. J. Am. Med. Assoc. 294 (2), 229–237.

Czarnik, R.E., Stone, K.S., Everhart, C.J., Preusser, B.A., 1991. Differential effects of continuous versus intermittent suction on tracheal tissue. Heart and Lung 20, 144–151.

D'Angio, C.T., et al., 2005. Pressure-regulated volume control ventilation vs synchronized intermittent mandatory ventilation for very low-birth-weight infants: a randomized controlled trial. Arch. Pediatr. Adolesc. Med. 159 (9), 868–875.

D'Angio, C.T., Sinkin, R.A., Stevens, T.P., et al., 2002. Longitudinal, 15-year follow-up of children born at less than 29 weeks' gestation after introduction of surfactant therapy into a region: neurologic, cognitive, and educational outcomes. Pediatrics 110 (6), 1094–1102.

Davies, H., Kitchman, R., Gordon, G., Helms, P., 1985. Regional ventilation in infancy. Reversal of the adult pattern. NEJM 313, 1627–1628.

Davis, P.G., Morley, C.J., Owen, L.S., 2009. Non-invasive respiratory support of preterm neonates with respiratory diseas : continuous positive airway pressure and nasal intermittent pos. ive pressure ventilation. Semin. Fetal Neonatal Med. 14 (1), 14–20.

De Leval, M., 1994a. Ventricular septal defects. In: Stark, J., De Leval, M. (Eds.), Surgery for Congenital Heart Defects, second ed. WB Saunders, Philadelphia, pp. 55–371.

De Leval, M., 1994b. Tricuspid valve. In: Stark, J., De Leval, M. (Eds.), Surgery for Congenital Heart Defects, second ed. WB Saunders, Philadelphia, Ch 23, pp. 453–466.

Deakers, T.W., Reynolds, G., Stretton, M., Newth, C.J., 1994. Cuffed endotracheal tubes in pediatric intensive care. J. Pediatr. 125, 57–62.

Demling, R.H., Riessen, R., 1993. Respiratory failure after cerebral injury. Crit. Care Med. 1, 440–446.

Depaepe, A., Dolk, A., Lechat, M.F., 1993. The epidemiology of tracheo-oesophageal fistula and oesophageal atresia in Europe. Arch. Dis. Child. 68, 743–748.

Dinwiddie, R., 1997. Aspiration syndromes. In: Dinwiddie, R. (Ed.), Diagnosis and Management of Paediatric Respiratory Disease, Churchill-Livingstone, London, 19, pp. 61–80.

Donn, S.M., Sinha, S.K., 2003. Invasive and non-invasive neonatal mechanical ventilation. Respir. Care 48 (4), 426–441.

Ehrenkranz, R.A., Walsh, M.C., Vohr, B.R., et al., 2005. National Institutes of Child Health and Human Development Neonatal Research Network. Validation of the National Institutes of Health consensus definition of bronchopulmonary dysplasia. Pediatrics 116 (6), 1353–1360.

Elliott, M., Hussey, J., 1995. Paediatric cardiac surgery. In: Prasad, S.A., Hussey, J. (Eds.), Paediatric Respiratory Care. Chapman & Hall, London, pp. 122–141.

Elmer, J., Wang, B., Melhem, S., et al., 2015. Exposure to high concentrations of inspired oxygen does not worsen lung injury after cardiac arrest. Critical Care 19, 105–114.

Engle, W.A., American Academy of Pediatrics Committee on Fetus and Newborn, 2008. Surfactant-replacement therapy for respiratory distress in the preterm and term neonate. Pediatrics 121 (2), 419–432. doi: 10.1542/peds.2007-3283.

Essouri, S., Chevret, L., Durand, P., et al., 2006. Non-invasive positive pressure ventilation: five years of experience in a pediatric intensive care unit. Pediatr. Crit. Care Med. 7 (4), 329–334.

Essouri, S., Durand, P., Chevret, L., et al., 2011. Optimal level of nasal continuous positive airway pressure in severe viral bronchiolitis. Intensive Care Med. 37, 2002–2007. doi: 10.1007/s00134-011-2372-4.

Farias, J.A., Alias, I., Retta, A., et al., 2002. An evaluation of extubation failure predictors in mechanically ventilated infants and children. Intensive Care Med. 28 (6), 752–757.

Feldman, Z., Kanter, M.J., Robertson, C.S., et al., 1992. Effect of head elevation on intracranial pressure and cerebral blood flow in head injured patients. J. Neurosurg. 59, 206–211.

Ferguson, N.D., et al., 2013. High-frequency oscillation in early acute respiratory distress syndrome. N. Engl. J. Med. 368 (9), 795–805.

Flenady, V.J., Gray, P.H., 2002. Chest physiotherapy for preventing morbidity in babies being extubated from mechanical ventilation. Cochrane Database Syst. Rev. (2), CD000283, doi: 10.1002/14651858.CD000283.

Frat, J.-P., et al., 2015. High-Flow Oxygen through Nasal Cannula in Acute Hypoxemic Respiratory Failure. NEJM 372 (23), 2185–2196.

Freed, D.H., Robertson, C.M., Sauve, R.S., et al., 2006. Intermediate-term outcomes of the arterial switch operation for transposition of great arteries in neonates: alive but well? J. Thorac. Cardiovasc. Surg. 132 (4), 845–852.

Gardner, S., Enzman-Hines, M., Dickey, L.A., 2011. Respiratory Diseases. In: Gardner, S.L., Carter, B.S., Enzman-Hines, M., Hernandez, J.A. (Eds.), Neonatal Intensive Care, seventh ed. Elsevier, Missouri.

Gattinoni, L., Caironi, P., Cressoni, M., et al., 2006. Lung recruitment in patients with the acute respiratory distress syndrome. NEJM 354 (17), 1775–1786.

Gattinoni, L., Pesenti, A., Bombino, M., et al., 1993. Role of extracorporeal circulation in adult respiratory distress syndrome management. New Horiz. 1, 603–612.

Gemma, M., Tommasino, C., Cerri, M., et al., 2002. Intracranial effects of endotracheal suctioning in the acute phase of head injury. J. Neurol. Anesthesiol. 14, 50–54.

Glass, C., Grap, M.J., Corley, M.C., Wallace, D., 1993. Nurses' ability to achieve hyperinflation and hyperoxygenation with a manual resuscitation bag during endotracheal suctioning. Heart Lung 22, 158–165.

Goldman, A.P., Kerr, S.J., Butt, W., et al., 1997. Extracorporeal support for intractable cardiorespiratory failure due to meningococcal disease. Lancet 349 (9050), 466–469.

Goodnough, S.K., 1985. The effects of oxygen and hyperinflation on arterial oxygen tension after endotracheal suctioning. Heart Lung 14, 11–17.

Gray, P.H., Flenady, V.J., Blackwell, L., 1999. Potential risks of chest physiotherapy in preterm infants. J. Pediatr. 135, 131.

Greenough, A., Kotecha, S., Vrijlandt, E. 2006 Bronchopulmonary dysplasia: current models and concepts. In: Frey U, Gerritsen J (eds) Respiratory diseases in infants and children. Eur. Respir. Monogr. 11: 217–229.

Gregson, R., Shannon, H., Main, E., et al., 2007a. The relationship between age and forces applied during chest physiotherapy in mechanically ventilated children. Physiotherapy 93, S517.

Gregson, R.K., Stocks, J., Petley, G.W., et al., 2007b. Simultaneous measurement of force and respiratory profiles during chest physiotherapy in ventilated children. Physiol. Meas. 28, 1017–1028.

Gregson, R.K., Shannon, H., Stocks, J., et al., 2012. The unique contribution of manual chest compression-vibrations to airflow during physiotherapy in sedated, fully ventilated children. Pediatr. Crit. Care Med. 13 (2), e97–e102.

Haddad, E., Lowson, S.M., Johns, R.A., Rich, G.F., 2000. Use of inhaled nitric oxide perioperatively and in intensive care patients. Anesthesiology 92, 1821–1825.

Hagler, D.A., Traver, G.A., 1994. Endotracheal saline and suction catheters: sources of lower airway contamination. Am. J. Crit. Care 3, 444–447.

Harding, J.E., Miles, F.K., Becroft, D.M., et al., 1998. Chest physiotherapy may be associated with brain damage in extremely premature infants. J. Pediatr. 132 (3 Pt 1), 440–444.

Harshbarger, S.A., Hoffman, L.A., Zullo, T.G., Pinsky, M.R., 1992. Effects of a closed tracheal suction system on ventilatory and cardiovascular parameters. Am. J. Crit. Care 1, 57–61.

Heaf, D.P., Helms, P., Gordon, I., Turner, H.M., 1983. Postural effects on gas exchange in infants. NEJM 308 (25), 1505–1508.

Henderson-Smart, D.J., Davis, P.G., 2003. Prophylactic methylxanthines for extubation in preterm infants. Cochrane Database Syst. Rev. (1), CD000139.

Hodge, D., Chetcuti, P.A.J., 2000. RSV: management of the acute episode. Paediatr. Respir. Rev. 1, 215–220.

Hoffman, J.I.E., Kaplan, S., 2002. The incidence of congenital heart disease. J. Am. Coll. Cardiol. 39 (12), 1890–1900.

Holloway, E., Ram, F.S.F., 2004. Breathing exercises for asthma. Cochrane Database Syst. Rev. (1), CD001277, pub2.

Hondras, M.A., Linde, K., Jones, A.P., 2000. Manual therapy for asthma (Cochrane Review). In: The Cochrane Library. Update Software, Oxford, p. 4.

Horiuchi, K., Jordan, D., Cohen, D., et al., 1997. Insights into the increased oxygen demand during chest physiotherapy. Crit. Care Med. 25, 1347–1351.

Hough, J.L., Johnston, L., Brauer, S.G., et al., 2012. Effect of body position on ventilation distribution in preterm infants on continuous positive airway pressure. Pediatr. Crit. Care Med. 13 (4), 446–451. doi: 10.1097/PCC.0b013e31822f18d9.

Huang, S.C., Wu, E.T., Chi, N.H., et al., 2007. Perioperative extracorporeal membrane oxygenation support for critical pediatric airway surgery. Eur. J. Pediatr. 166 (11), 1129–1133. doi: 10.1007/500431-006-0390-y.

Hudson, R.M., Box, R.C., 2003. Neonatal respiratory therapy in the new millennium: does clinical practice reflect scientific evidence? Aust. J. Physiother. 49 (4), 269–272.

Imle, P.C., Klemic, N., 1989. Methods of airway clearance: coughing and suctioning. In: Mackenzie, C.F., Imle, P.C., Ciesla, N. (Eds.), Chest Physiotherapy in the Intensive Care Unit. Williams and Wilkins, Baltimore, pp. 153–187.

Inwald, D., Roland, M., Kuitert, L., et al., 2001. Oxygen for all in acute severe asthma. Br. Med. J. 27, 722–729.

Jansson, T., Powell, T.L., 2007. Role of the placenta in fetal programming: underlying mechanisms and potential interventional approaches. Clin. Sci. (Lond.) 113 (1), 1–13. doi: 10.1042/CS20060339.

Jobe, A.H., 1993. Pulmonary surfactant therapy. N. Engl. J. Med. 328 (12), 861–868. doi: 10.1056/NEJM199303253281208.

Jobe, A.H., 2013. Good news for lung repair in preterm infants. Am. J. Respir. Crit. Care Med. 187 (10), 1043–1044. doi: 10.1164/rccm.201303-0485ED.

Jobe, A.H., Bancalari, E., 2001. Bronchopulmonary dysplasia. Am. J. Respir. Crit. Care Med. 163 (7), 1723–1729. doi: 10.1164/ajrccm.163.7.2011060.

Johnson, A.H., Peacock, J.L., Greenough, A., et al., 2002. United Kingdom Oscillation Study Group. High frequency oscillatory ventilation for the prevention of chronic lung disease of prematurity. NEJM 347, 633–642.

Kerem, E., Yatsiv, I., Goitein, K.J., 1990. Effect of endotracheal suctioning on arterial blood gases in children. Intensive Care Med. 16, 95–99.

Khine, H.H., Corddry, D.H., Kettrick, R.G., et al., 1997. Comparison of cuffed and uncuffed endotracheal tubes in young children during general anesthesia. Anesthesiology 86, 627–631.

Kim, C.S., Iglesias, A.J., Sackner, M.A., 1987. Mucus clearance by 2-phase gas–liquid flow mechanism: asymmetric periodic-flow model. J. Appl. Physiol. 62 (3), 959–971.

King, M., 1998. Experimental models for studying mucociliary clearance. Eur. Respir. J. 11 (1), 222–228.

Kinloch, D., 1999. Instillation of normal saline during endotracheal suctioning: effects on mixed venous oxygen saturation. Am. J. Crit. Care 8, 231–240.

Kinsella, J.P., Abman, S.H., 2000. Clinical approach to inhaled nitric oxide therapy in the newborn with hypoxemia. J. Pediatr. 136, 717–726.

Kleiber, C., Krutzfield, N., Rose, E.F., 1988. Acute histologic changes in the tracheobronchial tree associated with different suction catheter insertion techniques. Heart Lung 17, 10–14.

Kneyber, M.C., Plötz, F.B., Sibarani-Ponsen, R.D., Markhorst, D.G., 2005. High frequency oscillatory ventilation (HFOV) facilitates CO_2 elimination in small airway disease: the open airway concept. Respir. Med. 99 (11), 1459–1461.

Knight, D.B., Bevan, C.J., Harding, J.E., et al., 2001. Chest physiotherapy and porencephalic brain lesions in very preterm infants. Journal of Paediatric and Child Health 37 (6), 554–558.

Kotecha, S., 2000. Lung growth: implications for the newborn infant. Arch. Dis. Child. Fetal Neonatal Ed. 82, F69–F74.

Krastins, I., Corey, M.L., McLeod, A., et al., 1982. An evaluation of incentive spirometry in the management of pulmonary complications after cardiac surgery in a pediatric population. Crit. Care Med. 10, 525–528.

Krause, M.F., Hoehn, T., 2000. Chest physiotherapy in mechanically ventilated children: a review. Crit. Care Med. 28, 1648–1651.

Kuo, C.Y., Gerhardt, T., Bolivar, J., et al., 1996. Effect of leak around the endotracheal tube on measurements of pulmonary compliance and resistance during mechanical ventilation: a lung model study. Pediatr. Pulmonol. 22, 35–43.

Lassen, H.C., 1953. A preliminary report on the 1952 epidemic of poliomyelitis in Copenhagen with special reference to the treatment of acute respiratory insufficiency. Lancet 1 (1), 37–41.

Lindgren, S., Odenstedt, H., Olegard, C., et al., 2007. Regional lung derecruitment after endotracheal suction during volume- or pressure-controlled ventilation: a study using electric impedance tomography. Intensive Care Med. 33 (1), 172–180.

Lockridge, T., Taquino, L.T., Knight, A., 1999. Back to sleep: is there room in that crib for both AAP recommendations and developmentally supportive care? Neonatal Netw. 18 (5), 29–33. doi: 10.1891/0730-0832.18.5.29.

MacNaughton, P.D., Evans, T.W., 1999. Pulmonary function in the intensive care unit. In: Hughes, J.M.B., Pride, N.B. (Eds.), Lung Function Tests: Physiological Principles and Clinical Applications. WB Saunders, London, pp. 185–199.

Main, E., Castle, R., Newham, D., Stocks, J., 2004. Respiratory physiotherapy vs. suction: the effects on respiratory function in ventilated infants and children. Intensive Care Med. 30 (6), 1144–1151.

Main, E., Castle, R., Stocks, J., et al., 2001a. The influence of endotracheal tube leak on the assessment of respiratory function in ventilated children. Intensive Care Med. 27 (11), 1788–1797.

Main, E., Elliott, M.J., Schindler, M., Stocks, J., 2001b. Effect of delayed sternal closure after cardiac surgery on respiratory function in ventilated infants. Crit. Care Med. 29 (9), 1798–1802.

Manley, B.J., Owen, L.S., Doyle, L.W., et al., 2013. High-flow nasal cannulae in very preterm infants after extubation. N. Engl. J. Med. 369 (15), 1425–1433. doi: 10.1056/NEJMoa1300071.

Marcus, R.J., van der Walt, J.H., Pettifer, R.J., 2002. Pulmonary volume recruitment restores pulmonary compliance and resistance in anaesthetized young children. Paediatr. Anaesth. 12, 579–584.

McCabe, S.M., Smeltzer, S.C., 1993. Comparison of tidal volumes obtained by one-handed and two-handed ventilation techniques. Am. J. Crit. Care 2, 467–473.

McCarren, B., Alison, J.A., Herbert, R.D., 2006. Vibration and its effect on the respiratory system. Aust. J. Physiother. 52 (1), 39–43.

McKelvie, S., 1998. Endotracheal suctioning. Nurs. Crit. Care 3, 244–248.

Meessen, N.E., van der Grinten, C.P., Luijendijk, S.C., et al., 1994. Continuous negative airway pressure increases tonic activity in diaphragm and intercostal muscles in humans. J. Appl. Physiol. 77 (3), 1256–1262.

Menkes, H.A., Traystman, R.J., 1977. Collateral ventilation. Am. Rev. Respir. Dis. 116, 287–309.

Miske, L.J., Hickey, E.M., Kolb, S.M., et al., 2004. Use of the mechanical in-exsufflator in pediatric patients with neuromuscular disease and impaired cough. Chest 105 (3), 741–747.

Mok, Q., Ross-Russell, R., Mulvey, D., et al., 1991. Phrenic nerve injury in infants and children undergoing cardiac surgery. Br. Heart J. 65 (5), 287–292.

Moore, M., Little, P., 2006. Humidified air inhalation for treating croup. Cochrane Database Syst. Rev. (3), Art. No: CD002870, doi: 10.1002/14651858.CD002870.pub2.

Morini, F., Goldman, A., Pierro, A., 2006. Extracorporeal membrane oxygenation in infants with congenital diaghragmatic hernia. Eur. J. Pediatr. Surg. 16, 385–391.

Morley, C.J., Davis, P.G., Doyle, L.W., et al., 2008. Nasal CPAP or intubation at birth for very preterm infants. N. Engl. J. Med. 358 (7), 700–708. doi: 10.1056/NEJMoa072788.

Nassar, N., Leoncini, E., Amar, E., Arteaga-Vazquez, J., et al., 2012. Prevalence of esophageal atresia among 18 international birth defects surveillance programs. Birth Defects Res. A. Clin Mol. Teratol. 94 (11), 893–899. doi: 10.1002/bdra.23067.

Ng, G.Y.T., da Silva, O., Ohlsson, A., 2001. Bronchodilation for the prevention and treatment of chronic lung disease in preterm infants. Cochrane Database Syst. Rev. (23), CD003214.

Nicholas, K.J., Dhouibe, M.O., Marchall, T.G., et al., 1999. Physiotherapy in patients with bronchiolitis. Physiotherapy 85 (12), 669–674.

Norwood, W.I., Jacobs, M.L., 1994. Hypoplastic left heart syndrome. In: Stark, J., De Leval, M. (Eds.), Surgery for Congenital Heart Defects, second ed. WB Saunders, Philadelphia, pp. 587–598.

Ntoumenopoulos, G., 2005. Indications for manual lung hyperinflation (MHI) in the mechanically ventilated patient with chronic obstructive pulmonary disease. Chron. Respir. Dis. 2 (4), 199–207.

Nuysink, J., 2009. Supporting early development of infants with identified positional plagiocephaly. Phys. Occup. Ther. Pediatr. 29 (3), 236–238.

O'Donnell, C.P., Kamlin, C.O., Davis, P.G., Morley, C.J., 2006. Endotracheal intubation attempts during neonatal resuscitation:

success rates, duration, and adverse effects. Pediatrics 117 (1), e16–e21. doi: 10.1542/peds.2005-0901.

Panitch, H.B., 2006. Airway clearance in children with neuromuscular weakness. Curr. Opin. Pediatr. 18 (3), 277–281.

Pearson, G.A., Grant, J., Field, D., et al., 1993. Extracorporeal life support in paediatrics. Arch. Dis. Child. 68 (1), 94–96.

Peek, G.J., et al., 2009. Efficacy and economic assessment of conventional ventilatory support versus extracorporeal membrane oxygenation for severe adult respiratory failure (CESAR): a multicentre randomised controlled trial. Lancet 374 (9698), 1351–1363.

Pelosi, P., Brazzi, L., Gattinoni, L., 2002. Prone position in acute respiratory distress syndrome. Eur. Respir. J. 20 (4), 1017–1028.

Perrotta, C., Ortiz, Z., Roque, M., 2005. Chest physiotherapy for acute bronchiolitis in paediatric patients between 0 and 24 months old. Cochrane Database Syst. Rev. (2), Art. No: CD004873, pub2.

Peters, M.J., Tasker, R.C., Kiff, K.M., et al., 1998. Acute hypoxemic respiratory failure in children: case mix and the utility of respiratory severity indices. Intensive Care Med. 24 (7), 699–705.

Pettignano, R., Fortenberry, J.D., Heard, M.L., et al., 2003. Primary use of the venovenous approach for extracorporeal membrane oxygenation in pediatric acute respiratory failure. Pediatr. Crit. Care Med. 4 (3), 291–298.

Prasad, S.A., Tasker, R.C., 1990. Guidelines for physiotherapy management of critically ill children with acutely raised intracranial pressure. Physiother. 76 (4), 248–250.

Prasad, S.A., Tasker, R.C., 1995. Neurological intensive care. In: Prasad, S.A., Hussey, J. (Eds.), Paediatric Respiratory Care. Chapman & Hall, London, pp. 142–149.

Raguckas, S.E., Vandenbussche, H.L., Jacobs, C., Klepser, M.E., 2007. Pertussis resurgence: diagnosis, treatment, prevention, and beyond. Pharmacotherapy 27 (1), 41–52.

Ramsay, S., 1995. The Birmingham experience. Lancet 345, 510.

Randolph, A.G., Meert, K.L., O'Neil, M.E., et al., 2003. Pediatric Acute Injury Sepsis Investigators Network. The feasibility of conducting clinical trials in infants and children with acute respiratory failure. Am. J. Respir. Crit. Care Med. 167 (10), 1334–1340.

Randolph, A.G., Wypij, D., Venkataraman, S.T., et al., 2002. Pediatric Acute Lung Injury and Sepsis Investigators (PALISI) Network. Effect of mechanical ventilator weaning protocols on respiratory outcomes in infants and children: a randomized controlled trial. J. Am. Med. Assoc. 288 (20), 2561–2568.

Razmus, I., Wilson, D., 2006. Current trends in the development of sedation/ analgesia scales for the pediatric critical care patient. Pediatr. Nurs. 32, 435–441.

Ridling, D.A., Martin, L.D., Bratton, S.L., 2003. Endotracheal suctioning with or without instillation of isotonic sodium chloride solution in critically ill children. Am. J. Crit. Care 12 (3), 212–219.

Roberton, N.R.C., 1996. Intensive care. In: Greenough, A., Roberton, N.R.C., Milner, A. (Eds.), Neonatal Respiratory Disorders. Arnold, London, pp. 174–195.

Roberts, D., Dalziel, S., 2006. Antenatal corticosteroids for accelerating fetal lung maturation for women at risk of preterm birth.

Cochrane Database Syst. Rev. (3), CD004454, doi: 10.1002/14651858.CD004454.pub2.

Rojas-Reyes, M.X., Morley, C.J., Soll, R., 2012. Prophylactic versus selective use of surfactant in preventing morbidity and mortality in preterm infants. Cochrane Database Syst. Rev. 3, CD000510, doi: 10.1002/14651858.CD000510.pub2.

Russell, K., Wiebe, N., Saenz, A., et al., 2004. Glucocorticoids for croup. Cochrane Database Syst. Rev. (1), Art. No: CD001955, doi: 10.1002/14651858.CD001955.pub2.

Ryan, R.M., 2006. A new look at bronchopulmonary dysplasia classification. J. Perinatol. 26, 207–209.

Saigal, S., Doyle, L.W., 2008. An overview of mortality and sequelae of preterm birth from infancy to adulthood. Lancet 371 (9608), 261–269. doi: 10.1016/S0140-6736(08)60136-1.

Salt, A., Noble-Jameson, G., Barnes, N.D., et al., 1992. Liver transplantation in 100 children: Cambridge and King's College Hospital series. Br. Med. J. 304, 416–421.

Savian, C., Paratz, J., Davies, A., 2006. Comparison of the effectiveness of manual and ventilator hyperinflation at different levels of positive end-expiratory pressure in artificially ventilated and intubated intensive care patients. Heart Lung 35 (5), 334–341.

Schmidt, B., Roberts, R., Davis, P., et al., 2006. Caffeine Therapy for Apnea of Prematurity. N. Engl. J. Med. 345, 2112–2121.

Schreuder, F.M., Jones, U.F., 2004. The effect of saline instillation on sputum yield and oxygen saturation measurement in adult intubated patients: single subject design. Physiotherapy 90, 109.

Schultz, C.M., DiGeronimo, R.J., Yoder, B.A., Congenital Diaphragmatic Hernia Study Group, 2007. Congenital diaphragmatic hernia: a simplified postnatal predictor of outcome. J. Pediatr. Surg. 42 (3), 510–516. doi: 10.1016/j.jpedsurg.2006.10.043.

Scottish Intercollegiate Guidelines Network, 2006. Bronchiolitis in Children: A National Clinical Guideline. Scottish Intercollegiate Guidelines Network, Edinburgh.

Shah, A.R., Kurth, C.D., Gwiazdowski, S.G., et al., 1992. Fluctuations in cerebral oxygenation and blood volume during endotracheal suctioning in premature infants. J. Pediatr. 120, 769–774.

Shannon, H., Stocks, J., Gregson, R.K., et al., 2015a. Clinical effects of specialist and on-call respiratory physiotherapy treatments in mechanically ventilated children: a randomised crossover trial. Physiotherapy 101 (4), 349–356. doi: 10.1016/j.physio.2014.12.004.

Shannon, H., Stocks, J., Gregson, R.K., et al., 2015b. Differences in delivery of respiratory treatments by on-call physiotherapists in mechanically ventilated children: a randomised crossover trial. Physiotherapy 101 (4), 357–363. doi: 10.1016/j.physio.2014.12.001.

Shorten, D.R., Byrne, P.J., Jones, R.L., 1991. Infant responses to saline instillations and endotracheal suctioning. J Obstet. Gynecol. Neonatal Nurs. 20, 464–469.

Singer, M., Vermaat, J., Hall, G., et al., 1994. Hemodynamic effects of manual hyperinflation in critically ill mechanically ventilated patients. Chest 106, 1182–1187.

Slee-Wijffels, F.Y.A.M., van der Vaart, K.R.M., Twisk, J.W.R., et al., 2005. High-frequency ventilation in children: a single-center experience of 53 cases. Critical Care 9 (3), R274–R279.

Slutsky, A.S., Ranieri, V.M., 2013. Ventilator-induced lung injury. N. Engl. J. Med. 369 (22), 2126–2136.

Smith, N.P., Jesudason, E.C., Featherstone, N.C., et al., 2005. Recent advances in congenital diaghragmatic hernia. Arch. Dis. Child. 90, 426–428.

Sole, M.L., Byers, J.F., Ludy, J.E., et al., 2003. A multisite survey of suctioning techniques and airway management practices. Am. J. Crit. Care 12 (3), 220–230.

Southall, D.P., Samuels, M.P., 1992. Reducing risks in the sudden infant death syndrome. Br. Med. J. 304, 260–265.

Stark, A.R., Carlo, W.A., Tyson, J.E., et al., 2001. Adverse effects of early dexamethasone in extremely-low-birth-weight infants. National Institute of Child Health and Human Development Neonatal Research Network. N. Engl. J. Med. 344 (2), 95–101. doi: 10.1056/NEJM200101113440203.

Stark, J., Gallivan, S., Lovegrove, J., et al., 2000. Mortality rates after surgery for congenital heart defects in children and surgeons' performance. Lancet 355 (9208), 1004–1007.

Stevens, T.P., Blennow, M., Soll, R.F., 2004. Early surfactant administration with brief ventilation vs selective surfactant and continued mechanical ventilation for preterm infants with or at risk for respiratory distress syndrome. Cochrane Database Syst. Rev. (3), Art. No.: CD003063, doi: 10.1002/14651858.CD003063.pub2.

Stiller, K., 2000. Physiotherapy in intensive care: towards an evidence-based practice. Chest 118, 1801–1813.

Stone, K.S., 1990. Ventilator versus manual resuscitation bag as the method for delivering hyperoxygenation before endotracheal suctioning. AACN Clin. Issues Crit. Care Nurs. 1, 289–299.

Stone, K.S., Turner, B., 1989. Endotracheal suctioning. Annu. Rev. Nurs. Res. 7, 27–49.

Stone, K.S., Talaganis, S.A., Preusser, B., Gonyon, D.S., 1991. Effect of lung hyperinflation and endotracheal suctioning on heart rate and rhythm in patients after coronary artery bypass graft surgery. Heart Lung 20, 443–450.

Sutton, P.P., Lopezvidriero, M.T., Pavia, D., et al., 1985. Assessment of percussion, vibratory-shaking and breathing exercises in chest physiotherapy. Eur. J. Respir. Dis. 66, 147–152.

Swaniker, F., Kolla, S., Moler, F., et al., 2000. Extracorporeal life support outcome for 128 pediatric patients with respiratory failure. J. Pediatr. Surg. 35, 197–202.

Sweeney, J.K., Heriza, C.B., Blanchard, Y., 2009. Neonatal physical therapy. Part I: clinical competencies and neonatal intensive care unit clinical training models. Pediatr. Phys. Ther. 21 (4), 296–307. doi: 10.1097/PEP.0b013e3181bf75ee.

Sweeney, J.K., Heriza, C.B., Blanchard, Y., Dusing, S.C., 2010. Neonatal physical therapy. Part II. Practice frameworks and evidence-based practice guidelines. Pediatr. Phys. Ther. 22 (1), 2–16. doi: 10.1097/PEP.0b013e3181cdba43.

Symington, A., Pinelli, J., 2009. Developmental care for promoting development and preventing morbidity in preterm infants. Cochrane Database Syst. Rev. (2), CD001814, doi: 10.1002/14651858.CD001814.

Tannenbaum, E., Prasad, S.A., Dinwiddie, R., Main, E., 2007. Chest physiotherapy during anaesthesia for children with cystic fibrosis: effects on respiratory function. Pediatr. Pulmonol. 42 (12), 1152–1158.

Tasker, R.C., 2000a. Gender differences and critical medical illness. Acta Paediatr. 89 (5), 621–623.

Tasker, R.C., 2000b. Neurological critical care. Curr. Opin. Pediatr. 12 (3), 222–226.

Tasker, R.C., 2001. Neurocritical care and traumatic brain injury. Indian J. Paediatr. 68, 257–266.

Tasker, R.C., Gordon, I., Kiff, K., 2000. Time course of severe respiratory syncytial virus infection in mechanically ventilated infants. Acta Paediatr. 89 (8), 938–941.

Tasker, R.C., Morris, K.P., Forsyth, R.J., et al., 2006. Severe head injury in children: emergency access to neurosurgery in the United Kingdom. Emerg. Med. J. 23 (7), 519–522.

Teasdale, G., Jennett, B., 1974. Assessment of coma and impaired consciousness: a practical scale. Lancet 2, 81–84.

Thoresen, M., Cavan, F., Whitelaw, A., 1988. Effect of tilting on oxygenation in newborn infants. Arch. Dis. Child. 63, 315–317.

Tingay, D.G., Copnell, B., Mills, J.F., et al., 2007. Effects of open endotracheal suction on lung volume in infants receiving HFOV. Intensive Care Med. 33 (4), 689–693.

Toelle, B.G., Marks, G.B., 2005. The ebb and flow of asthma. Thorax 60 (2), 87–88.

Torres, A., Serra-Batlles, J., Ros, E., et al., 1992. Pulmonary aspiration of gastric contents in patients receiving mechanical ventilation: the effect of body position. Ann. Intern. Med. 116 (7), 540–543.

Tudehope, D.I., Bagley, C., 1980. Techniques of physiotherapy in intubated babies with RDS. Aust. Paediatr. J. 16, 226–228.

UK Collaborative ECMO Trial Group, 1996. UK collaborative randomised trial of neonatal extracorporeal membrane oxygenation. Lancet 348, 75–81.

van der Schans, C.P., Postma, D.S., Koeter, G.H., Rubin, B.K., 1999. Physiotherapy and bronchial mucus transport. Eur. Respir. J. 13 (6), 1477–1486.

Vaughan, R.S., Menke, J.A., Giacoia, G.P., 1978. Pneumothorax: a complication of endotracheal suctioning. J. Pediatr. 92, 633–634.

Vianello, A., Corrado, A., Arcaro, G., et al., 2005. Mechanical insufflation-exsufflation improves outcomes for neuromuscular disease patients with respiratory tract infections. Am. J. Phys. Med. Rehabil. 84 (2), 83–88.

Victorino, J.A., Borges, J.B., Okamoto, V.N., et al., 2004. Imbalances in regional lung ventilation: a validation study on electrical impedance tomography. Am. J. Respir. Crit. Care Med. 169 (7), 777–778.

Vincon, C., 1999. Potential risks of chest physiotherapy in preterm infants. Journal of Pediatrics 135, 131–132.

Wanner, A., 1984. Does chest physical therapy move airway secretions? Am. Rev. Respir. Dis. 130, 701–702.

Watkins, S.J., Peters, M.J., Tasker, R.C., 2000. One hundred courses of high frequency oscillatory ventilation: what have we learned? Eur. J. Pediatr. 159 (1–2), 134.

Webb, M.S.C., Martin, J.A., Cartlidge, P.H.T., et al., 1985. Chest physiotherapy in acute bronchiolitis. Arch. Dis. Child. 6, 1078–1079.

Weiss, M., et al., 2009. Prospective randomized controlled multi-centre trial of cuffed or uncuffed endotracheal tubes in small children #. Br. J. Anaesth. 103 (6), 867–873.

Wells, D.A., Gillies, D., Fitzgerald, D.A., 2005. Positioning for acute respiratory distress in hospitalised infants and children. Cochrane Database Syst. Rev. (2), CD003645, doi: 10.1002/14651858. CD003645.pub2.

Wenstrom, K.D., Weiner, C.P., Hanson, J.W., 1991. A five-year statewide experience with congenital diaphragmatic hernia. Am. J. Obstet. Gynecol. 165, 838–842.

Weston, E.J., Pondo, T., Lewis, M.M., et al., 2011. The burden of invasive early-onset neonatal sepsis in the United States, 2005-2008. Pediatr. Infect. Dis. J. 30 (11), 937–941. doi: 10.1097/INF.0b013e318223bad2.

Willson, D.F., Thomas, N.J., Markovitz, B.P., et al., (Pediatric Acute Lung Injury Sepsis Investigators), 2005. Effect of exogenous surfactant (calfactant) in pediatric acute lung injury: a randomized controlled trial. J. Am. Med. Assoc. 293 (4), 470–476.

Wong, W.P., Paratz, J.D., Wilson, K., Burns, Y.R., 2003. Hemodynamic and ventilatory effects of manual respiratory physiotherapy techniques of chest clapping, vibration, and shaking in an animal model. J. Appl. Physiol. 95 (3), 991–998.

Wood, B., 1987. Infant ribs: generalized periosteal reaction resulting from vibrator chest physiotherapy. Radiology 162, 811–812.

Wood, C.J., 1998. Endotracheal suctioning: a literature review. Intensive Crit. Care Nurs. 14, 124–136.

Yoder, B.A., Stoddard, R.A., Li, M., et al., 2013. Heated, humidified high-flow nasal cannula versus nasal CPAP for respiratory support in neonates. Pediatrics 131 (5), e1482–e1490. doi: 10.1542/peds.2012-2742.

Zahka, K.G., Patel, C.R., 2002. Congenital defects. In: Fanaroff, A., Martin, R.J. (Eds.), Neonatal–Perinatal Medicine: Diseases of the Fetus and Infant, seventh ed. Mosby, St Louis.

Zivanovic, S., et al., 2014. Late outcomes of a randomized trial of high-frequency oscillation in neonates. N. Engl. J. Med. 370, 1121–1130.

11

UPPER ABDOMINAL AND CARDIOTHORACIC SURGERY FOR ADULTS

DOA EL-ANSARY ■ JULIE C REEVE ■ LINDA DENEHY

with contributions from

SULAKSHANA BALACHANDRAN ■ MICHELLE MULLIGAN

CHAPTER OUTLINE

INTRODUCTION 513

PREOPERATIVE PHYSIOTHERAPY AND PREHABILITATION 514

THE SURGICAL PROCESS 515
General Anaesthesia 515
Management of Acute Postoperative Pain 516
Pharmacological Management of Postoperative Pain 516
Measurement of Pain 520
Effects of the Surgical Process on Respiratory Function 521

TYPES OF SURGERY 526
Abdominal Surgery 526
Bariatric Surgery 527

Evidence in Abdominal Surgery 532
Thoracic Surgery 532
Pneumothorax 539
Underwater Seal Drainage (UWSD) 543
Cardiac Surgery 545
Types of Surgery 546

SPECIAL CONSIDERATIONS FOLLOWING SURGERY 553

APPENDIX 555

REFERENCES 570

INTRODUCTION

Perioperative physiotherapy aims to prevent or minimize the adverse physiological changes associated with major surgical procedures and to facilitate a return to optimal function and a resumption of role within the community. In patients undergoing surgery, physiotherapy has played a significant role in minimizing the adverse effects of anaesthesia and the surgical process on the cardiorespiratory and neuromuscular systems for more than 50 years. The role of the physiotherapist in such patients has been investigated in clinical trials since 1947 and, for the most part, this evidence has advocated pre- and postoperative physiotherapy for all patients having major surgery, in order to reduce the incidence of postoperative pulmonary complications (PPCs) and thereby reduce patient morbidity and prolonged hospital admission (Denehy & Browning 2007).

Recent advances in the surgical process and pain management, the evolution of new forms of postoperative physiotherapy support and a reduction in the incidence of clinically significant PPCs have provided the stimulus for a re-evaluation of physiotherapy intervention following surgery. The incidence of PPCs has shown a gradual reduction over time in these patient populations. In part this is due to a change in the method for the measurement of PPCs, and because of improvements in anaesthetic and surgical access routes. More frequent use of epidural and

513

patient-controlled analgesic techniques has also had a profound impact on the incidence of PPCs (Liu et al 2007). The introduction of 'fast track' postoperative management and minimally invasive abdominal, thoracic and cardiac surgery has also impacted the physiotherapy management in these patient populations, and research in these areas is continuing to evolve. Despite these advances, there has been a concomitant increase in the age of patients undergoing surgery and an increase in the prevalence of comorbidities that have prompted physicians to evaluate such factors as frailty to assess whether surgery may lead to optimal patient outcomes. This presents ongoing challenges to healthcare professionals working in this area. Additionally, there is emerging evidence that prehabilitation may impact the incidence of PPCs, length of hospital stay and functional recovery. Further, while the focus of perioperative care has been the prevention of respiratory complications, current evidence for interventions that target postoperative pain, exercise capacity and functional recovery is growing.

This chapter outlines the effects of the surgical process, highlights current management of the surgical patient and considers the evidence for physiotherapy interventions in patients' undergoing abdominal and cardiothoracic surgery.

PREOPERATIVE PHYSIOTHERAPY AND PREHABILITATION

Traditionally the preoperative role of the physiotherapist has been based on assessment of risk (of developing a postoperative complication), education and advice regarding postoperative recovery. With the increase in same day surgical admissions and larger numbers of patients undergoing minimally invasive surgery, it is becoming difficult for physiotherapists to see patients preoperatively and the necessity for these interventions is unclear. Multidisciplinary preadmission clinics are becoming increasingly common and such clinics enable physiotherapists to identify and assess high-risk patients, and institute preoperative interventions aimed at reducing the risk of postoperative complications where necessary. It is important during the preoperative assessment to consider factors which have the potential to effect the patient's recovery and discharge plan postoperatively. These

include, patient age, comorbidities, general well-being, cognition, social support, falls history and risk and frailty. In addition, a patient's cultural background and language barriers should also be considered.

Preoperative interventions may consist of education and advice regarding postoperative care or may include the initiation of a preoperative exercise programme designed to improve preoperative fitness, increase respiratory muscle strength and decrease postoperative respiratory and musculoskeletal morbidity.

Education and advice in the preoperative period usually comprise an explanation of the role of the physiotherapist, augmenting information from other disciplines regarding the surgical procedure and likely postoperative management and progression, plus stressing the importance of adequate pain relief to ensure optimal postoperative recovery. The physiotherapist is especially likely to focus on the impact of anaesthesia, pain and surgery on the respiratory and cardiovascular systems and the associated importance of early respiratory care, upright positioning and ambulation.

Prehabilitation is a relatively new concept in surgical care and refers to strategies implemented prior to a planned intervention that aim to improve a patient's capacity to withstand anticipated stressors, improve postoperative outcomes, and reduce postoperative risk (Alkarmi et al 2010; Mayo et al 2011; Topp et al 2010). Prehabilitation may comprise whole body exercise training that incorporates strength and cardiovascular endurance training, breathing exercises, education, diet optimisation, and inspiratory muscle training (IMT) or any combination thereof. Prehabilitation programmes investigated in the literature vary widely in respect to frequency, intensity, duration, location and type of exercise. Thus, to date, the evidence supporting prehabilitation continues to accumulate but the optimum prehabilitation programme remains unclear. Commonly, prehabilitation is undertaken daily for between 2 and 4 weeks preoperatively, 3–7 days per week, and comprises aerobic and/or resistance work. Intensity varies throughout the studies but mostly commences at close to 60–65% of peak oxygen uptake (VO_{2peak}), at 30% of maximal inspiratory pressure (MIP) and at 60% of one repetition maximum (1RM).

Several systematic reviews have evaluated the effectiveness of prehabilitation interventions in reducing postoperative complications (Lemanu et al 2013; Olsen & Anzén 2012; Singh et al 2013; Valkenet et al 2011; Mans et al 2015). The studies included in these reviews enrolled patients across the spectrum of major surgery including upper abdominal, thoracic and cardiac surgery. Two of these studies included meta-analyses (Valkenet et al 2010, Mans et al 2015). Valkenet et al (2011) meta-analysed the effect of preoperative interventions, which included IMT, on PPCs in patients undergoing major cavity or orthopaedic surgery whereas Mans et al (2015) investigated the effect of preoperative IMT alone on postoperative outcomes. Both studies found that in patients undergoing abdominal or cardiac surgery, preoperative IMT and/or exercise training significantly reduced the risk of PPCs but not hospital length of stay (LOS). A further systematic review with meta-analysis of 17 trials by (Snowdon et al 2014) that evaluated the impact of preoperative intervention including education, IMT, exercise training or relaxation in people undergoing cardiac surgery reported significantly reduced times to extubation and relative risk of developing PPC.

Other systematic reviews also concluded that there were improvements in physiological outcomes, such as aerobic and functional capacity (Lemanu et al 2013; Olsen & Anzén 2012; Singh et al 2013).

Oesophagectomy is widely regarded as high-risk surgery with high rates of postoperative mortality and incidence of postoperative complications (Avendano et al 2001; Bailey et al 2003; Ferguson & Durkin 2002). Additionally, patients who develop a PPC have been shown to engage in less physical activity than those who do not (Feeney et al 2011). In patients undergoing oesophagectomy, two recent non-randomized studies investigated the effectiveness of prehabilitation and showed contrasting findings in respect of effectiveness on PPC and LOS (Dettling et al 2012; Inoue et al 2013). Further studies in this high-risk group are required.

Overall, prehabilitation confers benefit for some higher risk patients but, to date, the optimal type, duration and frequency of prehabilitation interventions remains unclear. Neither have the subgroups that would benefit most from prehabilitation been clearly identified. Adherence to prehabilitation programmes and the feasibility of training in the short time frame between diagnosis and surgery may limit the effectiveness of prehabilitation (Valkenet et al 2011).

THE SURGICAL PROCESS
General Anaesthesia
General anaesthesia (GA) provides the patient with unconsciousness, amnesia and analgesia and is the only type of anaesthesia suitable for major abdominal and thoracic surgery. Constant monitoring of the patient's vital signs allow these to be kept within physiological limits. GA can be divided into three different stages: induction, maintenance and reversal or emergence. Before induction an intravenous (IV) administration of a combination of an anxiolytic drug with amnesic power such as midazolam, together with a narcotic such as fentanyl, is often given. The narcotic given preoperatively helps to prevent nerve impulses, arising from intraoperative events, from sensitizing central neuronal structures and is called 'pre-emptive analgesia' (Katz 1993). There is some evidence that analgesia given before the painful stimulus reduces subsequent pain, but this remains controversial.

Induction of Anaesthesia
Anaesthesia is usually achieved by the IV administration of a short-acting, coma-inducing drug such as propofol or thiopental. Intubation may be performed if the surgery requires administration of muscle relaxants to cause paralysis (as is the case in major thoracic and abdominal surgical). Maintenance of anaesthesia is achieved using inhalational agents such as sevoflurane with nitrous oxide or air with a suitably high inspired oxygen concentration (FiO_2). Total IV anaesthesia using propofol may be used for maintenance and instead of an inhalation agent. During maintenance, muscle relaxants are often used to aid the surgical procedure and narcotics given for both intraoperative and postoperative analgesia. The process of reversal begins well before the surgeon has finished. Inspired anaesthetic concentrations are scaled back and drugs to reverse paralysis such as neostigmine or suggammadex are given. Analgesia is provided using narcotics or regional analgesia and extubation occurs once the patient is haemodynamically stable, can breath with an adequate tidal volume, protect their airway (gag reflex) and are conscious (Euliano & Gravenstein 2004).

Induction of anaesthesia causes unavoidable changes in lung mechanics, lung defences and gas exchange. The most profound effect on the lung of GA is the reduction in lung volumes, particularly functional residual capacity (FRC). These are discussed in a later section of this chapter.

Management of Acute Postoperative Pain

Adequate postoperative pain control is vital to: (1) minimize unwanted secondary physiological (sympathetic nervous system) effects, e.g. tachycardia or hypertension, which may impair haemodynamics; (2) minimize secondary respiratory dysfunction, by allowing increased tidal volumes and effective coughing and (3) allow patients to commence rehabilitation (Lemmer, Jr and Vlahakes 2010b). Inadequate analgesia may delay discharge from hospital, cause sleep disturbances and limit early mobilization.

Acute pain is defined as pain of recent onset and probable limited duration with an identifiable temporal and causal relationship to injury or disease. Chronic pain commonly exists beyond the time of healing of an injury and frequently there may not be any clearly identifiable cause (Ready & Edwards 1992). Increasingly it is recognized that acute and chronic pain may represent a continuum and in an individual patient, biological, psychological, environmental and social factors will all interact.

The complex neural processes underlying the encoding and processing of noxious stimuli are defined as 'nociception' and the perception and subjective experience is 'pain', which is multifactorial and subject to different psychological and environmental factors in every individual.

Nociception is complex and many sites have been identified from peripheral local tissue damage via the spinal cord to the cortex of the brain. Pharmacological intervention can occur at multiple sites along this pathway, e.g. non-steroidal anti-inflammatory drugs (NSAIDs) have peripheral action, epidurals are at the spinal cord level and opioids function to alter the central perception of pain.

Several factors may modify postoperative pain: these include the site and duration of surgery and the extent of the incision and surgical trauma, the physiological and psychological aspects of the patient and past pain experience. Postoperative pain is often accompanied by changes in autonomic activity that are sympathetically mediated and include hypertension, tachycardia, sweating and decreased gut motility (National Health and Medical Research Council 2005).

Pharmacological Management of Postoperative Pain

Many different methods of pain relief are available, using several different routes of administration. Opiates and derivatives (such as morphine, fentanyl, oxycodone) make up a large proportion of these drugs and morphine arguably remains the benchmark drug (Barrat 1997). Table 11-1 gives a summary of common routes of administration of drugs. In Table 11-2, a list of the common drugs used for postoperative pain is shown, together with their potential side effects. Drugs that have different sites of action are often used together, working synergistically to treat pain, while also minimizing harmful side effects; using paracetamol and NSAIDs can result in a 20–30% decrease in the opioid dose, thus decreasing the potential for dangerous respiratory depression.

Opioids are drugs that bind with specific opioid receptors. They mimic endogenous peptide transmitters involved in pain modulation and act principally within the central nervous system. NSAIDs such as indomethacin are also used in management of acute postoperative pain and can act as opioid sparing agents. They decrease production of prostaglandins that sensitize nociceptor nerve endings to inflammatory mediators and also have an antipyretic effect (reduce fever). Local anaesthetic agents such as bupivacaine and ropivacaine, block the initiation and propagation of action potentials by blocking sodium channels. They are used to produce nerve root blocks and to depress action potentials in sensory neurons, thereby reducing pain (NHMRC 2005). The use of multimodality analgesia rather than single analgesic administration is standard. Pain management teams led by specialists in anaesthetics and pain management and supported by expert nurses improve care.

Opiates have significant respiratory depression effects (Sabanathan et al 1999) and they are only partially effective in relieving pain. Richardson and Sabanathan (1997) report that since opioids may only relieve pain transmitted by C fibres, where opioid receptors exist, the sharp pain transmitted by A fibres still exists. More recently, use of local anaesthetics (bupivacaine, ropivacaine) by the epidural route has

TABLE 11-1
Common Routes of Drug Administration for Postoperative Analgesia

Route	Description	Drug Examples
Oral	Slow acting, drug is absorbed from the small intestine and therefore needs a working gut for absorption (often not the case immediately after major surgery).	Paracetamol NSAIDs Codeine
IM	Maximum blood concentrations in 15–60 minutes. Absorption variable. Given 3–4 hourly. May only provide adequate analgesia for 35% of the 4 hours. May be painful. Rarely used.	Morphine Pethidine Tramadol
SC	Maximum blood concentration 15–60 minutes. Absorption less variable. Less painful.	Morphine Pethidine
IV (infusion)	IV route provides a more rapid onset of action. Lower dose continuous infusion eliminates the peaks and troughs of IM administration. Need a loading bolus to reach analgesic blood concentration. Risk of respiratory depression is high with continuous IV opioids.	Morphine Fentanyl Ketamine Oxycodone
PCA	Self-administration of small doses of IV analgesics by patients when they feel pain. Microprocessor pumps triggered by depressing a button. Pump is programmed to deliver a pre-set bolus dose but has a minimum period between doses called 'lock-out interval'. Patients receive no drug if button is depressed during lock-out. Advantages: Patient autonomy, elimination of delay of delivery of pain relief, less total narcotic dose. Disadvantages: Some patients cannot use, improper programming.	Morphine Fentanyl Oxycodone
Epidural	Fine-bore catheter is inserted into the thoracic or lumbar epidural space (see Fig. 11-2) by the anaesthetist at time of operation. Insertion site is sealed with a dressing, and catheter is taped along its length up the patients back and over one shoulder. A pump is used to continuously infuse drugs via a bacterial filter. Nerves are blocked as they course from the spinal cord. Epidural can also be administered using a patient-controlled system (PCEA). The PCEA results in lower cumulative doses compared with continuous epidural infusions. Side effects: Hypotension, respiratory depression, total spinal block, causes motor and sensory block – patient unable to lift or feel legs. Block may be positional, nausea/vomiting, urinary retention, headache, neck stiffness.	Fentanyl Bupivacaine Ropivacaine Morphine Adjuvants (such as clonidine)
Peripheral blocks	Have the advantage of less central side effects such as drowsiness. Intercostal nerve blocks: Injection of local anaesthetic into main nerve supplying operative area or incision. Used for patients whose incisions are limited to thoracic dermatomes and are effective for incisional but not visceral pain. Intrapleural analgesia: Catheter is placed in the interpleural space and local anaesthetic is administered to produce unilateral pain relief as it spreads through parietal pleura. Best for surgery with intact pleura. Not commonly used.	Bupivacaine Ropivacaine Lignocaine

IM, Intramuscular; *IV*, intravenous; *NSAIDs*, non-steroidal anti-inflammatory drugs; *PCA*, patient-controlled analgesia; *PCEA*, patient-controlled epidural analgesia; *SC*, subcutaneous.

gained more favour in postoperative pain management, often used in combination with epidural opioids. The introduction of these multimodal methods has also seen an increase in the use of NSAIDs such as indomethacin. These are used as opioid sparing agents, but have also been shown to improve analgesia by a reduction in inflammation and stress inhibition (Richardson & Sabanathan 1997). There is level 1 evidence that oral administration of NSAIDs is as effective as IV (National Health and Medical Research

TABLE 11-2
Information About Commonly Used Analgesic Drugs

Drug	Dosage	Route of Administration	Analgesic Effect	Complications/Side Effects
Morphine Natural agonist opioid	0.1 mg/kg IM Weight dependent Also adjusted for age and tolerance	IM/SC: 0.1 mg/kg (may vary) Oral dose: 2–3 times IM dose IV: 1–2 mg bolus, 1–3 mg/hour as infusion Infusion delivers more constant pain relief	Peak effect 3–40 min Lasts 3–4 hours	Respiratory depression, nausea, vomiting, sedation, hypotension, pinpoint pupils, decreased cough reflex, decreased sensitivity to hypercapnia, hypoxaemia, renal excretion so potential for prolonged action and respiratory depression in renal impairment
Pethidine Synthetic agonist opioid	Mean range 1 mg/kg IM	IV: 20 mg bolus, 10–40 mg/hour infusion	Onset 10 min, lasts 2–4 hours, peak 20–30 min	As for all opioids. Toxic metabolite, norpethidine, which can accumulate, especially with renal impairment and cause grand mal seizures
Fentanyl Synthetic opioid agonist, structurally related to pethidine	20–30 μg IV boluses for PCA	Often used in epidurals May be administered transdermally for chronic pain as they take up to 12 hours to stop working once removed (e.g. cancer pain)	30 second onset, lasts 30–60 min Half-life 3 hours	Reported decreased nausea and hypotension compared with morphine/pethidine Suitable choice in renal failure Transdermal patches are not suitable for acute pain
Codeine Low-efficacy opioid (action is by conversion to morphine)	30–60 mg oral, SC, IM	500 mg paracetamol + 8 mg codeine phosphate (Panadeine) Adults: 1–2 tabs, 3–4 hourly PRN (maximum 8/day) or 500 mg paracetamol + 30 mg codeine (Panadeine Forte) Adults: 2 tabs, 4 hourly (maximum 8/day)	Most actions ⅙th those of morphine	Constipation Large doses have an excitatory effect compared with morphine 8–10% of Caucasian population do not metabolize codeine to morphine (therefore it will have no pain relief), while 5% are ultrafast metabolizers Prone to respiratory depression
Oxycodone A potent opioid agonist	Analgesic Oral 5–10 mg, 2–4 hourly Suppository 30 mg, 6–8 hourly	Oral (OxyContin: a slow release preparation, Endone) Suppository (Proladone)	Probably most effective opioid for gastrointestinal pain	As for morphine
Tramadol Synthetic opioid Has effect at μ-receptor as well as noradrenergic and serotonergic pathways ⅟₁₀th efficacy of morphine	50–100 mg, 4–6 hourly (maximum 600 mg/day)	Oral: immediate release or slow release (for chronic or persistent pain) and IV	1 hour (approximately) with peak effect 1–3 hours Half-life 4–6 hours	Less respiratory depression but nausea and dizziness **Precautions:** Renal and hepatic impairment, raised ICP **Drug interactions:** Can precipitate a serotonergic crisis in patients on serotonin antidepressants

TABLE 11-2
Information About Commonly Used Analgesic Drugs *(Continued)*

Drug	Dosage	Route of Administration	Analgesic Effect	Complications/Side Effects
NSAIDs Non-steroidal anti-inflammatory drugs	e.g. Indomethacin (Indocid) 50–200 mg daily	Suppository (100 mg) Oral (25 mg)	2–4 hours for full absorption (faster PR) Half-life 4.5 hours	GI ulcers/bleeding, tinnitus, oedema, dizziness, headache, rash, blurred vision, oedema Can have adverse renal effects especially if pre-existing renal dysfunction **Contraindicated if active GI bleed or ulcer**
Bupivacaine Local anaesthetic	Bupivacaine hydrochloride (maximum 2 mg/kg)	Epidural infusion Local blocks (e.g. intercostal block)	Anaesthetic agent	CNS, cardiovascular, respiratory and GI disturbances
Ketamine General anaesthetic and analgesic	Ketamine hydrochloride	IV or IM	Anaesthetic agent in large doses Analgesic in low doses Useful for short procedures and the prevention of chronic pain	Hypertension, arrhythmia, respiratory depression with rapid doses, psychosis
Paracetamol	1 g in 4–6 hours (maximum of 4 g in 24 hours)	Oral, suppository, IV	Analgesic	Liver toxicity in very high doses Inadequate alone for postoperative pain but can decrease opioid use by 30% when used regularly

CNS, central nervous system; *GI*, gastrointestinal; *ICP*, intracranial pressure; *IM*, intramuscular; *IV*, intravenous; *PCA*, patient-controlled analgesia; *PR*, per rectal; *PRN*, as necessary; *SC*, subcutaneous.

Council 2005). Oral paracetamol may also be added to these regimens. Multimodal analgesia has been developed in response to the commonly associated side effects of monotherapy, namely nausea, vomiting, paralytic ileus and respiratory depression in the case of opioids and urinary retention and motor block and hypotension in the case of local anaesthetic agents. Multimodal analgesia was also developed to allow early postoperative ambulation and enteral feeding, which minimize the respiratory and gut complications associated with use of opioids, leading to earlier patient discharge from hospital. The drugs are used in smaller doses than if used separately and provide effective pain relief as a result of their synergistic actions (Peeters-Asdourian & Gupta 1999).

The most common methods for pain control following abdominal surgery are patient-controlled analgesia (PCA) with IV opioids (Fig. 11-1) or continuous epidural analgesia delivering a combination of local anaesthetic and opioids (Fig. 11-2). In a recent systematic review it was concluded that continuous epidural analgesia is superior to PCA in relieving postoperative pain for up to 72 hours in patients undergoing intra-abdominal surgery. Similarly a large review of analgesia reports that all techniques of epidural analgesia provide better postoperative pain relief compared with parenteral opioid administration (NHMRC 2005). However, PCA remains a common method of analgesic delivery, as patients often prefer it (Werawatganon & Charuluxanun 2005). Continuous IV infusion may be associated with increased risk of respiratory depression compared with bolus IV administration and evidence for improved pain relief with continuous administration is lacking (NHMRC 2005).

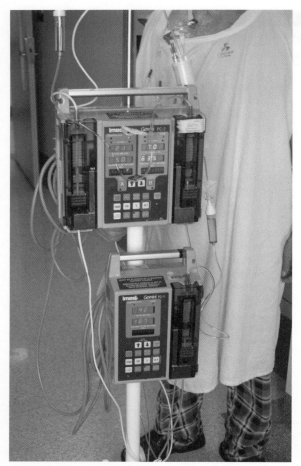

FIGURE 11-1 ■ A microprocessor pump (IMED) for delivery of patient-controlled analgesia (PCA).

Non-pharmacological methods for managing postoperative pain are generally perceived to be adjuncts to pharmacological methods, but there is growing evidence for the value of their contribution (National Health and Medical Research Council 2005). Education including providing procedural information about treatment (such as provided by physiotherapists preoperatively), combined with sensory information describing the sensory experiences a patient may expect and information regarding coping strategies, may be effective in reducing negative affect and pain medication use and in improving clinical recovery after surgery (National Health and Medical Research

Council 2005). Preoperative education may encourage a more positive attitude towards pain relief, although there is no evidence that preoperative education about pain has any effect on postoperative pain after cardiac surgery (National Health and Medical Research Council 2005). Implementation of an acute pain management service may also improve pain relief. Positioning and early postoperative mobilization, are also suggested to control postoperative pain (Sturgess et al 2014).

Measurement of Pain

Pain is difficult to measure, as it is a purely individual and sensory experience (Dodson 1985). The measurement of pain is often necessary to assess the results of an intervention or to measure intensity of pain, such as postoperative pain. Regular measurement of pain leads to improved acute pain management. Most measures of pain are based upon self-report but can provide sensitive and consistent results if performed properly (NHMRC 2005).

Several different instruments may be used to measure pain, these include:

- numerical rating scales (NRSs)
- verbal descriptor scales (VDSs)
- pain questionnaires (e.g. McGill)
- visual analogue scales (VASs).

Except for the McGill pain questionnaire, these methods only measure intensity of pain in absolute terms or changes in pain intensity. Verbal scales may use words that have different meanings for different people, such as 'mild', 'moderate' or 'severe' pain. These categorical scales are quick and simple but less sensitive than NRSs such as the VAS (National Health and Medical Research Council 2005). The McGill questionnaire uses 20 groups of two to six words and the patient is asked which word in each group best describes their pain. While this offers more valid information than a VDS, it is very time consuming and it not used extensively for the measurement of acute postoperative pain. Verbal rating scales are commonly used in clinical practice and use of the VAS is the most commonly used method. VASs usually consist of a straight line, 10 cm long, the extremes of which are taken to represent the limits of the subjective experience being measured. In the case of pain measurement,

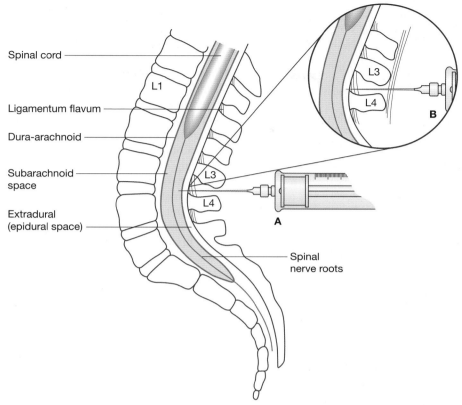

FIGURE 11-2 ■ Spinal and epidural anaesthesia. **(A)** Position of needle in subarachnoid space for spinal anaesthesia. **(B)** Position of needle in epidural space for epidural anaesthesia/analgesia.

one end of the line may be defined as 'no pain' and the other as 'severe pain' or 'worst possible pain'. The individual is asked to place a mark on the line corresponding to the severity of their pain. The distance from the mark to the end of the scale is taken to represent pain severity. The most common way to use a VAS in the study of postoperative pain is to ask the patient to score the pain they are experiencing at the time of completion of the VAS. VASs may also be used to obtain a pain score that reflects pain or pain relief over the preceding 24 hours. Commonly, physiotherapists ask patients to rate their pain on activity in the postoperative period to provide more meaningful information. The VAS has been shown to be a linear scale for patients with postoperative pain of mild to moderate intensity. Therefore results are equally distributed across the scale so that the difference between each

number on the scale is equal. It is reported that values greater than 70 mm are indicative of severe pain, while values between 45 and 74 mm represent moderate pain and those between 5 and 44 mm mild pain (National Health and Medical Research Council 2005). Box 11-1 provides the key points for physiotherapists in analgesia management.

Effects of the Surgical Process on Respiratory Function

The intra- and postoperative periods are frequently associated with alterations in pulmonary function (Craig 1981). Furthermore, altered physiological function of the respiratory system is an expected finding, especially after upper abdominal and thoracic surgery (Ford et al 1993). The combined effects of the GA, postoperative pain, recumbency, immobility and

BOX 11-1

PHYSIOTHERAPY KEY POINTS WITH REGARD TO ANALGESIA

■ Always assess the adequacy of pain relief before treatment.
■ Always note if the patient has pinpoint pupils and is drowsy.
■ Always check vital signs, particularly respiratory rate and blood pressure, as hypotension is a common side effect of pain management. Most important in position changes.
■ If a patient has had a spinal block or epidural, **always** assess motor and sensory function of the lower limbs, especially before upright mobilization.
■ Ask the patient if they need to use their PCA or PCEA before a physiotherapy treatment session or ask about a bolus dose of analgesia before treatment.
■ Always liaise with medical and nursing staff before treating the patient and know the local guidelines for mobilizing patients with an epidural in situ.

PCA, Patient-controlled analgesia; *PCEA*, patient-controlled epidural analgesia.

administration of drugs after surgery lead to several respiratory abnormalities.

Lung Volumes

The characteristic abnormality of respiratory mechanics following major surgery is a restrictive ventilatory defect manifest by changes in vital capacity (VC) and FRC (Wahba 1991). The VC can reduce to 40% of preoperative values, while the FRC may gradually reduce to be 70% of preoperative value at 24 hours postoperatively. These changes may persist for 5–10 days following surgery (Craig 1981). The timing of greatest reduction in FRC, while varying between studies, is generally on the first or second postoperative day. In morbidly and even mildly obese patients there is a significant reduction in FRC compared with patients within the ideal weight range (Jenkins & Moxham 1991). Although most other lung volumes also reduce following major surgery, it is thought that the reductions in FRC represent the most clinically important changes because of the functional consequences.

Functional Residual Capacity and Closing Capacity

An understanding of the relationship between FRC and closing capacity (CC) and the means by which

physical interventions may impact these is important in the early postoperative period, as they may have a profound outcome on postoperative recovery. FRC is the volume of air left in the lungs at the end of a quiet (passive) expiration. The FRC is linearly related to height and is 10% less in females for the same body height (Nunn 1993). The FRC is affected by gravity and therefore body position; it is highest in standing and reduces with recumbency (Fig. 11-3). In supine the abdominal contents push the diaphragm cephalad, reducing intrathoracic volume and FRC; in normal individuals supine positioning reduces the FRC by approximately 500–1000 mL (Macnaughton 1995). Postoperatively, compared with the supine position, sitting and standing improves postoperative pulmonary function including arterial blood gases (ABGs), FRC, arterial oxygen saturation (SaO_2) and spirometric values (Nielson et al 2003) Anaesthesia, surgery and recumbency reduce FRC with mechanical disruption of the thorax and abdomen, absence of spontaneous sighs, shallow breathing and pain and inhibition of diaphragmatic function being major contributors following upper abdominal surgery (UAS) (Wahba 1991). Abdominal distension, the presence of a nasogastric tube and the use of analgesics to control postoperative pain may also further impact ventilatory function (Nelson et al 2007, Smetana 2009).

CC is defined as the lung volume at which dependent airways begin to close, or cease to ventilate (Macnaughton 1995). The small airways (less than 1.0 mm diameter) in the periphery of the lung are not supported by cartilage and are therefore influenced by transmitted pleural pressures. Normally the transpulmonary pressure or distending pressure is less than atmospheric, producing a positive pressure, which distends the lungs. Breathing at lower lung volumes produces a higher pressure in gravity-dependent lung regions producing a negative distending pressure and causing small airways to narrow or close, resulting in reduced ventilation. The relationship between FRC and CC is an important determinant of dependent airway closure (Fig. 11-4). Normally FRC exceeds CC; hence small airways remain open at the end of quiet expiration. However, if the relationship between FRC and CC alters with FRC falling below CC or CC rising above FRC, then dependent lung regions hypoventilate, potentially resulting in ventilation–perfusion

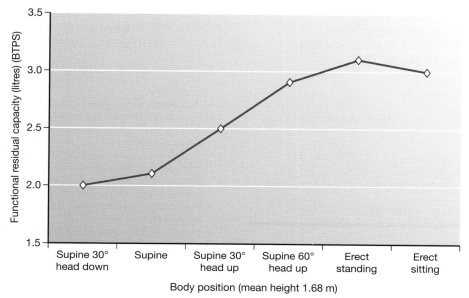

FIGURE 11-3 ▪ Functional residual capacity (FRC) in different body positions. BTPS, Body Temperature, ambient Pressure, Saturated. *(Adapted from Nunn 1993 p 55 with permission from Butterworth-Heinemann, Oxford.)*

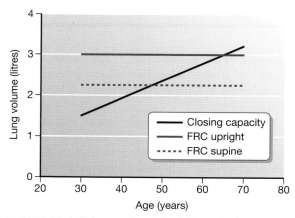

FIGURE 11-4 ▪ Lung volumes in different body positions and age groups. FRC, Functional residual capacity. *(Adapted from Nunn 1993 p 56 with permission from Butterworth-Heinemann, Oxford.)*

$\dot{V}/\dot{Q}$ mismatch and hypoxaemia. Such changes may account for the regional changes in ventilation that occur perioperatively and lead to reduced compliance, altered $\dot{V}/\dot{Q}$, arterial hypoxaemia and absorption atelectasis. Postoperative hypoxaemia and atelectasis are seen as inevitable consequences of major surgery, are usually subclinical and worst on the first and second postoperative days. The relationship between FRC and CC explains some of these alterations, and to counteract this supplemental oxygen, early upright positioning and mobilization are routinely administered postoperatively (Craig 1981; Fairshter & Williams 1987).

Mucociliary Clearance

Mucociliary clearance is a major function of the airway epithelium. This important function depends both on the biochemical properties of the airway mucus and on the activity of the cilia (Kim 1997). Anaesthesia, intubation, mechanical ventilation–reduced lung volumes and reduced cough effectiveness perioperatively present a significant insult to the mucociliary escalator (Box 11-2).

Respiratory Muscle Function

Diaphragmatic excursion has been shown in the research literature to be reduced following abdominal and thoracic surgery. Postoperative pain, the associated reduction in VC, a pattern of ventilation that is predominantly rib cage rather than abdominal movement, incisions and postoperative hypoxaemia may all

<table>
<tr><td>

BOX 11-2
FACTORS PROMOTING POSTOPERATIVE MUCOCILIARY DYSFUNCTION

- Anaesthetic agents
- Endotracheal intubation
- Pain medication
- Higher inspired oxygen concentrations and airway humidification
- Atelectasis
- Reduced lung volumes
- Reduced cough efficiency
- Increased viscosity of secretions

(Adapted from Denehy and van de Leur 2004)

</td><td>

BOX 11-3
KEY POINTS IN THE SURGICAL PROCESS

- Functional residual capacity (FRC) is reduced perioperatively as a result of anaesthesia, surgery and recumbency.
- FRC is increased in sitting and standing positions.
- The altered relationship between FRC and closing capacity is an important determinant of dependent airway collapse.
- Ventilation/perfusion $(\dot{V}/\dot{Q})$ mismatch and arterial hypoxaemia commonly occur after major surgery, although increases in carbon dioxide (CO_2) are rare unless patients are narcotized.
- Mucociliary clearance and cough effectiveness are reduced after surgery.
- Changes in pulmonary function after surgery generally resolve spontaneously with time from surgery.
- Clinically relevant postoperative pulmonary complications (PPCs) may develop in a subset of patients having major surgery.
- A combination of clinical signs and symptoms is used to diagnose a PPC.
- Assessment of risk factors for developing a PPC is important for the physiotherapist, as it allows prioritized respiratory care for high-risk patients.

</td></tr>
</table>

contribute to diaphragm dysfunction. This reduction in respiratory muscle function may last up to 1 week postoperatively. Reflex inhibition of the phrenic nerve may occur after UAS, but research findings are inconsistent. Phrenic nerve neuropraxia has been widely reported after cardiac surgery. The breathing pattern observed after abdominal surgery may act as a protective mechanism by splinting the abdomen, allowing faster healing of abdominal incisions and reducing the risk of peritoneal infection (Ford et al 1993). Key points in summary for the surgical process are provided in Box 11-3.

Postoperative Pulmonary Complications

PPCs following surgery are an important cause of postoperative morbidity and mortality, causing significant increases in LOS, use of resources and overall hospital costs (Taylor et al 1990; Varela, Ballesteros et al 2006; Zehr et al 1998). The pathogenesis of PPCs have been described above (e.g. alterations in mucociliary clearance, respiratory muscle dysfunction, alterations in $\dot{V}/\dot{Q}$ perfusion, small airway closure) yet many of these changes are considered inevitable following surgery, their natural progression being transient and self-limiting – one of spontaneous recovery requiring no specific therapy (Ford et al 1983; O'Donohue 1992). Thus any postoperative pulmonary changes that occur need to be clearly defined as being either those that will recover spontaneously or those that will adversely affect postoperative recovery, as this will help to determine the necessity for treatment. A clinically

significant PPC is described as '.... *a pulmonary abnormality that produces identifiable disease or dysfunction that adversely affects the clinical course*' (O'Donohue 1992).

While pulmonary changes occur regularly in patients undergoing major surgery, the exact mechanisms by which these combine to lead to clinically significant PPCs in only *some* patients is not currently well understood. The diagnosis of a clinically significant PPC may be made by using radiological and bacteriological criteria, clinical signs and symptoms, or a combination of these (Pasquina et al 2006) and usually include measures of oxygenation, fever, white cell count and presence of infection (e.g. abnormal sputum production or positive sputum microbiology). However, there are inconsistencies in not only which individual criteria comprise the PPC diagnosis but also how these are measured and combined, e.g. the variability of scales used to measure radiographic changes. Clearly, the method of defining a PPC impacts the reported incidence. For example, using only radiological evidence of atelectasis gives a higher incidence

BOX 11-4
MELBOURNE GROUP SCALE

Melbourne Group Scale (MGS)

A PPC will be diagnosed by presence of four or more of the following:

1. CXR report of atelectasis/consolidation
2. Fever as seen by raised oral temperature >38°C with no focus outside of the lungs
3. An otherwise unexplained WCC of >$11.2 \times 10^9 \text{ L}^{-1}$ **or** administration of respiratory antibiotics postoperatively (in addition to those administered routinely postoperatively)
4. SpO_2 <90% on room air.
5. Production of purulent (yellow or green) sputum differing from preoperative status
6. Positive signs of infection on sputum microbiology
7. Diagnosis of pneumonia/chest infection by attending physician
8. Readmission to the ICU/HDU with problems which are respiratory in origin or prolonged stay on the ICU/HDU (over 36 hours) with problems which are respiratory in origin*/Abnormal breath sounds on auscultation which differ from preoperative assessment[†]

CXR, Chest radiograph; *HDU*, high dependency unit; *ICU*, intensive care unit; *PPC*, postoperative pulmonary complication; *SpO₂*, percutaneous oxygen saturation; *WCC*, white cell count.
*MGS V1(thoracic surgery)
[†]MGS V2 (upper abdominal surgery).

of 'complications' than using a definition where factors are combined. Furthermore, incidence of PPC inevitably varies between centres and this is most likely due to local factors such as patient demographics, surgical approaches, postoperative care pathways, etc.

All of these factors make the *overall* incidence of clinically significant PPCs following major surgery difficult to determine. Recently, several studies investigating the efficacy of perioperative physiotherapy have investigated the incidence of PPCs using a scale called the Melbourne Group Scale (MGS) (Agostini et al 2013a, Reeve et al 2010a). This scale (Box 11-4) was originally designed for use in UAS (Browning et al 2007, Denehy et al 2001, Parry et al 2014) and adapted for use in thoracic surgery (Reeve et al 2008). It has been validated within the thoracic surgery population (Agostini et al 2011), has been shown to have high inter-rater and intra-rater reliability (Reeve 2010) and has been used widely in studies investigating

physiotherapy in UAS. To date it has not been used in studies investigating cardiac surgery. The MGS is an easy-to-use multidisciplinary tool but further research is required to validate its use across the major surgical spectrum.

Risk Factors for Postoperative Pulmonary Complications. Estimation of surgical risk is important for all health professionals involved in the management of surgical patients. Surgical risk is the probability of morbidity and mortality secondary to the presence of pre-, intra- and postoperative risk factors. This discussion will be limited to the development of PPCs, as this complication is that which is most often managed by physiotherapists. Assessment of risk of developing PPC is important for the physiotherapist to allow prioritized respiratory care for high-risk individuals and more appropriate use of increasingly scarce resources in physiotherapy staffing. Risk assessment for surgical complications such as wound breakdown, bleeding, renal failure and other respiratory problems such as pulmonary embolus (PE) will not be discussed in detail, although it should be noted that it is important to consider a PE in the differential diagnosis of a postoperative respiratory complication such as pneumonia, as similarities in respiratory presentation may exist.

Several patient characteristics are associated with an increased risk of developing complications. There is a large volume of literature published on this topic; for example in one systematic review (Fisher et al 2002), 40 variables were reported as possible risk factors for patients having non-thoracic surgery. Additionally, there have been attempts to develop risk factor prediction models to enable the prediction of complications in specific patient populations. The most common patient, operation and postoperative factors considered to increase risks of developing a PPC are described in this section. In physiotherapy research, a weighted model was developed to predict the risk of PPC in patients having UAS (Scholes et al 2006). This study determined that five main risk factors (all occurring together in one patient) predicted 82% of patients who developed a PPC in a population of 268 patients having UAS. Patients predicted as high risk were eight times more likely to develop a PPC than those predicted to be at low risk.

The risk factors identified were:

- duration of anaesthesia >180 minutes
- type of surgery performed (upper abdominal)
- presence of preoperative respiratory problems, e.g. chronic obstructive pulmonary disease (COPD)
- current smoking (within last 8 weeks)
- reduced level of preoperative activity (measured using a questionnaire).

In addition to this risk factor model, a systematic review of non-cardiopulmonary surgery (Smetana et al 2006) reported *good* evidence that the following risk factors increase the incidence of PPC:

- advanced age
- American Society of Anesthesiologists (ASA) classification of comorbidity of class 3–5 (American Society of Anesthesiologists, 1963)
- functional dependence
- respiratory and cardiac disease
- serum albumin <3 g/dL
- sleep apnoea.

Smetana et al (2006) reported *good* evidence that thoracic, abdominal, emergency and prolonged surgical procedures increased risk of PPC and *fair* evidence for significant intra-operative blood loss, oesophageal surgery and abnormal chest radiograph increasing the risk of PPC.

Importantly, Smetana et al (2006) also reported there was *good* evidence that the following were **not** important risk factors: obesity, asthma, hip and gynaecological surgery (lower abdominal surgery). These results challenge some traditional views, especially that of obesity being considered a risk factor. The results from this systematic review support the risk factors identified in the model by Scholes et al (2006). Further research on risk factor modelling across major surgical groups is ongoing.

The ASA score divides patients into six groups and collectively rates patient risk from undergoing anaesthesia. The score was developed as a standardized way for anaesthetists to convey information about the patients' overall health status and to allow outcomes to be stratified by a global assessment of their severity of illness. In practice, the ASA score may be the only overall documentation of preoperative condition that

is used widely. Generally, the attending anaesthetist ascribes a score to each patient upon preoperative assessment.

The classification of physical status recommended by the House of Delegates of the ASA (American Society of Anesthesiologists, 1963) is:

1. a normal healthy patient
2. a patient with mild to moderate systemic disease
3. a patient with a severe systemic disease that limits activity, but is not incapacitating
4. a patient with an incapacitating systemic disease that is a constant threat to life
5. a moribund patient not expected to survive 24 hours with or without operation
6. a declared brain-dead person whose organs are being removed for the purposes of donation.

The score is modified by the addition of 'E' denoting emergency, as emergency surgery and anaesthesia are associated with increased risk above that of the pre-existing condition.

TYPES OF SURGERY

Generally, surgical incisions are placed to optimize access to the target organ. Understanding surgery involves an appreciation of the anatomy of the abdominal and thoracic organs and the muscles and bony structures surrounding them. An appreciation of nomenclature also aids understanding descriptions of operations. The prefix of words can help to locate the surgery: for example, *enter-* relates to small intestine, *gaster-* to stomach and *pneum-* to lung. Surgical procedures may also be named for the person who first performed or reported them: for example, *Nissen* fundoplication, a wrap of fundus of the stomach around the intra-abdominal oesophagus; a *Whipple* procedure, a pancreaticoduodenectomy; and *Hartmann* procedure, a sigmoid colectomy with a colostomy. Understanding 'endings' of words also helps to work out the type of surgery (Table 11-3).

Abdominal Surgery

Understanding abdominal surgery requires an appreciation of the anatomy of abdominal organs. The abdomen is a cavity lined by peritoneum and surrounded by muscle and skin. Abdominal organs may

TABLE 11-3
Surgical Terminology

Suffixes

-ectomy	– removal of part, e.g. appendicectomy
-gram	– a radiographic picture, e.g. bronchogram
-graphy	– use of a radio-opaque contrast medium for radiography purposes, e.g. angiography
-itis	– inflammation, e.g. appendicitis
-oscopy	– visual examination of an interior of an organ (usually from externally), e.g. bronchoscopy
-osis	– disease, abnormal increase, e.g. cystic fibrosis
-ostomy	– formation of an artificial opening to the skin surface, e.g. colostomy
-otomy	– incision, e.g. laparotomy
-plasty	– tissue repair, remodelling, reconstruction, e.g. gastroplasty

Prefixes

Arthro-	– joint
Chol-	– bile
Cholecyst-	– gall bladder
Col-	– colon
Gastro-	– stomach
Ileo-	– ileum
Laparo-	– abdomen
Mast-	– breast

be intraperitoneal, and thus nourished via a mesentery (e.g. stomach), or extraperitoneal (e.g. pancreas). Some organs are both (e.g. liver).

Access to abdominal organs may be via their lumen, when there is one. This is called 'endoscopy' (Greek '*skopein*' = 'to look at'), where a fibre-optic telescope containing a light source and instruments are inserted. Examples are gastroscopy, colonoscopy and endoscopic retrograde choliangiopancreatography (ERCP). This may be used for diagnosis or therapy.

Laparoscopy involves insufflation of the peritoneal cavity with carbon dioxide (CO_2) gas (pneumoperitoneum), insertion of a camera through a 5–10 mm subumbilical incision and inspection of the abdominal contents using the transmitted picture and a monitor. Commonly, three ports are used to introduce the instruments and perform the procedure. The technique is performed under GA and the most common laparoscopic technique is for the removal of the gall bladder (cholecystectomy), but many other procedures are now performed this way, including hernia repair,

appendicectomy, splenectomy and oophorectomy (Harris 2006). The term 'minimal access surgery' has been used to reflect the fact that the operations themselves are the same, but the surgical approach is less invasive, which impacts the postoperative recovery of the patient. It has been well established in the literature that laparoscopic cholecystectomy is associated with a low incidence of PPC (Sharma et al 1996). Minimally invasive surgery is becoming more and more common globally with colorectal procedures increasingly performed using this form of surgery.

The addition of preoperative patient education, early feeding, enforced early mobilization, mobilization and optimized analgesia to minimal access surgery constitutes the basis of enhanced recovery after surgery (ERAS) pathways or 'fast track' surgery (Kehlet & Kennedy 2006). A meta-analysis of six randomized trials reported that adherence to fast track reduced morbidity by 52% and postoperative length of hospital stay by 2.5 days (Adamina et al 2011). The role of early mobility alone in this pathway has not been studied, although it is reported that failure to meet the (very aspirational) mobility pathway predicted poorer outcomes. There was very poor adherence to the pathway, with 40% not meeting the requirements to sit out of bed for 8 hours and walk four times daily for 60 m on the first postoperative day (Boulind et al 2011, Vlug et al 2011). Further research is clearly needed to assess outcomes from fast track surgery if a more achievable mobility regimen is used.

See Box 11-5 for diagrammatical representations of some of the common abdominal surgical procedures.

Bariatric Surgery

Obesity (defined as a body mass index of 30 or greater) is now recognized as a worldwide epidemic, affecting more than 1.7 billion people (Buchwald et al 2004). This has led to an increase in the development and performance of bariatric surgical techniques (Buchwald et al 2004; Sjöström et al 2007), including gastric bypass, gastroplasty, gastric banding and gastrectomy. It is well documented that open surgical procedures, combined with anaesthesia and mechanical ventilation, impair postoperative respiratory function and oxygenation; obesity exacerbates these postoperative changes (Barbalho-Moulim et al 2011, Casali et al 2011, Ebeo et al 2002, Gaszynski et al 2007,

Text continued on p. 532

BOX 11-5
COMMONLY PERFORMED ABDOMINAL SURGICAL PROCEDURES

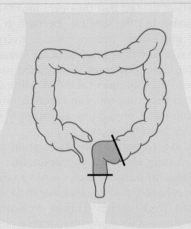

Anterior resection
Indication: Ca upper portion of rectum
Sigmoid colon to lower part of rectum

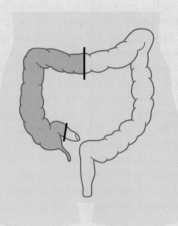

Right hemicolectomy
Indications: Ca right colon, terminal ileum
Incision: Right paramedian, midline, right oblique
Continuation restored by: Anastomosis of ileum to
   transverse colon

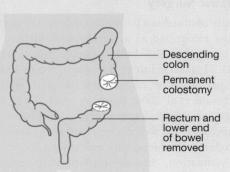

Descending
colon

Permanent
colostomy

Rectum and
lower end
of bowel
removed

Abdomino-perineal resection/sigmoid colostomy
Indication: Ca lower portion large bowel and rectum,
   ulcerative colitis
Incisions: Laparotomy and perineal

BOX 11-5
COMMONLY PERFORMED ABDOMINAL SURGICAL PROCEDURES *(Continued)*

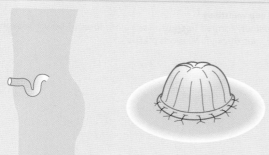

Ileostomy

Most are permanent (small bowel)

Indications: Ulcerative colitis, Crohn disease, Ca of bowel

Incision: Left paramedian or midline

Operation: Continent pouch ileostomy

Reservoir constructed out of distal ileum: removal of large colon and rectum

Outlet from reservoir is arranged as a valve so that fluid cannot escape on to the abdominal wall

Ileum brought through abdominal wall   Valve with sutures

Colostomy

May be temporary

Indications: Ca, trauma, Crohn disease, to rest bowel

Incision: Depends on site of colostomy

Operation: Stoma formed from colon; names according to section of colon it is situated in, e.g. ascending

Types of sigmoid colostomy permanent (performed for abdomino-perineal resection – Ca rectum)

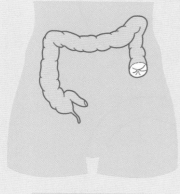

Single-barrelled colostomy

Permanent if bowel distal to colostomy is resected

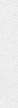

Double-barrelled colostomy

Both loop distal and proximal are opened, may be permanent or temporary depending on disease

Continued on following page

BOX 11-5

COMMONLY PERFORMED ABDOMINAL SURGICAL PROCEDURES *(Continued)*

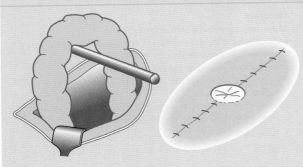

Loop colostomy
Usually formed in transverse colon; loop of bowel brought
out through incision, plastic

Before operation

After operation

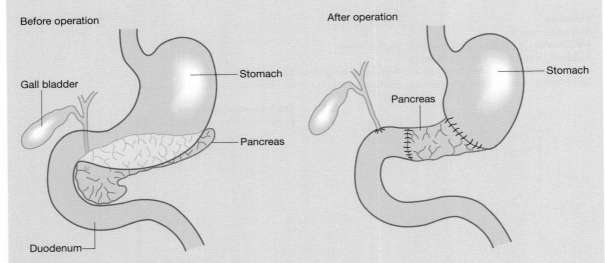

Whipple procedure (pancreaticoduodenectomy)
May be required when severe pancreatitis is confined to the head of the gland or in Ca
Resection of the distal stomach, common bile duct, duodenum, gall bladder and the pancreas to the mid-body

BOX 11-5
COMMONLY PERFORMED ABDOMINAL SURGICAL PROCEDURES *(Continued)*

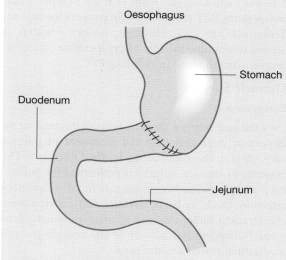

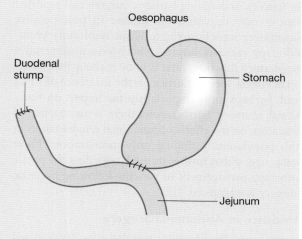

Gastrectomy
Removal of portions of the stomach
Indications: (partial) peptic ulcer, Ca distal stomach; (total) Ca
Incisions: Upper vertical – midline, paramedian, transverse or oblique
If thoracic extension for oesophagogastrectomy is involved, a left thoracotomy is performed
If upper oesophagus is involved, a right thoracotomy is used

Partial gastrectomy, Bill Roth I:
Anastomosis between severed end of duodenum with partially closed end of stomach
Partial gastrectomy, Bill Roth II:
Closes duodenal stump and joins resected stomach to jejunum

Ca, Cancer.
(Reproduced with permission, University of Melbourne School of Physiotherapy, 2006)

Neligan et al 2009). This may increase the incidence of PPCs' morbidity and mortality. The limited literature on the physiotherapy management of bariatric surgery patients has focused on the effects of respiratory exercises, including biphasic positive airway pressure (BiPAP), continuous positive airway pressure (CPAP) and IMT techniques (Barbalho-Moulim et al 2011, Casali et al 2011, Ebeo et al 2002, Gaszynski et al 2007, Neligan et al 2009). Ebeo et al (2002) suggested that the addition of BiPAP devices may minimize the decline in postoperative lung function, and oxygen saturation levels in patients undergoing bariatric surgery. Similar findings were reported in a study by Neligan et al (2009), which investigated the use of CPAP (via the Boussignac system) in patients following bariatric surgery, who were diagnosed with obstructive sleep apnoea. Gaszynski et al (2007) further reported that use of CPAP devices (via the Boussignac system) may improve postoperative blood oxygenation in bariatric surgical patients. With respect to IMT, a study by Casali et al (2011) suggested that such techniques may improve postoperative inspiratory muscle strength and endurance, and facilitate earlier recovery of respiratory function in this population. Barbalho-Moulim et al (2011) alternatively focused on preoperative IMT in females undergoing bariatric surgery and reported that it may minimize the decline in postoperative inspiratory muscle strength. While respiratory physiotherapy exercises improve short-term postoperative respiratory function, little is known about their long-term effects, their influence on the incidence of PPCs and, perhaps more importantly, the impact on functional recovery. Furthermore, there is an absence of literature on the effects of functional rehabilitation in this population, including early mobilization. These data suggest that further research regarding the physiotherapy management of patients following bariatric surgery is warranted.

Evidence in Abdominal Surgery

A review of the literature revealed nine randomized controlled trials (RCTs) took place from 2000 to 2013 in abdominal surgery. These provide levels 1b and 2b evidence (Sackett et al 2000) for the place of physiotherapy management and are summarized in Table A11-1 of the chapter appendix. Older data were not included because it was thought that these would no longer reflect current practice either in physiotherapy or pain and surgical management. Three studies evaluated prehabilitation interventions that have been discussed already. Other researchers have reported no benefit from the addition of deep breathing exercises to early mobilization in the postoperative period (Mackay et al 2005; Silva et al 2013). Similar findings have been reported with respect to the addition of prophylactic periodic CPAP (pCPAP) (Denehy et al 2001). The efficacy of pCPAP is however supported in a systematic review, although pCPAP should be reserved as a second-line treatment for patients with deteriorating hypoxaemia.

Four systematic reviews (Lawrence et al 2006, Overend et al 2001, Pasquina et al 2006, Thomas & McIntosh 1994) examined the role of postoperative physiotherapy in the prevention of PPCs in patients undergoing UAS. In summary, on the basis of the previously mentioned evidence, the role of prophylactic physiotherapy treatment in reducing PPC after UAS is supported, most particularly in higher risk patients. The techniques used to achieve this vary, with arguably the most important of these being early mobility (Haines et al 2013, Mackay et al 2005, Silva et al 2013), although these studies have small sample sizes. A recent meta-analysis (Mans et al 2015) reports that preoperative IMT reduced PPC in patients having cardiothoracic or UAS. However, further research is needed to examine the role of preoperative education and instruction alone in reducing PPC.

Thoracic Surgery

Background

Over the past century, thoracic surgery has become an important intervention in the treatment of pulmonary, pleural, chest wall or mediastinal disorders. The majority of thoracic surgery is performed for pulmonary malignancies, but management of pulmonary infection (such as bronchiectasis and tuberculosis), chest trauma, bullous disease, spontaneous or acquired pleural disorders and surgery of the oesophagus and mediastinal vessels are also seen.

Risk Assessment for Patients Undergoing Thoracic Procedures

Risk assessment of patients undergoing thoracic surgery has been widely investigated. With improvements in anaesthesia, surgical technique and pre- and post-operative management, higher risk patients than previously are undergoing lung resection and oesophageal surgery. In patients having oesophageal surgery, age, operation duration and location of tumour in the proximal oesophagus have been identified as risk factors for PPC (Law et al 2004). In order to undergo lung resection, patients are carefully evaluated to ensure they have sufficient respiratory capacity to undergo the level of resection required. The major areas for concern in terms of fitness for surgery are considered to be age, pulmonary function, cardiovascular fitness, nutritional and performance status (British Thoracic Society 2010, Berrisford et al 2005, Brunelli et al 2009, Colice et al 2007). Operability is determined by diagnosis and staging, neoadjuvant and adjuvant cancer therapy, disease advancement and type of tumour. Analysis of these risk factors and detailed pulmonary function, blood gas analysis, cardiopulmonary exercise and cardiovascular testing are performed according to practice guidelines developed by thoracic surgical bodies such as the British and American Thoracic Societies. If post-bronchodilator forced expiratory volume in 1 second (FEV_1) is less than required, more extensive lung function testing, resting SaO_2 on air, isotope perfusion scanning and cardiopulmonary exercise testing may be undertaken. A calculation of the estimated percentage of predicted postoperative FEV_1 and percentage of predicted post-operative TL_{CO} using either the lung scan for pneumonectomy or an anatomical equation for lobectomy (which accounts for lung segments to be resected) are considered. A VO_{2peak} of less than 15 mL/kg indicates high risk for surgery, and physiotherapists may be involved preoperatively in assessing and improving cardiovascular fitness in high-risk patients. While an increasing number of studies have recently investigated prehabilitation in this population, a number of these were non-randomized or had small sample sizes. Nonetheless, a body of evidence is developing that shows that high intensity exercise prior to lung resection can improve VO_{2peak}/exercise capacity and reduce postoperative morbidity (Benzo et al 2011, Bobbio et al 2008, Morano et al 2013, Pehlivan et al 2011). This may increase the surgical treatment options for high-risk patients requiring lung resection. Despite this, to date only small numbers of centres are offering prehabilitation to patients undergoing thoracic surgery (Agostini et al 2013a; Cavalheri et al 2013).

Surgical Approach

The standard surgical approach for thoracic surgery is the posterolateral thoracotomy (PLT), which involves the widest exposure for manipulation of the thoracic organs, but compared with other incision types increases postoperative pain, shoulder pain, and post-thoracotomy pain (Landreneau et al 1993, Li et al 2003, Sugi et al 1996). PLT is usually via the fifth or sixth intercostal space (see Fig. 11-5) and involves retraction of the ribs and muscular division of trapezius, latissimus dorsi, lower rhomboids, serratus anterior, the intercostals and erector spinae. Posterolateral thoracotomy is frequently associated with rib fracture and may include rib resection for better exposure (Campbell 2008). All thoracotomies require drainage with intercostal catheters and underwater seal drainage discussed subsequently in this chapter (Fig. 11-5).

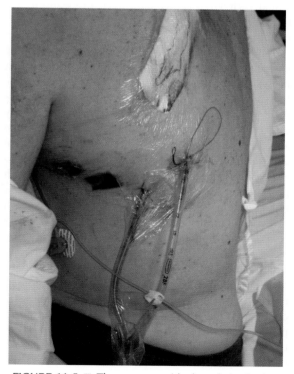

FIGURE 11-5 ■ Thoracotomy with chest drains in situ.

Video-assisted thoracoscopic surgery (VATS) involves several small (2 cm) thoracic incisions through which surgical instruments, cameras and light sources access the thoracic cavity. Studies have shown VATS provides better cosmesis, shorter hospital stay, earlier return to full function, reduced postoperative pain levels and improved preservation of pulmonary and early postoperative shoulder function compared with other thoracic approaches, but presents issues of greater technical feasibility (Landreneau et al 1993, Li et al 2003, McKenna and Houck 2005, Sugiura et al 1999, Yim 2002). VATS is now widely used for technically straightforward surgery, such as pleural surgery, lung biopsy and pneumothorax management, as it has a lower postoperative morbidity than PLT (Paul et al 2010). It is also becoming standard care for resection of early stage non–small cell lung cancer (NSCLC) in specialist centres, with the proportion of pulmonary resections via VATS now reaching between 25 and 50% in the United States (Farjah et al 2009, Paul et al 2010, Villamizar et al 2009). Superior oncological benefits have been suggested with VATS rather than open thoracotomy for lung cancer surgery (Whitson & D'Cunha 2010) but remain to be proven.

Other approaches to thoracic surgery include anterolateral and muscle sparing thoracotomy, which provide better cosmesis and potentially less postoperative shoulder dysfunction but less exposure to the thoracic viscera. Surgery of the oesophagus is usually undertaken via a variety of thoracic and/or abdominal approaches and may include thoracotomy and cervical and transhiatal incisions. Minimally invasive oesophageal resection remains relatively in its infancy, although prospective reviews have demonstrated significant reductions in PPCs and LOS, and equivalence with *early* oncological outcomes (Javidfar et al 2012; Sihag et al 2012). Minimally invasive oesophagectomy may be associated with higher surgical reintervention rates (Mamidanna et al 2012).

Following open thoracotomy, the use of a thoracic epidural catheters with opioid and local anaesthesia is considered the gold standard in post-thoracotomy pain management although alternatives such as intrathecal analgesia, thoracic paravertebral block, extrapleural analgesia, PCAs and intercostal blocks are also utilized (de Cosmo et al 2009).

Types of Surgery

Common thoracic surgical procedures and their implications for physiotherapy practice can be seen in Table 11-4.

Pulmonary resection. Pulmonary resection is most commonly performed for lung cancer and, while considered to be the best treatment for lung cancer, a recent Cochrane review determined there to be little compelling evidence that surgery improves survival compared with other forms of treatment for some types of lung cancer (Manser et al 2005). In addition to, or instead of, surgery, patients with lung cancer may undergo neo-adjuvant or adjuvant radiotherapy or chemotherapy and this may impact their physical presentation for surgery. Other types of therapy currently being trialled in association with surgery include photodynamic therapy, cryosurgery, laser surgery and chemoprevention. Other reasons for pulmonary resection include bronchiectasis, where surgery offers the best chance of cure for unilobar bronchiectasis and TB. Despite dramatic improvements in TB management since anti-TB drug regimens were introduced in the 1980s, a new global health crisis in the form of multidrug or extensively drug resistant TB has emerged (Mitnick et al 2008, Park et al 2009). Medical treatment in these types of TB has been reported to be unsatisfactory with a treatment failure rate of 40–70% (Sung et al 1999). As a result, in the past decade surgical intervention in the form of pulmonary resection has re-emerged as a treatment option for patients with TB (Park et al 2009, Sung et al 1999).

Pleural Surgery. Pleural surgery is commonly performed for recurrent pneumothoraxes, pleural biopsy, pleural effusion or management of empyema. VATS has been generally accepted as the preferred access route for pleural surgery (Yim et al 2001). LOS is usually short following these procedures, and return to work faster (Flores et al 2009). In addition analgesic requirements are reduced compared with open thoracotomy (Olavarrieta & Coronel 2009). Some patients undergoing pleural surgery via VATS may be admitted as day cases.

Oesophageal Surgery. Oesophageal surgery is normally undertaken for resection of carcinoma of the

TABLE 11-4

Common Pulmonary and Surgical Procedures and Their Implications for Physiotherapists

Operation	Procedure	Pre- and Postoperative Management and Implications for Physiotherapists
Pneumonectomy	Removal of an entire lung	■ Patient suitability to tolerate pneumonectomy assessed via: Post-bronchodilator FEV_1 >2 L (associated with less than 5% mortality) plus TL_{CO} if evidence of interstitial lung disease (BTS guidelines 2010). ■ Usual postop care: Patients should not normally lie on unoperated side (the operated side should be down if able to lie on side). This is to reduce risk of fluid moving onto the remaining lung and also causing break down the anastomosis of the bronchial stump. Physiotherapists must check with individual surgeons/units regarding local protocol for positioning in side lying. ■ Chest drain USUALLY inserted to control mediastinal shift for approximately 24 hours. Chest drain clamped but unclamped every hour to control in fluid pneumonectomy space and therefore mediastinal shift. Close monitoring of respiratory status and fluid balance essential. ■ Care must be taken with a high anastomosis, e.g. naso/oropharyngeal suction and high positive airway pressures should be avoided if possible.
Extrapleural pneumonectomy	Removal of lung with resection of pleura, diaphragm and/or pericardium	■ Performed for management of malignant mesothelioma. ■ High mortality and morbidity (Argote-Greene, Chang and Sugarbaker 2005; Sharifa, Zahida and Scarcib 2011). ■ Usual postop care: As pneumonectomy but side lying may be restricted if pericardium resected.
Lobectomy or bilobectomy	Removal of one or two lobes of the lung	■ Patient suitability to tolerate lobectomy assessed via: Post-bronchodilator FEV_1 >1.5 L (associated with less than 5% mortality) plus TL_{CO} if evidence of interstitial lung disease (BTS guidelines 2010). ■ Usual postop care: One or two chest drains inserted. Close monitoring of respiratory status. No contraindication to side lying or head-down tilt if necessary. Avoid high positive airway pressures where possible. Now increasingly performed using VATS.
Wedge or segmental resection	Removal of whole segment or wedge portion of the lung	■ Often via VATS. Usually low risk. ■ May be performed in patients with impaired pulmonary function where larger resection incurs greater risk. ■ Studies report an increase in local recurrence rates when compared with lobectomy (retrieved from http://www.cancer.gov/cancertopics/pdq/treatment/non-small-cell-lung/healthprofessional/page7).
Sleeve resection	Resection of upper lobe together with sleeve of main bronchus, to preserve lung tissue	■ Candidates for sleeve resection include patients with impaired pulmonary function, or patients who could not tolerate a pneumonectomy but in whom surgeon judges a complete resection is possible through a bronchoplastic procedure to conserve pulmonary function.
Pleurectomy	Partial stripping of parietal pleura	■ Most commonly via VATS but may be via open thoracotomy. ■ No contraindication to side lying or head-down tilt if necessary. ■ VATS pleurectomy comparable with open pleurectomy but may have increased rate of recurrence of pneumothorax (Qureshi et al, 2008; Vohra, Adamson and Weeden 2008).
Pleurodesis	Application of an irritant to the pleura	■ To prevent recurrent pleural effusion (e.g. malignant mesothelioma) or pneumothorax, or in unresolving pneumothorax. ■ Talc or chemical pleurodesis most commonly performed, inserted via chest drain or VATS.

Continued on following page

TABLE 11-4

Common Pulmonary and Surgical Procedures and Their Implications for Physiotherapists *(Continued)*

Operation	Procedure	Pre- and Postoperative Management and Implications for Physiotherapists
Drainage of empyema	Drainage of an infected pleural effusion	■ Via VATS or open drainage. ■ Usually successful via VATS when empyema in exudative or fibropurulent stages.
Decortication	Removal of thickened fibrous tissue/peel from visceral pleura ± drainage of pus (empyema)	■ When empyema in organized phase (usually 3+ weeks) decortication may be necessary due to denser adhesions. ■ Usually via VATS but conversion to open thoracotomy higher than other pleural procedures (Komanapalli and Sukumar, 2011)
LVRS	Reduction of emphysematous lung tissue allowing expansion of functioning lung tissue	■ May be via VATS or endobronchial approach. 　■ VATS: Removal of approximately 20–35% of lung tissue, mostly upper lobe. 　■ Endobronchial approach: Via introduction of one-way valve placed in a main airway to reduce air trapping and hyperinflation allowing for expansion of healthier lung. ■ Often preceded by period of prehabilitation and followed by postoperative rehabilitation to optimize outcomes.
Oesophagectomy and oesophagogastrectomy	Removal of part/all of the oesophagus or of the lower portion of the oesophagus and the stomach	■ Patients having oesophageal surgery are often undernourished preoperatively, which may affect anastomotic healing and postoperative progress. ■ The head-down position is avoided after oesophageal surgery to prevent gastric reflux and potential aspiration. Head-up positions are preferred. ■ Neck extension should be avoided in patients after oesophageal surgery that involves neck incisions. ■ Care must be taken with a high anastomosis, e.g. naso/oropharyngeal suction and high positive airway pressures should be avoided if possible.

FEV_1, Forced expiratory volume in 1 second; *LVRS*, lung volume reduction surgery; TL_{CO}, transfer factor for carbon monoxide; *VATS*, video-assisted thoracoscopic surgery.

oesophagus or oesophago-gastric junction. Adjuvant or neo-adjuvant therapy is common and surgery may be curative or palliative to provide symptom relief. Patients undergoing oesophageal resection are generally considered to be at high risk of postoperative complications due to the extent of the surgery, the (often) late presentation of the disease and the associated common symptoms, which include dysphagia and weight loss. The usual surgical approach for carcinoma of the middle and lower thirds of the oesophagus is by an Ivor Lewis oesophagectomy, which includes a laparotomy (to mobilize and prepare the stomach) and right thoracotomy (to resect the oesophagus). The stomach is delivered up into the thorax to anastomose with the remaining proximal oesophagus through the diaphragmatic hiatus. In carcinoma of the upper oesophagus, a neck incision is used in conjunction with the laparotomy and/or thoracotomy to allow anastomosis (Law & Wong 2006). Postoperatively, patients need to modify their lifestyle to eat small volume, well chewed meals regularly (up to six times daily), control reflux and avoid lying flat when sleeping. Impairments in respiratory and physical function have been found up to 2 years following oesophagectomy (Olsen et al 2005) and up to 50% of patients report procedure related chronic pain (Olsen et al 2009). Key points for thoracic surgery are in Box 11-6.

Chest Trauma. Approximately 25% of trauma deaths are due to thoracic injury and less than 10% of these require surgical intervention (Simon et al 2012), but nonetheless the need to ensure adequate ventilation and chest clearance is paramount. The majority of trauma to the chest is blunt and this causes injuries such as rib/sternal fracture, flail chest and potential injury to underlying tissues such as lung, pleural, heart and major vessels. Most blunt chest trauma is managed by non-surgical interventions such as intubation and ventilation, pain relief and chest drainage. Penetrating chest injuries often require surgery, usually rapidly. Surgery is normally via open thoracotomy or median sternotomy.

Sternal and rib fractures require effective pain relief to prevent hypoventilation and associated respiratory compromise. Flail chest (where 2 or more ribs are fractured in 2 or more places leading to a 'floating segment') causes paradoxical movement of the unstable portion of the chest wall. This causes severe pain, an asynchronous breathing pattern and a dramatic increase in the work of breathing. Poor ventilation of the underlying lung, which may have an associated pulmonary contusion, can lead to respiratory failure. Surgical stabilization in the form of rib splints and plates remain controversial but substantial benefits of fixation of flail segments in regards to mortality, pneumonia incidence and ICU LOS have been found (Fitzpatrick et al 2010). Randomized studies comparing endotracheal intubation and mechanical ventilation with (non-invasive) CPAP in patients with severe chest trauma showed positive outcomes in non-invasive ventilation (NIV) groups in terms of mortality and nosocomial pneumonia rates (Gunduz et al 2005) and necessity for intubation and length of hospital stay (Hernandez et al 2010). A recent meta-analysis found NIV significantly increased arterial oxygenation and was associated with a significant reduction in intubation rate and in the incidence of overall complications and infections (Chiumello et al 2013).

Guidelines for patients with flail chest recommend optimal analgesia and 'aggressive chest physiotherapy' (Simon et al 2012). Physiotherapists are actively engaged in attempting to ensure adequate ventilation, reduce the work of breathing and maintain adequate chest clearance in patients following chest trauma. For all patients, effective pain relief is imperative. Frequently patients will be managed with an epidural, but the use of nitrous oxide (Entonox) as an adjunct to pain relief for physiotherapy may be useful. Transcutaneous electrical nerve stimulation (TENS) may be useful in the treatment of simple rib fractures (Oncel et al 2002). Early ambulation, thoracic expansion exercises, effective supported coughing/huffing and postural advice from the main aspects of physiotherapy care. Key points from this section are given in Box 11-7.

Other Thoracic Surgery. Other thoracic surgery might include surgery of the major structures of the thorax such as the thoracic aorta, vena cavae, the sympathetic chain, thoracic duct/lymph nodes and heart and /or lung transplantation.

Evidence in Thoracic and Oesophageal Surgery

Recent surveys of practice have shown that prophylactic deep breathing exercises (DBEs) and coughing continues to form the basis of current practice with up to 84% of respondents administering these interventions prophylactically, predominately based upon established practice and personal experience rather than research evidence (Agostini et al 2013b, Reeve et al 2007, Cavalheri et al 2013). However, more high-quality studies have emerged over the past few years. RCTs investigating the effectiveness of physiotherapy interventions for the remediation of PPCs in this population can be seen in Table A11-2 of the appendix to this chapter. In summary, only one small RCT to date has evaluated the effectiveness of prophylactic targeted postoperative respiratory physiotherapy for patients undergoing lung resection (n = 42) compared with a control group (n = 34) who received standard nursing and medical care but no physiotherapy (Reeve et al 2010a). In this study there was a very low incidence of PPCs across both groups (4%) and no significant

difference in the development of PPCs between groups. In other RCTs, no significant differences in outcomes were found in patients who were administered incentive spirometry (IS) and standard care compared with those receiving standard care alone (which included respiratory physiotherapy) (Agostini et al 2013a, Gosselink et al 2000). The findings of each of these studies, whereby prophylactic respiratory physiotherapy and/or IS beyond standard care with early upright positioning and mobilization makes no significant difference to outcomes, echoes those in other major surgical groups (Freitas et al 2007, Guimarães et al 2009, Overend et al 2001, Pasquina et al 2003, Renault et al 2009). Despite this, physiotherapists regularly utilize DBE and IS in the care of patients following thoracic surgery (Agostini et al 2013b, Cavalheri et al 2013). Further studies should clarify whether early mobilization is sufficient, especially given advances in pain and medical management of these patients.

Two studies investigated the use of positive expiratory pressure (PEP) following lung resection and neither showed any significant benefit compared to sham PEP or inspiratory resistance-PEP (IR-PEP) (Frølund & Madsen 1986; Ingwersen et al 1993). A further study determined that the use of prophylactic pre- and postoperative NIV in patients undergoing pulmonary resection is safe and well tolerated, reduces LOS, improves pre- and postoperative ABGs and pulmonary function tests, but there was no significant difference in incidence of major atelectasis (Perrin et al 2009). Neither high frequency chest wall oscillation (HFCWO) nor NIV are currently considered routine interventions in the care of the patient undergoing thoracic surgery; rather they are second-line treatments once deterioration is identified (Allan et al 2009). Three further non-RCTs (Kaminski et al 2013, Novoa et al 2011, Varela et al 2006) report a difference in incidence of PPC when physiotherapy was implemented after thoracic surgery, including in a paediatric population (Kaminski et al 2013).

A recent longitudinal study compared the frequency of respiratory complications in patients undergoing oesophagectomy receiving chest physiotherapy compared to a no-treatment group (Lunardi et al 2011). Significantly less PPCs and a lower re-intubation rate were seen in the group receiving physiotherapy. Furthermore, postoperative deterioration in pulmonary function may be similar in patients undergoing thoracoscopic and open oesophagectomy and given this, authors recommend patients undergoing thoracoscopic surgery should continue to receive postoperative physiotherapy interventions to prevent postoperative complications (Nakatsuchi et al 2005). Further prospective RCTs are warranted to guide physiotherapy practice in this area.

To date, no studies have investigated the impact of physiotherapy on patients presenting with a PPC following thoracic surgery; thus no conclusions can be drawn about the effectiveness of physiotherapy interventions on the remediation of PPCs.

There have been limited studies investigating the effectiveness of physiotherapy involvement in the preoperative and postoperative rehabilitation of patients undergoing surgery for pleural disease. Both scopic and open pleural surgery have not been fully evaluated to date; thus the role of the physiotherapist with these patients remains unclear. Monitoring pulmonary function, early ambulation and ensuring full recovery of thoracic and shoulder function are believed to be important aspects of postoperative monitoring and treatment. Table 11-5 summarizes a sample progression for a patient following thoracic surgery.

RCTs investigating the efficacy of physiotherapy interventions to address the inpatient phase of postoperative rehabilitation of patients following thoracic and thoraco-abdominal surgery are given in Table A11-2 of the chapter appendix.

Postoperative Exercise Training. A small number of RCTs have investigated the impact of exercise training both in the immediate postoperative period following lung resection and following discharge from hospital. One study demonstrated that a daily progressive exercise programme commenced immediately postoperatively significantly reduced pain and improved shoulder function up to 3 months postoperatively (Reeve et al 2010b), while a further pilot RCT showed that early postoperative exercise continued for 3 months postoperatively assisted with maintaining quadriceps muscle force, but that this was not associated with improvements in exercise capacity or HRQoL benefits (Arbane et al 2011). Following their pilot study, Arbane et al (2014) investigated the effect of a combined hospital and home exercise programme

following lung resection. No significant differences between participants randomized to standard care or a postoperative exercise programme were found in quadriceps muscle strength, physical activity, exercise tolerance or HRQoL at 4 weeks postoperatively. Of note is that these studies included minimal clinical input after discharge from hospital.

More recently, studies have sought to determine the impact of supervised postoperative exercise programs after discharge from hospital (Cesario et al 2007, Granger et al 2011, Jones et al 2008, Spruit et al 2006, Stigt et al 2013). These studies are discussed in the section on oncology rehabilitation in Chapter 13.

Given the limited number of high quality studies investigating patients following thoracic and thoraco-abdominal surgery, additional studies, preferably RCTs, particularly focussing on higher risk patients, are required to confirm best practice. It is currently unclear who benefits from targeted respiratory physiotherapy interventions. Early upright positioning and ambulation appear to be sufficient for low-risk patients undergoing pulmonary resection, but it is unclear whether this translates to higher risk patients and to those undergoing thoraco-abdominal resection. Clarification of the role of the physiotherapist in the management of patients undergoing minimally invasive thoracic surgery and pleural surgery needs confirmation. In addition, the impact of prehabilitation and postoperative rehabilitation has not been sufficiently investigated to make practice recommendations for patients undergoing thoracic and thoraco-abdominal surgery, although safety and feasibility has been demonstrated. Further larger studies of exercise interventions are required to determine the impact of these interventions and to establish whether this translates to a reduction in surgical risk and an improvement in postoperative recovery and HRQoL.

Pneumothorax

Pneumothorax is defined as the presence of air in the pleural space. This may be spontaneous or acquired. Examples of acquired pneumothoraxes may be traumatic or following chest surgery. The common types of pneumothorax are primary spontaneous, secondary spontaneous, tension and traumatic (Smith 2006). *Primary spontaneous pneumothorax* is the most common and usually results from the rupture of a

TABLE 11-5

Sample Clinical Pathway for Physiotherapy for Patients Undergoing Thoracic and Cardiac Surgery

THORACIC SURGERY (THORACOTOMY)

	Assessment	Intervention
Preoperative Period	■ Preoperative respiratory status and risk of PPC ■ Preoperative mobility status ■ Preoperative upper limb function ■ Preoperative mobility status, including preoperative pulmonary function tests ■ Preoperative CPET ■ Muscle strength testing	■ Prehabilitation (exercise training; respiratory intervention; IMT) ■ Education (postoperative course of recovery) with written information (booklet)

Postoperative Period	■ Cardiorespiratory
	■ Mobility review
	■ Monitoring of pain management
	■ UWSD
	■ Upper limb function/ROM
	■ Postoperative pain levels
		■ Respiratory care as necessary, dependent upon identified problems
		■ Mobilization
		  ■ Day 0 /1: Sit out of bed
		  ■ Day 1: Commence ambulation
		  ■ Day 2: Gradual progression of ambulation distances and cadence including flight of stairs. Discharge Day 2 onwards
		■ UL function
		  ■ Day 1: Active assisted UL (unloaded) function as tolerated
		  ■ Day 2: Active UL aiming for full ROM asap
		  ■ Post UWSD removal check thoracic cage mobility

Pre–Hospital Discharge	■ Cardiorespiratory review ■ Shoulder and thoracic cage ROM review ■ UL and LL strength review ■ Mobility and exercise capacity review ■ Postoperative pain levels	■ Education regarding ADLs/ functional recovery ■ Activity and sport/leisure guidelines ■ Wound care guidelines ■ Referral to pulmonary rehabilitation if deemed necessary ■ Graduated home exercise and mobilization programme ■ Positioning advice (for pneumonectomy)

CARDIAC SURGERY (CABG AND/OR VALVE SURGERY)

	Assessment	Intervention
Preoperative Period*	■ Risk of PPC ■ Preoperative mobility status ■ Risk of sternal complication ■ Falls risk	■ Prehabilitation (exercise training; respiratory intervention; IMT) ■ Education (postoperative course of recovery) ■ Preoperative visit to intensive care
Postoperative Period*	■ Cardiorespiratory ■ Mobility review ■ Monitoring of pain management ■ Risk of sternal complications ■ Falls prevention plan if warranted	■ Cardiac rehabilitation – phase 1 ■ Respiratory care as necessary ■ Active exercises: upper limb and thorax ■ Sternal support, care and precautions ■ Gradual progression of mobility Day 1: 50–100 m or marching on the spot as tolerated with assistance Day 3 to 5: 100–400 m as tolerated ■ Stairs: 10–12 (pre-discharge from physiotherapy)

* Note: A patient may be discharged from physiotherapy prior to hospital discharge if mobilizing safely and independently and has no cardiorespiratory problems that warrant intervention. Patients who have cardiac valve surgery may be on anticoagulants (e.g. warfarin) and in hospital longer until they attain optimal International Normalized Ratio (INR) levels. Patients who are on a 'fast-track' pathway may be discharged earlier from hospital than detailed in this table.

TABLE 11-5
Sample Clinical Pathway for Physiotherapy for Patients Undergoing Thoracic and Cardiac Surgery *(Continued)*

CARDIAC SURGERY (CABG AND/OR VALVE SURGERY)

	Assessment	Intervention
Pre–Hospital Discharge	■ Sternal stability assessment ■ Cardiorespiratory review ■ Mobility review	■ Secondary prevention guidelines ■ Referral to cardiac rehabilitation – phase 2 and /or community support groups (Heart Support Australia) – phase 3 ■ Education ■ Sternal care (scar, pain management) ■ Self-monitoring and guidelines for seeking medical review/advice (angina, wound infection) ■ Graduated exercise and mobilization programme ■ Activity and sport/leisure guidelines

ADL, Activity of daily living; *CABG,* coronary artery bypass grafting; *CPET,* cardiopulmonary exercise testing, *IMT,* inspiratory muscle training, *LL,* lower limb, *PPC,* postoperative pulmonary complication, *ROM,* range of movement, *UL,* upper limb, *UWSD,* underwater seal drain.

tiny bleb at the apex of the lung. Clinical signs may include acute chest pain and shortness of breath or shortness of breath on exertion. It commonly occurs in tall, thin individuals of either sex. The size of the pneumothorax will usually dictate the management approach. This may include observation and repeat chest radiographs, needle aspiration of air directly from the pleural space or insertion of intercostal drainage. Spontaneous pneumothorax may be recurrent, with figures suggesting that about 30% recur. After a second episode, this figure increases to 70%. Surgical management is usually indicated after two pneumothoraxes on the same side and this most commonly involves pleurectomy or pleurodesis to allow the visceral pleura to adhere to the parietal, which thereby obliterates the 'potential' pleural space.

Secondary pneumothorax occurs as a result of underlying lung disease such as COPD or lung abscess. *Traumatic pneumothorax* occurs after penetrating trauma such as by a rib fracture, knife or gunshot wound. Traumatic pneumothoraxes are usually accompanied by *haemothorax,* which is defined as an accumulation of blood in the pleural space. Bleeding may be from the chest wall, heart, major vessels or lungs. When it occurs in conjunction with a pneumothorax, it is called a 'haemopneumothorax'. *Lung contusion* is also common in traumatic lung injury and involves injury to lung parenchyma, oedema and blood collecting in the alveoli and an inflammatory reaction to blood components in the lung. Gas exchange may be significantly affected by contusion, which may lead to acute respiratory distress syndrome (Trauma.org 2004).

Tension pneumothorax results when the site of air leak acts as a one-way valve so that air enters the pleural space during inspiration but cannot escape during expiration. The volume of air and pressure in the hemithorax increase, resulting in compression of the ipsilateral lung, mediastinal shift away from the side of pneumothorax including shift of the trachea, and possible kinking of the great vessels if the mediastinal shift is large. Clinical signs include deviation of the trachea, absent breath sounds, acute respiratory distress, raised jugular venous pressure and hypotension. Tension pneumothorax can be life-threatening and should be relieved as soon as possible by insertion of a large-bore needle to let the air escape under pressure followed by insertion of an intercostal drain (Smith 2006). Figure 11-6 shows different types of pneumothorax and flail chest.

Following open thoracic surgical procedures (including VATS), intercostal catheters (ICCs) are positioned in the pleural space before surgical closure and connected to a closed drainage system called 'underwater seal drainage (UWSD)'. UWSD units are systems used specifically to drain air and/or fluid from the thoracic cavity in order to regain and/or maintain re-expansion of the lung by re-establishing normal negative pressure in the pleural space.

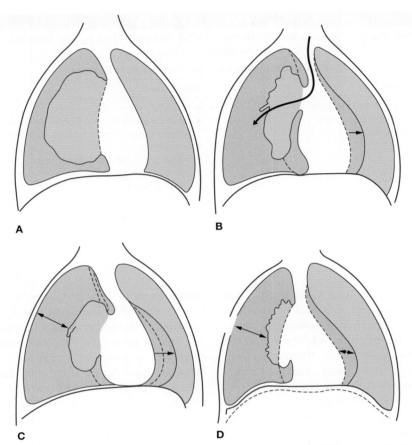

FIGURE 11-6 ■ **(A)** Partial pneumothorax. Partial collapse of the lung away from the chest wall but not under tension. **(B)** Tension pneumothorax allowing air to enter the pleural space with each inspiratory breath. **(C)** Tension pneumothorax on expiration. The hole in the lung closes on expiration, resulting in a build-up of pressure in the pleural space with mediastinal shift. **(D)** Open pneumothorax secondary to chest trauma, making respiration totally ineffective as air is sucked in and out of the open wound.

UWSD is indicated in the presence of any surgery or trauma where there has been a significant disruption to the integrity of the pleural space. The most common substances to enter the intrapleural space are air, blood, pus or an excess of pleural fluid. These may appear alone or in combination, and cause an increase in intrapleural pressure from negative to positive, thus terminating the suctioning effect and resulting in collapse of the lung.

Intercostal Catheters (ICCs)

A chest tube is generally made of clear pliable plastic into which a radio-opaque strip is incorporated. The diameter of the tube will vary depending on the size of the patient and on what is being drained. A smaller drain is usually employed to evacuate air, while a larger drain is used for fluids (Miller & Sahn 1987).

The location of the substance to be drained usually determines the placement of the tube. When the patient is upright, fluids in the pleural space will generally gravitate to the lower zones of the thorax, while air will usually rise to the apex. Therefore for drainage of a pneumothorax, the tube is usually inserted anteriorly in the mid-clavicular line into the second or third intercostal space or in the mid axillary line in the third to fifth space and is directed towards the apex of the

BOX 11-8

GENERAL CRITERIA FOR REMOVAL OF INTERCOSTAL CATHETERS AND UNDERWATER SEAL DRAINS

- Less than 100 mL of drainage in 24 hours
- Minimal swing
- Chest radiograph establishing full lung expansion
- Breath sounds present over the whole thorax on auscultation
- No air leak

thorax. When fluids are to be drained, the tube is usually inserted slightly lower, in the mid axillary line and the sixth space, and directed basally. Following surgery such as lobectomy or pleurectomy, two ICCs are inserted: one is usually directed apically and one basally. Criteria for removal of ICC are given in Box 11-8.

Underwater Seal Drainage (UWSD)

UWSD units normally consist of three components: gravity assisted drainage, an underwater seal and creation of a pressure gradient/suction.

Unobstructed Gravity Assisted Drainage

Fluids will drain into the drainage chamber by gravity. If the bottle is always kept below the level of the patients' chest, fluid will not spill back into the pleural space. If the bottle needs to be lifted above the chest (e.g. during a patient transfer), the tubing should be briefly double clamped as close to the patient as possible. The movement and unclamping should take place as quickly as possible to minimize clamping time. In general, clamping is avoided, as it increases the risk of tension pneumothorax.

The Underwater Seal

The distal end of the drain tube is submerged 2 cm under the surface level of water in the drainage (or collection) chamber. The underwater seal prevents air re-entering the pleural space. The positive pressure in the lungs during exhalation or coughing can push air out of the pleural space through the tubing, causing bubbling, but air cannot be drawn back up the tubing. Bubbling in the underwater seal chamber is associated with an air leak.

Creation of a Pressure Gradient

While normal intrapleural pressure is negative, if air or fluid enters the pleural space, the intrapleural pressure becomes positive. This creates a pressure gradient and facilitates air moving from higher (intrapleural) to lower (within the drainage chamber) pressure. The drainage chamber has a vent to allow air to escape the chamber and prevent pressure build up within it. The vent can be attached to low-grade suction if required. Suction may be applied to facilitate re-expansion of the lung and reduce the duration of air leaks. Patients may not be permitted to be disconnected from the suction, thus limiting ambulation and ADLs. Alternatively portable suction units may be used.

Types of Underwater Seal Drainage Systems

There are one-, two- and three-bottle UWSD systems but most commonly disposable (all-in-one) three-bottle systems are used. All systems drain both air and fluid. In the disposable system, one chamber collects fluid and one chamber has the underwater seal allowing air to escape from the chest. The third chamber controls suction, whereby either the height of the water in the chamber regulates the negative pressure applied to the system or a mechanical valve/regulator rather than an underwater seal is utilized to control the suction. These are accordingly called 'wet' or 'dry' systems.

Newer forms of chest drainage in use are integrated all-in-one disposable digitalized systems (Fig. 11-7). These newer systems are lightweight and portable, encouraging ambulation. They allow more immediate and continuous monitoring of suction pressures and air leaks, better reliability of reporting of air leaks and offer a more scientific rationale for the removal of chest drains (Cerfolio & Bryant 2008).

Implications for Physiotherapists

As part of a physiotherapy objective assessment, specific examination of a UWSD system should be performed. There are four important aspects of examination – swinging, bubbling, drainage, and suction. Bubbling and swinging rely on an intact underwater seal. When examining the UWSD system, ask the patient to take a deep breath and observe for swinging and bubbling. If there is no bubbling at this time, ask the patient to cough and observe for bubbling.

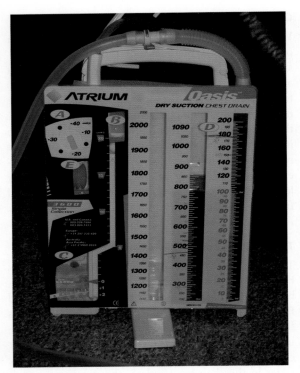

FIGURE 11-7 ▪ Underwater seal drainage (USWD) system.

Assessment for air leak (from the pleural space) must include observation of the underwater seal chamber during coughing.

Swing. Fluid in the tube (or water-sealed chamber) should move up and down with respiration, this is termed 'swing'. A small degree of swing (up to 5 cm) is usual in UWSDs and reflects usual changes in pleural pressure with respiration. Swinging may be a small movement during quiet breathing or a larger movement when the patient is coughing or during an increased respiratory effort. If the patient is attached to suction, pressure is more regulated and swing is reduced. If no swing is seen, the tubing may be occluded, obstructed, compressed, kinked or lying outside the pleural space. All of these require reporting and, potentially, urgent resolution.

Bubbling. The presence or absence of bubbling in the underwater seal chamber of the system should be determined. Bubbling in the underwater seal chamber

indicates an air leak (from the pleural space). It is important not to confuse the bubbling in the underwater seal chamber with the bubbling in the suction chamber. The bubbling in the suction chamber indicates suction is applied to the system at the correct level. No bubbling of the underwater seal indicates absence of an air leak, bubbling on coughing indicates a small air leak, bubbling on expiration indicates a moderate air leak, bubbling throughout inspiration and expiration indicates a large air leak.

Drainage. It is important to note the pattern of drainage of fluid from the chest drain. When drainage is reduced to 100 mL over 24 hours the tube may (usually) be removed. If large amounts of blood drain over a short period of time, this may indicate haemorrhage. Large amounts of haemoserous drainage may be associated with hypovolaemia, hypotension and low haemoglobin. It is not uncommon for some drainage to occur during patient movement, e.g. transfers and exercise. Generally, drainage of more than 100 mL per hour or a sudden increase in drainage is cause for concern and medical staff should be alerted.

Suction. Suction may or may not be applied. There is limited evidence of the benefits of suction following thoracic surgery (Deng et al 2010). Protocols for the use of suction vary from hospital to hospital and it is important to check care protocols for patient management if suction is applied; for example, it may not be possible to ambulate patients away from the bed space. When wall suction is applied, this should result in gentle bubbling only in the suction chamber. Vigorous bubbling will not increase the amount of suction applied to the patient and will cause evaporation of the water in the suction chamber. No bubbling in the suction chamber indicates that the wall suction is not sufficiently high enough and needs to be increased.

Persistent Air Leaks. A persistent air leak (PAL) is considered an air leak that fails to resolve before an expected length of time. It is a common complication for patients with emphysema undergoing thoracic surgery and is the most common condition that causes prolonged length of hospital stay, increased costs and patient dissatisfaction (Cerfolio & Bryant 2008). The optimal management of PAL, including the efficacy of

BOX 11-9
KEY POINTS FOR UNDERWATER SEAL DRAINAGE

- Underwater seal drainage (UWSD) devices normally have 3 chambers: a collection chamber, an underwater seal chamber and a suction chamber.
- The water seal must remain intact at all times. Therefore the water seal chamber must always be in an upright position. If the water seal chamber is tipped over such that the tip of the tube is above the water surface level, air can re-enter the pleural cavity.
- The drainage system must always be kept below the patient's chest or clamped briefly if it must be raised above this level.
- Air leaks should be regularly assessed and are usually documented as: continuous air leak, air leak with passive expiration, air leak with forced expiration, no air leak. This is assessed by the amount of bubbling occurring in the water seal chamber.
- If a patient with an air leak needs to lie on the drain tubing, it is important to ensure that air may continue to drain from the pleural space into the UWSD system, and that the weight of the patient does not result in occlusion of the tubing. If the latter were to occur, a tension pneumothorax could result.
- If the tubing becomes disconnected, it should be clamped by hand as close to the patient as possible. The drain may be immediately reconnected only if the ends of the tubing have avoided contact and contamination. A nurse should be called promptly to help with reconnection. The risk of this occurring can be minimized by checking all connections of the chest drain before moving the patient. When a patient is getting out of bed or moving around in the bed, care should be taken that the patient does not lean on the chest tubing.

- If the chest drain falls out, the wound should be covered immediately with a gloved hand and urgent assistance called for.
- If positive pressure therapies are being used in the presence of an air leak, the air leak needs to be constantly monitored as it may be exacerbated by these techniques. For example, during application, the air leak may be present on expiration when previously it was observed only on coughing.
- The pain from a chest drain can be severe and may limit the patient's ability to cooperate with physiotherapy treatment.
- Usually patients may move around with their chest drain in situ. They should be encouraged to keep the shoulder of the affected side moving, and generally discouraged from adopting protective postures.
- If suction is required, patients may be disconnected from suction and ambulated only following communication with the medical and nursing team. It is important to ensure that the UWSD system is kept below the level of the chest at all times.
- If the patient cannot be disconnected from suction, walking within the confines of the suction tubing or marching on the spot may be attempted.
- If a patient is being disconnected from suction, it is essential that the tubing from the collection chamber to the suction is disconnected rather than just switching the wall suction off. (If the patient is left connected to the wall suction with the suction switched off, there is no vent to the atmosphere through which air may escape from the pleural space and a tension pneumothorax may occur).

---

physiotherapy interventions to aid resolution, currently forms the basis of much debate. Non-resectional techniques for surgeries such as lung volume reduction surgery (LVRS), the use of pulmonary sealants and optimal chest drain management are amongst strategies used in an attempt to reduce PAL. The use of one-way valves (with or without reservoir drainage bags) and digital drainage systems allow for patients with PALs to be safely discharged from hospital with the drain remaining in situ and enable accurate monitoring of outpatient air leak data (Jenkins et al 2012). The impact of PAL on other PPCs has not been investigated and it is possible that patients with PAL are more susceptible to the development of PPCs. Clarification of whether and which physiotherapy interventions aid recovery of patients with PAL would

assist in optimizing patient management. See Box 11-9 for key points in management of UWSD.

Cardiac Surgery

Background

Open heart surgery (OHS) is defined as an operative procedure performed on or within the exposed heart, usually with cardiopulmonary bypass (CPB) (Stedman 2005). Despite advances in minimally invasive surgery and interventional cardiology with the advent of coronary stenting, OHS remains a more effective treatment in patients with multi-vessel disease and left main coronary artery stenosis (Taggart 2006). OHS is performed for both congenital and acquired heart diseases, most commonly for ischaemic heart disease and valvular disease. The standard surgical approach for

OHS is the median sternotomy, as it provides optimal access to the heart and is associated with excellent surgical outcomes (Tatoulis & Smith 2006).

The operative mortality for coronary artery surgery is 1%, with perioperative stroke, myocardial ischaemia, arrhythmias, cardiovascular instability, sternal infection and haemorrhage being the most common complications. Respiratory complications include low lung volumes, basal atelectasis and pleural effusion, which usually resolve. The long-term survival is excellent with 90–95% alive at 5 years and 80–85% at 10 years, but is significantly influenced by age at surgery, diabetes, left ventricular function and secondary risk factor modification after surgery (Tatoulis & Smith 2006).

Valvular heart disease primarily affects the aortic, mitral and occasionally the tricuspid valves. The most common form of valvular disease in Western countries is stenosis (narrowing), which is generally calcific, and incompetence/regurgitation occur as a result of degeneration and ageing. The two forms may occur together. The incidence of rheumatic heart disease (caused by rheumatic fever) has declined in Western countries but is still high in developing regions such as China, India and South America. The two most common presentations of valvular dysfunction are aortic stenoses and mitral regurgitation (Tatoulis & Smith 2006). Operative mortality is 1–3% in valve surgery and 3–5% for combined valve and coronary artery surgery, with long-term outcomes being reported as excellent. Morbidity of valve surgery is relatively low, with problems of anticoagulant-related haemorrhage, thromboembolism, endocarditis and perivalvular leaks occurring in 1% of patients annually. Please refer to Chapter 4 on cardiovascular disease for more details.

Types of Surgery

Minimally Invasive Heart Surgery. Minimally invasive techniques using endoscopy and robotics (avoiding a median sternotomy) are being utilized in some centres, particularly for valve surgery. Endoscopic harvesting of the saphenous vein to minimize incisions and pain is also performed.

Minimally invasive cardiac surgery encompasses a variety of operations performed through incisions that are substantially smaller and less traumatic than the standard sternotomy. Minimally invasive incisions measure about 8–10 centimetres compared to 20–25 centimetres for sternotomy incisions. Specialized handheld and robotic instruments are used to project the dexterity of the surgeon's hands through these small incisions in performing the operations.

Open Heart Surgery

Coronary Artery Bypass Grafting (CABG). Multiple severe coronary stenoses associated with unstable or uncontrolled angina may be treated with OHS and bypass grafting. This operation involves access via a median sternotomy and requires CPB, which is referred to as 'non-pulsatile OHS'. This procedure can also be performed 'off-pump' (OP). Please refer to the detailed description in the following section. Patients may achieve an excellent outcome with either type of procedure. To date, off-pump cardiopulmonary bypass (OPCPB) has been associated with trends that include less blood loss and need for transfusion, myocardial enzyme release up to 24 hours, early neurocognitive dysfunction and renal insufficiency (Sellke et al 2005). Fewer grafts tend to be performed using OP than with standard CABG. However, length of hospital stay, mortality rate, long-term neurological function and cardiac outcome are similar in the two groups (Sellke et al 2005).

For a sternotomy procedure the patient is commonly positioned supine on the operating table with the arms placed by the side (Sabiston & Spencer 1990). The vertical incision along the sternum starts one finger space below the suprasternal notch and extends caudally to a point approximately 3 cm below the xiphoid process (Sabiston & Spencer 1990). A sternal retractor with broad blades is placed in position, and opened to allow access to the heart (Figs 11-8 and 11-9). The preferred conduits for grafting are arteries, since they have a higher patency. The right internal mammary artery (IMA) is commonly anastomosed to the left anterior descending artery. The patency of the right mammary artery at 5 years is 96%, and at 10 years is still 95% compared with the saphenous vein (75%, reducing to 50% at 10 years) (Tatoulis & Smith 2006). Prior to closure of the chest, following the surgical procedure the patient is rewarmed and sinus rhythm is restored and pleural or mediastinal (if the pleural cavity has not been entered) drain tubes are inserted infero-laterally to the median sternotomy via stab incisions (Moghissi et al 2003, Shields et al

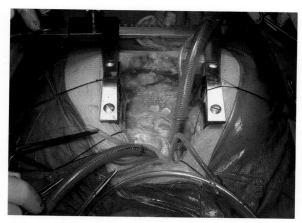

FIGURE 11-8 ■ Cardiac surgery–median sternotomy incision. A perioperative image with retractors, cannula and drain tubes in situ.

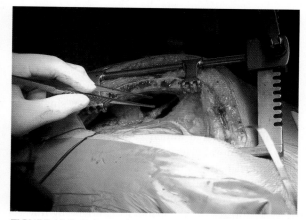

FIGURE 11-9 ■ Internal mammary artery (IMA) harvest with a Favalaro retractor in situ.

2004). Thereafter, the sternum is rewired back together by approximating the two divided sternal surfaces, most commonly by using interrupted wire sutures (Jamieson & Shumway 1986, Moghissi et al 2003, Shields et al 2004).

A typical operation usually takes 2–3 hours and the average number of vessels bypassed is three or four. The postoperative length of hospital stay is approximately 5–7 days for uncomplicated surgery and many patients are referred to outpatient cardiac rehabilitation after discharge from hospital. A sample clinical pathway depicting patient progression from the time

of surgery until hospital discharge is illustrated in Table 11-5.

Valve Surgery

AORTIC VALVE SURGERY. Aortic valve surgery involves OHS via a median sternotomy and CPB. A prosthetic valve replaces the diseased one and the operation takes approximately 3 hours with 80 minutes of CPB.

MITRAL VALVE SURGERY. Mitral stenosis may be treated by valvuloplasty, where a balloon is passed via catheterization of the femoral vein into the left atrium and mitral valve and then inflated. However, OHS is required for severe disease and may involve debridement of calcification and resection of portions of the thickened chordae, or may require replacement with a prosthetic valve. Mitral regurgitation is usually due to elongated and ruptured chordae, leading to a prolapsed and flail valve. In severe disease, valve replacement is necessary.

CARDIAC VALVE PROSTHESES. Both tissue and mechanical valves are used for valve replacement surgery. Mechanical valves (such as St Jude) are durable but the patient needs to continue on anticoagulation therapy for life. Tissue valves (bioprostheses) may be human allografts or xenografts from specially treated porcine or bovine valves. With these valves, anticoagulation is necessary only in the short-term period of postoperative care and the valves have long durability.

Patients undergoing valve surgery may have a longer hospitalization as they must attain therapeutic International Normalized Ratio (INR) (coagulation) levels prior to discharge. They require regular blood tests in the community to monitor their INR.

Cardiopulmonary Bypass (Non-Pulsatile Open Heart Surgery).

CPB ('heart–lung machine') was developed to allow operations on a still and empty heart. CPB involves the use of a mechanical pump and an oxygenating device to supply oxygenated blood to the body while the heart is still and empty. Blood is removed from the right atrium (using gravitational flow), oxygenated across a membrane and returned to the ascending aorta. A heat exchanger cools and rewarms blood and a centripetal pump or roller propels the blood (at 4–6 L/min) back into the aorta. Complete arrest of the heart requires cross clamping of the aorta, during which the myocardium is protected with hypothermia to reduce oxygen requirements. This is achieved by infusion of cold (4°C) cardioplegic solution (usually potassium with oxygenated blood and other products) into the coronary arteries, topical cold solution and using the heat exchanger on the CPB machine. The cardioplegic solution arrests the heart in diastole. The duration of CPB is usually between 1 and 2 hours, although up to 3 hours is possible. After 2 hours, problems such as blood cell destruction by the roller pump, coagulation problems and neurological, hepatic and renal dysfunction may occur.

Beating Heart or 'Off Pump' Coronary Artery Bypass Surgery (OPCAB).
Performance of surgery on a beating heart without the use of CPB is called 'beating heart bypass surgery' or OPCAB and its use is becoming more common in many cardiac units worldwide in an attempt to prevent some of the complications that may be associated with CPB such as air emboli. It is a technically more difficult procedure to perform especially when grafting the posterior surface of the heart (right coronary artery–posterior descending inter-ventricular artery), as the heart has to be lifted up from the chest cavity for access to the vessels.

Support Following Cardiac Surgery

HAEMODYNAMIC MANAGEMENT. Cardiac surgery places significant stress on the cardiac, vascular and renal body systems that are primarily responsible for haemodynamic 'homoeostasis'. The primary goal of haemodynamic management after OHS is to maintain adequate end-organ perfusion and oxygen delivery, while minimizing unnecessary cardiac demand (Khalpey et al 2008). Haemodynamic stability is achieved through assessment and manipulation of multiple codependent factors, including 'volume status (preload), peripheral vascular tone (afterload), cardiac pump function, heart rate and rhythm and blood oxygen-carrying capacity' (Khalpey et al 2008, p. 465). In the initial postoperative period (12 to 24 hours postoperatively), invasive monitoring via peripheral and/or pulmonary arterial catheterization and central venous catheterization, electrocardiography (ECG) and peripheral pulse oximetry allow for continuous haemodynamic assessment (Lemmer & Vlahakes 2010b). Medications are frequently used to

1) provide inotropic support, i.e. to enhance cardiac ventricular systolic function; 2) promote positive lusitropy, i.e. myocardial relaxation; 3) alter venous and arterial vascular resistance; and 4) treat cardiac arrhythmias (Walcot & Marchbank 2007, Khalpey et al 2008). Cardiac pacing may be used to increase heart rate and improve cardiac synchrony. Mechanical circulatory support, e.g. resumption of CPB or intra-aortic balloon counterpulsation, may be used along with inotropic therapy to treat myocardial failure (Walcot & Marchbank 2007). Pacing wires may be inserted at the time of the operation and the patient is returned to the cardiothoracic intensive care with ECG, blood pressure, right atrial pressure, pulmonary artery pressure and cardiac and urine output monitoring. The patient is initially mechanically ventilated (4–12 hours), then weaned and supported with oxygen therapy. Some patients require inotropic circulatory support, including dopamine and afterload reducing agents such as nitroprusside. In cases where the function of the left ventricle is poor postoperatively, an intra-aortic balloon pump (IABP) may be required to support the heart.

The IABP is a circulatory device providing support for the left ventricle. It consists of a single- or multi-chamber balloon attached to an external pump console via a large lumen catheter, and is inserted into the femoral artery with the balloon positioned in the aorta between the subclavian and renal arteries. The balloon is inflated during diastole and deflated during systole. Inflation and deflation of the balloon is synchronized to the patient's cardiac rhythm via the ECG trace. The physiological aims of the IABP are to improve myocardial perfusion and reduce afterload, resulting in a reduction in myocardial oxygen demand, improved cardiac contractility and decreased risk of ongoing myocardial ischaemia. These aims are achieved by increasing the blood flow through the coronary arteries from the counter pressure exerted by the inflated balloon during coronary filling. This in turn reduces the volume of blood in the aortic arch, thus decreasing the work of the left ventricle to eject the cardiac output. Patients usually begin on a cycle of 1 : 1 (i.e. inflation/deflation every heart contraction) and are weaned from IABP by reducing the ratio of assisted beats, reducing the balloon augmentation or both usually over a period of several days.

Patients with the IABP in situ should only be treated by physiotherapists as indicated following discussion with the ICU consultant. Their myocardial dysfunction may result in circulatory shock, an inability of oxygen supply to meet demand. Interventions that put these patients under greater physiological stress (i.e. activities that increase the work of the myocardium) should be carefully assessed and often be avoided. If the patient requires repositioning, great care should be taken not to flex the IABP catheter to avoid kinking or migration of the catheter. Usually hip flexion beyond 90 degrees is forbidden. Additionally, aggressive anticoagulation is required while the IABP is in situ and this, together with their cardiovascular status, prevents patients ambulating while the IABP is in situ and for 24 hours following removal of the pump. Ventricular assist devices (VADs), which perform the work of the left ventricle, are used when inotropes and balloon pump are insufficient to maintain adequate circulation.

Respiratory Management. OHS is associated with acute postoperative alterations in respiratory function. The pathogenesis of these respiratory alterations is complex, and inevitably results from a combination of factors related to the procedure, perioperative management, the use of CPB and individual patient factors (Wynne & Botti 2004). Respiratory management after CABG holds two primary aims, being to: 1) maintain adequate gas exchange (adequate arterial oxygenation); and 2) reduce the risk and/or impact of PPCs (Lemmer & Vlahakes 2010b).

During OHS procedures, mediastinal drains are positioned and connected to a UWSD system to prevent postoperative accumulation of intrathoracic air, blood and fluid. Positive pressure mechanical ventilation (commenced prior to the cessation of CPB) is routinely maintained following surgery to promote alveolar re-expansion and gas exchange. The fraction of inspired oxygen (FiO_2) is titrated to maintain arterial oxygenation, and endotracheal suction is employed to remove airway secretions. Early weaning from mechanical ventilation and extubation is recommended where possible, following which physiotherapy aimed at reducing the incidence of PPCs is usually commenced. Early mobilization out of bed, usually on the **first** postoperative day, is encouraged. Supplemental oxygen with a mask or nasal cannula is commenced following extubation and continued as indicated to achieve the desired levels of peripheral oxygen saturation (SpO_2) (Lemmer & Vlahakes 2010b).

Postoperative Management

'Fast-Track'. Rapid sustained recovery, or 'fast-track' protocols are increasingly recommended to reduce postoperative length of hospital stay and the attendant healthcare costs (Cheng 1998). Fast-track protocols incorporate short-acting anaesthetic agents and reduced opiate analgesia so as to allow early postoperative extubation, early discharge from the ICU and early ambulation (Myles & McIlroy 2005). The use of fast-track protocols after CABG are safe, insofar as their use does not increase 30-day mortality or major morbidity (Myles et al 2003), and may reduce acute care hospital readmission time (Cheng et al 2003).

Post-Sternotomy Pain

Median sternotomy, incisions for graft harvesting, retraction of the chest wall, mediastinal drains and prolonged surgical positioning all contribute to pain after CABG (Lemmer & Vlahakes 2010b). The incidence of post-sternotomy pain remains high with approximately 30% of patients developing musculoskeletal complications that affect shoulder, chest and/or upper limb function for up to 3 months following surgery (El-Ansary et al 2000a, Stiller et al 1997). In particular, a significant association between harvesting of the IMA and anterior chest wall pain has been reported (El-Ansary et al 2000a). It is postulated that this may be due to the mechanical demands of the procedure, as harvest of the IMA necessitates retraction and eversion of the upper ribs asymmetrically at an angle varying from 20 degrees to 70 degrees from the horizontal plane (e.g. Ruletract, Favalaro) (see Fig. 11-9). The International Association for the Study of Pain (IASP) recognized 'Internal Mammary Artery Syndrome' in 1999. This is classified by the presence of:

■ numbness +/− allodynia anterior intercostal nerves T1–T2 and T5–T6
■ constant pain and shooting intermittent pain on harvest side
■ tenderness on palpation of manubrium, sternocostal joints and anterior rib cage

Chronic post-sternotomy pain has also been reported in 28% of patients at 6–12 months postoperatively (Kalso et al 2001, Meyerson et al 2001). King et al (2008) documented incision or breast pain 12 months following surgery in 47% of women and found that increasing chest circumference and harvesting of bilateral IMAs were associated with ongoing pain (see Fig. 11-9). The prescription of a programme of progressive thoracic exercises was reported to significantly reduce sternal pain, and improve patient perception of change and wellness (Sturgess et al 2014). In addition, patients with persistent pain or dysfunction of musculoskeletal origin (e.g. thoracic spine pain, scar hyperalgesia) may require individual physiotherapy intervention that targets the musculoskeletal system on discharge from hospital. They can be referred for assessment and management in the community or access specialized outpatient physiotherapy services.

Sternal Management. There have been recent innovations in sternal closure that aim to prevent sternal complications by targeting patients that present with comorbidities that comprise bone healing. One such innovation is 'Kryptonite', which is a biocompatible adhesive polymer that prevents pathologic sternal displacement (up to 600 N) (Fedak et al 2010). Such a procedure may make sternal precautions redundant. There have also been developments in acute pain management that involve the direct infusion of local anaesthesia such as ropivacaine into the sternal region (Hong et al 2013).

Evidence in Cardiac Surgery

Prevention of Postoperative Pulmonary Complications. Following cardiac surgery, the evidence obtained from a large body of research clearly challenges the traditional approach of prophylactic postoperative respiratory physiotherapy intervention. A search of the physiotherapy evidence database (PEDro) using 'cardiac surgery' reveals four systematic reviews regarding the place of respiratory physiotherapy for patients having cardiac surgery (Brooks et al 2001, Jonasson & Timmermans 2001, Moore 1997, Pasquina et al 2003) in addition to numerous clinical trials. The most recent systematic review concluded that there is *no* clear evidence that prophylactic respiratory physiotherapy reduces the incidence of PPC

following cardiac surgery (Pasquina et al 2003). In addition, a plethora of studies evaluating interventions aiming to reduce the incidence of PPC and improve pulmonary function have emerged (see Table A11-3, Appendix). The literature to date supports the conclusion that prophylactic respiratory physiotherapy after cardiac surgery is no longer warranted (Pasquina et al 2003; Freitas et al 2007; Savci et al 2006; Renault et al 2007).

Postoperative Exercise Training. Physiotherapists are routinely involved in the in-hospital management (or phase I cardiac rehabilitation). Exercise is generally accepted as an important physical intervention to promote recovery after CABG (phase 1). Patients undergoing CABG may be deconditioned prior to surgery, and exercise capacity is further compromised postoperatively. Patients are encouraged to mobilize with the assistance of a physiotherapist on day one following surgery if they are medically stable. They will be guided to gradually progress their mobility within safe limits until they can negotiate a flight of stairs (e.g. 12 to 14 steps) independently prior to hospital discharge. The 'stair test' assesses their orthopaedic safety while ensuring that they are also stable from a cardiovascular perspective by screening for arrhythmia in response to exercise.

The restoration of functional capacity is one of the key indications for cardiac surgery, and exercise has proven benefits in secondary prevention of congenital heart disease, yet uptake of formal exercise programs after cardiac surgery remains suboptimal. There is limited research investigating the potential benefits of physiotherapy-prescribed and supervised phase I exercise in recovery after cardiac surgery, and specifically the optimal dose (mode, frequency, intensity and duration) of exercise. Busch et al (2012) reported significant improvement in functional capacity in a group of patients aged 75 years and over following a programme of upper and lower limb resistance exercises and balance training. Similar findings were reported following progressive treadmill training and treadmill training in a virtual outdoor environment respectively (Chuang et al 2005, Wu et al 2012).

A better understanding of the trajectory of functional recovery following cardiac surgery would assist physiotherapists in optimizing pre- and postoperative care to ensure timely access to rehabilitation programs following discharge from hospital and a return to optimal function.

The clinician should also consider the multiple physiological factors that may reduce exercise capacity in the early postoperative period. These may include:

- anaemia
- impaired autonomic cardiac modulation
- impaired ventricular function
- deconditioning from bed-rest and/or limited physical activity (both before and after surgery)
- alterations in respiratory function
- fatigue, including as a result of sleep deprivation
- postoperative pain and
- sternal or leg wound complications.

Recently Hirschhorn et al (2012) conducted a RCT comparing the effects of stationary cycling to walking. Moderate intensity stationary cycling was reported to be as effective as moderate intensity walking with respect to postoperative functional exercise capacity independent of mode of exercise testing (see Table A11-3, Appendix). Stationary cycling is a safe alternative to walking for patients who may have neuromotor impairment (Hirschhorn et al 2012, Macchi et al 2007). Hirschhorn et al (2012) also identified a 6-minute cycle test that quantifies work output that can be used as an outcome measure of exercise functional capacity.

The standard 6-minute walk test (6MWT) or modified 6-minute walk assessment (6MWA) are two feasible options for the assessment of exercise capacity at hospital discharge. If a walk test has been performed prior to surgery, a repeat walk test at hospital discharge will give information which can be used to benchmark early and relative recovery of exercise capacity.

The provision of rehabilitation for cardiac surgery patients is supported by evidence and constitutes best practice (see Table A11-3). Further information regarding cardiac rehabilitation can be found in Chapter 12. Additionally a small but significant number of patients may also require specific physiotherapy intervention to target musculoskeletal problems and functional limitations that are outside the scope of cardiac rehabilitation (El-Ansary el al 2000a, LaPier & Schenk 2002).

BOX 11-10

KEY POINTS IN PHYSIOTHERAPY TREATMENT TECHNIQUES

- To date no specific treatment techniques have been found to be superior to any another.
- Preoperative treatment allows physiotherapists to assess patient risk factors and may be an effective treatment in its own right.
- The additional value of incentive spirometry over other forms of postoperative prophylaxis has not been supported in surgical patients.
- Continuous positive airway pressure is most commonly used as a second-line treatment intervention for prevention of deteriorating hypoxaemia in the management of surgical patients.
- Mobilization of patients is now considered the first line treatment for surgical prophylaxis.
- The effectiveness of physiotherapy in the postoperative rehabilitation and fast tracking of surgical patients needs further clarification.

A summary of the evidence for physiotherapy treatment techniques in abdominal, thoracic and cardiac surgery is provided in Box 11-10.

Sternal Precautions. Historically, in an attempt to prevent the development of sternal complications, many patients are routinely asked to observe sternal precautions that limit the use of the upper limbs and trunk (Adams et al 2006, Adams et al 2008, Brocki et al 2010, Cahalin et al 2011, Parker et al 2008, Tuyl et al 2012). However, there is no evidence to support this assumption and it seems that sternal precautions or rather 'restrictions' have been drawn from expert opinion, institutional protocols and limited studies on cadaver/replica models (Balachandran et al 2014, Cahalin et al 2011, Casha et al 1999, Dasika et al 2003, Losanoff et al 2004, McGregor et al 1999, Robicsek et al 2000, Tuyl et al 2012). There is significant variation in the clinical application of sternal precautions among institutions worldwide, with no consensus on the type (e.g. use of one arm; use of no arms, use of both arms) and duration of time for which they are applied, which can range from 4 weeks to 3 months (Balachandran et al 2014, Overend et al 2010, Tuyl et al 2012). Given that the majority of patients post median sternotomy heal without any sternal complications the setting of restrictions may delay recovery and

TABLE 11-6

Risk Factors Associated with Sternal Wound Complications

Primary Risk Factors	Secondary Risk Factors
■ Obesity/high BMI	■ OP
■ COPD	■ Longer ICU LOS
■ IMA grafts (bilateral)	■ Time of surgery
■ Diabetes	■ Staple use for skin closure
■ Resternotomy	■ Impaired renal function
■ Smoking	■ Immunocompromised function
■ Prolonged MV	
■ Large chest circumference	■ Septic shock
■ PVD	■ ACE inhibitor
■ Prolonged cardiopulmonary bypass time	■ Depressed LV function
	■ Inadvertent (off centre line) median sternotomy
■ Increased blood loss/transfused units	■ Antibiotic admin >2 hours pre-surgery
■ Higher disability classification (NYHA/CCS)	■ Closure by non-CV surgeon
■ Female gender with large breasts	■ Use and duration of pacing wires

ACE, Angiotensin-converting enzyme; BMI, basal metabolic index; COPD, chronic obstructive pulmonary disease; CV, cardiovascular; ICU, intensive care unit; IMA, internal mammary artery; LOS, length of stay; LV, left ventricle; MV, mechanical ventilation; NYHA/CCS, New York Heart Association/Canadian Cardiovascular Society; OP, osteoporosis; PVD, peripheral vascular disease.

TABLE 11-7

Sternal Instability Scale (SIS)

Grades of Motion	Modified Sternal Instability Scale
0	*Clinically stable sternum* (no detectable motion) – normal
1	*Minimally separated sternum* (slight increase in motion upon special testing* – upper limb, trunk)
2	*Partially separated sternum – regional* (moderate increase in movement upon special testing*)
3	*Completely separated sternum – entire length* (marked increase in motion upon special testing*)

*Special testing may include shoulder flexion (unilateral/bilateral), trunk rotation, lateral flexion, coughing and opposing movements of the upper limb (e.g. flexion, abduction and external rotation of one upper limb accompanied by extension, adduction and internal rotation of the other upper limb).

mobilization (Cahalin et al 2011, LaPier 2007). It may be more appropriate to modify sternal precautions according an individual's risk for sternal complications (Table 11-6), physical examination of sternal stability (Sternal Instability Scale (SIS)) and their response to exercise (Cahalin et al (2011).

Sternal Instability. Sternal instability refers to excessive movement of the two sternal halves due to disruption of the wires connecting the surgically divided sternum (El-Ansary et al 2007a, Robicsek et al 2000). It has a documented incidence of 0.4% to 8% (Losanoff et al 2002, Olbrecht et al 2006, Ramzisham et al 2009, Robicsek et al 2000). A range of risk factors are thought to contribute to the development of this complication (Abid et al 2001, Bitkover et al 1998, El-Ansary et al 2007b, King et al 2009, McDonald et al 1989, Olbrecht et al 2006, Robicsek et al 2000, Vymazal et al 2009). Cahalin et al (2011) categorized these risks as primary or secondary in order to guide the clinician in the prescription of sternal precautions (see Table 11-6).

If sternal complications are identified early, timely medical management can reduce the risk of further progression to mediastinitis, which has an associated mortality of up to 50% (Grevious et al 2014, Robicsek et al 2000).

Assessment of sternal stability following sternotomy constitutes best practice in postoperative care. As most sternal wound complications are identified after discharge from hospital by health professionals, it is imperative to assess and screen patients in cardiac rehabilitation and community settings (El-Ansary et al 2000b, Ridderstolpe et al 2001).

The SIS is a physical examination test that has been developed to identify and grade instability. This scale is a four-point numeral scale that ranges from 0 (no detectable sternal motion) to 3 (complete sternal instability) (Table 11-7). The SIS is valid and reliable with reported intra-rater and inter-rater reliability of 0.98 and 0.99 respectively (El-Ansary et al 2000a). It is important that sternal instability be reported to the cardiothoracic surgeon or medical practitioner caring for the patient to ensure optimal management (surgical or conservative).

Sternal Instability Management. Treatment of sternal instability usually requires surgical re-wiring, but at times this is not an option if patients have

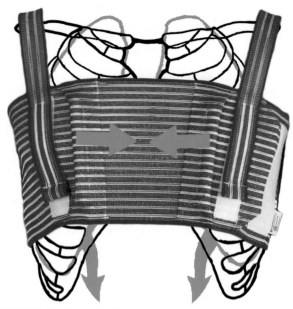

FIGURE 11-10 ■ QualiBreath sternal support device – an orthopaedic stabilization brace for a median sternotomy. *(Image courtesy of Qualiteam s.r.l., 2015, www.qualiteam.com.)*

confounding risk factors. As such, clinicians are often consulted about activity and exercise guidelines for patients with sternal instability. It has been suggested that bilateral upper limb movements result in less sheer at the sternal edges and this explains why patients tolerate these symmetrical movements of the upper limb preferentially (El-Ansary et al 2007b). Activity modification to include bilateral upper limb movements and care with trunk motion may further facilitate bone healing. Recently, non-surgical management options of sternal instability have emerged, including the use of supportive devices (e.g. QualiBreath) to minimize patient symptoms (Fig. 11-10). Supportive devices may also be used as an interim measure, prior to surgical repair or to prevent the progression of a minimally unstable sternum (El-Ansary et al 2008). In patients with chronic sternal instability, specific trunk stabilization exercises that facilitated the recruitment of the muscles of the abdominal wall performed for 10 minutes twice a day over a 6-week period resulted in less sternal separation and in a significant reduction in pain with activity (El-Ansary et al 2007c).

Specific Considerations for Women Undergoing Cardiac Surgery. Following cardiac surgery women are reported to have greater disruption to functional activities yet resume household tasks earlier than men (King 2001). In women there is a significant correlation between chest circumference and sternal complications as well as ongoing incisional pain (King et al 2008). As such, it may be appropriate that women wear a supportive bra (with wide straps and no underwire) early in the postoperative period to ensure support of their breasts to prevent sternal wound breakdown (e.g. Qualibra Advanced). They may also benefit from rehabilitation that targets functional tasks and education about pain and scar management. Key points in cardiac surgery are given in Box 11-11.

SPECIAL CONSIDERATIONS FOLLOWING SURGERY

The key points in managing drips and drains can be found in Box 11-12.

BOX 11-12
KEY POINTS FOR THE PHYSIOTHERAPIST IN MANAGING DRIPS AND DRAINS

- Ensure there is adequate tubing to roll, sit up and ambulate the patient without pulling lines.
- Note dosage/rate of drugs being delivered, especially by infusion pumps. For patient-controlled analgesia (PCA), note if the system is in patient 'lock-out mode'. Patients will be unable to use delivery button until the lockout signal is cleared.
- For pumps, note the alarm silence button. If the alarm sounds, contact the nursing staff.
- All pumps can run on battery, but ensure cords are plugged into wall supply when patients are non-ambulant.
- All pumps can be transferred to mobile intravenous poles. Nursing staff may need to assist with some types of PCA pump transfer, as they need to be unlocked with keys.
- Care and consultation is required if you plan to use the head-down position with a patient who is being enterally fed.
- For patients with a colostomy or ileostomy, observe for leakages before moving the patient. If full of air or fluid, the bag will require emptying before mobilizing or rolling the patient.
- Ensure a nasogastric tube is always supported after positioning a patient so there is no traction on the patient's nose to reduce the risk of disconnecting the tubing. Dislodging a nasogastric tube may lead to aspiration and may not be possible to replace the tube for example following oesophageal surgery.
- In relation to drips and drains, the following points are not your specific responsibility but should be noted.
  - Check patency of drip: Is it running?
  - Is there blood tracking in the tubing? This is a sign that the drip may be too slow, hence not causing enough pressure to resist blood flow. Notify nursing staff.
  - Has the IV line tissued? The entrance point is allowing fluid to enter subcutaneously rather than intravenously. If the skin around the insertion site becomes swollen and tender notify nursing staff.

Postoperative prevention of venous thromboembolism (VTE): VTE encompasses the clinical conditions of deep vein thrombosis (DVT) and pulmonary embolism (PE). Further details of VTE can be found in Chapter 4. Typically, prevention of VTE following major surgery consists of pharmacological and mechanical thromboprophylaxis, including the use of graduated compression stockings, intermittent pneumatic compression devices, foot pumps and early ambulation. Major abdominal, cardiothoracic and vascular surgeries increase the risk of VTE, and therefore thromboprophylaxis is recommended for all patients undergoing these surgeries (NHMRC 2009). Physiotherapists working with patients following major surgery should be aware of strategies to reduce the risk of VTE. Two meta-analyses of interest to physiotherapists have considered the effects of early ambulation on VTE. Both of these meta-analyses suggest that prescribing early ambulation as part of the early management of patients following surgery both presenting with DVT and/or PE or in the prevention of DVT and PE is safe (Aissaouil et al 2009, Anderson et al (2009).

Acknowledgements

We wish to thank our physiotherapy colleagues Ms Meave Sorohan and Dr Andrew Hirchhorn for their suggestions and input. Additionally, we would like to acknowledge the clinicians of the University of Melbourne Clinical Schools in Australia who jointly contributed the information presented from the cardiorespiratory practice manuals of the Department of Physiotherapy.

APPENDIX

TABLE A11-1
Randomized Controlled Trials of Physiotherapy in Upper Abdominal Surgery (Since 2000–2013) in Order of Physiotherapy Evidence Database (PEDro) Score (www.pedro.org.au)

Primary Author (Year) PEDro Score	Patient Population (Sample Size)	Intervention/s	Results	Conclusions
Carneiro et al (2013) 3/10	Abdominal surgery patients (n = 75)	■ Control: Usual care. No breathing exercises. ■ Intervention: Sustained deep inspiration breathing exercises (×1 daily, 24 hours preop, POD 1 and POD 2). Three sets of 10 breaths.	■ No significant differences for: 1) pulmonary function, 2) endocrine or immune responses and 3) incidence of PPC between groups. However, the intervention group demonstrated a trend towards fewer PPCs.	■ Intervention shows no improvement in pulmonary function, endocrine or immune responses and incidence of PPC.
Kulkarni et al (2010) 5/10	Major abdominal surgery (n = 66)	■ Control: No intervention. ■ Intervention 1: DBE. ■ Intervention 2: IS. ■ Intervention 3: IMT. ■ Participants in intervention groups asked to perform breathing exercises (over 2 week postop period, 15-minute duration, ×2 daily).	■ IMT group demonstrated a significant increase in MIP during the intervention period, which was maintained postoperatively (POD 1–7).	■ Preop IMT may improve postop MIP in patients undergoing major abdominal surgery.
Soares et al (2013) 5/10	Upper abdominal surgery patients (n = 32)	■ Control: Usual care: Postop physiotherapy (POD 1–7, 45 minute duration, ×1 daily). Supervised sessions. DBE, huffing/coughing techniques, early mobilization and active UL/LL exercises. Participants encouraged to continue respiratory and limb exercises independently (×1 daily). ■ Intervention: Usual care + preop physical therapy programme 2–3 weeks preop. Preop programme (50 minute duration, ×2/week. Supervised sessions. Respiratory muscle training (IMT, 15-minute duration, active UL/LL exercises, walking). Participants encouraged to continue respiratory muscle training and walking independently (×4/week).	■ Intervention group demonstrated a significantly: 1) greater MIP and respiratory muscle endurance in the preop period, 2) greater MIP, respiratory muscle endurance, functional independence and 6MWT distance at POD 7 and 3) lower incidence of PPC compared to the control group.	■ Preop IMT and exercise improve pulmonary and functional recovery.

Continued on following page

TABLE A11-1

Randomized Controlled Trials of Physiotherapy in Upper Abdominal Surgery (Since 2000–2013) in Order of Physiotherapy Evidence Database (PEDro) Score (www.pedro.org.au) *(Continued)*

Primary Author (Year) PEDro Score	Patient Population (Sample Size)	Intervention/s	Results	Conclusions
Kindgen-Milles et al (2005) 6/10	Thoracoabdominal aortic aneurysm repair (n = 50)	■ Postop physiotherapy: Respiratory physiotherapy (manual vibration), positioning and early mobilization. ■ Intervention 1: Humidified oxygen via facemask (flow = 25 L/min) and intermittent nCPAP (every 4–10 hours post-extubation). Expiratory pressure = 10 cmH$_2$O. ■ Intervention 2: Continuous nCPAP (12–24 hours post-extubation). Humidified air/oxygen, flow = 65 L/min, expiratory pressure = 10 cmH$_2$O.	■ Intervention 2 demonstrated a significant: 1) increase in PaO$_2$/FiO$_2$ ratio, 2) decrease in incidence of PPC and 3) decrease in hospital length of stay compared to intervention 1. ■ No significant differences in haemodynamic measures between interventions and oxygen transfer was similar between groups once intervention 2 ceased.	■ Continuous nCPAP may lead to a transient improvement in oxygen transfer and reduce the incidence of PPC and hospital length of stay in patients post-thoracoabdominal aortic aneurysm repair.
Dronkers et al (2008) 7/10	Abdominal aortic aneurysm surgery patients at high risk of PPC (n = 20)	■ Control: Usual care: Preoperative education on diaphragmatic breathing, deep inspiration, IS and cough/FET. ■ Intervention 1: Usual care + preop IMT (15-minute duration over at least 2-week preop period, ×1/week with supervision, ×5/week independently). Commenced at 20% MIP. ■ All participants received same postop physical therapy: deep inspiration +/− IS, diaphragmatic inspiration and cough/FET and encouragement to SOOB/mobilize early.	■ No significant differences between groups for: 1) incidence of PPC, 2) inspiratory muscle strength and 3) VC. ■ Preop IMT well tolerated by participants and there was a trend towards: 1) faster recovery of inspiratory muscle strength and 2) decreased incidence of PPC for participants in this group.	■ Although well tolerated by participants, the addition of preop IMT does not decrease the incidence of PPC or improve pulmonary function in patients at high risk of PPC following abdominal aortic aneurysm surgery.
Forgiarini et al (2009) 7/10	Open abdominal surgery patients (n = 36)	■ Intervention 1: Physical therapy in recovery room (not standardized, but included diaphragmatic proprioception, inflating respiratory patterns, forced expiratory manoeuvres, expiratory delay and supported cough) and infirmary (included addition of early mobilization). ■ Intervention 2: Physical therapy in infirmary alone.	■ Compared to preop measures, there was a: 1) significant decrease in FVC and FEV$_1$ in intervention 2 and 2) significant decrease in MEP in both intervention groups.	■ Early physical therapy (in the recovery room) minimizes the decrease in pulmonary function and respiratory muscle strength.

Randomized Controlled Trials of Physiotherapy in Upper Abdominal Surgery (Since 2000–2013) in Order of Physiotherapy Evidence Database (PEDro) Score (www.pedro.org.au) *(Continued)*

Primary Author (Year) PEDro Score	Patient Population (Sample Size)	Intervention/s	Results	Conclusions
Silva et al (2013) 7/10	Open upper abdominal surgery patients at high risk of PPC (n = 86)	■ Postop physiotherapy (POD 1 to discharge from acute physiotherapy, ×1 daily). ■ Intervention 1: Moderate intensity, early mobilization (commenced POD 1). Moderate intensity. ■ Intervention 2: Moderate intensity, early mobilization + breathing exercises with supervision: four sets of 5 deep breaths. ■ Intervention 3: Moderate intensity, delayed mobilization (commenced post-POD 3) + breathing exercises with supervision. ■ Participants encouraged to mobilize as tolerated and continue breathing exercises hourly, while awake.	■ Intervention 1 had a significantly reduced hospital length of stay compared to the other interventions (Note: Participants in intervention 2 had a greater incidence of PPC compared to intervention 1). ■ No significant differences between the interventions for: 1) the incidence of PPC and 2) days until discharge from acute physiotherapy.	■ The addition of breathing exercises to an early mobilization programme does not reduce the incidence of PPC in patients post open upper abdominal surgery who are at high risk of PPC.
Denehy et al (2001) 8/10	Upper abdominal surgery patients (n = 50)	■ Postop physiotherapy (POD 1–3, minimum 10-minute duration, ×2 daily). ■ Control: Usual care: DBE, FET, supported cough and early mobilization. Participants also encouraged to continue hourly DBE independently. ■ Intervention 1: Usual care + PCPAP (15-minute duration, ×4 daily). PEEP = 10 cmH$_2$O, FiO$_2$ = 30%, flow rate = 30 L/min. ■ Intervention 3: Usual care + PCPAP (30 minute duration, ×4 daily). PEEP = 10 cmH$_2$O, FiO$_2$ = 30%, flow rate = 30 L/min.	■ No significant differences between groups for: 1) FRC, VC and SpO$_2$, 2) pain, 3) incidence of PPC and 4) length of hospital stay. ■ There was a trend towards: 1) faster recovery of FRC and 2) decreased incidence of PPC in the PCPAP groups.	■ The addition of PCPAP did not have any significant benefits on physiological and clinical outcomes for patients following upper abdominal surgery.
Mackay et al (2005) 8/10	Open abdominal patients at high risk of developing PPC (n = 50)	■ Postop physiotherapy (×3 daily POD 1–2, ×2 daily POD 3–4, ×1 daily until participants mobilized independently AND had a clear chest assessment). ■ **Control:** Usual care of early mobilization + ankle exercises ■ **Intervention:** Usual care + DBE	■ No significant differences in the incidence of PPC or the restoration of mobility between groups.	■ The addition of deep breathing and coughing exercises to an early mobilization programme did reduce the incidence of PPC in high-risk patients

6MWT, 6-Minute walk test; *DBE,* deep breathing exercises; *FET,* forced expiration technique; *FEV$_1$,* forced expiratory volume in 1 second; *FiO$_2$,* fraction of inspired oxygen; *FRC,* functional residual capacity; *FVC,* forced vital capacity; *IMT,* inspiratory muscle training; *IS,* incentive spirometry; *LL,* lower limb; *MEP,* maximal expiratory pressure; *MIP,* maximal inspiratory pressure; *n,* number; *nCPAP,* nasal continuous positive airway pressure; *PaO$_2$,* partial pressure of oxygen; *PCPAP,* periodic continuous positive airway pressure; *PEEP,* positive end-expiratory pressure; *POD,* postoperative day; *Postop,* postoperative; *PPC,* postoperative pulmonary complication; *Preop,* preoperative; *SOOB,* sitting out of bed; *SpO$_2$,* oxygen saturation; *UL,* upper limb; *VC,* vital capacity.

TABLE A11-2

Randomized Controlled Trials of Physiotherapy in Thoracic Surgery (Since 2000–2013) in Order of Physiotherapy Evidence Database (PEDro) Score (www.pedro.org.au).

Primary Author (Year) PEDro Score	Patient Population (Sample Size)	Intervention/s	Results	Conclusions
Ludwig et al (2011) 2/10	Lung resection patients (n = 135)	■ Control: Pressure expiration, diaphragmatic breathing, posture correction, stretching and shoulder girdle exercises. ■ Treatment: Control + IPPB (×3 daily; 15–20 mmHg).	■ No significant differences between groups for the incidence of PPC or any other outcomes.	■ The addition of IPPB did not appear to improve patient outcomes following lung resection surgery.
Olsen et al (2002) 5/10	Thoracoabdominal resection patients (n = 70)	■ Intervention 1: Breathing exercises by IR-PEP. ■ Intervention 2: Breathing exercises by CPAP	■ Both groups demonstrated a significant decrease in respiratory variables. ■ Intervention 1 demonstrated a significantly higher rate of re-intubation. ■ No other significant differences between groups (LOS and morbidity).	■ The addition of CPAP may prevent the rate of re-intubation in patients post thoracoabdominal resection surgery.
Park et al (2012) 5/10	Lung resection patients (n = 90)	■ Control: Routine percussive chest physiotherapy (×4 daily, performed by nursing staff). ■ Intervention: HFCWO (every 8 hours for 15 minutes)	■ Intervention group demonstrated a significant improvement in: 1) FEV_1 on POD 3 and POD 5 and 2) arterial oxygenation on POD 1 compared to the control group.	■ HFCWO appears to facilitate faster recovery of pulmonary function in patients following lung resection.
Gosselink et al (2000) 6/10	Thoracic surgery patients (n = 67)	■ Control: Postop CPT only. ■ Intervention: Postop CPT with IS.	■ No significant differences between groups for: 1) incidence of PPC (even after breakdown of surgery type), 2) LOS and 3) FEV_1 recovery.	■ The addition of IS does not appear to improve patient outcomes post thoracic surgery.
Agostini et al (2013a) 6/10	Lung resection surgery patients (n = 181)	■ Control: Usual care including TEE, supported cough, early ambulation and shoulder exercises ■ Intervention: Control (minus TEE) + IS.	■ No significant differences between groups for: 1) incidence of PPC (for high-and low-risk groups), 2) FEV_1 drop, 3) LOS, 4) insertion of 'rescue' mini-tracheostomy and 5) in-hospital mortality.	■ The addition of IS does not appear to improve patient outcomes post-lung resection. ■ Further research in the high-risk population may be warranted.

TABLE A11-2

Randomized Controlled Trials of Physiotherapy in Thoracic Surgery (Since 2000–2013) in Order of Physiotherapy Evidence Database (PEDro) Score (www.pedro.org.au) (Continued)

Primary Author (Year) PEDro Score	Patient Population (Sample Size)	Intervention/s	Results	Conclusions
Arbane et al (2011) 7/10	Lung resection patients (n = 53)	■ Control: Standard care. ■ Intervention: Control + postop strength and mobility training (×2 daily). 12-week home exercise programme with three home visits from therapist.	■ Significant difference in change in quadriceps strength between groups at POD 5 (decrease in strength in control group and increase in strength in intervention group). No significant differences between groups at 12 weeks. ■ Both groups demonstrated a significant decrease in 6MWT distance at POD 5, but returned to preop levels at 12 weeks. ■ No other significant differences between groups (LOS, postop complications, HRQoL)	■ While postop strength and mobility training appears to minimize the loss of quadriceps strength immediately following lung resection surgery, there were no significant benefits at 12 weeks.
Reeve et al (2010a) 8/10	Lung resection patients (n = 76)	■ Control: Standard care + no physiotherapy. ■ Intervention: Standard care + respiratory physiotherapy (daily).	■ No significant differences between groups for: 1) incidence of PPC and 2) LOS.	■ Respiratory physiotherapy does not appear to improve patient outcomes in patients following lung resection surgery.
Reeve et al (2010b) 8/10	Lung resection patients (n = 76)	■ Control: Standard care + no physiotherapy. ■ Intervention: Supervised shoulder and mobilization exercises (daily). Discharge exercise sheet.	■ Intervention group demonstrated significantly: 1) less shoulder pain and total pain at discharge and 2) improved shoulder function and HRQoL at 3 months, compared to the control group. ■ No significant differences between groups for: 1) shoulder ROM and 2) shoulder strength.	■ The addition of a shoulder exercise programme appears to reduce pain and improve HRQoL in patients post lung resection surgery.
Bonde et al (2002) No score	High-risk lung resection surgery patients (n = 102)	■ *Control:* Standard care (including postop CPT). ■ *Intervention:* Control + mini-tracheostomy.	■ Intervention group demonstrated significantly fewer incidences of postop sputum retention compared to the control group. ■ No significant differences between groups for: 1) chest infection, 2) physiotherapy visits/day, 3) sputum-related life-threatening incidents. ■ Trend towards fewer sputum-related deaths in intervention group, compared to the control group.	■ The insertion of a mini-tracheostomy may lead to fewer incidences of sputum retention in high-risk patients following lung resection surgery.

6MWT, 6-Minute walk test; *CPAP*, continuous positive airway pressure; *CPT*, chest physiotherapy; *FEV₁*, forced expiratory volume in 1 second; *HFCWO*, high frequency chest wall oscillation; *HRQoL*, health related quality of life; *IPPB*, intermittent positive pressure breathing; *IR-PEP*, inspiratory resistance positive expiratory pressure; *IS*, incentive spirometry; *LOS*, length of stay; *POD*, postoperative day; *postop*, postoperative; *PPC*, postoperative pulmonary complication; *preop*, preoperative; *ROM*, range of motion; *TEE*, thoracic expansion exercise.

TABLE A11-3				
Randomized Controlled Trials of Physiotherapy in Cardiac Surgery (Since 2000–2013) in Order of PEDro Score				
Primary Author (Year) PEDro Score	**Patient Population (Sample Size)**	**Intervention/s**	**Results**	**Conclusions**
Renault et al (2009) 2/10	CABG surgery patients (n = 36)	▪ Postop physiotherapy (commenced 24 hours post extubation, ×2 daily in ICU, ×1 daily on ward). ▪ Intervention 1 (DBE): Three sets of 10 DBE (focus on diaphragmatic breathing) and assisted cough and/or huff and early mobilization. ▪ Intervention 2 (IS): Three sets of 10 DBE with IS + assisted cough and/or huff and early mobilization.	▪ Both interventions demonstrated a: 1) significant decrease in FVC and FEV_1, 2) partial recovery of maximal respiratory pressures and 3) complete recovery of oxygen saturations at POD 7. ▪ No significant differences between two interventions for FVC, FEV_1, maximal respiratory pressures and oxygen saturation.	▪ DBE, with and without IS, appears to have similar effects during the early postoperative period following CABG surgery. ▪ The benefit of these exercises remains unclear.
Macchi et al (2007) 3/10	Cardiac surgery patients (n = 300)	▪ Inpatient CR (3 week duration): Physical therapy (×2 hours daily). Cycle ergometry, callisthenics exercises with resistance and passive stretching. ▪ Intervention 1 (Early CR): Commenced within second postop week. ▪ Intervention 2 (Late CR): Commenced within fourth postop week.	▪ Significantly greater occurrence of new-onset AF in intervention 1. ▪ No significant differences between two interventions for mortality rate, occurrence of non-fatal events, 6MWCT, control of cardiovascular risk factors and HRQoL at 1 year follow-up.	▪ Apart from the greater occurrence of new-onset AF in early CR, both interventions appear to have similar benefits on patients following CABG surgery at 1 year follow-up.
Franco et al (2011) 3/10	CABG surgery patients (n = 26)	▪ Postop physiotherapy. ▪ Control (CRT): Diaphragmatic breathing, cough/sputum clearance techniques and UL/LL exercises (performed ×2 daily). ▪ Intervention: CRT + BiPAP (30-minute duration, ×2 daily). Spontaneous mode, inspiratory pressure = 8–12 cmH_2O; expiratory pressure = 6 cmH_2O.	▪ Both groups demonstrated a/an: 1) significant decrease in MV, TV, VC, expiratory PF, MIP and MEP, 2) significant increase in RR and 3) occurrence of PPC post extubation. ▪ Intervention group demonstrated a significantly greater recovery of VC than control group.	▪ The addition of BiPAP may aid in the quicker recovery of pulmonary function in patients following cardiac surgery.
Westerdahl et al (2005) 4/10	CABG surgery patients (n = 90)	▪ Control: Usual care: Preop education and postop physiotherapy ×1–2 daily. Early mobilization, coughing technique, active shoulder girdle/upper back exercises. No breathing exercises prescribed. ▪ Intervention: Usual care + breathing exercises with positive expiratory pressure blow bottle (POD 1–4, ×1 hourly during day). 30 deep breaths, expiratory pressure = 10 cmH_2O.	▪ Intervention group demonstrated a significantly smaller: 1) increase in atelectatic area and 2) decline in FVC and FEV_1 compared to the control group at POD 4. ▪ No significant differences between groups for PaO_2, $PaCO_2$, incidence of fever and ICU/hospital length of stay.	▪ The addition of a positive expiratory pressure blow bottle may facilitate improved recovery of pulmonary function and incidence of PPC after CABG surgery.

TABLE A11-3
Randomized Controlled Trials of Physiotherapy in Cardiac Surgery (Since 2000–2013) in Order of PEDro Score *(Continued)*

Primary Author (Year) PEDro Score	Patient Population (Sample Size)	Intervention/s	Results	Conclusions
Chuang et al (2005) 4/10	CABG surgery patients (n = 32)	■ Incremental treadmill training (30 minute duration, ×2/week over 3 months in hospital). Intensity = 70–80% max HR, 60–75% VO_2 max, 11–15 on BORG scale. ■ Intervention 1: Without VR. ■ Intervention 2: With VR.	■ Intervention 2 achieved a significantly higher: 1) peak VO_2, 2) peak METS and 3) VO_2 at anaerobic threshold than intervention 1.	■ Inpatient CR with VR may improve oxygen consumption and exercise capacity in patients following CABG surgery.
Borghi-Silva et al (2005) 4/10	Cardiac surgery patients (n = 24)	■ Control: Usual care: Postop physiotherapy (POD 1 to discharge from hospital, 30-minute duration, ×2 daily. Breathing exercises, airway clearance, active UL/LL exercises and early mobilization. ■ Intervention: Usual care + breathing exercises with expiratory positive airway pressure mask (×2 daily). Three sets of 20 breaths, expiratory pressure = 10 cmH_2O.	■ Control group demonstrated a significant decline in VC, FEV_1, FEF 25–75%, FVC and PF at POD 5. ■ Intervention group only demonstrated a significant decline in VC at POD 5. ■ Decline in PF was significantly greater in control group, compared to intervention group. ■ MIP declined significantly in both groups at POD 1. However, by POD 5, only the control group demonstrated a significant decline in MIP compared to preop.	■ The addition of breathing exercises with expiratory positive airway pressure may facilitate better recovery of pulmonary function and inspiratory muscle strength after cardiac surgery.
Mendes et al (2010) 5/10	CABG surgery patients (n = 47)	■ Postop physiotherapy. ■ Control: Usual care: DBE (×1 daily with supervision, participants encouraged to continue same every hour, while awake). Four sets of 10 breaths and supported huff/cough. ■ Intervention: Usual care + exercise programme encouraging early mobilization (×1 daily with supervision).	■ Intervention group demonstrated significantly higher: 1) parasympathetic HR variability and 2) R-R interval at discharge from hospital, compared to the control group.	■ Early mobilization may improve autonomic cardiac function in the short-term in patients following CABG surgery.

Continued on following page

TABLE A11-3				
Randomized Controlled Trials of Physiotherapy in Cardiac Surgery (Since 2000–2013) in Order of PEDro Score *(Continued)*				
Primary Author (Year) PEDro Score	Patient Population (Sample Size)	Intervention/s	Results	Conclusions
Ferreira et al (2010) 5/10	CABG surgery patients (n = 16)	■ Postop physiotherapy (POD 1 to discharge from hospital). Control: Usual care: early mobilization, DBE and cough technique. ■ Intervention: Usual care + IS with expiratory positive airway pressure (15-minute duration, ×2 daily with supervision, ×2 daily independently). Expiratory pressure commenced at 5 cmH$_2$O. Participants encouraged to continue IS with expiratory positive airway pressure independently (×2 daily over 4-week period post discharge from hospital).	■ 18 months postop, there were no significant differences in: 1) pulmonary function, 2) 6MWT distance and 3) physical activity levels between groups. ■ Intervention group demonstrated a significantly: 1) lower sensation of perceived effort post 6MWT, 2) lower sensation of dyspnoea post 6MWT and 3) higher HRQoL (for limitations of physical aspects) compared to the control group, 18 months postop.	■ The addition of IS with expiratory positive airway pressure may reduce perceived effort and dyspnoea as well as increase HRQoL in patients following CABG surgery.
Urell et al (2011) 5/10	OHS patients (n = 107)	■ Postop physiotherapy: circulation exercises, coughing techniques, early mobilization and shoulder girdle exercises + breathing exercises with positive expiratory pressure device (POD 1–2, hourly during day). Expiratory pressure = 10–15 cmH$_2$O. ■ Intervention 1: One set of 10 breathing exercises with positive expiratory pressure device. Intervention 2: Three sets of 10 breathing exercises with positive expiratory pressure device.	■ Intervention 2 demonstrated significantly higher PaO$_2$ and SpO$_2$ levels than intervention 1. ■ No significant differences for: 1) pulmonary function and 2) postop pain between groups.	■ Higher frequency breathing exercises with a positive expiratory pressure device may improve PaO$_2$ and SpO$_2$ levels in patients post OHS.
Smith et al (2011) 5/10	CABG surgery patients (n = 144)	■ CR (30–50-minute duration, ×3/week). 60–80% target HR reserve. Education also provided on general exercise guidelines (minimum of 20-minute duration, ×5–7/week). ■ Intervention 1: Independent home-based CR: Walking and customized exercises according to environment/equipment available. ■ Intervention 2: Supervised hospital based CR: Treadmill training, stationary cycling, arm ergometry, stair climbing.	■ At 6-year follow-up, home-based CR group demonstrated a significantly higher: 1) mean peak VO$_2$ and 2) PASE score compared to the hospital based CR group.	■ Home-based CR appears to lead to better long-term benefits to exercise capacity and physical activity than hospital based CR, in patients post CABG.

TABLE A11-3

Randomized Controlled Trials of Physiotherapy in Cardiac Surgery (Since 2000–2013) in Order of PEDro Score *(Continued)*

Primary Author (Year) PEDro Score	Patient Population (Sample Size)	Intervention/s	Results	Conclusions
Moholdt et al (2012) 5/10	CABG surgery patients (n = 30)	■ Intervention 1: Conventional supervised inpatient CR programme (4-week duration). Endurance-type exercises including walking, skiing, cycling, ball games and strength training. Participants encouraged to continue exercise training independently over remaining 5 months. ■ Intervention 2: Unsupervised, home-based aerobic interval training (×3/week, 6-month duration). ×4 4-minute high intensity intervals at 85–95% max HR. ×3 min moderate intensity intervals in between at 70% max HR. Exercises included walking, cycling, jogging and swimming.	■ At 6 months follow-up, both groups demonstrated a significant improvement in: 1) VO_2 peak and 2) HRQoL. ■ No significant differences between groups for any of the outcome measures.	■ Home-based aerobic interval training appears to have similar benefits to conventional inpatient CR in patients following CABG surgery at 6 month follow-up.
Matte et al (2000) 6/10	CABG surgery patients (n = 98)	■ Postop physiotherapy (POD 1 post extubation to POD 2). Coughing exercises, aerosol therapy and mobilization. ■ Intervention 1: Usual care + IS (one set every 2 hours). 20 deep breaths. ■ Intervention 2: Usual care + intermittent CPAP (1 hour every 3 hours). Expiratory pressure = 5 cmH_2O. ■ Intervention 3: Usual care + intermittent BiPAP (1 hour every 3 hours). Expiratory pressure = 5 cmH_2O, Inspiratory pressure = 12 cmH_2O.	■ All groups demonstrated a significant decrease in: 1) VC and FEV_1 and 2) SpO_2 at POD 1. ■ Interventions 2 and 3 demonstrated a significant: 1) increase in VC and FEV_1, 2) increase in SpO_2 and 3) decrease in venous admixture compared to intervention 1. ■ No significant differences in: 1) incidence of PPC, 2) CO and 3) length of ICU stay between groups.	■ The use of CPAP or BiPAP may reduce the decline in pulmonary function and oxygen saturation in patients following CABG surgery.

Continued on following page

	TABLE A11-3			
Randomized Controlled Trials of Physiotherapy in Cardiac Surgery (Since 2000–2013) in Order of PEDro Score *(Continued)*				
Primary Author (Year) PEDro Score	**Patient Population (Sample Size)**	**Intervention/s**	**Results**	**Conclusions**
Wu et al (2006) 6/10	CABG surgery patients (n = 54)	■ Control: Usual care: No formal CR programme post discharge from hospital. ■ Intervention 1: Inpatient CR post discharge from hospital (12-week duration). Supervised aerobic exercise programme: stationary bicycle or treadmill jogging (30–60-minute duration, ×3/week). 60–85% peak HR. ■ Intervention 2: Home-based CR post discharge from hospital (12-week duration). Unsupervised aerobic exercise programme: fast walking or jogging (30–60-minute duration, ×3/week). 60–85% peak HR.	■ Both groups demonstrated a significant improvement in HR recovery. ■ Intervention 1 demonstrated a significant increase in HR recovery compared to the control group. ■ No significant differences in HR recovery between: 1) inpatient and home-based CR groups and 2) home-based CR and control groups.	■ Inpatient CR appears to significantly improve HR recovery in patients following CABG surgery. ■ Further research into home-based CR is warranted.
Savci et al (2006) 6/10	CABG surgery (n = 60)	■ Postop physiotherapy: DBE, coughing and huffing techniques, early mobilization, active UL/thorax exercises. ■ Intervention 1: Usual care + ACBT (15-minute duration, ×2 daily POD 1–2, ×1 daily POD 3). 3 deep breaths + SMI + FET/huffing and breathing control. ■ Intervention 2: Usual care + IS (15-minute duration, ×2 daily POD 1–2, ×1 daily POD 3). Three deep breaths + SMI + huffing and breathing control.	■ Both groups demonstrated a significant: 1) decrease VC, FVC, FEV_1 and PEF, 2) decrease in 6MWT distance and 3) increase in SpO_2. ■ No significant differences between groups for: 1) VC, FVC, FEV_1 and PEF, 2) arterial blood gas values, 3) 6MWT distance, 4) postop pain and 5) incidence of PPC.	■ ACBT and breathing exercises with IS both appear to have similar effects on patients following CABG. ■ The benefit of these exercises remain unclear.
Haeffener et al (2008) 6/10	CABG surgery patients (n = 34)	■ Control: Usual care: Education regarding DBE, coughing technique and early mobilization. ■ Intervention: Postop IS training and expiratory positive airway pressure (15–20-minute duration, ×2 daily. Performed under supervision. Expiratory pressure commenced at 5 cmH_2O. Participants encouraged to continue above on discharge (15-minute duration, ×2 daily, independently).	■ Intervention group demonstrated a significantly: 1) increased MIP and MEP, 2) greater recovery of pulmonary function, 3) increased 6MWT distance 4) decreased length of hospital stay and 5) decreased incidence of PPC compared to the control group. ■ At 1 year postop, the intervention group still had a significantly greater MIP, pulmonary function and 6MWT distance.	■ Postop IS training and expiratory positive airway pressure appears to improve MIP, MEP, pulmonary function and walking capacity in patients following CABG surgery. ■ It may also reduce length of hospital stay and the incidence of PPC in this population.

TABLE A11-3

Randomized Controlled Trials of Physiotherapy in Cardiac Surgery (Since 2000–2013) in Order of PEDro Score *(Continued)*

Primary Author (Year) PEDro Score	Patient Population (Sample Size)	Intervention/s	Results	Conclusions
Moholdt et al (2009) 6/10	CABG surgery patients (n = 48)	■ Inpatient rehabilitation 4–16 weeks postop (5 days/week, 4-week duration): Aerobic exercise training programme. ■ Intervention 1: Aerobic interval training (×4 4-minute intervals of treadmill training at 90% maximum HR. Active rests of 3 minute intervals at 70% maximum HR. ■ Intervention 2: Moderate continuous treadmill training. Continuous training at 70% maximum HR. ■ Additional exercises similar across interventions. At discharge, all participants advised to continue exercise at same intensity (×3–4/ week).	■ Both interventions demonstrated a significant increase in: 1) VO_2 peak, 2) HR recovery and 3) HRQoL following a 4-week period of inpatient rehabilitation. ■ At 6 months post discharge from inpatient rehabilitation: 1) intervention 1 demonstrated a further significant increase in VO_2 peak and 2) the increase in HR recovery and HRQoL were maintained in both groups.	■ Aerobic exercise training appears to improve VO_2 peak, HR recovery and HRQoL in the short term in patients post CABG. ■ Aerobic interval training may lead to better long-term improvements in VO_2 peak in this population.
Wright et al (2002) 6/10	CABG surgery patients (n = 22)	■ Control: No inpatient CR. ■ Intervention: Inpatient CR approximately 6 weeks postop (×1/week, 6-week duration). 12 aerobic exercises performed under supervision. Repetitions/workload gradually increased.	■ Peak VO_2 improved significantly in both groups. ■ Intervention group demonstrated a significant: 1) decrease in rate of ventilation/VO_2 and rate of ventilation/VCO_2 and 2) increase in peak CO, cardiac power output and cardiac reserve. ■ No significant differences in all outcome measures between groups.	■ Even low intensity inpatient CR may improve cardiac and pulmonary function in patients post CABG surgery. ■ Further research on optimal dosage is required.
Savci et al (2011) 6/10	CABG surgery patients (n = 43)	■ Control Usual care: Postop physiotherapy (×1 daily). Early mobilization, UL/LL active exercises and breathing exercises/ coughing techniques). ■ Intervention 1: Usual care + IMT (5 days preop and 5 days postop; 30-minute duration, ×2 daily. Performed under supervision. Resistance commenced at 15% of inspiratory muscle strength.	■ Both groups demonstrated a significant decrease in FEV_1 and FVC at discharge from hospital. ■ Inspiratory muscle strength improved significantly from preop to discharge in the intervention group. ■ Intervention group demonstrated a significant: 1) decrease in ICU length of stay, 2) increase in 6MWT distance, 3) increase in HRQoL for sleep and 3) decrease in anxiety compared to the control group.	■ IMT (preop and postop) may facilitate quicker recovery of inspiratory muscle strength and function, HRQoL and anxiety in patients post CABG surgery. It may also reduce postop ICU length stay in this population.

Continued on following page

TABLE A11-3				
Randomized Controlled Trials of Physiotherapy in Cardiac Surgery (Since 2000–2013) in Order of PEDro Score *(Continued)*				
Primary Author (Year) PEDro Score	**Patient Population (Sample Size)**	**Intervention/s**	**Results**	**Conclusions**
Kodric et al (2013) 6/10	Patients who developed diaphragm paralysis after major cardiac surgery (n = 52)	■ Control: Sham IMT (device with no resistance). ■ Intervention: IMT (commenced within 4 weeks postop until 1 year postop; ×1 daily). Resistance started at 30% of MIP.	■ No significant differences in FEV_1, VC, FEV_1/VC, FEF 25–75%, TLC, IC and RV between groups 1 year postop. ■ Intervention group demonstrated a significant increase in MIP and greater recovery of diaphragm mobility at 1 year follow-up compared to the control group.	■ IMT may facilitate postop recovery of inspiratory muscle strength and diaphragm mobility in patients with diaphragm paralysis after major cardiac surgery.
Arthur et al (2000) 7/10	CABG surgery patients (n = 208)	■ Control: Usual care. ■ Intervention: 8-week preop programme: Exercise programme (×2/week). Education/ reinforcement, nurse telephone follow-up (×1 monthly). ■ Postop treatment similar for both groups.	■ Intervention group had significantly shorter length of ICU and hospital stay, compared to the control group. ■ Intervention group had a significantly greater increase in HRQoL (physical composite summary score). This was maintained 6 months postop.	■ A preop programme during the waiting period (including an exercise programme), may reduce length of ICU and hospital stay and improve HRQoL in patients following CABG surgery.
Westerdahl et al (2001) 7/10	CABG surgery patients (n = 98)	■ Preop education + postop physiotherapy: Breathing + coughing exercises, early mobilization and active UL/thorax exercises (POD 1-4, ×1-2 daily). ■ Intervention 1: Conventional breathing exercises (×1 hourly during day). Three sets of 10 breaths and coughing/huffing. ■ Intervention 2: Breathing exercises with inspiratory resistance + positive expiratory pressure mask (×1 hourly during day). Three sets of 10 breaths and coughing/ huffing. Inspiratory pressure = −5 cmH_2O, expiratory pressure = 10 cmH_2O. ■ Intervention 3: Blow bottle device (×1 hourly during day). Three sets of 10 breaths and coughing/ huffing. Expiratory peak pressure = 10 cmH_2O.	■ No significant differences in: 1) postop pain and 2) incidence of PPC between groups. ■ Pulmonary function declined significantly in all groups postop. However, TLC declined significantly less in the blow bottle group compared to the conventional breathing exercises group.	■ While there were no significant differences in postop recovery between the three intervention groups, the blow bottle technique may minimize loss of TLC in patients following CABG surgery.

		TABLE A11-3			
		Randomized Controlled Trials of Physiotherapy in Cardiac Surgery (Since 2000–2013) in Order of PEDro Score *(Continued)*			

Primary Author (Year) PEDro Score	Patient Population (Sample Size)	Intervention/s	Results	Conclusions
Brasher et al (2003) 7/10	OHS patients (n = 198)	■ Preop education and postop physiotherapy (POD 1–POD 3). ■ Control: Usual care: Early mobilization. ■ Intervention: Usual care + breathing exercises. Four sets of 5 deep breaths with supervision/ hands on facilitation and supported cough). Participants encouraged to continue breathing exercises independently every hour, while awake.	■ No significant differences between groups for: 1) pulmonary function, 2) oxygen saturation, 3) incidence of PPC, 4) postop pain and 5) length of hospital stay.	■ The addition of breathing exercises to an early mobilization programme does not appear to improve the recovery of patients post OHS.
Hulzebos et al (2006) 7/10	CABG surgery patients at high risk for PPC (n = 279)	■ Control: Usual care: Education on DBE, coughing and early mobilization 1 day preop. ■ Intervention: Preop IMT (20-minute duration, ×1 daily for at least 2 weeks preop, included ×1 weekly session with supervision). Resistance started at 30% MIP (mouth). Education also provided on IS, ACBT, FET). ■ No differences in postop treatment for both groups.	■ Intervention group demonstrated a significant: 1) improvement in mean inspiratory muscle strength and endurance, 2) decrease in incidence of PPC and 3) decrease in postop hospitalization period compared to the control group.	■ Preop IMT appears to improve pulmonary function and decrease the incidence of PPC and postop hospitalization period in CABG patients who are at high risk of developing PPC.
El-Ansary et al (2007c) 7/10	CABG surgery patients who developed chronic SI (n = 9)	■ Control: Usual care. ■ Intervention: Trunk stabilization exercises (10-minute duration, ×2/week over 6 weeks). Exercises performed independently and progressed weekly.	■ Intervention group demonstrated a significant decrease in: 1) sternal separation and 2) pain during UL/trunk tasks compared to the control group.	■ The addition of trunk stabilization exercises may reduce sternal separation and pain during UL/trunk tasks in patients with SI post CABG surgery.

Continued on following page

TABLE A11-3

Randomized Controlled Trials of Physiotherapy in Cardiac Surgery (Since 2000–2013) in Order of PEDro Score *(Continued)*

Primary Author (Year) PEDro Score	Patient Population (Sample Size)	Intervention/s	Results	Conclusions
Hirschhorn et al (2008) 7/10	CABG surgery patients (n = 92)	■ Preop education + postop physiotherapy (POD 1 to discharge from hospital). ■ Control: Usual care: Supervised gentle, early mobilization (×1 daily). ■ Intervention 1: Supervised moderate-intensity walking programme (×1 daily). ■ Intervention 2: Supervised moderate-intensity walking programme + respiratory (IS, five sets of 4 breaths) and musculoskeletal (DBE combined with UL/thorax ROM exercises, 10 reps of 3 movements) exercise programme (×1 daily). Participants encouraged to continue respiratory exercises independently every hour, while awake.	■ Two intervention groups demonstrated a significant increase in 6MWT distances at discharge from hospital, compared to the control group. ■ No significant differences in 6MWT distances between groups at 4 month post discharge from hospital. ■ No significant differences in VC and HRQoL between groups at discharge from hospital and 4 month post discharge from hospital.	■ A supervised moderate intensity inpatient walking programme may improve walking capacity in patients following CABG surgery, at discharge from hospital. The addition of respiratory and musculoskeletal exercises does not appear to improve patient outcomes in this population.
Zarbock et al (2009) 7/10	Patients admitted to ICU post-cardiac surgery (n = 468)	■ Intervention 1: Usual care: Oxygen therapy, drug therapy and physiotherapy + intermittent nCPAP following extubation (10-minute duration every 4 hours). Expiratory pressure = 10 cmH$_2$O. ■ Intervention 2: Usual care + continuous nCPAP following extubation (6 hour duration at least). Expiratory pressure = 10 cmH$_2$O.	■ Compared to intervention 1, there was a significant decrease in the: 1) occurrence of PPC and 2) rate of readmission to ICU/MICU for intervention 2. ■ Intervention 2 also demonstrated a significant improvement in arterial oxygenation.	■ Continuous nCPAP immediately following extubation appears to improve arterial oxygenation, reduce the incidence of PPC and decrease the rate of readmissions to ICU/MICU, in patients following cardiac surgery.
Patman et al (2001) 8/10	Patients admitted to ICU post cardiac surgery (n = 210)	■ Control: No physiotherapy intervention during the postop intubation period. ■ Intervention: Physiotherapy during the intubation period. Not standardized, but included positioning, manual hyperinflation, endotracheal suctioning, thoracic expansion and UL exercises.	■ No significant differences between groups for length of intubation period, length of ICU stay, length of postop hospital stay, incentive spirometry values and incidence of PPC.	■ Physiotherapy during the postop intubation may not be indicated for all patients following cardiac surgery (namely, routine, uncomplicated patients).

TABLE A11-3				
Randomized Controlled Trials of Physiotherapy in Cardiac Surgery (Since 2000–2013) in Order of PEDro Score *(Continued)*				
Primary Author (Year) PEDro Score	Patient Population (Sample Size)	Intervention/s	Results	Conclusions
Busch et al (2012) 8/10	CABG surgery patients ≥75 years of age (n = 173)	▪ Control: Usual inpatient CR programme (5 days/week, 3-week duration). Walking, callisthenics and cycle ergometer. ▪ Intervention: Usual inpatient CR programme + UL/LL resistance training (×1 daily, 60% RM) and balance training (×1 daily in small groups).	▪ Significant improvements in 6MWT distance, CPET, TUG time, QF isometric muscle strength and HRQoL for both groups. ▪ Improvements significantly greater in intervention group compared to control group for 6MWT distance, TUG time and relative workload.	▪ Inpatient CR appears to improve the functional capacity and HRQoL in patients ≥75 years of age, following CABG surgery. ▪ The addition of resistive and balance training may lead to greater improvements in functional capacity in this population.
Wu et al (2012) 8/10	CABG surgery patients (n = 61)	▪ Control: Usual care: Routine check-ups and education on coronary risk factors, diet, stress management and physical activities. ▪ Intervention: Usual care + outpatient exercise programme. Treadmill training (30 minute duration, ×3/week). 60% HR reserve. Programme also included stretching or ROM exercises.	▪ Significant improvement in VO_2 peak in intervention group compared to control group, regardless of a diagnosis of DM.	▪ Exercise training 3 months following CABG surgery leads to significant improvements in exercise capacity in patients with and without DM.
Pasquina et al (2004) 9/10	Cardiac surgery patients who developed atelectasis (n = 150)	▪ Intervention 1: CPAP (tracheal extubation to SICU discharge, 30-minute duration, ×4 daily). Expiratory pressure = 5 cmH$_2$O. ▪ Intervention 2: NIPSV (tracheal extubation to SICU discharge, 30-minute duration, ×4 daily). Expiratory pressure = 5 cmH$_2$O.	▪ Significant improvement in RAS in intervention group compared to control group. ▪ No significant differences between control and intervention groups for PaO$_2$/FiO$_2$, pulmonary function tests and length of stay.	▪ While NIPSV results in radiological improvements of atelectasis, it does not appear to have any additional clinical benefits compared to CPAP for the treatment of atelectasis in patients following cardiac surgery.

Continued on following page

TABLE A11-3				
Randomized Controlled Trials of Physiotherapy in Cardiac Surgery (Since 2000–2013) in Order of PEDro Score *(Continued)*				
Primary Author (Year) PEDro Score	Patient Population (Sample Size)	Intervention/s	Results	Conclusions
Hirschhorn et al (2012) 9/10	CABG surgery patients (n = 64)	■ Postop physiotherapy (POD 3 to discharge from hospital, 10-minute duration, ×2 daily. Moderate intensity exercise. ■ ***Intervention 1:*** Walking exercise programme. ***Intervention 2:*** Stationary cycling programme.	■ No significant differences between two interventions for 6MWT distance, 6MCW, HRQoL, postop length of stay and compliance.	■ A moderate intensity stationary cycling programme is an appropriate alternative to a moderate intensity walking programme during the early postop period following CABG surgery.

6MCW, 6-minute cycle work; *6MWCT*, 6-minute walk corridor test; *6MWT*, 6-minute walk test; *ACBT*, active cycle of breathing techniques; *AF*, atrial fibrillation; *BiPAP*, bi-level positive airway pressure; *CABG*, coronary artery bypass graft; *CO*, cardiac output; *CPAP*, continuous positive airway pressure; *CPET*, cardiopulmonary exercise test; *CR*, cardiac rehabilitation; *CRT*, conventional respiratory therapy; *DBE*, deep breathing exercises; *DM*, diabetes mellitus; *FEF 25–75%*, forced expiratory flow at 25–75% of forced vital capacity; *FET*, forced expiratory technique; *FEV₁*, forced expiratory volume in 1 second; *FiO₂*, fraction of inspired oxygen; *FVC*, forced vital capacity; *HR*, heart rate; *HRQoL*, health related quality of life; *IC*, inspiratory capacity; *ICU*, intensive care unit; *IMT*, inspiratory muscle training; *IS*, incentive spirometry; *LL*, lower limb; *MEP*, maximal expiratory pressure; *METS*, metabolic equivalent of tasks; *MICU*, medical intensive care unit; *MIP*, maximal inspiratory pressure; *MV*, minute volume; *NIPSV*, non-invasive pressure support ventilation; *n*, number; *nCPAP*, nasal continuous positive airway pressure; *OHS*, open heart surgery; *PaCO₂*, partial pressure of carbon dioxide; *PaO₂*, partial pressure of oxygen; *PASE*, physical activity scale for the elderly; *PEF*, peak expiratory flow; *PF*, peak flow; *Postop*, postoperative; *POD*, postoperative day; *PPC*, postoperative pulmonary complication; *Preop*, preoperative; *QF*, quadratis femoris; *RAS*, radiological atelectasis score; *RM*, repetition maximum; *ROM*, range of movement; *RR*, respiratory rate; *R-R*, time between two consecutive R waves; *RV*, residual volume; *SICU*, surgical intensive care unit; *SMI*, sustained maximal inspiration; *SpO₂*, oxygen saturation; *SI*, sternal instability; *TLC*, total lung capacity; *TUG*, timed up and go test; *TV*, tidal volume; *UL*, upper limb; *VC*, vital capacity; *VCO₂*, carbon dioxide elimination; *VO₂*, oxygen consumption; *VR*, virtual reality.

REFERENCES

Abid, Q., Podila, S., Kendall, S., 2001. Sternal dehiscence after cardiac surgery and ACE inhibitors. Eur. J. Cardiothorac Surg. 20 (1), 203–204.

Adamina, M., Kehlet, H., Tomlinson, G., et al., 2011. Enhanced recovery pathways optimize health outcomes and resource utilization: a meta-analysis of randomized controlled trials in colorectal surgery. Surgery 149 (6), 830–837.

Adams, J., Cline, M.J., Hubbard, M., et al., 2006. A new paradigm for post-cardiac event resistance exercise guidelines. Am. J. Cardiol. 97 (2), 281–286.

Adams, J., Pullum, G., Stafford, P., et al., 2008. Challenging traditional activity limits after coronary artery bypass graft surgery: a simulated lawn-mowing activity. J. Cardiopulm. Rehabil. Prev. 28 (2), 118–121.

Agostini, P., Naidu, B., Cieslik, H., et al., 2011. Comparison of recognition tools for postoperative pulmonary complications following thoracotomy. Physiotherapy 97 (4), 278–283. doi:10.1016/j.physio.2010.11.007.

Agostini, P., Naidu, B., Cieslik, H., et al., 2013a. Effectiveness of incentive spirometry in patients following thoracotomy and lung resection including those at high risk for developing pulmonary complications. Thorax 68, 580–585. doi:10.1136/thoraxjnl-2012-202785.

Agostini, P., Reeve, J., Dromard, S., et al., 2013b. A survey of physiotherapeutic provision for patients undergoing thoracic surgery in the U.K. Physiotherapy 99 (1), 56–62. doi:10.1016/j.physio.2011.11.001.

AIHW (Australian Institute of Health and Welfare) & AACR (Australasian Association of Cancer Registries), 2007. Cancer in Australia: an overview, 2006. Cancer series no. 37. Cat. no. CAN 32. <www.aihw.gov.au/publications/can/ca06/ca06.pdf> (Accessed July 23 2007).

Aissaoui, N., Martins, E., Mouly, S., et al., 2009. A meta-analysis of bed rest versus early ambulation in the management of pulmonary embolism, deep vein thrombosis, or both. Int. J. Cardiol. 137 (1), 37–41. doi:10.1016/j.ijcard.2008.06.020.

Alkarmi, A., Thijssen, D.H.J., Albouaini, K., et al., 2010. Arterial prehabilitation: can exercise induce changes in artery size and function that decrease complications of catheterization. Sports Med. 40 (6), 481–492. 10.2165/11531950-000000000-00000.

Allan, J.S., Garrity, J.M., Dean, M., Donahue, D.M., 2009. High-frequency chest-wall compression during the 48 hours following thoracic surgery. Respir. Care 54 (3), 340–343.

American Society of Anesthesiologists (ASA), 1963. New classification of physical status. Anesthesiology 24, 111.

Anderson, C.M., Overend, T.J., Godwin, J., et al., 2009. Ambulation after Deep Vein Thrombosis: A Systematic Review. Physiother. Can. 61 (3), 133–140. doi:10.3138/physio.61.3.133.

Arbane, G., Tropman, D., Jackson, D., Garrod, R., 2011. Evaluation of an early exercise intervention after thoracotomy for non-small cell lung cancer (NSCLC), effects on quality of life, muscle strength and exercise tolerance: randomised controlled trial. Lung Cancer 71, 229–234.

Arbane, G., Douiri, A., Hart, N., et al., 2014. Effect of postoperative physical training on activity after curative surgery for non-small cell lung cancer: a multicentre randomised controlled trial. Physiotherapy 100 (2), 100–107. doi:10.1016/j.physio.2013.12.002.

Argote-Greene, L.M., Chang, M.Y., Sugarbaker, D.J., 2005. Extrapleural pneumonectomy for malignant pleural mesothelioma. Multimed. Man. Cardiothorac. Surg. 2005: mmcts.2004.000133 doi:10.1510/mmcts.2004.000133. Published online January 1, 2005.

Arthur, H.M., Daniels, C., McKelvie, R., et al., 2000. Effect of preoperative intervention on preoperative and postoperative outcomes in low-risk patients awaiting elective coronary artery bypass graft surgery: a randomized controlled trial. Ann. Intern. Med. 133, 253–262.

Avendano, C.E., Flume, P.A., Silvestri, G.A., et al., 2001. Pulmonary complications after oesophagectomy. Ann. Thorac. Surg. 73, 922–926.

Bailey, S.H., Bull, D.A., Harpole, D.H., et al., 2003. Outcomes after esophagectomy: a ten-year prospective cohort. Ann. Thorac. Surg. 75, 217–222.

Balachandran, S., Lee, A., Royse, A., et al., 2014. Upper limb exercise prescription following cardiac surgery via median sternotomy: A web survey. J. Cardiopulm. Rehabil. Prev. 34, 390–395.

Barbalho-Moulim, M.C., Miguel, G.P.S., Forti, E.M.P., et al., 2011. Effects of preoperative inspiratory muscle training in obese women undergoing open bariatric surgery: respiratory muscle strength, lung volumes, and diaphragmatic excursion. Clinics 66, 1721–1727.

Barrat, S., 1997. Advances in acute pain management. Int. Anesthesiol. Clin. 35, 27–33.

Benzo, R., Wigle, D., Novotny, P., et al., 2011. Preoperative pulmonary rehabilitation before lung cancer resection: results from two randomized studies. Lung Cancer 74 (3), 441–445.

Berrisford, R., Brunelli, A., Rocco, G., et al., 2005. The European Thoracic Surgery Database project: modelling the risk of in-hospital death following lung resection. Eur. J. Cardiothorac. Surg. 28, 306–311.

Bitkover, C.Y., Gardlund, B., 1998. Mediastinitis after cardiovascular operations: a case-control study of risk factors. Ann. Thorac. Surg. 65 (1), 36–40.

Bobbio, A., Chetta, A., Ampollini, L., et al., 2008. Preoperative pulmonary rehabilitation in patients undergoing lung resection for non-small cell lung cancer. Eur. J. Cardiothorac Surg. 33 (1), 95–98.

Bonde, P., Papachristos, I., McCraith, A., et al., 2002. Sputum retention after lung operation: prospective, randomized trial shows superiority of prophylactic minitracheostomy in high-risk patients. Ann. Thorac. Surg. 74, 196–203.

Borghi-Silva, A., Mendes, R.G., Costa, F.D.M., et al., 2005. The influences of positive end expiratory pressure (PEEP) associated with physiotherapy intervention in phase 1 cardiac rehabilitation. Clinics 60, 465–472.

Boulind, C.E., Yeo, M., Burkhill, C., et al., 2011. Factors predicting deviation from an enhanced recovery programme and delayed discharge after laparoscopic colorectal surgery. Colorectal Dis. 14, e103–e110.

Brasher, P., McClelland, K., Denehy, L., et al., 2003. Does removal of deep breathing exercises from a physiotherapy program including pre-operative education and early mobilization after cardiac surgery alter patient outcomes? Austr. J. Physiother. 49, 165–173.

British Thoracic Society and the Society for Cardiothoracic Surgery in Great Britain and Ireland, Lim, E., Baldwin, D., et al., 2010. Guidelines on the radical management of patients with lung cancer. Thorax 65 (Suppl. III), 1–27. doi:10.1136/thx.2010.145938.

Brocki, B.C., Thorup, C.B., Andreasen, J.J., 2010. Precautions related to midline sternotomy in cardiac surgery: a review of mechanical stress factors leading to sternal complications. Eur. J. Cardiovasc. Nurs. 9 (2), 77–84.

Brooks, D., Crowe, J., Kelsey, C., et al., 2001. A clinical practice guideline on peri-operative physical therapy. Physiother. Can. 53, 9–25.

Browning, L., Denehy, L., Scholes, R.L., 2007. The quantity of early upright mobilisation performed following upper abdominal surgery is low: an observational study. Aust. J. Physiother. 53 (1), 47–52.

Brunelli, A., Charloux, A., Bolliger, C.T., et al., 2009. ERS/ESTS clinical guidelines on fitness for radical therapy in lung cancer patients (surgery and chemo-radiotherapy). Eur. Respir. J. 34 (1), 17–41.

Buchwald, H., Avidor, Y., Braunwald, E., et al., 2004. Bariatric surgery: a systematic review and meta-analysis. J. Am. Med. Asso. 12, 1724–1737.

Busch, J.C., Lillou, D., Wittig, G., et al., 2012. Resistance and balance training improves functional capacity in very old participants attending cardiac rehabilitation after coronary bypass surgery. J. Am. Geriatr. Soc. 60, 2270–2276.

Cahalin, L.P., LaPier, T.K., Shaw, D.K., 2011. Sternal precautions: is it time for a change? Precautions versus restrictions: a review of literature and recommendations for revision. Cardiopulm. Phys. Ther. J. 22 (1), 5–15.

Campbell, D.B., 2008. Thoracic incisions. Oper. Tech. Gen. Surg. 10 (2), 77–86.

Carneiro, E.M., Ramos Mde, C., Terra, G.A., et al., 2013. Evaluation of breathing exercise in hormonal and immunological responses in patients undergoing abdominal surgery. Acta. Cir. Bras. 28, 385–390.

Casali, C.C., Pereira, A.P., Martinez, J.A., et al., 2011. Effects of inspiratory muscle training on muscular and pulmonary function after bariatric surgery in obese patients. Obes. Surg. 21, 1389–1394.

Casha, A.R., Yang, L., Kay, P.H., et al., 1999. A biomechanical study of median sternotomy closure techniques. Eur. J. Cardiothorac Surg. 15 (3), 365–369.

Cavalheri, V., Jenkins, S., Hill, K., 2013. Physiotherapy practice patterns for patients undergoing surgery for lung cancer: a survey of hospitals in Australia and New Zealand. Intern. Med. J. 43 (4), 394–401. doi:10.1111/j.1445-5994.2012.02928.x.

Cerfolio, R.J., Bryant, A.S., 2008. The benefits of continuous and digital air leak assessment after elective pulmonary resection: a prospective study. Ann. Thorac. Surg. 86 (2), 396–401.

Cesario, A., Ferri, L., Galetta, D., et al., 2007. Postoperative pulmonary rehabilitation after lung resection for non-small cell lung cancer. Lung Cancer 57 (2), 177–180.

Cheng, D.C., 1998. Fast track cardiac surgery pathways: early extubation, process of care, and cost containment. Anesthesiology 88, 1429–1433.

Cheng, D.C., Wall, C., Djaiani, G., et al., 2003. Randomized assessment of resource use in fast-track cardiac surgery 1-year after hospital discharge. Anesthesiology 98, 651–657.

Chiumello, D., Coppola, S., Froio, S., et al., 2013. Noninvasive ventilation in chest trauma: systematic review and meta-analysis. Intensive Care Med. 39 (7), 1171–1180. doi:10.1007/s00134-013 -2901-4.

Chuang, T.Y., Sung, W.H., Lin, C.Y., 2005. Application of a virtual reality-enhanced exercise protocol in patients after coronary bypass. Arch. Phys. Med. Rehabil. 86, 1929–1932.

Colice, G.L., Shafazand, S., Griffin, J.P., et al., 2007. Physiologic evaluation of the patient with lung cancer being considered for resectional surgery: ACCP evidenced-based clinical practice guidelines. Chest 132 (3 Suppl.), 161S–177S.

Craig, D.B., 1981. Postoperative recovery of pulmonary function. Anesth. Analg. 60, 46–52.

Dasika, U.K., Trumble, D.R., Magovern, J.A., 2003. Lower sternal reinforcement improves the stability of sternal closure. Ann. Thorac. Surg. 75 (5), 1618–1621.

de Cosmo, G., Aceto, P., Gualtieri, E., Congedo, E., 2009. Analgesia in thoracic surgery: review. Minerva Anestesiol. 75 (6), 393–400.

Denehy, L., Browning, L., 2007. Abdominal surgery: the evidence for physiotherapy intervention. In: Partridge, C. (Ed.), Recent Advances in Physiotherapy. John Wiley and Sons, Chichester.

Denehy, L., Carroll, S., Ntoumenopoulos, G., Jenkins, S., 2001. A randomized controlled trial comparing periodic mask CPAP with physiotherapy after abdominal surgery. Physiother. Res. Int. 6, 236–250.

Denehy, L., van de Leur, J., 2004. Postoperative mucus clearance. In: Rubins, B., van der Schans, C. (Eds.), Therapy for Mucus-Clearance Disorders. Marcel Dekker, New York.

Deng, B., Tan, Q.Y., Zhao, Y.P., et al., 2010. Suction or non-suction to the underwater seal drains following pulmonary operation: meta-analysis of randomised controlled trials. Eur. J. Cardiothorac. Surg. 38 (2), 210–215. doi:10.1016/j.ejcts.2010.01.050.

Dettling, D.S., Van der Schaaf, M., Blom, R.L., et al., 2012. Feasibility and effectiveness of pre-operative inspiratory muscle training in patients undergoing oesophagectomy: a pilot study. Physiother. Res. Int. 18, 16–26.

Dodson, M., 1985. The Management of Postoperative Pain. Edward Arnold Ltd, London.

Dronkers, J., Veldman, A., Hoberg, E., et al., 2008. Prevention of pulmonary complications after upper abdominal surgery by preoperative intensive inspiratory muscle training: a randomized controlled pilot study. Clin. Rehabil. 22, 134–142.

Ebeo, C.T., Benotti, P.N., Byrd, R.P. Jr., et al., 2002. The effect of bi-level positive airway pressure on postoperative pulmonary function following gastric surgery for obesity. Respir. Med. 96, 672–676.

El-Ansary, D., Adams, R., Ghandi, A., 2000a. Musculoskeletal and neurological complications following coronary artery bypass graft surgery: a comparison between saphenous vein and internal mammary artery grafting. Austr. J. Physiother. 46 (1), 19–25.

El-Ansary, D., Adams, R., Toms, L., Elkins, M., 2000b. Sternal instability following coronary artery bypass grafting. Physiother. Theory Pract. 16 (1), 27–33.

El-Ansary, D., Waddington, G., Adams, R., 2007a. Measurement of non-physiological movement in sternal instability by ultrasound. Ann. Thorac. Surg. 83 (4), 1513–1517.

El-Ansary, D., Waddington, G., Adams, R., 2007b. Relationship between pain and upper limb movement in patients with chronic sternal instability following cardiac surgery. Physiother. Theory Pract. 23 (5), 273–280.

El-Ansary, D., Waddington, G., Adams, R., 2007c. Trunk stabilisation exercises reduce sternal separation in chronic sternal instability after cardiac surgery: a randomised cross-over trial. Austr. J. Physiother. 53, 255–260.

El-Ansary, D., Waddington, G., Adams, R., 2008. Control of non-physiological movement in sternal instability by supportive devices: a comparison of a fastening brace, compressive garment and sports tape. Arch. Phys. Med. Rehabil. 89 (9), 1775–1781.

Euliano, T., Gravenstein, J., 2004. Essential Anaesthesia: From Science to Practice. Cambridge University Press, Cambridge.

Fairshter, R., Williams, J., 1987. Pulmonary physiology in the postoperative period. Crit. Care Clin. 3, 286–306.

Farjah, F., Wood, D.E., Mulligan, M.S., et al., 2009. Safety and efficacy of video-assisted versus conventional lung resection for lung cancer. J. Thorac. Cardiovasc. Surg. 137, 1415–1421.

Fedak, P.W., Kolb, E., Borsato, G., et al., 2010. Kryptonite bone cement prevents pathologic sternal displacement. Ann. Thorac. Surg. 90, 979–985.

Feeney, C., Reynolds, J.V., Hussey, J., 2011. Preoperative physical activity levels and postoperative pulmonary complications post-esophagectomy. Dis. Esophagus 24 (7), 489–494.

Ferguson, M.K., Durkin, A.E., 2002. Preoperative prediction of the risk of pulmonary complications after esophagectomy for cancer. J. Thorac. Cardiovasc. Surg. 123 (4), 661–669.

Ferreira, G.M., Haeffner, M.P., Barreto, S.S., Dall'Ago, P., 2010. Incentive spirometry with expiratory positive airway pressure brings benefits after myocardial revascularization. Arq. Bras. Cardiol. 94, 246–251.

Fisher, B., Majumdar, S., McAllister, F., 2002. Predicting pulmonary complications after non-thoracic surgery: a systematic review of blinded studies. Am. J. Med. 112, 219–225.

Fitzpatrick, D.C., Denard, J.P., Phelan, D., et al., 2010. Operative stabilization of flail chest injuries: review of literature and fixation options. Eur. J. Trauma Emerg. Surg. 36 (5), 427–433. doi:10.1007/s00068-010-0027-8.

Flores, R.M., Park, B.J., Dycoco, J., et al., 2009. Lobectomy by video-assisted thoracic surgery (VATS) versus thoracotomy for lung cancer. J. Thorac. Cardiovasc. Surg. 138 (1), 11–18. doi:10.1016/j.jtcvs.2009.03.030.

Ford, G.T., Rosenal, T.W., Clergue, F., et al., 1993. Respiratory physiology in upper abdominal surgery. Clin. Chest Med. 14, 237–252.

Ford, G.T., Whitelaw, W.A., Rosenal, T.W., et al., 1983. Diaphragm function after upper abdominal surgery in humans. Am. Rev. Respir. Dis. 127, 431–436.

Forgiarini, L.A., Carvalho, A.T., Ferreira Tde, S., et al., 2009. Physical therapy in the immediate postoperative period after abdominal surgery. J. Bras. Pneumol. 35, 455–459.

Franco, A.M., Torres, F.C., Simon, I.S., et al., 2011. Assessment of noninvasive ventilation with two levels of positive airway pressure in patients after cardiac surgery. Rev. Bras. Cir. Cardiovasc. 26, 582–590.

Freitas, E., Soares, B., Cardoso, J., Atallah, A., 2007. Incentive spirometry for preventing pulmonary complications after coronary artery bypass graft. Cochrane Database Syst. Rev. (3), CD004466, doi:10.1002/14651858.CD004466.pub2; Retrieved from Cochrane Database of Systematic Reviews.

Frølund, L., Madsen, F., 1986. Self-administered prophylactic postoperative positive expiratory pressure in thoracic surgery. Acta Anaesthesiol. Scand. 30 (5), 381–385.

Gaszynski, T., Tokarz, A., Piotrowski, D., Machala, W., 2007. Boussignac CPAP in the postoperative period in morbidly obese patients. Obes. Surg. 17, 452–456.

Gosselink, R., Schrever, K., Cops, P., et al., 2000. Incentive spirometry does not enhance recovery after thoracic surgery. Crit. Care Med. 28 (3), 679–683.

Granger, C., McDonald, C., Berney, S., et al., 2011. Exercise intervention to improve exercise capacity and health related quality of life for patients with Non-small cell lung cancer: a systematic review. Lung Cancer 72, 139–153.

Grevious, M.A., Henry, G.I., Ramaswamy, R., Grubb, K.J., 2014. Chest reconstruction, sternal dehiscence. Web site. <http://emedicine.medscape.com/article/1278627-overview> (Accessed January 1, 2015).

Guimarães, M.M.F., El Dib, R., Smith, A.F., Matos, D., 2009. Incentive spirometry for prevention of postoperative pulmonary complications in upper abdominal surgery. Cochrane Database Syst. Rev. (3), CD006058.

Gunduz, M., Unlugenc, H., Ozalevli, M., et al., 2005. A comparative study of continuous positive airway pressure (CPAP) and intermittent positive pressure ventilation (IPPV) in patients with flail chest. Emerg. Med. J. 22, 325–329. doi:10.1136/emj.2004.019786.

Haeffener, M.P., Ferreira, G.M., Barreto, S.S., et al., 2008. Incentive spirometry with expiratory positive airway pressure reduces pulmonary complications, improves pulmonary function and 6-minute walk distance in patients undergoing coronary artery bypass graft surgery. Am. Heart J. 156, 900e1–900e8.

Haines, K.J., Skinner, E.H., Berney, S., 2013. Association of postoperative pulmonary complications with delayed mobilisation following major abdominal surgery: an observational cohort study. Physiotherapy 99 (2), 119–125.

Harris, J., 2006. Disorders of the arterial system. In: Tjandra, J., Clunie, G., Kaye, A., Smith, J. (Eds.), Textbook of Surgery. Blackwell Publishing, Massachusetts.

Hernandez, G., Fernandez, R., Lopez-Reina, P., et al., 2010. Noninvasive ventilation reduces intubation in chest trauma-related hypoxemia: a randomized clinical trial. Chest 137 (1), 4–80.

Hirschhorn, A.D., Richards, D., Mungovan, S.F., et al., 2008. Supervised moderate intensity exercise improves distance walked at hospital discharge following coronary artery bypass graft surgery: a randomized controlled trial. Heart Lung Circ. 17, 129–138.

Hirschhorn, A.D., Richards, D.A., Mungovan, S.F., et al., 2012. Does the mode of exercise influence recovery of functional capacity in the early postoperative period after coronary artery bypass graft surgery? A randomized controlled trial. Interact. Cardiovasc. Thorac. Surg. 15, 995–1003.

Hong, S.S., Alison, J.A., Milrose, M.A., Dignan, R., 2013. Does local anaesthesia after coronary artery bypass graft surgery improve pain control and walking distance? APA conference proceedings, Melbourne, 2013.

Hulzebos, E.H., Helders, P.J., Favie, N.J., et al., 2006. Preoperative intensive inspiratory muscle training to prevent postoperative pulmonary complications in high-risk patients undergoing CABG surgery: a randomized clinical trial. J. Am. Med. Assoc. 296, 1851–1857.

Ingwersen, U.M., Larsen, K.R., Bertelsen, M.T., et al., 1993. Three different mask physiotherapy regimens for prevention of postoperative pulmonary complications after heart and pulmonary surgery. Intensive Care Med. 19 (5), 294–298.

Inoue, J., Ono, R., Makiura, D., et al., 2013. Prevention of postoperative pulmonary complications through intensive preoperative respiratory rehabilitation in patients with esophageal cancer. Dis. Esophagus 26, 68–74. doi:10.1111/j.1442-2050.2012.01336.x.

Jamieson, S.W., Shumway, N.E. (Eds.), 1986. Rob and Smith's Operative Surgery: Cardiac Surgery, fourth ed. Butterworths, Sevenoaks.

Javidfar, J., Bacchetta, M., Yang, J.A., et al., 2012. The use of a tailored surgical technique for minimally invasive esophagectomy. J. Thorac. Cardiovasc. Surg. 143 (5), 1125–1129. doi:10.1016/j.jtcvs.2012.01.071.

Jenkins, S., Moxham, J., 1991. The effects of mild obesity on lung function. Respir. Med. 85, 309–311.

Jenkins, W.S.A., Hall, D.P., Dhaliwal, K., et al., 2012. The use of a portable digital thoracic suction Thopaz drainage system for the management of a persistent spontaneous secondary pneumothorax in a patient with underlying interstitial lung disease. BMJ Case Rep. 2012, doi:10.1136/bcr.02.2012.5881.

Jonasson, B., Timmermans, C., 2001. The effect of incentive spirometry on postoperative pulmonary complications: a systematic review. Chest 120, 971–978.

Jones, L., Eves, N., Peterson, B., et al., 2008. Safety and feasibility of aerobic training on cardiopulmonary function and quality of life in postsurgical nonsmall cell lung cancer patients. Cancer 113 (12), 3430–3439.

Kalso, E., Mennander, S., Tasmuth, T., Nilsson, E., 2001. Chronic post-sternotomy pain. Acta Anaesthesiol. Scand. 45 (8), 935–939.

Kaminski, P.N., Forgiarini, L.A., Andrade, C.F., 2013. Early respiratory therapy reduces postoperative atelectasis in children undergoing lung resection. Respir. Care 58 (5), 805–809. doi:10.4187/respcare.01870.

Katz, J., 1993. Preoperative analgesia for postoperative pain. Lancet 342, 65–66.

Kehlet, H., Kennedy, R., 2006. Laparoscopic colonic surgery: mission accomplished or work in progress. Colorectal Dis. 8, 514–517.

Khalpey, Z.I., Ganim, R.B., Rawn, J.D., 2008. Postoperative care of cardiac surgery patients. In: Cohn, L. (Ed.), Cardiac Surgery in the Adult, third ed. Mc-Graw-Hill, New York, pp. 465–486.

Kim, W.D., 1997. Lung mucus: a clinician's view. Eur. Respir. J. 10, 1914–1917.

Kindgen-Milles, D., Muller, E., Buhl, R., et al., 2005. Nasal-continuous positive airway pressure reduces pulmonary morbidity and length of hospital stay following thoracoabdominal aortic surgery. Chest 128, 821–828.

King, K.B., 2001. Emotional and Functional Outcomes in Women with Coronary Heart Disease. J. Cardiovasc. Nurs. 15, 54–70.

King, K., McFetridge-Durdle, J., LeBlanc, P., et al., 2009. A descriptive examination of the impact of sternal scar formation in women. Eur. J. Cardiovasc. Nurs. 8 (2), 112–118.

King, K., Parry, M., Southern, D., et al., 2008. Women's recovery from sternotomy-extension (WRESTE) study: examining long-term pain and discomfort following sternotomy and their predictors. Heart 94 (4), 493–497.

Kodric, M., Trevisan, R., Torregiani, C., et al., 2013. Inspiratory muscle training for diaphragm dysfunction after cardiac surgery. J. Thorac. Cardiovasc. Surg. 145, 819–823.

Komanapalli, C.B., Sukumar, M.S., 2011. Thoracoscopic Decortication. Retrieved from <http://www.ctsnet.org/sections/clinicalresources/thoracic/expert_tech-33.html>.

Kulkarni, S.R., Fletcher, E., McConnell, A.K., et al., 2010. Preoperative inspiratory muscle training preserves postoperative inspiratory muscle strength following major abdominal surgery: a randomized pilot study. Ann. R. Coll. Surg. Engl. 92, 700–705.

Landreneau, R.J., Hazelrigg, S.R., Mack, M.J., et al., 1993. Postoperative pain-related morbidity: video-assisted thoracic surgery versus thoracotomy. Ann. Thorac. Surg. 56 (6), 1285–1289.

LaPier, T.K., 2007. Functional status of patients during subacute recovery from coronary artery bypass surgery. Heart Lung 36 (2), 114–124.

LaPier, T., Schenk, R., 2002. Thoracic musculoskeletal considerations following open-heart surgery. Cardiopulm. Phys. Ther. J. 13, 16–20.

Law, S., Wong, J., 2006. Tumours of the oesophagus. In: Tjandra, J., Clunie, G., Kaye, A., Smith, J. (Eds.), Textbook of Surgery. Blackwell Publishing, Massachusetts.

Law, S., Wong, K., Kwok, K., et al., 2004. Predictive factors for postoperative pulmonary complications and mortality after esophagectomy for cancer. Ann. Surg. 240, 791–800.

Lawrence, V., Cornell, J., Smetana, G., 2006. Strategies to reduce postoperative pulmonary complications after noncardiothoracic surgery: systematic review for the American College of Physicians. Ann. Intern. Med. 144, 596–608.

Lemanu, D.P., Singh, P.P., MacCormick, A.D., et al., 2013. Effect of preoperative exercise on cardiorespiratory function and recovery after surgery: a systematic review. World J. Surg. 37, 711–720. doi:10.1007/s00268-012-1886-4.

Lemmer, J.H. Jr., Vlahakes, G.J., 2010b. Postoperative management. In: Lemmer, J.H., Jr., Vlahakes, G.J. (Eds.), Handbook of Patient Care in Cardiac Surgery, seventh ed. Lippincott Williams & Wilkins, Philadelphia, pp. 81–135.

Li, W., Lee, R., Lee, T., et al., 2003. The impact of thoracic surgical access on early shoulder function: video-assisted thoracic surgery versus posterolateral thoracotomy. Eur. J. Cardiothorac Surg. 23 (3), 390–396.

Liu, S.S., Wu, C.L., 2007. Effect of postoperative analgesia on major postoperative complications: a systematic update of the evidence. Anesth. Analg. 104, 689–702.

Losanoff, J.E., Collier, A.D., Wagner-Mann, C.C., et al., 2004. Biomechanical comparison of median sternotomy closures. Ann. Thorac. Surg. 77 (1), 203–209.

Losanoff, J.E., Richman, B.W., Jones, J.W., 2002. Disruption and infection of median sternotomy: a comprehensive review. Eur. J. Cardiothorac. Surg. 21, 831–839.

Ludwig, C., Angenendt, S., Martins, R., et al., 2011. Intermittent positive-pressure breathing after lung surgery. Asian Cardiovasc. Thorac. Ann. 19 (1), 10–13.

Lunardi, A.C., Cecconello, I., Carvalho, C.R.F., 2011. Postoperative chest physical therapy prevents respiratory complications in patients undergoing esophagectomy. Rev. Bras. Fisioter. 15 (2), 160–165.

Macchi, C., Fatttirolli, F., Lova, R.M., et al., 2007. Early and late rehabilitation and physical training in elderly patients after cardiac surgery. Am. J. Phys. Med. Rehabil. 86, 826–834.

Mackay, M., Ellis, E., Johnston, C., 2005. Randomized clinical trial of physiotherapy after open abdominal surgery in high risk patients. Austr. J. Physiother. 51, 151–159.

Macnaughton, P.D., 1995. Posture and lung function in health and disease. Int. J. Intensive Care Winter, 133–137.

Mamidanna, R., Bottle, A., Aylin, P., et al., 2012. Short-term outcomes following open versus minimally invasive esophagectomy for cancer in England: a population-based national study. Ann. Surg. 255 (2), 197–203. doi:10.1097/SLA.0b013e31823e39fa.

Mans, C.M., Reeve, J.C., Elkins, M.R., 2015. Postoperative outcomes following preoperative inspiratory muscle training in patients undergoing cardiothoracic or upper abdominal surgery: a systematic review and meta analysis. Clin. Rehabil. 29 (5), 426–438. doi:10.1177/0269215514545350; [Epub 2014 Aug 26]; 2015 May.

Manser, R., Wright, G., Hart, D., et al., 2005. Surgery for local and locally advanced non-small cell lung cancer. Cochrane Database Syst. Rev. (1), Art. No.: CD004699, doi:10.1002/14651858.CD004699.pub2.

Matte, P., Jacquet, L., Van Dyck, M., Goenen, M., 2000. Effects of conventional physiotherapy, continuous positive airway pressure and non-invasive ventilatory support with bilevel positive airway pressure after coronary artery bypass grafting. Acta Anaesthesiol. Scand. 44, 75–81.

Mayo, N.E., Feldman, L., Scott, S., et al., 2011. Impact of preoperative change in physical function on postoperative recovery: argument supporting prehabilitation for colorectal surgery. Surgery 150 (3), 505–514.

McDonald, W., Brame, M., Sharp, C., Eggerstedt, J., 1989. Risk factors for median sternotomy dehiscence in cardiac surgery. South. Med. J. 82 (11), 1361–1364.

McGregor, W.E., Trumble, D.R., Magovern, J.A., 1999. Mechanical analysis of midline sternotomy wound closure. J. Thorac. Cardiovasc. Surg. 117 (6), 1144–1149.

McKenna, R., Houck, W., 2005. New approaches to the minimally invasive treatment of lung cancer. Curr. Opin. Pulm. Med. 11 (4), 282–286.

Mendes, R.G., Simoes, R.P., De Souza Melo Costa, F., et al., 2010. Short-term supervised inpatient physiotherapy exercise protocol improves cardiac autonomic function after coronary artery bypass graft surgery: a randomized controlled trial. Disabil. Rehabil. 32, 1320–1327.

Meyerson, J., Thelin, S., Gordh, T., Karlsten, R., 2001. The incidence of chronic post-sternotomy pain after cardiac surgery: a prospective study. Acta Anaesthesiol. Scand. 45 (8), 940–944.

Miller, K., Sahn, S., 1987. Chest tubes. Chest 91, 258–264.

Mitnick, C.D., Shin, S.S., Seung, K.J., et al., 2008. Comprehensive treatment of extensively drug-resistant tuberculosis. NEJM 359 (6), 563–574. doi:10.1056/NEJMoa0800106.

Moghissi, K., Thorpe, J.A.C., Ciulli, F. (Eds.), 2003. Moghissi's Essentials of Thoracic and Cardiac Surgery, second ed. Elsevier, Amsterdam.

Moholdt, T., Amundsen, B.H., Rustad, L.A., et al., 2009. Aerobic interval training versus continuous moderate exercise after coronary artery bypass surgery: a randomized study of cardiovascular effects and quality of life. Am. Heart J. 158, 1031–1037.

Moholdt, T., Vold, M.B., Grimsmo, J., et al., 2012. Home-based aerobic interval training improves peak oxygen uptake equal to residential cardiac rehabilitation: a randomized, controlled trial. PLoS ONE 7, 1–6.

Moore, S., 1997. Effects of interventions to promote recovery in coronary artery bypass surgical patients. J. Cardiovasc. Nurs. 12, 59–70.

Morano, M.T., Araújo, A.S., Nascimento, F.B., et al., 2013. Preoperative pulmonary rehabilitation versus chest physical therapy in patients undergoing lung cancer resection: a pilot randomized controlled trial. Arch. Phys. Med. Rehabil. 94 (1), 53–58. doi:10.1016/j.apmr.2012.08.206.

Morran, C., Finlay, I., Mathieson, M., et al., 1983. Randomized controlled trial of physiotherapy for postoperative pulmonary complications. Br. J. Anaesth. 55, 1113–1116.

Myles, P.S., Daly, D.J., Djaiani, G., et al., 2003. A systematic review of the safety and effectiveness of fast-track cardiac anesthesia. Anesthesiology 99, 982–987.

Myles, P.S., McIlroy, D., 2005. Fast-track cardiac anesthesia: choice of anesthetic agents and techniques. Semin. Cardiothorac. Vasc. Anesth. 9, 5–16.

Nakatsuchi, T., Otani, M., Osugi, H., et al., 2005. The necessity of chest physical therapy for thoracoscopic oesophagectomy. J. Int. Med. Res. 33 (4), 434–441.

National Health and Medical Research Council, 2005. Acute pain management: scientific evidence. <www.nhmrc.gov.au/publications/synopses/cp104syn.htm> (accessed 16 July 2007).

National Health and Medical Research Council, 2009. Clinical practice guideline for the prevention of venous thromboembolism (deep vein thrombosis and pulmonary embolism) in patients admitted to Australian hospitals. National Health and Medical Research Council, Melbourne.

Neligan, P.J., Malhotra, G., Fraser, M., et al., 2009. Continuous positive airway pressure via the Boussignac system immediately after extubation improves lung function in morbidly obese patients with obstructive sleep apnea undergoing laparoscopic bariatric surgery. Anesthesiology 110, 878–884.

Nelson, R., Edwards, S., Tse, B., 2007. Prophylactic nasogastric decompression after abdominal surgery. Cochrane Database Syst. Rev. (18), CD004929, doi:10.1002/14651858.CD004929.pub3.

Nielsen, K., Holte, K., Kehlet, H., 2003. Effects of posture on postoperative pulmonary function. Acta Anaesthesiol. Scand. 47, 1270–1275.

Novoa, N., Ballesteros, E., Jiménez, M., et al., 2011. Chest physiotherapy revisited: evaluation of its influence on the pulmonary morbidity after pulmonary resection. J. Cardiothorac. Surg. 40, 130–135.

Nunn, J., 1993. Nunn's Applied Respiratory Physiology. Butterworth-Heinemann, Oxford.

O'Donohue, W., 1992. Postoperative pulmonary complications. Postgrad. Med. 91, 167–175.

Olavarrieta, J.R., Coronel, P., 2009. Expectations and patient satisfaction related to the use of thoracotomy and video-assisted thoracoscopic surgery for treating recurrence of spontaneous primary pneumothorax. J. Bras. Pneumonol. 35 (2), 122–128.

Olbrecht, V., Barreiro, C., Bonde, P., et al., 2006. Clinical outcomes of noninfectious sternal dehiscence after median sternotomy. Ann. Thorac. Surg. 82 (3), 902–908.

Olsen, M.F., Anzén, H., 2012. Effects of training interventions prior to thoracic or abdominal surgery: a systematic review. Physical Therapy Reviews 17 (2), 124–131. doi:10.1179/1743288x11y.0000000054.

Olsen, M.F., Grell, M., Linde, L., Lundell, L., 2009. Procedure-related chronic pain after thoracoabdominal resection of the esophagus. Physiother. Theory Pract. 25 (7), 489–494. doi:10.3109/09593980902813432.

Olsen, M.F., Larsson, M., Hammerlid, E., Lundell, L., 2005. Physical function and quality of life after thoracoabdominal oesophageal resection. Dig. Surg. 22, 63–68. doi:10.1159/000085348.

Olsen, M., Wennberg, E., Johnsson, E., et al., 2002. Randomised clinical study of the prevention of pulmonary complications after thoracoabdominal resection by 2 different breathing techniques. Br. J. Surg. 89 (10), 1228–1234.

Oncel, M., Sencan, S., Yildiz, H., Kurt, N., 2002. Transcutaneous electrical nerve stimulation for pain management in patients with uncomplicated minor rib fractures. Eur. J. Cardiothorac. Surg. 22 (1), 13–17.

Overend, T.J., Anderson, C.M., Jackson, J., et al., 2010. Physical therapy management for adult patients undergoing cardiac surgery: a Canadian practice survey. Physiother. Can. 62 (3), 215–221.

Overend, T.J., Anderson, C.M., Lucy, S.D., et al., 2001. The effect of incentive spirometry on postoperative pulmonary complications: a systematic review. Chest 120 (3), 971–978.

Park, H., Park, J.S., Woo, S.Y., et al., 2012. Effect of high-frequency chest wall oscillation on pulmonary function after pulmonary lobectomy for non-small cell lung cancer. Crit. Care Med. 40, 2583–2589.

Park, S.K., Kim, J.H., Kang, H., et al., 2009. Pulmonary resection combined with isoniazid and rifampin based drug therapy for patients with multidrug-resistant and extensively drug-resistant tuberculosis. Int. J. Infect. Dis. 13 (2), 170–175.

Parker, R., Adams, J.L., Ogola, G., et al., 2008. Current activity guidelines for CABG patients are too restrictive: comparison of the forces exerted on the median sternotomy during a cough vs. lifting activities combined with Valsalva maneuver. Thorac. Cardiovasc. Surg. 56 (4), 190–194.

Parry, S., Denehy, L., Berney, S., Browning, L., 2014. Clinical application of the Melbourne risk prediction tool in a high-risk upper abdominal surgical population: an observational cohort study. Physiotherapy 100 (1), 47–53.

Pasquina, P., Merlani, P., Granier, J.M., Ricou, B., 2004. Continuous positive airway pressure versus noninvasive pressure support ventilation to treat atelectasis after cardiac surgery. Anesth. Analg. 99, 1001–1008.

Pasquina, P., Tramer, M., Granier, J., et al., 2006. Respiratory physiotherapy to prevent pulmonary complications after abdominal surgery: a systematic review. Chest 130, 1887–1899.

Pasquina, P., Tramer, M.R., Walder, B., 2003. Prophylactic respiratory physiotherapy after cardiac surgery: systematic review. Br. Med. J. 327 (7428), 1379–1381.

Patman, S., Sanderson, D., Blackmore, M., 2001. Physiotherapy following cardiac surgery: is it necessary during the intubation period? Austr. J. Physiother. 47, 7–16.

Paul, S., Altork, N.K., Sheng, S., et al., 2010. Thoracoscopic lobectomy is associated with lower morbidity than open lobectomy: a propensity-matched analysis from the STS database. J. Thorac. Cardiovasc. Surg. 139, 366–378.

Peeters-Asdourian, C., Gupta, S., 1999. Choices in pain management following thoracotomy. Chest 115, 122S–124S.

Pehlivan, E., Turna, A., Gurses, A., Gurses, H.N., 2011. The effects of preoperative short-term intense physical therapy in lung cancer patients: a randomized controlled trial. Ann. Thorac. Cardiovasc. Surg. 17 (5), 461–468.

Perrin, C., Julliena, V., Venissac, N., et al., 2009. Prophylactic use of noninvasive ventilation in patients undergoing lung resectional surgery. Respir. Med. 101, 1572–1578.

Qureshi, R., Nugent, A., Hayat, J., et al., 2008. Should surgical pleurectomy for spontaneous pneumothorax be always thoracoscopic? Interact. Cardiovasc. Thorac. Surg. 7 (4), 569–572.

Ramzisham, A.R., Raflis, A.R., Khairulasri, M.G., et al., 2009. Figure-of-eight vs. interrupted sternal wire closure of median sternotomy. Asian Cardiovasc. Thorac. Ann. 17 (6), 587–591.

Ready, L.B., Edwards, W.T. (Eds.), 1992. Management of Acute Pain: A Practical Guide. Taskforce on Acute Pain, IASP Publications, Seattle.

Reeve, J.C., 2010. The physiotherapy management of the patient undergoing thoracic surgery (Doctoral Thesis). University of Melbourne, Victoria, Australia. Retrieved from: <http://repository.unimelb.edu.au/10187/8590>.

Reeve, J., Nicol, K., Stiller, K., et al., 2008. Does physiotherapy reduce the incidence of postoperative complications in patients following pulmonary resection via thoracotomy? A protocol for a randomised controlled trial. J. Cardiothorac. Surg. 3 (48).

Reeve, J., Nicol, K., Stiller, K., et al., 2010a. Does physiotherapy reduce the incidence of postoperative pulmonary complications following pulmonary resection via open thoracotomy? A preliminary randomized single-blind clinical trial. Eur. J. Cardiothorac. Surg. 37 (5), 1158–1167.

Reeve, J.C., Stiller, K., Nicol, K., et al., 2010b. A postoperative shoulder exercise program improves function and decreases pain following open thoracotomy: a randomized trial. J. Physiother. 56 (4), 245–252.

Renault, J., Costa-Val, R., Rosseti, M., Houri Neto, M., 2009. Comparison between deep breathing exercises and incentive spirometry after CABG surgery. Rev. Bras. Cir. Cardiovasc. 24 (2), 165–172.

Richardson, J., Sabanathan, S., 1997. Prevention of respiratory complications after abdominal surgery. Thorax 52, S35–S40.

Ridderstolpe, L., Gill, H., Granfeldt, H., et al., 2001. Superficial and deep sternal wound complications: incidence, risk factors and mortality. Eur. J. Cardiothorac. Surg. 20, 1168–1175.

Robicsek, F., Fokin, A., Cook, J., Bhatia, D., 2000. Sternal instability after midline sternotomy. Thorac. Cardiovasc. Surg. 48 (1), 1–8.

Sabanathan, S., Shah, R., Tsiamis, A., et al., 1999. Oesophagogastrectomy in the elderly high-risk patients: role of effective regional analgesia and early mobilization. J. Cardiovasc. Surg. (Torino) 40, 153–156.

Sabiston, D.C. Jr., Spencer, F.C. (Eds.), 1990. Surgery of the Chest, fifth ed. WB Saunders, Philadelphia.

Sackett, D., Strauss, S., Richardson, W., et al., 2000. Evidence-Based Medicine. Churchill Livingstone, Edinburgh.

Samnani, S.S., Umer, M.F., Mehdi, S.H., Farid, F.N., 2014. Impact of preoperative counseling on early postoperative mobilization and its role in smooth recovery. International Scholarly Research Notices Volume 2014, Article ID 250536 5 pages <http://dx.doi.org/10.1155/2014/250536>.

Savci, S., Degirmenci, B., Saglam, M., et al., 2011. Short-term effects of inspiratory muscle training in coronary artery bypass graft surgery: a randomized controlled trial. Scand. Cardiovasc. J. 45, 286–293.

Savci, S., Sakinc, S., Inal Ince, D., et al., 2006. Active cycle of breathing techniques and incentive spirometer in coronary artery bypass graft surgery. Fizyoterapi Rehabilitasyon 17, 61–69.

Scholes, R., Denehy, L., Sztendur, E., et al., 2006. Development of a risk assessment model to predict pulmonary risk following upper abdominal surgery. Austr. J. Physiother. 52, S26.

School of Physiotherapy University of Melbourne, 2006. Cardiorespiratory physiotherapy 1 student clinical Manual. Parkville.

Sellke, F.W., DiMaio, J.M., Caplan, L.R., et al., 2005. Comparing on-pump and off-pump coronary artery bypass grafting: numerous studies but few conclusions: a scientific statement from the American Heart Association council on cardiovascular surgery and anesthesia in collaboration with the interdisciplinary working group on quality of care and outcomes research. Circulation 111, 2858–2864.

Sharifa, S., Zahida, I., Routledge, T., Scarcib, M., 2011. Extrapleural pneumonectomy or supportive care: treatment of malignant pleural mesothelioma? Interact. Cardiovasc. Thorac. Surg. 12, 1040–1045.

Sharma, K., Brandstetter, R., Brensilver, J., et al., 1996. Cardiopulmonary physiology and pathophysiology as a consequence of laparoscopic surgery. Chest 110, 810–815.

Shields, T.W., LoCicero, J., Ponn, R.B., Rusch, V.W. (Eds.), 2004. General Thoracic Surgery, sixth ed. Lippincott Williams and Wilkins, Philadelphia.

Sihag, S., Wright, C.D., Wain, J.C., et al., 2012. Comparison of perioperative outcomes following open versus minimally invasive Ivor Lewis oesophagectomy at a single, high-volume centre. Eur. J. Cardiothorac. Surg. 42 (3), 430–437. doi:10.1093/ejcts/ezs031.

Silva, Y.R., Li, S.K., Rickard, M.J., 2013. Does the addition of deep breathing exercises to physiotherapy-directed early mobilization alter patient outcomes following high-risk open upper abdominal surgery? Cluster randomized controlled trial. Physiotherapy 99, 187–193.

Simon, B., Ebert, J., Bokhari, F., et al., 2012. Management of pulmonary contusion and flail chest: an Eastern Association for the Surgery of Trauma practice management guideline. J. Trauma Acute Care Surg. 73 (5 Suppl. 4), S351–S361. doi:10.1097/TA.0b013e31827019fd.

Singh, F., Newton, R.U., Galvão, D.A., et al., 2013. A systematic review of pre-surgical exercise intervention studies with cancer patients. Surg. Oncol. 22, 92–104. doi:10.1016/j.suronc.2013.01.004.

Sjostrom, L., Narbro, K., Sjöström, C.D., et al., 2007. Effects of bariatric surgery on mortality in Swedish obese subjects. NEJM 23, 741–752.

Smetana, G., Lawrence, V., Cornell, J., 2006. Preoperative pulmonary risk stratification for non-cardiothoracic surgery: systematic review for the American college of physicians. Ann. Intern. Med. 144, 581–595.

Smetana, G.W., 2009. Postoperative pulmonary complications: an update on risk assessment and reduction. Cleve. Clin. J. Med. 76, S60–S65.

Smith, J., 2006. Common topics in thoracic surgery. In: Tjandra, J., Clunie, G., Kaye, A., Smith, J. (Eds.), Textbook of Surgery, third ed. Blackwell Publishing, Massachusetts.

Smith, K.M., McKelvie, R.S., Thorpe, K.E., Arthur, H.M., 2011. Six-year follow-up of a randomized controlled trial examining hospital versus home-based exercise training after coronary artery bypass graft surgery. Heart 97, 1169–1174.

Snowdon, D., Haines, T.P., Skinner, E.H., 2014. Preoperative intervention reduces postoperative pulmonary complications but not length of stay in cardiac surgical patients: a systematic review. J. Physiother. 60 (2), 66–77. doi:10.1016/j.jphys.2014.04.002.

Soares, S.M., Nucci, L.B., de Silva, M.M., Campacci, T.C., 2013. Pulmonary function and physical performance outcomes with preoperative physical therapy in upper abdominal surgery: a randomized controlled trial. Clin. Rehabil. 27, 616–627.

Spruit, M., Janssen, P., Willemson, S., et al., 2006. Exercise capacity before and after an 8 week multidisciplinary inpatient rehabilitation program in lung cancer patients: a pilot study. Lung Cancer 52 (2), 257–260.

Stedman, T.L. (Ed.), 2005. Stedman's medical dictionary for the health professions and nursing, twenty-eighth ed. Lippincott Williams and Wilkins, Philadelphia.

Stigt, J.A., Uil, S.M., van Riesen, S.J., et al., 2013. A randomised controlled trial of postthoracotomy pulmonary rehabilitation in patients with resectable lung cancer. J. Thorac. Oncol. 8 (2), 214–221.

Stiller, K., McInnes, M., Huff, N., et al., 1997. Do exercises prevent musculoskeletal complications after cardiac surgery? Physiother. Theory Pract. 13 (2), 117–126.

Sturgess, T., Denehy, L., Tully, E., El-Ansary, D., 2014. A pilot thoracic exercise programme reduces early (0-6 weeks) sternal pain post open heart surgery. Int. J. Ther. Rehabil. 21, 110–117.

Sugi, K., Nawata, S., Kaneda, Y., et al., 1996. Disadvantages of muscle-sparing thoracotomy in patients with lung cancer. World J. Surg. 20 (5), 551–555.

Sugiura, H., Morikawa, T., Kaji, M., et al., 1999. Long-term benefits for the quality of life after video-assisted thoracoscopic lobectomy in patients with lung cancer. Surg. Laparosc. Endosc. Percutan. Tech. 9 (6), 403–408.

Sung, S.W., Kang, C.H., Kim, Y.T., et al., 1999. Surgery increased the chance of cure in multi-drug resistant pulmonary tuberculosis. Eur. J. Cardiothorac. Surg. 16 (2), 187–193.

Tatoulis, J., Smith, J., 2006. Principles and practice of cardiac surgery. In: Tjandra, J., Clunie, G., Kaye, A., Smith, J. (Eds.), Textbook of Surgery, third ed. Blackwell Publishing, Massachusetts.

Taggart, D.P., 2006. Coronary artery bypass grafting is still the best treatment for multivessel and left main disease, but patients need to know. Ann. Thorac. Surg. 82, 1966–1975.

Taylor, G.J., Mikell, F.L., Moses, H., 1990. Determinants of hospital charges for coronary artery bypass surgery: The economic consequences of post operative complications. Am. J. Cardiol. 65 (5), 309–313.

Thomas, J., McIntosh, J., 1994. Are incentive spirometry, intermittent positive pressure breathing, and deep breathing exercises effective in the prevention of postoperative pulmonary complications after upper abdominal surgery? A systematic overview and meta-analysis. Phys. Ther. 74, 3–16.

Thrombosis, 2009. A Systematic Review. Physiother. Can. 61, 133–140.

Topp, R., Ditmyer, M., King, K., et al., 2010. The effect of bed rest and potential for prehabilitation on patients in the intensive care unit. AACN Clin. Issues 13 (2), 263–276.

Trauma.org, 2004. Pulmonary contusion. <www.trauma.org/index.php?/main/article/398/> (Accessed 16 July 2007).

Tuyl, L., Mackney, J.H., Johnston, C.L., 2012. Management of sternal precautions following median sternotomy by physical therapists in Australia: a web-based survey. Phys. Ther. 92 (1), 83–97.

Urell, C., Emtner, M., Hedenstrom, H., et al., 2011. Deep breathing exercises with positive expiratory pressure at a higher rate improve oxygenation in the early period after cardiac surgery: a randomized controlled trial. Eur. J. Cardiothorac Surg. 40, 162–167.

Valkenet, K., van de Port, I.G.L., Dronkers, J.J., et al., 2011. The effects of preoperative exercise therapy on postoperative outcome: a systematic review. Clin. Rehabil. 25 (2), 99–111.

Varela, G., Ballesteros, E., Jiménez, M.F., et al., 2006. Cost-effectiveness analysis of prophylactic respiratory physiotherapy in pulmonary lobectomy. Eur. J. Cardiothorac Surg. 29 (2), 216–220.

Villamizar, N.R., Darrabie, M.D., Burfeind, W.R., et al., 2009. Thoracoscopic lobectomy is associated with lower morbidity compared with thora-cotomy. J. Thorac. Cardiovasc. Surg. 138, 419–425.

Vlug, M.S., Wind, J., Hollman, M., et al., 2011. Laparoscopy in combination with fast track multimodal management is the best perioperative strategy in patients undergoing colonic surgery (LAFA study). Ann. Surg. 254 (6), 868–875.

Vohra, H.A., Adamson, L., Weeden, D.F., 2008. Does video-assisted thoracoscopic pleurectomy result in better outcomes than open pleurectomy for primary spontaneous pneumothorax? Interact. Cardiovasc. Thorac. Surg. 7 (4), 673–677. doi:10.1510/icvts .2008.176081.

Vymazal, T., Horácek, M., Durpekt, R., et al., 2009. Is allogeneic blood transfusion a risk factor for sternal dehiscence following cardiac surgery? A prospective observational study. Int. Heart J. 50 (5), 601–607.

Wahba, R., 1991. Perioperative functional residual capacity. Can. J. Anaesth. 38, 384–400.

Walcot, N., Marchbank, A., 2007. Postoperative care of adult cardiac surgery patients. Surgery 25 (5), 211–214.

Werawatganon, T., Charuluxanun, S., 2005. Patient-controlled intravenous opioid analgesia versus continuous epidural analgesia for pain after intra-abdominal surgery. Cochrane Database Syst. Rev. (1), Art. No: CD004088, doi:10.1002/14651858. CD004088.pub2.

Westerdahl, E., Lindmark, B., Eriksson, T., et al., 2005. Deep-breathing exercises reduce atelectasis and improve pulmonary function after coronary bypass surgery. Chest 128, 3482–3488.

Westerdahl, E., Lindmark, B., Almgren, S.O., Tenling, A., 2001. Chest physiotherapy after coronary artery bypass graft surgery: a comparison of three different deep breathing techniques. J. Rehabil. Med. 33, 79–84.

Whitson, B.A., D'Cunha, J., 2010. Video-assisted thoracoscopic surgical lobectomy: the potential oncological benefit of surgical immunomodulation. Semin. Thorac. Cardiovasc. Surg. 22, 113–115.

Wright, D.J., Williams, S.G., Riley, R., et al., 2002. Is early, low level, short term exercise cardiac rehabilitation following coronary bypass surgery beneficial? A randomized controlled trial. Heart 88, 83–84.

Wu, S.K., Lin, Y.W., Chen, C.L., Tsai, S.W., 2006. Cardiac rehabilitation vs. home exercise after coronary artery bypass graft surgery: a comparison of heart rate recovery. Am. J. Phys. Med. Rehabil. 85, 711–717.

Wu, Y.T., Wu, Y.W., Hwang, C.L., Wang, S.S., 2012. Changes in diastolic function after exercise training in patients with and without diabetes mellitus after coronary artery bypass surgery: a randomized controlled trial. Eur. J. Phys. Rehabili. Med. 48, 351–360.

Wynne, R., Botti, M., 2004. Postoperative pulmonary dysfunction in adults after cardiac surgery with cardiopulmonary bypass: clinical significance and implications for practice. Am. J. Crit. Care 13 (5), 384–393.

Yim, A., 2002. VATS major pulmonary resection revisited: controversies, techniques and results. Ann. Thorac. Surg. 74 (2), 615–623.

Yim, A.P., Lee, T.W., Izzat, M.B., Wan, S., 2001. Place of video-thoracoscopy in thoracic surgical practice. World J. Surg. 25 (2), 157–161.

Zarbock, A., Mueller, E., Netzer, S., et al., 2009. Prophylactic nasal continuous positive airway pressure following cardiac surgery protects from postoperative pulmonary complications: a prospective, randomized, controlled trial in 500 patients. Chest 135, 1252–1259.

Zehr, K.J., Dawson, P.B., Yang, S.C., Heitmiller, R.F., 1998. Standardized clinical care pathways for major thoracic cases reduce hospital costs. Ann. Thorac. Surg. 66 (3), 914–919.

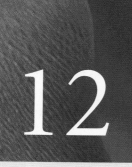

12

PHYSICAL ACTIVITY AND REHABILITATION

Physical Activity and Physical Fitness in Health and Disease

CHRIS BURTIN ■ VASILEIOS ANDRIANOPOULOS ■ MARTIJN A SPRUIT

Pulmonary Rehabilitation

KATY MITCHELL ■ FABIO PITTA ■ ANNE E HOLLAND ■ ANNEMARIE L LEE ■ LINDA DENEHY

Cardiac Rehabilitation

JULIE REDFERN ■ JENNIFER JONES

■ ■

CHAPTER OUTLINE

PHYSICAL ACTIVITY AND PHYSICAL FITNESS IN HEALTH AND DISEASE 580
Physical Activity Versus Physical Fitness 580
Physical Activity, Physical Fitness and Health 581
Strategies to Improve and Maintain Physical Fitness 582
    General Principles 582
    Chronic Organ Failure 583
    Strategies to Improve Long-Term Activity Behaviour in Health and Disease 584

PULMONARY REHABILITATION 586
Introduction 586
Aims of Rehabilitation in Chronic Obstructive Pulmonary Disease 586
Exercise Prescription 587
The Training Programme 587
    Duration 587
    Frequency 587
    Intensity 587

Training Modality 588
    Respiratory Muscle Training 589
Education and Self-Efficacy 589
    Neuromuscular Electrical Stimulation 590
    Balance Training 590
    Whole Body Vibration (WBV) 590
Timing of Rehabilitation 591
    Disease Stability 591
    Post-Exacerbation 591
    Peri-Exacerbation 591
Non-COPD Populations 592
    Rehabilitation for Interstitial Lung Disease 592
    Rehabilitation for Bronchiectasis 592
    Asthma 593
Practical Aspects of Training 593
    Location 593
    Equipment 593
    Supplemental Oxygen 593
    Non-Invasive Ventilation 595
    Safety Issues in Rehabilitation 596

Breathing Techniques 596
Nutrition 596
Long-Term Effects of Pulmonary Rehabilitation – Is
Benefit Maintained? 596
Conclusions 597
CARDIAC REHABILITATION 597
Introduction 597
Cardiac Rehabilitation – Past, Present and Future
Directions 598
Cardiac Rehabilitation and Secondary Prevention –
Evidence of Effectiveness 600
To Whom Should Secondary Prevention Programmes Be
Made Available? 601
By Whom Should Secondary Prevention Be
Delivered? 601
How Should Secondary Prevention Be
Delivered? 602
Emergence of Contemporary Models to Broaden
Delivery 603
Exercise Training in Secondary Prevention
Programmes 604
Benefits of Exercise Training 605
Improved Exercise Capacity 605

Recommended Levels of Physical Activity and
Exercise 606
Exercise Prescription 607
Principles of Exercise Prescription 607
Frequency of Exercise 607
Intensity of Exercise 608
Type of Training 610
Format of a Typical Exercise Session 610
Progression of Exercise Training 613
Programme Implementation 614
In-Hospital Activity Component 614
Immediate Post-Discharge Phase 614
The First 3 Months 615
Assessment and Risk Stratification 615
Safe Delivery and Programme Management 616
Exercise Considerations for Special Cardiac
Groups 623
Transition of Patients to Long-Term Community-Based
Exercise Provision 626
Conclusion 627
References 627

Physical Activity and Physical Fitness in Health and Disease

PHYSICAL ACTIVITY VERSUS PHYSICAL FITNESS

In recent years, the importance of physical activity behaviour as a strategy to maintain long-term health has been emphasized. Indeed there is reported to be a global physical inactivity pandemic (Kohl et al 2012). National and international guidelines on the appropriate dose of physical activity have been published and gain increasing attention of caregivers around the world (Garber et al 2011). When discussing physical activity behaviour, the terms 'physical activity' and 'physical fitness' are often interchanged, but they constitute different concepts.

Physical activity is defined by the World Health Organization (WHO) as any bodily movement produced by skeletal muscles that results in energy expenditure beyond resting energy expenditure (http://www.who.int/topics/physical_activity/en/). Physical activity is undertaken in different contexts or domains, which are related to daily routines (e.g. domestic activities), occupational activities and leisure activities (e.g. sports and exercise). Physical activity is frequently quantified as the active energy expenditure that has been spent in a specific time period (which is dependent of both amount and intensity of performed activities). The intensity of a performed activity can be easily transformed in metabolic equivalent of tasks (METs), which is the ratio of the task-related energy expenditure over resting metabolic rate, the latter equalling an oxygen consumption of 3.5 mL O_2/min kg^{-1} (= 1 MET).

A compendium of physical activities has been developed, assigning MET-levels to a range of frequently performed physical activities (Ainsworth et al 2011). As an example, walking at a speed of 3 miles/hour is associated with a mean energy expenditure of 3.3 METs, which equals 3.3 times the resting metabolic rate. Since MET levels reflect only the intensity of performed activities, the concept of MET-minutes (i.e.

performing an activity with an intensity of 1 MET for 1 minute equals 1 MET-min) has been introduced to consider both the amount and intensity of activities. When a person walks at the same speed of 3 miles/hour, as mentioned before, for 30 minutes, the associated energy expenditure can be quantified as 99 MET-minutes (3.3 METs × 30 min).

Physical fitness is a set of attributes that are either health- or skill-related. Health-related fitness includes the attributes of cardiorespiratory fitness, muscle strength, muscle endurance, flexibility, and body composition (weight in relation to height, body fat and lean muscle percentage, bone structure) (Caspersen et al 1985, Chen et al 2002). Skill-related fitness includes features of agility, balance, coordination, power, speed and reaction time (Caspersen et al 1985). The degree to which people have these attributes can be measured with specific fitness tests.

Although they are different concepts, physical activity and physical fitness are closely related, with higher doses of physical activity leading to larger increases in physical fitness (Church et al 2007).

PHYSICAL ACTIVITY, PHYSICAL FITNESS AND HEALTH

In 1953, Dr. Jeremy Morris and colleagues reported that middle-aged bus drivers in London had a higher incidence of coronary heart disease (CHD) compared to the conductors working in the same busses (Morris et al 1953). Indeed, the conductors had a lower early case fatality and a lower early mortality rate. The investigators linked this phenomenon to the clear difference in occupational physical activity level. So, regular physical activity prolongs life. Multiple studies have confirmed this hypothesis. For example, Wen and colleagues (2011) showed a close association between the level of physical activity and mortality risk in 416 715 Taiwanese individuals. Physically *active* showed a 14% reduction in mortality risk compared to physically *inactive* individuals. The reduction in mortality was 35% in physically *very active* individuals. Nowadays, physical inactivity is established as the fourth leading risk factor for global mortality, with 6% of worldwide deaths being attributed to it (WHO 2009).

Globally, 31% of adults aged 15 years or over were insufficiently active in 2008, with the highest prevalence in the individuals aged 60 years and older (Hallal et al 2012, WHO 2009). Moreover, 41% spend over 4 hours per day sitting (Hallal et al 2012). A dose–response relationship has been identified between the amount of physical activity and cardiovascular risk factors (Klenk et al 2013), cardiovascular morbidity (Vanhees et al 2012) and all-cause mortality (Samitz et al 2011). Moreover, there is strong evidence that sufficient physical activity reduces the rates of depression and falls, and increases cardiorespiratory and muscular fitness, results in healthier body mass and composition, improves bone health and increases functional health and cognitive function (Kohl et al 2012).

Similarly, cardiorespiratory fitness, assessed using maximal exercise testing, is related to long-term development of cardiovascular disease (CVD) (Vanhees et al 2012), even in patients with a low risk profile (Barlow et al 2012) and low cardiovascular and total mortality (Vigen et al 2012). Numerous mechanisms are proposed to be involved in this process. Importantly, physical activity and exercise training improve blood lipid profile, lower blood pressure, increase insulin sensitivity, improve C-reactive protein and other biomarkers of chronic heart disease (de Torres et al 2006, Vanhees et al 2012) and enhance the immune system (Pedersen 1991). Furthermore, physical activity is an essential component of weight management, as combining physical activity with dietary interventions increases the chance of success (Goldberg et al 2007).

Evidence also emerges that regular physical activity plays a protective role in the onset of several types of cancer, including colon cancer, breast cancer, prostate cancer, endometrial cancer and lung cancer (Anzuini et al 2011). Interestingly, physical activity levels also appear to influence lung function decline and risk to develop chronic obstructive pulmonary disease (COPD) in 'healthy' smokers (Garcia-Aymerich et al 2007). Moreover, high sensitivity C-reactive protein can be used as a marker for impaired energy metabolism, functional capacity, and distress due to respiratory symptoms in COPD (Broekhuizen et al 2006).

Among medical treatment, weight management and smoking cessation, sufficient physical activity levels and exercise training play an important role in secondary prevention in patients with atherosclerotic diseases (Moyna et al 2004, Piepoli et al 2010, Smith et al 2006). Indeed, increased levels of physical activity and fitness in males and females may reduce the cardiovascular-related mortality by about 20% to 35% (Macera et al 2003).

Whereas optimal physical activity behaviour plays an important role in the prevention of chronic diseases, it is also an important target for intervention in patients with established chronic disease. Indeed, lower-limb muscle weakness (Hulsmann et al 2004, Swallow et al 2007), exercise intolerance (Cote et al 2007, Ingle 2008, Polkey et al 2013, Spruit et al 2012) and low levels of daily physical activity (Waschki et al 2011) are independent predictors of mortality in patients with chronic diseases, like COPD or chronic heart failure (CHF). Therefore interventions focussing on increasing physical fitness and daily physical activity levels (e.g. rehabilitation and/or activity counselling (Spruit et al 2013, Vaes et al 2014) are of great clinical and societal importance.

STRATEGIES TO IMPROVE AND MAINTAIN PHYSICAL FITNESS

General Principles

Currently established guidelines on individualized exercise prescription have been based on large epidemiologic and clinical trials (Garber et al 2011, Nelson et al 2007). A comprehensive exercise programme mostly includes cardiorespiratory or aerobic exercise, resistance exercise, flexibility exercise and neuromotor exercise. Obviously, exercise training should be tailored to address the individuals' goals, considering the main limiting factors of exercise performance and regular daily physical activity.

The American College of Sports Medicine recommends that adults engage in moderate intense cardiorespiratory exercise training for more than 30 minutes on at least 5 days per week or vigorous cardiorespiratory exercise training for more than 20 minutes on at least 3 days per week to achieve optimal physical fitness and health (Garber et al 2011). Improvement in maximal oxygen uptake (VO_{2max}) is directly related to frequency, intensity and duration. It is also possible to combine training at moderate and vigorous intensity, to achieve a total energy expenditure exceeding 500 to 1000 MET-minutes per week. The observation that the exercise above a minimal intensity threshold is necessary to obtain results in terms of physical fitness and health confirms the overload principle of training. The training should have a 20- to 60-minute duration and be performed in bouts of at least 10 minutes, and should consist of continuous and rhythmic exercises that involve large muscle groups. The proposed training activities are additional to routine activities of daily life.

Moderate intense exercise equals a training zone range of 40–59% of heart rate reserve (HRR)/oxygen uptake (VO_2) reserve or 64–76% of maximal heart rate. Maximal heart rate is often estimated based on age (common formulas: $220 - age$ or $208 - (0.7 \times age)$) (Tanaka et al 2001) or response to submaximal exercise testing (Johnson et al 1991). As these estimations are based on linear regression analysis, clinicians should realize that these prediction formulas have a standard error in individual persons exceeding 10 beats per minute (bpm) (Nes et al 2013). Consequently, to ensure an adequate training intensity, it is recommended to combine exercise prescriptions based on heart rate with subjective parameters. Moderate intense activity is generally experienced as fairly light to somewhat hard (Borg 1982). People should be able to speak but not sing comfortably during exercise. The kind of activities that are considered moderately intense changes with increasing age. As maximal exercise tolerance decreases with increasing age, the relative intensity of performed activities increases simultaneously. As an example, walking 4 mph on a flat surface (equalling an intensity of 5 METs) is considered a mild to moderately intense activity in young adults (<40 years), whereas it is categorized as a vigorous activity in healthy elderly (>65 years).

Vigorous intense exercise is determined by a training zone between 60% and 89% of HRR/VO_2 reserve or 77–95% of maximal heart rate. The rate of perceived exertion ranges from somewhat hard to very hard. Table 12-1 provides an overview of parameters corresponding to exercise training of moderate and vigorous intensity.

A gradual progression of exercise volume (i.e. duration, frequency and intensity) is recommended until the desired goal of the exercise programme has been reached. At that moment, the goal of the exercise programme is to maintain the achieved results.

TABLE 12-1

An Overview of Parameters Corresponding to Exercise Training of Moderate and Vigorous Intensity

	Moderate Intensity	Vigorous Intensity
%HRR/%VO$_2$R	40–59	60–89
%HR$_{max}$	64–76	77–95
Rate of perceived exertion (6–20) (Borg 1982)	Fairly light to somewhat hard (12–13)	Somewhat hard to very hard (14–17)
METs	3.0–5.9	6.0–8.7
METs in young adults (20–40 yrs)	4.8–7.1	7.2–10.1
METs in middle-aged adults (40–65 yrs)	4.0–5.9	6.0–8.4
METs in elderly (65+ yrs)	3.2–4.7	4.8–6.7
Examples of activities for elderly	Level walking 2.5–3.5 mph Stair climbing (slow pace) Stationary cycling 30–90 Watts	Level walking 3.5–4.5 mph Walking 3.0–3.5 mph uphill (1–5°) Stationary cycling 80–100 Watts

Adapted from Garber et al 2011 and Ainsworth et al 2011.
HR, Heart rate; HRR, heart rate reserve; MET, metabolic equivalent; VO$_2$R, oxygen uptake reserve.

The general recommendations on resistance training advice is to train each major muscle group with a frequency of two to three times per week. Two to four sets of eight to 12 repetitions at an intensity of 60–70% of the one-repetition maximum (1-RM) are proposed when aiming to improve muscular strength. Rest intervals of 2–3 minutes between sets are sufficient. A higher intensity can be used in experienced athletes. In elderly and sedentary people who initiate a training programme, it is appropriate to initially decrease training intensity (40–50% of 1-RM) and increase the number of repetitions per set (10–15 repetitions), inserting an endurance component into the strength training programme. A gradual increase of the resistance (guided by the change in 1-RM) is necessary to ensure sufficient training intensity during the course of the programme (Kraemer et al 2002).

Static stretching of the major muscle–tendon units improves joint range of motion (ROM). Although the guidelines are to perform this exercise at least two to three times per week, it is most effective when performed daily. A static stretch of 10–30 consecutive seconds is recommended in adults, but a longer stretch (30–60 seconds) may be more efficient in the elderly. The greatest change in ROM with a static stretch occurs between 15 and 30 seconds (Bandy et al

1994, McHugh et al 1992). The proposed target is to stretch each muscle–tendon unit for 60 seconds in total. Additionally, neuromotor exercises are recommended at least two to three times per week in elderly people. Neuromotor exercises involve motor skills (e.g. balance, coordination), proprioceptive training and multifaceted activities (e.g. yoga, Tai Chi). An important goal of these exercise is to improve physical function and outcomes such as improved balance and reduced falls incidence.

Chronic Organ Failure

In patients with CHF or COPD, exercise training programmes are generally considered the cornerstone of multidisciplinary rehabilitation programmes (Corra et al 2010, Spruit et al 2013). Exercise training improves lower-limb muscle function, exercise tolerance and quality of life, and reduces symptoms of dyspnoea and fatigue, and the number of hospitalizations (Spruit et al 2013, O'Connor et al 2009). In CHF, exercise training is also associated with a modest reduction in all-cause and cardiovascular mortality (O'Connor et al 2009).

Although general exercise training recommendations are largely applicable in these patients, training intensity during aerobic exercise warrants some specific attention. Even though moderately intense activities are associated with lower absolute MET levels compared to healthy elderly, due to the observed decrease in exercise tolerance, the targeted relative intensity of aerobic training is comparable (i.e. 40–60% of VO_2 reserve). Whereas in healthy individuals, heart rate could be used as a surrogate parameter to describe exercise intensity, this is in most cases not appropriate in patients with CHF or COPD. Patients with CHF often have chronotropic incompetence and widely used β-blockers influence both resting heart rate and maximal heart rate (Beale et al 2010). Most patients with COPD are primarily limited by their ventilatory system or by gas exchange abnormalities during maximal exercise and the majority of patients do not reach their maximal heart rate (Palange et al 2007). Because the increase in ventilation and ventilatory symptoms during progressive exercise is non-linear, in contrast with heart rate, the latter cannot be used to ensure adequate training intensity. The maximal workload during incremental cycling exercise can be used to titrate the intensity of stationary cycle training (e.g. 60–70% of maximal workload for endurance exercise) (Troosters et al 2000, Neder et al 2000). In patients with CHF, intensities corresponding to a rate of perceived exertion <13 (somewhat hard) are usually well tolerated and have been successfully applied (Keteyian et al 1996). In patients with COPD, the modified Borg score (0–10) for symptoms of dyspnoea and fatigue is most commonly used in clinical practice. A Borg score of 4–6 is considered equivalent to moderately intense exercise (Chida et al 1991, Horowitz et al 1996) and is frequently used to define the training load. For resistance training exercises, the 1-RM is most commonly used to determine training load (Spruit et al 2002, Spruit et al 2009). The same approach can be used by healthy elderly as described.

Strategies to Improve Long-Term Activity Behaviour in Health and Disease

Given the beneficial health effects of regular physical activity, a change of physical activity behaviour and subsequently long-term adherence to this change is of utmost importance. However, physical activity behaviour is a complex concept which is attenuated by individual, interpersonal, environmental, regional, national and global factors (Fig. 12-1).

Commonly reported barriers that prevent elderly people from engaging in physical activity are lack of time, logistical problems, lack of energy, lack of experience with physical activity, issues related to intrinsic motivation, the presence of illness or injuries and low self-efficacy (Brawley et al 2003, Schutzer et al 2004). The presence or the lack of social support constitutes an important enabler or barrier towards engagement in physical activity (Thorpe et al 2012). Climatological circumstances also have a major impact on activity behaviour (Sumukadas et al 2009). Weather conditions may affect physical activity with temperature, wind speed, precipitation and humidity being strong determinants of walking duration in elderly people (Klenk et al 2012).

Individually tailored activity behaviour programmes induce short-term increases in daily physical activity (Kahn et al 2002, Hillsdon et al 2005). Behavioural strategies such as goal setting, social support, reinforcement, problem solving and relapse prevention should be incorporated in these interventions (Kahn et al 2002). Techniques of motivational interviewing have been successfully used to obtain lifestyle changes in several health behaviours including physical activity (Bennett et al 2007). In terms of physical activity behaviour, this patient-centred technique focuses on the identification of personal barriers precluding an increase in daily physical activity and stimulates the patients to actively search for solutions to overcome these barriers. Enhancing self-efficacy plays a central role in this process. The use of a pedometer to provide direct feedback on the amount of steps results in an acute 30% increase in physical activity levels (Bravata et al 2007). Therefore it might be interesting to incorporate direct feedback on physical activity into activity counselling programmes in a variety of healthy and patient populations.

Despite the short-term effectiveness of individual activity programs, long-term adherence is low (van der Bij et al 2002). Continued contact and social support might play a crucial role in the prevention of dropout from activity (Castro et al 2001). Use of telephone and e-mail have been proven effective in this context (Castro et al 2001, Goode et al 2012) and the ongoing development of smartphone applications and wearable activity monitors opens a new avenue of possibilities for prolonged follow-up (Fanning et al 2012).

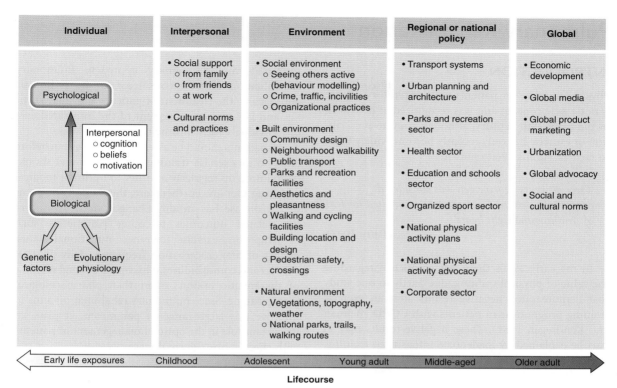

Individual	Interpersonal	Environment	Regional or national policy	Global

Psychological
 	
Interpersonal
○ cognition
○ beliefs
○ motivation
 	
Biological
 	
Genetic factors   Evolutionary physiology
	• Social support
	  ○ from family
	  ○ from friends
	  ○ at work
	
	• Cultural norms and practices
		• Social environment
		  ○ Seeing others active (behaviour modelling)
		  ○ Crime, traffic, incivilities
		  ○ Organizational practices
		
		• Built environment
		  ○ Community design
		  ○ Neighbourhood walkability
		  ○ Public transport
		  ○ Parks and recreation facilities
		  ○ Aesthetics and pleasantness
		  ○ Walking and cycling facilities
		  ○ Building location and design
		  ○ Pedestrian safety, crossings
		
		• Natural environment
		  ○ Vegetations, topography, weather
		  ○ National parks, trails, walking routes
			• Transport systems
			
			• Urban planning and architecture
			
			• Parks and recreation sector
			
			• Health sector
			
			• Education and schools sector
			
			• Organized sport sector
			
			• National physical activity plans
			
			• National physical activity advocacy
			
			• Corporate sector
				• Economic development
				
				• Global media
				
				• Global product marketing
				
				• Urbanization
				
				• Global advocacy
				
				• Social and cultural norms

Early life exposures   Childhood   Adolescent   Young adult   Middle-aged   Older adult

Lifecourse

FIGURE 12-1 ■ Factors influencing physical activity behaviour. *(Reproduced with permission from Bauman et al 2012.)*

In patients with chronic diseases, changes in health status (e.g. exacerbations), health beliefs and professional support have an additional influence on health behaviour (Thorpe et al 2012). In light of this, it is not surprising that structured outpatient rehabilitation programs are not associated with a consistent increase in daily physical activity levels (Cindy Ng et al 2012). Even though these programs induce clinically relevant increases in exercise tolerance, this change in physical fitness is not automatically translated in all cases into a change in physical activity behaviour outside the context of the rehabilitation programme. Overcoming the barriers to exercise in order to obtain long-term adherence to physical activity provides an important challenge for professionals within the field of rehabilitation (Soicher et al 2012). For example, one-third of the patients with COPD have concerns to perform physical activity, including shortness of breath, leg fatigue and a 'low oxygen level' (Danilack et al 2014).

In patients with CHF and COPD, individual activity counselling has the potential to induce a short-term increase in daily physical activity levels, both within and outside the context of multidisciplinary rehabilitation (Altenburg et al 2015, Ferrier et al 2011). The implementation of structured, self-monitored home-based exercises in the course of or following a rehabilitation programme also has the potential to translate the short-term increase in physical fitness into a long-term adherence to activity (Strijbos et al 1996).

In summary, physical activity and fitness are important aspects of everyday life in both healthy and diseased populations. Increased levels of both can impact risks for developing chronic diseases, morbidity and, indeed, mortality. Maintenance of longer-term adherence to increases gained in rehabilitation programs is a challenge for health professionals. The inclusion of techniques to address adherence to increase levels of physical activity are recommended.

Pulmonary Rehabilitation

INTRODUCTION

Physical training for patients with respiratory disease is not a new concept and was recognized as beneficial in the early 19th century, although routine prescription of exercise has only recently become widely used. In fact, as Thomas Petty puts it:

'Over 40 years ago, oxygen was considered contraindicated, and exercise was prohibited for fear of straining the right heart'

(Petty 1993).

In the early 1980s there was scepticism regarding the value of physical training, due partly to one study that demonstrated negative results after an exercise training programme in patients with COPD (Belman and Kendregan 1981). These negative results may in part be explained by inadequate intensity of training. Fortunately, scientific advances have led to widespread recognition of the value of exercise in COPD. There is now a strong body of evidence showing that exercise training by itself or as part of a pulmonary rehabilitation (PR) programme results in improvements in disease-related problems of dyspnoea, exercise capacity, muscle weakness and health-related quality of life (Lacasse et al 2006).

Pulmonary rehabilitation is defined as:

'a comprehensive intervention based on a thorough patient assessment followed by patient tailored therapies that include, but are not limited to, exercise training, education, and behaviour change, designed to improve the physical and psychological condition of people with chronic respiratory disease and to promote the long-term adherence to health-enhancing behaviours'

(Spruit et al 2013).

Pulmonary rehabilitation programs are ideally delivered by an interdisciplinary team whose structure varies according to the patient population, programme budget and availability of team members (Spruit et al 2013). Physiotherapists are an important part of this resource's multidisciplinary approach. Pulmonary rehabilitation is now considered to be a holistic approach to the treatment of patients and their families and is a major component of the integrated care of individuals with chronic respiratory disease.

All patients should be assessed by a physician before entry to an exercise training programme and should be followed up regularly in order to optimize medical and drug therapy. Furthermore, the therapeutic focus of the disease has steadily changed from expiratory flow-related outcomes to other parameters such as symptoms, exercise tolerance, nutritional status, quality of life, exacerbation frequency, daily physical activity and comorbidities. This opens a broad window of therapeutic options other than pharmacological therapy alone. Since pulmonary rehabilitation aims to improve this large range of parameters, it plays an important role in the optimal management of patients with chronic obstructive disease.

AIMS OF REHABILITATION IN CHRONIC OBSTRUCTIVE PULMONARY DISEASE

COPD is a major cause of morbidity and mortality worldwide, and individuals with COPD constitute the largest proportion of patients referred for pulmonary rehabilitation. The disease-specific clinical signs and symptoms for different respiratory diseases are given in Chapter 5 and provide the rationale for pulmonary rehabilitation. In brief, these are dyspnoea: reduction in exercise tolerance and health-related quality of life, cardiac dysfunction, gas exchange limitations, pre-existing levels of cardiovascular fitness and peripheral muscle dysfunction. Outcome measures used in PR such as field walking tests and health-related quality of life (HR-QoL) questionnaires are described in detail in Chapter 6.

The aims of pulmonary rehabilitation are to (Spruit et al 2013):

- reduce symptom burden
- maximize exercise capacity
- promote autonomy

- improve participation in activities of daily living (ADLs)
- enhance HR-QoL
- promote health behaviour change.

EXERCISE PRESCRIPTION

Exercise training is considered the cornerstone of a pulmonary rehabilitation programme (Lacasse et al 2006). Reconditioning of patients with respiratory disease reflects the same principles as those applied in healthy individuals, although programmes should be adapted to the individual limitations of the patient and take into consideration ventilatory, cardiovascular and muscular abnormalities (Troosters et al 2005). It is now widely accepted that exercise training is beneficial to patients with chronic respiratory diseases. It is also known that the training effects depend on different factors including duration and frequency of the training programme, training intensity and training modality (Vogiatzis 2008). Maximizing medical management, including treatment of comorbidities will assist effectiveness of rehabilitation (Spruit et al 2013).

THE TRAINING PROGRAMME

Duration

There is as yet no consensus as to the optimal duration of an exercise training programme for patients with COPD. Twenty sessions of pulmonary rehabilitation have been shown to produce better results than 10 sessions in outcomes such as exercise tolerance and HR-QoL (Rossi et al 2005). While one study has shown that a 4-week programme was as effective as a 7-week programme at 6 months (Sewell et al 2006), several other studies have demonstrated that exercise programmes lasting at least 7 weeks (7–12 weeks) result in greater benefits than those of shorter duration (Bendstrup et al 1997, Carrieri-Kohlman et al 2005, Green et al 2001, Lake et al 1990). It has therefore been suggested that programmes with a minimum duration of 8 weeks are advisable to achieve substantial positive effects on exercise performance and quality of life (Spruit et al 2013). Programmes of 6 months or longer may result in better long-term effects (Berry et al 2003, Guell et al 2000, Salman et al 2003, Troosters et al 2000).

Frequency

Ideal training frequency is also a topic that is much debated but there is as yet insufficient evidence to identify the optimal frequency. The scarce evidence available suggests that patients should exercise at least three times per week, and that regular supervision is fundamental (Puente-Maestu et al 2000, Ringbaek et al 2000, Wadell et al 2005). However, many programmes with twice-weekly supervision and encouragement of 'home exercise' have shown good results (Lacasse et al 2006). A small pilot study (n = 30) and a randomized controlled trial (RCT) of once versus twice weekly supervised training for 8 and 6 weeks respectively were conducted (Liddell & Webber 2010, O'Neill et al 2007). Although neither were adequately powered, there was less convincing improvement in HR-QoL and exercise performance in those who trained only once weekly.

Intensity

A further element of exercise prescription concerns the intensity of exercise. Before considering appropriate levels of intensity, it is necessary to revisit relevant assessment tools. Several common methods of prescribing intensity are used: symptom-limited exercise prescription and physiological testing derived from maximal (or peak) oxygen consumption. In the first method, patients are instructed to exercise to a prescribed symptom level, for example 'moderately or somewhat short of breath' (scores of 4–6) on the Borg breathlessness score (Borg 1982, Horowitz et al 1996). Although this provides an effective training stimulus for most patients, problems may occur when patients demonstrate very high levels of dyspnoea, thus limiting the intensity of training (Killian et al 1992, O'Donnell 1994). Dyspnoea is a subjective perception, meaning that fear and anxiety at the start of a programme may heighten scores. If this method is used, it may be necessary to reassess dyspnoea levels halfway through the programme and set a higher training target if appropriate. Calculating the exercise intensity from VO_{2max} is more reliable and is easily performed using cycle ergometry or derived from an associated measure such as the shuttle walk or 6-minute walk test (6MWT) (Dyer et al 2002). However, for patients with COPD, a true VO_{2max} may be unattainable due to ventilatory limitations. An effective compromise is to determine the initial exercise prescription at 70–80% of the derived VO_{2max} or VO_{2peak} and then to use breathlessness scores to monitor the training and adjust accordingly (Mahler et al 2003). A further method for calculating walking distance is to use the distance walked in the 6MWT. Devise the 1-minute distance from this and then set walking distance to 80% of that value for the required time. Although the 6MWT and the incremental shuttle walk test (ISWT) both provoke a VO_2 similar to that seen on a cardiopulmonary exercise test (CPET), the ISWT may be better for prescribing an exercise regimen as a percentage of peak performance because responses to exercise are more incremental (Holland et al 2014). Another option to determine training intensity is using a percentage of the maximal heart rate. Caution is necessary because this may result in inadequate training stimulus (Brolin et al 2003, Pitta et al 2004, Zacarias et al 2000). This inadequacy may occur because maximal exercise capacity is often not affected by the cardio-circulatory system in COPD patients, and heart rate is also influenced by various medications commonly prescribed to COPD patients.

Several studies (Casaburi et al 1997, Gimenez et al 2000, Maltais et al 1997, Puente-Maestu et al 2000) found higher intensity exercise to be effective in COPD. They recommend training intensities of 60–80% of peak work rate or maximal oxygen consumption in order to achieve the greatest effects. Low-intensity training has also been shown to result in significant improvements in symptoms and quality of life (Normandin et al 2002) and even in exercise tolerance (Clark et al 1996, Roomi et al 1996). Wedzicha and colleagues (1998) reported that the improvement in exercise performance and health status following an exercise programme depends on the initial degree of dyspnoea. Therefore a cautionary note concerns the relative severity of the patients. Findings from a systematic review highlight the fact that in very severe patients, there is a lack of evidence to indicate that high-intensity exercise is the ideal mode of training. (Puhan et al 2005). Applicability of high-intensity training in these most severe and symptomatic COPD patients requires further study. In cases where high-intensity exercise is advocated for the more symptomatic patients with severe COPD, interval training may prove to be more comfortable (Vogiatzis et al 2005), since it allows higher training intensities while generating less dyspnoea.

Training Modality

A variety of training modalities is employed in the management of patients with COPD, all with generally good results. Most programmes use **continuous** (or endurance) exercise training (Spruit et al 2013), incorporating an element of walking and/or cycling for 20–30 minutes per session. These are optimal exercise modalities, as they are functional, especially walking. An alternative approach is **interval training,** where the 20- or 30-minute exercise session is divided into short bouts of high-intensity exercise for 30 seconds to 2–3 minutes, interspersed with periods of rest and lower intensity exercise. Interval training may allow more severe patients to achieve higher work rates and to exercise for longer with fewer symptoms, due to less dynamic hyperinflation and a higher stable ventilation (Sabapathy et al 2004, Vogiatzis et al 2004). Both training methods demonstrate improvements in clinically relevant outcomes but further research is necessary in comparing the two modalities in other chronic respiratory diseases (Spruit et al 2013).

The optimal **strength (resistance) training** protocol in COPD is yet to be established. However, strength training is an important component of rehabilitation since it is aimed at the systemic effects of COPD and improves muscle strength, which may impact falls, balance and function and reduce osteoporosis. Strength training needs to meet physiological training principles including being performed 2–3 times weekly at 60–70% of the 1-RM at a dosage of around 1 to 3 sets of 8–12 repetitions (American College of Sports Medicine 2013) and must be progressively increased over time to ensure progressive overload is achieved. Probst and colleagues (2006) showed that a major advantage of strength training is that the cardiopulmonary stress during this kind of exercise is lower than during whole-body endurance exercise and results in fewer symptoms. Guidelines for pulmonary rehabilitation in COPD patients currently recommend a combination of endurance and strength training (Bolton et al 2013, Spruit et al 2013).

Additional Training Considerations

Upper Limb Training. Although the focus of most studies of exercise training in COPD patients has been the lower limbs, the upper limbs are important since many activities of daily life require upper limb involvement (Franssen et al 2005). Therefore exercises that reflect ADLs such as resistance training targeting the biceps, triceps and pectoral muscles and arm cycle ergometry are included in programmes (O'Shea et al 2004). To date, research is equivocal regarding the effect of upper limb training on improving HR-QoL and other important patient outcomes (Spruit 2013).

Water-Based Training

There are two trials that have investigated the efficacy of water-based exercise training (McNamara et al 2013, Wadell et al 2004), as well as a recent Cochrane review (McNamara et al 2013). While there has been concern around the safety of people with COPD exercising in water due to increased chest wall pressure, no adverse events to training have been reported in studies. Furthermore, of the two RCTs comparing water-based training to land-based training and no training, there are clear benefits in exercise performance and HR-QoL from this modality of training. McNamara et al (2013) suggest this may be a particularly useful method for people with COPD who have other physical comorbidities which restrict their ability to participate in traditional land-based exercise.

Other Training Methods

Other methods of training include Tai Chi, Nordic walking and non-linear periodic training. One RCT of a 3-month Nordic walking intervention compared with usual care demonstrated significant gains in walking performance following the intervention, which were maintained up to 9 months later (Breyer et al 2010). A systematic review of Tai Chi for COPD included eight RCTs, involving 544 patients (Yan et al 2013). Meta-analyses showed there were significant gains in exercise performance, HR-QoL and dyspnoea following a Tai Chi programme compared with usual care. Studies that were included largely reported the short-term impact (around 12 weeks), and the longer-term effectiveness is unclear regarding improvement in exercise capacity and HR-QoL. Also interestingly, Leung et al reported that Tai Chi exercise for individuals with COPD was moderate level exercise that had a high level of adherence and satisfaction for participants (Leung et al 2013; Leung et al 2014). Another recent RCT used periodic, non-linear training and

found improved cycle endurance and HR-QoL outcomes in patients with more severe COPD (Klijn et al 2013). Alternative forms of training are important for broadening the options of training modalities, which may better be able to meet the needs of each individual across different continents (Andrianopoulos et al 2014).

Respiratory Muscle Training

In theory, by improving the strength or endurance of the diaphragm, greater inspiratory loads may be tolerated, thereby prolonging exercise tolerance and reducing dyspnoea. Inspiratory muscle training (IMT) can be performed using inspiratory resistive training, threshold loading and normocapnic hyperpnoea, but currently there is insufficient evidence to support one method over another of IMT added to whole-body exercise training. Meta-analyses of IMT, compared with sham IMT or no intervention, in individuals with COPD demonstrate significant improvements al 2011, Spruit et al 2013). Improvements have been demonstrated in walk distance, and small improvement in HR-QOL (Belman & Shadmehr 1988, Budweiser et al 2006). However, current evidence indicates that IMT used in isolation is questionable. It is conceivable that IMT might be useful when added to whole-body exercise training, especially in individuals with marked inspiratory muscle weakness or those unable to participate in cycling or walking, but this requires further evaluation.

EDUCATION AND SELF-EFFICACY

The focus of educating the patient has evolved over the years from single lectures to a self-management approach that encourages and teaches skills involved in disease control: namely, health behaviour modification and improved self-efficacy. To educate the patient should be a shared responsibility between the family and all health professionals involved. More information relating to health behaviour modification can be found in Chapter 8.

There are few trials specifically evaluating the benefit of education programmes as part of pulmonary rehabilitation. Collaborative self-management as a core component of pulmonary rehabilitation is well accepted (Bourbeau et al 2006, Wagg 2012). Self-management support should guide individuals in generic self-management skills such as goal-setting, problem-solving, decision-making and utilizing resources (Lorig et al 2003). Furthermore, there are many disease-specific skills such as chest clearance, breathing strategies, nutritional control and energy conservation which can be optimized through pulmonary rehabilitation (Spruit et al 2013).

Since the prevalence of depression and anxiety in COPD patients is very high (Janssen et al 2010), psychological counselling in addition to pulmonary rehabilitation renders additional benefits to patients with these characteristics (i.e. 20–40% of the patients) (Nguyen & Carrieri-Kohlman 2005, Withers et al 1999). Behaviour-oriented approaches to pulmonary rehabilitation such as goal setting may improve adherence and task performance and lead to improved ability to undertake exercise after completion of programmes (Locke et al 1981).

Neuromuscular Electrical Stimulation

Using transcutaneous low-intensity currents, muscle contraction can be induced by neuromuscular electrical stimulation (NMES) and specific muscle groups can be trained. In stable patients with muscle weakness, NMES applied to the lower limb muscles improved muscle strength, exercise tolerance and peak oxygen uptake (Bourjeily-Habr et al 2002, Neder et al 2002, Sillen et al 2014). The use of NMES has also been reported to result in a fast functional recovery in severely disabled patients receiving mechanical ventilation who were bedbound for more than 30 days (Zanotti et al 2003). In patients with well-preserved functional status, however, the results were very modest (Dal Corso et al 2007). The use of NMES as an adjunct to rehabilitation in severely disabled patients with low body mass index (BMI) has been shown to result in improvements in dyspnoea, exercise tolerance and muscle strength (Vivodtzev et al 2006). This suggests that NMES may provide an additional stimulus for changes in muscle physiology for malnourished patients or those with severe ventilatory limitation. The intervention was provided early following discharge from a hospital admission for acute exacerbation. It is possible that malnourished patients show greater hospital-induced sarcopenia than those with adequate BMI and that this may have contributed to the improved effects found in this study. In summary, NMES may be a promising modality for use in more severely disabled patients but it is unclear if there are effects in patients with higher levels of functional exercise capacity and in populations other than COPD.

Balance Training

Emerging evidence identifies altered postural balance control as an important secondary impairment in COPD, which may directly increase risk of falling (Roig et al 2009). Currently, balance retraining and fall risk assessment are not included in international guidelines for COPD or PR programmes (Beauchamp et al 2010, Johnston et al 2011, Ries et al 2007). Furthermore, standard pulmonary rehabilitation alone does not improve balance performance in COPD (Beauchamp et al 2009). Exercise training for older adults may provide an excellent model to further broaden exercise prescription for COPD patients, because, as with the elderly, people with COPD are now being identified to have a high relative risk of falls (Beauchamp et al 2009, Oliveira et al 2015). Further, individuals with COPD are shown to have a high fear of falling (Oliveira et al 2015). This may impact their physical activity levels; this is important since low physical activity is associated with mortality in COPD. A recent randomized trial has shown that incorporation of a specific balance re-education programme alongside standard exercise training is feasible and improves balance in people with COPD (Beauchamp et al 2013). The effect of impaired balance and other COPD-specific impairments such as lung hyperinflation and hypoxaemia on the incidence of falls in COPD has not yet been reported.

Whole Body Vibration (WBV)

Two studies have investigated the additional benefits of training on a WBV plate. One study compared a 6-week training programme with no training (Pleguezuelos et al 2013) and another study compared a 3-week intensive inpatient training programme with conventional exercise (Gloeckl et al 2012). WBV training appears to show significant benefits in walking distance compared with no exercise training, and these benefits may be greater than conventional training alone. These are small studies, and further research to confirm findings and understand the optimal WBV training parameters is required. Guidelines for exercise

BOX 12-1

GUIDELINES FOR EXERCISE IN PULMONARY REHABILITATION FOR PATIENTS WITH COPD

- A training programme consisting of between 16 and 24 sessions, supervised at least twice a week, should be offered; longer programmes generally result in better long-term effects.
- Encourage patients to exercise independently at home in addition to supervised sessions.
- Both continuous and interval training approaches can be used. Interval training may deliver equivalent training loads with less symptoms.
- A combination of endurance and strength training is recommended in rehabilitation programmes.
- Progression of the training load should be based on the patient's tolerance (symptom scores).
- Both upper and lower extremities should be trained.
- Training can improve outcomes across the range of disease severity in COPD.
- A comprehensive, supervised rehabilitation programme commenced immediately after an AECOPD may improve exercise capacity and reduce hospital re-admissions.
- Rehabilitation during an AECOPD may hasten recovery.
- Alternative exercise methods such as water-based and Tai Chi exercise are effective modalities.
- Health behaviour modification may improve longer-term outcomes for patients.
- Rehabilitation is effective for patients with bronchiectasis and interstitial lung diseases.

AECOPD, acute exacerbation of chronic obstructive pulmonary disease; *COPD*, chronic obstructive pulmonary disease.

prescription in pulmonary rehabilitation for patients with COPD are outlined in Box 12-1.

TIMING OF REHABILITATION

Disease Stability

COPD is usually defined as 'stable' if the patient has been exacerbation free for 8 weeks. The majority of the evidence for pulmonary rehabilitation has been carried out in people who are considered stable. Given the substantial evidence of the effectiveness of pulmonary rehabilitation in this population, it is recommended in several sets of international guidelines

that pulmonary rehabilitation be offered to patients with COPD who are considered to be functionally disabled by their disease (Bolton et al 2013, NICE 2010, Spruit et al 2013).

Post-Exacerbation

There is now an accumulating body of evidence to suggest that pulmonary rehabilitation delivered in the immediate period following hospitalization from an acute exacerbation can be superior to usual care. A Cochrane review of RCTs investigating the impact of post-exacerbation rehabilitation found 9 trials, which included 432 patients up to 2011 (Puhan et al 2011). The review concluded that pulmonary rehabilitation delivered immediately post exacerbation significantly improved hospital re-admission, mortality, HR-QoL and exercise capacity. Furthermore, of the three trials which specifically recorded adverse events, no increased risk from the intervention was shown, suggesting rehabilitation following exacerbation is safe. Based on these findings, guidelines now recommend that patients discharged from hospital with an acute exacerbation of COPD be offered pulmonary rehabilitation within 1 month of discharge (Bolton et al 2013). There may, however, be difficulties around the practicalities and feasibility of delivering this kind of intervention to large numbers of patients at this point. In the study by Seymour et al (2010), it took 3 years to recruit 60 participants, suggesting uptake was low. Additionally, data are reported that highlight the difficulties of referring and retaining patients in this service, with only 9% of all patients discharged from hospital with an exacerbation of COPD actually completing rehabilitation (Jones et al 2013). Rehabilitation programmes that are closed courses, with fixed start and end dates may find post-exacerbation pulmonary rehabilitation particularly challenging to deliver within the 1 month time-frame (Bolton et al 2013).

Peri-Exacerbation

There is a limited amount of work investigating the effects of exercise training during hospitalization for an acute exacerbation of COPD. There is evidence to suggest that while patients with COPD are hospitalized with an acute exacerbation, both peripheral muscle strength and physical activity levels are markedly reduced (Pitta et al 2006). The aim of physical training during hospitalization is to prevent, or minimize, this decline. Troosters et al (2010) demonstrated that resistance training in people with COPD during a hospitalization significantly improved quadriceps muscle force at 10 days, that was maintained at 30 days compared to a control with no training. A recent large RCT reported that there were no between group differences in re-admission rates between those receiving an intervention commenced within 48 hours of admission with an acute exacerbation chronic obstructive pulmonary disease (AECOPD) and a usual care group. A cautionary note from this trial was that the intervention group had a higher 1-year mortality, although this was not able to be explained. The authors suggest that early intervention is unnecessary but that future work should monitor this patient group carefully (Greening et al 2014).

NON-COPD POPULATIONS

Rehabilitation for Interstitial Lung Disease

Although the pathophysiology of interstitial lung disease (ILD) differs significantly from COPD (Chapter 5), patients present with similar signs and symptoms, including dyspnoea on exertion, fatigue, reduced peripheral muscle strength and low levels of physical activity. With the emergence of new treatments that slow disease progression but do not provide cure, pulmonary rehabilitation has an increasingly important role in maximizing functional capacity and improving well-being for people with ILD (NICE guidelines 2013). A Cochrane review examining pulmonary rehabilitation for ILD included nine RCTs with a total of 386 participants, including 153 with idiopathic pulmonary fibrosis (IPF) (Dowman et al 2014). Pulmonary rehabilitation resulted in clinically meaningful improvements in 6-minute walk distance (weighted mean difference 44 metres, 95% confidence interval (CI) 26–64 metres) and quality of life (standardized mean difference 0.59, 95% CI 0.2–0.98). Effect sizes are similar to those documented in COPD (McCarthy et al 2015) and people with IPF experienced a similar magnitude of improvement to those with other forms of ILD (Dowman et al 2014). A traditional pulmonary rehabilitation format has been used, with a median programme duration of 10 weeks, two sessions each week and 30 minutes of aerobic training in each

session (Holland et al 2015). Most programmes also use resistance training and some include other non-exercise components such as education, nutritional advice and stress management. Because people with ILD often experience profound oxygen desaturation on exertion and may have significant pulmonary hypertension, it is recommended that programmes take place in a setting where supplemental oxygen can be delivered (Spruit et al 2013). The benefits of rehabilitation may diminish in the 6–12 months following programme completion, particularly in those with progressive disease (Holland et al 2008, Holland et al 2012, Vainshelboim et al 2015); as a result, the NICE guidelines recommend that patients with IPF are reassessed for rehabilitation every 6–12 months (NICE guidelines 2013).

Rehabilitation for Bronchiectasis

International guidelines recommend the inclusion of people with bronchiectasis in pulmonary rehabilitation to improve functional capacity and HR-QoL. Retrospective studies which explored the effects of the standard pulmonary rehabilitation model (cardiovascular and strength training with or without education) had encouraging findings of similar benefits in exercise capacity and HR-QoL as those observed in COPD (Ong et al 2011, van Zeller et al 2012). There have been three randomized controlled trials of pulmonary rehabilitation in this patient population. Eight weeks of endurance training with or without IMT were examined in a group of 32 patients. While exercise capacity increased irrespective of this additional intervention, IMT was associated with greater HR-QoL and sustained improvement in exercise capacity at 3 months follow-up (Newall et al 2005). A combination of 8 weeks of pulmonary rehabilitation and airway clearance therapy using oscillatory positive expiratory pressure was associated with greater improvement in exercise capacity and quality of life immediately following the intervention and at 3 months follow-up compared to airway clearance therapy alone (Mandal et al 2012). In the only study which incorporated longer-term follow-up, a twice weekly, 8-week cardiovascular and strength training programme was associated with short-term gains in exercise capacity and reduced dyspnoea and fatigue and fewer acute exacerbations of bronchiectasis over 12 months (Lee et al

2014). This current evidence suggests that people with bronchiectasis may benefit from pulmonary rehabilitation, with further trials necessary to determine the optimal components of a programme.

Asthma

A Cochrane review evaluated the impact of exercise training in people with asthma over the age of 8 years old, who had trained at least twice weekly for a minimum of 4 weeks (Carson et al 2013). Twenty-one studies were included, and the review concluded that exercise training was safe and conferred significant improvements in exercise performance compared with no training. There was no impact on measures of pulmonary function, and in four of the five studies which evaluated HR-QoL, there were statistical and clinically significant gains.

PRACTICAL ASPECTS OF TRAINING

Location

There are arguments in favour of rehabilitation in a number of settings, from the hospital inpatient setting to the outpatient (Fig. 12-2), home or community setting. A recent Cochrane systematic review reported on 39 studies that were hospital based and 25 that were community based. Results from sub-analyses demonstrated a significant difference in treatment effect between subgroups for all domains of the Chronic Respiratory Disease Questionnaire (CRQ), with higher mean values, on average, in the PR group in hospital than in the community-based groups. However, in recognition of patient wishes and significant under-resourcing of pulmonary rehabilitation programmes, future developments may need to make greater use of community facilities (Garrod and Backley 2006). Physiotherapists are ideally placed to lead the way with referrals, support and training of local members.

It may be that patients with moderate to severe disease and exercise hypoxaemia may require assessment and training at a specialist centre with a view to oxygen requirements and adequate monitoring during exercise. However, patients with mild to moderate disease may perform all aspects of training at home or in the community, requiring only initial supervision from a physiotherapist. Further research comparing home- and community-based programmes with hospital-based programmes are thus warranted.

Equipment

As mentioned previously, functional exercise programmes are of the utmost importance to the success of pulmonary rehabilitation. Simple exercises aid clarity, and practical measures to include exercise in daily life may aid long-term adherence. Moreover, for older patients with COPD, exercise must be seen as 'appropriate'; for patients with less severe disease, swimming, bike riding, golfing, bowling and walking are all appropriate forms of exercise. The type of equipment will depend primarily on the type of training to be performed and local financial resources. Equipment requirements may be as simple as a mat for floor exercises, dumbbells or hand weights (see Fig. 12-2A) and space to perform aerobic training. Where endurance training is the main objective, equipment such as cycle ergometry (see Fig. 12-2B) and a treadmill may be helpful. However, walking practice, devices to simulate stair climbing or actual stairs have high functional applicability. In order to improve walking ability, a rollator may be a useful option (see Fig. 12-2C). A rollator is a walker with four wheels, equipped with swivel castors on the front wheels, brakes, a basket for carrying objects and a seat that allows sitting for rest. An alternative is a three-wheeled walker.

In order to achieve long-term benefits, patients must be able to continue exercising effectively after the programme has ended. For strength training, a multi-gym may be ideal but simple hand and ankle weights will also be useful.

Supplemental Oxygen

The use of supplemental oxygen during training remains a complex question, one that in many cases is further complicated by the issue of available resources. Further detailed information on oxygen therapy can be found in Chapter 7. It is widely thought that oxygen supplementation leads to significant acute improvement in exercise tolerance in hypoxaemic patients (O'Donnell et al 2001), even in patients without appreciable exercise desaturation (Somfay et al 2001). Despite this, studies in which oxygen was provided during an exercise training programme have not shown additional benefits directly linked to oxygen

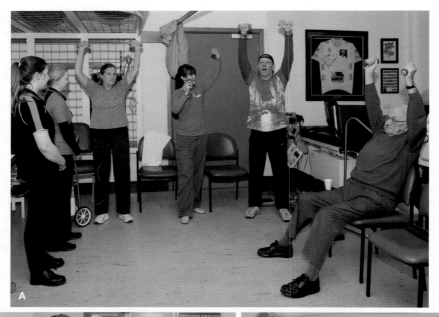

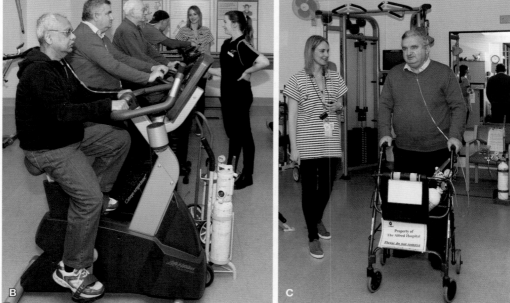

FIGURE 12-2 ■ Patients exercising during pulmonary rehabilitation (PR). **(A)** Hand weights for upper limb exercises. **(B)** Group exercise using a cycle ergometer. **(C)** A patient using a walker and oxygen therapy.

supplementation. One randomized study investigated the role of oxygen in patients with severe COPD and exercise desaturation (Garrod et al 2000a). This showed an improvement in dyspnoea after rehabilitation that was greater in the patients who trained with oxygen compared with those who did not. However, as in an earlier study (Rooyackers et al 1997), there was no difference in the changes in exercise tolerance between the two groups. This suggests that although additional oxygen may augment desensitization to dyspnoea, it does little to enhance changes in exercise tolerance. Further data showed similar results and concluded there were minimal benefits of oxygen as a training adjunct (Wadell et al 2001).

Emtner and colleagues (2003) performed a randomized evaluation of the effects of oxygen on training in 29 non-hypoxaemic COPD patients. Breathing oxygen significantly increased endurance time compared with the air-trained group. Furthermore, the rate of improvement was greater in the oxygen-trained patients. These data support previous observations that supplemental oxygen has a greater effect on submaximal exercise, improving endurance rather than intensity and reinforcing the likelihood that oxygen benefits are accrued largely through reductions in dynamic hyperinflation rather than correction of hypoxia per se (Somfay et al 2001). A recent RCT compared training with oxygen against compressed air cylinders during a 6-week rehabilitation programme in people with COPD who had exercise-induced desaturation (Dyer et al 2012). The study found there were significantly greater improvements in walking endurance performance measured by the endurance shuttle walk test (ESWT) in those who had trained on oxygen compared with those trained on compressed air. A key aspect of this study was that patients were selected on the basis that they had demonstrated at least a 10% improvement in ESWT at baseline when walking with correctly titrated oxygen compared with no oxygen. This suggests it may be possible to identify responders to supplemental oxygen during training by evaluating their response at a baseline assessment. Additionally a recent randomised trial (Spielmanns et al 2015) evaluated the effects of training in individuals with COPD who were normoxaemic at rest and during exercise. The authors concluded that the endurance training with oxygen 3 times/week resulted in significant improvements in quality of life and exercise capacity in individuals with moderate to severe COPD within the initial 12-week programme.

At the present time it is prudent to advise that patients who are on long-term oxygen therapy (LTOT) should exercise with supplemental oxygen. In addition, training with oxygen both for hypoxaemic and non-hypoxaemic patients may allow them to exercise at higher intensity and with less dyspnoea, although more research is still needed.

The routine use of oxygen during pulmonary rehabilitation has implications. Instruction to exercise with supplemental oxygen during rehabilitation for patients not already prescribed LTOT or ambulatory oxygen could relay a confused message. This may adversely affect adherence both to the rehabilitation programme and the use of oxygen. Patients with exercise desaturation, even without resting daytime hypoxaemia, should ideally have saturation levels monitored throughout training. Where desaturation occurs and a clear benefit is shown, they should train with oxygen and be provided with ambulatory oxygen for home use.

Non-Invasive Ventilation

The role of non-invasive ventilation (NIV) as an adjunct to rehabilitation is based on the theory that unloading of the respiratory muscles during activity will enable higher work intensities to be reached, accruing greater benefit from exercise. For many patients with severe problems, dyspnoea may significantly limit the ability to exercise and NIV may be a valuable addition to rehabilitation. In a systematic review, rehabilitation experts from the Netherlands pooled data from seven critically appraised studies (van't Hul et al 2002) and found there was a significant benefit related to exercise-induced dyspnoea and endurance time when NIV was applied during an acute exercise test.

However, there are practical difficulties to providing ventilation during a training session in terms of limiting the type of exercise and adherence to exercise. In an RCT of overnight application of non-invasive positive pressure ventilation (NIPPV) plus daytime non-assisted rehabilitation, significant improvements in exercise tolerance and quality of life were found after rehabilitation in the home-ventilated group compared with a non-ventilated group (Garrod et al 2000b). Improvement in exercise tolerance may have resulted from overnight relief of low-level fatigue of respiratory muscles caused during exhaustive exercise. Valid criticisms of this work concern the relatively short period of time spent using the ventilator (mean 2.5 hours) and the lack of placebo ventilation. In a more recent randomized trial of 28 patients with COPD, Borghi-Silva et al (2010) tested administration of NIV against supplemental oxygen during PR. The authors found NIV to be superior in improving endurance walking distance in patients who desaturated on exertion with a positive acute response to ambulatory oxygen at baseline. Further information regarding NIV can be found in Chapter 7.

Safety Issues in Rehabilitation

Many elderly people perceive exercise at 'their age' to be dangerous (O'Brien et al 1995). Issues of safety are obviously compounded in older people with respiratory disease and considerable reassurance may be required concerning safety. The issues of safety are somewhat unknown in the field of pulmonary rehabilitation. Although full exercise testing with electrocardiography (ECG) heart monitoring is recommended as routine for patients with COPD (Spruit et al 2013), a maximal incremental cycle ergometry test is unrealistic for many patients with severe disease and in many units due to cost and staffing limitations. Even unloaded cycling can be exhausting for these patients, while adding incremental loads may cause distressing dyspnoea, ultimately preventing further exercise and disheartening the patient.

Most programmes exclude patients with unstable angina. For most patients, a field walking test with pulse oximetry and heart rate monitoring will identify oxygen needs and enable prescription of exercise intensity (Holland et al 2014). In the hospital setting, resuscitation equipment and oxygen should be readily available, and the personnel involved trained in the use of this equipment. However, a more pragmatic approach is required in the community setting where patients may be exercising at home or in local centres. There is evidence that patients with COPD demonstrate oxygen desaturation during routine activities. The long-term effects of temporary falls in pulse saturation are unknown and warrant further investigation

(Schenkel et al 1996). Patients with COPD often demonstrate ventilatory limitation or report fatigue before there is significant cardiovascular stress. However, this will not be the same for all groups of patients with respiratory disease and further research is required in this area. Anecdotally the only complications of exercise in these patients have been related to minor musculoskeletal injuries.

Breathing Techniques

Breathing control is defined as:

> '... gentle breathing using the lower chest with relaxation of the upper chest and shoulders; it is performed at normal tidal volume, at a natural rate and expiration should not be forced'
> *(Partridge et al 1989)*

More information on breathing techniques can be found in Chapter 7.

A recent Cochrane review (Holland et al 2012) concluded that breathing exercises may improve functional exercise capacity in those people with COPD unable to undertake exercise training, but did not provide additional benefit to exercise training. In addition, the effect of breathing exercises on dyspnoea was inconsistent. Currently, there is not strong evidence for breathing exercises in COPD.

Nutrition

A systematic review of randomized controlled trials showed no significant effects of nutritional supplementation on anthropometric measures, lung function or exercise capacity in patients with stable COPD (Ferreira et al 2005). Recent RCTs (Leong et al 2015, Shepherd et al 2015) also conclude that no benefit was found with dietary nitrate supplementation. Although there may be subgroups of patients who benefit, more research should be undertaken exploring these (Creutzberg et al 2000).

LONG-TERM EFFECTS OF PULMONARY REHABILITATION – IS BENEFIT MAINTAINED?

Many studies have assessed the short-term benefits of pulmonary rehabilitation. These studies have shown that patients can gain significant benefits in exercise capacity, health status and dyspnoea immediately following a rehabilitation programme. However, full assessment of pulmonary rehabilitation requires an evaluation of the long-term benefits of such programmes. One of the ways to obtain longer-lasting effects is to increase the programme's duration and another is to provide a follow-up programme.

Berry and co-workers (2003) studied two groups: a follow-up programme comprising exercise sessions three times per week for 15 months, and an exercise advice programme for the same period of time. The exercise group showed superior results, demonstrating the value of long-term follow-up including regular exercise training. Further, participation in regular walking, after completing a pulmonary rehabilitation programme, is associated with slower declines in overall HR-QoL and walking self-efficacy as well as less progression of dyspnoea during ADLs (Heppner et al 2006). Repeated short-term programmes report a reduction in exacerbation rates (Foglio et al 2001) but no improvements in functional outcomes. Regular telephone support and monthly visits or meetings with health professionals report modest effects (Brooks et al 2002, Ries et al 2003).

Overall the literature in this area is conflicting and the available evidence does not allow definitive conclusions to be drawn on the ideal design of a follow-up programme, although periodic supervised exercise sessions seem advisable.

CONCLUSIONS

Pulmonary rehabilitation is an effective therapy with level I evidence in COPD, and level 2 evidence in bronchiectasis and ILD. There is evidence to support that pulmonary rehabilitation programmes result in:

- improvement in exercise tolerance
- improvement in the sensation of dyspnoea
- improvement in the ability to perform routine ADLs
- improvement in HR-QoL
- improvement in muscle strength, endurance and mass
- reductions in number of days spent in hospital.

There is little information on cost effectiveness of PR programmes, and cost and resources will remain obstacles to overcome, with waiting lists for PR in many countries. In the future, improving access to pulmonary rehabilitation by developing new models of delivery may improve participation; self-management and health behaviour change may improve longer-term outcomes. Further, it is recommended that no further trials are needed to assess efficacy of PR but that future research should focus on identifying which components of pulmonary rehabilitation are essential, the ideal length and location (hospital versus community), the degree of supervision and intensity of training required and length of treatment effects (McCarthy et al 2015).

Cardiac Rehabilitation

INTRODUCTION

Cardiovascular Disease (CVD) encompasses all disorders of the heart and blood vessels and is the leading cause of global mortality; accounting for over 17 million deaths each year (WHO, 2011). Specifically, chronic heart disease (CHD) is the most common type of heart disease. According to the WHO, CHD accounted for 12.9% of all deaths (seven million deaths) and 5.8% of total disability-adjusted life years globally in 2011 (WHO, 2014). In low- to middle-income countries there is a growing epidemic where coronary events and mortality rates are rapidly increasing. In high-income countries, although mortality rates have been declining over the last thirty years, CHD still remains the leading single disease burden. Advances in diagnosis, revascularisation, pharmacotherapy and treatment of acute illness have contributed to these reductions in mortality. A growing population of people surviving acute cardiac events and living longer with chronic long-term conditions such as heart failure (Ford et al 2007, Unal et al 2004). This places a growing and unsustainable burden on healthcare resources and consequently the demand for effective secondary prevention is intensifying (Redfern and Briffa 2011). Availability of interventions that complement standard medical care and aim to reduce further events in those with established disease is now a pressing and urgent priority.

Cardiac rehabilitation is considered an integral part of the regular medical management of patients with CHD and is widely recommended in international guidelines (Anderson et al 2011, Aroney et al 2006, Steg et al 2012). Without systematic access to cardiac rehabilitation, these individuals may experience multiple recurrent acute care events and suffer unnecessarily premature death (Clark et al 2010, Davies et al 2010, Heran et al 2011). Survivors are at very high risk of a recurrence, with one-quarter likely to be readmitted to hospital within 1 year of the index event (Briffa et al 2009, Chew et al 2008, Rothwell et al 2005, Steg et al 2007). Participation in cardiac rehabilitation is associated with fewer unplanned and costly readmissions (Anderson and Taylor 2014, Clark et al 2005, Lam et al 2011, Lawler et al 2011, McAlister et al 2004), which translates to important reductions in the growing economic burden on healthcare services.

Exercise therapy is recognized as the 'glue' of cardiac rehabilitation. Systematic reviews and meta-analyses of RCTs consistently support that the exercise component of a rehabilitation programme as essential, and better outcomes are achieved when this component is included (Anderson and Taylor 2014, Taylor et al 2004). Consequently physiotherapists play a vital role within the multidisciplinary team (MDT) delivering comprehensive cardiac rehabilitation. This section focuses on the physical activity and exercise component of cardiac rehabilitation and aims to present an overview of the evidence base, the current status and future directions in service implementation and, most importantly, guide physiotherapists in effectively supporting their cardiac patients to be physically active and embrace activity as part of a range of lifestyle improvement measures. This requires knowledge and skills in assessing each individual's clinical condition, physical activity status and fitness, and interpreting clinical exercise test results, as well as the ability to then synthesize assessment findings into safe and effective exercise and physical activity plans, sensitive to each individual patient's physical, psychosocial (cognitive and behavioural) capabilities and needs. The majority of patients attending cardiac rehabilitation typically also present with a range of other non-cardiac conditions such as arthritis, diabetes, joint replacements, stroke and respiratory problems. Consequently the physiotherapist working in cardiac rehabilitation must draw upon extensive background knowledge in pathophysiology in order to adapt exercises to patients with comorbidities, thus individualizing the exercise to be both clinically effective as well as sensitive to these limitations.

CARDIAC REHABILITATION – PAST, PRESENT AND FUTURE DIRECTIONS

Since the 1960s, early prevention programmes, termed *'cardiac rehabilitation'*, have been the traditional model for delivery of secondary prevention for patients with CHD (Balady et al 2000). Early programmes focussed on supervised exercise to counter de-conditioning following bypass surgery and to improve exercise capacity following myocardial infarction (MI) (Balady et al 2000). These programmes later evolved to include an educational component (usually in a group format) aimed at educating patients about the importance of lowering multiple risk factors, including smoking, diet and psychosocial well-being (Marlow and Stoller 2003, Thompson et al 1999).

Our knowledge about which cardiovascular risk factors to modify (Yusuf et al 2004) and methods available for modifying them have greatly expanded (Abraham and Michie 2008, Clark et al 2007). Consequently, comprehensive cardiac rehabilitation is more than exercise training for patients with coronary artery disease and now includes all aspects of secondary prevention (Briffa et al 2013). Definitions for contemporary cardiac rehabilitation include growing emphasis on prevention and chronic disease based strategies (BACPR 2012a, Balady et al 2007, Wenger 2008). Exercise is an important sub-component of lifestyle risk factor management, with the other main components being psychosocial health, medical risk factor management, cardio-protective therapies and, central to all these, health behaviour change and education (BACPR, 2012a) (Fig. 12-3). Efficient and cost-effective

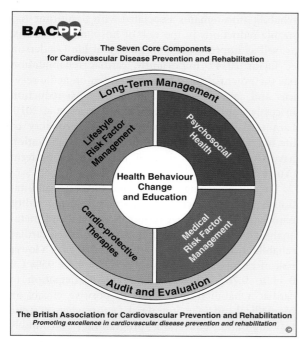

FIGURE 12-3 ■ Definition and core components of cardiac rehabilitation. *(Reproduced with permission from BACPR.)*

cardiac rehabilitation is tailored to a patient's medical condition, risk factor evaluation, and vocational status.

What Is Cardiac Rehabilitation?

'The coordinated sum of activities required to influence favourably the underlying cause of cardiovascular disease, as well as to provide the best possible physical, mental and social conditions, so that the patients may, by their own efforts, preserve or resume optimal functioning in their community and through improved health behaviour, slow or reverse progression of disease.'

(BACPR 2012a)

Although there are class IA recommendations for cardiac rehabilitation in the American Heart Association (AHA) and American College of Cardiology (ACC) management guidelines and performance measures, only around 20% of eligible patients are apparently referred (Menezes et al 2014). Earlier studies from multiple countries reported an average referral rate of approximately 30% in Canada, the

United States and the United Kingdom and a little higher at around 50% in the rest of Europe (Aragam et al., 2011). Even among patients who are appropriately and/or automatically referred to cardiac rehabilitation, participation rates remain concerningly low. Surveys across nine European countries show within 1 and 6 months after acute MI, only 29% and 48% of referred patients participated in cardiac rehabilitation (EUROASPIRE I and II, 2001). Predictors of suboptimal participation include poor functional status, higher BMI, tobacco use, depression, low health literacy and long travel distances (Menezes et al 2014). Further, international data show unacceptable levels of modifiable risk factors at follow-up in the majority of people with CHD and other vascular disease (Kotseva et al 2009, Steg et al 2007). Moreover, non-attendees are less likely to believe that rehabilitation is necessary (Cooper et al 2007) yet have higher baseline risk and poorer risk factor knowledge than those who attend (Redfern et al 2007).

In efforts to increase participation there is recognition of the need to 'rebrand and reinvigorate' cardiac rehabilitation (Sandesara et al 2015). Efforts include reducing specific barriers to referral and participation, offering choice (e.g. home-based, evening sessions etc.) and the use of modern technologies (Internet, phone and other communication tools). Commencing programme orientation within 10 days of discharge and initiating structured activity early are associated with increased uptake and improved patient outcomes (Aamot et al 2010, Haykowsky et al 2011, Pack et al 2013). Regarding the use of innovative strategies to bring exercise-based cardiac rehabilitation to more patients, new delivery models must be adopted, especially for patients at low or low-to-intermediate risk. These include the use of telemedicine as well as Internet-based, home-based (including smartphone–based home-care models) and community-based programmes to provide alternatives to conventional, medically supervised, facility-based programmes (Clark et al 2015, Varnfield et al 2014). Moving traditional cardiac rehabilitation out of the hospital setting and into community-based venues may increase accessibility and provides an environment removed from acute illness, thereby promoting health and well-being. Consequently, it is essential for physiotherapists and the MDT to also be equipped to deliver and rigorously evaluate novel approaches in prevention and rehabilitation. Physiotherapists need to draw on the evidence base and contribute to driving vital high-quality research in CVD prevention and rehabilitation. Experimental delivery models for should not be widely adopted until they have been shown to be both clinically effective and cost effective (Balady et al 2011).

Cardiac rehabilitation programmes are evolving to become 'chronic disease management programmes' treating atherosclerosis as a single disease. For example in the United Kingdom, the Cardiovascular Outcomes Strategy (Department of Health 2013) calls for service integration and the inclusion of different clinical presentations beyond CHD, such as transient cerebral ischaemia, stroke and peripheral arterial disease to be included. These different clinical presentations are associated with a common pathology of atherosclerosis and common underling risk factors, particularly smoking, high blood pressure, elevated cholesterol, diabetes, obesity and unhealthy lifestyle. Many patients present with one clinical manifestation of CVD but also have disease in other territories. Physiotherapists are ideally placed in delivering exercise interventions, given their extensive knowledge in pathophysiology and training to adapt exercises to patients with a wide array of comorbidities.

Cardiac Rehabilitation and Secondary Prevention – Evidence of Effectiveness

Good quality systematic reviews and meta-analyses of RCT data since the 1980s demonstrate that survivors of acute coronary syndrome who participate in cardiac rehabilitation have significant reductions in mortality, and combined with hospital readmissions, may reduce such events by up to 45% within 1 year, thereby improving quality of life significantly (Clark et al 2005, Taylor et al 2004). However, there have also been major advances in cardiology practice together with improvements in public health which have contributed to lower mortality rates following acute coronary syndromes. As a consequence, the influence that cardiac rehabilitation post MI or revascularization may have on mortality in contemporary practice is limited. A more recent systematic review encompassing 148 RCTs in 98 093 people who experienced heart attack, had undergone heart surgery or had CHF showed that while the benefits for mortality are now less, cardiac rehabilitation remains associated with significant and sizable reductions in the risk of hospital admissions, as well as improvements in quality of life (Anderson & Taylor 2014). Importantly, cardiac rehabilitation has the potential to reduce the burden on acute services and save money through a 28–56% reduction in costly unplanned readmissions (Davies et al 2010, Lam et al 2011). The improvements in quality of life following a short course of cardiac rehabilitation have also been shown in RCT data to last long term (Yu et al 2004).

There is emerging evidence that cardiac rehabilitation is also associated with a reduction in morbidity, namely recurrent MI. A systematic review and meta-analysis of 34 RCTs showed that exercise-based cardiac rehabilitation programmes are associated with a lower risk of re-infarction (odds ratio (OR): 0.53; 95% CI: 0.38 to 0.76) (Lawler et al 2011). Participation in cardiac rehabilitation extends to positive effects on biomedical and behavioural risk factors where exercise training and education programmes favourably modify lipid levels, blood pressure, insulin sensitivity and glucose homoeostasis, weight and smoking rates (Chow et al 2010, Clark et al 2005, Leon et al 2005). Further, cardiac rehabilitation improves functional capacity and perceived quality of life while also supporting early return to work and the development of self-management skills (Yohannes et al 2010).

Notably, cardiac rehabilitation is a complex and multifaceted intervention and therefore it is difficult to ascertain whether effects are due to a single component or a combination of components. Reviews have questioned whether the benefits are due to aggressive risk factor modification, psychosocial counselling or exercise training (Anderson & Taylor 2014). There is evidence to support the former, with a recent study indicating that approximately half of the 28% reduction in cardiac mortality achieved with exercise-based cardiac rehabilitation may be attributed to reductions in major risk factors, particularly smoking (Taylor et al 2006). Interestingly, modelling of the determinants in the primary prevention of CHD suggest risk factor modification accounts for half of the decline in fatal coronary events (Ford et al 2007, Unal et al 2004). This reiterates the important emphasis on implementing the recommended targets for CVD prevention as a key priority.

A more recent systematic review of meta-analyses of RCTs in cardiac rehabilitation clearly shows the importance of the exercise component as core. Psychological- and education-based interventions without the addition of an exercise intervention appear to have little impact on mortality or morbidity but may improve HR-QoL (Anderson & Taylor 2014). This large systematic review also revealed that home- and centre-based programmes are equally effective in improving HR-QoL at similar costs.

While there is a limited data pertaining to cost-effectiveness trials (Briffa et al 2005), systematic reviews indicate that cardiac rehabilitation is cost-effective (compared to standard medical care) (Oldridge et al 2008, Papadakis et al 2008). The diversity of programmes and client groups makes it difficult to determine the cost-effectiveness of cardiac rehabilitation and this is compounded by differences in health provision among countries where this has been investigated. A survey within the UK calculated the cost per patient to be of the order of £490 (Beswick et al 2004), while an American review had higher average costs of $2054 and determined that participation prolonged survival by an additional 1.82 years at a cost of $1773 per/life-year saved (Georgiou et al 2001). It has been suggested that cardiac rehabilitation is more cost-effective than thrombolytic therapy and coronary bypass surgery (Ades et al 1997).

To Whom Should Secondary Prevention Programmes Be Made Available?

Cardiac rehabilitation should be offered to all cardiac patients who would benefit. Traditionally, programmes have been targeted at post MI and coronary artery bypass graft (CABG) patients with limited and variable service provision for patients following percutaneous coronary intervention (PCI), with angina or CHF or who have undergone cardiac transplantation. Uptake of service is often poor among women, multipathology patients, some ethnic groups and the elderly. As a consequence, issues relating to access, distance, timing and flexibility of cardiac rehabilitation programmes are crucial considerations when trying to optimize service provision for such under-represented groups.

Programmes should aim to offer cardiac rehabilitation to the following patient groups irrespective of age, sex, ethnic group and clinical condition. Inclusion and re-inclusion to cardiac rehabilitation also apply following any stepwise alteration in any of the conditions listed below:

- acute coronary syndrome
- following revascularisation
- stable heart failure
- stable angina
- following implantation of cardiac defibrillators and resynchronisation devices
- heart valve repair/replacement
- heart transplantation and ventricular assist devices
- grown-up congenital heart disease (GUCH)
- other atherosclerotic diseases, e.g. peripheral arterial disease, transient ischaemic attack.

It is also recognized that asymptomatic people, including those with diabetes, identified at high cardiovascular risk require the same professional lifestyle intervention and appropriate risk factor and therapeutic management. Existing cardiac rehabilitation services are in a strong position to evolve to provide care to include a wider spectrum of patient groups. Non-communicable diseases such as cancer and COPD also share commonalities offering even greater widespread opportunities for service integration.

By Who Should Secondary Prevention Be Delivered?

A broad spectrum of care requires the combined skills and close collaboration of a MDT of professionals. Practitioners who lead each of the core components (see Fig. 12-3) must be able to demonstrate that they have appropriate training, professional development, qualifications, skills and competency for the component(s) for which they are responsible. The team must include a senior clinician who has responsibility for coordinating, managing and evaluating the service. The composition of each team may differ but collectively the team must have the necessary knowledge, skills and competences to meet the standards and deliver all the core components. Typically the team may include the following: a cardiologist, nurse, physiotherapist, dietitian, occupational therapist, pharmacist and psychology staff, who have specialist training in cardiology and prevention. Additional input may be required from social services and vocational guidance staff. Continuation of care in the community includes the primary healthcare team (principally general practitioner and practice nurse), long-term risk factor monitoring and management, coupled with a regular activity programme should be continually promoted to reinforce the need for ongoing secondary prevention.

The exercise component should be delivered by a team of clinical and exercise specialists who are skilled in cardiovascular assessment, risk stratification, patient monitoring, exercise prescription, goal setting and behavioural management. The team needs to be able to deal with concurrent medical and psychosocial issues and combine the art and science of exercise prescription and delivery, i.e. the art of integrating strategies for behaviour change in order to enhance exercise compliance and long-term adherence, with the science of exercise prescription (American College of Sports Medicine 2013). Physiotherapists are key members of the team as they have specialist skills in the assessment, exercise prescription and rehabilitation management of multi-pathology patients, as well as being health educators and exercise advisors (Jolliffe et al 2000). The Association of Chartered Physiotherapists in Cardiac Rehabilitation (ACPICR) in the UK has developed guidelines for practice (Association of Chartered Physiotherapists in Cardiac Rehabilitation 2015) and a competency document outlining the physiotherapist's role and required knowledge, skills and standard of performance in cardiac rehabilitation (BACPR 2012b).

How Should Secondary Prevention Be Delivered?

In most countries, patients attend rehabilitation facilities, mostly in hospitals, to participate in 6- to 8-week programmes of health education, supervised exercise and psychosocial support (Wenger 2008). Facilities generally, but not always, require gym equipment and space for the exercise and education sessions, with some programmes providing transport and 'after hours' programmes which increase cost (Redfern & Briffa 2011). However, as previously alluded, traditional facility-based cardiac rehabilitation is facing substantial challenges in terms of access, appeal and cost. Indeed, improving access to and equity of disease management services is vital to its future and

achieving better health outcomes. Despite the proven benefits of cardiac rehabilitation programmes and knowledge of low and unequal access for nearly 2 decades, utilization of these facility-based preventive interventions remains unacceptably low at 15–30% of those eligible (Beswick et al 2004, Scott et al 2003, Suaya et al 2007). Overall, provision and uptake remains inconsistent (Beswick et al 2004, Bittner and Sanderson 2006, Brodie et al 2006).

Barriers to uptake of facility-based cardiac rehabilitation have been extensively studied and are multifactorial (Beswick et al 2004, Daly et al 2002, Higgins et al 2008, Scott et al 2003). Examples include patients' indifferent perceptions of such programmes, failure of clinicians to refer patients, insufficient organizational support, lack of flexibility, distance from secondary prevention services and fragmented funding. Several strategies have been recommended to facilitate the uptake of programmes, including automatic referral processes, encouragement to attend by treating doctors, and flexible interventions in a variety of settings (Ades 2007, Briffa et al 2009, Clark et al 2007, Redfern et al 2011).

Conceivably, a further issue is the inherent structure of cardiac rehabilitation programmes in our changing society (finite resourcing, changing employment needs and access to information). Revascularization is generally achieved today with a day-only hospital stay and workers often return to employment within 1–2 days. Consequently, people are having increasing difficulty attending 6–8 week structured and facility-based programmes. In addition, economic changes (finite resources) in society today have resulted in the need to explore new and cost-effective ways of delivering programmes, potentially with more community engagement (Redfern & Briffa 2011).

Therefore despite evidence for facility-based rehabilitation in terms of attenuating risk, it is limited by incomplete uptake. Health systems are seeking ways to provide secondary prevention to more people for the same or less money. It would appear that implementing strategies to increase referral and physician engagement and reduce geographical and language barriers may go some way to improving access but these changes would be costly and are unlikely to completely narrow the evidence-practice gap. The development of contemporary models that have inherent flexibility and that utilize existing community services may be another alternative. As a result, cardiac rehabilitation programmes are evolving into flexible multifaceted preventive interventions to provide maximal clinical benefits to a majority of patients with a variety of conditions (Ades 2007).

Emergence of Contemporary Models to Broaden Delivery

Contemporary programmes have became more inclusive but also more diverse, and this growth in programme diversity continues today. From a single service model around a single risk factor in a specific setting, CHD management has evolved into a complex web of differing models offered by various professionals to diverse patient populations (Redfern et al 2011). This evolution is supported by contemporary scientific evidence showing that effective secondary prevention can be achieved through a range of different models in addition to facility-based rehabilitation (Clark et al 2005).

Meta-analyses of secondary prevention programmes, including contemporary alternatives to rehabilitation (e.g. coaching, clinics and home based) suggest that centrally coordinated, brief and personalized management of risk factors in consultation with the patient's treating doctor(s) is effective (Clark et al 2005, Clark et al 2007). Importantly, these programmes are safe, appear to benefit patients of all ages, are considered cost-effective compared with other approaches to disease management and lead to improved clinical markers and behavioural changes (Ades 2001, Briffa et al 2009, Clark et al 2005, Clark et al 2007, Wenger 2008).

Many trials reporting outcomes of contemporary models for delivery of secondary prevention have been investigated and common components or features of these programmes include their individualized approach, the inclusion of telehealth strategies for ongoing support, the provision of supplementary materials and the potential for community or home-based delivery. Most, if not all, contemporary models are based on individualized or case-management approaches. This differs from the traditional model of CR, which tends to be delivered in a group-format. Also, a large number of the programmes include supplementary telephone support (Dalal et al 2007,

DeBusk et al 1994, Haskell et al 1994, Hanssen et al 2007, Lear et al 2003, Redfern et al 2010, Vale et al 2003). In addition, Internet-based programmes have also been used to deliver ongoing support (Southard et al 2003). Many contemporary programmes also include the provision of supplementary written materials (Mittag et al 2006, Sinclair et al 2005), a 'heart manual' (Dalal et al 2007, Lewin et al 2002), written health records (Wister et al 2007, Wood et al 2008) or audiotapes (Lewin et al 2002, Taylor et al 1997) for patients and their families. Finally, numerous programmes have formal arrangements designed to facilitate coordinated care with specialists and family physicians (Lear et al 2003, Redfern et al 2009, Vale et al 2003, Young et al 2003). In terms of setting, contemporary programmes can be delivered in hospital, at a patient's home or in community health facilities based on local resources and patient preference. Several programmes provide specific advice (Haskell et al 1994, Lear et al 2003, Vale et al 2003), while others are patient-centred, inviting choice and shared decision-making (Dalal et al 2007, Redfern et al 2009). Importantly, there is no clear evidence at this stage suggesting one model is more effective than another and there are no reported effect sizes for differing components and formats.

Overall, there is a strong case for expansion of community-based programmes where ongoing prevention is better integrated with primary care-based services, with the aim of increasing access, uptake and support over the long term (Thompson & Clark 2009). Community-based cardiac rehabilitation programmes appear to be effective at increasing enrolment, reducing risk and containing cost (Harris and Record 2003). Some patients, particularly those who are employed and have time constraints, may prefer home-based programmes and see participation as more viable (Brubaker 2005, Grace et al 2005). Other evidence suggests that home-based rehabilitation can also improve exercise capacity and HR-QoL in patients after surgery (Smith et al 2004) and MI (Dalal et al 2010, Jolly et al 2006), as well as cost-benefit ratios (Jolly et al 2006) similarly to hospital-based programmes. The provision of telehealth models also offers a viable and attractive option that could help increase the uptake of formal cardiac rehabilitation by those who currently do not access it (Neubeck et al

2009). Thompson and Clark (2009) conclude, in their recent review, by stating that patients should be routinely offered an informed choice of home- or hospital- or telehealth-based cardiac rehabilitation.

Moving forwards, in order to optimize uptake of secondary prevention, and appeal to non-attenders, alternative models of programme delivery should continue to be explored and evaluated to identify what works for whom, when and where (Clark et al 2007). Contemporary evidence suggests preventive interventions must be flexible and tailored to the individual's preferences, needs and values. Moving forwards, our problem lies in the challenge of untangling the web of trial and review evidence into practical information that is evidence-based, locally relevant and clinically deliverable (Redfern et al 2010). Our challenge in the future, as clinicians, researchers and policymakers is to decipher the evidence and provide programmes that are both structured and evidence-based but also are inherently flexible. We are challenged with a changing society and making evidence-based changes to the way we deliver ongoing preventative management to patients with chronic disease.

The optimal model of rehabilitation or prevention is largely dependent on the availability of local resources, a patient's clinical condition, circumstances and what a patient agrees to. For example, patients who have advanced coronary disease or psychosocial impairment accompanying heart disease are more likely suited to facility group programmes, if feasible. In contrast, the majority of patients with clinically stable coronary disease are more likely to be better suited if there is a variety of programmes from which they can select. Overall, each intervention should be evidence based, informed by national guidelines, and include individual goals and strategies that underpin long-term secondary prevention, role resumption and return to paid work if appropriate. Programmes should also include evaluation and a review of outcomes, together with continuous quality improvement.

Exercise Training in Secondary Prevention Programmes

Research suggests the inclusion of exercise training is a key element in eliciting benefits both in facilitating return to function and secondary prevention (Leon et al 1991, National Institute for Clinical Excellence 2013; Taylor et al 2004). There is considerable variation across and between patient groups in the type and setting of exercise training (Hansen et al 2005). Many studies have concentrated on aerobic exercise owing to concerns regarding the effects of resistance training on cardiac function, but there is growing evidence that a mix of endurance and strength exercises are both safe and optimize the benefits (Adams et al 2006, Delagardelle et al 2002, Jonsdottir et al 2005, Levinger et al 2005).

Concern that some patients may develop myocardial remodelling as a result of participating in early activity (Jugdutt et al 1988, Kloner & Kloner 1983) has been alleviated by other work indicating that exercise does not contribute to the onset of remodelling (Cannistra et al 1999, DuBach et al 1997, Giannuzzi et al 1993, Myers et al 2000). The benefits of low-intensity exercise in the early stages of a programme are thought be similar to those of higher intensity (Blumenthal et al 1988, Goble et al 1991, Worcester et al 1993) and adoption of low-intensity exercise would facilitate both adherence and safety.

The duration of the period of exercise training is influenced by many factors, such as physiological and psychological state (Kovoor et al 2006), objectives and adherence. Secondary prevention requires a prolonged period of training (Brubaker et al 2000) and adherence and uptake to a programme may be influenced by social support (Husak et al 2004), age, gender (Todaro et al 2004) and location of training (Grace et al 2005). The lack of consensus on an optimal period of exercise training for different groups of patients and an absence of a robust prediction model to determine the magnitude of benefit each patient may receive from a rehabilitation programme (Pierson et al 2004, Shen et al 2006) places an emphasis on assessment, joint goal setting and regular re-evaluation of response. Few studies have included a prolonged follow-up period, but any benefits appear to be quickly lost on cessation of regular exercise training.

Overall, cardiac rehabilitation is safe and well tolerated. Although there is a perception that exercise training could be dangerous, the evidence is that rehabilitation programmes result in very few complications and the incidence of major cardiac events, including MI and resuscitated cardiac arrest, occurred in 1 in 50 000 to 100 000 patient-hours of supervised

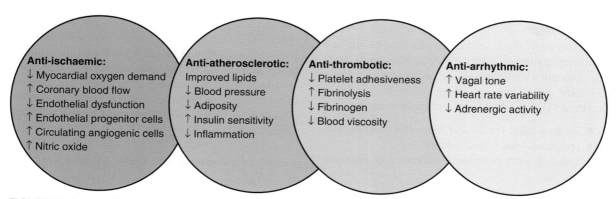

FIGURE 12-4 ■ Cardioprotective mechanisms associated with regular exercise training. *(Adapted from Franklin & Gordon, 2009.)*

exercise, with only 2 fatalities reported for 1.5 million patient-hours of supervised exercise (Franklin et al 1998, Leon et al 2005, Thompson et al 2007). The respect of indications and contraindications and proper risk stratification are key to safety. Patients considered most at risk are those with residual ischaemia, complex ventricular arrhythmia and severe left ventricular dysfunction (ejection fraction of less than 35%), especially New York Heart Association (NYHA) class III or IV. In spite of this there has not been any reported increase in adverse events during either supervised or unsupervised exercise training following the inclusion of people who were previously considered a high risk, i.e. CHF and implantable cardioverter defibrillators (ICDs) (Davids et al 2005, Fitchet et al 2003, Pashkow et al 1997). However, there is a paucity of information on the occurrence of adverse events outside research studies, which usually include highly selected patients who undergo formal exercise tests.

BENEFITS OF EXERCISE TRAINING

Supporting evidence of causative relationships has demonstrated multiple plausible cardioprotective biological mechanisms that explain the association between structured physical activity and reduced incidence of CVD. These include direct anti-atherosclerotic effects by improving artery endothelial function and reducing inflammation, and indirectly by modification of other risk factor components of the metabolic syndrome, by reducing risk of a coronary thrombotic occlusion (anti-thrombotic effects), by decreasing myocardial

oxygen demands and increasing its vascular supply (anti-ischaemic effects) and by improving cardio-myocyte electrical stability and autonomic nervous system adaptations (anti-arrhythmic effects) (Golbidi and Laher 2011, Leon 2009). These underlying cardioprotective mechanisms associated with regular physical activity offer explanation as to why activity-based interventions are fundamental to contemporary CVD prevention and rehabilitative practice (Fig. 12-4). The following summarizes the key benefits associated with exercise training in secondary prevention.

Improved Exercise Capacity

The development of cardiovascular endurance is the primary objective for CHD patients. Endurance training, defined as any activity which uses large muscle groups, can be sustained for a prolonged period and is rhythmic and aerobic in nature, results in an increase in maximal oxygen uptake (VO_{2max}), i.e. the highest rate of oxygen consumption attainable during maximal exercise. VO_{2max} is limited:

- centrally by cardiac output (CO), which is a function of heart rate (HR) and stroke volume (SV)
- peripherally, in particular by the capacity of skeletal muscle to extract oxygen from the blood. This is represented as the difference between the oxygen content of arterial blood and mixed venous blood (arterio-venous oxygen difference ($a\text{-}vO_{2diff}$)). Consequently an increase in VO_{2max} depends on the potential for inducing central and/or peripheral adaptations.

Central Changes

In healthy individuals, endurance training results in a significant increase in maximal CO. Maximum heart rate does not alter with training and so the increase in CO must arise from a training-induced increase in maximal SV. This is achieved primarily through:

- increased left ventricular mass and chamber size
- increased total blood volume
- reduced total peripheral resistance at maximal exercise.

Peripheral Changes

Training-induced changes within skeletal muscle, which contribute to increased extraction and utilization of oxygen, include:

- increased number and size of mitochondria
- increased oxidative enzyme activity
- increased capillarization
- increased myoglobin.

In cardiac patients, the increase in VO_{2max} is attributed predominantly to peripheral adaptation. Central changes are associated with prolonged periods of high-intensity training and although in selected patients, central changes have been provoked (Ehsani et al 1986, Schuler et al 1992), the high intensity of the training regimen would be inappropriate for the heterogeneous group of patients eligible for cardiac rehabilitation programmes.

Consequences of an Increase in Maximal Oxygen Uptake

The significance of an increase in VO_{2max} for cardiac patients is not that it permits a higher level of maximal effort (as this is rarely demanded in everyday life) but that repeated submaximal ADLs constitute a smaller percentage of the increased maximal capacity and therefore impose relatively less physiological stress. This is reflected in a reduction in heart rate (attributed to both increased vagal tone and reduced sympathetic outflow), blood pressure and plasma catecholamine concentrations at rest and at submaximal workloads. Since myocardial oxygen consumption (MVO_2) is determined by heart rate and systolic blood pressure (referred to as 'rate pressure product (RPP)' or 'double

product'), a reduction in either or both delays the onset of ischaemia and lessens the potential for arrhythmias. A further benefit of the training-induced bradycardia is that at any reference submaximal work load, the period of diastole is extended and, since 80% of coronary blood flow occurs during the relaxation phase of the cardiac cycle, myocardial perfusion is significantly enhanced.

Benefits of Exercise on Risk Factor Modification

In cardiac patients exercise may have an important secondary prevention role. The rationale for aggressive risk factor modification, as part of optimal care of CHD patients, is based on the premise that the factors that contribute to initial development of disease will also influence the progression of established disease and the likelihood of future events. The 'acute' effects of each bout of exercise in healthy people include:

- a raised post-exercise metabolic rate
- changes in lipoprotein metabolism with consequent increased synthesis of high-density lipoprotein (HDL)
- improved insulin sensitivity
- decreased blood pressure.

These effects all relate to local changes in the previously exercised muscle and are evident even after light to moderate exercise, suggesting that a general increase in physical activity is likely to contribute to the patient's continued well-being and to the reduced mortality and morbidity associated with exercise rehabilitation.

In addition, exercise training is known to reduce triggers for cardiac events including:

- preventing thrombus formation
- improving endothelial function
- reducing potential for serious arrhythmias.

RECOMMENDED LEVELS OF PHYSICAL ACTIVITY AND EXERCISE

Essentially there are two sets of recommendations – those that deal with increasing physical activity levels for public health and those that target increasing physical fitness. Recommendations for increasing physical activity are expressed in different ways; for example achieving a particular target of minutes of a particular intensity of activity (i.e. 150 minutes per week of moderate intensity activity), kilocalorie expenditure over the week (>1000 kcal/wk) or steps per day (>10 000 steps per day). Being 'active' does not necessarily result in gains in physical fitness. To gain increases in physical fitness, structured activity that provides a physiological stimulus, which exceeds what the body is normally accustomed to, is required. This is known as 'overload'. In the context of CVD prevention and recovery we know that people with a higher cardiorespiratory fitness have significantly fewer events. Consequently, structured activity, specifically aerobic in nature that provokes this overload stimulus, should be built into the week.

The physiotherapist should consequently encourage an increase in overall levels of sustained physical activity and avoidance of prolonged sedentary behaviour, as these are important for reduction of CVD risk. Emphasise walking, cycling and other aerobic physical daily activities, at moderate intensity, as part of an active lifestyle, for at least 150 minutes per week in bouts of at least 10 minutes and include muscle-strengthening activities performed on at least two occasions per week. Importantly, exercise training, incorporating a warm-up and cool-down period, should be performed at moderate to high intensity two to three times per week for 30 to 40 minutes each time. The mode of exercise should be aerobic and, where possible, continuously allowing for a steady progression in effort. The time spent exercise training contributes to meeting the 150 minutes per week physical activity recommendation.

EXERCISE PRESCRIPTION

The main objective of the exercise programme is to increase cardiorespiratory fitness through a cardiovascular and muscular endurance training programme. Patients report that the consequent improvement in functional capacity and strength enables them to perform activities with less effort, fewer symptoms, more confidence and an enhanced quality of life. The evidence and related pathophysiology, for endurance training in higher-risk patients with poor functional capacity, is that this is best achieved by increasing peripheral stimulus while minimizing cardiovascular stress (Swedberg et al 2005).

Principles of Exercise Prescription

When individual bouts of exercise are repeated regularly, and in accordance with established principles of training, a series of longer-term cardiovascular and metabolic adaptations occur; for instance, as described earlier, an increase in VO_{2max} results from aerobic endurance training.

The principles of exercise training are:

Individuality – Heredity plays a major part in how quickly and to what extent an individual's body adapts to a training programme: i.e. no two individuals (other than identical twins) will exhibit the same adaptations in response to the same training programme.

Progressive overload – Overload refers to placing greater demands on the body than it is accustomed to, thereby provoking adaptations. In order to continue to stimulate training adaptations, the overload must be progressively increased.

Regression or reversibility – This principle is often referred to as the principle of 'use it or lose it': i.e. if the stimulus to change (the overload) is withdrawn, the adaptations conferred will diminish until the level of functional capacity is once again sufficient to meet only the demands imposed by general activities of daily life.

Specificity – The adaptations conferred by training are highly specific to:

- the volume of training, which includes the **F**requency
- the **I**ntensity of training
- the mode or **T**ype of training
- The duration (or **T**ime) of training.

The effectiveness and appropriateness of all exercise prescriptions will depend upon manipulation of the **FITT** principle: i.e. the frequency, intensity, time and type of training (Tables 12-2 and 12-3).

Frequency of Exercise

The frequency should be adjusted according to individual needs, although the ultimate goal is for all people to be physically active every day. Exercise training (or structured activity targeting cardiorespiratory fitness) should be performed on at least 2–3 days per week (ACSM 2013).

TABLE 12-2		
The FITT Principle for Increasing Aerobic Capacity		
F	Frequency	Two to three times weekly (e.g. two rehabilitation classes and one home circuit) Other days – walk/leisure activities
I	Intensity	Dependent on assessment findings* $HRR/VO_{2max}/MET_{max} = 40–70\%$ RPE 2–4 (CR 0–10 Borg scale), 11–14 RPE (Borg scale) $HR_{max} = 60–80\%$
T	Time	20–30 minutes conditioning period (not inclusive of warm-up and cool-down periods)
T	Type	Aerobic endurance training

CR, Cardiac rehabilitation; HR_{max}, maximal heart rate; *HRR*, heart rate reserve; *MET*, metabolic equivalent; *RPE*, rating of perceived exertion; VO_2R, oxygen uptake reserve.
*Benefits may occur at lower intensities (e.g. 35% HRR/VO_{2max} in deconditioned patients).

TABLE 12-3		
Strength Training and Resistance Exercise Prescription		
F	Frequency	Minimum 2 times per week
I	Intensity	Upper body *30–40% 1 rep max Lower body *50–60% 1 rep max
T	Time	1 set min (2–4 sets optimal) of 10–15 reps
T	Type	8–10 different muscle groups

Adapted from AHA (Williams et al 2007), ACSM (Pollock et al 2010).
*After 1st 5 reps RPE should be <15 (CR10 <7), if higher recommended repetitions likely not to be achievable.

Type or Mode of Exercise

The type and mode of exercise should be varied and functional and should also be based on individual need, preference and availability of locations and equipment. In essence the aim is to include a variety of the following:

- Aerobic and muscular strength and endurance training that involves large muscle groups in dynamic movement, e.g. walk, cycle, circuit training.
- Initial adoption of an interval approach with eventual progression to low/moderate intensity continuous aerobic exercise.

- Caution should be exercised over:
  - The introduction of resistance training; exercises should be relatively low in resistance and high in repetitions (American College of Sports Medicine 2013). Debilitated, higher-risk heart failure patients may require seated or very low intensity alternative exercises during the conditioning component.
  - Abrupt posture shifts, e.g. upright work to recumbent position and recumbent to upright.
  - Excessive use of arm/upper body exercise relative to leg work, as arm work (at a given workload) results in a higher systolic and diastolic BP than when the same work is performed by a larger muscle mass such as the legs.

Intensity of Exercise

The intensity of exercise is a critical issue because vigorous activity carries a greatly increased risk of precipitating adverse events such as MI or arrhythmias (Willich et al 1993). Frequent, moderate-intensity exercise is recommended for CHD patients since it will optimize benefits without increasing the risk of adverse events (Dafoe & Huston 1997). For individuals with greatly diminished functional capacity, several short bouts (as little as 5–10 minutes) throughout the day may be advisable. There are a number of established methods for prescribing and monitoring intensity, which may be used separately or in combination with one another.

Use of Rating of Perceived Exertion

Cardiorespiratory and metabolic variables are strongly related to perceived exertion, which is accepted as a practical, valid and reproducible indicator of the intensity of steady-state exercise. Physiotherapists and exercise specialists working in a cardiac rehabilitation setting are recommended to familiarize themselves with the scales of perceived exertion developed by Borg (1998). The Borg 15-point scale and the Borg CR10 scale of perceived exertion, together with patient instructions, are published in the appendix of *Borg's Perceived Exertion and Pain Scales* (1998). In order to preserve the validity and reproducibility of these scales, their format should not be altered and the patient instructions should be closely followed.

On the 15-point scale, a rating of 11 (equivalent to 2 on the Borg CR10 scale) corresponds to approximately 40% of HRR or VO_{2max} (60% of maximal heart rate (HR_{max})). A rating of 13–14 on the 15-point scale (equivalent to between 3.5 and 4.5 on the Borg CR10 scale) corresponds to approximately 70% of HRR or VO_{2max} (80% HR_{max}).

Use of Heart Rate

Where a maximal test has been achieved, training heart rate should be set at 60–80% of HR_{max}. If the test was symptom limited, training intensity should be set at 10–20 bpm below the heart rate at which symptoms were apparent and the patient's heart rate should be monitored throughout each exercise session. ECG test information is, however, not always available to health professionals and is becoming less common in the management of CVD. When these tests are available, it is not uncommon for the test end point to be the achievement of a predicted maximal heart rate. Hence, true maximal heart rate may still be unknown. In the absence of test data other methods for establishing appropriate training intensity have to be used. Age-adjusted predicted maximal rates can be used (220 bpm minus age in years is one formula) and the training heart rate set at 60–80% of the predicted maximum; this is equivalent to 40–70% VO_{2max}. Cardiac rehabilitation practitioners also need to be able to adjust appropriately where patients are taking chronotropic medications such as β-blockade therapy. While a simple formula, the standard deviation (SD) for maximal heart rate during exercise is 10 bpm and some individuals will, therefore, have an actual maximum heart rate 20 bpm higher or lower (2 SD above or below the population mean) than predicted. There is also evidence to suggest this method provides an underestimate of true HR_{max} (Robergs and Landwehr, 2002). In this review the Tanaka et al (2001) method was found to provide a better estimate of HR_{max} in people under the age of 30 years of age ($208 - (0.7 \times age)$) and the Inbar et al (1994) method ($205.8 - (0.685 \times age)$) in those over the age of 45 years of age.

The preferred more individualized approach is to prescribe training at 40–70% of HRR (the difference between resting and maximal heart rate). This HRR approach (also known as the 'Karvonen method') is convenient since it is known that 40–70% of HRR is equivalent to about 40–70% of VO_{2max} (60–80% of HR_{max}) although, across the entire range of fitness levels, it is more closely linked to the percentage of oxygen uptake reserve (VO_2R), i.e. the difference between resting oxygen consumption and maximal oxygen consumption (American College of Sports Medicine 2013). It is important to note that this formula is intended for use with known maximal heart rates. In the absence of these data, the substitution of age-adjusted predicted maxima introduces the same potential for error as previously mentioned. Consequently, any prescription that is based on predicted maximal heart rates should be used in conjunction with a rating of perceived exertion (RPE) scale.

Use of Metabolic Equivalent Values (METs)

Exercise may also be regulated by choice of activities according to their known MET (metabolic equivalent) values (for which tables are available in most exercise physiology texts). If an individual assesses walking at 3 mph as 12–13 on the Borg RPE scale (corresponding to around 60% of VO_{2max}), then activities of comparable MET value can be prescribed in the knowledge that they will present an appropriate training stimulus. Knowledge of MET values is also important in terms of excluding those activities that might pose a risk to certain individuals. Skipping (8–12 METs) or freestyle swimming (9–10 METs), for example, would be entirely inappropriate for someone with a peak capacity of 7 METs.

Some activities have a wide range of MET values, while others are relatively constant between individuals, mainly because they permit little variation in individual execution, e.g. there is very little difference in the way individuals walk or cycle. In contrast, there can be great variation in the way 'free-moving' activities such as dancing, skipping or rebounding on a mini-trampoline are executed. Because precise control of the exercise prescription in a cardiac population is necessary (particularly in early recovery post event and for stable angina patients) activities that can be maintained at prescribed workloads and which permit uniform modification, e.g. altering the speed of walking or jogging or the resistance on a cycle ergometer, are preferred to those that are not amenable to standardized prescription.

Regardless of the objective method used for monitoring intensity, it is important to observe individuals for signs of excessive breathlessness, loss of quality of movement, unusual pallor or excessive sweating, all of which are inappropriate responses to moderate levels of exertion. Indications for ceasing exercise and contraindications to initiating exercise are included in the section on programme implementation.

Type of Training

The inclusion of a variety of training modes within the individual prescription or the class format will minimize the incidence of overuse injuries, maximize peripheral adaptation (as, for example, when activities which require a contribution from both upper and lower body musculature are included) and increase patient motivation and adherence. It is well documented that CHD patients who expend about 250–300 kcal per session and 1000–1500 kcal per week in additional physical activity will improve their aerobic capacity by 15–30% over a 4- to 6-month period (Balady et al 1994). There appears to be a continuous gradient in the benefits conferred and there is evidence that a minimum of 1600 kcal per week may halt the progression of CHD, whereas atherosclerotic regression may be achieved with a weekly energy expenditure of about 2200 kcal (Hambrecht et al 1994). Within the recommended ranges of frequency, intensity and time (or duration) of training, similar conditioning effects can be expected from any programme that realizes comparable weekly energy expenditure. Consequently the FITT components may be adjusted to provide an optimal prescription for individuals of varying cardiovascular and general medical status.

Format of a Typical Exercise Session

Warm-Up

Preparation for activity in older adults and especially in the cardiac population must be more gradual than for apparently healthy individuals. Fifteen minutes devoted to the warm-up component is recommended (Association of Chartered Physiotherapists in Cardiac Rehabilitation 2015). Low-impact, dynamic movements which use large muscle groups and which take all major joint complexes through their normal ROM should be incorporated. A gradual increase in the size and range of movements performed will delay the onset of ischaemia by allowing adequate time for coronary blood flow to increase in response to the greater myocardial demand. Gradual increments in myocardial workload will also lessen the risk of arrhythmias, which can be a consequence of abrupt increases in demand and concomitant elevated sympathetic activity. As a guideline, individuals should be within 20 bpm below the lower end of their prescribed training heart rate range at the end of the warm-up or, if RPE is used in place of heart rate monitoring, a rating no higher than 2 on the Borg CR10 scale or 10–11 on the original scale.

AEROBIC CONDITIONING. The type of aerobic activity used for conditioning may adopt a continuous or interval approach. Continuous training, as the name implies, involves uninterrupted activity usually performed at a constant submaximal intensity. Its advantage is the ease with which intensity may be prescribed and monitored. Walking, jogging, cycling, rowing, bench stepping and swimming all lend themselves to a continuous approach. Interval training entails bouts of relatively intense work separated by periods of rest or less intense activity. Its main advantage is that, especially for debilitated patients, the total volume of work accomplished is generally greater than when exercise is continuous; consequently the stimulus to physiological change is greater. In an older cardiac population, the transition from one activity to another also provides a time for social interaction and support, which probably aids long-term adherence.

In group exercise sessions, various approaches to circuit training have proved popular; an activity is undertaken for a fixed period of time after which participants all move on to a different activity. Depending on cardiac status and individual functional capacity, participants may be prescribed an interval approach in which relatively intense periods of activity are followed by a period of less intense exercise, or alternatively, they may undertake activities all of which are of similar intensity. Circuits can be performed using little or no equipment or, if sufficient equipment is available to accommodate the whole group, cycles, rowing machines, treadmills, etc., can be used throughout the exercise session.

Two approaches to group training are provided; Box 12-2 presents a circuit design that requires only

BOX 12-2
CIRCUIT DESIGN WITH MINIMAL EQUIPMENT

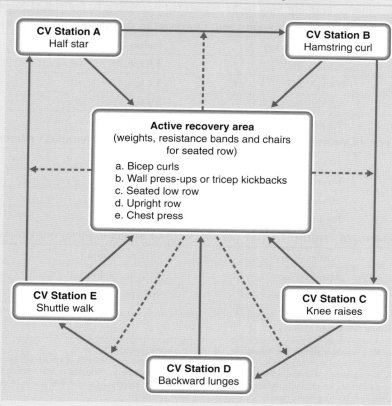

Aerobic stations are denoted as 'CV' and active recovery as 'AR'.

- ***Level 1 performs one CV station and one AR station*** i.e. starting at CV station A, the sequence is CV,A; AR,a; CV,B; AR,b; CV,C; AR,c; CV,D; AR,d; CV,E; AR,e and start again at CV,A.
- Based on a 1 : 1 ratio of CV/AR; during a 24-minute conditioning component a level 1 participant will complete a total CV exercise time of 12 minutes and a total AR time of 12 minutes.
- ***Level 2 performs two CV stations and one AR station*** i.e,. starting at CV station B, the sequence will be CV,B; CV,C; AR,c; CV,D; CV,E; AR,e; etc.
- Based on a 2 : 1 ratio of CV/AR; during a 24-minute conditioning component, a level 2 participant will complete a total CV exercise time of 16 minutes and a total AR time of 8 minutes.
- ***Level 3 performs three CV stations and one AR station*** i.e. starting at CV station C, the sequence will

be CV,C; CV,D; CV,E; AR,e; CV,A; CV,B; CV,C; AR,c; etc.
- Based on a 3 : 1 ratio of CV/AR; during a 24-minute conditioning component, a level 3 participant will complete a total CV exercise time of 18 minutes and a total AR time of 6 minutes.
- ***Level 4 performs four CV stations and one AR station*** i.e. starting at CV station D, the sequence will be CV,D; CV,E; CV,A; CV,B; AR,b; CV,C; CV,D; CV,E; CV,A; AR,a; etc.
- Based on a 4 : 1 ratio of CV/AR; during a 24-minute conditioning component, a level 4 participant will complete a total CV exercise time of 20 minutes and a total AR time of 4 minutes.
- ***Level 5 performs only the CV stations*** i.e. starting at CV,E, a level 5 participant will complete 24 minutes of continuous CV exercise.

TABLE 12-4		
An Example of Circuit Training Using Gym Equipment in Which Both Interval and Continuous Training May Be Incorporated According to Individual Need		
TREADMILL FOR 6 MINUTES – SPEED (KPH) AND GRADIENT (% GRADE) IS INDIVIDUALLY PRESCRIBED		
	Patient 1 (70 kg)	Patient 2 (70 kg)	Patient 3 (70 kg)
Minute 1, 2	3.2 kph, 0%	4.8 kph, 0%	4.8 kph, 2.5%
Minute 3	2.5 kph, 0%	3.2 kph, 0%	4.8 kph, 2.5%
Minute 4, 5	3.2 kph, 0%	4.8 kph, 0%	4.8 kph, 2.5%
Minute 6	2.5 kph, 0%	3.2 kph, 0%	4.8 kph, 2.5%
CYCLE FOR 6 MINUTES AT 50–60 RPM – RESISTANCE (WATTS) INDIVIDUALLY PRESCRIBED		
Minute 1, 2	30 watts	50 watts	60 watts
Minute 3	No resistance	30 watts	60 watts
Minute 4, 5	30 watts	50 watts	60 watts
Minute 6	No resistance	30 watts	60 watts
STEPPING FOR 3 MINUTES – HEIGHT OF STEP (m) AND RATE OF STEPPING (RPM) INDIVIDUALLY PRESCRIBED		
Minute 1	0.10 m, 12 rpm	0.15 m, 16 rpm	0.15 m, 20 rpm
Minute 2	March on spot	0.15 m, 12 rpm	0.15 m, 20 rpm
Minute 3	0.10 m, 12 rpm	0.15 m, 16 rpm	0.15 m, 20 rpm

Repeat each activity to achieve a total conditioning period of 30 minutes or repeat selected activities in accordance with individual needs and abilities

rpm, Rate per minute in cycles (1 cycle of stepping is 4 footfalls, i.e. up, up, down, down).
Note: On a treadmill and during stepping, relative VO_2 (mL O_2/min) may be estimated on the basis of speed and gradient or speed and height of stepping, respectively, because the individual is carrying his own bodyweight and this contributes to the amount of work performed. On a cycle, body weight has no influence on the cycle workload. It is important to start exercise at a relatively low level and to adjust the prescription in accordance with training heart rates and rating of perceived exertion.

minimal equipment and Table 12-4 provides an example of how a group circuit might operate when extensive equipment is available. In the design shown in Box 12-2, participants spend an increasing duration at 'aerobic/cardiovascular (CV)' stations and either rest or perform a lower intensity activity before moving on to the next aerobic station. The lower intensity or 'active recovery' (AR) stations are usually designed to increase the strength and endurance of specific muscle groups (muscle strength endurance), e.g. triceps, pectorals, trapezius, used in ADLs.

Individualization of the cardiovascular component of the programme is achieved through variation in:

- the duration at each CV station
- the intensity (by changing the resistance or the speed or range of movement)
- the period of rest between stations
- the overall duration of conditioning.

In general, the duration of activity is extended before increasing the intensity.

Exercises involving recumbent positions are discouraged because:

- some older participants have difficulty in getting up and down
- following vigorous activity, the increase in venous return on lying down enhances preload and thereby myocardial workload, which increases the risk of arrhythmias and angina in some individuals
- on return to an upright position the potential for orthostatic hypotensive episodes is dramatically

increased in cardiac patients, most of whom are on medication that lowers blood pressure, e.g. β-blockers and angiotensin-converting enzyme (ACE) inhibitors. Consequently, it is recommended that any recumbent work (e.g. for the abdominals or erector spinae) should be performed after completion of the circuit and a cool-down period.

Resistance Training

Traditionally, training to increase strength (as opposed to endurance) of specific muscle groups was considered to be inappropriate for individuals with established heart disease. This was because resistance training is associated with an increase in arterial blood pressure, which increases myocardial workload. However, studies have generally reported that cardiovascular and haemodynamic responses to resistance training in CHD patients and in normal individuals are similar and, because of increased diastolic pressure, may even enhance myocardial perfusion (Squires et al 1991, Williams 1994). With an ageing population, the relevance of resistance training is growing, as it is associated with enhancement and maintenance of muscle strength and power, leading to an improvement in functional ability, stimulation in bone formation and reduction in bone loss. It has also been shown to improve glucose, reduce blood pressure and maintain weight (Williams et al 2007). Resistance training can be used as either an independent session or as part of the active recovery component or cool-down of an aerobic circuit; when undertaken after the CV component, a partial cool-down is necessary prior to resistance work. Resistance work should be followed by a final cool-down.

Selection of the appropriate weight is important in order to achieve the recommended guidelines (see Table 12-3). These levels should result in moderate fatiguing of the muscle. In some cases intensity may need to be lowered, and therefore exercises should be adjusted to involve higher repetitions and lower resistance. To avoid injury ensure correct technique. Avoid isometric exercises and breath holding due to the risk of exaggerated increases in blood pressure. If the participant performs the exercise while standing, instruct them to keep the feet moving to encourage venous return. Even moving the toes or contracting

the calf (gastrocnemius) muscles will help to maintain venous return. Caution should be taken with patients that present with sternal instability. Bilateral upper limb resistance exercises are better tolerated than unilateral loaded exercises in these patients (El-Ansary et al 2007).

Cool-Down

A period of 10 minutes is recommended for cool-down at the end of the cardiovascular component. This is because:

- There is an increased risk of hypotension in this group – for some this is a specific side effect of their medication. In addition, there is an age-related slowing of baroreceptor responsiveness which increases the risk of venous pooling following sustained exercise.
- In older adults, heart rates take longer to return to pre-exercise rates.
- Raised sympathetic activity during vigorous exercise increases the risk of arrhythmias during the immediate period following cessation of exercise.

The cool-down should incorporate movements of diminishing intensity and passive stretching of the major muscle groups used during the conditioning phase. Patient observation for up to 30 minutes after the exercise session is recommended. Many traditional programmes follow the exercise session with an education or relaxation component, which affords the opportunity for extended observation and supervision of participants.

Progression of Exercise Training

The duration, frequency or intensity of training can be increased in order to maintain the training stimulus. Ideally serial exercise testing will form the basis on which the prescription is modified, in order to ensure that it provokes physiological adaptation. In the absence of exercise testing, heart rate monitoring and RPE, at reference workloads, may be used to establish the appropriateness of increasing any of the three variables, either singly or in combination with one another. The way in which exercise prescription is progressed and the rate at which it is progressed will be highly variable between individuals with CHD and will be a function of many factors including age, severity of disease, motivation, dual pathology and compliance. Ideally it should always be remembered that the ultimate goal of the exercise component of a secondary prevention programmes is to facilitate lifelong increased physical activity.

PROGRAMME IMPLEMENTATION

In-Hospital Activity Component

Graduated mobilization of cardiac patients following acute MI, CABG or unstable heart failure is initiated by nursing or physiotherapy staff on acute units as part of overall patient care. Patients are encouraged to sit out of bed, take short walks, shower and dress as soon as possible, depending on their cardiac status. For primary PCI, in the mainstay this is the same day with many being discharged within 48 hours, while for patients who have had CABG the typical length of stay is around 5 days. Although the physiotherapist may be involved in the earlier stages with a multi-pathology patient, their customary role is to supervise the patient's mobilization plan, e.g. pre-discharge walk or stair assessments to determine individual exercise capacity, symptoms and/or limitations. By discharge, all patients should be conversant with the signs and symptoms of excessive exertion and be able to rate level of effort using, for example, the validated Borg scale (Borg 1998) or a locally developed scale. Both the patient and family should be advised on how to manage chest pain and symptoms of overexertion and be encouraged to keep symptom diaries to discuss with staff at follow-up appointments.

A home exercise programme, which gives guidance on convalescence and household activities during the initial discharge period and written advice on specific 'do and don't activities', should be provided. Walking is recommended as the main mode of exercise and means of increasing functional capacity. An individual schedule suggesting distance/speed ratios and progressions and a home activity diary should be incorporated.

Although the starting level and progression of activity is always dependent on individual clinical status, symptoms and medical history, the following exercise prescription may be used as a guideline at discharge:

- *Type/mode* – An interval rather than a continuous approach may be required initially; encourage walking and performance of sitting/standing functional activities, including active, non-resisted general arm and leg exercises.
- *Frequency and Timing* – Initially, short intermittent bouts of 5–10 minutes of activity interspersed with rest periods, 2–3 times per day; overall duration of activity may be progressed from 5 to 20 minutes, 1–2 times per day.
- *Intensity* – RPE <11 (6–20 Borg scale) or to individual tolerance.

During the admission, it is ideal if patients also receive some basic information about heart disease and secondary prevention, including the importance of lifestyle change and medication adherence. All patients should also receive a referral to a formal secondary prevention or rehabilitation programme. At discharge, communication should be provided to the patient's general practitioner, summarizing inpatient outcomes, CHD risk factor status and secondary prevention options and plans.

Immediate Post-Discharge Phase

The immediate post-discharge phase is a time of high anxiety for patients and families, and unfortunately rehabilitation services vary considerably and range from either no or limited contact to regular phone follow-up and home visits in some areas. A home programme for MI and CABG patients in the form of a workbook or exercise videos (e.g. *Cardiac Rehabilitation* – a British Heart Foundation publication, https://www.bhf.org.uk/search/publications?keyword=road%20to%20recovery&lang=english&showAdv=1&page=4 Accessed April 19 2016) may be used as either a complete rehabilitation package or as an interim measure or adjunct to a programme. Contact with the patient's primary care provider and ideally a secondary prevention programme at this stage provides the opportunity to answer questions, discuss symptoms and reinforce home exercises and daily walking as appropriate; e.g. uncomplicated post-MI and CABG patients should have increased the duration and frequency of activities and may be achieving up to 30 minutes of walking once or twice daily. Telephone contact also facilitates the review of risk factor modification goals and achievements.

The First 3 Months

The onset and duration of outpatient rehabilitation programmes vary considerably and are usually dependent on local resources. There is strong evidence to support that patients should attend orientation to cardiac rehabilitation within 10 days of discharge (NICE 2013, Pack et al 2013). Some may not be ready to participate in the supervised exercise component (e.g. unstable sternotomy) and in these instances they should progress with their management across other core components as relevant, such as health-behaviour change, psychosocial health and medical risk factor management (see Fig. 12-3). Programmes typically last for up to 6–12 weeks and include patients at different stages in their recovery. More information on immediate postopertive and postdischarge management can be found in Chapter 11.

The challenge for the exercise professional is to devise a safe and effective training programme that enables a patient to achieve a gradual transition from low-level convalescence activity through to an incremental exercise prescription. Indeed, if agreed guidelines and protocols for exercise training that relate to assessment, risk stratification, health and safety, patient induction, management and exercise prescription are implemented, then a safe, systematic approach, which minimizes risk and maximizes benefit, may be achieved (American Association of Cardiovascular and Pulmonary Rehabilitation 2013, American College of Sports Medicine 2013, Association of Chartered Physiotherapists in Cardiac Rehabilitation 2015).

Assessment and Risk Stratification

Local protocols referring patients for exercise training should include appropriate screening and consent from a hospital physician or cardiologist. The following information should be available to the rehabilitation health professional as part of the assessment and risk stratification process:

- current clinical status, symptoms, progress since discharge and any complications

- current cardiac status, e.g. site and size of the infarct, revascularization details, results of investigations, e.g. exercise tolerance test, echocardiogram
- cardiac history and relevant previous medical history, e.g. musculoskeletal problems, respiratory or neurological conditions
- risk stratification, to enable appropriate patient management and exercise prescription
- current medication and CHD risk factor profile.

Clinical risk stratification, i.e. determining the prognosis and relative risk of future cardiac events and complications, as well as the risk of complications during exercise, should be carried out in accordance with American Association of Cardiovascular and Pulmonary Rehabilitation (AACVPR) guidelines (AACVPR 2013). The stratification of patients into low-, medium- or high-risk groups for the occurrence of events during exercise depends on their current cardiac status, including cardiac damage, complications and associated signs and symptoms. Patients who have a low ejection fraction consistent with impaired left ventricular function, serious arrhythmias or left ventricular failure are at greater risk of complications and future cardiac events and would be classified as high risk. Also the prognosis for these patients is much poorer than for the general cardiac patient; 50% of heart failure patients die within 4 years and in patients with severe heart failure 50% of those will die within 1 year (Swedberg et al 2005), compared with the mortality for patients in the first 4 weeks post MI of 10–15% and 5% annually thereafter.

Patient safety during exercise is the main consideration for health professionals. The main risk to cardiac patients attending an exercise programme is ventricular fibrillation. When 'predicting' risk from clinical evidence and exercise assessment, the patients who have suffered extensive cardiac damage have residual ischaemia and demonstrate ventricular arrhythmias on exercise; for example, a patient with a significantly positive exercise ECG test (exercise tolerance test) or poor functional capacity and low VO_{2max} would be considered to be at higher risk of cardiac events and consequently prescribed a lower-level, more cautious rehabilitation exercise programme. Limits for exercise prescription may be determined by onset of symptoms during the exercise tolerance test, e.g. breathlessness or fatigue, and, very importantly, by evidence of ischaemia, with or without the presence of angina (silent ischaemia). Peak exercise prescription should always be set at least 10 bpm below the ischaemic threshold (American Association of Cardiovascular and Pulmonary Rehabilitation 2013, American College of Sports Medicine 2013). Distance achieved during a 6MWT has also been used in risk assessment and exercise prescription, with a walking distance of less than 335 m associated with poorer short-term survival (Andrianopoulos et al 2015, Spruit et al 2012). Please see page 587 and 588 in this chapter for more information on exercise prescription using the 6MWT.

In addition to the initial screening and risk stratification on entry to the programme, there should be ongoing clinical assessment before each exercise session. Patients should be screened by the rehabilitation professional for changes and/or compliance with medication, symptoms and home activity levels. It is recommended that patients should not exercise if they are generally unwell, symptomatic or clinically unstable on arrival (Fletcher et al 2001), e.g. if they present with:

- fever and acute systemic illness
- unresolved/unstable angina
- resting blood pressure (BP) systolic >200 mmHg and diastolic >110 mmHg
- significant unexplained drop in blood pressure
- symptomatic hypotension
- resting or uncontrolled tachycardia (HR >100 bpm)
- uncontrolled atrial or ventricular arrhythmias
- new or recurrent symptoms of breathlessness, lethargy, palpitations, dizziness
- unstable heart failure, e.g. swelling of ankles and/ or weight gain >2 kg over 2 days
- unstable/uncontrolled diabetes.

If any of these signs or symptoms is present, the patient should be seen by their general practitioner and/or cardiologist. Home activity and exercise goals should be adjusted appropriately and reviewed by rehabilitation staff before the patient restarts the exercise programme. For guidance on medication commonly used and prescribed for cardiac patients and its associated relevance to exercise, see Table 12-5.

Safe Delivery and Programme Management

Safe delivery of exercise also depends on patient supervision, appropriate education, induction and observance of health and safety protocols.

Patient Supervision and Staffing for Group Exercise Sessions

- There should be an appropriate skill mix of staff with specialist training to lead and supervise exercise and deal with medical problems and emergencies.
- In the UK there should be a minimum of two trained staff present with staff:patient ratio dependent on the risk stratification of patients in the group. Current recommended ratio to ensure safe monitoring/management of patients is 1 : 5; inclusion of higher-risk patients may require a higher ratio (Association of Chartered Physiotherapists in Cardiac Rehabilitation 2015, Coats et al 1995, Scottish Intercollegiate Guidelines Network 2002). However, these guidelines may differ in different countries and should be checked.
- All staff should be skilled in monitoring the patient's HR, BP, symptoms and pacing of exercise.
- All staff should be competent and regularly updated in basic life support and be able to access and use an automated external defibrillator (AED). Preferably one professional should have advanced life support training.

Patient Induction

An induction and education session should be conducted with each patient and cover:

- the aims of the exercise programme
- use of equipment
- importance of safety, self-monitoring and pacing of exercise
- setting exercise goals and maintaining a home exercise and activity log book.

Patients and their families should also be advised on educational issues such as:

- signs and symptoms of exertion, e.g. 'listen to your body'

Text continued on p. 623

TABLE 12-5

Exercise Considerations for Medications

Drug Group or Name	When Used	How They Work	Side Effects	Exercise Considerations
ACE Inhibitors				
Captopril Enalapril Fosinopril Lisinopril Perindopril Ramipril Trandolapril	**Standard drug therapy for post-MI patients, especially those who are at increased risk of deteriorating LV function and heart failure.** ◼ Hypertension ◼ Heart failure ◼ Post MI to improve LV function and as secondary prevention	ACE plays a crucial role in the regulation of BP by the kidneys. ACE inhibitors prevent the formation of angiotensin II, a vasoconstrictor that raises BP and causes fluid retention. By blocking constriction and preventing fluid retention the heart can pump more easily because ◼ afterload is reduced ◼ circulating volume is reduced.	◼ Dry annoying cough ◼ Hypotension ◼ Skin rash ◼ Metallic taste ◼ Reduced kidney function ◼ Allergic reaction involving swelling of the lips and tongue (angio-oedema)	◼ Possible increase in exercise capacity in individuals with heart failure ◼ Rapid changes in posture or abrupt cessation of exercise will increase risk of hypotension
α-Blockers				
Doxazosin Indoramin Prazosin	◼ Hypertension (not controlled by other drugs)	α-Receptors in vascular smooth muscle respond to noradrenaline by vasoconstricting. By blocking this response, peripheral arteries remain more dilated and so BP is reduced.	◼ Postural hypotension ◼ Headache ◼ Palpitations	◼ Fatigue
Angiotensin Receptor Blockers				
Candesartan Irbesartan Losartan Telmisartan Valsartan	◼ Hypertension (often used when the dry cough associated with ACE inhibitors cannot be tolerated) ◼ Heart failure	While ACE inhibitors inhibit the formation of angiotensin II, this group of drugs directly blocks the angiotensin II receptors, preventing the vasoconstrictor action of angiotensin II.	◼ Fatigue ◼ Hypotension ◼ Taste disturbance ◼ Skin rash	◼ Rapid changes in posture or abrupt cessation of exercise will increase risk of hypotension.
Anti-Arrhythmics				
	Arrhythmias	Drugs in this group will all affect the conduction system of the heart at various points. They are used to correct fast and often irregular heartbeats. Anti-arrhythmic effects are also obtained from other groups of drugs including β-blockers and calcium channel blockers (see under separate sections of this table).		

Continued on following page

TABLE 12-5
Exercise Considerations for Medications (*Continued*)

Drug Group or Name	When Used	How They Work	Side Effects	Exercise Considerations
Amiodarone Digoxin	■ Atrial fibrillation ■ Atrial flutter ■ Ventricular arrhythmias ■ Atrial fibrillation ■ Limited use in heart failure	Prolongs the refractory period of the heart, i.e. when there is no electrical activity. This suppresses arrhythmias, increases myocardial contraction and reduces conductivity within the AV node, thereby preventing rapid atrial rates from being transmitted to the ventricles, increasing cardiac efficiency.	■ Photosensitivity (avoid direct sun on skin) ■ Night glare ■ Metallic taste ■ Nightmares ■ Thyroid disorders ■ Nausea, vomiting ■ Loss of appetite ■ Fatigue ■ Slow pulse ■ Ventricular arrhythmias ■ Vision disturbances	■ Possible slower heart rate response to exercise ■ Reduced exercise capacity due to depressant effect on myocardium
Anti-Coagulants Warfarin New oral anti-coagulants (NOACs) Apixaban Dabigatran Rivaroxaban	Reduce the risk of embolism forming in: ■ Atrial fibrillation ■ Valve disease ■ Valve surgery (taken for life if mechanical valve used and for about 3 months if tissue valve used) ■ Following large anterior MI if, as a consequence of poor ventricular contraction, there is a risk of thrombus formation within the left ventricle ■ Reduce the risk of embolism forming but only indicated in AF in the absence of valve disease.	Prevent the blood from clotting by interfering with the synthesis of clotting proteins in the liver.	■ Haemorrhage as a result of external damage, e.g. cuts ■ Internal bleeding, e.g. gastro-intestinal (Note: severe bleeding on warfarin can be rapidly reversed with vitamin K. There is no antidote to NOACs.)	■ Care with equipment to avoid accidents ■ Avoid contact sports or sports where there is a high risk of injury. Note: Unless under medical advice, patients should not take products containing aspirin when taking anticoagulants.

Anti-Platelets

Aspirin
Clopidogrel
Prasugrel
Ticagrelor

Standard drug therapy for all patients with CVD

Also used in acute phase of MI

- Acute coronary syndrome
- Standard therapy post PCI for limited period

Decrease platelet aggregation (or stickiness) that may stop clots forming in the arterial side of the circulation similar action to aspirin.

- Gastro-intestinal upset/ bleed
- Bronchospasm in susceptible individuals
- Other internal haemorrhage
- Lower incidence of gastro-intestinal upset/ bleed than with aspirin
- Blood disorders

β-Blockers

Atenolol
Bisoprolol*
Carvedilol*
Metoprolol
Nebivolol*
Propranolol
Sotalol
Timolol

Standard drug therapy for post-MI patients who are at increased risk of further MI and sudden cardiac death.

- Hypertension
- Angina
- Arrhythmias
- Tachycardia
- Heart failure

Block β-receptors to decrease sympathetic activity. As a result:

- Myocardial oxygen demand is reduced due to reduced HR, BP and strength of myocardial contraction.
- Reduced HR extends the period of diastole and, since most coronary blood flow occurs during diastole, myocardial blood flow is improved.
- Suppresses arrhythmias – especially fast atrial arrhythmias – by slowing the conducting impulse (mainly through the AV node).
- Slows down the remodelling process and reduces myocardial workload in HF.

- Reduced pulse rate
- Reduced BP
- Dizziness
- Tiredness/lethargy
- Airway constriction
- Cold fingers/toes
- Male impotence
- Sleep disturbance/ nightmares

Note: β-blockers should not be stopped suddenly without medical advice as this may lead to rebound angina and possibly MI.

- Rapid changes in posture or abrupt cessation of exercise will increase risk of hypotension.
- Unless a training HR has been established from an ECG exercise tolerance test done 'on medication', appropriate training intensity is best determined using a combination of RPE and HR responses.
- Estimated HR$_{max}$ rate will be 20–30 bpm lower than for those not on β-blockers.

Continued on following page

TABLE 12-5

Exercise Considerations for Medications (*Continued*)

Drug Group or Name	When Used	How They Work	Side Effects	Exercise Considerations
Calcium-Channel Blockers				
Type 1 Verapamil	■ Angina ■ Hypertension ■ Arrhythmias	Release of calcium into cells precedes contraction in cardiac, skeletal and smooth muscle. Different groups of CC blockers reduce calcium influx into specific types of cells, which reduces the strength of contraction.	–	■ Possible reduced HR response to exercise in verapamil and diltiazem.
Type 2 Amlodipine Felodipine Nicardipine Nifedipine	Amlodipine is used when the radial artery is used in CABGS, as it helps to maintain vasodilatation of the grafted vessel.	■ Suppresses arrhythmias by suppressing conduction through the AV node.	■ Hypotension ■ Facial flushing ■ Palpitations ■ Pounding headaches ■ Mild ankle swelling (mostly nifedipine, amlodipine)	■ Rapid changes in posture or abrupt cessation of exercise will increase risk of hypotension.
Type 3 Diltiazem		■ Reduces myocardial contractility and may slow heart rate. ■ Relaxes smooth muscle in walls of systemic arteries, reducing BP and, therefore afterload combines the actions of both the other groups.	■ Constipation (mostly verapamil)	■ Type 2, e.g. nifedipine, may cause a reflex increase in HR in response to reduced BP.
Diuretics				
Thiazide diuretics (*'weaker' diuretics*) Bendroflumethiazide Hydrochlorothiazide Metolazone	■ Heart failure ■ Hypertension ■ Oedema	This group acts on the kidneys and increases the volume of urine excreted by:	■ Loss of potassium (in some types) ■ Ventricular arrhythmias ■ Tiredness ■ Muscle weakness and/cramps	■ Dehydration effects – Keep encouraging fluids during exercise, especially in hot weather.
Loop diuretics (*'strong' diuretics*) Bumetanide Furosemide Torasemide	Any of the above situations where there is increased risk of potassium loss	■ removing salt and, thereby, water from the circulation ■ dilating arterioles.	■ Elevated cholesterol and triglycerides ■ Loss of appetite	■ Dehydration increases potential for hypotension.
Potassium-sparing diuretics Amiloride Co-amilofruse Eplerenone Moduretic Spironolactone Triamterene		The reduction in circulating fluid and vasodilatation reduces blood pressure (afterload) and, therefore the work of the myocardium.	■ Gout ■ Diabetes ■ Impotence	■ Aching legs and/or tiredness may affect exercise capacity.

Lipid-Lowering Drugs

Drug	Action / Use	Side effects
Statins Atorvastatin Fluvastatin Pravastatin Rosuvastatin Simvastatin	**Standard drug therapy for all CVD patients and anyone at high risk of developing CHD or other vascular disease.** Hyperlipidaemia ■ Potent at lowering LDL-C ■ Moderate increase in HDL-C ■ Moderate reduction in elevated triglyceride levels in Control levels of cholesterol and triglycerides in the blood by inhibiting enzymes involved in cholesterol synthesis, especially in the liver.	■ Possible aching legs
Ezetimibe	combination with statin therapy when further reduction of LDL-C is sought or on their own in patients who do not tolerate statin therapy mainly elevated triglyceride Prevents cholesterol absorption	■ Gastro-intestinal upsets
Fibrates Bezafibrate Clofibrate Fenofibrate Gemfibrozil	■ Also to reduce LDL-C levels and raise HDL-C stimulate enzymes that initiate the breakdown of triglycerides. Its use has declined since the introduction of statins.	■ Muscle pain ■ Headache ■ Gallstones ■ Rash ■ Acute pain in calf or thigh muscle if kidney function is impaired

Nitrates

Drug	Action / Use	Side effects
Isosorbide dinitrate Isosorbide mononitrate Glyceryl trinitrate (tablets or spray)	■ Angina Longer-acting nitrates are given to prevent angina. ■ 'Breakthrough' angina When, despite the use of long acting nitrates, angina occurs, GTN is used to alleviate the angina. GTN can also be used to prevent angina, e.g. prior to exercise. Vasodilatation of blood vessels ■ Dilates coronary arteries to improve coronary blood flow. ■ Dilates great veins which reduces venous return and preload and consequently myocardial work. ■ Dilates the large arteries in the systemic circulation which decreases vascular resistance (afterload) and consequently myocardial work.	■ Hypotension ■ Facial flushing ■ Headache ■ Dizziness ■ Nausea ■ Possible severe interaction with sildenafil (Viagra) and other medication used for erectile dysfunction ■ Rapid changes in posture or abrupt cessation of exercise will increase risk of hypotension. ■ Improved exercise tolerance as the ischaemic threshold is improved. Clients must never exercise with or through an episode of angina, as it may indicate the onset of MI.

Continued on following page

TABLE 12-5
Exercise Considerations for Medications (Continued)

Drug Group or Name	When Used	How They Work	Side Effects	Exercise Considerations
Potassium-Channel Activators				
Nicorandil	■ Angina (especially when angina is resistant to other medication)	Potassium is essential in the transmission of nerve impulses and for the stimulation and action of muscle. Promotes dilatation of the large coronary arteries (which improves coronary blood flow) and systemic arteries and veins (which reduces both preload and afterload).	■ Dizziness ■ Headaches ■ Hypotension ■ Tachycardia ■ Interaction with sildenafil (Viagra) as described for nitrates	■ Rapid changes in posture or abrupt cessation of exercise will increase risk of hypotension. ■ Possible tachycardia
Sinus Node Inhibitor				
Ivabradine	■ Angina ■ Heart failure	Slows sinus heart rate (thus of no use in atrial arrhythmias)	■ Bradycardia ■ Headache ■ Dizziness ■ Gastro-intestinal effects ■ Luminous phenomena in eyes (mostly resolves with ongoing use)	Unless a training HR has been established from an ECG exercise tolerance test done while taking drug, training intensity is best determined by using both RPE and HR responses. Estimated HR$_{max}$ rate will be about 20-30 bpm lower than those not on ivabradine.

(From BACPR Exercise Instructor Training Manual 2015. BACR Instructor manual and DVD can be purchased from http://www.bacpr.com/pages/page_box_contents.asp?pageid=851&navcatid=182 accessed April 19 2016.)

ACE, Angiotensin-converting enzyme; AF, atrial fibrillation; AV, atrioventricular; BP, blood pressure; CABGS, coronary artery bypass graft surgery; CC, calcium channel; CHD, coronary heart disease; CVD, cardiovascular disease; ECG exercise tolerance test, electrocardiography exercise tolerance test; GTN, glyceryl trinitrate; HDL-C, high-density lipoprotein cholesterol; HF, heart failure; HR, heart rate; HR$_{max}$, maximal heart rate; LDL-C, low-density lipoprotein cholesterol; LV, left ventricular; MI, myocardial infarction; PCI, percutaneous coronary intervention; RPE, rating of perceived exertion.
*Licensed for use in heart failure.

- warm-up and cool-down advice
- caution with isometric activities
- relative haemodynamic responses to arm work versus leg work
- environmental issues, e.g. excessive heat/cold, dehydration
- avoiding exercise after a heavy meal, during systemic illness and when fatigued
- the importance of remaining until surveillance of all patients in the immediate post-exercise period (for up to 30 minutes) is completed.

Health and Safety Protocols

Relevant considerations:

- There should be a local written policy, clearly displayed, for managing emergency situations, e.g. collapse of patient, and management of medical problems, e.g. chest pain, hypoglycaemic episode.
- There should be rapid access to an emergency team either in hospital or via ambulance, with access to a telephone for raising emergency help.
- Appropriate emergency equipment should be available. It should be regularly maintained in accordance with local protocols and staff should have regular practice in emergency drills and procedures.
- Exercise equipment should be regularly checked and maintained by staff.
- Drinking water and glucose drinks or supplements should be available for patients as required.
- Venue access, emergency exits, toilet and changing facilities, lighting, floor surface and room space should be checked by staff to be safe and appropriate. There should be adequate space for a free exercise area and patient traffic around exercise room, and safe placement of equipment meeting recommended requirements, e.g. floor space for aerobic exercise of 1.8–2.3 m^2 per patient and 0.6 m^2 of space per individual using equipment (American Association of Cardiovascular and Pulmonary Rehabilitation 2013, Tharrett & Peterson 1997).

- Temperature and ventilation of the room should be maintained at 18–23°C (65–72°F) and humidity at 65%.

Programme Outcome Measures

Outcome measures are essential, not only to determine risk stratification and functional capacity but also to set and evaluate the effectiveness of an exercise training programme, provide objective feedback to the patient and facilitate evidence-based practice. These measures can be used both as a baseline, entry assessment tool and as an exit outcome measure. They may include heart rate and blood pressure at rest, during exercise and at recovery and comparative RPEs, BMI and waist circumference measures, as well as measures of nutritional status, medication adherence, sternal stability (Sternal Instability Scale, SIS), smoking status and functional capacity. Indirect submaximal measures of functional capacity may be derived from the 6MWT (Steele 1994), shuttle walk test (Singh et al 1992) or Chester step test (Sykes & Roberts 2004). Further information on outcome measures can be found in Chapter 6.

Exercise Considerations for Special Cardiac Groups

Considerations for prescribing and delivering exercise for various groups within the CHD population, e.g. patients with diabetes, hypertension and peripheral vascular disease, are summarized in Table 12-6. Exercise issues for specific cardiac patient groups, i.e. patients with heart failure, implantable cardioverter defibrillators and following a median sternotomy (e.g. CABG and/valve surgery) are described in the following sections. Further guidelines for other conditions, such as cardiac transplantation, pacemakers and left ventricular assist devices, are easily accessible (Association of Chartered Physiotherapists in Cardiac Rehabilitation 2015).

Heart Failure

Systematic reviews of exercise-based cardiac rehabilitation in individuals in stable heart failure have confirmed the safety and effectiveness of exercise as an intervention (Davies et al 2010, Rees et al 2010, Taylor et al 2014). Benefits reported are a reduction in hospitalization rates, decreased symptoms and improved

TABLE 12-6

Considerations for Prescribing Exercise for Special Groups Within the Coronary Heart Disease Population

	Management	Precautions/Other Considerations

Diabetes	■ Diabetes must be stable.
	■ Blood sugar levels should be checked twice before exercising: 30 minutes prior to exercise and again immediately before commencement of exercise. 20–30 g of additional carbohydrate should be ingested if pre-exercise blood glucose is <5.5 mMol/L.
	■ If new to exercise or increasing the intensity or duration of exercise, levels should be monitored every 30 minutes during exercise.
	■ Check blood glucose levels at least twice after exercise to ensure that hypoglycaemia is not developing.
	■ Those on insulin medication may experience 'exercise-induced hyperglycaemia'. Exercise should not be commenced if pre-exercise blood glucose levels are >13 mMol/L. If glucose levels pre-exercise are >10 mMol/L, check again 10 minutes after starting exercise and only continue to exercise if the level has fallen.
		■ Carry medical information about condition in case of adverse incidents.
		■ 'Silent' ischaemia is more common in diabetics.
		■ Insulin may need to be reduced on exercise days.
		■ Insulin uptake may be increased if it is injected into exercising limbs, e.g. use the abdomen rather than the thigh.
		■ Have rapid-acting glucose source available.
		■ Late evening exercise is inadvisable.
		■ Autonomic neuropathy may lead to abnormal HR and BP responses.
		■ Peripheral neuropathy may cause sensory loss, impaired balance and coordination.
		■ Peripheral neuropathy highlights the need for good foot care. Patients should check their feet before and after exercise.
		■ The effect of a single bout of exercise on blood glucose levels lasts less than 72 hours, so exercise needs to be frequent and regular.
		■ Specific benefits of aerobic exercise for diabetic patients include:
		  ■ improved glycaemic clearance
		  ■ increased insulin sensitivity
		  ■ reduction in body fat while preserving lean muscle mass.

Hypertension	■ Do not exercise if SBP >200 mmHg and DBP >110 mmHg
	■ Follow FITT principles but adopt lower end of training intensity with compensatory increase in the frequency and/or duration.
	■ Reduce resistance and increase number of repetitions for muscular strength and endurance exercises.
		■ Medication is likely to lead to hypotension. Ensure that:
		  ■ during upright exercise, feet are constantly moving to aid venous return
		  ■ there is an extended post-exercise recovery period.
		■ Avoid Valsalva manoeuvre.
		■ Avoid high-intensity arm work and overgripping of equipment, e.g. cycle handlebars.
		■ A specific benefit of exercise for hypertensive patients is that total peripheral resistance is reduced for several hours following a single bout of exercise. Consequently, an increase in frequency of exercise ensures that the overall time spent in a relative 'hypotensive' state is increased.

Peripheral vascular disease	■ Promote daily walking and other weightbearing exercise.
	■ Increase duration before intensity.
	■ Interval training may be better tolerated than continuous exercise.
	■ Use supplementary non-weightbearing exercise, e.g. cycling, if pain is severe and/or motivation is poor and an adequate CV dose is unlikely to be achieved through weightbearing exercises alone.
	■ Reassure and support patient to exercise despite discomfort and teach PVD scale of discomfort (ACSM 2013).
		■ Cold weather, leading to vasoconstriction, may worsen symptoms; encourage extended warm-up period, e.g. slow walking gradually increasing to individually prescribed pace.
		■ Monitor for injuries to legs that could lead to leg ulcers or gangrene.
		■ Specific benefits of weightbearing exercise for patients with PVD may include:
		  ■ increase in peripheral blood flow and oxygen delivery
		  ■ improved oxygen extraction
		  ■ changed gait and, thereby, efficiency, i.e. less effort at same workload.

TABLE 12-6

Considerations for Prescribing Exercise for Special Groups Within the Coronary Heart Disease Population *(Continued)*

	Management	Precautions/Other Considerations
Ageing population	▪ FITT principles apply for CV training but at lower intensity until ability is established. ▪ Extended warm-up and cool-down is required. ▪ Promote strength work for major muscle groups used in activities of daily living. ▪ Include flexibility and general mobility work within the programme.	▪ Avoid exercises in extreme temperatures. ▪ Monitor hydration, especially if diuretics have been prescribed. ▪ Avoid using partners for support or in resistance work. ▪ Instructions must be especially clear/precise/unhurried and should be enhanced by good visual demonstration. ▪ Avoid exercises that might exacerbate urinary incontinence.

BP, blood pressure; *CV*, cardiovascular; *DBP*, diastolic blood pressure; *FITT*, frequency, intensity, type and time of training; *HR*, heart rate; *PVD*, peripheral vascular disease; *SBP*, systolic blood pressure.

quality of life. Heart failure patients are among those deemed at highest risk of further cardiac events during exercise according to the AACVPR stratification criteria (AACVPR 2013), fulfilling one of the essential criteria for high-risk patients of an ejection fraction of less than 40%, but may additionally present with other criteria, e.g. significant symptoms at low levels of activity of less than 5 METs or the presence of abnormal haemodynamics with exercise testing. Quantifying functional capacity further stratifies relative risk: a peak VO_2 of less than 10 mL of oxygen per kilogram of bodyweight per minute (10 mL/kg min^{-1}) is associated with a relatively higher risk; a peak VO_2 of 18 mL/kg min^{-1} categorizes a patient at lower risk, while a walking distance of 300 m in the 6MWT is associated with poorer short-term survival (Cahalin et al 1996, Likoff et al 1987, Lipkin et al 1986, Swedberg et al 2005). When undertaking exercise training with higher-risk patients, rigorous patient assessment, individual exercise prescription and monitoring, coupled with safe management and delivery of exercise, are paramount (Hunt et al 2005, Pina et al 2003).

In addition to the previously discussed exercise contraindications and cautions that apply to cardiac patients, heart failure patients should report:

▪ significant weight gain of >2 kg over 2 days
▪ deterioration in exercise tolerance or increased breathlessness on exertion
▪ any recent ICD event or change in pacemaker status
▪ significant ischaemia during low-intensity exercise (<2 METs)
▪ new-onset atrial fibrillation/atrial flutter.

Issues relating to the monitoring and safety of exercise include:

▪ Staff:patient supervision ratio should be reviewed dependent on higher risk stratification.
▪ Rigorous monitoring of individual patient's heart rate, blood pressure and use of RPE (i.e. Borg CR 0–10 scale) and dyspnoea scales is required.
▪ Exercise heart rate for individuals will be approximately 10–20 beats lower than in individuals without heart failure (Beale et al 2010). To account for this the Keteyian et al (2012) method is recommended to estimate maximal heart rate.
▪ For those with ICDs, heart rate thresholds should be incorporated into the exercise prescription.

Additional training considerations include:

▪ Aim for low/moderate intensity of training; may be as low as 40% of VO_2R/HRR and/or 11–13 RPE.
▪ Adopt an interval training approach with initial work phases of 1–6 minutes of activity and rest phases of 1–2 minutes (American College of Sports Medicine 2013).
▪ Include respiratory and posture training; very deconditioned patients may suffer gross fatigue with arm and upper body exercise and accessory muscle use compromises breathing pattern.

Exercise Issues Following Implantation of a Cardioverter Defibrillator

Exercise rehabilitation plays an important part in enabling patients to regain the confidence to resume activity following implantation of an ICD device (Lampman & Knight 2000). Significant benefits in cardiorespiratory fitness, confidence and psychological well-being have been demonstrated in patients participating in rehabilitation following implantation of an ICD device (Fitchet et al 2003). The following specific points should be considered when prescribing and delivering exercise for ICD patients:

- knowledge of ICD heart rate settings
- knowledge of ICD therapy settings
- knowledge of medication used to control heart rate, e.g. β-blockade
- avoidance of excessive shoulder range of movement and/or highly repetitive vigorous shoulder movement.

Exercise Following a Median Sternotomy (e.g. CABG and/or Valve Surgery)

Cardiac rehabilitation forms standard best practice postoperative care for patients who undergo cardiac surgery. Several studies have documented the impact of a sternotomy on patient functional status. Zimmerman et al (2002) examined symptoms in patients 2, 4 and 6 weeks after cardiac surgery and found that shortness of breath, fatigue and pain were all common and were related to function. In a separate study, they also found that an education intervention using telehealth technology focusing on self-efficacy and strategies to manage prospective situations (for 6 weeks post discharge from hospital) reduced symptom influence with physical activity in patients recovering after cardiac surgery (Zimmerman et al 2004). In addition, 2 months following CABG surgery many patients have reported deficits in performing home chores needing assistance (36%), having difficulty (56%), and/or experiencing pain (44%) (LaPier 2003, LaPier 2007, LaPier et al 2008). Other studies by the same authors found that patients who had undergone CABG surgery in the past 6 months frequently reported chest incision tenderness/irritation (69%), chest incision numbness/tingling (50%), and waking multiple times at night (75%) (LaPier & Wilson 2006, LaPier & Wilson 2007, LaPier 2006). It was also noted that 1 year after CABG surgery, 36% of patients subjectively reported their functional status was 'unsatisfactory' (Falcoz et al 2003).

The following specific points should be considered when prescribing and delivering exercise for cardiac surgery patients who have a median sternotomy:

- Optimal pain control is important so as to ensure a positive exercise experience.
- Should pain and discomfort be moderate to severe (rating >5/10) and/or interfere with everyday tasks, patients should consult their medical practitioner.
- Localized pain of musculoskeletal origin may require assessment and treatment by a physiotherapist.
- The programme should incorporate thoracic exercises as they reduce sternal pain.
- Sternal stability should be screened and assessed (e.g. SIS, subjective questions) prior to the commencement and for the duration of the programme.
- Patients with sternal instability should be referred to the surgical/medical team for a review of their management.
- Patients with sternal instability should be prescribed bilateral upper limb exercises where possible, as unilateral loaded upper limb exercises may provoke symptoms of pain and discomfort.

Transition of Patients to Long-Term Community-Based Exercise Provision

When medically and psychologically stable, CHD patients should progress from the clinically supervised rehabilitation environment to a community-based, long-term exercise programme. They should demonstrate:

- significant improvement in functional capacity (achieving approximately 5 METs is recommended)
- psychological adaptation to chronic disease
- the foundation of behavioural and lifestyle changes required for continued risk factor modification.

Rehabilitation staff discharging the patient to their general practitioner and trained and certified exercise instructors should be satisfied that the patient is able to:

- exercise safely and effectively, according to an individual exercise prescription

- monitor own heart rate or use scale of perceived exertion effectively
- recognize warning signs and symptoms and take appropriate action (e.g. stop/reduce exercise level, take glyceryl trinitrate)
- identify specific goals for long-term maintenance of lifestyle change and risk factor reduction, relating to own personal history
- take responsibility to monitor risk factors (i.e. smoking, blood pressure, cholesterol and diabetes) with their general practitioner and the practice nurse
- report results of any ongoing investigations and possible implications for exercise prescription to the phase IV instructor.

CONCLUSION

Secondary prevention, including cardiac rehabilitation and exercise training, is an effective form of management for people with cardiac disease and is endorsed by numerous clinical guidelines. It has a large and increasing evidence base to support its implementation in a variety of settings and for a variety of cardiac conditions. Challenges remain to increase the uptake of all people who would benefit from participation in programmes and to ensure programmes and research evidence reflect changes in the medical management of this group of people. The availability of flexible models of ongoing prevention is likely to improve access and equity and ultimately ensure the ongoing evolution of CR with the changing needs of society.

REFERENCES

Aamot, I., Moholdt, T., Amundsen, B., et al., 2010. Onset of exercise training 14 days after uncomplicated MI: a randomized controlled trial. Eur. J. Cardiovasc. Prev. Rehabil. 17 (14), 387–392.

Abraham, C., Michie, S., 2008. A taxonomy of behavior changes techniques used in interventions. Health Psychol. 27, 379–387.

Adams, J., Cline, M.J., Hibbard, M., et al., 2006. A new paradigm for post-cardiac event resistance exercise guidelines. Am. J. Cardiol. 97, 281–286.

Ades, P.A., 2001. Cardiac rehabilitation and secondary prevention of coronary heart disease. N. Engl. J. Med. 345, 892–902.

Ades, P., 2007. Individualized preventive care in cardiac rehabilitation. J. Cardiopulm. Rehabil. Prev. 27, 130–134.

Ades, P.A., Pashkow, F.J., Nestor, J.R., 1997. Cost-effectiveness of cardiac rehabilitation after myocardial infarction. J. Cardiopulm. Rehabil. 17, 222–231.

Ainsworth, B.E., Haskell, W.L., Herrmann, S.D., et al., 2011. Compendium of Physical Activities: a second update of codes and MET values. Med. Sci. Sports Exerc. 43 (8), 1575–1581.

Altenburg, W.A., ten Hacken, N.H., Bossenbroek, L., et al., 2015. Short- and long-term effects of a physical activity counselling programme in COPD: a randomized controlled trial. Respir. Med. 109 (1), 112–121.

American Association of Cardiovascular and Pulmonary Rehabilitation, 2013. Guidelines for Cardiac Rehabilitation and Secondary Prevention Programmes, fifth ed. Human Kinetics, Champaign, IL.

American College of Sports Medicine, 2013. ACSMs Guidelines for Exercise Testing and Prescription, ninth ed. Williams and Wilkins, Baltimore.

Anderson, J.L., Adams, C.D., Antman, E.M., et al., 2011. ACCF/AHA focused update incorporated into the ACC/AHA 2007 Guidelines for the Management of Patients with Unstable Angina/Non–ST-elevation myocardial infarction: a report of the American College of Cardiology Foundation/American Heart Association Task Force on Practice Guidelines. Circulation 123, e426–e579.

Anderson, L., Taylor, R.S., 2014. Cardiac rehabilitation for people with heart disease: an overview of Cochrane systematic reviews (Protocol). Cochrane Database Syst. Rev. (8), Art. No.: CD011273, doi:10.1002/14651858.CD011273.

Andrianopoulos, V., Klijn, P., Franssen, F.M., Spruit, M.A., 2014. Exercise training in pulmonary rehabilitation. Clin. Chest Med. 35 (2), 313–322.

Andrianopoulos, V., Wouters, E.F., Pinto-Plata, V.M., et al., 2015. Prognostic value of variables derived from the six-minute walk test in patients with COPD: results from the ECLIPSE study. Respir. Med. 109 (9), 1138–1146.

Anzuini, F., Battistella, A., Izzotti, A., 2011. Physical activity and cancer prevention: a review of current evidence and biological mechanisms. J. Prev. Med. Hyg. 52 (4), 174–180.

Aragam, K.G., Moscucci, M., Smith, D.E., et al., 2011. Trends and disparities in referral to cardiac rehabilitation after percutaneous coronary intervention. Am. Heart J. 161, 544–551.e2.

Aroney, C.N., Aylward, P., Kelly, A.M., for the Acute Coronary Syndrome Guidelines Working Group, et al., 2006. Guidelines for the management of acute coronary syndromes 2006. Med. J. Aust. 184, S1–S30.

Association of Chartered Physiotherapists in Cardiac Rehabilitation, 2015. Standards for Physical Activity and Exercise in the Cardiovascular Population, third ed. CSP, London.

Balady, G.J., Ades, P.A., Comoss, P., et al., 2000. Core components of cardiac rehabilitation/secondary prevention programs. Circulation 102, 1069–1073.

Balady, G.J., Fletcher, B.J., Froelicher, E.S., et al., 1994. Cardiac rehabilitation programs: a statement for healthcare professionals from the American Heart Association. Circulation 90, 1602–1610.

Balady, G.J., Williams, M.A., Ades, P.A., et al., 2007. American Heart Association Exercise, Cardiac Rehabilitation, and Prevention Committee; the Council on Clinical Cardiology; American Heart Association Council on Cardiovascular Nursing; American

Heart Association Council on Epidemiology and Prevention; American Heart Association Council on Nutrition, Physical Activity, and Metabolism; American Association of Cardiovascular and Pulmonary Rehabilitation Core components of cardiac rehabilitation/secondary prevention programs. 2007 update: a scientific statement from the American Heart Association Exercise, Cardiac Rehabilitation, and Prevention Committee, the Council on Clinical Cardiology; the Councils on Cardiovascular Nursing, Epidemiology and Prevention, and Nutrition, Physical Activity, and Metabolism; and the American Association of Cardiovascular and Pulmonary Rehabilitation. Circulation 115, 2675–2682.

Bandy, W.D., Irion, J.M., 1994. The effect of time on static stretch on the flexibility of the hamstring muscles. Phys. Ther. 74 (9), 845–850.

Balady, G.J., Ades, P.A., Bittner, V.A., et al., 2011. American Heart Association Science Advisory and Coordinating Committee. Referral, enrollment, and delivery of cardiac rehabilitation/secondary prevention programs at clinical centers and beyond: a presidential advisory from the American Heart Association. Circulation 124, 2951–2960.

Barlow, C.E., Defina, L.F., Radford, N.B., et al., 2012. Cardiorespiratory fitness and long-term survival in 'low-risk' adults. J. Am. Heart Assoc. 1 (4), e001354.

Bauman, A.E., Reis, R.S., Sallis, J.F., et al., 2012. Correlates of physical activity: why are some people physically active and others not? Lancet 380 (9838), 258–271.

Beale, L., Silberbauer, J., Lloyd, G., et al., 2010. Exercise heart rate guidelines overestimate recommended intensity for chronic heart failure patients. Br. J. Cardiol. 17 (3), 133–137.

Beauchamp, M.K., Brooks, D., Lloyd, G., et al., 2010. Deficits in postural control in individuals with COPD: emerging evidence for an important secondary impairment. Multidiscip. Respir. Med. 5 (6), 417–421.

Beauchamp, M.K., Hill, K., Goldstein, R.S., et al., 2009. Impairments in balance discriminate fallers from non-fallers in COPD. Respir. Med. 103 (12), 1885–1891.

Beauchamp, M.K., Janaudis-Ferreira, T., Parreira, V., et al., 2013. A randomized controlled trial of balance training during pulmonary rehabilitation for individuals with COPD Chest. Aug 22. doi:10.1378/chest.13–1093.

Beauchamp, M.K., O'Hoski, S., Goldstein, R.S., et al., 2010. Effect of pulmonary rehabilitation on balance in persons with chronic obstructive pulmonary disease. Arch. Phys. Med. Rehabil. 91 (9), 1460–1465.

Belman, M.J., Kendregan, B.A., 1981. Exercise training fails to increase skeletal muscle enzymes in patients with chronic obstructive pulmonary disease. Am. Rev. Respir. Dis. 123, 256–261.

Belman, M.J., Shadmehr, R., 1988. Targeted resistive muscle training in COPD. J. Appl. Physiol. 65, 2726–2735.

Bendstrup, K.E., Ingemann, J.J., Holm, S., et al., 1997. Out-patient rehabilitation improves activities of daily living, quality of life and exercise tolerance in COPD. Eur. Respir. J. 10, 2801–2806.

Bennett, J.A., Lyons, K.S., Winters-Stone, K., et al., 2007. Motivational interviewing to increase physical activity in long-term cancer survivors: a randomized controlled trial. Nurs. Res. 56 (1), 18–27.

Berry, M.J., Rejeski, W.J., Adair, N.E., et al., 2003. A randomized controlled trial comparing long-term and short-term exercise in patients with COPD. J. Cardiopulm. Rehabil. 23, 60–68.

Beswick, A.D., Rees, K., Griebsch, I., et al., 2004. Provision, uptake and cost of cardiac rehabilitation programmes: improving services to under-represented groups. Health Technol. Assess. 8, 1–152.

Bittner, V., Sanderson, B., 2006. Cardiac rehabilitation as a secondary prevention centre. Coron. Artery Dis. 17, 211–218.

Blumenthal, J.A., Rejeski, W.J., Walsh-Riddle, M., et al., 1988. Comparison of high- and low-intensity exercise training early after acute myocardial infarction. Am. J. Cardiol. 61, 26–30.

Bolton, C., Bevan-Smith, E.F., Blakey, J.D., et al., 2013. BTS guideline on pulmonary rehabilitation in adults. Thorax 68, ii1–ii30.

Borg, G.A., 1982. Psychophysical bases of perceived exertion. Med. Sci. Sports Exerc. 14 (5), 377–381.

Borg, G., 1998. Borg's Perceived Exertion and Pain Scales. Human Kinetics, Champaign, IL.

Borghi-Silva, A., Mendes, R.G., Toledo, A.C., et al., 2010. Adjuncts to physical training of patients with severe COPD: oxygen or noninvasive ventilation? Respir. Care 55, 885–894.

Bourbeau, J., Collet, J.P., Schwartzman, K., et al., 2006. Economic benefits of self-management education in COPD. Chest 130 (6), 1704–1711.

Bourjeily-Habr, G., Rochester, C., Palermo, F., et al., 2002. Randomized controlled trial of transcutaneous electrical muscle stimulation of the lower extremities in patients with chronic obstructive pulmonary disease. Thorax 57, 1045–1049.

Bravata, D.M., Smith-Spangler, C., Sundaram, V., et al., 2007. Using pedometers to increase physical activity and improve health: a systematic review. JAMA 298 (19), 2296–2304.

Brawley, L.R., Rejeski, W.J., King, A.C., 2003. Promoting physical activity for older adults: the challenges for changing behavior. Am. J. Prev. Med. 25 (3 Suppl. 2), 172–183.

Breyer, M., Breyer-Kohansal, R., Funk, G., et al., 2010. Nordic walking improves daily physical activities in COPD: a randomised controlled trial. Respir. Res. 11, 112.

Briffa, T.G., Chow, C.K., Clark, A.M., Redfern, J., 2013. Improving outcomes after acute coronary syndrome with rehabilitation and secondary prevention. Clin. Ther. 35 (8), 1076–1081.

Briffa, T.G., Eckermann, S.D., Griffiths, A.D., et al., 2005. Cost-effectiveness of rehabilitation after an acute coronary event: a randomized controlled trial. Med. J. Aust. 183, 450–455.

Briffa, T.G., Kinsman, L., Maiorana, A.J., et al., 2009. An integrated and coordinated approach to preventing recurrent coronary heart disease events in Australia: a policy statement from the Australian cardiovascular health and rehabilitation association. Med. J. Aust. 190, 683–686.

Briffa, T., Tonkin, A.M., Hickling, S., Hobbs, M., 2009. High rates of recurrent ischaemic heart disease necessitate better secondary prevention. Circulation 120, S497.

British Association for Cardiovascular Prevention and Rehabilitation, 2012a. The BACPR Standards and Core Components for Cardiovascular Disease Prevention and Rehabilitation 2nd

Edition. British Association for Cardiovascular Prevention and Rehabilitation, London.

British Association for Cardiovascular Prevention and Rehabilitation, 2012b. Core Competences for the Physical Activity and Exercise Component: For Cardiovascular Prevention and Rehabilitation Services. British Association for Cardiovascular Prevention and Rehabilitation, London.

Brodie, D., Bethell, H., Bren, S., 2006. Cardiac rehabilitation in England: a detailed national survey. Eur. J. Cardiovasc. Prev. Rehabil. 13, 122–128.

Broekhuizen, R., Wouters, E.F., Creutzberg, E.C., Schols, A.M., 2006. Raised CRP levels mark metabolic and functional impairment in advanced COPD. Thorax 61 (1), 17–22.

Brolin, S.E., Cecins, N.M., Jenkins, S.C., 2003. Questioning the use of heart rate and dyspnea in the prescription of exercise in subjects with chronic obstructive pulmonary disease. J. Cardiopulm. Rehabil. 23 (3), 228–234.

Brooks, D., Krip, B., Mangovski-Alzamora, S., et al., 2002. The effect of post-rehabilitation programmes among individuals with chronic obstructive pulmonary disease. Eur. Respir. J. 20 (1), 20–29.

Brubaker, P.H., 2005. Is home-based cardiac rehabilitation a preferred and viable option? J. Cardiopulm. Rehabil. 25, 30–32.

Brubaker, P.H., Rejeski, W.J., Smith, M.J., et al., 2000. A home-based maintenance exercise program after centre-based cardiac rehabilitation: effects on blood lipids, body composition and functional capacity. J. Cardiopulm. Rehabil. 20, 50–56.

Budweiser, S., Moertl, M., Jörres, R.A., et al., 2006. Respiratory muscle training in restrictive thoracic disease: a randomized controlled trial. Arch. Phys. Med. Rehabil. 87 (12), 1559–1565.

Cahalin, L.P., Mathier, M.A., Semigran, M.J., et al., 1996. The six minute walk test predicts peak oxygen uptake and survival in patients with advanced heart failure. Chest 110, 325–332.

Cannistra, L.B., Davidoff, R., Picard, M.H., Balady, G.J., 1999. Moderate-high intensity exercise training after myocardial infarction: effect on left ventricular remodeling. J. Cardiopulm. Rehabil. 19, 373–380.

Carrieri-Kohlman, V., Nguyen, H.Q., Doneski-Cuenco, D., et al., 2005. Impact of brief or extended exercise training on the benefit of a dyspnea self-management program in COPD. J. Cardiopulm. Rehabil. 25 (5), 275–284.

Carson, K.V., Chandratilleke, M.G., Picot, J., 2013. Physical training for asthma. Cochrane Database Syst. Rev. (9), CD001116.

Casaburi, R., Porszasz, J., Burns, M.R., et al., 1997. Physiologic benefits of exercise training in rehabilitation of patients with severe COPD. Am. J. Respir. Crit. Care Med. 155, 1541–1551.

Caspersen, C.J., Powell, K.E., Christenson, G.M., 1985. Physical activity, exercise, and physical fitness: definitions and distinctions for health-related research. Public Health Rep. 100 (2), 126–131.

Castro, C.M., King, A.C., Brassington, G.S., 2001. Telephone versus mail interventions for maintenance of physical activity in older adults. Health Psychol. 20 (6), 438–444.

Chen, W., Lin, C.C., Peng, C.T., et al., 2002. Approaching healthy body mass index norms for children and adolescents from health-related physical fitness. Obes. Rev. 3 (3), 225–232.

Chew, D.P., Amerena, J.V., Coverdale, S.G., et al., 2008. Invasive management and late clinical outcomes in contemporary Australian management of ACS: observations from the ACACIA registry. Med. J. Aust. 188, 691–697.

Chida, M., Inase, N., Ichioka, M., et al., 1991. Ratings of perceived exertion in chronic obstructive pulmonary disease: a possible indicator for exercise training in patients with this disease. Eur. J. Appl. Physiol. Occup. Physiol. 62 (6), 390–393.

Chow, C.K., Jolly, S., Rao-Melacini, P., et al., 2010. Association of diet, exercise, and smoking modification with risk of early cardiovascular events after acute coronary syndromes. Circulation 121, 750–758.

Church, T.S., Earnest, C.P., Skinner, J.S., Blair, S.N., 2007. Effects of different doses of physical activity on cardiorespiratory fitness among sedentary, overweight or obese postmenopausal women with elevated blood pressure: a randomized controlled trial. JAMA 297 (19), 2081–2091.

Cindy Ng, L.W., Mackney, J., Jenkins, S., Hill, K., 2012. Does exercise training change physical activity in people with COPD? A systematic review and meta-analysis. Chron. Respir. Dis. 9 (1), 17–26.

Clark, C.J., Cochrane, L., Mackay, E., 1996. Low intensity peripheral muscle conditioning improves exercise tolerance and breathlessness in COPD. Eur. Respir. J. 9 (12), 2590–2596.

Clark, R.A., Conway, A., Poulsen, V., et al., 2015. Alternative models of cardiac rehabilitation: a systematic review. Eur. J. Prev. Cardiol. 22 (1), 35–74.

Clark, A.M., Hartling, L., Vandermeer, B., McAlister, F.A., 2005. Secondary prevention program for patients with coronary artery disease: a meta-analysis of randomized control trials. Ann. Intern. Med. 143, 659–672.

Clark, A., Hartling, L., Vandermeer, B., McAlister, F., 2007. Secondary prevention programmes for coronary heart disease: a meta-regression showing the merits of shorter, generalist, primary care-based interventions. Eur. J. Cardiovasc. Prev. Rehabil. 14, 538–546.

Clark, A.M., Haykowsky, M., Kryworuchko, J., et al., 2010. A meta-analysis of randomized control trials of home-based secondary prevention programs for coronary artery disease. Eur. J. Cardiovasc. Prev. Rehabil. 17, 261–270.

Coats, A., McGee, H., Stokes, H., Thompson, D., 1995. BACR Guidelines for Cardiac Rehabilitation. Blackwell Science, Oxford.

Cooper, A.F., Weinman, J., Hankins, M., et al., 2007. Assessing patients' beliefs about cardiac rehabilitation as a basis for predicting attendance after acute myocardial infarction. Heart 93, 53–58.

Corra, U., Piepoli, M.F., Carre, F., et al., 2010. Secondary prevention through cardiac rehabilitation: physical activity counselling and exercise training: key components of the position paper from the Cardiac Rehabilitation Section of the European Association of Cardiovascular Prevention and Rehabilitation. Eur. Heart J. 31 (16), 1967–1974.

Cote, C.G., Dordelly, L.J., Celli, B.R., 2007. Impact of COPD exacerbations on patient-centered outcomes. Chest 131 (3), 696–704.

Creutzberg, E.C., Schols, A.M., Weling-Scheepers, C.A., et al., 2000. Characterization of nonresponse to high caloric oral nutritional therapy in depleted patients with COPD. Am. J. Respir. Crit. Care Med. 161 (3 Pt 1), 745–752.

Dafoe, W., Huston, P., 1997. Current trends in cardiac rehabilitation. Can. Med. Assoc. J. 156, 527–532.

Dal Corso, S., Nápolis, L., Malaguti, C., et al., 2007. Skeletal muscle structure and function in response to electrical stimulation in moderately impaired COPD patients. Respir. Med. 101 (6), 1236–1243.

Dalal, H.M., Evans, P.H., Campbell, J.L., et al., 2007. Home-based versus hospital-based rehabilitation after myocardial infarction: a randomized trial with preference arms. Cornwall Heart Attack Rehabilitation Management Study (CHARMS). Int. J. Cardiol. 192, 202–211.

Dalal, H., Zawada, A., Jolly, K., et al., 2010. Home based versus centre based cardiac rehabilitation: Cochrane systematic review and meta-analysis. Br. Med. J. 340, b5631.

Daly, J., Sindone, A.P., Thompson, D.R., et al., 2002. Barriers to participation in and adherence to cardiac rehabilitation programs: a critical literature review. Prog. Cardiovasc. Nurs. 17, 8–17.

Danilack, V.A., Weston, N.A., Richardson, C.R., et al., 2014. Reasons persons with COPD do not walk and relationship with daily step count. COPD 11 (3), 290–299.

Davids, J.S., McPherson, C.A., Early, C., et al., 2005. Benefits of cardiac rehabilitation in patients with implantable cardioverter-defibrillators: a patient survey. Arch. Phys. Med. Rehabil. 86, 1924–1928.

Davies, E.J., Moxham, T., Rees, K., et al., 2010. Exercise training for systolic heart failure: Cochrane systematic review and meta-analysis. Eur. J. Heart Fail. 12 (7), 706–715.

de Torres, J.P., Cordoba-Lanus, E., Lopez-Aguilar, C., et al., 2006. C-reactive protein levels and clinically important predictive outcomes in stable COPD patients. Eur. Respir. J. 27, 902–907.

DeBusk, R.F., Miller, N.H., Superko, H.R., et al., 1994. A case-management system for coronary risk factor modification after acute myocardial infarction. Ann. Intern. Med. 120, 721–729.

Delagardelle, C., Feiereisen, P., Autier, P., et al., 2002. Strength/endurance training versus endurance training in congestive heart failure. Med. Sci. Sports Exerc. 34, 1868–1872.

Department of Health, 2013. Cardiovascular Disease Outcomes Strategy: Improving Outcomes for People with or at Risk of Cardiovascular Disease. DH, London.

Dowman, L., Hill, C.J., Holland, A.E., 2014. Pulmonary rehabilitation for interstitial lung disease. Cochrane Database Syst. Rev. (10), CD006322.

DuBach, P., Myers, J., Dziekan, G., et al., 1997. Effect of exercise training on myocardial remodeling in patients with reduced left ventricular function after myocardial infarction. Circulation 95, 2060–2067.

Dyer, F., Callaghan, J., Cheema, K., et al., 2012. Ambulatory oxygen improves the effectiveness of pulmonary rehabilitation in selected patients with chronic obstructive pulmonary disease. Chron. Respir. Dis. 9 (2), 83–91.

Dyer, C.A., Singh, S.J., Stockley, R.A., et al., 2002. The incremental shuttle walking test in elderly people with chronic airflow limitation. Thorax 57, 34–38.

Ehsani, A.A., Biello, D.R., Schultz, J., et al., 1986. Improvement of left ventricular contractile function in patients with coronary artery disease. Circulation 74, 350–388.

El-Ansary, D., Waddington, G., Adams, R., 2007. Relationship between pain and upper limb movement in patients with chronic sternal instability following cardiac surgery. Physiother. Theory Pract. 23 (5), 273–280.

Emtner, M., Porszasz, J., Burns, M., et al., 2003. Benefits of supplemental oxygen in exercise training in nonhypoxemic chronic obstructive pulmonary disease patients. Am. J. Respir. Crit. Care Med. 168, 1034–1042.

EUROASPIRE I and II Group, European Action on Secondary Prevention by Intervention to Reduce Events, 2001. Clinical reality of coronary prevention guidelines: a comparison of EUROASPIRE I and II in nine countries. EUROASPIRE I and II Group. European Action on Secondary Prevention by Intervention to Reduce Events. Lancet 357, 995–1001.

Falcoz, P.E., Chocron, S., Stoica, L., et al., 2003. Open heart surgery: one-year self-assessment of quality of life and functional outcome. Ann. Thorac. Surg. 76, 1598–1604.

Fanning, J., Mullen, S.P., McAuley, E., 2012. Increasing physical activity with mobile devices: a meta-analysis. J. Med. Internet Res. 14 (6), e161.

Ferreira, I.M., Brooks, D., Lacasse, Y., et al., 2005. Nutritional supplementation for stable chronic obstructive pulmonary disease. Cochrane Database Syst. Rev. 2002; (1), CD000998.

Ferrier, S., Blanchard, C.M., Vallis, M., Giacomantonio, N., 2011. Behavioural interventions to increase the physical activity of cardiac patients: a review. Eur. J. Cardiovasc. Prev. Rehabil. 18 (1), 15–32.

Fitchet, A., Doherty, P.J., Bundy, C., et al., 2003. Comprehensive cardiac rehabilitation programme for ICD patients: a randomized controlled trial. Heart 89, 155–160.

Fletcher, G.F., Balady, G.J., Amsterdam, E.A., et al., 2001. Exercise standards for testing and training: a statement for healthcare professionals from the American Heart Association. Circulation 104, 1694–1781.

Foglio, K., Bianchi, L., Ambrosino, N., 2001. Is it really useful to repeat outpatient pulmonary rehabilitation programs in patients with chronic airway obstruction? A 2-year controlled study. Chest 119, 1696–1704.

Ford, E.S., Ajani, U.A., Croft, J.B., et al., 2007. Explaining the decrease in US deaths from coronary disease, 1980–2000. N. Engl. J. Med. 356, 2388–2398.

Franklin, B.A., Bonzheim, K., Gordon, S., Timmis, G.C., 1998. Safety of medically supervised outpatient cardiac rehabilitation exercise therapy: a 16 year follow-up. Chest 114, 902–906.

Franklin, B.A., Gordon, N.F., 2009. Contemporary Diagnosis and Management in Cardiovascular Exercise. Handbooks in Health Care Company, Newtown (PA).

Franssen, F.M., Broekhuizen, R., Janssen, P.P., et al., 2005. Limb muscle dysfunction in COPD: effects of muscle wasting and exercise training. Med. Sci. Sports Exerc. 37 (1), 2–9.

Garber, C.E., Blissmer, B., Deschenes, M.R., et al., 2011. American College of Sports Medicine position stand. Quantity and quality of exercise for developing and maintaining cardiorespiratory, musculoskeletal, and neuromotor fitness in apparently healthy adults: guidance for prescribing exercise. Med. Sci. Sports Exerc. 43 (7), 1334–1359.

Garcia-Aymerich, J., Lange, P., Benet, M., et al., 2007. Regular physical activity modifies smoking-related lung function decline and reduces risk of chronic obstructive pulmonary disease: a population-based cohort study. Am. J. Respir. Crit. Care Med. 175 (5), 458–463.

Garrod, R., Backley, J., 2006. Community-based pulmonary rehabilitation: meeting demand in chronic obstructive pulmonary disease. Phys. Ther. Rev. 11, 57–61.

Garrod, R., Mikelsons, C., Paul, E.A., Wedzicha, J.A., 2000b. Randomized controlled trial of domiciliary noninvasive positive pressure ventilation and physical training in severe chronic obstructive pulmonary disease. Am. J. Respir. Crit. Care Med. 162 (41), 1335–1341.

Garrod, R., Paul, E.A., Wedzicha, J.A., 2000a. Supplemental oxygen during pulmonary rehabilitation in patients with COPD and exercise hypoxaemia. Thorax 55, 539–543.

Georgiou, D., Chen, Y., Appadoo, S., et al., 2001. Cost-effectiveness analysis of long-term moderate exercise training in chronic heart failure. Am. J. Cardiol. 87, 984–988.

Giannuzzi, I., Tavazzi, L., Temporelli, P.L., for EAMI, et al., 1993. Long-term physical training and left ventricular remodeling after anterior myocardial infarction: results of the Exercise in Anterior MI (EAMI) trial. J. Am. Coll. Cardiol. 22, 1821–1829.

Gimenez, M., Serverra, E., Vergara, P., et al., 2000. Endurance training in patients with COPD: a comparison of high versus moderate intensity. Arch. Phys. Med. Rehabil. 81, 102–109.

Gloeckl, R., Heinzelmann, I., Baeuerle, S., et al., 2012. Effects of whole body vibration in patients with chronic obstructive pulmonary disease: a randomized controlled trial. Respir. Med. 106, 75–83.

Goble, A.J., Hare, D.L., MacDonald, P.S., et al., 1991. Effect of early programmes of high and low intensity exercise on physical performance after transmural acute myocardial infarction. Br. Heart J. 65, 126–131.

Golbidi, S., Laher, I., 2011. Molecular Mechanisms in Exercise-Induced Cardioprotection. Cardiol. Res. Pract. 2011, 972807. [Online] Article ID.

Goldberg, J.H., King, A.C., 2007. Physical activity and weight management across the lifespan. Annu. Rev. Public Health 28, 145–170.

Goode, A.D., Reeves, M.M., Eakin, E.G., 2012. Telephone-delivered interventions for physical activity and dietary behavior change: an updated systematic review. Am. J. Prev. Med. 42 (1), 81–88.

Grace, S.L., McDonald, J., Fishman, D., et al., 2005. Patient preferences for home-based versus hospital-based cardiac rehabilitation. J. Cardiopulm. Rehabil. 25, 24–29.

Green, R.H., Singh, S.J., Williams, J., et al., 2001. A randomized controlled trial of 4 weeks versus 7 weeks of pulmonary rehabilitation in COPD. Thorax 56, 143–145.

Greening, N.J., Williams, J.E.A., Hussain, S.F., et al., 2014. An early rehabilitation intervention to enhance recovery during hospital admission for an exacerbation of chronic respiratory disease: randomised controlled trial. BMJ 349, g4315. doi: http://dx.doi.org/10.1136/bmj.g4315, (Published 08 July 2014).

Guell, R., Casan, P., Belda, J., et al., 2000. Long-term effects of outpatient rehabilitation of COPD: a randomized trial. Chest 117, 976–983.

Hallal, P.C., Andersen, L.B., Bull, F.C., et al., 2012. Global physical activity levels: surveillance progress, pitfalls, and prospects. Lancet 380 (9838), 247–257.

Hambrecht, R., Niebauer, J., Marburger, C., et al., 1994. Various intensities of leisure time physical activity in patients with coronary atherosclerotic lesions. J. Cardiopulm. Rehabil. 14, 167–168.

Hansen, D., Dendale, P., Berger, J., Meeusen, R., 2005. Rehabilitation in cardiac patients: what do we know about training modalities. Sports Med. 35, 1063–1084.

Hanssen, T.A., Nordrehaug, J.E., Eide, G.E., Hanestad, B.R., 2007. Improving outcomes after myocardial infarction: a randomized controlled trial evaluating effects of a telephone follow-up intervention. Eur. J. Cardiovasc. Prev. Rehabil. 14, 429–437.

Harris, D.E., Record, N.B., 2003. Cardiac rehabilitation in community settings. J. Cardiopulm. Rehabil. 23, 250–259.

Haskell, W.L., Alderman, E.L., Fair, J.M., et al., 1994. Effects of intensive multiple risk factor reduction on coronary atherosclerosis and clinical cardiac events in men and women with coronary artery disease. The Stanford Coronary Risk Intervention Project (SCRIP). Circulation 89, 975–990.

Haykowsky, M., Scott, J., Esch, B., et al., 2011. A meta-analysis of the effects of exercise training on left ventricular remodeling following myocardial infarction: start early and go longer for greatest exercise benefits on remodeling. Trials 12, 92.

Heppner, P.S., Morgan, C., Kaplan, R.M., et al., 2006. Regular walking and long-term maintenance of outcomes after pulmonary rehabilitation. J. Cardiopulm. Rehabil. 26 (1), 44–53.

Heran, B.S., Chen, J.M.H., Ebrahim, S., et al., 2011. Exercise-based cardiac rehabilitation for coronary heart disease. Cochrane Database Syst. Rev. (7), Art. No: CD001800, doi:10.1002/14651858.CD001800.pub2.

Higgins, R.O., Murphy, B.M., Goble, A.J., et al., 2008. Cardiac rehabilitation program attendance after coronary artery bypass surgery: overcoming the barriers. Med. J. Aust. 188, 712–714.

Hillsdon, M., Foster, C., Thorogood, M., 2005. Interventions for promoting physical activity. Cochrane Database Syst. Rev. (1), CD003180.

Holland, A.E., Dowman, L.M., Hill, C.J., 2015. Principles of rehabilitation and reactivation: interstitial lung disease, sarcoidosis and rheumatoid disease with respiratory involvement. Respiration 89 (2), 89–99.

Holland, A.E., Hill, C.J., Conron, M., et al., 2008. Short term improvement in exercise capacity and symptoms following exercise training in interstitial lung disease. Thorax 63 (6), 549–554.

Holland, A.E., Hill, C.J., Glaspole, I., et al., 2012. Predictors of benefit following pulmonary rehabilitation for interstitial lung disease. Respir. Med. 106, 429–435.

Holland, A.E., Spruit, M.A., Troosters, T., et al., 2014. An official European Respiratory Society/American Thoracic Society technical standard: field walking tests in chronic respiratory disease. Eur. Respir. J. 44 (6), 1428–1446.

Horowitz, M.B., Littenberg, B., Mahler, D.A., 1996. Dyspnea ratings for prescribing exercise intensity in patients with COPD. Chest 109 (5), 1169–1175.

Hulsmann, M., Quittan, M., Berger, R., et al., 2004. Muscle strength as a predictor of long-term survival in severe congestive heart failure. Eur. J. Heart Fail. 6 (1), 101–107.

Hunt, S.A., Abraham, W.T., Chin, M.H., et al., 2005. A report of the American College of Cardiology and American Heart Association (ACC/AHA) Task Force on Practice Guidelines 'Guideline Update for the Diagnosis and Management of Chronic Heart Failure in the Adult: Summary Article'. J. Am. Coll. Cardiol. 46, 1116–1143.

Husak, L., Krumholz, H.M., Qiutin, Z., et al., 2004. Social support as a predictor of participation in cardiac rehabilitation after coronary artery bypass surgery. J. Cardiopulm. Rehabil. 24, 19–25.

Inbar, O., Oten, A., Scheinowitz, M., et al., 1994. Normal cardiopulmonary responses during incremental exercise in 20–70-yr-old men. Med. Sci. Sport Exerc. 26 (5), 538–546.

Ingle, L., 2008. Prognostic value and diagnostic potential of cardiopulmonary exercise testing in patients with chronic heart failure. Eur. J. Heart Fail. 10 (2), 112–118.

Janssen, D.J., Spruit, M.A., Leue, C., et al., 2010. Symptoms of anxiety and depression in people entering pulmonary rehabilitation. Chron. Respir. Dis. 7 (3), 147–157.

Johnson, J.H., Prins, A., 1991. Prediction of maximal heart rate during a submaximal work test. J. Sports Med. Phys. Fitness 31 (1), 44–47.

Johnston, C.L., Maxwell, L.J., Alison, J.A., 2011. Pulmonary rehabilitation in Australia: a national survey. Physiotherapy 97 (4), 284–290.

Jolliffe, J.A., Rees, K., Taylor, R.S., et al., 2000. Exercise-based rehabilitation for coronary heart disease. Cochrane Database Syst. Rev. (1), Art. No.: CD001800, doi:10.1002/14651858.CD001800.

Jolly, K., Taylor, R.S., Lip, G.Y., et al., 2006. Home-based cardiac rehabilitation compared with centre-based rehabilitation and usual care: a systematic review and meta-analysis. Int. J. Cardiol. 111, 343–351.

Jones, S.E., Green, S.A., Clark, A.L., et al., 2013. Pulmonary rehabilitation following hospitalisation for acute exacerbation of COPD: referrals, uptake and adherence Thorax Aug 14. doi:10.1136/thoraxjnl-2013-204227.

Jonsdottir, S., Anderson, K.K., Sigurosson, A.F., Sigurosson, S.B., 2005. The effect of physical training in chronic heart failure. Eur. J. Heart Fail. 8, 97–101.

Jugdutt, B.I., Michorowski, B.L., Kappagoda, C.T., 1988. Exercise training after anterior Q wave myocardial infarction: importance of regional left ventricular function and topography. J. Am. Coll. Cardiol. 12, 362–372.

Kahn, E.B., Ramsey, L.T., Brownson, R.C., et al., 2002. The effectiveness of interventions to increase physical activity: a systematic review. Am. J. Prev. Med. 22 (4 Suppl.), 73–107.

Keteyian, S.J., Kitzman, D., Zannad, F., et al., 2012. Predicting maximal HR in heart failure patients on β-blockade therapy. Med. Sci. Sports Exerc. 44 (3), 371–376.

Keteyian, S.J., Levine, A.B., Brawner, C.A., et al., 1996. Exercise training in patients with heart failure: a randomized, controlled trial. Ann. Intern. Med. 124 (12), 1051–1057.

Killian, K.J., Leblanc, P., Martin, D.H., et al., 1992. Exercise capacity and ventilatory, circulatory, and symptom limitation in patients with chronic airflow limitation. Am. Rev. Respir. Dis. 146, 935–940.

Klenk, J., Buchele, G., Rapp, K., et al., 2012. Walking on sunshine: effect of weather conditions on physical activity in older people. J. Epidemiol. Community Health 66 (5), 474–476.

Klenk, J., Denkinger, M., Nikolaus, T., et al., 2013. Association of objectively measured physical activity with established and novel cardiovascular biomarkers in elderly subjects: every step counts. J. Epidemiol. Community Health 67 (2), 194–197.

Klijn, P., van Keimpema, A., Legemaat, M., et al., 2013. Nonlinear exercise training in advanced chronic obstructive pulmonary disease is superior to traditional exercise training. A randomized trial. Am. J. Respir. Crit. Care Med. 188 (2), 193–200.

Kloner, R.A., Kloner, J.A., 1983. The effect of early exercise on myocardial infarct scar formation. Am. Heart J. 106 (5 Pt 1), 1009–1013.

Kohl, H.W., Craig, C.L., Lambert, E.V., et al., 2012. The pandemic of physical inactivity: global action for public health. Lancet 380 (9838), 294–305.

Kotseva, K., Wood, D., De Backer, G., et al., 2009. EUROASPIRE III: a survey on the lifestyle, risk factors and use of cardioprotective drug therapies in coronary patients from 22 European countries. Eur. J. Cardiovasc. Prev. Rehabil. 16, 121–137.

Kovoor, P., Lee, A.K., Carrozzi, F., et al., 2006. Return to full normal activities including work after acute myocardial infarction. Am. J. Cardiol. 97, 952–958.

Kraemer, W.J., Ratamess, N.A., French, D.N., 2002. Resistance training for health and performance. Curr. Sports Med. Rep. 1 (3), 165–171.

Lacasse, Y., Goldstein, R., Lasserson, T.J., et al., 2006. Pulmonary rehabilitation for chronic obstructive pulmonary disease. Cochrane Database Syst. Rev. (4), Art. No.: CD0003793.

Lake, F., Henderson, K., Briffa, T., et al., 1990. Upper limb and lower limb exercise training in patients with chronic airflow obstruction. Chest 97, 1077–1082.

Lam, G., Snow, R., Shaffer, L., et al., 2011. The effect of a comprehensive cardiac rehabilitation program on 60-day hospital readmissions after an acute myocardial infarction. J. Am. Coll. Cardiol. 57, 597–604.

Lampman, R.M., Knight, B.P., 2000. Prescribing exercise training for patients with defibrillators. Am. J. Phys. Med. Rehabil. 79 (3), 292–297.

LaPier, T.L., 2003. Functional status during acute recovery following hospitalization for coronary artery disease. J. Cardiopulm. Rehabil. 23, 203–207.

LaPier, T.L., 2006. Psychometric evaluation of the Heart Surgery Symptom Inventory in patients recovering from coronary artery bypass surgery. J. Cardiopulm. Rehabil. 26, 101–106.

LaPier, T.K., 2007. Functional status of patients during subacute recovery from coronary artery bypass surgery. Heart Lung 36 (2), 114–124.

LaPier, T.L., Wilson, B., 2006. Functional deficits at the time of hospital discharge in patients following coronary artery bypass surgery. Cardiopulm. Phys. Ther. J. 17, 144.

LaPier, T.L., Wilson, B., 2007. Prevalence and severity of symptoms in patients recovering from coronary artery bypass surgery. Acute Care Perspectives 16 (3), 10–15.

LaPier, T.L., Wintz, G., Holmes, W., et al., 2008. Analysis of activities of daily living performance in patients recovering from coronary artery bypass surgery. J. Phys. Occupational Ther. Geriatrics. 27 (1), 16–35.

Lawler, P.R., Filion, K.B., Eisenberg, M.J., 2011. Efficacy of exercise-based cardiac rehabilitation post-myocardial infarction: a systematic review and meta-analysis of randomized controlled trials. Am. Heart J. 162, 571–584.

Lear, S.A., Ignaszewski, A., Linden, W., et al., 2003. The Extensive Lifestyle Management Intervention (ELMI) following cardiac rehabilitation trial. Eur. Heart J. 24, 1920–1927.

Lee, A.L., Hill, C.J., Cecins, N., et al., 2014. The short and long term effects of exercise training in non-cystic fibrosis bronchiectasis – a randomised controlled trial. Respir. Res. 15, 44.

Leon, A.S., 2009. Biological mechanisms for the cardioprotective effects of aerobic exercise. Am. J. Lifestyle Med. 3 (1), 32–34.

Leon, A.S., Certo, C., Comoss, P., et al., 1991. Scientific evidence of the value of cardiac rehabilitation services with emphasis on patients following myocardial infarction. J. Cardiopulm. Rehabil. 10, 79–87.

Leon, A.S., Franklin, B.A., Costa, F., et al., 2005. Cardiac rehabilitation and secondary prevention of CHD: American Heart Association scientific statement. Circulation 111, 369–376.

Leong, P., Basham, J.E., Yong, T., et al., 2015. A double blind randomized placebo control crossover trial on the effect of dietary nitrate supplementation on exercise tolerance in stable moderate chronic obstructive pulmonary disease. BMC Pulm. Med. 15 (1), 52. doi:10.1186/s12890-015-0057-4.

Leung, R.W., McKeough, Z.J., Peters, M.J., Alison, J.A., 2013. Short-form Sun-style T'ai Chi as an exercise training modality in people with COPD. Eur. Respir. J. 41 (5), 1051–1057.

Leung, R.W., McKeough, Z.J., Peters, M.J., Alison, J.A., 2014. Experiences and perceptions of the short-form Sun-style Tai Chi training in Caucasians with COPD. European Journal of Integrative Medicine. <http://dx.doi.org/10.1016/j.eujim.2014.11.005>.

Levinger, I., Bronks, R., Cody, D.V., et al., 2005. Resistance training for chronic heart failure patients on beta-blocker medications. Int. J. Cardiol. 102, 493–499.

Lewin, R.J.P., Furze, G., Robinson, J., et al., 2002. A randomized controlled trial of a self-management plan for patients with newly diagnosed angina. Br. J. Gen. Pract. 52, 194–201.

Liddell, F., Webber, J., 2010. Pulmonary rehabilitation for chronic obstructive pulmonary disease: a pilot study evaluating a once-weekly versus twice-weekly supervised programme. Physiotherapy 96 (1), 68–74.

Likoff, M.J., Chandler, S.L., Kay, H.R., 1987. Clinical determinants of mortality in chronic congestive heart failure secondary to idiopathic dilated or ischaemic cardiomyopathy. Am. J. Cardiol. 59, 634–638.

Lipkin, D.P., Scriven, A.J., Crake, T., Poole-Wilson, P.A., 1986. Six minute walking test for assessing exercise capacity in chronic heart failure patients. Br. Med. J. 292, 653–655.

Locke, E., Shaw, K., Sari, L., et al., 1981. Goal setting and task performance 1969–1980. Psychol. Bull. 90 (1), 125–152.

Lorig, K.R., Holman, H., 2003. Self-management education: history, definition, outcomes, and mechanisms. Anns. Behav. Med. 26 (1), 1–7.

Macera, C.A., Hootman, J.M., Sniezek, J.E., 2003. Major public health benefits of physical activity. Arthritis Rheum. 49 (1), 122–128.

Mahler, D.A., Ward, J., Mejia-Alfaro, R., 2003. Stability of dyspnea ratings after exercise training in patients with COPD. Med. Sci. Sports Exerc. 35 (7), 1083–1087.

Maltais, F., Leblanc, P., Jobin, J., et al., 1997. Intensity of training and physiologic adaptation with COPD. Am. J. Respir. Crit. Care Med. 155, 555–561.

Marlow, S.P., Stoller, J.K., 2003. Smoking cessation. Respir. Care 48 (12), 1238–1254.

McAlister, F.A., Stewart, S., Ferrua, S., McMurray, J.J., 2004. Multi-disciplinary strategies for the management of heart failure patients at high risk for admission: a systematic review of randomized trials. J. Am. Coll. Cardiol. 44 (4), 810–819.

McCarthy, B., Casey, D., Devane, D., et al., 2015. Pulmonary rehabilitation for chronic obstructive pulmonary disease. Cochrane Database Syst. Rev. (2), CD003793, doi:10.1002/14651858 .CD003793.pub3.

McHugh, M.P., Magnusson, S.P., Gleim, G.W., Nicholas, J.A., 1992. Viscoelastic stress relaxation in human skeletal muscle. Med. Sci. Sports Exerc. 24 (12), 1375–1382.

McNamara, R.J., McKeough, Z.J., McKenzie, D.K., et al., 2013. Water-based exercise in COPD with physical comorbidities: a randomised controlled trial. Eur. Respir. J. 41 (6), 1284–1291.

McNamara, R.J., McKeough, Z.J., McKenzie, D.K., Alison, J.A., 2013. Water-based exercise training for chronic obstructive pulmonary disease. Cochrane Database Syst. Rev. (12), CD008290, doi:10 .1002/14651858.CD008290.pub2.

Menezes, A.R., Lavie, C.J., Milani, R.V., et al., 2014. Cardiac rehabilitation in the United States. Prog. Cardiovasc. Dis. 56, 522–529.

Mittag, O., China, C., Hoberg, E., et al., 2006. Outcomes of cardiac rehabilitation with versus without a follow-up intervention rendered by telephone (Luebeck follow-up trial): overall and gender-specific effects. Int. J. Rehabil. Res. 29, 295–302.

Morris, J.N., Heady, J.A., Raffle, P.A., et al., 1953. Coronary heart-disease and physical activity of work. Lancet 265 (6795), 1053–1057.

Moyna, N.M., Thompson, P.D., 2004. The effect of physical activity on endothelial function in man. Acta Physiol. Scand. 180 (2), 113–123.

Myers, J., Goebbels, U., Dzeikan, G., 2000. Exercise training and myocardial remodelling in patients with reduced ventricular function: one-year follow-up with magnetic resonance imaging. Am. Heart J. 139, 252–261.

National Institute for Clinical Excellence, 2010. Clinical Guideline 101.

National Institute for Clinical Excellence, 2013. Clinical Guideline Idiopathic pulmonary fibrosis: the diagnosis and management of suspected idiopathic pulmonary fibrosis.

National Institute of Health and Care Excellence (NICE), 2013. CG172 Secondary Prevention Post Myocardial Infarction. Royal College of Physicians, London.

Neder, J.A., Jones, P.W., Nery, L.E., et al., 2000. Determinants of the exercise endurance capacity in patients with COPD: the power-duration relationship. Am. J. Respir. Crit. Care Med. 162, 497–504.

Neder, J.A., Sword, D., Ward, S.A., et al., 2002. Home based neuromuscular electrical stimulation as a new rehabilitative strategy for severely disabled patients with chronic obstructive pulmonary disease (COPD). Thorax 57 (4), 333–337.

Nelson, M.E., Rejeski, W.J., Blair, S.N., et al., 2007. Physical activity and public health in older adults: recommendation from the American College of Sports Medicine and the American Heart Association. Circulation 116 (9), 1094–1105.

Nes, B.M., Janszky, I., Wisloff, U., et al., 2013. Age-predicted maximal heart rate in healthy subjects: The HUNT fitness study. Scand. J. Med. Sci. Sports 23 (6), 697–704.

Neubeck, L., Redfern, J., Fernandez, R., et al., 2009. Telehealth interventions for the secondary prevention of CHD: a systematic review. Eur. J. Cardiovasc. Prev. Rehabil. 16, 281–289.

Newall, C., Stockley, R.A., Hill, S.L., 2005. Exercise training and inspiratory muscle training in patients with bronchiectasis. Thorax 60, 943–948.

Nguyen, H.Q., Carrieri-Kohlman, V., 2005. Dyspnea self-management in patients with chronic obstructive pulmonary disease: moderating effects of depressed mood. Psychosomatics 46 (5), 402–410.

Normandin, E.A., McCusker, C., Connors, M., et al., 2002. An evaluation of two approaches to exercise conditioning in pulmonary rehabilitation. Chest 121 (4), 1085–1091.

O'Brien Cousins, S., Keating, N., 1995. Life cycle patterns of physical activity among sedentary and older women. J. Ageing Phys. Act. 3, 340–359.

O'Connor, C.M., Whellan, D.J., Lee, K.L., et al., 2009. Efficacy and safety of exercise training in patients with chronic heart failure: HF-ACTION randomized controlled trial. JAMA 301 (14), 1439–1450.

O'Donnell, D., 1994. Breathlessness in patients with chronic airflow limitation. Chest 106, 905–912.

O'Donnell, D.E., D'Arsigny, C., Webb, K.A., 2001. Effects of hyperoxia on ventilatory limitation in advanced COPD. Am. J. Respir. Crit. Care Med. 163, 892–898.

O'Neill, B., McKevitt, A., Rafferty, S., et al., 2007. A comparison of twice- versus once-weekly supervision during pulmonary rehabilitation in chronic obstructive pulmonary disease. Arch. Phys. Med. Rehabil. 88, 167–172.

O'Shea, S.D., Taylor, N.F., Paratz, J., 2004. Peripheral muscle strength training in COPD: a systematic review. Chest 126, 903–914.

Oldridge, N., Furlong, W., Perkins, A., et al., 2008. Community or patient preferences for cost-effectiveness of cardiac rehabilitation: does it matter? Eur. J. Cardiovasc. Prev. Rehabil. 15, 608–615.

Oliveira, C.C., Lee, A.L., McGinley, J., et al., 2015. Falls by individuals with chronic obstructive pulmonary disease: A preliminary 12-month prospective cohort study. Respirology 20 (7), 1096–1101.

Ong, H.K., Lee, A.L., Hill, C.J., et al., 2011. Effects of pulmonary rehabilitation in bronchiectasis: a retrospective study. Chronic. Respir. Dis. 8 (1), 21–30.

Pack, Q.R., Mansour, M., Barboza, J.S., et al., 2013. An early appointment to outpatient cardiac rehabilitation at hospital discharge improves attendance at orientation: a randomized, single-blind, controlled trial. Circulation 127 (3), 349–355.

Palange, P., Ward, S.A., Carlsen, K.H., et al., 2007. Recommendations on the use of exercise testing in clinical practice. Eur. Respir. J. 29 (1), 185–209.

Papadakis, S., Reid, R.D., Coyle, D., et al., 2008. Cost-effectiveness of cardiac rehabilitation program delivery models in patients at varying cardiac risk, reason for referral, and sex. Eur. J. Cardiovasc. Prev. Rehabil. 15, 347–353.

Partridge, C., Pryor, J., Webber, B., 1989. Characteristics of the forced expiration technique. Physiotherapy 73 (3), 193–194.

Pashkow, F.J., Schweikert, R.A., Wilkoff, B.L., 1997. Exercise testing and training in patients with malignant arrhythmias. Exerc. Sport Sci. Rev. 25, 235–269.

Pedersen, B.K., 1991. Influence of physical activity on the cellular immune system: mechanisms of action. Int. J. Sports Med. 12 (Suppl. 1), S23–S29.

Petty, T.L., 1993. Pulmonary rehabilitation in chronic respiratory insufficiency. 1. Pulmonary rehabilitation in perspective: historical roots, present status, and future projections. Thorax 48 (8), 855–862.

Piepoli, M.F., Corra, U., Benzer, W., et al., 2010. Secondary prevention through cardiac rehabilitation: from knowledge to implementation. A position paper from the Cardiac Rehabilitation Section of the European Association of Cardiovascular Prevention and Rehabilitation. Eur. J. Cardiovasc. Prev. Rehabil. 17 (1), 1–17.

Pierson, L.M., Miller, L.E., Herbert, W.G., 2004. Predicting exercise training outcome from cardiac rehabilitation. J. Cardiopulm. Rehabil. 24, 113–118.

Pina, I.L., Apstein, C.S., Balady, G.J., et al., 2003. Exercise and heart failure: a statement from the American Heart Association Committee on Exercise, Rehabilitation and Prevention. Circulation 107 (8), 1210–1229.

Pitta, F.O., Brunetto, A.F., Padovani, C.R., et al., 2004. Effects of isolated cycle ergometer training on patients with moderate-to-severe chronic obstructive pulmonary disease. Respiration 71 (5), 477–483.

Pitta, F., Troosters, T., Probst, V.S., et al., 2006. Physical activity and hospitalization for exacerbation of COPD. Chest 129, 536–544.

Pleguezuelos, E., Pérez, M.E., Guirao, L., 2013. Effects of whole body vibration training in patients with severe chronic obstructive pulmonary disease. Respirology 18 (6), 1028–1034.

Polkey, M.I., Spruit, M.A., Edwards, L.D., et al., 2013. Six-minute-walk test in chronic obstructive pulmonary disease: minimal clinically important difference for death or hospitalization. Am. J. Respir. Crit. Care Med. 187 (4), 382–386.

Pollock, M., Gaesser, G., Butcher, J., et al., 2010. ACSM Position Stand: The Recommended Quantity and Quality of Exercise for Developing and Maintaining Cardiorespiratory and Muscular Fitness, and Flexibility in Healthy Adults. Medscape.

Probst, V.S., Troosters, T., Pitta, F., et al., 2006. Cardiopulmonary stress during exercise training in patients with COPD. Eur. Respir. J. 27 (6), 1110–1118.

Puente-Maestu, L., Sanz, M., Sanz, P., et al., 2000. Comparison of effects of supervised versus self-monitored training programmes in patients with chronic obstructive pulmonary disease. Eur. Respir. J. 15 (3), 517–525.

Puhan, M.A., Gimeno-Santos, E., Scharplatz, M., et al., 2011. Pulmonary rehabilitation following exacerbations of chronic obstructive pulmonary disease. Cochrane Database Syst. Rev. (10), CD005305.

Puhan, M.A., Schunemann, H.J., Frey, M., et al., 2005. How should COPD patients exercise during respiratory rehabilitation? Comparison of exercise modalities and intensities to treat skeletal muscle dysfunction. Thorax 60 (5), 367–375.

Redfern, J., Briffa, T., 2011. Cardiac rehabilitation: moving forward with new models of care. Phys. Ther. Rev. 16 (1), 31–38.

Redfern, J., Briffa, T., Ellis, E., Freedman, S.B., 2009. Choice of secondary prevention improves risk factors after acute coronary syndrome: 1-year follow-up of the CHOICE (Choice of Health Options In prevention of Cardiovascular Events) randomised controlled trial. Heart 95, 468–475.

Redfern, J.R., Ellis, E.R., Briffa, T., Freedman, S.B., 2007. High-risk factor level and prevalence and low-risk factor knowledge in patients not accessing cardiac rehabilitation after acute coronary syndrome. Med. J. Aust. 186, 21–25.

Redfern, J., Maiorana, A., Neubeck, L., et al., 2011. Achieving coordinated secondary prevention of coronary heart disease for all in need (SPAN). Int. J. Cardiol. 146 (1), 1–3.

Rees, K., Taylor, R.R.S., Singh, S., et al., 2010. Exercise based rehabilitation for heart failure (review). Cochrane Database Syst. Rev. (4), Art. No. CD003331.

Ries, A.L., et al., 2007. Pulmonary rehabilitation: joint ACCP/AACVPR evidence-based clinical practice guidelines. Chest 131 (5 Suppl.), 4S–42S.

Ries, A.L., Kaplan, R.M., Myers, R., et al., 2003. Maintenance after pulmonary rehabilitation in chronic lung disease: a randomized trial. Am. J. Respir. Crit. Care Med. 167 (6), 880–888.

Ringbaek, T.J., Broendum, E., Hemmingsen, L., et al., 2000. Rehabilitation of patients with chronic obstructive pulmonary disease: exercise twice a week is not sufficient! Respir. Med. 94, 150–154.

Roberts, R.A., Landwehr, R., 2002. The surprising history of the HRmax = 220 − age equation. JEPonline 5 (2), 1–10.

Roig, M., et al., 2009. Falls in patients with chronic obstructive pulmonary disease: a call for further research. Respir. Med. 103 (9), 1257–1269.

Roomi, J., Johnson, M.M., Waters, K., et al., 1996. Respiratory rehabilitation, exercise capacity and quality of life in chronic airways disease in old age. Age. Ageing 25, 12–16.

Rooyackers, J.M., Dekhuijzen, P.N., Van Herwaarden, C.L., Folgering, H.T., 1997. Training with supplemental oxygen in patients with COPD and hypoxaemia at peak exercise. Eur. Respir. J. 10 (6), 1278–1284.

Rossi, G., Florini, F., Romagnoli, M., et al., 2005. Length and clinical effectiveness of pulmonary rehabilitation in outpatients with chronic airway obstruction. Chest 127, 105–109.

Rothwell, P.M., Coull, A.J., Silver, L.E., et al., 2005. Population-based study of event-rate, incidence, case fatality, and mortality for all acute. Lancet 366 (9499), 1773–1783.

Sabapathy, S., Kingsley, R.A., Schneider, D.A., et al., 2004. Continuous and intermittent exercise responses in individuals with chronic obstructive pulmonary disease. Thorax 59 (12), 1026–1031.

Salman, G.F., Mosier, M.C., Beasley, B.W., et al., 2003. Rehabilitation for patients with chronic obstructive pulmonary disease. J. Gen. Intern. Med. 18, 213–221.

Samitz, G., Egger, M., Zwahlen, M., 2011. Domains of physical activity and all-cause mortality: systematic review and dose-response meta-analysis of cohort studies. Int. J. Epidemiol. 40 (5), 1382–1400.

Sandesara, P.B., Lambert, C.T., Gordon, N.F., et al., 2015. Cardiac rehabilitation and risk reduction: time to 'rebrand and reinvigorate'. J. Am. Coll. Cardiol. 65 (4), 389–395.

Schenkel, N.S., Muralt, B.B., Fitting, J.W., 1996. Oxygen saturation during daily activities in chronic obstructive pulmonary disease. Eur. Respir. J. 9, 2584–2589.

Schuler, G., Hambrecht, R., Schlierf, G., et al., 1992. Regular physical exercise and low-fat diet: effects on progression of coronary artery disease. Circulation 86, 1–11.

Schutzer, K.A., Graves, B.S., 2004. Barriers and motivations to exercise in older adults. Prev. Med. 39 (5), 1056–1061.

Scott, I.A., Lindsay, K.A., Harden, H.E., 2003. Utilisation of outpatient cardiac rehabilitation in Queensland. Med. J. Aust. 179, 341–345.

Sewell, L., Singh, S.J., Williams, J.E.A., 2006. How long should outpatient pulmonary rehabilitation be? A randomised controlled trial of 4 weeks versus 7 weeks. Thorax 61, 767–771.

Seymour, J.M., Moore, L., Jolley, C.J., et al., 2010. Outpatient pulmonary rehabilitation following acute exacerbations of COPD. Thorax 65 (5), 423–428.

Shen, B.J., Myers, H.F., McCreary, C.P., 2006. Psychological predictors of cardiac rehabilitation quality-of-life outcomes. J. Psychosom. Res. 60, 3–11.

Shepherd, A.I., Wilkerson, D.P., Dobson, L., et al., 2015. The effect of dietary nitrate supplementation on the oxygen cost of cycling, walking performance and resting blood pressure in individuals with chronic obstructive pulmonary disease: A double blind placebo controlled, randomised control trial. Nitric Oxide 48, 31–37.

Sillen, M.J., Franssen, F.M., Delbressine, J.M., et al., 2014. Efficacy of lower-limb muscle training modalities in severely dyspnoeic individuals with COPD and quadriceps muscle weakness: results from the DICES trial. Thorax 69 (6), 525–531.

Sinclair, A., Conroy, S., Davies, P., 2005. Post-discharge home-based support for older cardiac patients: a randomised controlled trial. Age. Ageing 34, 338–343.

Singh, S.J., Morgan, M.D.L., Scott, S., et al., 1992. Development of a shuttle walking test of disability in patients with chronic airways obstruction. Thorax 47, 1019–1024.

Smith, S.C., Allen, J., Blair, S.N., et al., 2006. AHA/ACC guidelines for secondary prevention for patients with coronary and other atherosclerotic vascular disease: 2006 update: endorsed by the National Heart, Lung, and Blood Institute. Circulation 113 (19), 2363–2372.

Smith, K.M., Arthur, H.M., McKelvie, R.S., et al., 2004. Differences in sustainability of exercise and health-related quality of life outcomes following home or hospital-based cardiac rehabilitation. Eur. J. Cardiovasc. Prev. Rehabil. 11, 313–319.

Soicher, J.E., Mayo, N.E., Gauvin, L., et al., 2012. Trajectories of endurance activity following pulmonary rehabilitation in COPD patients. Eur. Respir. J. 39 (2), 272–278.

Somfay, A., Porszasz, J., Lee, S.M., et al., 2001. Dose-response effect of oxygen on hyperinflation and exercise endurance in nonhypoxaemic COPD patients. Eur. Respir. J. 18, 77–84.

Southard, B., Southard, D., Nuckolls, C.W., 2003. Clinical trial of an Internet-based case management system for secondary prevention of heart disease. J. Cardiopulm. Rehabil. Prev. 23, 341–348.

Spielmanns, M., Fuchs-Bergsma, C., Winkler, A., et al., 2015. Effects of Oxygen Supply During Training on Subjects With COPD Who Are Normoxemic at Rest and During Exercise: A Blinded Randomized Controlled Trial. Respir. Care 60 (4), 540–548. doi:10.4187/respcare.03647; [Epub 2014 Dec 16].

Spruit, M.A., Eterman, R.M., Hellwig, V.A., et al., 2009. Uszko-Lencer NH. Effects of moderate-to-high intensity resistance training in patients with chronic heart failure. Heart 95 (17), 1399–1408.

Spruit, M.A., Gosselink, R., Troosters, T., et al., 2002. Resistance versus endurance training in patients with COPD and peripheral muscle weakness. Eur. Respir. J. 19 (6), 1072–1078.

Spruit, M.A., Polkey, M.I., Celli, B., et al., 2012. Predicting outcomes from 6-minute walk distance in chronic obstructive pulmonary disease. J. Am. Med. Dir. Assoc. 13 (3), 291–297.

Spruit, M.A., Singh, S.J., Garvey, C., et al., 2013. An official American Thoracic Society/European Respiratory Society statement: key concepts and advances in pulmonary rehabilitation. Am. J. Respir. Crit. Care Med. 188 (8), e13–e64.

Squires, R.W., Muri, A.J., Anderson, L.J., et al., 1991. Weight training during phase II (early outpatient) cardiac rehabilitation: heart rate and blood pressure responses. J. Card. Rehabil. 11, 360–364.

Steele, B., 1994. The six minute walk. In: AACVPR Proceedings 9th Annual Meeting Portland, OR. AACVPR, Chicago, pp. 383–388.

Steg, P.G., Bhatt, D.L., Wilson, P.W.F., et al., 2007. One-year cardiovascular event rates in outpatients with atherothrombosis. JAMA 297, 1197–1206.

Steg, P.G., James, S.K., Atar, D., et al., 2012. ESC guidelines for the management of acute myocardial infarction in patients presenting with ST-segment elevation: the task force on the management of ST-segment elevation acute myocardial infarction of the European Society of Cardiology (ESC). Eur. Heart J. 33, 2569–2619.

Strijbos, J.H., Postma, D.S., van Altena, R., et al., 1996. A comparison between an outpatient hospital-based pulmonary rehabilitation program and a home-care pulmonary rehabilitation program in patients with COPD. A follow-up of 18 months. Chest 109 (2), 366–372.

Suaya, J.A., Shepard, D., Normand, S., et al., 2007. Use of cardiac rehabilitation by Medicare beneficiaries after myocardial infarction or coronary bypass surgery. Circulation 116, 1653–1662.

Sumukadas, D., Witham, M., Struthers, A., McMurdo, M., 2009. Day length and weather conditions profoundly affect physical activity levels in older functionally impaired people. J. Epidemiol. Community Health 63 (4), 305–309.

Swallow, E.B., Reyes, D., Hopkinson, N.S., et al., 2007. Quadriceps strength predicts mortality in patients with moderate to severe chronic obstructive pulmonary disease. Thorax 62 (2), 115–120.

Swedberg, K., Cleland, J., Dargie, H., 2005. Task Force for the Diagnosis and Treatment of Chronic Heart Failure of the European Society of Cardiology Guidelines for the diagnosis and treatment of chronic heart failure: full text (update 2005). Eur. Heart J. 26, 1115–1140.

Sykes, K., Roberts, A., 2004. The Chester step test: a simple yet effective tool for the prediction of aerobic capacity. Physiotherapy 90, 183–188.

Tanaka, H., Monahan, K.D., Seals, D.R., 2001. Age-predicted maximal heart rate revisited. J. Am. Coll. Cardiol. 37 (1), 153–156.

Taylor, R.S., Brown, A., Ebrahim, S., et al., 2004. Exercise-based rehabilitation for patients with coronary heart disease: a systematic review and meta-analysis of randomized controlled trials. Am. J. Med. 11, 682–692.

Taylor, C.B., Miller, N.H., Smith, P.M., DeBusk, R.F., 1997. The effect of a home-based, case managed, multifactorial risk-reduction program on reducing psychological distress in patients with cardiovascular disease. J. Cardiopulm. Rehabil. Prev. 17, 157–162.

Taylor, R.S., Sagar, V.A., Davies, E.J., et al., 2014. Exercise-based rehabilitation for heart failure. Cochrane Database Syst. Rev. (4), Art. No.: CD003331, doi:10.1002/14651858.CD003331.pub4.

Taylor, R.S., Unal, B., Critchley, J.A., Capewell, S., 2006. Mortality reductions in patients receiving exercise-based cardiac rehabilitation: how much can be attributed to cardiovascular risk factor improvements? Eur. J. Cardiovasc. Prev. Rehabil. 13 (3), 369–374.

Tharrett, S.J., Peterson, J.A., 1997. ACSM's Health/Fitness Facility Standards and Guidelines. Human Kinetics, Champaign, IL.

Thompson, D.R., Clark, A.M., 2009. Cardiac Rehabilitation: into the future. Heart 95, 1897–1900.

Thompson, D.R., De Bono, D.P., 1999. How valuable is cardiac rehabilitation and who should get it? Heart 82, 545–546.

Thompson, P.D., Franklin, B.A., Balady, G.J., 2007. Exercise and acute cardiovascular events placing the risks into perspective: a scientific statement from the American Heart Association Council on Nutrition, Physical Activity, and Metabolism and the Council on Clinical Cardiology. Circulation 115, 2358–2368.

Thorpe, O., Johnston, K., Kumar, S., 2012. Barriers and enablers to physical activity participation in patients with COPD: a systematic review. J. Cardiopulm. Rehabil. Prev. 32 (6), 359–369.

Todaro, J.F., Shen, B.J., Niaura, R., et al., 2004. Do men and women achieve similar benefits from cardiac rehabilitation. J. Cardiopulm. Rehabil. 24, 45–50.

Troosters, T., Casaburi, R., Gosselink, R., et al., 2005. Pulmonary rehabilitation in chronic obstructive pulmonary disease (state of the art). Am. J. Respir. Crit. Care Med. 172, 19–38.

Troosters, T., Gosselink, R., Decramer, M., 2000. Short- and long-term effects of outpatient rehabilitation in patients with chronic obstructive pulmonary disease: a randomized trial. Am. J. Med. 109 (3), 207–212.

Troosters, T., Probst, V.S., Crul, T., et al., 2010. Resistance training prevents deterioration in quadriceps muscle function during acute exacerbations of chronic obstructive pulmonary disease. Am. J. Respir. Crit. Care Med. 181 (10), 1072–1077.

Unal, B., Critchley, J.A., Capewell, S., 2004. Explaining the decline in coronary heart disease mortality in England and Wales between 1981 and 2000. Circulation 109, 1101–1107.

Vaes, A.W., Garcia-Aymerich, J., Marott, J.L., et al., 2014. Changes in physical activity and all-cause mortality in COPD. Eur. Respir. J. 44 (5), 1199–1209.

Vainshelboim, B., Oliveira, J., Fox, B.D., et al., 2015. Long-term effects of a 12-week exercise training program on clinical outcomes in idiopathic pulmonary fibrosis. Lung 193 (3), 345–354. published online March 3rd.

Vale, M.J., Jelinek, M.V., Best, J.D., et al., 2003. for the Coach Study Group. Coaching patients on achieving cardiovascular health (COACH): a multicenter randomized trial in patients with coronary heart disease. Arch. Int. Med. 163, 2775–2783.

van der Bij, A.K., Laurant, M.G., Wensing, M., 2002. Effectiveness of physical activity interventions for older adults: a review. Am. J. Prev. Med. 22 (2), 120–133.

van Zeller, M., Mota, P.C., Amorim, A., 2012. Pulmonary rehabilitation in patients with bronchiectasis: pulmonary function, arterial blood gases, and the 6-minute walk test. J. Cardiopulm. Rehabil. Prev. 32 (5), 278–283.

van't Hul, A., Kwakkel, G., Gosselink, R., 2002. The acute effects of noninvasive ventilatory support during exercise on exercise endurance and dyspnea in patients with chronic obstructive pulmonary disease. J. Cardiopulm. Rehabil. 22, 290–297.

Vanhees, L., De, S.J., Geladas, N., et al., 2012. Importance of characteristics and modalities of physical activity and exercise in defining the benefits to cardiovascular health within the general population: recommendations from the EACPR (Part I). Eur. J. Prev. Cardiol. 19 (4), 670–686.

Varnfield, M., Karunanithi, M., Lee, C.K., et al., 2014. Smartphone-based home care model improved use of cardiac rehabilitation in postmyocardial infarction patients: results from a randomised controlled trial. Heart 100 (22), 1770–1779.

Vigen, R., Ayers, C., Willis, B., et al., 2012. Association of cardiorespiratory fitness with total, cardiovascular, and noncardiovascular mortality across 3 decades of follow-up in men and women. Circ. Cardiovasc. Qual. Outcomes 5 (3), 358–364.

Vivodtzev, I., Pepin, J.L., Vottero, G., et al., 2006. Improvement in quadriceps strength and dyspnea in daily tasks after 1 month of electrical stimulation in severely deconditioned and malnourished COPD. Chest 129 (6), 1540–1548.

Vogiatzis, I., 2008. Prescription of exercise training in patients with COPD. Curr. Op. Resp. Med. Rev. 4, 291–297.

Vogiatzis, I., Nanas, S., Kastanakis, E., et al., 2004. Dynamic hyperinflation and tolerance to interval exercise in patients with advanced COPD. Eur. Respir. J. 24, 385–390.

Vogiatzis, I., Terzis, G., Nanas, S., et al., 2005. Skeletal muscle adaptations to interval training in patients with advanced COPD. Chest 128, 3838–3845.

Wadell, K., Henriksson-Larsen, K., Lundgren, R., 2001. Physical training with and without oxygen in patients with chronic obstructive pulmonary disease and exercise-induced hypoxaemia. J. Rehabil. Med. 33 (5), 200–205.

Wadell, K., Henriksson-Larsen, K., Lundgren, R., et al., 2005. Group training in patients with COPD: long-term effects after decreased training frequency. Disabil. Rehabil. 27 (10), 571–581.

Wadell, K., Sundelin, G., Henriksson-Larsén, K., et al., 2004. High intensity physical group training in water: an effective training modality for patients with COPD. Respir. Med. 98 (5), 428–438.

Wagg, K., 2012. Unravelling self-management for COPD: what next? Chron. Respir. Dis. 9 (1), 5–7.

Waschki, B., Kirsten, A., Holz, O., et al., 2011. Physical activity is the strongest predictor of all-cause mortality in patients with COPD: a prospective cohort study. Chest 140 (2), 331–342.

Wedzicha, J.A., Bestall, J.C., Garrod, R., et al., 1998. Randomized controlled trial of pulmonary rehabilitation in severe chronic obstructive pulmonary disease patients, stratified with the MRC scale. Eur. Respir. J. 12, 363–369.

Wen, C.P., Wai, J.P., Tsai, M.K., et al., 2011. Minimum amount of physical activity for reduced mortality and extended life expectancy: a prospective cohort study. Lancet 378 (9798), 1244–1253.

Wenger, N., 2008. Current status of cardiac rehabilitation. J. Am. Coll. Cardiol. 51, 1619–1631.

WHO, 2009. Global health risks: mortality and burden of disease attributable to selected major risks.

Williams, M.A., 1994. Exercise Testing and Training in the Elderly Cardiac Patient: Current Issues in Cardiac Rehabilitation Series. Human Kinetics, Champaign, IL.

Williams, M.A., Haskell, W.L., Ades, P.A., et al., 2007. Resistance exercise in individuals with and without cardiovascular disease: 2007 update: a scientific statement from the American Heart Association Council on Clinical Cardiology and Council on Nutrition, Physical Activity, and Metabolism. Circulation 116 (5), 572–584.

Willich, S.N., Lewis, M., Lowel, H., et al., 1993. Physical exertion as a trigger of acute myocardial infarction. NEJM 329, 1684–1690.

Wister, A., Loewen, N., Kennedy-Symonds, H., et al., 2007. One-year follow-up of a therapeutic lifestyle intervention targeting cardiovascular disease risk. C. Med. Assoc. J. 177, 859–865.

Withers, N.J., Rudkin, S.T., White, R.J., 1999. Anxiety and depression in severe COPD: the effects of pulmonary rehabilitation. J. Cardiopulm. Rehabil. 19, 362–365.

Wood, D.A., Kotseva, K., Connolly, S., et al., 2008. On behalf of EUROACTION Study Group. Nurse-coordinated multidisciplinary, family-based cardiovascular disease prevention programme (EUROACTION) for patients with coronary heart disease and asymptomatic individuals at high risk of cardiovascular disease: a paired, cluster randomised controlled trial. Lancet 371, 1999–2012.

Worcester, M.C., Hare, D.L., Oliver, R.G., et al., 1993. Early programmes of high and low intensity exercise and quality of life after acute myocardial infarction. Br. Med. J. 307, 1244–1247.

World Health Organization, 2011. Global Atlas On Cardiovascular Disease Prevention and Control. WHO, Geneva.

World Health Organization, 2014. World Health Statistics. WHO, Geneva.

Yan, J.H., Guo, Y.Z., Yao, H.M., et al., 2013. Effects of Tai Chi in patients with chronic obstructive pulmonary disease: preliminary evidence. PLoS ONE 8 (4), e61806.

Yohannes, A.M., Doherty, P., Bundy, C., Yalfani, A., 2010. The long-term benefits of cardiac rehabilitation on depression, anxiety, physical activity and quality of life. J. Clin. Nurs. 19 (19–20), 2806–2813.

Young, W., Rewa, G., Goodman, S.G., et al., 2003. Evaluation of a community-based inner-city disease management program for postmyocardial infarction patients: a randomized controlled trial. C. Med. Assoc. J. 169, 905–910.

Yu, C.M., Lau, C.P., Chau, J., et al., 2004. A short course of cardiac rehabilitation program is highly cost effective in improving long-term quality of life in patients with recent myocardial infarction or percutaneous coronary intervention. Arch. Phys. Med. Rehabil. 85 (12), 1915–1922.

Yusuf, S., Hawken, S., Ounpuu, S., et al., 2004. Effect of potentially modifiable risk factors associated with MI in 52 countries (INTERHEART): case-control study. Lancet 364, 937–952.

Zacarias, E.C., Neder, J.A., Cendom, S.P., et al., 2000. Heart rate at the estimated lactate threshold in patients with COPD: effects on the target intensity for dynamic exercise training. J. Cardiopulm. Rehabil. 20, 369–376.

Zanotti, E., Felicetti, G., Maini, M., et al., 2003. Peripheral muscle strength training in bedbound patients with COPD receiving mechanical ventilation: effect of electrical stimulation. Chest 124, 292–296.

Zimmerman, L., Barnason, S., Brey, B.A., et al., 2002. Comparison of recovery patterns for patients undergoing coronary artery bypass grafting and minimally invasive direct coronary artery bypass in the early discharge period. Prog. Cardiovasc. Nurs. 17, 132–141.

Zimmerman, L., Barnason, S., Nieveen, J., Schmaderer, M., 2004. Symptom management intervention in elderly coronary artery bypass graft patients. Outcomes Manag. 8, 5–12.

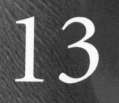

13

CARDIORESPIRATORY MANAGEMENT OF SPECIAL POPULATIONS

LINDA DENEHY ▪ ELEANOR MAIN

with contributions from

Acute Management of Burn Patients

SARAH SMAILES ▪ ANITA PLAZA ▪ JENNIFER PARATZ

Head Injury Management

LEANNE WILLIAMS

Liver Disease

CLAIRE BRADLEY ▪ JACQUELINE L LUKE

Spinal Cord Injury

JACQUELINE ROSS ▪ BROOKE WADSWORTH

Thoracic Organ Transplantation

KATE J HAYES ▪ PRUE E MUNRO ▪ PAUL AURORA

Trauma

HELENA VAN ASWEGEN

Paediatrics

CRAIG A WILLIAMS ▪ SARAH RAND

Exercise Training in Cancer Populations

CATHERINE L GRANGER

Rehabilitation for Survivors of Intensive Care

SUE BERNEY ▪ AMY NORDON-CRAFT ▪ LINDA DENEHY

CHAPTER OUTLINE

ACUTE MANAGEMENT OF BURN PATIENTS 641
Introduction 641
  Classification of Burns 642
  Burn Surgery 645
  Pathophysiological Response to Major Burn Injury 645
  Smoke Inhalation Injury 650
  Cardiorespiratory Physiotherapy Assessment of Major
    Burn/Smoke Inhalation Patients 653
  Cardiorespiratory Physiotherapy Treatment of Major
    Burn/Smoke Inhalation Patients 654
  Physical Rehabilitation Following Burn Injury 655
  Summary 658

HEAD INJURY MANAGEMENT 658
Introduction 658
  Types of Brain Injury 658
  Intracranial Hypertension Management 659
  Respiratory Consequences in Severe Acquired Brain
    Injury 660
  Physiotherapy Management 660

LIVER DISEASE 661
Introduction 661
  Signs and Symptoms of Liver Disease 661
  Chronic Liver Disease 662
  Hepatopulmonary Syndrome (HPS) 663
  Fulminant Hepatic Failure (FHF) 664
  Conclusion 667

SPINAL CORD INJURY 667
Introduction 667
Acute Spinal Cord Injury and Respiration 668
  Effects of Spinal Cord Injury 668
  Neurological Level and Completeness 669
  Orthopaedic Management 669
  Cardiovascular and Autonomic Impact on
    Respiration 670
  Pulmonary Oedema and Pulmonary Embolism 671
  Lung Volumes 672
  Positioning 673
  Cough 673
  Sleep-Disordered Breathing and Sleep Apnoea
    Syndrome 673
Respiratory Assessment 674
Physiotherapy Treatment 674
  Secretion Clearance 675
  Mechanical Aids for Assisted Coughing 675
  Maximize Lung Volumes 678
  Abdominal Binders 678
  Increase Muscle Strength 679
  Airway Management and Weaning from
    Ventilation 679

Long-Term Respiratory Management 680
  Long-Term Ventilation 680
  Readmissions to Hospital with a Chest
    Infection 681
  Treatment of Obstructive Sleep Apnoea 681
  Electrical and Magnetic Stimulation of Breathing 682
Conclusion 682

THORACIC ORGAN TRANSPLANTATION 682
Introduction 682
History 682
Selection of Candidates 683
Indications for Transplantation 683
Contraindications to Transplantation 684
Assessment 684
  Physiotherapy Assessment 685
Surgical Procedures 685
  Orthotopic Heart Transplantation 685
  Lung Transplantation 686
Key Concepts 686
  Organ Donation 686
  Immunosuppression and Rejection 687
  Infection 690
  Denervation 690
Preoperative Rehabilitation 691
  Exercise Training 691
  Pre-Transplant Exercise Guidelines 693
  Education 693
  Bridge to Transplant 693
Postoperative Management 694
  Management in the Intensive Care Unit 695
  Ward Management 695
Outpatient Rehabilitation 696
Exercise Limitation and Function Post
Transplant 697
Long-Term Management 699
Specific Considerations for Paediatric Patients 699
Conclusion 699

TRAUMA 700
Introduction 700
Causes and Mechanisms of Injury 700
Complications Related to Traumatic Injury 701
  Circulatory Deficits 701
  Deficits in Oxygenation 701
  Systemic Inflammatory Response Syndrome, Sepsis and
    Muscle Weakness 701
Medical and Surgical Management of Patients
with Traumatic Injury 702
  Primary Survey and Resuscitation of Vital
    Functions 702

Secondary Survey 702
  Definitive Care 702
Physiotherapy Intervention for the Trauma
Patient 705
  Complications That May Develop Due to
    Immobility 706
Quality of Life after Traumatic Injury 708
Conclusion 709

PAEDIATRICS 709
Introduction 709
Rehabilitation in Special Paediatric
Populations 711
Cystic Fibrosis 711
Asthma 712
Other Respiratory Conditions 715
  Interstitial Lung Disease 715
  Non-CF Bronchiectasis 715
  Lung Transplant 716
Obesity 716
Heart Disease 717
  Congenital Heart Disease 717
  Acquired Heart Disease 718
  Ventricular Assist Devices 719
  Heart Transplant 720
Exercise Prescription 721

EXERCISE TRAINING IN CANCER
POPULATIONS 722
Introduction 722
Physical Activity for Cancer Prevention 722

Medical Treatment of Cancer and the Associated
Side Effects 723
Lack of Physical Activity after a Diagnosis of
Cancer 725
Physical Activity Guidelines for People Living with
Cancer 727
The Role of Exercise Training in the Management
of Cancer 728
Delivery and Timing of Exercise Training for
Individuals with Cancer 728
Evaluation of Exercise Training for Individuals with
Cancer 729
Exercise Prescription for Individuals with
Cancer 730
Monitoring during Exercise for Individuals with
Cancer 731
Strategies for Adherence to Increased Physical
Activity for Individuals with Cancer 731

REHABILITATION FOR SURVIVORS OF
INTENSIVE CARE 733
Definition and Mechanisms of Muscle Weakness
in ICU 734
Patients Who Are Unconscious/Sedated 737
Conscious and Stable Patients 738
  Early Mobilization 738
Neurocognitive Interventions 739
Resources 740
Summary 740
References 740

Acute Management of Burn Patients

INTRODUCTION

Over the last 50 years there have been significant improvements in the survival of patients after severe burn injuries. One of the most important developments over this time has been the establishment of specialized burn centres leading to advances in critical care management such as appropriate fluid resuscitation, early surgical management, improved ventilation strategies and early management of infection.

With improved survival there is now more emphasis on rehabilitation and quality of life outcomes requiring a coordinated approach to management from a multi-disciplinary burn team in which physiotherapy plays a vital role (Johnson 1984, Wright 1984). The physiotherapist's role within the burn team is to facilitate appropriate physical rehabilitation to return the patient to full independence with focus on areas such as

- optimizing cardiorespiratory function
- weaning and extubation assessments
- exercise prescription for prevention of contracture, improvement of strength and cardiovascular endurance
- scar management
- functional retraining.

	TABLE 13-1			
	Multi-Organ Dysfunction after a Burn Injury			
Organ/System	**Typical Dysfunction after Burn Injury**		**Organ/System**	**Typical Dysfunction after Burn Injury**
Cardiovascular system	1st 48 hours ■ Generalized oedema: increased vascular permeability, extravasation of fluid and plasma protein (in greater than 15% TBSA) ■ Hypovolaemia, decreased cardiac output, tachycardia ■ >48 hours ■ Increased cardiac output ■ Increased cardiac work		Immune system	■ Suppression of immune function: increases susceptibility to infections
			Bones	■ Demineralization of bones: osteopenia/osteoporosis ■ Heterotopic ossification ■ Growth retardation in children
Metabolism	■ Hypermetabolic response 　■ 100–150% increase above resting energy expenditure 　■ Catabolism of body protein stores ■ Insulin resistance		Nervous system	■ Direct damage to nerves by burn injury especially electrical injury ■ Compartment syndrome leading to compression of nerves and ischaemic changes ■ Prolonged positioning: prolonged stretch/tension on nerves ■ Critical illness polyneuropathy post ICU admission
Renal	■ Decreased urine output ■ Haemoglobinuria/myoglobinuria: as a result of tissue damage leading to discolouration of urine ■ Acute renal failure		Muscle	■ Direct damage by burn injury, especially electrical injury ■ Compartment syndrome leading to muscle ischaemia ■ Catabolism of muscle: decreased muscle strength/endurance
Pulmonary	■ Inhalation injury ■ Pneumonia: ventilator acquired ■ ARDS		Skin	■ Loss of thermoregulatory function of skin ■ Loss of barrier to infection ■ Inflammatory and proliferative response to heal wound
Gastro-intestinal	■ Ileus ■ Gastric and/or duodenal ulceration ■ Abdominal compartment syndrome		Psychosocial	■ Depression ■ Anxiety ■ Altered body image ■ Post-traumatic stress syndrome
Endocrine	■ Increase catecholamines and cortisol ■ Impaired glucose tolerance ■ Decreased testosterone			
Liver	■ Vitamin deficiency: derangement of vitamin absorption ■ Liver failure secondary to ischaemia			

ARDS, Acute respiratory distress syndrome; *ICU,* intensive care unit; *TBSA,* total body surface area.

When discussing management of burn injuries, it is important to remember that a burn is a multi-system injury involving all organ systems. Table 13-1 details the responses of each organ system to a burn injury. Patients with burn injuries are at risk of common complications related to an intensive care stay which include intensive care unit (ICU)–acquired weakness (AW), ventilator-associated pneumonia, ventilator-induced lung injury, secondary infections from the use of invasive monitoring and delirium. They are also at risk of additional problems arising from the burn or smoke inhalation injury or from the patient's responses to these injuries.

This section provides a broad overview of burns and smoke inhalation injuries and the physiotherapy management of these conditions.

Classification of Burns

Significant improvements in survival of patients with burns have been made in recent years due to advancements in the emergency and early management of this injury (Roberts et al 2012). Most patients survive the early 'resuscitation' phase and the principle cause of mortality is multiple organ failure due to sepsis later on in the post-burn course. Survival following burn injury is directly related to patient age, burn size (percentage of total body surface area (TBSA) burnt), depth of burn injury and presence of smoke inhalation injury. Comorbidity is also predictive of patient outcome, and this probably explains the smaller improvement in survival of elderly burn patients despite clinical advancements (Krishnan et al 2013). Depth of burn injury is possibly the most important determinant of patient outcome and also dictates the patient's course of treatment. Burns are most commonly classified by their depth and these are summarized in Table 13-2.

Spontaneously Healing Wounds

Erythema (sunburn) spontaneously heals within 7 days, while superficial partial thickness wounds (Fig. 13-1) heal within 3 weeks of injury without residual scarring or alteration of skin function. Deep dermal wounds often heal without the need for surgical intervention, but healing may be prolonged and while the wound is open, infection, pain and, ultimately, hypertrophic scarring are significant problems. Therefore some deep dermal wounds require surgical excision and skin grafting to optimize healing and scarring.

After patients have arrived at the burn centre an initial wound assessment is performed to ascertain burn size (% TBSA) and depth. Subsequently, the wounds are cleaned and dressed, and limbs are elevated to reduce local burn oedema. Patient management is centred on preventing wound infection and providing ideal conditions for healing, i.e. adequate warmth, nutrition, effective analgesia and appropriate dressings with frequent wound inspection and cleaning. The greatest risk for all burn patients is infection

TABLE 13-2
Burn Depth Classification

Type of Burn	Skin Structures Damaged	Appearance and Sensation	Healing / Implications for Scar and Contracture	Common Cause
Superficial burns	■ Epidermis	■ Red ■ Good blanching and capillary return ■ Sensation intact and painful	■ Heals in 7–10 days ■ Minimal chance of hypertrophic scar ■ Minimal chance of contracture	Radiation (sunburn)
Superficial partial thickness burns	■ Epidermis ■ Superficial dermis ■ Sparing of epidermal appendages, e.g. hair follicles	■ Red to pink, blisters ■ Good blanching and capillary return ■ Sensation intact and painful	■ Heals in 14 days ■ Very low chance of hypertrophic scar ■ Very low chance of contracture	Hot water scalds
Deep partial thickness (deep dermal)	■ Epidermis ■ Deep into dermis ■ Sparing of hair follicles and sweat glands	■ White, oedematous ■ Pseudo-membranous film over wound ■ Delayed capillary return after blanching but still present ■ Sensation intact but decreased light touch and pain sensation	■ Heals in 2–3 weeks ■ May require skin graft to achieve complete healing & better outcome ■ High risk of hypertrophic scar ■ High risk of contracture	Flames, contact burns
Full thickness	■ Epidermis ■ Dermis ■ All epidermal appendages, e.g. hair follicles, sweat glands ■ Fascia, muscle and bone	■ Charred brown, marbled white or deep red ■ Dry, leather-like ■ Thrombosed vessels visible below skin ■ No capillary return or blanching ■ No sensation from the skin only deeper structures	■ Granulates from wound edges and often requires a skin graft to heal wound ■ Hypertrophic scar and contracture formation after injury	■ Flames, hot oil, electrical conduction

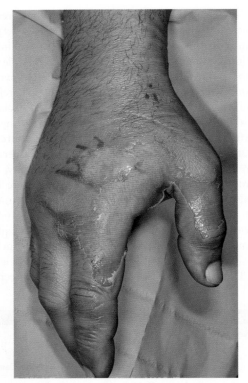

FIGURE 13-1 ■ Superficial partial thickness burn after blisters have been debrided. *(© Mid Essex Hospitals NHS Trust. Permission is granted for first publication in* Cardiorespiratory Physiotherapy: Adults and Paediatrics, *5th edition, 2016.)*

of the wounds, which impairs healing and may have the effect of deepening the wound, 'converting' it to full thickness. Also invasive wound infection may lead to secondary infections of other organ systems. Therefore strict infection prevention procedures are in place at the burn centre.

Full Thickness Wounds

Deep dermal and full thickness burns can be modest in size and these patients can usually be managed on a low-dependency ward. However, burn wounds of most patients in the ICU are full thickness and may involve a significant area of the body. Major burn injury (>20% TBSA) is a catastrophic injury and results in pathophysiological changes which cause homoeostatic imbalance and the need for organ support, often over a prolonged period of time until the wound is closed. The full thickness burnt tissue is termed 'eschar' and it lacks the elasticity of normal skin since the dermis, the elastic component, is not viable. The eschar of a patient with burns caused by fire has a blackened, charred appearance (Fig. 13-2) and a distinctive odour.

If the eschar extends to cover the circumference of the chest, abdomen, neck or a limb, an escharotomy must be performed early in the post-burn course. Escharotomy describes a procedure where vertical incisions are made through the eschar to relieve the

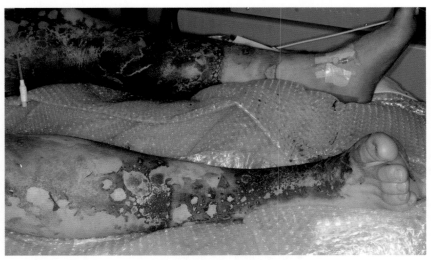

FIGURE 13-2 ■ Extensive full thickness burn. *(© Mid Essex Hospitals NHS Trust. Permission is granted for first publication in* Cardiorespiratory Physiotherapy: Adults and Paediatrics, *5th edition, 2016.)*

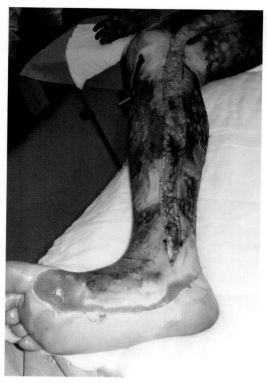

FIGURE 13-3 ■ Escharotomy for circumferential full thickness wounds. (© *Mid Essex Hospitals NHS Trust. Permission is granted for first publication in* Cardiorespiratory Physiotherapy: Adults and Paediatrics, *5th edition, 2016.*)

pressure of the accumulating burn oedema beneath, thus facilitating lung ventilation and perfusion of abdominal organs and limbs (Fig. 13-3). Escharotomy is performed as an emergency procedure in the hours following burn injury to preserve life and limb (Pruitt et al 1968).

Burn Surgery

Full thickness wounds do not have the potential to heal and so surgical excision of the eschar and skin grafting are necessary to close the wound. Over the last 25 years the practice of early total excision of the eschar has become widespread because there is convincing evidence that patient survival is improved (Herndon et al 1989). Therefore patients with full thickness injuries should be transferred to a specialist burn centre as soon as possible following their burn injury. The

principles of burn surgery are to completely excise the eschar and to close the wound as soon as possible.

Unless the patient is too unstable, burn eschar excision is undertaken within 24 hours of admission to the burn centre. The burn eschar is excised down to healthy, bleeding tissue, the wound bed. Perioperative blood loss can be significant at times, necessitating replacement blood transfusions. Subsequently, the wound is closed using the patient's skin, the 'autograft' which is removed from an unburnt area of skin, the 'donor site'. The autograft is usually meshed so that a larger wound area can be covered by donor skin; this is a particularly useful practice for patients with major burns where it is desirable to cover as much open wound as possible. However, widely meshed autografts are very vulnerable to shearing forces in the days after application. If there is insufficient donor skin to cover the wound in one sitting, cadavaric allograft is commonly used to temporarily cover the wound until the donor site can be reharvested once it is healed (after approximately 2 weeks). The autograft is secured to the wound bed with sutures, staples or glue and covered with a bulky dressing to protect it against shearing until it is stable at approximately 5 days after application. During this period it is important to immobilize all joints involved or near to the skin graft with splints to minimize the risk of autograft loss. Figure 13-4 shows a patient with newly applied autografts, and also part of the donor site can be seen on the lower aspect of the right side of the chest. A summary of burn surgery and its implication for physiotherapy management is given in Table 13-3.

Pathophysiological Response to Major Burn Injury

Early management of critically ill burns patients is directed at effective fluid resuscitation, optimum airway management, avoidance of infection, early debridement and grafting and adequate nutrition (Latenser 2009). This all has important implications for physiotherapy management. Patients with thermal injury are frequently admitted to intensive care (Kasten et al 2011). Reasons for admission include:

■ need to complete fluid resuscitation in a monitored environment
■ haemodynamic instability

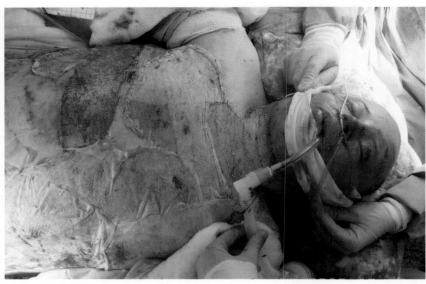

FIGURE 13-4 ■ Newly applied autografts. (*© Mid Essex Hospitals NHS Trust. Permission is granted for first publication in* Cardiorespiratory Physiotherapy: Adults and Paediatrics, *5th edition, 2016.*)

- decreased immune response (linear flow cubicle)
- >20% TBSA, necessitating frequent grafting
- a threatened airway including facial oedema and burns around the face or neck
- heavy sedation requiring mechanical ventilation
- inhalational injury
- concomitant injuries
- pre-morbid conditions
- extremes of age
- monitoring of cardiac function after electrical injuries.

A major burn injury affects all organ systems and results in severe homoeostatic imbalance. These pathophysiological responses necessitate patients to be nursed in isolation in individual temperature- and humidity-controlled rooms. Typical responses to injury include:

1. significant fluid shifts
2. hypermetabolism
3. systemic inflammatory response syndrome (SIRS).

Significant Fluid Shifts

Immediately following burn injury, inflammatory mediators, endogenous catecholamines and cortisol are released so that systemic levels of these increase by several fold. There is a transient reduction in cardiac output which lasts approximately 48 hours, and disruption of the integrity of the microcirculation leading to capillary leak and significant shifts of fluid from the circulating plasma to the interstitial spaces. In patients with major burn injuries, this results in rapid accumulation of oedema at the burn wound site but also in unburnt tissues, reducing circulating blood volume and leading to 'burn shock', a state also characterized by increased vascular resistance (Demling 1987, Warden 1992). Consequently, these patients have considerably increased fluid requirements following injury and receive 'fluid resuscitation' immediately after rescue and for the first 24 hours after injury. The TBSA threshold for which fluid resuscitation is commenced is ≥15% for adults and ≥10% for children and elderly patients. Substantial fluid resuscitation is required at this stage, with requirements often exceeding 20 L in the first 24 hours. This resuscitation and its effectiveness has important implications for haemodynamic stability and secondary respiratory problems. A delay or inadequate fluid resuscitation can result in fatal hypovolaemic shock or organ failure and necrosis of viable burn tissue, while over-resuscitation can result in pulmonary oedema, abdominal or limb

TABLE 13-3

Surgical Intervention for Burn Wounds and Implications for Physiotherapy Management

Type of Skin Graft/Skin Substitute	Description	Implications for Physiotherapy
Autografts		
Split thickness skin grafts (SSG)	Donor skin taken from any area of own body (usually antero-lateral thigh if available) and used to cover area of defect 0.008–0.012 inch in thickness so only transplants epidermis and small part of dermis **Meshed SSG** ■ Can be meshed and spread up to ratio of 4 : 1 to allow coverage of larger surface areas ■ Allows drainage of haematoma/exudate through mesh so initially better adherent graft **Non-meshed SSG** ■ Maintains better cosmetic result and used for visible areas of face and hands ■ More fragile in early stages as less ability to drain haematoma/exudate from beneath graft	■ Thinner graft with less dermis present increases the risk of contracture. ■ Needs initial immobilization of underlying joints for 3–5 days to allow adherence of skin graft*. ■ Manual respiratory techniques (e.g. percussion and vibrations need to cease for 3–5 days post SSG to chest wall to allow adherence of skin graft*. ■ Standing and mobility can commence day 3–5 post lower limb SSG but appropriate compression bandaging must be in situ*. ■ All SSG will lead to hypertrophic scar and require scar management.
Full thickness skin grafts (FTG)	Donor area taken from own body but includes entire dermal and epidermal layers. 0.025–0.03 inches in thickness Donor site is now also a full thickness deficit and is unable to heal on its own, requiring an SSG. Used if %TBSA is small or in reconstructive procedures	■ Thicker graft with dermal elements has less risk of contracture than an SSG. ■ Needs initial immobilization of underlying joints for 5 days to allow adherence of skin graft*. ■ Manual respiratory techniques (e.g. percussion and vibrations need to cease for a minimum 5 days post FTG to chest wall to allow adherence of skin graft*. ■ Standing and mobility can commence day 5–7 post lower limb FTG but appropriate compression bandaging must be in situ*. ■ All FTG will lead to hypertrophic scar and require scar management.
Cultured Autografts		
Cultured epithelial autografts (CEA)	Cell biopsy taken early post injury, cells cultured in the laboratory to produce cell sheets (takes 2–3 weeks) or cells in suspension (5–7 days) Used in major burns where donor sites are scarce to aid in survival	■ More fragile grafts with high susceptibility to shear forces, increased skin blistering ■ Needs initial immobilization of underlying joints for 5–7 days to allow adherence of CEA* ■ Manual respiratory techniques (e.g. percussion and vibrations need to cease for 5–7 days post CEA to chest wall to allow adherence of skin graft*. ■ Standing and mobility can commence day 5–7 post CEA but appropriate compression bandaging must be in situ*. ■ All CEA will lead to hypertrophic scar and require scar management. ■ Fragile nature of skin long term may lead to modification of pressure garment design for scar management.

Continued on following page

TABLE 13-3		
Surgical Intervention for Burn Wounds and Implications for Physiotherapy Management (Continued)		
Type of Skin Graft/Skin Substitute	**Description**	**Implications for Physiotherapy**
Allografts		
Human cadaver allograft	Human cadaver skin harvested and stored for use as a temporary coverage Used as a SSG and becomes vascularized from underlying wound bed. Remains adherent until immunologically rejected or removed (≈2–3 weeks).	■ Needs initial immobilization of underlying joints for 3–5 days to allow adherence of skin graft as per SSG* ■ Manual respiratory techniques (e.g. percussion and vibrations need to cease for 3–5 days post application to chest wall to allow adherence of skin graft*. ■ Standing and mobility can commence day 3–5 post lower limb cadaver skin SSG but appropriate compression bandaging must be in situ*. ■ Only temporary skin coverage and will need a SSG for permanent wound coverage
Skin Substitutes		
Biobrane	Synthetic product of nylon fabric coated with porcine collagen embedded into silicone film Temporary synthetic skin substitute which forms adherent bond with wound bed until epithelialization has occurred (or it is removed to replace with a permanent SSG) Can be used for the following: ■ Clean superficial partial thickness wounds that will heal on their own under the Biobrane ■ Fresh non-infected wounds free of eschar while awaiting definitive grafting ■ Coverage for widely meshed autografts to promote healing ■ Coverage of donor sites to promote healing.	■ Needs initial immobilization of underlying joints for 48–72 hours to allow adherence of Biobrane* ■ Manual respiratory techniques (e.g. percussion and vibrations need to cease for 48–72 hours post application to chest wall to allow adherence of Biobrane*. ■ Standing and mobility can commence day 3–5 post Biobrane application but appropriate compression bandaging must be in situ*. ■ Only temporary coverage and will need a SSG for permanent wound coverage
Integra	Bi-layered skin substitute ■ Silicone epidermal component ■ Dermal component: neodermis of bovine and shark cartilage and glycosaminoglycans Temporary skin substitute that allows the patient's own dermis to grow on the neodermal structure Will require a second operation 2–3 weeks after application for removal of silicone layer and replacement with thin SSG Used in major burns where donor sites are scarce to aid in survival. Allows time for healing and reharvesting of donor sites Useful in deep wounds to muscle/tendon as augments dermal thickness	■ Needs initial immobilization of underlying joints for 5–7 days or longer to allow adherence of Integra* ■ Manual respiratory techniques (e.g. percussion and vibrations) need to cease for 5–7 days or longer post application to chest wall to allow adherence of Integra*. ■ Standing and mobility can commence from day 7 or later after lower limb Integra but appropriate compression bandaging must be in situ*. ■ Will need an SSG for permanent wound coverage after 2–3 weeks and therefore further immobilization time as per SSG protocols ■ Will still lead to hypertrophic scar and contracture and requires scar management

TBSA, Total body surface area.
*Important points to note.

compartment syndrome and increased depth of burn injuries. Effectiveness of resuscitation is demonstrated by a urine output of >30 mL/hr, a decrease in haemoglobin (Hb) towards normal levels and a decrease in blood lactate. The goal of fluid resuscitation is to maintain intravascular volume and end-organ perfusion. Use of continuous cardiac output monitoring to evaluate response to fluid therapy has been shown to optimize fluid volumes titrated and improve patient outcome in paediatric burn patients (Kraft et al 2013). Indeed, critical care monitoring is necessary for all burn patients receiving fluid resuscitation to minimize the complications of under-resuscitation and also over-resuscitation, so-called 'fluid creep' (Cartotto 2009, Faraklas et al 2012, Saffle 2007). Another important source of intravascular fluid (and heat) loss is evaporation through the open wound. Evaporative losses in severely burnt patients account for ongoing increased fluid requirements and electrolyte disturbances until the wounds are closed.

Hypermetabolism

Initially, for the first 48 hours after burn injury, there is a reduction in the patient's basal metabolic rate called the 'ebb' phase and this is followed by an extreme and sustained elevation of the basal metabolic rate leading to increased resting energy expenditure, the 'flow' phase (Rojas et al 2012). The magnitude of the hypermetabolic response exhibited following burn injury is far in excess of any other injury or disease and can be considered to be a variant of the stress response. The patient's basal metabolic rate is elevated in proportion to the size of the burn and can still be in evidence 3 years after injury with increased resting energy expenditure of up to 140% predicted (Jeschke et al 2011). Hypermetabolic severely burnt patients exhibit a hyperdynamic circulation, increased respiratory rate, oxygen consumption and carbon dioxide production and increased core temperature (hyperthermia). Hypermetabolism is thought to be an appropriate response to major burn injury, but the magnitude of it seems to predict patient outcome. This was illustrated by Jeschke et al (2013) who demonstrated that burnt children who did not survive exhibited vastly elevated hypermetabolic responses above survivors with similar burn injuries and these exaggerated responses were associated with organ dysfunction and sepsis.

To sustain the hypermetabolic response rates of lipolysis, proteolysis, glycogenolysis and glucose consumption are elevated and these increase the patient's need for nutrition. A requirement of up to 4000 kcal/day to maintain a stable body mass is not unusual. Mortality is increased if patients become overly catabolic and lose lean body mass, as this invariably leads to wound breakdown, impaired immune responses and subsequent susceptibility to infection (Rojas et al 2012). Therefore all patients with major burns are fed enterally not only to sustain their lean body mass but also to facilitate wound healing. Early placement of feeding tubes into the jejunum is beneficial so that starvation periods are avoided before wound care procedures. Many patients also require parenteral nutrition during periods of sepsis when gastrointestinal tract absorption is affected. Use of parenteral nutrition is not without risk but judicious use of it has been shown to be safe in severely burnt children (Dylewski et al 2013).

Systemic Inflammatory Response Syndrome (SIRS)

Nearly all patients with major burns meet the criteria used to diagnose SIRS. SIRS in the context of major burns is a systemic, non-specific over-activation of the immune system caused by release of inflammatory mediators and over-activation of the complement cascade. The resultant extensive capillary endothelium damage leads to ongoing capillary leak, increased fluid requirements and generalized body oedema (Hogan et al 2012). These changes occur not only within the first 24 hours after injury but also with each episode of sepsis and following every inflammatory insult, e.g. burn surgery. Pulmonary oedema may also result leading to increased ventilator dependence. Mechanical ventilation strategies vary between burn centres, but most aim at a lung protective strategies, limiting tidal volumes (6 mL/kg) and peak inspiratory pressures (<30 cmH$_2$O) (The ARDS Network 2000). The airway is managed very proactively (Ipaktchi and Arbabi 2006). With the large amount of fluid resuscitation required, it is very likely that facial and airway oedema will occur. The hypopharynx, epiglottis and aryepiglottic folds are specifically prone to oedema. The patient will be intubated early, before the oedema can cause obstruction (Fig. 13-5). Meticulous care is required with handling the airway as accidental extubation can be fatal.

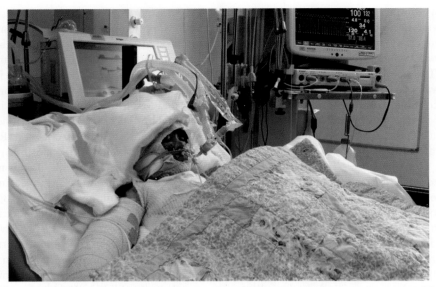

FIGURE 13-5 ■ An intubated child with major burns. *(© Mid Essex Hospitals NHS Trust. Permission is granted for first publication in Cardiorespiratory Physiotherapy: Adults and Paediatrics, 5th edition, 2016.)*

Burn patients are susceptible to sepsis because of loss of skin, a viable physical barrier to infection, and immunosuppression. Sepsis further increases the hypermetabolic response and leads to exaggerated SIRS responses hyperpyrexias and increased need for cardiovascular and respiratory support (American Burn Association Consensus on Burn Sepsis and Infection Group 2007). Pulmonary sepsis is common especially following major burn and/or smoke inhalation injury and aggressive airway clearance is one of the key therapies available to patients (Cancio 2009). Ventilator-associated pneumonia (VAP) and acute respiratory distress syndrome (ARDS) are common complications in burn patients. Development of VAP is associated with an increase in mortality (Huzar et al 2011, Mosier et al 2009). Further, if pulmonary oedema occurred early during fluid resuscitation, this is often a precursor to ARDS. In addition, excision and grafting of the chest and abdomen can lead to a restrictive ventilator defect due to dense fibrous tissue formation and scar contraction. This loss of lung chest wall elasticity and effective lung volume can lead to later respiratory failure (Boots et al 2009).

Regular and thorough physiotherapy assessments and airway clearance are therefore required throughout the patient's hospital stay to optimize respiratory function.

As well as inhalation injuries and VAP, the factors after a burn injury can make the patient more susceptible to respiratory compromise (Box 13-1).

Smoke Inhalation Injury

Smoke inhalation injury accounts for the majority of deaths in house fires and it increases morbidity and mortality of burn patients. Smoke inhalation injury increases mortality by up to 20% in burn patients, but if inhalation injury is complicated by pneumonia, expected mortality increases by up to 60% (Colohan 2010, Shirani et al 1987). The current understanding of the pathophysiology of smoke inhalation injury describes three distinct processes which can occur in isolation but more commonly in combination:

1. thermal injury
2. chemical injury
3. systemic intoxication.

Thermal Injury

Thermal injury is caused by inhalation of superheated gases that cause burning of predominantly the upper

BOX 13-1
FACTORS AFTER A BURN INJURY THAT INCREASE SUSCEPTIBILITY TO RESPIRATORY COMPROMISE

- Repeated general anaesthetics for multiple skin grafting procedures, especially when the injury is greater than 20% total body surface area (TBSA). This increases the risk of development of atelectasis and pneumonia.
- Prolonged bed rest ± sedation, mechanical ventilation from extended intensive care unit (ICU) stay or due to immobilization post grafting procedures. Increases the risk of atelectasis, pneumonia and deconditioning.
- Relative immunosuppression
- Leakage of plasma into the lung parenchyma
- Pre-existing respiratory pathology. The presence of chronic pulmonary conditions and a smoking history will increase the risk of atelectasis and pneumonia.
- Circumferential chest wall burns. This may limit thoracic expansion and contribute to increased risk of atelectasis.

airway, thus the effects of thermal injury usually do not extend below the carina. This is because heat is absorbed by the efficient heat-exchanging mechanisms of the upper airway and dissipated rapidly because of the low thermal capacity of smoke, and there is reflex closure of the larynx. Inhalation of super-heated steam causes thermal injury to the lower airways because steam has a much higher thermal capacity and thus retains its heat for longer. Thermal injury results in immediate and progressive upper airway oedema, erythema and ulceration. The tongue and epiglottis swell rapidly and these threaten patency of the airway. Once mucosal healing is underway airway casts are sloughed off increasing the risk of plugging of lower airways (Dries & Endorf 2013).

Clinical signs: face/lip oedema, hoarse voice, stridor, face/neck burn, intra-oral burn/oedema, increased work of breathing.

Chemical Injury

Smoke contains by-products of burning materials and these are toxic and irritant to the respiratory tract. Inhalation of these chemicals causes extensive inflammation in the lower airways leading to acid/alkali corrosion, bronchospasm, hyperaemia, bronchiolar swelling and shedding of bronchial epithelium. Muco-

ciliary transport mechanisms are damaged, leading to poor clearance of bacteria and other inhaled substances. There is also accumulation of initially 'foamy' secretions in the airways which clot and cause obstruction after several hours, and hypersecretion by goblet cells. Carbonaceous particulate matter containing toxic by-products of combustion is deposited throughout the respiratory tree or adhered to the tracheobronchial mucosa, increasing the risk of obstruction and further corrosion. Changes in the lung parenchyma resemble those of acute lung injury (ALI) or ARDS with the development of alveolar and interstitial oedema due to capillary leak and small airway/alveolar atelectasis due to loss of surfactant (Dries & Endorf 2013, Herndon et al 1986, Pruitt et al 1975).

Clinical signs: face burns, cough, bronchospasm, increased work of breathing, soot stained sputum, decreased partial pressure of oxygen in arterial blood (PaO_2) : fraction of inspired oxygen (FiO_2) ratio.

Systemic Intoxication

Systemic intoxication is caused by the systemic effects of inhalation of toxic chemicals contained within smoke, most notably carbon monoxide and hydrogen cyanide. These result in death in victims who are not rescued from the scene of the fire and morbidity in burn patients. The pathophysiology of carbon monoxide poisoning relates to the strong affinity of carbon monoxide for the haemoglobin molecule and the resultant displacement of oxygen from the oxyhaemoglobin molecule and formation of carboxyhaemoglobin. In turn, there is reduced oxygen-carrying capacity of the blood and a left shift of the oxygen dissociation curve, causing inefficient dissociation of oxyhaemoglobin at the cellular level. Additionally, carbon monoxide inhibits the cytochrome oxidase system in the mitochondria, thereby inhibiting cellular oxidation, and these result in acidosis, tissue hypoxia and the inability to utilize oxygen. Carboxyhaemoglobin has a half-life of approximately 4 hours but this is shortened to around 45 minutes if 100% O_2 is administered. Hydrogen cyanide also inhibits the cytochrome oxidase system and may have a synergistic effect with carbon monoxide (Dries & Endorf 2013, Goldbaum et al 1976, Herndon et al 1986).

Clinical signs: patient confusion, reduced consciousness level, persisting metabolic acidosis, increased levels of carboxyhaemoglobin, inability to extract oxygen at the cellular level – mixed venous oxygen saturation and arterial oxygen saturation are equal.

Management of Smoke Inhalation Injury

Principles of emergency management include securing the patient's airway to prevent obstruction, administering 100% oxygen (until carboxyhaemoglobin levels normalize) and analgesia, and commencing fluid resuscitation. Antidotes to cyanide poisoning should be used early after the patient is rescued from the scene of the fire. Once the patient has arrived at hospital the priority is to definitively diagnose smoke inhalation injury. Diagnosis is based upon the presence of three factors:

1. history of entrapment with fire/smoke
2. clinical signs and symptoms
3. fibre-optic bronchoscopy (FOB).

FOB has two key functions: definitive diagnosis of smoke inhalation injury by visualization of the airway and lavage of toxic carbonaceous secretions, particularly from the larger airways. Commonly FOB is performed promptly after the patient is admitted to the burn centre and approximately 24 hours afterwards to evaluate the progress of the airway injury. Attempts have been made to measure the severity of smoke inhalation by bronchoscopic grading in order to predict patient morbidity and mortality. Although mortality has been found to be higher in the most severe injuries as graded by FOB in one study, the grading systems did not definitively predict extent of pulmonary dysfunction, development of ARDS or other clinical outcomes (Endorf & Gamelli 2007, Mosier et al 2012). It appears that admission computerized tomography (CT) chest scans in conjunction with bronchoscopy may more accurately predict lung dysfunction following smoke inhalation injury (Oh et al 2012).

Ongoing medical management for patients with major burns and smoke inhalation injury is largely supportive with utilization of protective lung ventilation strategies, VAP prevention care bundles, high-frequency oscillatory ventilation (after toxic particulate matter has been removed), active humidification and regular and thorough tracheobronchial toilet (Cancio 2009). Non-invasive positive pressure ventilation (NIPPV) is not widely used, as it is contraindicated in patients with full thickness face burns and in those who cannot protect their airway, cough or clear secretions after the administration of sedatives for wound care procedures. Tracheostomy is frequently indicated for airway management, especially for patients with full thickness face burns (Aggarwal et al 2009). High-flow humidified oxygen systems are well tolerated in self-ventilating patients with face burns and facilitate airway clearance, a major benefit for newly extubated patients or for those following sedated procedures.

There is little evidence supporting other medical treatments for smoke inhalation injury apart from the use of nebulized agents with the potential to attenuate lung injury. Several animal studies have evaluated the use of various nebulized agents where the aim is to reduce bronchoconstriction and bronchial hyperaemia (Lange et al 2011), anticoagulate fibrin (loosen secretions and reduce airway obstruction) (Enkhbaatar et al 2004) and reduce inflammation (Yamamoto et al 2012), and these have generated favourable results. Currently, a triple regimen of nebulized salbutamol, heparin and N-acetylcysteine is widely used in patients with smoke inhalation injury, based on studies where there were favourable survival results in children (Desai et al 1998) and a reduction in progression to ARDS in adults (Miller et al 2009).

Cardiorespiratory physiotherapy is a fundamental part of the management of smoke inhalation injury because of the key role it has to offer with respect to clearance of toxic particulate matter in the early stages after injury, and mucosal slough, bronchial casts and infective secretions in the later stages. For these reasons patients with smoke inhalation injury receive frequent assessments by a cardiorespiratory physiotherapist. Table 13-4 outlines the indicators of an inhalation injury and these factors should be included as part of a thorough patient examination to determine if an inhalation injury is likely to have occurred.

Additionally, there is a very high incidence of pneumonia because of necrosis of the tracheobronchial mucosa leading to exposure to pathogens (Shirani et al 1987), and so frequent collection of sputum specimens for microbiological surveillance is mandatory to enable early identification and treatment of infection.

TABLE 13-4	
Indicators of an Inhalation Injury	
Assessment	**Indicators**
History	■ Entrapped in a smoke filled enclosed space ■ Explosions at the fire scene ■ Altered LOC at the time of the injury ■ Under the influence of alcohol or drugs which alters LOC ■ Patients with slower reaction times to escape fire, e.g. elderly patients, patients with physical disabilities e.g. cerebral palsy
Physical examination	■ Signs of respiratory distress: dyspnoea, tachypnoea ■ Burns to the face, lips, nose and/or pharynx ■ Singed nasal hair ■ Hoarse voice ■ Signs of bronchospasm: stridor, wheeze ■ Carbonaceous sputum ■ Soot in the oropharynx/nasopharynx ■ Decreased LOC and confusion
Investigations	■ Arterial blood gases: low PaO₂ ■ Elevated carboxyhaemoglobin levels ■ Bronchoscopy: soot in airways, erythema of bronchial mucosa ■ Chest radiography changes: pulmonary oedema and later patchy atelectasis, collapse and consolidation of lung segments

LOC, Level of consciousness; *PaO₂*, partial pressure of oxygen in arterial blood.

Cardiorespiratory Physiotherapy Assessment of Major Burn/Smoke Inhalation Patients

The components of the physiotherapy assessment of burn ICU patients are similar to that of any other ICU patient. However, the patients' physiological responses to major burn impact on the physiotherapist's assessment such that 'normal' values for many vital signs differ from most ICU patients (outlined in the following sections). The physiotherapist should be able to interpret vital parameter variables in the context of these physiological processes and consider these to be 'normal adaptive responses' to injury.

Core and Peripheral Temperature. A core temperature of 38–38.5°C should be considered as normal in patients with major burn injury because of generation of the hypermetabolic response. Additionally, patients are generally not screened for sepsis unless their core temperature rises to approximately 39.5°C. The

peripheral temperature is also elevated above 'normal' and is maintained approximately 2°C below the core temperature so that there is adequate perfusion to the peripheries and wounds to facilitate healing. It must be noted that patients with extensive skin loss rapidly lose heat if bed linen, warming devices and dressings are removed, and so this should be considered when performing physiotherapy assessments and treatments.

Cardiovascular System. The cardiovascular responses to injury include reduced contractility and 'normal' heart rate initially following injury (for approximately 48 hours). This is followed by a sustained increased cardiac output and profound tachycardia such that a pulse rate of 130 beats per minute is not uncommon in an adult patient.

Respiratory System. The respiratory rate and minute ventilation of burn patients is elevated in the first days and weeks after injury to prevent the development of hypercapnia and respiratory acidosis caused by increased cellular carbon dioxide production. Carbon monoxide toxicity may result in a falsely elevated oxygen saturation on pulse oximetry. These factors should be taken into consideration when weaning the patient from ventilation and assessing readiness for extubation.

Fluid Balance. In the first days after injury, the 24-hour fluid balance measurement is unreliable because of fluid shifts, since evaporative fluid losses and extravasation of fluid into interstitial tissues cannot be accurately measured. In addition, surgical wound manipulation is usually required frequently in the first few days after injury and these complicate analysis of the fluid balance charts. To ascertain the patient's fluid status more accurately other observations should be relied upon:

1. continuous cardiac output studies
2. urine output
3. chest radiographs to assess for the presence of pulmonary oedema
4. visual observation and palpation of the patient
5. capillary refill time.

Auscultation. This essential component of the cardiopulmonary assessment is made more difficult where there are full thickness burns/skin grafts/dressings to the patient's chest. Auscultation over dressings is possible using a sterile glove over the diaphragm of your stethoscope to listen to the chest wall over the graft site. This skill becomes easier with experience but the physiotherapist may also need to rely on other components of the assessment to more accurately assess the patient's respiratory status, e.g. chest radiography, FOB recording, palpation, ventilator observations.

Cardiorespiratory Physiotherapy Treatment of Major Burn/Smoke Inhalation Patients

Firstly, it is worthy of note that there is a prolonged and ongoing risk of pulmonary sepsis until wounds are healed, a process that can take months to occur. Therefore during this time patients require regular cardiorespiratory physiotherapy assessments and treatments to optimize function. Special considerations for treatment of intubated and self-ventilating patients with burns are outlined in the following list:

1. **Pain control:** Patients with burn injuries suffer with severe pain especially during interventions and therefore it is important that the physiotherapist works closely with nursing and medical staff to optimize patients' pain relief. Physiotherapy treatment should be planned so that it is administered after analgesia.

2. **Newly applied autografts to the chest wall:** It is desirable to adopt a 'hands off' approach to administering manual techniques to the chest wall for approximately 5 days after application of autografts in order to minimize the risk of autograft loss by shearing forces. Vibrations and shaking should not be used at this stage. Additionally, it is important that extra attention is given to manual handling when moving or turning a burn patient with fresh autografts to avoid shearing the newly grafted surfaces.

3. **Smoke inhalation injury:** Patients with smoke inhalation may have copious toxic carbonaceous secretions in the distal airways which are not removed by FOB, and so these should be treated with physiotherapy at the earliest opportunity after admission to intensive care. Additionally, during periods of airway sloughing, physiotherapy should be scheduled so that it is administered regularly throughout the 24-hour period involving on-call services as necessary. In non-intubated patients, active humidification and nebulizers should be routinely used and the timing of physiotherapy should coordinate with nebulizers, i.e. 30 minutes after bronchodilators and mucolytic agents and prior to heparin/antibiotic nebulizers. If the patient's cough is ineffective, it may be necessary to use either nasopharyngeal or oropharyngeal suction to assist with secretion removal. In ventilated patients, regular suction via endotracheal tube or tracheostomy is mandatory to clear secretions. The amount of endotracheal secretions present, indicated by the frequency of suction required, is an independent predictor of extubation outcome for the ventilated burn patient (Smailes et al 2013b). Those patients with abundant secretions requiring suction every hour or more frequently were eight times more likely to fail extubation than those requiring less frequent suction (Smailes et al 2013b). Hyperinflation techniques may be appropriate in these patients while intubated (Chapter 9).

   Suction pressures should be closely monitored to avoid secondary injury to the airway. There is a very high incidence of pneumonia and so patients usually require frequent airway clearance techniques.

4. **Self ventilating patients:** Since wound healing is dependent on regular and thorough cleaning, patients with major burns are exposed to changes of dressings and wound hygiene every 24–48 hours. These procedures are very painful, and so the patient requires sedation or anaesthesia and this increases the potential for atelectasis and sputum retention (Smailes et al 2009a, b). Careful planning and teamwork is necessary to maintain active mobilization of the patient by undertaking rehabilitation before sedation is administered, passive range of motion (ROM) of joints by carrying out passive movements during the procedure and cardiorespiratory assessment and treatment afterwards. An effective cough is necessary to promote clearance of mucous and fibrin casts (in the case of inhalation injury) from the tracheobronchial tree. If the patient's cough is

impaired for any reason this will result in retained secretions, possible bronchial obstruction, atelectasis and increased risk of pneumonia. Cough strength can be easily measured objectively using a peak flow meter (Smailes et al 2013b). Cough peak flow (CPF) is strongly associated with extubation outcome in patients after burn injury. This study showed that patients with a CPF of ≤60 L/min were nine times more likely to fail extubation as those with a CPF of ≥60 L/min (Smailes et al 2013b). Regular physiotherapy assessments, treatments and early usage of adjuncts to increase functional residual capacity and assist with airway clearance are often required, e.g. high-flow humidified oxygen and continuous positive airway pressure (CPAP).

5. **Sepsis:** Burn patients with sepsis have increased inotrope requirements and are less tolerant to physiotherapy intervention, and so it is important that having identified an indication for cardiorespiratory intervention from an assessment, the physiotherapist must balance the risk of the negative effects of poor tolerance to physiotherapy treatment against the risk of further deterioration if treatment is not carried out.

Readiness for Extubation. Physiotherapy also has an extended role assisting with decisions regarding the timing of extubation of patients. Burn patients present many challenges with achieving this goal because of the pathophysiology of injury coupled with the need for regular general anaesthetics or sedation for wound care procedures and these impair respiratory function and airway clearance. Use of the spontaneous breathing trial protocol as an objective method of determining burn patients' readiness for extubation leads to a shorter duration of ventilation (Smailes et al 2009a, b) and is therefore recommended. Indeed, use of weaning protocols in ICU in all patients groups are shown to be more effective in achieving extubation success. Positive pressure techniques (Chapter 7) (intermittent positive pressure breathing (IPPB), bi-level positive airway pressure (BiPAP) and CPAP) post extubation may reduce the work of breathing, facilitate lung expansion and reduce the risk of reintubation but non-invasive techniques are contraindicated with patients with face burns.

Physical Rehabilitation Following Burn Injury

Physical Rehabilitation for burn patients is grounded in the same principles as that for other conditions with emphasis on early active exercises and functional activities (see Rehabilitation for survivors of intensive care in this chapter). Special considerations for burn injury are explored in this section and principally relate to the formation of scar and contractures, which are inelastic structures, and if allowed to develop unhindered, result in significant physical morbidity.

The success of a physical rehabilitation programme for burn patients depends upon:

1. adequate preparation for active exercise
2. involvement of the patient and family in rehabilitation goals
3. provision of a daily rehabilitation programme.

Preparation for active exercise involves three key factors: consistent education, adequate pain relief and appropriate psychological support.

Education for the patient and their family/network of support regarding the benefits of exercise and the complications of inactivity, i.e. pressure sores, contractures, respiratory complications, should begin early following burn injury. As part of the education process, rehabilitation goals with deadlines should be set with the patient and their family so that all parties are aware of the aims of physical rehabilitation at any particular time.

Provision of adequate analgesia prior to active and passive exercise is paramount in gaining the trust and motivation of burn patients. Background analgesia should be supplemented by interventional shorter acting analgesia before exercise sessions with patients with open wounds. The physiotherapist should assess whether the analgesia provided is adequate for the rehabilitation session and feedback to other team members as necessary.

Since burn injury affects psychological functioning, psychotherapy and counselling should be available to all burn patients and their families from admission to hospital and for as long as it is needed. Psychotherapy assists with psychological rehabilitation though various stages of anxiety, depression and loss of control, and provides support to allow adjustment to injury. This empowers patients to take responsibility for their own recovery and participate fully in exercise programmes.

Contractures

A healed full thickness burn forms a scar in the weeks and months after autografting. The scar is unlike normal skin, as it lacks its elasticity and is therefore vulnerable to the development of contractures through long-term shrinkage. Contractures develop over the course of months through the presence of fibroblasts in the wound. The fibroblasts probably contract to further shrink the wound and this force, if left unopposed through patient inactivity, pulls the underlying joints into non-functional positions, leading to joint contractures, deformity and dysfunction (Greenhalgh 2007, Harrison et al 2008). Therefore joint deformity through contracture formation is especially prevalent where burns and autografts extend over joint surfaces.

Exercise Prescription

Physiotherapy exercise programs should commence early following burn injury and be continued for a minimum of 6 months to reduce the need for surgical releases of contractures and other reconstructive procedures (Celis et al 2003, Paratz et al 2012). Active or active assisted exercises with end of range holds are ideal to provide a sustained stretch in the opposite direction to potential skin contracture. Active ROM exercises can commence from the time of admission and are performed both with and without dressings in situ to ensure that full excursion of the joints and skin are maintained. Passive ROM exercises are only performed if the patient requires assistance to achieve full ROM or if the patient is sedated in ICU and unable to perform active movements.

Similar to all ICU patients, early mobilization and functional activities should commence as early as possible after admission while patients are receiving organ support as appropriate and with monitoring of vital signs. Activities such as sitting on the edge of the bed, use of the tilt table, standing marching and walking provide a gradual progression of activities according to muscle power and endurance. Compression bandages should be applied to the lower limbs before upright positioning to provide support to autografts. Appropriate measures to assess treatment outcomes should be incorporated into management (Chapter 6).

Anti-contracture positions (Table 13-5) facilitate extension of the joints to stretch the healing tissues and therefore discourage contracture formation. Joints near or under newly applied autografts should be immobilized in anti-contracture positions for short periods after autografting procedures (usually 5 days) and then progressed back to full ROM.

Once autografts are stable, combined joint active and active assisted movements with end of range holds provide a sustained stretch in the opposite direction to potential scar contractures and are recommended for all burn patients unless there are tendon injuries which require protected movements. Active ROM exercises are performed both with and without dressings in situ to ensure that full excursion of the joints and scar are maintained. Passive ROM exercises are performed if the patient requires assistance to achieve full ROM or for unconscious patients. Table 13-5 outlines some of the typical exercises used to prevent contractures dependent on the area burnt. Contracture prevention also requires regular scar moisturization and massage. Major burn injury results in overwhelming catabolism, which leads to deconditioning and lean muscle mass loss (Rojas et al 2012), but rehabilitation should progress as tolerated with aerobic and strength training in the gym. Theraband or light weights can be utilized as well as cycling, treadmills and rowing machines. The majority of burns patients should have a normal cardiorespiratory response to exercise training (Stockton et al 2012).

Box 13-2 lists the benefits of resistance and aerobic exercise programs in both adults and children.

Objective physical function scores are useful to index patients' functional ability, thus increasing patient motivation and assisting with decisions regarding discharge outcome. The Functional Assessment for

---

BOX 13-2

BENEFITS OF RESISTANCE AND AEROBIC EXERCISE PROGRAMS FOR ADULTS AND CHILDREN

- Increase lean muscle mass and muscle strength (Paratz et al 2012, Suman et al 2001, 2003)
- Improve pulmonary function, increase aerobic capacity and peak oxygen consumption (de Lateur et al 2007, Paratz et al 2012, Suman et al 2003)
- Reduce the need for surgical interventions for contracture release (Celis et al 2003, Paratz et al 2012)
- Improve health-related quality of life (Paratz et al 2012)

TABLE 13-5

Positioning and Exercise to Prevent Contractures

Area of Burn	Potential Contractures	Exercise	Anti-Contracture Position
Face	■ Eyelid contracture (ectropion) and inability to close eyes ■ Loss of facial expression ■ Difficulty closing mouth ■ Decreased mouth opening (microstomia)	■ Active facial expressions ■ Combine face exercises with neck movements	■ Mouth guards and microstomia splints ■ Taping for eyelids to assist closure
Neck	■ Anterior burns: flexion contracture with poor lower lip closure ■ Lateral burns: limitation to rotation and lateral flexion	■ Neck extension in combination with face exercises ■ Lateral flexion and rotation exercises	■ Neck extension pillow, use of towel/pillow under thoracic spine, no pillow under head in supine ■ Neck extension over edge of bed ■ Prone positioning
Trunk	■ Anterior trunk: shoulder protraction, kyphosis, decreased shoulder range, decreased trunk rotation ■ Posterior trunk: limitation to shoulder horizontal flexion, shoulder flexion	■ Shoulder flexion, abduction, external rotation, trunk extension, lateral flexion and rotation	■ Prone positioning, side lying over pillows or wedge with shoulder abduction
Axilla	■ Anterior axilla: limitations to shoulder abduction, horizontal abduction, external rotation, scapula retraction and trunk rotation ■ Posterior axilla: limitations to shoulder flexion, internal rotation and horizontal adduction	■ Scapula stability exercises, shoulder elevation: flexion/abduction, shoulder horizontal flexion, trunk rotation ■ Reciprocal pulleys, weighted stick, wall stretches	■ Prone lying with shoulders elevated ■ Hanging from overhead monkey bars/wall ladder ■ Supine with shoulders at 90-degree abduction with 20-degree forwards flexion ■ Use of axilla splints
Elbow	■ Elbow flexion contracture: limitation to full extension	■ Elbow extension, supination combined with wrist extension ■ Weight-bearing exercises, e.g. 4-point kneeling	■ Weight-bearing positions: 4-point kneeling, prone on elbows ■ Use of elbow splints
Wrist	■ Wrist flexion contracture: limitation to wrist extension	■ Wrist extension activities, e.g. prayer position, weight bearing on flat hands e.g. 4-point kneeling	■ Wrist extension splints
Hands	■ Dorsal hooding: increased webbing at finger web spaces ■ Palmar cupping ■ Little finger F/ABD/Ext Rot ■ Boutonniere deformities ■ Swan neck deformities ■ Intrinsic minus contracture: MCP extension, PIP/DIP flexion	■ Finger flexion isolated and combined, finger extension, thumb opposition, thumb extension and abduction, web space stretches especially for 1st web space ■ Functional hand activities ■ Grip strength, coordination, desensitization	■ Hand splinting ■ Use of pillows to elevate hands to decrease oedema
Hip	■ Hip flexion contractures	■ Hip extension, mobilization, walking backwards	■ Prone lying
Knee	■ Knee flexion contractures	■ Knee extension exercises, mobilization, walking backwards, walking on heels, exercise bike, calf stretches	■ Knee extension splint ■ Prone lying
Ankle and foot	■ Plantar flexion contractures ■ Toe extension contractures	■ Ankle dorsiflexion exercises, ambulation, wobble boards, calf stretches, squatting activities ■ Toe flexion exercises	■ Foot drop splints, pillows or wedges to keep feet at plantar grade position ■ Use of splints or moulds to extend toes

DIP, Distal interphalangeal joint; *F/ABD/Ext Rot,* Flexion, Abduction, External Rotation; *MCP,* metacarpophalangeal joint; *PIP,* proximal interphalangeal joint.

Burns (FAB) score is such a measure and has been shown to accurately predict patient discharge outcome early in the patient's course of treatment (Smailes et al 2013a, 2016).

Summary

The physiotherapist plays a very important role in the management of the patient with burn injuries, working as part of the multidisciplinary team to optimize cardiovascular, neuromuscular and functional outcomes. The physiotherapist is uniquely placed to follow the patient from the critical care management in the ICU through the long rehabilitation process to the outpatient follow-up several years after the initial injury to ensure optimal functional outcomes are achieved after such a devastating injury.

Head Injury Management

INTRODUCTION

There are a number of ways acquired brain injury may occur, most commonly due to stroke, subarachnoid haemorrhage or trauma. A severe traumatic brain injury (TBI) can be defined by a Glasgow Coma Scale (GCS) score between 3 and 8. The pathophysiology of TBI can be described in terms of primary and secondary brain injury. Primary brain injury is the initial damage of tissue or vessels at the time of the event and is irreversible. This can either be from focal contusions, intracerebral haematomas or diffuse axonal injury. Secondary brain injury is a process of a complex cascade of events which lead to further neuronal damage. This can be further exacerbated by hypoxaemia, hypercapnia, hypotension and intracranial hypertension. With expert critical care management these additional complications can be prevented or minimized. Within the critical care setting, maintenance of cerebral haemodynamics and oxygenation to the remaining brain tissue is essential (Haddad & Arabi 2012).

Types of Brain Injury

Cerebral Contusions

These are areas of 'bruising' in the brain tissue where the maximum effects of swelling and bleeding may not be seen until 72 hours following injury. The effects of the contusion will depend on its location and size.

Diffuse Axonal Injury

This is caused by rapid deceleration of the brain within the skull and produces widespread damage to axons. The CT scan shows a loss of grey and white differentiation (Fig. 13-6).

Extradural Haematoma

This occurs from damage to the middle meningeal artery which is outside of the extradural layer of the

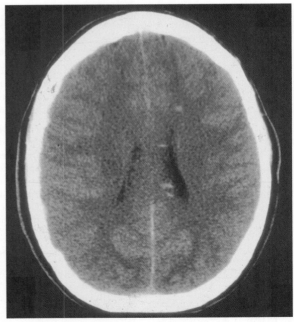

FIGURE 13-6 ■ Diffuse axonal injury. The CT scan demonstrates small haemorrhagic diffuse axonal injuries in the deep white matter and corpus callosum. *(Reproduced with permission from Wasenko & Hochhauser 2009.)*

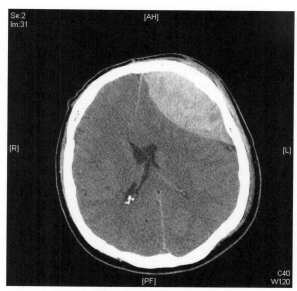

FIGURE 13-7 ■ Extradural haematoma. The CT scan demonstrates a lens-shaped lesion. *(Reproduced with permission from Rosenfeld, J 2012.)*

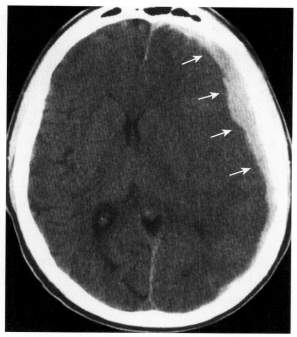

FIGURE 13-8 ■ Subdural haematoma. The CT scan shows a crescent-shaped lesion. *(Reproduced with permission from Myburgh, JA 2009.)*

meninges. This leads to a significant blood clot which can compress the brain. This requires urgent surgical evacuation as death is likely due to the high pressure of the arterial bleed. The CT scan will demonstrate a lens shape (Fig. 13-7).

Subdural Haematoma

This is usually venous in origin and occurs within the subdural space leading to compression of the brain. Acute injuries will require urgent surgical evacuation. Chronic haematomas are more commonly seen in the elderly and post–initial injury symptoms may develop in the following weeks. The CT scan will show a crescent shape (Fig. 13-8).

Intracranial Hypertension Management

Intracranial pressure (ICP) is defined as the pressure exerted with the cranial cavity. ICP is measured by insertion of a catheter through the skull into the lateral ventricle or by a subdural bolt. Within the critical care setting, ICP measurement and mean arterial pressure (MAP) are used to calculate cerebral perfusion pressure (CPP), which relates closely to cerebral blood flow

(CBF) and therefore oxygen and metabolite delivery: CPP = MAP–ICP. Therefore to enhance perfusion and to reduce the risk of further cerebral ischaemia following TBI, the ICP should be less than 20 mmHg (Normal ICP is 10–15 mmHg) and CPP should be maintained between 50 and 70 mmHg (Dunn & Smith 2008).

The partial pressure of carbon dioxide (PCO_2) has the most significant influence on CBF, where changes in PCO_2 will lead to alteration in vascular resistance. A rise in PCO_2 results in an increase in CBF due to vasodilatation, which will increase ICP. Traditionally, the management was to prophylactically hyperventilate to reduce PCO_2, leading to vasoconstriction and therefore reducing CBF and ICP. Evidence now suggests that hyperventilation can further compromise the perfusion of the brain, leading to further cerebral ischaemia and should only be used as a temporary measure. A PCO_2 target of 4.5–5.0 kPa should be used unless ICP is greater than 20 mmHg; then 4.0–4.5 kPa could be considered (Dunn & Smith 2008).

Further critical care ICP management strategies (Dutton & McCunn 2003) are listed:

- nursing 30 degrees head up to aid venous drainage
- head and neck to remain in neutral position to improve cerebral venous drainage and reduce ICP
- avoiding compression of internal and external jugular veins from a tight cervical collar
- sedation and paralysis in early stage to prevent ICP increases from coughing and painful stimulus and to decrease brain metabolism
- barbiturate coma for uncontrollable ICP
- anti-seizure prophylaxis for high-risk patients
- decompressive craniectomy for uncontrollable ICP.

Respiratory Consequences in Severe Acquired Brain Injury

Pneumonia is a common complication of the brain-injured patient in the early stages of their intensive care stay and can occur in up to 60% of patients. Several factors can put patients at risk of pneumonia, including aspiration of stomach contents, restricted movement and heavy sedation in the first few days. There is also a significant risk of ARDS, with an incidence of 10–30% (Lee & Rincon 2012).

Physiotherapy Management

Safe and effective treatment should be based on careful assessment with consideration of factors such as ICP, CPP, chest radiography and arterial blood gases (ABGs). It is essential to have good communication with the multi-disciplinary team (MDT) and several questions need to be considered to weigh up the benefits of treatment (Roberts 2002).

- Is respiratory physiotherapy indicated? How will treatment impact CPP and ICP?
- How does the patient tolerate nursing interventions such as positioning and how quickly does any increase in ICP return to baseline?
  Short bursts of increases in ICP may be acceptable within some critical care settings.
- Is the timing of physiotherapy intervention most optimal?
  Coordinate management so the patient does not receive multiple interventions in quick succession.

Patient should be treated in maximally sedated state.

There is evidence that respiratory physiotherapy may be beneficial in this patient group when indicated but **should not be carried out routinely.** Discussed in the following list are the effects of physiotherapeutic intervention on ICP. More information on manual and ventilator hyperinflation (VHI) is available in Chapter 7.

- There is conflicting evidence for the effects of manual hyperinflation (MHI). It is important to consider the rate of hyperinflation as this may have an impact on PCO_2 levels; i.e. if it is too slow, then this can lead to a rise in PCO_2 and vasodilatation. The effects of VHI have not been reported within the literature on this patient group.
- Ferreira et al (2013) completed a systematic review on the effects of respiratory physiotherapy (manual techniques and endotracheal suctioning) on ICP. They concluded that the evidence demonstrates there is an increase in ICP but no effect on CPP.
- Endotracheal suctioning has been shown to increase ICP and it is suggested that a bolus of sedation maybe required. However, if the patient is paralyzed, then the cough is suppressed and therefore does not impact ICP (Ersson et al 1990).

In the acute management of the acquired brain injury patient it is necessary for the physiotherapist to consider the following:

- maintenance of range of movement and monitoring changes of tone through passive movements (Williams, 1990)
- the provision of a 24-hour positioning programme which may include splinting; commencement of anti-spasticity medication for significant increases in tone
- when the patient is stable, consideration of early rehabilitation which may include mobilization, seating and standing on the tilt table. The aim is to preserve the integrity of the musculoskeletal system, stimulate the reticular system (regulating wakefulness), provide somatosensory stimulus and regain motor control.

Liver Disease

INTRODUCTION

The liver is the largest organ in the body. It plays a major role in metabolism and the maintenance of homoeostasis, carrying out a wide range of functions including storage of glycogen, decomposition of red blood cells, production of plasma proteins, hormone production and detoxification of the blood. The liver is the only organ in the body that has the ability to regenerate itself and can maintain a degree of function with up to 80–90% of its cells damaged. Liver failure occurs when the liver becomes damaged beyond repair and is therefore no longer able to function adequately. Insults to the liver result in inflammation and scaring which progress onto fibrosis and the development of cirrhosis with time.

The liver can fail acutely and rapidly due to viral insults or drug use. This is known as 'fulminant hepatic failure (FHF)'. The most common cause of FHF in the UK is paracetamol overdose, accounting for 70% of all acute cases. Liver disease may also occur more progressively and chronically, commonly due to cirrhosis secondary to alcohol consumption and chronic hepatitis.

Chronic liver disease (CLD) accounts for 98% of patients in the general population with liver failure. Towards the end stages of the disease, patients often require assessment for suitability for liver transplantation. FHF only accounts for 2% of patients with liver disease, but despite its less common presentation presents more complexities in terms of management.

Signs and Symptoms of Liver Disease

The signs and symptoms of liver failure vary between individuals but the most common ones include:

Jaundice: The most easily recognized symptom of liver failure evident by a yellowish discoloration of the skin and sclera due to a build up of bilirubin in the blood and extracellular fluid.

Encephalopathy: The occurrence of confusion, altered mental state and in severe cases coma due to the accumulation of toxic substances, in particular ammonia that are normally removed by the liver. Encephalopathy is another frequently seen symptom of liver disease and can be categorized into 4 grades ranging from mild confusion, disorientation and forgetfulness through to coma (Table 13-6). In more severe cases of hepatic encephalopathy (grades 3–4) patients may require intubation to enable further medical management of the condition, protecting and maintaining an airway.

Ascites: The accumulation of extra-cellular fluid in the peritoneal cavity. Portal hypertension combined with sodium and water retention alters interstitial capillary pressure and permeability, favouring transudation of fluid into the peritoneal cavity where it accumulates as ascites (Moore & Aithal 2006). The volume of ascites can range from minimal to several litres of fluid in the abdomen. Larger volumes of fluid result in a restrictive pattern of ventilation, hypoxia, breathlessness on exertion and reduced exercise tolerance. The treatment of ascites includes dietary sodium restriction, diuretics and paracentesis (drainage of the fluid from the peritoneal cavity).

Hepatic hydrothorax: An hepatic hydrothorax is a pleural effusion >500 mL that is a direct result of ascites. The low protein transudates flow into the pleural space via small diaphragmatic defects due to the pressure gradient created. This occurs in 5–10% of patients with ascites (Sargent 2006) and is also treated with sodium restriction, diuretics and paracentesis. Trans-jugular

TABLE 13-6	
Grades of Encephalopathy	
Grade of Encephalopathy	**Presentation**
Grade 1	Mild confusion, forgetfulness, irritability, inverted sleep wake cycle
Grade 2	Lethargy, disorientation, inappropriate behaviour, personality changes
Grade 3	Confusion, agitation, gross disorientation, somnolence (responsive to verbal stimuli)
Grade 4	Coma (unresponsive to pain or verbal stimuli)

intrahepatic portosystemic shunt (TIPSS) may be indicated for a difficult to control hydrothorax (Krowka 2000).

Oedema: Peripheral and pulmonary oedema occur due to the reduced ability of the damaged liver to synthesis plasma proteins such as albumin. This results in a fluid shift, with fluid being drawn from the vessels into the tissues and interstitial spaces via osmosis.

Muscle wasting: Patients with CLD display a marked decrease in muscle bulk resulting from a combination of a catabolic state and reduced activity levels (Stockton 2001, Vintro et al 2002). Protein malnutrition frequently develops in patients with end stage liver disease as carbohydrate stores are depleted, leading to the breakdown of muscle protein to provide energy (Larson & Curtis 2006, Stockton 2001). There may be a role for rehabilitation to maintain muscle mass, regain strength and maintain activity levels (Larson & Curtis 2006).

Fatigue: Fatigue is a common symptom of liver disease, closely related to the protein malnourishment of patients, muscle wasting, weakness and general malaise (Larson & Curtis 2006). Fatigue is often worsened by the reduced activity levels associated with CLD. However, there is no correlation between degree of fatigue and disease duration or severity (Wu et al 2011).

Pruritus: Itching of the skin associated with the build up of waste products.

Coagulopathy: The liver is responsible for producing clotting factors and proteins. Impairment of the clotting systems, along with reduced number and function of platelets mean patients with liver disease are more prone to bleeding, especially with invasive treatment techniques. Care should therefore be taken with any invasive procedures such as nasopharyngeal airway insertion or suction, and close monitoring of platelet levels is imperative. It may be appropriate for a patient to be given clotting products prior to invasive treatment techniques to minimize chances of severe bleeding occurring.

Oesophageal varices: Portal hypertension leads to the development of oesophageal varices, treatment of which aims to decompress the hypertensive portal vein and return blood to the systemic circulation. These engorged veins are susceptible to rupturing which can be life-threatening. Varices are treated with band ligation via gastroscopy which significantly decreases the risk of bleeding.

Hepatorenal syndrome (HRS): HRS is a result of CLD with portal hypertension. The local increased renal vascular resistance decreases renal perfusion and is associated with a decreased glomerular filtration rate and sodium ion (Na^{2+}) excretion. Vasopressins such as terlipressin are used to decrease renal vascular resistance and increase renal blood flow and glomerular filtration rate.

Osteoporosis: Osteoporosis occurs in up to 40% of CLD patients (Vintro et al 2002). There is abnormal bone metabolism, poor diet ± malnutrition, reduced physical activity and use of corticosteroids that further contribute to low bone mineral density.

Chronic Liver Disease

Liver disease usually develops progressively over the course of years and remains largely undetectable until scaring and cirrhosis become severe, resulting in irreversible damage. Patients present with many of the signs and symptoms above and may require frequent hospital admissions to treat the side effects of liver damage. As the degree of liver damage increases, patients may need to be assessed for suitability for liver transplantation.

Transplant assessment is carried out at regional transplant centres and is multi-factorial in nature. As well as assessing the degree of liver damage, transplant assessment also includes consideration of the patient's pre-morbid functional status, exercise tolerance, other comorbidities, social support networks, modification of any lifestyle factors (patients requiring transplantation for alcohol-related liver disease must be abstinent from drinking alcohol for 6 months prior to listing for transplant) and the ability to cope with the demands of a postoperative immunosuppressive drug regimen.

Throughout the assessment process and during the build-up to transplantation, patients have continued access to transplant coordinators who monitor progress and provide patients with relevant information and support.

Considerations for Physiotherapists

Patients with CLD will fluctuate in their clinical state and presentation. Recurrent episodes of encephalopathy, ascites and peripheral oedema impact the patients' level of function and ability to comply with treatment and exercise training.

Following assessment by a hepatologist, dietician and physiotherapist, dietary advice, exercise and weight reduction if indicated have the potential to reduce the risk factors associated with the progression of liver disease, improve quality of life and, in a proportion of patients, improve histological features of liver disease (Hickman et al 2004). It is recommended that rehabilitation programmes be individually tailored to meet patients' specific needs and should include a cool down to improve lactate clearance (Cassaburi & Oi, 1989).

Peripheral oedema may further impact patients mobility and functional levels. It may be necessary to consider the provision of walking aids or adaptive equipment to assist patient function until the oedema improves.

Cardiorespiratory abnormalities present in most patients with advanced liver disease, many of which are extra-pulmonary in origin. Arterial hypoxaemia is present in 30–70% of patients with cirrhosis (Moller & Henriksen 2006) and is often multifactorial in nature due to ascites, pleural effusions, pulmonary vasodilatations and fluid overload.

Moderate to severe ascites results in a restrictive pattern of ventilation characterized by rapid shallow respirations, dyspnoea, limited activity and variable degrees of hypoxaemia (Rosado & Banner 1996). An increase in intra-abdominal pressure results in increased rigidity of the abdominal wall and elevation of the diaphragm, reducing chest wall compliance and increasing energy consumption and work of breathing (Rosado & Banner 1996, Stockton 2001). Severe ascites also changes the patient's centre of gravity and affects their balance, which increases their risk of falls.

Pleural effusions cause further respiratory compromise on top of that already imposed by the presence of ascites (Stockton 2001). This often limits patient's ability to mobilize and exercise to an appropriate intensity.

Patients with liver disease present with a hyperdynamic circulation; resting tachycardia, bounding pulse, peripheral vasodilatation and arterial hypotension despite an increase in cardiac output and plasma volume due to the over-production of inflammatory cytokines (Sargent 2006, Stockton, 2001).

Consideration and advice should be given on positioning and pacing to help relieve symptoms of breathlessness and reduced exercise tolerance due to compromise of the cardiorespiratory system.

Hepatopulmonary Syndrome (HPS)

Hepatopulmonary syndrome (HPS) may occur in CLD and is characterized by a triad of conditions: liver disease, intrapulmonary vascular dilatations and hypoxaemia. It affects 15–30% of patients with cirrhosis and is associated with poorer outcomes and survival rates. There is no correlation between liver disease severity and severity of HPS (Gupta et al 2010, Martinez et al 2001).

The mechanism of pulmonary vessel dilatation is unknown but occurs predominantly in the bases of the lungs, possibly due to increased production or reduced hepatic clearance of vasodilators. These dilatations lead to over-perfusion in relation to ventilation, resulting in hypoxia and breathlessness which worsen when moving from supine to sitting as ventilation–perfusion ($\dot{V}/\dot{Q}$) matching is reduced in the upright position.

Platypnoea: increasing shortness of breath (SOB) when moving from lying to sitting.

Orthodeoxia: a reduction in oxygen saturations of 10% or more when moving from lying to sitting (Martinez et al 2001).

Clinical assessment and diagnosis of HPS includes ABGs and arterial oxygen saturation (SaO_2) in lying and sitting to assess for changes in the partial pressure of oxygen (PO_2) and an increase in alveolar–arterial oxygen gradient while breathing room air. The shunt can also be assessed while breathing on FiO_2 of 1. The gold standard diagnosis of HPS involves bubble echocardiography. Aggravated normal saline containing microbubbles (>10 μm) is injected into the jugular vein. These bubbles, normally trapped and absorbed by the small diameter pulmonary capillaries, readily transit the dilated vessels in HPS and are visible in the left ventricle on echocardiography.

Management of HPS involves supplementary oxygen for hypoxia and symptom relief, although there is no available evidence to support this. The only treatment to cure the syndrome is liver transplantation. A diagnosis of HPS increases a patients priority for liver transplant, as outcomes worsen with progression of the syndrome. Following transplant, signs and symptoms of HPS usually resolve within 2–3 months but have been reported to take up to 2 years in some cases (Fallon & Abrahams 2000). A complete resolution or significant improvement in gas exchange occurs in over 85% of patients with HPS post liver transplant (Lang & Stoller 1996).

Considerations for Physiotherapists

Due to reduced $\dot{V}/\dot{Q}$ matching in the upright position, patients may require an increase in supplementary oxygen when going from lying to the upright position.

Breathlessness often limits mobility, which can be improved with increased oxygen flow rates and advice on pacing and breaking up activities. Hypoxia during exercise is a significant problem, as further increases to an already elevated cardiac output reduces the transit time further and worsens oxygenation through formation of a greater functional shunt. (Thorens & Junod 1992). Strength training can be performed in supine to enable higher intensities while minimizing the oxygen (O_2) desaturation that occurs. These symptoms should improve post liver transplant.

Fulminant Hepatic Failure (FHF)

As previously mentioned, the liver more commonly fails progressively over the course of years. In fulminant hepatic failure, however, the problems develop over a much quicker time frame, usually a matter of days to weeks.

It is characterized by the rapid development of hepatocellular dysfunction, jaundice, coagulopathy and encephalopathy in a patient without known previous liver disease (Gotthardt et al 2007). The onset of encephalopathy usually occurs within 8 weeks of the first symptoms of liver failure, although it should be noted FHF itself can be further subdivided into hyperacute, acute and sub-acute stages.

Patients with FHF present with multi-organ failure which is phenotypically similar to severe septic shock. They frequently require ventilation and sedation, vaso-

pressor support to maintain an adequate blood pressure and renal replacement therapy to support kidney function and facilitate removal of ammonia. Cerebral oedema is a potential and serious complication of FHF. Its pathophysiology is not fully understood but thought to be multifactorial in origin. As the liver acutely fails, ammonia levels in the body rise. This rapid and subsequent hyperammonemia causes cerebral irritation and swelling. This is also combined with a loss of autoregulation in the brain, resulting in an increase in CBF and increased ICP. Raised ICP remains a significant clinical problem in FHF and is associated with poor overall outcome (Jalan et al 2004, O'Grady et al 1989).

Intracranial Dynamics

The Monro-Kellie doctrine states the cranial compartment is relatively incompressible and the volume inside the cranium therefore relatively fixed. The cranium and its constituents (blood, cerebrospinal fluid (CSF) and brain tissue) create a state of dynamic volume equilibrium such that any increase in volume of one of the cranial constituents must be compensated for by a relative decrease of another.

Increase in ICP due to FHF will initially result in a reduction in cerebral spinal fluid in an attempt to decrease ICP. This is followed by a reduction in blood flow as a secondary measure. If pressure within the skull remains increased, herniation of brain tissue through the foramen magnum occurs, leading to 'coning' and brain stem death.

A healthy brain will autoregulate, maintaining a constant rate of CBF by regulating cerebral vascular resistance. With the MAP in a normal range, the vasculature vasoconstrict or dilate to regulate a consistent CBF. If MAPs go outside of normal range, the brain loses the ability to autoregulate, with CPP becoming directly proportional to flow (Fig. 13-9). The loss of autoregulation presents the greatest risk of damage to brain tissue either due to ischaemia or increased ICP. An injured brain, as in the case of FHF, will be less able to autoregulate as the curve shifts to the right and thus becomes more sensitive to changes in MAP.

Measuring Intracranial Pressure.
The simplest indication of raised ICP is the monitoring of a patient's pupils. Pupils should constrict when a light is shone in the eyes. Dilated and sluggish pupils indicate the

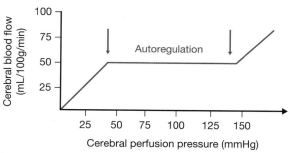

FIGURE 13-9 ■ Autoregulation of blood flow in the brain.

TABLE 13-7	
Neuroprotective Treatment of Fulminant Hepatic Failure	
Sedation	Maintain sedation level so patient unrousable
Position	Head of the bed elevated 15–30 degrees, head mid-line
Hypertonic saline infusion	Maintain sodium at 145–155 mmol
CVS support	Noradrenaline to maintain MAP and CPP
Therapeutic hypothermia	Core body temperature of 35–36°C.
Optimize ventilation	PCO_2 4.5–5 kPa (34–38 mmHg). PO_2 11–13 kPa (85–98 mmHg).
Haemodiafiltration	Decreases ammonia

CPP, Central perfusion pressure; *CVS*, cardiovascular system; *MAP*, mean arterial pressure; *PCO2*, partial pressure of carbon dioxide; *PO2*, partial pressure of oxygen.

presence of cerebral oedema with resultant pressure on the optic nerve. Pupillary response is a very crude indication of raised ICP, indicating presence but not the degree of cerebral oedema.

Jugular venous saturation of oxygen ($SjvO_2$) can be used to indirectly assess the brains ability to extract and metabolize oxygen, enabling further assessment of cerebral oedema (White & Baker 2002). Normal jugular venous saturations should be 60–75%. A reading obtained in excess of this indicates the potential presence of CBF in excess of metabolic demand. Low $SjvO_2$ suggests inadequate blood flow for demand.

The most accurate means to measure ICP and hence the degree of cerebral oedema is to place an ICP bolt directly into the brain parenchyma or subdural space. This provides a continuous and acute reading of pressure within the skull. Being an invasive monitoring technique, ICP bolt insertion is not without associated complications, including haemorrhage and infection: therefore the risk/benefit ratio should be calculated by the medical team prior to insertion (Lidofsky et al 1992).

ICP readings greater than 15 mmHg are indicative of intracranial hypertension.

Intracranial hypertension may also compromise CPP given their relationship: CPP = MAP–ICP.

Management of Fulminant Hepatic Failure

Initial management of patients with FHF involves neuroprotective strategies to minimize ICP and prevent secondary complications (Table 13-7).

Patients are maintained fully sedated and unrousable in the acute stages to prevent stimulation and subsequent increases in ICP. As a result, minimal intervention is recommended to avoid unnecessary surges

in ICP. Patients will typically be nursed with the head of the bed elevated 15–30 degrees, with the head kept in a neutral alignment to facilitate venous drainage.

Hypertonic saline (3–30%) is administered as a continuous infusion in an attempt to increase serum sodium levels to 145–155 mmol. This acts as an osmotic diuretic, drawing excess fluid out of the brain parenchyma and back into the circulation, subsequently reducing cerebral oedema and ICP.

Mild to moderate hypothermia to a core body temperature of 35–36°C is targeted with the aim of reducing cerebral metabolic rate and ICP (Stravitz & Larsen 2009) and decreasing the production of ammonia (Warrillow & Bellomo 2014). While there is insufficient data to strongly support recommendation of this approach for reducing mortality, prophylactic hypothermia may achieve more favourable neurological outcomes (Brain Trauma Foundation Guidelines for the Management of Severe Traumatic Brain Injury 2007).

FHF results in systemic vasodilatation and subsequent reduction in blood pressure. Cardiovascular support is often provided in the form of vasopressors to artificially increase MAP, maintaining autoregulation and CPP, and offsetting any increase in ICP. Care must be taken with patients not autoregulating, where increased blood pressure will lead to increased CBF and possible increased ICP.

Ventilation can also be manipulated to mange ICP. Ventilator settings are adjusted to maintain a PCO_2 of 4.5–5 kPa (34–38 mmHg). Carbon dioxide is a potent vasodilator; therefore any increase in PCO_2 will potentially increase CBF and ICP. By maintaining a PCO_2 towards the lower end of normal, increases to ICP are minimized while still maintaining adequate blood flow and perfusion to the brain. Hyperventilation should be avoided unless an acute emergency, as lowering PCO_2 levels below normal, may result in excessive vasoconstriction and secondary brain hypoxia (Stravitz et al 2007).

The FiO_2 delivered to the patient should be adequate to maintain a PO_2 between 11 and 13 kPa. Hypoxia will similarly result in vasodilatation with the subsequent increase in CBF, potentially raising ICP (Fig. 13-10).

On admission to intensive care and during their early clinical course, patients admitted with FHF are assessed as to the need for liver transplant. Assessment occurs against criteria that include: a lactate of more than 3.5 mmol, pH less than 7.3, an unsupported International Normalized Ratio (INR) of more than 6.5, renal failure and the presence of grade 3–4 encephalopathy prior to intubation. If these criteria are met and the patient deemed appropriate, urgent listing for liver transplant occurs.

Those not meeting criteria or deemed inappropriate for transplant due to other psychosocial reasons continue to receive supportive medical management while allowing the liver the opportunity to spontaneously regenerate and regain function in time.

Considerations for Physiotherapists

FHF presents many challenges to management due to the potential for increased ICP and its subsequent deleterious consequences.

Initially patients present with few respiratory problems, as intubation has been initiated to facilitate further medical management rather than underlying chest pathology. Over time, chest complications may

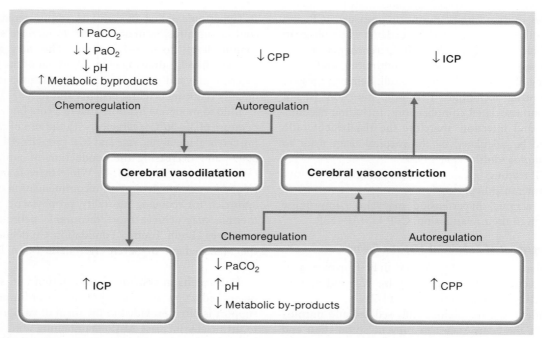

FIGURE 13-10 ■ Chemoregulation and autoregulation of intracranial pressure (ICP). *CPP,* Cerebral perfusion pressure; *PaCO₂,* arterial partial pressure of carbon dioxide; *PaO₂,* arterial partial pressure of oxygen.

arise due to progressive basal atelectasis and a $\dot{V}/\dot{Q}$ mismatch secondary to prolonged positioning in a semi-recumbent position. ARDS is a common complication of FHF due to the systemic inflammatory response from the damaged hepatocytes. Protective ventilation strategies may be usefully employed in such cases, albeit with close monitoring and manipulation of the associated hypercapnia.

The maintenance of deep sedation to minimize surges in ICP will result in the suppression of the cough reflex. This potentially impacts on the clearance of secretions and subsequent impairment in gas exchange which may affect ICP.

Any treatment needs to weigh up the benefits of treating the chest against the potentially deleterious effects on cerebral status and may require close liaison with the medical team. Please see Chapter 9, Adult Intensive Care, for further information on physiotherapy management in ICU and management of ICP.

During recovery, physiotherapy issues often relate to those associated with ICU-AW following prolonged ICU admission (see the section on rehabilitation for survivors of intensive care in this chapter).

Conclusion

Patients with liver disease are a challenging group of patients to manage. The majority of patients present with CLD characterized by a fluctuating picture of recurrent encephalopathy, ascites, oedema, muscle wasting and fatigue. Physiotherapy intervention for this population primarily centres on functional rehabilitation and management of symptoms associated with CLD. While cardiorespiratory abnormalities present in most patients with advanced liver disease, many of these are extra-pulmonary in origin and therefore not primarily amenable to physiotherapy interventions. Many symptoms of CLD may, however, directly impact physiotherapy treatment.

FHF is less common in occurrence but presents more complexities to management. Patients presenting with FHF and raised ICP should be managed using neuroprotective strategies. Interventions should be kept to the necessary minimum and treatment will often involve MDT discussion to weigh up the benefits of treating the patient's chest while preserving cerebral status. Rehabilitation after prolonged ICU admission is also important for these patients.

Spinal Cord Injury

INTRODUCTION

In North America, Western Europe and Australia, spinal cord injury (SCI) most commonly occurs as a result of motor vehicle accidents, with falls from trees and rooftops being the most frequent cause in South-East Asia and Oceania (Cripps et al 2011). A worldwide survey showed the average person with traumatic SCI is likely to be male, in his early 30s with a 70% chance of being paraplegic and a 50% likelihood of having a complete lesion (Wyndaele & Wyndaele 2006). SCI may also be secondary to non-traumatic causes such as vascular abnormalities, tumours or infection (New & Sundararajan 2008). The incidence of traumatic SCI is 15 per million per year in Australia, 16 in Europe and 40 in North America (Lee et al 2013).

The prognosis of a person sustaining SCI was poor until the latter part of the twentieth century. Although survival rates for those who sustain an SCI in developed countries continue to improve (Kemp & Krause 1999), tetraplegia remains a life-threatening condition with low survival rates in developing countries (Cripps et al 2011). In sub-Saharan Africa the occurrence of a SCI is likely to be fatal within a year (Cripps et al 2011). In Australia, Middleton et al (2012) found that 8.2% of those with tetraplegia died within the first year compared to 4.1% of those with paraplegia. Yeo et al (1998) found a projected mean life expectancy of 84% of normal for paraplegia and 70% for tetraplegia.

Respiratory complications remain the most common cause of mortality following SCI (DeVivo et al 1999, Fishburn et al 1990, NSCISC Report 2013). Patients are most vulnerable to respiratory illness in the first year after injury, but continue to suffer from respiratory complications throughout life. The number of respiratory complications suffered during initial admission is more important than level of injury in determining length of stay and hospital costs (Winslow et al 2002).

ACUTE SPINAL CORD INJURY AND RESPIRATION

Effects of Spinal Cord Injury

The ability to breathe deeply and cough forcefully is impaired to varying degrees depending on the level and completeness of the SCI, with greater dysfunction seen at higher injury levels (Linn et al 2000, Vazquez et al 2013). Figure 13-11 lists the muscles of respiration and their level of innervation. Immediately following a traumatic SCI, there is a period of spinal shock resulting in flaccid paralysis of the muscles below the level of injury, which lasts for a period of weeks to months (Ditunno et al 2004). Flaccid paralysis of the intercostal muscles creates an unstable chest wall so that the negative intrathoracic pressure occurring during inspiration causes paradoxical inward depression of the ribs (Lucke 1998, Menter et al 1997) (Fig. 13-12). These forces favouring airway closure may lead to microatelectasis and increased work of breathing (Fishburn et al 1990). The major factor favouring opening of the airways is the negative pressure generated during inspiration. This force is greatly reduced due to paralysis. Mucus can block the inflow of air, and the paralyzed patient has trouble keeping the airways free of mucus because of weakness of the cough. It is during this time that patients are most likely to require intubation and ventilation for respiratory support (Claxton et al 1998).

Initially those with a lesion level at or above C4 are more likely to develop pneumonia, with lower cervical injuries developing atelectasis (Jackson and Groomes 1994). Ventilatory failure has been shown to occur most frequently in the first 4.5 ± 1.2 days after injury (Jackson & Groomes 1994). Decreased lung expansion, increased volume of pulmonary secretions (Slack & Shucart 1994) and decreased surfactant production (Wong et al 2012) may explain the reduction in lung compliance seen acutely. The long-term picture of respiratory impairment is a restrictive defect characterized by low lung volumes resulting from loss of inspiratory muscle strength (De Troyer & Heilporn 1980; Scanlon et al 1989) and impaired cough secondary to loss of expiratory muscles, including the abdominal muscles, expiratory intercostals, pectorals and latissimus dorsi (De Troyer & Estenne 1991; Fujiwara

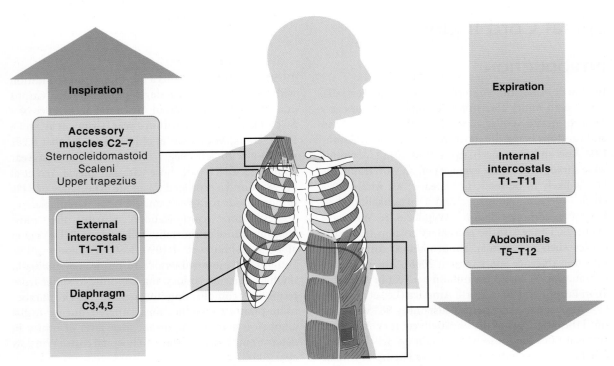

FIGURE 13-11 ■ Innervation of respiratory muscles.

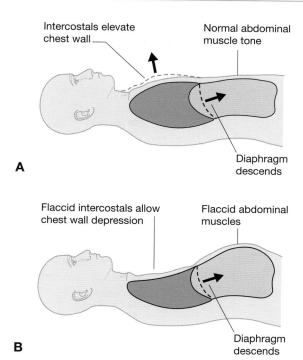

Intercostals elevate chest wall

Normal abdominal muscle tone

Diaphragm descends

A

Flaccid intercostals allow chest wall depression

Flaccid abdominal muscles

Diaphragm descends

B

FIGURE 13-12 ■ Paradoxical breathing in supine.

et al 1999). Obstructive respiratory changes have also been noted secondary to reduction in sympathetic innervation of those with lesions above T6 (Urdaneta & Layon 2003) (see Table 13-9).

With time, the tendons, ligaments and joints of the ribcage stiffen as a result of decreased active movement. This, together with spasticity of the intercostals, will stabilize the ribcage, so that paradoxical breathing lessens (Axen et al 1985; Mansel & Norman 1990). The resolution of spinal shock generally results in improved lung volumes.

Neurological Level and Completeness

The American Spinal Injury Association (ASIA) has established a neurological classification testing procedure, now internationally endorsed as the ASIA Impairment Scale (AIS) (Fig. 13-13). This scale provides clinicians with a common language for the description of neurological function by assessing sensory and motor function at key dermatomes and myotomes. The level of completeness of the damage is also reported. Further information can be found at http://www.asia-spinalinjury.org/elearning/elearning .php (accessed 12 Jan 2016).

The risk of respiratory failure is directly associated with injury level. Patients may lose up to one AIS level within the first few days of injury as a result of cord swelling or bleeding, making this a high-risk period (Como et al 2005). A patient with a complete injury above C5 will have impaired diaphragm function. They are likely to require endotracheal intubation and mechanical ventilation on presentation (Hassid et al 2008). A C5 injury level may also involve diaphragm weakness but is more likely to be associated with the ability to breathe independently. Impaired inspiration, lack of cough strength and no movement of the hands, trunk and lower limbs are seen. A patient with a complete T12 classification will have no observable inspiratory or expiratory impairment, full upper body strength, good trunk strength and balance, but no movement of the lower limbs. An understanding of this classification allows the clinician to predict the likely needs and respiratory management of their patient (Table 13-8).

Incomplete injuries have some feeling and often movement preserved below the level of injury. The degree of incompleteness will indicate the remaining function of the muscles and systems below the lesion. Hence early neurological testing is important. Neurological testing may also need to incorporate an assessment for brain injury, as TBI occurs in 24% of patients with a primary diagnosis of cervical SCI (Michael et al 1989). Traumatic SCI may also result in thoracic cage trauma, including rib fractures and damage to internal organs such as liver and spleen lacerations. Immediate full body screening will allow timely diagnosis and ensure any respiratory intervention takes this into account.

Orthopaedic Management

The level and completeness of the neurological dysfunction dictates the most appropriate orthopaedic management after acute spinal cord injury. Traumatic injuries to the spinal column require stabilization. Stabilization may initially be achieved by immobilizing the patient and using skulls tongs and traction for cervical injuries to maintain alignment and provide relative decompression. Conservative management by immobilization for up to 12 weeks was the most common management worldwide up until 20 years ago (El Masri 2010). Surgical decompression and fixation is now utilized in most specialist centres, with

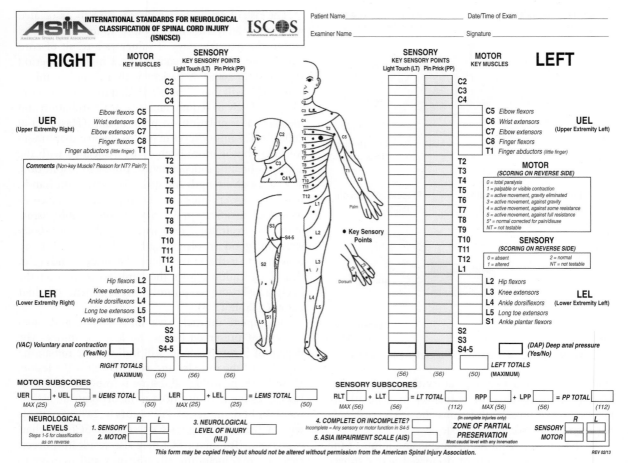

FIGURE 13-13 ■ American Spinal Injury Association (ASIA) International Standards Worksheet.

surgery performed as soon as possible after injury (Fehlings et al 2012). However, in less well resourced countries, conservative management is more likely due to the surgical cost (Shamim et al. 2011).

Goals of surgical management in patients with traumatic SCI are (1) to decompress neural tissue and (2) to prevent further cord injury by ensuring mechanical stability of the spine (Stevens et al 2003). For cervical injury, surgery is usually via an anterior approach with the need to also fix posteriorly being less common. Potential complications from an anterior approach include transient sore throat, dysphagia, hoarseness, dysphonia, recurrent laryngeal nerve paralysis, oesophageal perforation and respiratory insufficiency as a result of upper airway obstruction (Sagi et al 2002). Patients

with acute cervical SCI are predisposed to swallowing abnormalities. Chaw et al (2012) identified dysphagia in 30.9% of a prospective cohort of 68 individuals with acute cervical SCI. Predictive risk factors included tracheostomy, mechanical ventilation and presence of a nasogastric tube. There was also a significant increase in the incidence of pneumonia in the dysphagic group, indicating the need for early identification and management of those with impaired swallow.

Cardiovascular and Autonomic Impact on Respiration

In the acute post-injury period of spinal shock, not only is there flaccid paralysis of the muscles below the injury, in lesions above T6 there is also a reduction in

Muscle Function Grading

0 = total paralysis

1 = palpable or visible contraction

2 = active movement, full range of motion (ROM) with gravity eliminated

3 = active movement, full ROM against gravity

4 = active movement, full ROM against gravity and moderate resistance in a muscle specific position

5 = (normal) active movement, full ROM against gravity and full resistance in a functional muscle position expected from an otherwise unimpaired person

5* = (normal) active movement, full ROM against gravity and sufficient resistance to be considered normal if identified inhibiting factors (i.e. pain, disuse) were not present

NT = not testable (i.e. due to immobilization, severe pain such that the patient cannot be graded, amputation of limb, or contracture of > 50% of the normal range of motion)

Sensory Grading

0 = Absent

1 = Altered, either decreased/impaired sensation or hypersensitivity

2 = Normal

NT = Not testable

Non Key Muscle Functions (optional)

May be used to assign a motor level to differentiate AIS B vs. C

Movement	Root level
Shoulder: Flexion, extension, abduction, adduction, internal and external rotation **Elbow:** Supination	C5
Elbow: Pronation **Wrist:** Flexion	C6
Finger: Flexion at proximal joint, extension. **Thumb:** Flexion, extension and abduction in plane of thumb	C7
Finger: Flexion at MCP joint **Thumb:** Opposition, adduction and abduction perpendicular to palm	C8
Finger: Abduction of the index finger	T1
Hip: Adduction	L2
Hip: External rotation	L3
Hip: Extension, abduction, internal rotation **Knee:** Flexion **Ankle:** Inversion and eversion **Toe:** MP and IP extension	L4
Hallux and Toe: DIP and PIP flexion and abduction	L5
Hallux: Adduction	S1

ASIA Impairment Scale (AIS)

A = Complete No sensory or motor function is preserved in the sacral segments S4-5

B = Sensory Incomplete Sensory but not motor function is preserved below the neurological level and includes the sacral segments S4-5 (light touch or pin prick at S4-5 or deep anal pressure) AND no motor function is preserved more than three levels below the motor level on either side of the body

C = Motor Incomplete Motor function is preserved below the neurological level**, and more than half of key muscle functions below the neurological level of injury (NLI) have a muscle grade less than 3 (Grades 0-2)

D = Motor Incomplete Motor function is preserved below the neurological level**, and at least half (half or more) of key muscle functions below the NLI have a muscle grade ≥ 3

E = Normal If sensation and motor function as tested with the ISNCSCI are graded as normal in all segments, and the patient had prior deficits, then the AIS grade is E. Someone without an initial SCI does not receive an AIS grade

** For an individual to receive a grade of C or D, i.e. motor incomplete status, they must have either (1) voluntary anal sphincter contraction or (2) sacral sensory sparing with sparing of motor function more than three levels below the motor level for that side of the body. The International Standards at this time allow even non-key muscle function more than 3 levels below the motor level to be used in determining motor incomplete status (AIS B versus C)

NOTE: When assessing the extent of motor sparing below the level for distinguishing between AIS B and C, the **motor level** on each side is used; whereas to differentiate between AIS C and D (based on proportion of key muscle functions with strength grade 3 or greater) the **neurological level of injury** is used

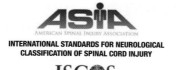

INTERNATIONAL STANDARDS FOR NEUROLOGICAL CLASSIFICATION OF SPINAL CORD INJURY

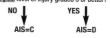

Steps in Classification

The following order is recommended for determining the classification of individuals with SCI

1. Determine sensory levels for right and left sides.
The sensory level is the most caudal, intact dermatome for both pin prick and light touch sensation

2. Determine motor levels for right and left sides.
Defined by the lowest key muscle function that has a grade of at least 3 (on supine testing), providing the key muscle functions represented by segments above that level are judged to be intact (graded as a 5)
Note: In regions where there is no myotome to test, the motor level is presumed to be the same as the sensory level, if testable motor function above that level is also normal

3. Determine the neurological level of injury (NLI)
This refers to the most caudal segment of the cord with intact sensation and antigravity (3 or more) muscle function strength, provided that there is normal (intact) sensory and motor function rostrally respectively
The NLI is the most cephalad of the sensory and motor levels determined in steps 1 and 2

4. Determine whether the injury is Complete or Incomplete.
(i.e. absence or presence of sacral sparing)
If voluntary anal contraction = No AND all S4-5 sensory scores = 0 AND deep anal pressure = No, then injury is Complete
Otherwise, injury is Incomplete

5. Determine ASIA Impairment Scale (AIS) Grade:

Is injury Complete?   If YES, AIS=A and can record
NO ↓   ZPP (lowest dermatome or myotome on each side with some preservation)

Is injury Motor Complete?   If YES, AIS=B
NO ↓   (No=voluntary anal contraction OR motor function more than three levels below the motor level on a given side, if the patient has sensory incomplete classification)

Are at least half (half or more) of the key muscles below the neurological level of injury graded 3 or better?
NO ↓   YES ↓
AIS=C   AIS=D

If sensation and motor function is normal in all segments, AIS=E
Note: AIS E is used in follow-up testing when an individual with a documented SCI has recovered normal function. If at initial testing no deficits are found, the individual is neurologically intact; the ASIA Impairment Scale does not apply

FIGURE 13-13, cont'd

---

sympathetic nervous system activity (Ditunno et al 2004) and an unopposed expression of parasympathetic activity via the vagus nerve (Berlly & Shem 2007, Bravo et al 2001, Garstang & Miller-Smith 2007, Yardley et al 1989) (Table 13-9).

Impaired control of the autonomic nervous system seen in individuals with high thoracic and cervical SCI can lead to hypotension and cardiac arrhythmias. The most common arrhythmia seen is bradycardia. Higher, more complete injuries will result in more significant arrhythmias and these are most common in the first 14 days (Lehmann et al 1987).

Additional associated cardiovascular concerns in SCI include deep vein thrombosis (DVT) and long-term risk for coronary heart disease. DVT incidence is high after SCI, at up to 27.6%, and has been shown to correlate with an absence of spasticity (Do et al 2013).

Pulmonary Oedema and Pulmonary Embolism

Pulmonary oedema can affect as many as 50% of individuals with acute tetraplegia (Lanig & Peterson 2000). The causes are multifactorial and include excessive fluid resuscitation in the presence of hypotension in the acute post-injury setting. The physiotherapist needs to be aware of this, as medical staff balance the need for maintenance of adequate blood pressure and potential respiratory compromise.

The risk of pulmonary embolism (PE) is increased following acute SCI with an incidence of 4.6% (Waring

TABLE 13-8
Neurological Level for Complete SCI and Expected Respiratory Dysfunction

Neurological Level	Dysfunction
C1-C3	Likely dependent on ventilator full time for breathing as diaphragm either completely paralyzed or significantly impaired. May have the ability to come off the ventilator for short periods of time if able to perform frog/glossopharyngeal breathing. Potential candidate for diaphragm pacing.
C3-C4	Diaphragm function will be impaired, reducing tidal volume and vital capacity. Periods of ventilator-free time possible, may manage with nocturnal ventilation alone if lung volumes high enough during day in sitting and supine.
C5	Independent respiration possible in long term. May require initial period of ventilator assistance. Diaphragm function intact but intercostal and abdominal muscle paralysis leads to ↓ lung volume and ↓cough strength.
C6-8	Independent respiration. Lesions closer to C8 and below have the ability to augment inspiration and cough with accessory muscles, particularly pectoralis major and minor.
T1-T4	Intercostal activity will ↑ inspiratory capacity and forced expiration. Abdominal activity unlikely to be present at this level to ↑ cough.
T5-T12	Significantly more intercostal and abdominal activity present with descending lesion levels. Minimal disruption to autonomic dysfunction affecting the cardiovascular system with lesions below T6 (see Table 13-9).
T12	Respiratory function essentially comparable to that of an able-bodied person.

Brown et al 2006, Chiodo et al 2008, Hassid et al 2008, Jackson and Groomes 1994.
SCI, Spinal cord injury.

TABLE 13-9
Impact of Autonomic Disruption in Lesions Above T6

Impact of Autonomic Disruption in Lesions Above T6	References
Bradycardia	Garstang & Walker 2011
	Heary et al 2011
Bronchial hyperreactivity which responds to bronchodilator therapy	Mateus et al 2006
	Barratt et al 2012
	Schilero et al 2005
Hypersecretion of bronchial mucus	Bhaskar et al 1991
Hypotension	Garstang & Walker 2011
	Heary et al 2011

and Karunas 1991), and is not infrequent in chronic SCI with an incidence of 0.4% identified in a review by Frisbie and Sharma in 2012. The clinical signs of PE, tachypnea, tachycardia and hypoxia often combined with a raised core temperature, may initially be noted by the physiotherapist. Awareness of the diagnosis can facilitate timely treatment and resolution of the symptoms of what can be a life-threatening complication (Ragnarrson 2012).

Lung Volumes

Lung function and respiratory muscle pressure generating capacity change over time and are correlated with lesion level (Mueller et al 2008). Repeated measurements of vital capacity provide an indication of trends developing in respiratory function (Lucke 1998). Vital capacity may fall over the first few days following injury owing to muscle and/or patient fatigue, sputum retention or oedema, which may result in a rise in neurological level (Alderson 1999). Lucke (1998) reported initial vital capacities of 24% of predicted normal values in mid-cervical injuries and 31% in lower cervical injuries. Baydur et al (2001) reported a mean FVC of 57% in acute tetraplegic individuals and 86% in paraplegic individuals compared to predicted values in patients with chronic SCI. Improvement is usually seen as oedema resolves and respiratory function stabilizes (Axen et al 1985, Ledsome & Sharp 1981). Vital capacity values of less than 15 mL per kilogram of bodyweight may, in conjunction with clinical assessment, indicate the need for ventilation (Thomas & Paulson 1994). Total lung capacity and functional residual capacity are also reduced. Residual volume may remain the same or increase slightly, although this increase is not associated with an increase in total lung capacity (Stepp et al 2008).

Positioning

Positional changes affect the respiratory function of the tetraplegic and high paraplegic individual differently than the able bodied person. In supine, the weight of the abdominal contents forces the diaphragm to a higher resting level so that contraction produces greater excursion of the diaphragm. The diaphragm will function more effectively when starting from a more cephalad position due to the orientation of its fibres (Fig. 13-14). In sitting or standing, the abdominal contents move inferiorly and anteriorly, resulting in a lower and flatter position of the diaphragm, decreasing effectiveness and restricting available excursion in those patients without functioning abdominal

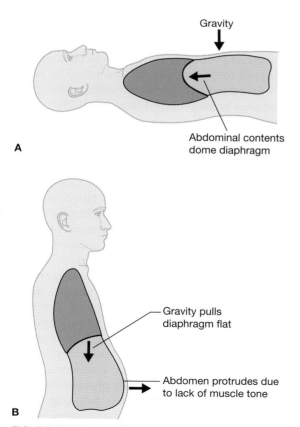

A

Gravity

Abdominal contents dome diaphragm

B

Gravity pulls diaphragm flat

Abdomen protrudes due to lack of muscle tone

FIGURE 13-14 ■ Diaphragm and the effect of position.

muscles (Chen et al 1990, Lucke 1998). Chen et al (1990) recorded a 14% drop in predicted vital capacity and Linn et al (2000) showed a statistically significant decrease in FVC in the tetraplegic person on changing from supine to sitting or standing. Conversely, vital capacity of the tetraplegic person rises by 6% when the bed is tipped 15 degrees head down from supine (Cameron et al 1955). Further evidence for the use of Trendelenburg (head-down) positioning is reported prolongation of spontaneous breathing trials in ventilated patients with low cervical SCI (Gutierrez et al 2010). Head-down position must be used with caution to prevent the risk of reflux and vomiting.

Patients do report less breathlessness in supine compared to sitting during the acute stage after high SCI (Arora et al 2012). Positioning should be considered when a patient is experiencing breathlessness or weaning from ventilation, as the use of supine positioning may seem counter-intuitive based on experience in other patient groups.

Cough

The ability to produce an effective cough is severely impaired in patients with cervical or high thoracic SCI (Roth et al 1997, Wang et al 1997). This is most marked during spinal shock when the muscles are flaccid and the ribcage is at its most mobile. Patients who have loss of innervation to the abdominal muscles and the internal intercostals lose the ability to produce a forced expiration (Gouden 1997). De Troyer & Estenne (1991) have shown that patients with injuries at C5–8 can utilize the clavicular portion of pectoralis major to generate an expulsive force, although the extent to which this is functional is not clear. Linn et al (2000) found that in a group of patients with high tetraplegia, peak expiratory flow rate was less than 50% of predicted normal values. The most effective peak cough flows can be achieved with a positive pressure–supported inspiration followed by expiration augmented by a manually assisted cough (Bach 1993).

Sleep-Disordered Breathing and Sleep Apnoea Syndrome

The most significant sleep-related respiratory problems post SCI are sleep hypoventilation and obstructive sleep apnoea (OSA) (Castriotta et al 2012). OSA has a prevalence of 40–83% post cervical SCI

(Berlowitz et al 2005, Burns et al 2000, Leduc et al 2007, Stockhammer et al 2002, Tran et al 2010). In the general population, untreated sleep disorders are associated with cardiovascular disease and impaired cognition (Punjabi 2008). Neurocognitive impairments including decreased memory and attention have also been linked to nocturnal hypoxia in tetraplegic individuals with untreated OSA (Sajkov et al 1998). Studies in chronic SCI have found a positive correlation with age, body mass index (BMI) and neck circumference (Burns et al 2000, McEvoy et al 1995, Stockhammer et al 2002). In contrast, Berlowitz et al (2005) noted that the usual risk factors for OSA do not appear to be important in acute tetraplegia. An individual with acute tetraplegia and undiagnosed or untreated OSA may struggle to participate in the demanding process of rehabilitation. Ongoing cognitive impairment will also be of significance for an individual whose future employment opportunities are skewed towards computer and desk-based tasks.

RESPIRATORY ASSESSMENT

Assessment is discussed in Chapter 2; Post SCI; particular note should be made of the following:

1. Neurological examination: Determines respiratory muscle innervation and hence likely function (Roth et al 1997).
2. Associated injuries: Rib fractures, flail segments, pneumothorax and pulmonary contusions are often associated with thoracic SCI. Patients involved in diving accidents may aspirate. Thoracic and intra-abdominal trauma or complications such as paralytic ileus, acute gastric dilatation or gastrointestinal bleeding will require modification of the techniques used by the physiotherapist, especially manually assisted coughing.
3. Visual assessment of breathing pattern: Identifies paradoxical or unequal movement of the chest wall. Determines whether intercostal activation present by way of lateral ribcage movement.
4. Assessment of diaphragm function: View the patient in supine from the foot of the bed to assess symmetry. Inspect and palpate the upper abdomen. Ask the patient to sniff which selectively recruits the diaphragm.

5. Cough: Listen to the sound of the cough and observe the abdomen for signs of muscle activity. Assess ability to take a deep breath, hold and then expel forcefully; note what components are affected.
6. Lung function testing: Forced vital capacity (FVC) should be measured at the time of admission and subsequently to monitor for signs of respiratory deterioration. Forced expiratory volume in 1 second (FEV_1) will identify any obstructive impairment and peak cough flow should be measured to quantify cough strength.
7. Psychological state: Major psychological adjustment is required by the patient with SCI, not only to the injury itself but also to the necessary treatment procedures. Sensory deprivation, enforced immobilization, fragmented sleep and limited communication can lead to anxiety or contribute to delirium.

PHYSIOTHERAPY TREATMENT

Until the mid 90s, traumatic cervical SCI was managed with skull tongs, traction and bed rest. The past 20 years have seen early surgical stabilization of the spine being widely adopted (Fehlings et al 2010, 2012). Patients are intubated for surgery and admitted to intensive care postoperatively on ventilation. Once surgically stabilized, patients are cleared to sit out of bed. Upright positioning while a patient is in spinal shock may lead to increased work of breathing and hypotension. Use of an abdominal binder and anti-hypotensive medication may to some extent counteract this, but the physiotherapist must proceed cautiously, monitoring for signs of fatigue and dizziness.

Secretion and ventilation management of individuals with acute cervical SCI differs from that required by individuals with pulmonary dysfunction secondary to non-neurological injuries (Wong et al 2012). Secretions accumulate secondary to increased production (Bhaskar et al 1991), poor cough and, in some instances, aspiration of saliva. Atelectasis leads to impaired aeration, infection and pneumonia (Berlly & Shem 2007). A literature review of respiratory management during the first 6 weeks following cervical SCI showed a protocol using a combination of techniques which may include IPPB, manually assisted coughing, respiratory muscle resistance training, non-invasive ventilation (NIV) and/or a clinical pathway is most likely to provide positive outcomes (Berney et al 2011a).

Injuries above the level of C5 with AIS A classification have the highest incidence of intubation and ventilation with rates of up to 90% (Como et al 2005, Hassid et al 2008). Early intervention with a non-invasive ventilatory technique may avoid progression of respiratory failure and the need for sedation, intubation and invasive mechanical ventilation (Bach 2012, Tromans et al 1998). However, failure to intubate in a timely way in the presence of tetraplegia can lead to the need for emergency airway intervention (Ball 2001, Como et al 2005) or catastrophic airway loss and death (Hassid et al 2008). In a generalist unit not familiar with SCI specific management, intubation and invasive ventilation followed by the use of a tracheostomy to facilitate weaning from ventilation, may provide the safest option for the patient.

Physiotherapy goals for treatment of the ventilated patient are the same as those for the non-ventilated patient. Treatment may include postural drainage, volume augmentation with manual or VHI, and suction or exsufflation to remove secretions (Berney et al 2011a, b, Wong et al 2012). Patients requiring ventilation due to complications from SCI are often not sedated and a system of communication must be established before physiotherapy is started.

Frequent brief treatments are desirable, as acutely injured patients will tire quickly. Treatment must be effective, using two physiotherapists if necessary. Where possible, linking with planned position changes will optimize efficiency and allow rest between procedures.

Secretion Clearance

Assisted Coughing

A large inspiratory effort followed by a quick and forceful expiration is required in order to achieve a successful cough. Utilizing techniques to increase inspiratory volume outlined in the following paragraphs will allow more efficient airway clearance. Expiratory assistance is provided by the application of a compressive force directed inwards and upwards under the diaphragm and compression of the ribcage, thus replacing the work of the abdominal and internal intercostal muscles (Fig. 13-15). The sound of the resultant cough is the best indicator of the force required. Pressure directed down through the abdomen must be avoided in the acute patient, in the presence of abdominal injury or with paralytic ileus. Care should also be taken in the presence of rib fractures or other chest injuries and therapists should position their hands away from the problem area to perform an assisted cough.

Frownfelter and Massery (2006) describe various methods of achieving assisted cough. The technique needs to be relatively forceful and it is advisable for the therapist to lower the bed to gain the most advantageous position from which to perform the technique. The spinal stability of the patient must be carefully considered and a shoulder hold should be used to counter any movement of an unstable cervical spine (see Fig. 13-15D and E). The therapist must synchronize the applied compressive force with the expiratory effort of the patient. Once the cough is completed, pressure must be lifted momentarily from the ribs and abdomen, enabling the patient to initiate the next breath. Patients should be encouraged to cough 3–4 times per day or more where indicated, with nursing staff and/or family involved in this process. Patients should also be taught self-assisted coughing when in a wheelchair (Figs 13-15F and 13-16).

Mechanical Aids for Assisted Coughing

Mechanical insufflation–exsufflation devices to assist coughing have been documented in the literature as being effective with patients with neuromuscular disorders and respiratory muscle weakness (Bach 1993, Chatwin et al 2003, Sancho et al 2004, Vianello et al 2005, Whitney et al 2002). Whitney et al (2002) suggest using pressures in the range of +25 cmH$_2$O positive pressure and −30 cmH$_2$O negative pressure, while Chatwin & Simonds (2002) have reported effective coughs at pressures of +10 to +30 cmH$_2$O and −10 to −30 cmH$_2$O. Winck et al (2004) and Tzeng & Bach (2000) have suggested that pressures of 40 cmH$_2$O or more may be required.

The range of cough assistance devices has recently expanded (Fig. 13-17) (Porot and Guerin 2013). Much lighter and with an internal battery, the Philips E70 device has inspiratory and expiratory oscillation modes and a memory card for data management. It

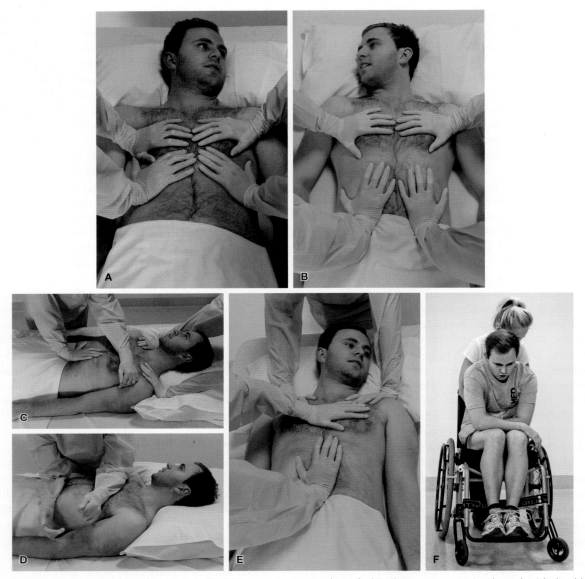

FIGURE 13-15 ■ Assisted cough variations. **(A, B)** Two-person assisted cough. **(C, E)** Two-person assisted cough with shoulder stabilization. **(D)** One-person assisted cough. **(F)** Assisted cough with carer providing abdominal compression.

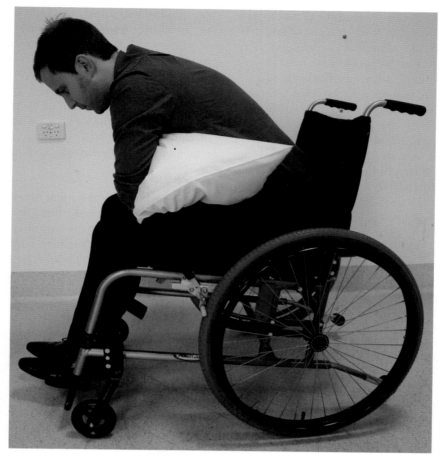

FIGURE 13-16 ■ Self-assist cough.

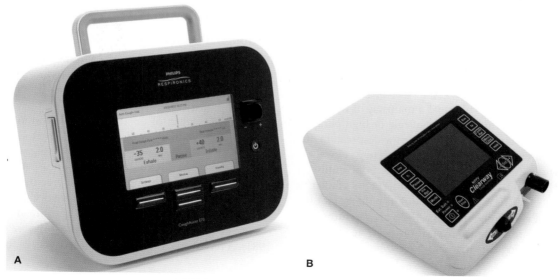

FIGURE 13-17 ■ Cough assistance devices.

also has a feature allowing the machine to synchronize with the user's breathing. Nippy 'Clearway' has IPPB and time limited NIV capabilities in addition to an oscillation mode. These features of both machines are in addition to the insufflation–exsufflation mode.

Nasopharyngeal suction may be used as a last resort. Care must be taken, as pharyngeal suction can cause stimulation of the parasympathetic nervous system via the vagus nerve, resulting in bradycardia and even cardiac arrest. Hyperoxygenation of the patient with 100% oxygen before treatment will help to minimize this possibility (Wicks & Menter 1986). Atropine or an equivalent drug may be used to treat profound bradycardia. As the left main stem bronchus branches off at a much more acute angle than the right, it is more challenging to introduce a suction catheter to clear the left lung. Fishburn et al (1990) reported increased incidence of left-sided pneumonia in SCI, making an insufflation–exsufflation device which targets both lungs, a potentially preferred option for airway clearance. Occasionally FOB may be necessary to treat unresolved lung or lobar collapse. Insertion of a mini-tracheostomy may also be considered for patients with problems of retained secretions (Wright 2003).

An increasing body of literature describes using electrical stimulation of the abdominal muscles to assist coughing either via implanted or surface electrodes (Langbein et al 2001, Lin et al 1998, Linder 1993, Stanic et al 2000, Taylor et al 2002, Zupan et al 1997). Implantable electrical stimulation has been shown to restore cough effectiveness to near able-bodied levels (DiMarco et al 2009). However, its use has yet to be trailed more globally.

Maximize Lung Volumes

Positive Pressure Treatments

Restoration of lung volume is a mainstay of treatment for the person with acute tetraplegia or high paraplegia. While the use of IPPB has been widespread in SCI management for years, the evidence as to its efficacy is of low quality. When studied as a sole intervention, it failed to yield clinically significant results (Stiller & Huff 1999). This may not discount its potential for use as part of a treatment package. IPPB via a mouthpiece/face mask to support inspiration prior to manually assist coughing can augment lung volume to increase the speed of exhalation. Similarly insufflation using an insufflation–exsufflation device will also boost inspiratory volumes prior to assisted coughing or exsufflation (Bach 1993). Both IPPB and insufflation–exsufflation can be delivered via a variety of interfaces including mouthpiece, face mask and tracheostomy connector. The introduction of many new ventilators for NIV has overcome some of the limitations of IPPB machines such as lack of choice of interface and requirement for pressurized gas (Bott et al 1992).

Breath Stacking

Breath stacking is a technique where a resuscitation bag is used with a mouth piece or face mask and a one-way valve to deliver two or more breaths prior to exhalation in order to augment lung volume and aid in secretion clearance. This low-cost treatment can be provided at home or in the subacute environment (Armstrong 2009, Mc Kim 2008, Torres-Castro 2014).

Glossopharyngeal Breathing

Glossopharyngeal breathing (GPB) (Chapter 7) can be used to increase lung volumes and assist secretion clearance in the person with high tetraplegia (Pryor 1999). Vital capacity may be increased by as much as 1000 mL (Alvarez et al 1981). Bach refers to the technique for use in patients with neuromuscular disorders to the extent that they can achieve a vital capacity of up to 1.7 L (Bach 1993, Bach & McDermott 1990, Bach et al 1993). In ventilator users, GPB can provide security in case of ventilator failure and independence from the ventilator for periods of time.

Abdominal Binders

Patients without functioning abdominal muscles present with a prominent abdomen when they assume upright positioning. Elasticated abdominal binders are used on patients with high SCI when mobilizing to minimize the effect of postural hypotension and aid respiration (Goldman et al 1986, McCool et al 1986, Scott et al 1993, Wadsworth et al 2009) (Fig. 13-18). The decrease in abdominal compliance with the abdominal binder is thought to restore pressure transference across the thorax and abdominal chambers, allowing the diaphragm to assume a more normal resting position in the upright posture (Alvarez et al 1981). A recent study by Wadsworth et al (2012) found

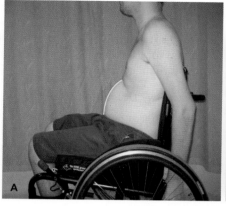
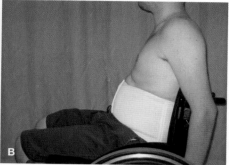

FIGURE 13-18 ■ Abdominal binder.

that not only does an abdominal binder improve vital capacity, FEV_1, peak expiratory flow and maximal inspiratory pressure, but also increases the time the patient can sustain voice. The cosmetic impact of eliminating the 'pot belly' should not be underestimated in this patient group.

Increase Muscle Strength

Respiratory Muscle Training

Although a review by Brooks & O'Brien (2005) could not recommend routine use of respiratory muscle training for tetraplegic patients, Van Houtte et al (2006) concluded in their review that respiratory muscle training tended to improve expiratory muscle strength, vital capacity and residual volume. They reported lack of sufficient data on inspiratory muscle strength training. Mueller et al (2013) found inspiratory muscle training to be better than placebo and isocapnic hyperpnoea training at strengthening the inspiratory muscles at a surprisingly low training volume of 10 minutes four times per week. As with any training, the effect is soon lost when training ceases, so this must be a lifelong commitment for any long-term benefit to be maintained.

Airway Management and Weaning from Ventilation

Extubation

Readiness for weaning from mechanical ventilation is indicated by a vital capacity of 15 mL/kg or greater (Chevrolet & Deleamont 1991, Mahanes & Lewis

2004), a decreasing sputum load, ability to cooperate, a patent upper airway, a relatively clear chest radiograph with no new changes and reduction in the requirement for ventilator assistance (Ball 2001, Berlly & Shem 2007, Wallbom et al 2005). Extubation should be followed by intensive physiotherapy treatment to ensure adequate secretion clearance and volume maintenance/restoration (Berney et al 2002). If not managed by an experienced team, SCI patients may be extubated prematurely, resulting in respiratory failure due to secretion retention (Berlly & Shem 2007). Extubation failure has been associated with increased mortality, increased tracheostomy rate and increased length of hospital stay (Epstein 2004, Harrop et al 2004).

Tracheostomy

Tracheostomy may be required in some instances to facilitate weaning. The incidence of tracheostomy following cervical SCI has been reported to be as high as 59.7% by Berney et al in a prospective study of an Australian cohort in 2011 and as low as 10.03% by Yugue et al in 2012 in a retrospective study of Japanese patients. Both authors found that FVC was an important predictor of the need for tracheostomy: Berney <830 mL and Yugue ≤500 mL. Berney also found volume of pulmonary secretions and gas exchange to be predictive of airway management. Yugue did not record these, but found completeness of lesion and age >69 years to be associated with tracheostomy. Level of lesion is also important, with Como et al (2005) reporting a tracheostomy rate of 81–83% in patients with a complete SCI above the level of C5. Tracheostomy may be performed as early as day 4 following anterior cervical surgery with no increase in the incidence of wound or implant infection (Berney et al 2008).

Weaning

Weaning from ventilation is best performed with the patient supine (Chen et al 1990, Mansel & Norman 1990, Wallbom et al 2005) or with a head-down tip (Gutierrez et al 2010) to optimize diaphragm function. Cohn (1993) suggests that weaning should be thought of as a conditioning process for the diaphragm and warns that fatigue of the muscle should be avoided. Wallbom et al (2005) suggests a regime of twice-daily trials with a 3–4 hour rest period in between trials and gradual increases for each session until weaning is achieved. An evidence-based protocol to guide weaning of ventilator-dependent cervical SCI has also been shown to increase mean maximal inspiratory and expiratory pressure, mean vital capacity, mean off-ventilator breathing times (Gutierrez et al 2003).

Measurement of respiratory muscle strength by way of recording static mouth maximum inspiratory and expiratory pressures can be useful in directing extubation (Arora et al 2012) and also weaning from ventilation (Chiodo et al 2008, Wallbom et al 2005).

Speech Options with a Tracheostomy

When a patient has a tracheostomy, enabling speech can be achieved by close coordination between the speech pathologist and other team members (Brown et al 2006, Cameron et al 2009, MacBean et al 2009). Full or partial tracheostomy cuff deflation during ventilation can enable speech by allowing air to pass across the vocal folds during the inspiratory cycle of the ventilator.

Increasing tidal volume, positive end expiratory pressure and inspiratory time will facilitate speech by compensating for leak and allowing the patient to remain stable on ventilation even in the acute post-injury phase (Brown et al 2006). An alternative method of speech production is to incorporate a one-way speaking valve into the ventilation circuit to redirect all exhaled air across the vocal folds during cuff deflation; similar ventilation adjustments are used. In those patients who have a tracheostomy and who are not ventilated, cuff deflation may also allow for use of a one-way speaking valve (Suiter et al 2003). Speaking valve use may increase work of breathing and monitoring for fatigue is required.

Tracheostomy Decannulation

Assessing the optimal time to decannulate the SCI patient requires particular attention to cough effectiveness, airway patency and airway protection (Cameron et al 2009, Ross & White 2003). The physiotherapist must establish an effective method for secretion clearance before tracheostomy removal. As the incidence of aspiration is moderately high in acute tetraplegia, 35% identified by Abel et al (2004) and 16% by Seidl et al (2010), speech pathology assessment is required. Speaking valve use during oral intake has been shown to decrease aspiration risk in non-ventilated patients, potentially as a result of increased pharyngeal pressures and may be a useful strategy (Prigent et al 2012). The presence of persistent aspiration following cervical SCI may not be an obstacle to decannulation if a carefully considered risk-management approach is taken (Ross & White 2003). Cameron et al (2009) showed that management of the SCI patient by a specialist multidisciplinary tracheostomy team decreased total cannulation time and acute length of stay with associated cost savings.

LONG-TERM RESPIRATORY MANAGEMENT

Long-Term Ventilation

For the patient on long-term ventilation, a ventilator with an internal battery is attached to the wheelchair to enable mobility (Fig. 13-19). With increased survival after high SCI owing to greater public awareness of resuscitation skills, long-term ventilation is now more prevalent (Alderson 1999, Carter 1993). Planning must start early in conjunction with the patient's local hospital and community services to facilitate timely discharge to an appropriate location. Comprehensive training is needed for the family and care team to minimize the risks of being fully ventilator dependent within the community. Annual medical evaluations of the patient's ability to breathe may identify delayed diaphragm recovery (Oo et al 1999).

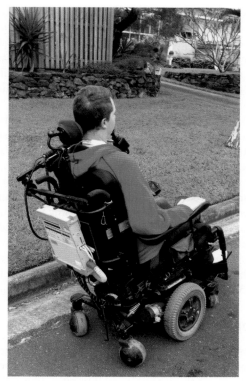

FIGURE 13-19 ■ Ventilated person in power wheelchair.

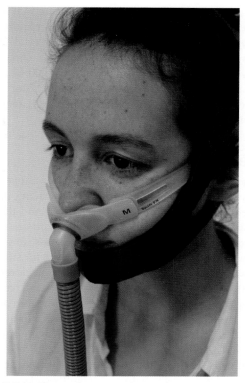

FIGURE 13-20 ■ Obstructive sleep apnoea treatment: nasal pillows with a chin strap.

Readmissions to Hospital with a Chest Infection

As survival of individuals following SCI increases, the impact of ageing on respiratory health and well-being has become more evident with an increase in hospital readmission for chest infection noted (Burns et al 2004, Capoor & Stein 2005). Postma et al (2009) found that pulmonary function tests were a stronger predictor of respiratory infection in the first year following injury than lesion level or completeness. Patients with a vital capacity of less than 2 L are at greatest risk of developing late-onset respiratory failure (Peterson & Kirshblum 2002). Patients with chronic SCI will not exhibit the marked paradoxical chest wall movement seen in the period of spinal shock. They will also have existing strategies for independent secretion clearance, which they can share with their treating therapist. They may present with undiagnosed obstructive sleep apnoea and potentially benefit from CPAP treatment, as not only will this treat their airway obstruction, but will also provide ongoing lung volume support. Some

patients with long-standing SCI chronically hypoventilate and develop a raised partial pressure of carbon dioxide in the blood leading to decreased chemoreceptor sensitivity (Stockhammer et al 2002). Consequently for these patients, high concentrations of oxygen may result in respiratory suppression.

Treatment of Obstructive Sleep Apnoea

The gold standard for treatment of OSA remains noninvasive positive pressure therapy (Burns et al 2001). The acceptance of this treatment is varied in the SCI population (Stockhammer et al 2002) and is complicated by tetraplegic individuals potentially being unable to independently don and doff their masks, necessitating either an increase in care hours or adaptations to their interfaces. Nasal interfaces and sturdier chin straps may be more attractive, as they allow the possibility of speech and drinking while wearing the mask without excessive mouth leakage of pressure during sleep (Fig. 13-20). The less claustrophobic nature of nasal pillows also means they are well suited to tetraplegic users. The lower pressures required by many tetraplegic CPAP users (Le Guen et al 2012) allows for greater flexibility in interface choice, as leak is less likely at lower pressures. It should be noted that CPAP is not an adequate treatment for sleep hypoventilation and that bi-level therapy is required (Guillemenault et al 1998).

Electrical and Magnetic Stimulation of Breathing

A paralyzed diaphragm can be stimulated via a phrenic nerve pacer or by direct motor point pacing of the diaphragm if the phrenic nerve is intact and the cell bodies of C3, C4 and C5 at the spinal cord are viable (Jarosz et al 2012). Full preoperative assessment is required to ascertain a patient's suitability for stimulation (DiMarco 2005). Stimulation is achieved by means of a radio transmitter placed over the receiver. Early postoperative training can be commenced on the ventilator in assist control mode in order to achieve adequate volumes, which can be challenging initially due to diaphragm atrophy. Extensive postoperative training is necessary to increase diaphragmatic endurance and to teach the patient, his family and carers the necessary skills and understanding of the device. The conditioning period may be complicated by initial feelings of dyspnoea, particularly when the patient has

previously been ventilated to induce hyperventilation and reduce bicarbonate stores (Jarosz et al 2012). For some patients, phrenic nerve pacing will provide a full-time alternative to the ventilator and the tracheostomy will no longer be required, but for others the ventilator and tracheostomy will be required for additional hours during the day or night (Onders et al 2010).

Benefits include greater wheelchair mobility, elimination of the fear of accidental ventilator disconnection, loss of social stigma associated with being attached to a ventilator, improved speech, no noise from the ventilator, reduced need for carer input and improved well-being and overall health, particularly when decannulation of the tracheostomy has occurred (DiMarco 1999 2005, Onders et al 2010, Wolfe 2013). Disadvantages include the need for major surgery involving thoracotomy, risk of surgical damage to the phrenic nerve and failure of the implanted device (Gay 2013, DiMarco 2005).

CONCLUSION

Greater understanding of the respiratory dysfunction accompanying SCI has led to continuing improvements in morbidity and mortality rates. Physiotherapists provide a vital contribution to the respiratory well-being and care of individuals with SCI in both the acute and chronic phases.

Thoracic Organ Transplantation

INTRODUCTION

Thoracic organ transplantation is a well-established treatment for patients with end-stage heart and lung disease. It aims to improve the quality of life and survival of those patients who are already managed optimally, often with maximal medical therapy. Physiotherapists are key members of the transplant team, providing expertise in the physical and functional assessment, respiratory management and rehabilitation of patients both before and after surgery.

This section discusses the physiotherapy management before and after heart, heart–lung and lung transplantation. The historical context, assessment

and selection of appropriate candidates, surgical procedures, key concepts of immunosuppression, rejection, infection and denervation are also considered. Issues specific to paediatric patients are identified.

HISTORY

A long history of experimental and clinical advances has led to the current successes of thoracic transplantation. In 1967 Christiaan Barnard (Cape Town, South Africa) performed the first human-to-human orthotopic heart transplant. More than a hundred heart transplants were performed in 1968–1969, but almost all patients died within 60 days. The 1980s heralded a

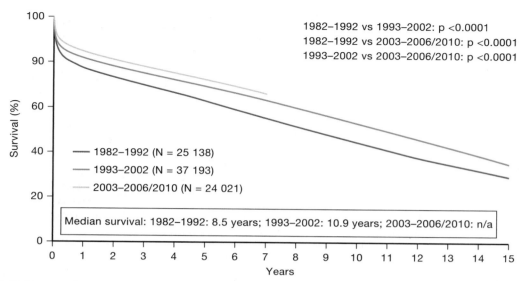

FIGURE 13-21 ■ Kaplan–Meier survival curves for adult heart transplant recipients. *(Reproduced with permission from Stehlik et al 2012.)*

new era in thoracic organ transplantation with the first long-term survivors of heart–lung (Reitz et al 1982), single lung (Cooper et al 1987) and double lung (Patterson et al 1988) transplantation. The advent of cyclosporin (Borel 1980) as the principal immunosuppressant, with a greater ability to prevent acute rejection, was considered pivotal to improved survival outcomes.

Over the last 30 years, significant advances have been made in all aspects of the care of thoracic organ transplant recipients. There have been improvements in operative techniques, organ preservation and cross matching. New, less toxic immunosuppressants have been developed. There is a greater understanding of immunology and a greater ability to bridge to transplant with mechanical support devices.

In the current era, approximately 4000 heart transplants, 3500 lung transplants and 90 heart–lung transplants are performed internationally in adults each year (Christie et al 2012, Stehlik et al 2012). The number of paediatric transplants is much smaller, with approximately 530 heart transplants, 130 lung transplants and less than 10 heart–lung transplants performed (Benden et al 2012, Kirk et al 2012). Adult lung transplant activity has continued to grow in the past decade, perhaps in part due to advances in widening the lung donor pool, while the annual adult heart transplant volume has been relatively constant reflecting donor shortages. Current survival outcomes for patients receiving heart transplantation are more favourable than for lung transplantation (Figs 13-21 and 13-22). Outcomes in children are similar to those in adults.

SELECTION OF CANDIDATES

A variety of criteria have been developed to identify patients who will live longer and function better with transplantation than with medical therapy. Through a rigorous evaluation process, the transplant team assesses the patient's severity of organ failure, screens for comorbidities that may negatively affect survival and assesses psychosocial variables necessary for successful outcomes following transplantation.

INDICATIONS FOR TRANSPLANTATION

Thoracic organ transplantation is indicated in patients with various end-stage diseases where survival is limited and quality of life poor (Table 13-10).

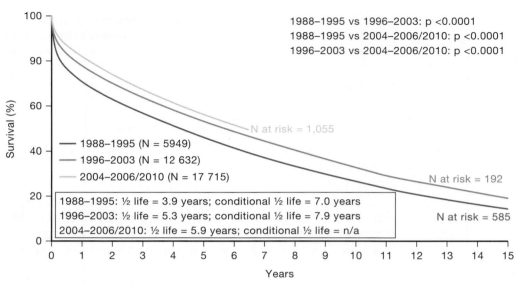

FIGURE 13-22 ■ Kaplan–Meier survival curves for adult lung transplant recipients. *NA,* not available. *(Reproduced with permission from Christie et al 2012.)*

TABLE 13-10		
Indications for Thoracic Organ Transplantation		
Heart	Non-ischaemic cardiomyopathy (54%)	
	Ischaemic cardiomyopathy (37%)	
	Valvular disease (3%)	
	Congenital heart disease (3%)	
	Allograft failure requiring retransplantation (3%)	
Heart–lung	Congenital heart diseases (36)%	
	Pulmonary arterial hypertension (28%)	
	Cystic fibrosis (14%), acquired heart disease (5%)	
	COPD/emphysema (4%), idiopathic pulmonary fibrosis (4%)	
Single lung	COPD/emphysema (46%)	
	Pulmonary fibrosis (37%), α_1-antitrypsin deficiency (6%)	
	Allograft failure requiring retransplantation (3%)	
Bilateral lung	COPD/emphysema (27%)	
	Cystic fibrosis (26%), pulmonary fibrosis (20%)	
	α_1-antitrypsin deficiency (6%), pulmonary arterial hypertension (5%)	
	Bronchiectasis (5%), sarcoidosis (3%)	

Adapted from Christie et al 2012, Stehlik et al 2012.
COPD, Chronic obstructive pulmonary disease.

CONTRAINDICATIONS TO TRANSPLANTATION

Patients with comorbidities that may seriously compromise the outcome of transplantation are excluded. There are few absolute contraindications to thoracic organ transplantation, and consideration of relative contraindications is usually made on an individual basis (Box 13-3).

ASSESSMENT

Potential recipients are assessed by an experienced multidisciplinary team at a transplant centre (Box 13-4). This process involves extensive physiological, functional and psychological assessment in order to:

- evaluate the severity of cardiac and/or pulmonary dysfunction (e.g. pulmonary function testing, echocardiography, right heart catheter)
- identify contraindications to transplantation (see Box 13-3)
- assess immunological status (ABO group, tissue typing)
- identify previous exposure to potentially complicating infection: cytomegalovirus (CMV),

BOX 13-3
POTENTIAL CONTRAINDICATIONS FOR THORACIC ORGAN TRANSPLANTATION

- Irreversible dysfunction of other organ systems (e.g. hepatic, renal)
- Malignancy with a high risk of recurrence
- Older than 65 years
- Complicated diabetes mellitus
- Active systemic infection
- Active systemic illness that would significantly limit survival or rehabilitation
- Peripheral or cerebrovascular disorders
- Active substance abuse including cigarette smoking, alcohol and illicit drugs
- Severe psychiatric disorders
- Non-adherence with medical regimen
- Body mass index outside the healthy weight range
- Inadequate social supports
- Severely limited functional status with poor rehabilitation potential
- Significant chest wall or spinal deformity, or severe osteoporosis

BOX 13-4
MULTIDISCIPLINARY TRANSPLANT TEAM

- Physician
- Surgeon
- Transplant coordinator
- Physiotherapist
- Nurse
- Social worker
- Psychiatrist
- Dietitian
- Occupational therapist

toxoplasmosis, hepatitis B, hepatitis C, methicillin-resistant *Staphylococcus aureus* (MRSA), Epstein-Barr virus (EBV) and human immunodeficiency virus (HIV)
- evaluate nutritional status
- evaluate psychological status
- assess exercise capacity and functional status.

The assessment is usually performed as an inpatient over a 2–3 day period. Once the evaluation has been compiled, all members of the transplant team meet to discuss the findings and come to a consensus regarding the patient's appropriateness for listing considering the individual's risk–benefit profile.

Physiotherapy Assessment

Physiotherapy assessment of the potential transplant candidate is similar to that of any cardiorespiratory medical or surgical patient (Chapter 2). It focuses on the impact of cardiac, respiratory and musculoskeletal limitations on exercise, functional capacity and social performance. Particular attention should be paid to anticipated issues that may arise during post-transplantation rehabilitation.

A detailed subjective and objective assessment is required. The medical history and the available results of relevant investigations (e.g. imaging, ABGs, lung function, angiography) should be reviewed before seeing the patient so that the patient's unique pathophysiology and clinical status is understood.

At the completion of the assessment, the physiotherapist will have formed an opinion regarding the patient's current level of function, limitations and quality of life. Most importantly, opportunities to further optimize their physical status with physiotherapy intervention/s in preparation for transplant are identified and a plan to address these factors can be developed.

At the time of assessment, patients and their carers are provided with information regarding physiotherapy during the acute postoperative course and the commitment required for rehabilitation pre and post transplant.

Close collaboration with the patient's local physiotherapist or treating team is needed. It is very useful to discuss the candidate's response to any previous rehabilitation or regularly performed interventions (e.g. airway clearance for those with cystic fibrosis (CF)). These clinicians can often provide additional insight into knowledge and practice deficits in disease self-management, clinical course and local available supports.

SURGICAL PROCEDURES

Orthotopic Heart Transplantation

Preparation of the heart transplant recipient is similar to that for any patient undergoing cardiac surgery (anaesthesia, median sternotomy and cardiopulmonary bypass). There has been minimal changes in surgical technique since the 1960s, except for the introduction of the bicaval technique, which better preserves the sinus node and the anatomic integrity of the donor right atrium, resulting in lower incidence of conduction disturbances and tricuspid regurgitation (Davies et al 2010). When the donor heart is present in the recipient theatre and has passed a final inspection, the recipient heart is excised, leaving behind a 2–3 cm right atrial cuff around the superior and inferior vena cava (cavoatrial cuff) and a small left atrial cuff around the four pulmonary veins. The donor left atrium is sutured to the recipient left atrial cuff before the superior and inferior vena cava are then sutured to the recipient cavoatrial cuff, along with end-to-end aortic and pulmonary anastomoses.

Heterotopic transplantation, a 'piggyback' procedure where the recipient heart is left in place and the donor heart is positioned in the right chest, is now very rarely performed.

Lung Transplantation

Single Lung Transplantation

Single lung transplantation (SLTx) is performed via a postero-lateral thoracotomy through the fourth or fifth intercostal space. The recipient's lung is removed and the donor lung positioned in the chest. The bronchial anastomosis is performed first, followed by the pulmonary artery anastomosis. After completion of these anastomoses, the lung is reinflated and perfusion is re-established. Following resumption of ventilation to the donor lung, haemostasis is obtained, two intercostal catheters are placed (apical and basal) and the chest is closed. Following reintubation with a single lumen tube, flexible bronchoscopy is performed to inspect the bronchial anastomosis and clear the airway of blood or residual secretions. Cardiopulmonary bypass is rarely needed during this operation. SLTx can only be performed in the absence of contralateral sepsis. It is ideal for restrictive lung disease, as both ventilation and perfusion are directed towards the transplanted lung.

Double Lung/Bilateral Sequential Lung Transplantation

Bilateral sequential lung transplantation (BSLTx) is performed via bilateral anterolateral thoracotomies through the fourth or fifth intercostal space. This can be combined with a transverse sternotomy (often termed a 'clamshell incision'), but many surgeons now leave the sternum intact, particularly when transplanting adults. Avoidance of sternal division has been associated with fewer complications and improved respiratory function postoperatively (Bittner et al 2011, Venuta et al 2003). A minimally invasive approach to BSLTx has also been reported (Fischer et al 2001).

Heart–Lung Transplantation

This operation can be performed via a median sternotomy or a clamshell incision. Following the institution of cardiopulmonary bypass, the heart and lungs are excised separately, allowing identification and protection of the phrenic, recurrent laryngeal and vagus nerves. The heart is removed first, followed by the left and then right lungs (following stapling of the bronchi to minimize the risk of contaminating the area) and the trachea is divided. The donor heart–lung block is implanted, starting with the tracheal, then the cardiac and great vessel anastomoses. Ventilation is established (ensuring the patency of the airway anastomosis) and the heart resuscitated (Jamieson et al 1984). This procedure is only performed rarely now, and only in patients with combined cardiac and respiratory failure (see Table 13-10).

Other Lung Techniques

The scarcity of donor lungs, especially for small and paediatric recipients, has led to the development of operations that allow larger lungs to be downsized. These techniques are not considered standard practice. The *split-lung technique* (Couetil et al 1997) utilizes individual lobes from the donor. It may be indicated if there is localized pathology in one lobe of the donor lung or if the donor organ is larger than expected.

KEY CONCEPTS

Organ Donation

Organ donation for transplantation is most commonly performed in the setting of brain death. Brain death is defined as a complete and irreversible cessation of brain activity. The main causes are severe head injury from physical trauma, often from road traffic accidents and from subarachnoid haemorrhage. In most countries, consent from family members or next of kin is required. It is normal practice for consent to be sought even if the brain-dead individual had expressed the wish to donate. In some countries (e.g. Spain, Belgium, Poland, France) potential donors are presumed to have given consent, although jurisdictions allow opting out from the system. Once consent is obtained, the non-living donor is kept on ventilatory support until the organs have been surgically removed. The donor is given expert medical and nursing care to optimize organ performance. Physiotherapists sometimes assist in the removal of retained lung secretions and help to optimize ventilation (Gabbay et al 1999).

Donation after cardiac death (DCD) provides an additional pathway to organ donation for patients who do not meet the brain death criteria and for whom further medical intervention is futile. In this circumstance, the donor organs are rapidly retrieved after certification of death following withdrawal of support and asystole. Recipient survival rates after DCD lung transplantation have been shown to be comparable to rates in recipients who received donations after brain death (De Oliveira et al 2010). This strategy is used to expand the donor pool.

A very small number of living donors are used for lung transplantation internationally. *Living donor lobar lung transplantation* (Starnes et al 1999) typically involves two donors (usually relatives), each donating a single lobe (usually lower lobe) for bilateral lung transplantation. It is most often performed as a life-saving procedure for the critically ill who cannot wait for cadaveric transplantation (Date 2011). Living donor lobar transplantation remains a second-line treatment due to the inevitable risk of lobectomy to the donors. It is applicable to smaller recipients, such as children and adolescents.

Timing of organ retrieval and implantation is important and necessitates a high level of coordination between the donor and recipient transplant teams. Organ procurement occurs at the hospital where the donor is managed. The organ is kept in preservation solution while it is transported to the transplant centre for implantation into the selected recipient. Most cardiac teams aim for an ischaemic time of less than 4 hours, from the time of cross-clamping the aorta in the donor to reperfusing the organ in the recipient. Lung teams aim for less than 8 hours. Longer ischaemic times are associated with poorer early graft function (Del Rizzo et al 1999, Thabut et al 2005).

Ex vivo heart and lung perfusion, using a modified cardiopulmonary bypass circuit, may be used to improve graft function prior to implantation and extends the viable preservation time, allowing more remote donor organs to be utilized (Cypel et al 2012, Wagner 2011).

The recipient team selects the appropriate recipient based upon:

- blood group
- size (weight and height)
- CMV serological status (lungs)
- prospective cross matching
- clinical status.

Organ allocation systems vary worldwide. Severity of illness and medical urgency are taken into account.

Immunosuppression and Rejection

Rejection is a specific immune response to the donor tissue (allograft) and is part of the normal host defence system against foreign antigens. The response can occur by humoral (B lymphocyte) or cell-mediated (T lymphocyte) immune mechanisms. Immunosuppression is required to manage rejection.

Immunosuppression protocols vary widely from centre to centre. The majority of thoracic organ transplant recipients remain on two or three lifelong maintenance immunosuppressive agents. Most commonly, one of these will be a calcineurin inhibitor (e.g. tacrolimus, cyclosporin), one will be a cell-cycle inhibitor (e.g. mycophenolate mofetil, azathioprine) and the third will be a corticosteroid (e.g. prednisolone). The use of a proliferation signal inhibitor or mammalian target of rapamycin inhibitor (e.g. sirolimus, everolimus) as part of a long-term immunosuppressive regimen has increased (Stehlik et al 2012), especially in circumstances of nephrotoxicity where a calcineurin inhibitor may need to be avoided or reduced.

Immunosuppressants have a number of specific side effects, which are listed in Table 13-11. It is important that physiotherapists working with thoracic organ transplant recipients are familiar with these side effects. Many agents impact the musculoskeletal system and may cause bone morbidities such as avascular necrosis, osteoporosis and reduced tissue healing. Side effects of some agents affect the patient's ability to participate in exercise training (e.g. hypertension,

TABLE 13-11
Immunosuppression and Side Effects

Immunosuppressant	Side Effects
Calcineurin Inhibitors	
Tacrolimus	Nephrotoxicity, hypertension, diabetes, tremor, headache, diarrhoea, nausea
Cyclosporin	Nephrotoxicity, hepatic dysfunction, hirsutism, tremor, hypertension, gingival hyperplasia, dyslipidaemia, skin lesions (e.g. acne)
Cell Cycle Inhibitors	
Mycophenolate mofetil (MMF)	Diarrhoea, nausea and vomiting, bone marrow suppression, opportunistic infection (especially invasive CMV)
Azathioprine	Bone marrow suppression, hepatic dysfunction, nausea and vomiting, anorexia, mouth ulceration, increased risk of malignancies
Proliferation Signal Inhibitors/Mammalian Target of Rapamycin Inhibitors	
Sirolimus	Impaired wound healing, interstitial pneumonitis, hyperlipidaemia, diarrhoea, haematological disturbances, arthralgia,
Everolimus	Haematological disturbances, opportunistic infection (PJP, CMV), gastro-intestinal upset, hepatic dysfunction, hyperlipidaemia, hypertension, hyperglycaemia, oral mucositis
Corticosteroids	
Prednisolone	Sodium and fluid retention, hypokalaemia, hyperglycaemia, dyspepsia, myopathy, osteoporosis, skin fragility, increased appetite, mood changes, adrenal suppression

CMV, Cytomegalovirus; PJP, Pneumocystis jiroveci pneumonia.

nausea) or have practical implications (e.g. fine hand tremor affecting writing ability and difficulty fitting into footwear due to fluid retention).

Immunosuppressive therapy must be carefully balanced to prevent rejection without the development of serious adverse effects of the immunotherapy itself. Excessive immunosuppression increases the risk of infection, kidney and liver dysfunction and malignancies. Inadequate immunosuppression may result in rejection.

Graft rejection can be divided into three subcategories: hyperacute, acute and chronic rejection. The discrimination between acute and chronic rejection refers to the persistence of the dysfunction rather than the time post transplant. Acute rejection resolves spontaneously or with treatment. The dysfunction resulting from chronic rejection does not resolve.

Hyperacute Rejection

Hyperacute rejection usually occurs within the first 72 hours postoperatively. The presenting features of the heart transplant recipient may be similar to a patient in cardiogenic shock, while the features of the lung transplant recipient may be similar to a patient with ARDS. Both may require total mechanical support in the form of extracorporeal membrane oxygenation (ECMO). Hyperacute rejection is relatively rare, and a more common cause of graft dysfunction in the early period is primary graft dysfunction, which is related to ischaemia reperfusion injury.

Acute Rejection

Acute cellular rejection (Fig. 13-23) is characterized by a host T-cell response towards the transplanted organ and is a common complication in the first year following transplant. The diagnosis is based on both clinical and histological criteria. Often, mild to moderate rejection is not associated with any reliable signs or symptoms.

Routine endomyocardial biopsies via right heart catheter are the mainstay for monitoring acute cellular rejection in heart transplant recipients. Criteria for grading these biopsies are based on the two key elements of acute rejection: the presence of lymphocytes and myocyte injury. Standardized grading criteria (Stewart et al 2005) include four levels of rejection (Table 13-12). At most institutions, a grade of 0R or 1R does not require further treatment, while a higher grade is treated with augmented anti-rejection therapy. Heart transplant recipients with moderate to severe rejection may present with arrhythmias, hypotension, fever, increased weight/fluid retention, malaise or dyspnoea.

In lung transplant recipients, acute rejection often mimics an upper respiratory tract infection or bronchitis. The spectrum of clinical features is non-specific and includes dyspnoea, fever, non-productive cough

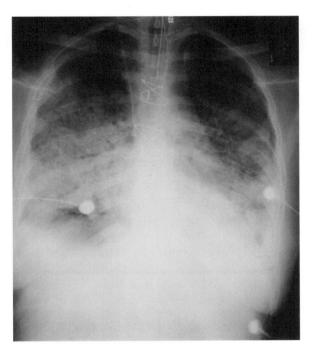

FIGURE 13-23 ■ A chest radiograph showing acute pulmonary rejection in a heart–lung recipient.

TABLE 13-12

Acute Cellular Rejection Grading Scheme in Heart Transplant Recipients

Grade	Histopathologic Findings
0R, none	None
1R, mild	Interstitial and/or perivascular lymphocyte infiltrate with up to 1 focus of myocyte damage
2R, moderate	Two or more foci of infiltrate with associated myocyte damage
3R, severe	Diffuse infiltrate with multifocal myocyte damage ± oedema ± haemorrhage ± vasculitis

Stewart et al 2005.

or malaise. New infiltrates or pleural effusion may be seen on chest radiograph. There may be hypoxia and a drop in lung function. As it is difficult to differentiate rejection and infection on the basis of clinical, radiological or physiological criteria, bronchoscopy with bronchoalveolar lavage (BAL) and transbronchial biopsy (TBB) are required. Acute lung rejection is graded from A0 (none) to A4 (severe) (Stewart et al

TABLE 13-13

Classification and Grading of Pulmonary Allograft Rejection

A: Acute Rejection	
Grade 0	None
Grade 1	Minimal
Grade 2	Mild
Grade 3	Moderate
Grade 4	Severe

B: Airway Inflammation	
Grade 0	None
Grade 1	Low grade
Grade 2	High grade
Grade X	Ungradable

C: Chronic Airway Rejection	Obliterative Bronchiolitis
0	Absent
1	Present

D: Chronic Vascular Rejection	Accelerated Graft Vascular Sclerosis

Stewart et al 2007.

2007). In addition, the presence of airway inflammation is graded (Table 13-13). Early acute rejection is generally treated with pulsed intravenous methylprednisolone and augmented immunosuppression.

The diagnosis of antibody-mediated humoral rejection (AMR) in heart and lung transplant recipients remains controversial and continues to evolve. The most commonly used marker is positive immunoperoxidase staining for C4d. The incidence of AMR is much lower than acute cellular rejection, but is highly variable between centres. The treatment of AMR is also controversial, but many centres use plasmaphoresis.

Chronic Graft Dysfunction

Chronic graft dysfunction, sometimes called 'chronic rejection', commonly presents as bronchiolitis obliterans syndrome (BOS) in lung transplant recipients and cardiac allograft vasculopathy (CAV) in cardiac recipients. In both cases the causes are not completely understood, but are likely to be a result of scarring following acute rejection, infection and other triggers combined with chronic low-grade inflammation.

In the lung, BOS is clinically defined by an irreversible fall in lung function as measured by FEV_1 from a stable post-transplant baseline when other causes have been excluded. It is graded from BOS 0 where FEV_1 > 90% baseline to BOS 3 where FEV_1 ≤ 50% baseline (Estenne et al 2002). It has a prevalence of 48% by 5 years and 76% by 10 years after transplantation (Christie et al 2012). As the disease progresses, the lung transplant recipient develops exertional dyspnoea, cough and wheezing, and can suffer frequent respiratory tract infections and respiratory failure. Chronic lung allograft dysfunction remains very difficult to treat and is largely responsible for diminished quality of life and relatively poor long-term survival of lung transplant recipients (Christie et al 2012). Some improvements in outcome have been obtained with early gastric fundoplication for patients with gastro-oesophageal reflux disease in order to prevent allograft injury from aspiration (Cantu et al 2004), and the use of the macrolide antibiotic azithromycin (Vos et al 2010). Retransplantation is sometimes performed.

CAV is one of the main causes of late graft failure and death in heart transplant recipients (Stehlik et al 2012). The coronary arteries develop a progressive concentric hyperplasia, leading to vessel lumen obliteration. Its evolution is often rapid and diffuse and remains mostly silent because of the denervation of the transplanted heart (Stark et al 1991). Coronary angiography remains the standard for screening and is usually performed annually, although is relatively insensitive compared to intravascular ultrasound (Schmauss & Weis 2008). Other non-invasive techniques (e.g. multislice CT) are also being explored (Barthelemy et al 2012). The cause of the process is unclear, although long graft ischaemic time, recurrent rejection episodes and viral infections, along with classic cardiovascular risk factors (hypertension, diabetes, hyperlipidaemia) which are associated with the immunosuppressive regimen have been identified as contributing factors (Schmauss & Weis 2008). Treatment options are limited, although statin therapy may be of some benefit (Grigioni et al 2006) and is therefore now prescribed to all heart transplant recipients, including those with no evidence of vasculopathy. Angioplasty may be undertaken for diseased vessels if there is a discrete lesion, but is considered palliative and has not been shown to alter the natural history of CAV (Jonas et al 2006). The use of proliferation signal inhibitors (e.g. sirolimus, everolimus) as part of the immunosuppressive regimen may be protective and

---

BOX 13-5
INFECTIOUS ORGANISMS IN THORACIC ORGAN TRANSPLANT RECIPIENTS

- Bacterial
  - Gram negative
  - Gram positive
  - Atypical
- Viral
  - Cytomegalovirus (CMV)
  - Herpes simplex virus (HSV)
- Fungal
  - *Aspergillus*
  - *Candida albicans*
  - *Pneumocystis jiroveci*
- Mycobacteria
  - Tuberculosis
  - Atypical

---

slow the progression of CAV (Manito et al 2010). The only definitive therapy is retransplantation.

Infection

Chronic immunosuppression renders transplant recipients more susceptible to infections (Box 13-5). The frequency of bacterial infections tends to peak within the first 3 months, while immunosuppressive therapy is often at a maximum level. The most frequent sites of infection are the lungs and blood. Regular dental check-ups and hygiene are important, as the teeth and gums can also be sources of infection. It is recommended that antibiotics be given prior to dental procedures because of susceptibility of the heart to endocarditis with blood-borne bacteria.

Infection is a major cause of morbidity and mortality in both the early and late post-transplant periods.

Denervation

Cardiac Denervation

The pathophysiology of the transplanted heart is unique. The denervation of the organ makes it dependent on its intrinsic rate. It will therefore have a higher than normal resting heart rate secondary to the lack of inhibitory vagal influence. An alteration in the physiological response to exercise is also seen. In the normally innervated heart it is predominantly changes in heart rate that account for the increase in cardiac output in response to dynamic exercise. In contrast, the denervated heart increases cardiac output by increasing stroke volume (based on the Frank-Starling mechanism). The heart rate rises more gradually following the start of exercise, does not reach a similar peak and slows more gradually once exercise is stopped, and is primarily the result of changing levels of circulating catecholamines (i.e. adrenaline and noradrenaline). Peak heart rate early post heart transplantation has been shown to be reduced to 60–70% of aged matched normal individuals, and is closely correlated with a similarly reduced peak rate of oxygen consumption (VO_2) (Mettauer et al 2005). This appears to improve over time, suggesting possible autonomic reinnervation in some patients (Gullestad et al 1996). In addition, transmission of ischaemic pain is prevented in the denervated heart (Weber 1990). Although partial reinnervation occurs in some recipients, the majority of patients will not experience anginal symptoms and should be advised against unsupervised exercise at high intensities for long periods. This is especially important if angiography indicates the presence of CAV (Hosenpud 1999, Kavanagh 1996).

Lung Denervation

Similarly, lung and heart–lung transplantation involves denervation of the lungs below the airway anastomosis, with associated loss of all pulmonary innervation except post-ganglionic efferent nerves. Although the laryngeal expiration reflex is preserved, the cough response is severely impaired (Higenbottam et al 1989). In addition, ciliary function in the graft is abnormal, at least in the early post-transplant period (Thomas et al 2012). Taken together, these two defects predispose the recipient to retained airway secretions and lower respiratory tract infection, particularly in the early postoperative period.

PREOPERATIVE REHABILITATION

Pre-transplant rehabilitation aims to optimize physical and functional performance and quality of life. Addressing the deconditioning that results from the preoperative disease state is considered important for survival to transplant and recovery afterwards (Langer et al 2012b, Martinu et al 2008).

As cardiac and pulmonary rehabilitation programs are increasingly recognized as part of best practice management of patients with chronic heart failure (Selig et al 2010) and a growing number of chronic respiratory diseases (Nici et al 2006), many patients assessed for transplant will have participated in a rehabilitation programme before transplant assessment. Exercise training, education, nutritional intervention and psychosocial support are key components of pre-transplant rehabilitation for thoracic transplant candidates.

Most transplant centres require that where safe, transplant candidates participate in an ongoing supervised exercise training programme while they are on the waiting list. Most large adult centres offer dedicated, supervised preoperative exercise training classes 2–3 times a week. Exercise training classes are often a key referral point for care from other members of the multidisciplinary team.

Patients and carers experience high levels of stress during the waiting period. Regular contact with other candidates and the transplant team is ideal, as it can help support self-management behaviours, maintain patient motivation and improve psychosocial outcomes (Rosenberger et al 2012).

Patients who cannot access the transplant centre (e.g. live too far away) will usually participate in a programme locally. When a patient attends another institution, their progress should be regularly reported back to the transplant team. The physiotherapist from the transplant unit is a useful resource, often providing advice and practical support to clinicians in the community.

Exercise Training

The heterogeneous nature of transplant candidates means that the individual patient's unique pathophysiology, time in clinical course, symptoms, needs, goals and response to exercise must be taken into consideration when undertaking exercise training. All patients waiting for heart, heart–lung and lung transplants are encouraged to remain as active as possible. A careful assessment is required to ensure that each patient is safe to exercise. Physiotherapists working in this area may be exposed to conditions rarely seen. Caution must be taken with all patients. Patients who demonstrate profound desaturation despite oxygen therapy, hypotension or any other markedly abnormal response may not be able to exercise, or will be restricted to gentle stretches or ADLs only. Overall, the vast majority of patients are safe to participate in an exercise training programme.

General guidelines for exercise training in cardiac rehabilitation and pulmonary rehabilitation have been discussed (see Chapter 12). There is a growing evidence base regarding the safety, efficacy and feasibility of exercise training programs in lung disease populations other than chronic obstructive pulmonary disease (COPD), including interstitial lung disease (Garvey 2010, Holland & Hill 2008) and pulmonary arterial hypertension (de Man et al 2009, Fox et al 2011, Mereles et al 2006).

In lung transplant candidates, many factors may contribute to exercise limitation including ventilatory limitations, gas exchange abnormalities, skeletal muscle dysfunction and respiratory muscle dysfunction. It has been shown that patients with severe chronic respiratory disease can sustain the necessary training intensity and duration for skeletal muscle adaptation (Maltais et al 1996, Whittom et al 1998).

Close monitoring of symptoms, particularly SOB, in addition to oxygen saturation and heart rate is required. An appropriate target for oxygen saturation during exercise for each individual should be determined before starting exercise. Supplemental oxygen is often required. It is clinical practice to maintain oxygen saturation at greater than 85–90% during exercise. Exact thresholds will vary depending on the patient's native disease and clinical state. This may require discussion with the primary respiratory physician.

Some disease groups have unique features that must be taken into consideration when planning and conducting exercise training programs. Patients who experience dynamic hyperinflation may benefit from using a four-wheeled frame to support their upper limbs during lower limb training (Solway et al 2002). Care must be taken if prescribing upper limb exercises above shoulder level, as dysynchronous breathing may occur in some individuals (Mathur et al 2009). The prevention of cross-infection and ensuring an adequate salt intake is essential for patients with CF (Lands et al 1999, Saiman & Siegel 2004). Patients with interstitial lung disease often experience significant dyspnoea but may be able to perform interval training

regimens with high-flow oxygen. Interval training is often better tolerated than continuous training in those who experience high levels of dyspnoea and has been shown to achieve similar improvements in exercise capacity (Beauchamp et al 2010, Gloeckl et al 2012). NIV may help achieve a greater training intensity by unloading the respiratory muscles in some patients (Hoo 2003, van 't Hul et al 2006). High-intensity exercise is generally not recommended for patients with pulmonary arterial hypertension (Nici et al 2006) and interval training is avoided because of rapid changes in pulmonary dynamics and risk of syncope.

Cardiac transplant candidates are generally able to exercise within the limits of standard haemodynamic guidelines. Close monitoring of symptoms, in particular dyspnoea, dizziness, light-headedness and chest pain, in addition to heart rate and blood pressure, is required. An increase of more than 1–2 kg in body weight over the previous few days may indicate fluid retention and along with worsening of heart failure symptoms, should be reported back to the transplant clinic. If they have an inappropriate response to exercise (e.g. a decrease in systolic blood pressure >10 mmHg with an increased workload), exercise should be ceased (Selig et al 2010).

Exercise capacity in heart failure patients is poorly correlated with the degree of cardiac dysfunction (Franciosa et al 1981, Myers et al 1998). The major limitation to exercise capacity stems from secondary, peripheral adaptations. These include impaired muscle structure and function, and vascular and metabolic abnormalities (Clark et al 1996). The positive effect of endurance training on peak VO_2 in patients with heart failure is well recognized (Lloyd-Williams et al 2002, Mandic et al 2009); however, it is known that endurance training alone does not enhance skeletal muscle strength (Feiereisen et al 2007). Resistance training has been shown to be safe and is recommended for patients with stable heart failure, as it directly targets the peripheral impairments (Braith and Beck, 2008, Selig et al 2010). A combined model of training would appear to be superior to either isolated endurance or resistance training, with improvements in peak VO_2, muscle strength, endurance, vascular function and quality of life (Gary et al 2011, Maiorana et al 2000, Piepoli et al 2011, Servantes et al 2012).

Pre-Transplant Exercise Guidelines

- Supervision of exercise training by an experienced clinician where possible, 2–3 times per week; home exercise programme 2–3 times per week
- Combination of endurance and resistance training
- *Closely monitor relevant signs and symptoms*
- Blood pressure (BP), heart rate (HR), oxyhaemoglobin saturation by pulse oximeter (SpO_2), Borg SOB, rating of perceived exertion (RPE)
- Training duration and intensity performed according to patient's signs and symptoms
- Endurance training:
  - Heart patients: gradual progression to 45–60 minutes where able; aim for Borg RPE 11–14.
  - Lung patients: progress to cumulative total of 30 minutes where able; rate dyspnoea and leg fatigue separately to ensure that limitation to exercise is adequately monitored. Aim for Borg 3–4 for dyspnoea or Borg RPE 12–15 for leg fatigue.
  - Consider interval training.
- Resistance training:
  - Heart patients: aim for 40–50% 1 repetition maximum (RM) or RPE 10–15, 5–15 repetitions per set, 1–2 sets, depending on symptoms and New York Heart Association (NYHA) class.
  - Lung patients: aim for 8–10 repetitions at 8–10 RM, 1–3 sets depending on tolerance.
- Stretch/maintain muscle length, particularly calf, hamstrings, iliopsoas, pectorals
- Maintain range of movement of shoulders and chest wall, with a focus on facilitating normal posture
- Include functional exercises (e.g. step ups, squats).

Education

Pre-transplant education is facilitated by various members of the multidisciplinary team. Some units have a structured, group education programme while others provide one-to-one (individual patients and carer) education.

Topics may include:

- keeping active
- nutrition
- practical aspects of being on the waiting lists (notification, what to bring to hospital, how to get to hospital)
- understanding the patient's role in transplantation
- appliances to assist with activities of daily living (ADLs) and energy conservation strategies
- constructive use of time to improve quality of life while awaiting transplant
- stress management.

Timing to transplantation is variable and can range from weeks to years. Once on the waiting list, patients are monitored closely by the transplant team to ensure that candidates continue to meet selection criteria. Periodic review also allows for fine-tuning of patient management.

Bridge to Transplant

In an effort to optimize therapy and improve survival while on the waiting list, a number of management strategies including pharmacological therapies, device therapies and surgical intervention are considered.

Device therapies have been shown to decrease mortality and improve cardiac function in patients with end-stage heart failure. Device therapies used in cardiac transplant candidates include implantable cardioverter–defibrillators (ICDs), cardiac resynchronization therapy (CRT) and mechanical assist devices.

Mechanical cardiac assist devices have been increasingly utilized as a bridge to transplant with over one-third of patients being on mechanical support at the time of heart transplant (Stehlik et al 2012). The vast majority of these patients are supported with a left ventricular assist device (LVAD). Increased knowledge about patient selection, the timing of implantation and improved patient management has resulted in improved outcomes with decreasing adverse events. There is a paucity of studies examining the effect of exercise training after LVAD implantation. Previous research has demonstrated that insertion of the mechanical pump alone improves exercise capacity and quality of life (Kugler et al 2011). Haemodynamic, ventilatory and neurohormonal measures have been shown to improve post insertion of an LVAD (Branch et al 1994, Jaski et al 1997, Mancini et al 1998). Other studies have reported significant improvements in sub-maximal exercise capacity following LVAD implantation (Foray et al 1996, Morrone et al 1996). However, patients continue to have significant functional limitations, with exercise capacity below that reported for patients following heart transplantation (Jaski et al 1999, Kugler et al 2011) and significantly lower than those reported for the normal population (Kugler et al 2011).

These patients are sometimes in a moribund state prior to LVAD implantation and physiotherapy goals are centred on improving exercise capacity prior to receiving a transplant. Despite evidence that exercise capacity improves after insertion of a LVAD, it remains unclear whether exercise training has additional benefits on cardiovascular fitness. Several studies (Morrone et al 1996, Reedy et al 1992) have demonstrated that early submaximal exercise is not only safe in this population but improves morbidity and mortality. Improvements in peak and functional exercise capacity and quality of life with a structured exercise training programme have been demonstrated in several small studies (Hayes et al 2012, Laoutaris et al 2011). Despite the need for larger trials to determine the ideal type, timing, duration and intensity of exercise training post LVAD implantation, international guidelines recommend that all patients with a mechanical cardiac assist device participate in exercise training and undergo regular testing of functional capacity (Feldman et al 2013).

In lung transplant candidates, surgery, pharmaceutical agents and mechanical support are also used. Lung volume reduction surgery may be used to delay the need for transplant in highly selected patients with emphysema (Cordova & Criner 2002). Inhaled nitric oxide or intravenous prostacyclin may be used in the setting of severe pulmonary hypertension (Olsson et al 2005, Yung et al 2001) and NIV for those with hypercapnic respiratory failure (British Thoracic Society 2002) and CF (Madden et al 2002). As outcomes in patients supported pre-transplantation with ECMO have traditionally been poor, its use as a bridge to lung transplantation has been quite limited. There have been some promising reports of using ECMO in awake, non-intubated patients, allowing them to actively participate in airway clearance techniques and safely ambulate and potentially be in better physical condition by the time of transplant (Fuehner et al 2012, Turner et al 2011).

POSTOPERATIVE MANAGEMENT

The aim of medical management in the early transplant period is to initiate effective immunosuppression, to minimize the risk of infection and to protect other organ systems such as the renal system.

Post-transplant physiotherapy management is similar to that of other thoracic surgery patients. Subjective and objective assessment findings must be reviewed along with the latest microbiology results, ABGs, chest radiograph and cardiovascular measures. Treatment choice, frequency and duration will depend on the individual patient presentation. Patients vary according to a number of factors, including:

- graft function
- pain control
- preoperative physical condition
- presence of comorbidities (diabetes, unstable blood sugar levels)
- emotional adjustment
- postoperative complications (Box 13-6).

Physiotherapy treatment in the postoperative period aims to:

- optimize ventilation
- clear retained lung secretions
- promote independent function (i.e. bed mobility, transfers, ambulation)
- improve fitness/activity tolerance
- facilitate self-management.

BOX 13-6
POSTOPERATIVE COMPLICATIONS IMPACTING REHABILITATION

- Pain control
- Acute rejection
- Chest infection
- Renal insufficiency
- Steroid myopathy
- Psychiatric disturbance secondary to steroid therapy
- Persistent air leak*
- Phrenic nerve injury*
- Poor healing airway anastomosis*

---

*Lung transplant.

Management in the Intensive Care Unit

The physiotherapy programme is initiated in the ICU as early as the first postoperative day. Acutely, the goals are to prevent perioperative complications of bedrest. Airway clearance techniques, joint ROM and positioning are implemented as indicated. Once the cardiovascular and respiratory systems are stabilized, the patient is rapidly weaned from the ventilator and extubated. Delay in extubation can occur for a number of reasons, including primary graft dysfunction. As the intubation period increases, so too does the risk of nosocomial pneumonia. Non-invasive ventilatory support may be useful in assisting patients who have experienced difficulties in weaning and extubation.

Lung transplant patients often have a poor ability to perceive the presence of secretions and this may persist in the long term. It is common for lung and heart–lung transplant recipients to expectorate old blood and slough from the bronchial/tracheal anastomosis. Secretions may also originate from the donor (donor-acquired infection) or recipient's native airways (common in CF). If sputum retention becomes a problem for a recipient, inhalation therapy and an airway clearance technique should be instituted, and this should be considered early in the postoperative course. Positioning, combined with an airway clearance technique (e.g. active cycle of breathing techniques), are the primary forms of initial treatment.

Once extubated and stable, the emphasis is on early mobilization, with patients assisted to sit out of bed and commence ambulation, often within 1–2 days post operatively (Fig. 13-24). It is important for patients to have sufficient analgesia to allow effective huffing, coughing and for early mobilization. The length of stay in ICU can be as short as 1 day or extend to prolonged periods, depending on complications.

Ward Management

On the ward, physiotherapy treatment focuses on achieving independence with ADLs, increasing endurance (walking, stationary cycling, stair climbing) and exercises addressing any specific musculoskeletal deficits. Stationary cycling in the patient's room is

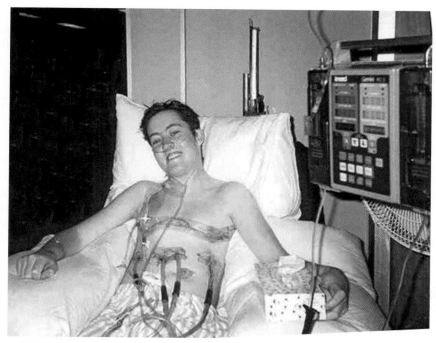

FIGURE 13-24 ■ Sitting out of bed soon after bilateral sequential lung transplantation (BSLTx).

particularly useful in the early stages following lung and heart–lung transplant when intercostal drains (ICDs) are on suction. Once drain tubes are removed, bilateral upper limb elevation and trunk ROM is performed within patient comfort. Postural re-education is also often required. Motivation and self-management may be enhanced by using charts and exercise diaries to provide a measure of improvement in function.

In lung transplant recipients, routine bronchoscopy is used to assess airway anastomotic healing and patency, the presence of infection (from BAL) and rejection (from TBB). Bronchoscopic findings are very useful to the physiotherapist and assist in clinical decision making to determine appropriate treatments. Significant ischaemia can occur at the site of bronchial anastomosis where healing is inherently slow. Most lung transplant recipients still have slough at the bronchial anastomoses at 1 month post transplant (Munro et al 2008). This does not require active physiotherapy treatment. In the setting of sputum retention, airway clearance techniques are utilized. Treatments involving high levels of positive pressure (e.g. NIV, positive expiratory pressure (PEP) therapy) are generally avoided if the recipient has a significant defect in a bronchial anastomosis.

Chest wall/sternal precautions may vary between institutions, surgeons and individual patients. In general, a conservative approach is taken due to slow tissue healing and considerable morbidity associated with sternal instability. Patients are often advised not to lift greater than a total of 5 kg for 10–12 weeks.

The average length of hospital stay following heart or lung transplantation is 2–3 weeks. Some patients are discharged as early as 1–2 weeks postoperatively, while others may spend weeks to months in hospital secondary to complications.

Before discharge from hospital, patients must have a good understanding of the signs and symptoms of rejection and infection, and their medications. Rehabilitation usually continues on an outpatient basis at the transplant centre.

OUTPATIENT REHABILITATION

Many transplant units require recipients to participate in a formal rehabilitation programme comprising 8–12 weeks of supervised exercise training (Fig. 13-25)

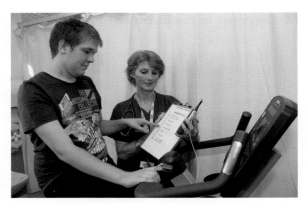

FIGURE 13-25 ■ Post-transplant gym class.

and an education programme at the transplant centre following discharge.

The primary goals in the rehabilitation phase are to:

- improve physical condition – functional performance, strength and endurance
- achieve competency in self-management – lifelong medication, monitoring and maintenance of health, regular follow-up
- facilitate active engagement and participation in social, recreational and employment activities
- provide the recipient with sufficient psychological support for adjustment to new health status.

By approximately 12 weeks, most patients require less frequent review by the transplant team and are discharged from physiotherapy with a maintenance home exercise programme to be undertaken independently. Patients are encouraged to maintain an active lifestyle (Fig. 13-26). Those who require further rehabilitation are referred to a programme in their local area where access is more convenient.

The optimal protocols for exercise training (frequency, duration, intensity of exercise) are yet to be established; however; the best available evidence supports the inclusion of both endurance and resistance training for both heart transplant (Hsieh et al 2011, Pina et al 2003) and lung transplant recipients (Langer et al 2012a, Wickerson et al 2010).

Special considerations for exercise training are outlined in Box 13-7.

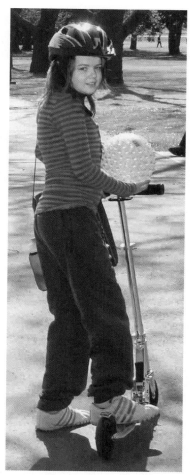

FIGURE 13-26 ■ An active lifestyle is strongly encouraged.

Rehabilitation programs for children must also meet their individual developmental needs. Age-appropriate activities such as hopping, jumping and running are introduced in a graded fashion. Play-based activities including indoor and outdoor ball games and bike riding can be incorporated to facilitate the acquisition of balance and coordination skills. They also promote confidence in participating in recreation and sports with family and peers. Interactive video games are particularly popular with children and adolescents, and can provide a high level of motivation with immediate feedback and rewards for physical activity (Burton et al 2009).

Education continues for the patient and carer in the outpatient setting facilitated by the multidisciplinary team. Common topics include:

- medication
- recognizing rejection and infection
- getting fit and staying active
- food hygiene
- returning to work
- organ donation.

Regular medical follow-up continues until most patients can be reviewed on a 6–12 monthly basis. Improvements in functional exercise capacity and quality of life reflect the multimodal nature of the management of the transplant recipient (e.g. surgery, rehabilitation, lifestyle changes). Specific outcome measures for physiotherapy interventions should relate to each physiotherapy goal. It has been suggested that functional exercise capacity, level of activity, strength and health-related quality of life (HRQoL) be measured before and after postoperative rehabilitation and then yearly as a minimum.

EXERCISE LIMITATION AND FUNCTION POST TRANSPLANT

Exercise capacity improves significantly after heart, heart–lung and lung transplantation; however, it remains below normal predicted values.

Heart transplant recipients demonstrate a reduced peak heart rate and peak VO_2 of 60–70% of age-matched normal individuals, particularly in the first 2 years following transplant (Gullestad et al 1996). The main determinants of this lower exercise capacity appear to be a combination of chronotropic and inotropic incompetence, both consequences of cardiac denervation (Andreassen 2008). Peripheral factors (endothelial and muscular impairments) secondary to the immunosuppressive regimen and muscle atrophy/deconditioning also contribute to this reduction in exercise capacity (Mettauer et al 2005). With high intensity, long-term endurance training programs, some heart transplant recipients have demonstrated improvements up to 95% of predicted peak HR and peak VO_2 late after transplantation (Braith & Edwards 2000). A combination of endurance and resistance training may improve peak VO_2 and muscle strength

BOX 13-7
REHABILITATION GUIDELINES POST THORACIC TRANSPLANTATION

Type of exercise: combination of endurance and resistance training
Frequency: supervised 3× weekly. In addition, home exercise programme 2–3×/week
Training duration: Progression to 30–45 minutes endurance training for 8–12 weeks
Training intensity: moderate intensity guided by symptoms

CLOSELY MONITOR SIGNS AND SYMPTOMS

- Heart transplant: BP, HR, Borg SOB, RPE
- Lung transplant: HR, SpO_2, Borg SOB, RPE
- Transplant complications (e.g. rejection, infection) often manifest as a reduction in exercise tolerance or abnormal exercise response. Concerns should be reported immediately to the transplant unit.

HEART TRANSPLANT RECIPIENTS HAVE AN ABNORMAL RESPONSE TO EXERCISE DUE TO DENERVATION

- Do not use HR as the primary indicator of response to exercise. Restrict exercise intensity to a level that elicits an RPE 11–14, or a HR response of <20 beats greater than resting levels (Braith 1998).
- Ensure adequate warm-up to allow adequate time for the effects of catecholamine levels on cardiac output (Andreassen 2008, Braith 1998, Mettauer et al 2005).
- Hypotension during resistance exercise is common, particularly with above heart level exercises (Braith 1998). Strategies to reduce this include: alternate upper and lower limb exercises to reduce venous pooling, walk for 2 minutes between exercises or do seated calf raises, and ensure minimum 5-minute cool down at low intensity.

CONSIDER THE MUSCULOSKELETAL SIDE EFFECTS OF IMMUNOSUPPRESSANT DRUGS

Observe Chest Wall Precautions

- Sternal stability may be assessed using the sternal instability scale (SIS) (El-Ansary et al 2007). A SIS score of greater than 0, or reports of ongoing pain and deformity (Macchiarini et al 1999) may require

surgery or other management such as external bracing (Fuller et al 2012, Karnak et al 2006).

Bone Morbidity: Osteoporosis, Pathological Fracture and Avascular Necrosis are Common

- Progressive resistance training should be included to optimize bone mineral density and reverse corticosteroid mediated muscle atrophy (Braith 1998; Braith et al 1996, 2007; Mitchell et al 2003). Be conservative with initial resistances and ensure a very gradual progression, especially in patients with advanced osteoporosis.
- Pathological fracture (particularly vertebral compression) and avascular necrosis (commonly head of femur) should be considered as potential causes of pain (Shane et al 1993). Imaging techniques such as bone scan may be required so that appropriate management is undertaken (Henderson et al 1997).

Care Must be Taken When Progressing Activity

- Most patients are unaccustomed to exercise and are at risk of overuse injuries if activity is progressed too rapidly (e.g. Achilles tendinitis, shin splints).

Modify Exercise during Episodes of Acute Rejection

- Mild rejection: continue with close monitoring of patient's signs and symptoms.
- Moderate rejection: patients should not exercise during the short period in which they are receiving high-dose corticosteroids due to the heightened risk of a coronary event and catabolic effects of the corticosteroids on bone and skeletal muscle (Braith 1998). Exercise should be gradually increased and symptom-limited when recommenned.
- Severe rejection: no exercise; activity limited to self-care only

Ensure Adequate Infection Control Due to Immunosuppression

- Handwashing before and after attendance at exercise class
- Cleaning of exercise equipment
- Individuals with active infection should not attend group exercise classes

---

BP, Blood pressure; *HR*, heart rate; *RPE*, rate of perceived exertion; *SOB*, shortness of breath; *SpO₂*, oxyhaemoglobin saturation by pulse oximeter.

---

and decrease the side effects of the immunosuppressive drugs and control risk factors for CAV (Hsieh et al 2011, Marconi & Marzorati 2003).

Substantial exercise limitation is also seen in lung transplant recipients. Leg fatigue is commonly reported as the predominant symptom at exercise

termination on cardiopulmonary exercise testing and with functional activities. Numerous studies have shown a reduced peak VO_2 of 40–60% of age-matched norms (Levy et al 1993, Reinsma et al 2006, Williams et al 1992). This is mostly unrelated to ventilation or cardiac limitations. Abnormal peripheral circulation and abnormal skeletal muscle structure and function have been shown (Lands et al 1999, McKenna et al 2003, Tirdel et al 1998, Wang et al 1999). Multiple factors are thought to be responsible, including myotoxic effects of immunosuppressants, pre-operative lung disease and deconditioning.

A small number of studies have evaluated exercise training programs following lung transplant. Improvements have been demonstrated in functional (Langer et al 2012a) and maximal exercise capacity (Stiebellehner et al 1998), skeletal muscle function (Guerrero et al 2005) and strength (Langer et al 2012a). In addition, improvements have been demonstrated in bone mineral density (Braith et al 2007) and HRQoL (Munro et al 2009). Exercise training is an important therapeutic tool in the long-term management of thoracic organ transplant recipients and may also have an important role in reducing the incidence of common transplant comorbidities such as hypertension and diabetes (Langer et al 2012a).

LONG-TERM MANAGEMENT

Improved survival outcomes have led to significant growth in the demand for physiotherapy management of long-term morbidity. Long-term survivors experience a range of problems requiring hospital admission or outpatient follow-up. These include:

- acute rejection
- chronic graft dysfunction
- steroid myopathy
- renal dysfunction
- acute or chronic infection
- hypertension
- hyperlipidaemia
- malignancy.

Many transplant recipients maintain near-normal function for many years post transplant. Others develop complications that require long-term medical or physiotherapy input. Physiotherapists commonly address problems such as:

- respiratory tract infection
- musculoskeletal morbidities
- reduced functional mobility
- declining exercise capacity
- changes in social and vocational roles.

In such cases, there is a need to set realistic goals and to assist the patient and family to adjust to the change in functional performance. Optimizing quality of life remains the primary goal. Inevitably, the care of these patients shifts away from acute medical management towards chronic disease management and palliative care. This transition is often difficult for both the patient and the healthcare team.

SPECIFIC CONSIDERATIONS FOR PAEDIATRIC PATIENTS

Most of the information presented above applies to both paediatric and adult heart and lung transplant recipients. However, there are a few additional issues that are specific to children. These are listed in Table 13-14.

CONCLUSION

Over the past 4 decades, thoracic organ transplantation has changed from a highly experimental surgical procedure to a common treatment for management of end-stage cardiac and pulmonary failure. Continuing advances in all aspects of pre- and post-transplant management have led to significant improvements in morbidity and mortality. As long-term survival improves, there is greater recognition of the importance of optimizing the physical condition of potential candidates pre-transplant and the need to actively manage long-term comorbidities. Physiotherapists have a key and enduring role in the management of these patients that extends from pre-transplant assessment through to the palliative care of long-term survivors. Patients undergoing thoracic organ transplantation present with a broad range of complex medical issues which necessitate management by a highly specialized team. Physiotherapists are an integral part of that team, and as such require a high level of knowledge and a range of specialist skills in the management of cardiorespiratory, orthopaedic and neurological pathologies.

Acknowledgement

The authors would like to thank Catherine E Bray for the sections taken from 'Cardiopulmonary Transplantation' in the third edition of *Physiotherapy for Respiratory and Cardiac Problems*.

TABLE 13-14	
Specific Considerations for Children Undergoing Heart or Lung Transplantation	
Lung function testing	All lung transplant recipients use spirometry to monitor lung function. This is possible in all children aged 4 years or more, though techniques may need to be modified. Different lung function techniques are needed for children less than 4 years.
Biopsy	Endocardial and transbronchial biopsies are essential for detecting graft rejection. In all children these procedures are performed under general anaesthetic, rather than sedation. They are technically more difficult in younger children.
Infections	Many children will not have had previous exposure to common viruses, and the incidence of primary infection is much higher than for adults. It is therefore essential that immunization status is optimized prior to listing for transplantation.
Malignancy	Post-transplant lymphoproliferative disease (PTLD) is far more common in children than in adults. Other tumours, especially skin and lung, are more rare in children.
Psychosocial issues	Many children coming to transplant are physically and emotionally immature because of their chronic illness. A successful transplant allows a child to transform their life and to catch up on many of the activities that were previously denied to them. Some children find this change in lifestyle difficult, particularly if it coincides with puberty. Non-adherence to therapy is an important cause of poor outcome, especially in teenage patients, and appears worst in those who have a chronic illness such as cystic fibrosis. Most centres stress that adolescents should steadily take more responsibility for their own care and are given practical assistance to boost adherence to therapy.

Trauma

INTRODUCTION

People in the prime of their economically productive lives are often involved in traumatic injury as a result of road traffic accidents, injuries sustained at work, interpersonal violence or even attempted suicide. Traumatic injury contributes largely to the burden of diseases worldwide, as severe trauma often leads to long-term disability which negatively impacts trauma survivors' HRQoL (World Health Organization 2011). For the purpose of this section, 'trauma' refers to damage to any body part as a result of physical impact or accident. Severity of injury can range from mild to life-threatening. Blunt or penetrating injuries to the thoracic cage and/or abdominal organs often result from motor vehicle or pedestrian–vehicle accidents, falls from a height or intentional injury such as physical abuse, gunshot or stab wounds. Those who are involved in high-energy impact injury may also present with fractures of the pelvic girdle or extremities. This section focuses on the management of the polytrauma patient who sustained abdominal, thoracic and/or pelvic injuries. These are the types of patients that physiotherapists often encounter in the ICU and may feel less confident to handle due to the severity of their injuries.

CAUSES AND MECHANISMS OF INJURY

The use of drugs and a positive blood alcohol level remain the highest risk factors for motor cycle, motor vehicle and pedestrian–vehicle crashes as well as intentional injury caused to others or oneself (Brady & Li 2013, Carrasco et al 2012). High-energy injury often results in pelvic fractures, although the elderly may develop pelvic fracture from a simple fall. Forces distributed over a large area (deceleration injury such as fall from a height) often result in blunt injury. Forces distributed over a small area by penetrating objects (gunshot or stab wounds, shrapnel) injure the organs that lie along the path of the penetrating object. In gunshot-related injury, high-velocity bullets cause damage to the organs in the path of the bullet but also to remote organs (blood vessels, nerves and bone) through shock waves that radiate from the missile tract. Tissues are forced forwards and outward by the shock waves and a cavity is formed which may be larger than the penetrating bullet. A vacuum forms which sucks air and bacteria from the environment and debris into the missile tract before the cavity collapses during a period of milliseconds after bullet penetration, and this often becomes a source of infection (Hauer et al 2011, Maiden 2009). Penetrating abdominal injury is only life-threatening if a major blood vessel is damaged. In contrast, penetrating thoracic injury is immediately life-threatening, as it often results in severe respiratory distress due to loss of negative intrapleural pressures and lack of oxygen delivery to tissues due to blood loss and parenchymal damage (Livingstone & Hauser 2004).

COMPLICATIONS RELATED TO TRAUMATIC INJURY

Circulatory Deficits

Traumatic injury results in haemorrhage. Blunt and penetrating injury often lead to damage to internal organs and blood vessels, leading to contusion and loss of intravascular blood volume into the surrounding tissues or to the external environment. The pelvis is rich in blood supply and fracture of the pelvis is associated with significant internal blood loss (Mejaddam & Velmahos 2012). Loss of intravascular volume leads to decreases in venous return, cardiac output, stroke volume and eventually systemic blood pressure. When up to a third of total blood volume is lost, the patient presents with elevated heart rate and diastolic blood pressure. Blood loss of more than 40% total blood volume results in bradycardia and in some situations un-recordable blood pressure, which is immediately life-threatening (Garrioch 2004). Severe traumatic injury often leads to the development of shock due to massive blood loss, myocardial contusion, cardiac tamponade and tension pneumothorax. Shock signifies circulatory failure and inadequate tissue perfusion and due to the lack of oxygen delivery at cellular level, end organ injury may develop. Individuals who suffered thoracic trauma are at risk of the development of cardiogenic shock due to ventricle contusion; those who lost a large amount of blood due to abdominal, thoracic or pelvic injury are at risk of developing hypovolemic shock (Kumar & Parrillo 2008).

Deficits in Oxygenation

Blunt or penetrating thoracic injury causes damage to the lung parenchyma and capillaries and results in contusion and blood loss into the pleural cavity. Loss of the negative intrapleural pressure due to blood or air accumulation in the pleural cavity is associated with lung volume loss due to the development of pneumo- and/or haemothorax. These factors give rise to $\dot{V}/\dot{Q}$ mismatch and the development of hypoxaemia. Less oxygen is extracted from inhaled air due to lung volume loss and therefore less oxygen is available for delivery at cellular level. The reduction in cardiac output, stroke volume and systemic blood pressure described also contributes to the lack of oxygen delivery at cellular level. Both these factors give rise to the development of hypoxia. As a compensatory measure, the patient's respiratory rate increases. Fast and shallow respiration leads to further lung volume loss. Hyperventilation accompanies the metabolic acidosis that develops due to the shocked state of the patient. ARDS may develop as a result of SIRS, which results in severe hypoxaemia (Schroeder et al 2009).

Systemic Inflammatory Response Syndrome, Sepsis and Muscle Weakness

Inflammation develops in patients who are in low perfusion states due to inadequate restoration of blood volume after the traumatic event. SIRS develops when the body is subjected to severe clinical insults such as traumatic injury, burns, ischaemia or inflammation but is not associated with infection (Schroeder et al 2009). Sepsis is diagnosed in the presence of the systemic response to Gram negative or positive bacterial or fungal infection. Sepsis in the presence of cardiovascular failure is defined as septic shock (Nguyen et al 2006). As the patient's immune system attempts to fight the infection, white blood cells and macrophages are released, and vascular endothelial damage occurs and gives rise to leakage of fluid into the extravascular compartments. Multiple chemicals such as cytokines, reactive oxygen species, nitric oxide, platelet activating factor and vasodilators are released into the blood stream. Endotoxins and exotoxins are also released and together with the aforementioned chemicals cause microvascular injury, vasodilatation of the capillary bed, thrombosis and tissue ischaemia

(Nguyen & Smith 2007, Nguyen et al 2006). These systemic changes lead to multiple organ dysfunction and the development of disseminated intravascular coagulation which is associated with poor patient outcome (Nguyen & Smith 2007, Nguyen et al 2006).

In sepsis, circulating cytokine balance is disturbed. The unbalanced cytokine activity together with immobility that results from traumatic injury leads to the development of musculoskeletal abnormalities. Elevated levels of pro-inflammatory cytokines and decreased levels of anti-inflammatory cytokines have been reported in patients who suffer from critical illness and traumatic injury (Jawa et al 2011). Pro-inflammatory cytokines such as interleukin (IL)-1 and tumour necrosis factor α contribute to muscle protein breakdown, cell death and reduction in muscle mass. Persistently high levels of IL-6 lead to increased patient mortality. Excessive inflammation and muscle damage is associated with persistently low levels of anti-inflammatory cytokines such as IL-10 (Callahan & Supinski 2009, Winkelman et al 2007, Winkelman 2004). High levels of reactive oxygen species in circulating blood of patients with critical illness is associated with myofilament dysfunction and muscle weakness (Callahan & Supinsky 2009). The resulting muscle weakness involves the peripheral and respiratory muscles and often leads to difficulty with weaning patients off mechanical ventilation, poor functional activity and decreased exercise endurance.

MEDICAL AND SURGICAL MANAGEMENT OF PATIENTS WITH TRAUMATIC INJURY

Any patient who presents to the casualty department with traumatic injury is managed according to three steps: namely, primary survey and resuscitation of vital functions, secondary survey and definitive care. Each of these steps is discussed in the following sections.

Primary Survey and Resuscitation of Vital Functions

The primary survey is conducted according to 'airway, breathing, circulation, disability and exposure' in order to stabilize the patient's condition, also known as the ABCDE approach to basic life support (Thim et al 2012). 'Disability' refers to assessment of level of consciousness and 'exposure' refers to the removal of clothes to visualize the skin and identify injuries. Life-threatening injuries that are not visible are identified with the use of ultrasound technology, chest radiography and CT scans. During the primary survey, care is provided to the patient in the form of oxygen therapy, placement of an artificial airway if indicated, placement of nasogastric tube, peripheral intravenous lines (analgesic and fluid administration) and a urinary catheter. In the presence of pneumothorax or haemothorax, an ICD is placed to drain excess air and/or blood from the pleural cavity. As soon as the patient's condition is stabilized the secondary survey commences.

Secondary Survey

This is a head-to-toe evaluation of the patient that is guided by suspicion of missed injuries during the primary survey. It includes a complete neurological and physical examination, as well as detailed history-taking from the patient and/or the emergency response team members. Arterial and central venous lines are placed for the patient and further CT investigations are done to identify internal organ injuries that may have been missed during the primary survey. On identification of all injuries sustained, decisions are made regarding definitive care.

Definitive Care

Definitive care may involve admission to ICU for monitoring and therapy for stable patients with traumatic injury or operative management for those who are haemodynamically unstable.

Abdominal Injury

Patients who suffered blunt abdominal trauma and who are in a stable condition are admitted to ICU for management as mentioned. Those with blunt abdominal trauma and shock are taken to theatre immediately for exploratory laparotomy in order to identify the extent of internal bleeding. An exploratory laparotomy is also performed on patients who suffered penetrating abdominal trauma and present with haemodynamic instability (Van der Vlies et al 2011). After wound closure, these patients are admitted to ICU for monitoring, therapy and close observation, especially for the development of abdominal compartment

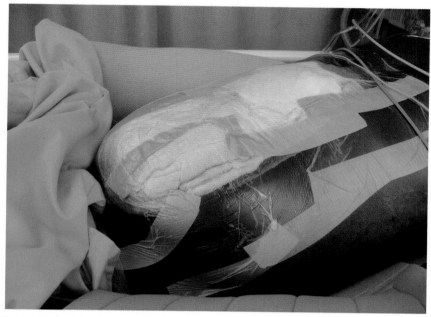

FIGURE 13-27 ■ Damage control surgery for traumatic abdominal injury (open packed abdomen).

syndrome. Damage control surgery is used in the case of severely unstable patients with abdominal injuries (Fig. 13-27). This concept involves an initial exploratory laparotomy to control bleeding from large organ tears. The abdominal cavity is then left open, packed with dressings, and the patient is admitted to ICU for stabilization. A re-look laparotomy is performed 48 hours later to repair smaller organ tears. The patient may even be taken back to theatre a third or fourth time if indicated prior to abdominal wound closure (Cirocchi et al 2013, Kirkpatrick et al 2006).

In cases where abdominal sepsis develops, the use of negative pressure wound therapy is well supported (Roberts et al 2012a, b). Negative pressure wound therapy assists with rapid removal of infective material from the wound bed and stimulates growth of granulation tissue. It also assists with pulling the wound edges closer to facilitate wound closure (Roberts et al 2012a, b) (Fig. 13-28).

Thoracic Injury

Patients with myocardial contusion are closely monitored in ICU through electrocardiography and blood enzyme levels. Those with airway or great vessel injury that are stable are closely monitored in ICU. Non-operative management is indicated for patients with pulmonary contusion. Pain management, accurate fluid administration, bronchopulmonary hygiene therapy and NIPPV (if appropriate) are important components of the ICU care provided for these patients (Cohn & DuBose 2010). Fractures of the ribs or sternum are usually managed conservatively through adequate administration of analgesia, NIPPV (if appropriate) and optimization of lung volumes. Patients with flail rib injuries managed with NIPPV showed better outcomes related to nosocomial infection and mortality rates than those managed with intubation and mechanical ventilation (Gunduz et al 2005). Patients with flail rib injuries who suffer with poor oxygenation despite optimal mechanical ventilation may undergo operative stabilization of the ribcage (Fitzpatrick et al 2010) (Fig. 13-29).

Operative management of patients who present with haemodynamic instability following thoracic injury includes median sternotomy to repair injuries to the great vessels, airways, oesophagus or heart and for surgical stabilization of overlapping sternal fractures. Laparotomy is performed for most patients

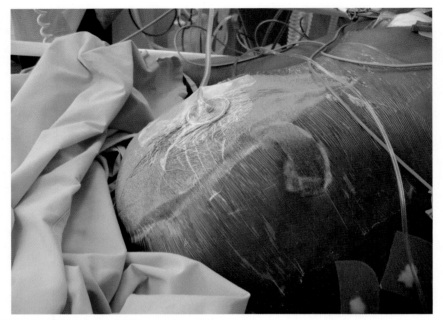

FIGURE 13-28 ▪ Septic abdominal wound managed with negative pressure wound therapy.

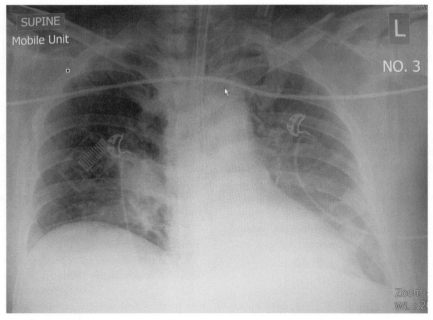

FIGURE 13-29 ▪ Chest radiograph. Multiple rib fractures (left ribs 2–6) with left-sided haemothorax and clavicle fracture following motorcycle accident.

who present with diaphragm laceration. In some cases, thoracotomy is performed to repair lacerations to the right hemi-diaphragm (Chughtai et al 2009). Surgical debridement of soft-tissue injuries that result from gunshot wounds is performed to remove necrotic tissue in order to prevent the development of infection.

Pelvic Injury

Surgical management of patients with orthopaedic injuries has evolved over the years and now focuses on the concept of damage control orthopaedics. This approach uses little operative intervention after injury until patients are physiologically stable enough to be taken to theatre for surgical stabilization. Improved patient outcomes are reported using this approach to orthopaedic management of the polytrauma patient (Mejaddam & Velmahos 2012). In the case of pelvic fractures, external fixators are placed to obtain optimal alignment while the patient is stabilized in ICU prior to theatre. If such patients present with excessive haemorrhage, they will be taken to theatre immediately in order to control bleeding surgically (Mejaddam & Velmahos 2012).

PHYSIOTHERAPY INTERVENTION FOR THE TRAUMA PATIENT

Any patient who suffered traumatic injury should receive an individualized assessment to identify problems and set appropriate goals for physiotherapy management in ICU and the trauma ward setting. The National Institute of Health and Care Excellence (NICE) clinical practice guidelines promotes the use of specific, measurable, achievable, results-focused and time-bound (SMART) goals for patient care (NICE 2009). Involvement of patients and their families in goal setting for physiotherapy management throughout their hospital stay is recommended (NICE 2009). Rehabilitation should commence in ICU and each patient's condition should be re-assessed before discharge to the trauma ward to ensure modification of rehabilitation interventions for each patient as indicated. Re-assessment of the trauma patient's condition before discharge from hospital is of utmost importance to ensure appropriate goal setting and rehabilitation on return to the community (NICE 2009).

Care for any patient with critical illness should be based on early rehabilitation in ICU as previously stated. The same approach should be used for patients with critical illness as a result of traumatic injury. Clinical management algorithms are available to guide the physiotherapist through clinical decision making regarding when and how to start rehabilitation interventions for patients in ICU (Hanekom et al 2011, Morris et al 2008). Although these algorithms were not written specifically for patients with traumatic injuries, the same principles can be applied to their rehabilitation. The physiotherapist's willingness to start early rehabilitation in ICU for patients with traumatic injuries may be hampered by the severity of these patients' conditions. Safety issues that need to be considered prior to and during rehabilitation of acutely ill patients have been described in the literature (Stiller 2007) and these are applicable to the trauma population as well. Specific precautions and contraindications related to the management of patients who suffered abdominal, thoracic and/or pelvic injuries are outlined in Boxes 13-8 and 13-9 and Table 13-15.

BOX 13-8

PRECAUTIONS AND CONTRAINDICATIONS FOR THE MANAGEMENT OF PATIENTS WITH TRAUMATIC INJURY TO THE ABDOMEN

ABDOMINAL TRAUMA

- Manual chest therapy techniques should be avoided over the anterior basal lung segments after laparotomy or in case of an open abdomen due to abdominal swelling and pain induced by the procedure.
- Manual support should be provided to the laparotomy site or open packed abdomen (on sides of abdomen) during coughing to reduce induced pain.
- Upright sitting should be done only to 20 degrees for someone with an open abdomen.
- Upright sitting beyond 20 degrees as well as mobilization of the patient with an open abdomen may **only** be done after consultation with the trauma surgeon.
- An abdominal corset must be worn by patients with open abdomens when sitting or mobilizing in order to provide support to the abdominal contents.
- Abdominal strengthening exercises may only be initiated at 6 weeks after wound closure to allow adequate time for wound healing.

BOX 13-9

PRECAUTIONS AND CONTRAINDICATIONS FOR THE MANAGEMENT OF PATIENTS WITH THORACIC INJURY

THORACIC TRAUMA

- Support any thoracic surgical site manually during coughing to reduce the amount of pain induced.
- Avoid chest shaking and vibrations over rib fracture sites, as chest compression during the performance of these techniques can cause inwards movement of the fracture segments and resultant damage to the underlying lung tissue and other pulmonary structures.
- In the presence of acute pulmonary oedema, the use of manual chest clearance techniques and airway suctioning is contraindicated, as it contributes to lung volume loss due to the removal of surfactant from the airways.
- No chest therapy techniques should be used around the insertion site of the intercostal drainage (ICD) tubing into the chest wall, as it causes discomfort for the patient.
- Underwater sealed drainage precautions should be taken as per outlined in Chapter 11.

TABLE 13-15

Precautions and Contraindications for the Management of Patients with Pelvic Injury

Pelvic Injury	
Tile type A	■ Bed rest is prescribed as necessary according to the patient's symptoms. Weight bearing and mobilization is allowed according to the patient's tolerance of pain.
Tile type B1	■ Bed rest is prescribed for 4 weeks. After this period, mobilization using partial or full weight bearing may commence.
Tile types B2 and B3	■ Such injuries are managed with external fixation or with the use of a pelvic sling. Those managed with external fixation may only sit up to 45 degrees for the first 4 weeks; those managed with a sling are not allowed to sit up for 4 weeks. After this period of bed rest, mobilization through partial or full weight bearing may commence.
Tile type C	■ External fixation is used as management. Bed rest is prescribed for 6 weeks and the patient is only allowed to sit up to 45 degrees hip flexion after 3 weeks. Gait is non-weight bearing for a further 6 weeks following the initial bed rest period.

Complications That May Develop Due to Immobility

The patient who suffered traumatic injury to the abdomen, thorax and/or pelvis is often severely injured and undergoes prolonged immobilization due to the frequent need for repeated surgical procedures and the effect of critical illness itself on the patient's system. These patients are at risk of developing complications such as lung volume loss, decreased lung compliance and increased airways resistance, excessive secretion accumulation, poor cough effort due to pain or weakness and development of respiratory tract infections. Musculoskeletal complications include shortening of two-joint muscles, muscle weakness and atrophy, decreased participation in functional activities and resultant reduction in exercise endurance. ROM of peripheral joints, thoracic cage and neck may become restricted due to long periods of immobility (head turned towards the ventilator for prolonged periods) and injury-associated or postoperative pain. In order to prevent the onset of these complications there are a variety of interventions that may be utilized by the physiotherapist.

Unresponsive Patient with Traumatic Injury

The unresponsive patient is at particular risk for the development of the previously mentioned complications. Interventions such as manual chest clearance techniques used together with gravity-assisted body positioning (where possible), MHI, ventilator hyperinflation (VHI)–supported cough manoeuvres and airway suctioning can be used to clear excessive airway secretions, restore lung volumes, improve lung compliance and reduce airflow resistance (Choi & Jones 2005, Paratz et al 2002). See Chapter 7 for more information on these techniques. If the aim of treatment is to treat pathology in the left basal lung segments, the patient should preferably not be treated in the supine position. A recent cross-over randomized trial showed that through the use of technetium administration and γ camera imaging, that airflow distribution through a patient's airways using either the Mapleson-C or Laerdal MHI circuit was least in the left lower zones in supine (Van Aswegen et al 2013).

Muscle length and joint ROM may be improved or maintained through the use of passive muscle stretches, passive/active ROM exercises and cycling using a supine cycle (but not with pelvic fractures). Twenty minutes of daily passive cycling in longer-stay critically ill patients improved functional activity participation and exercise endurance when re-assessed prior to hospital discharge (Burtin et al 2009). The use of neuromuscular electrical stimulation (NMES) in an attempt to preserve muscle fibre integrity in critically ill patients is a topic of debate. Several small trials with conflicting results have been published recently and evidence from large randomized trials that supports or refutes the use of NMES in the critical care population is awaited (Gosselink et al 2008). Regular 2–4 hourly body position changes out of the supine position are important in order to maintain skin integrity and to optimize oxygenation through $\dot{V}/\dot{Q}$ matching. The use of splints should be considered if patients present with shortening of two-joint muscles such as finger flexors and ankle plantarflexors. Splints should be removed for periods during the day to prevent pressure sore formation.

Responsive Intubated Patient with Traumatic Injury

As soon as the patient regains consciousness, active rehabilitation should form part of the physiotherapist's approach to patient management. Active deep breathing exercises (such as active cycle of breathing techniques) and active coughing should form part of the patient's bronchopulmonary hygiene routine even while intubated. The patient should be educated on correct methods of wound support during coughing in order to increase cough effectiveness. Functional activities should be encouraged in bed in line with the precautions and contraindications listed in Boxes 13-8 and 13-9 and Table 13-15. If patients are stable enough, they should be sat up over the edge of the bed with feet firmly supported on the floor to perform active lower and upper limb strengthening exercises against gravity. Special attention should be given to achieve active end-of-range movements of the shoulder joint on the side of the ICD in patients with pneumothorax or haemothorax and/or rib fractures. Active ROM exercises of the neck and trunk should also be performed in this position. Early mobilization out of bed is vitally important for patients with ICD to assist with drainage of excess air and/or fluid from the pleural cavity. If the postoperative patient remains stable mobilization out of bed to a chair should be encouraged from day two after surgery. Progression of management should include mobiliza-

tion away from the bedside in ICU or marching on the spot if walking is not possible. Walking can be achieved by connecting the intubated patient to a portable ventilator or MHI circuit attached to a portable oxygen cylinder. Assistive devices such as walking or rollator frames may be used to provide additional support to the patient while mobilizing. Early mobilization away from the bedside frequently during the day reduces the risk of development of postoperative pulmonary complications three-fold for patients who underwent upper abdominal surgery (Haines et al 2013).

Responsive Patient with Traumatic Injury and Prolonged ICU Stay

Those patients who are responsive but undergo prolonged stay in ICU due to complications such as sepsis may develop general muscle weakness, as discussed previously. This often delays the weaning process off mechanical ventilation. Such patients may benefit from respiratory muscle training interventions in addition to the management described above. An inspiratory muscle trainer device (Threshold IMT, Phillips Respironics, Texas, USA or PowerBreathe, Warwickshire, UK) may be attached to the patient's artificial airway to allow for short periods of spontaneous breathing against resistance. Longer periods of spontaneous breathing through this device should be encouraged as the patient's respiratory muscle strength improves. Further discussion of intensive care acquired weakness can be found in the section on rehabilitation for survivors of intensive care in this chapter.

Structured active whole body exercises (within limitations posed by the presence of fractures) are important for such patients to further improve their chances of weaning success from mechanical ventilation. A similar approach is also necessary to avoid deconditioning of patients with pelvic fractures who undergo a period of enforced immobility. Pre-gait exercise training, especially for patients with pelvic fractures, should focus on strength training of gluteus, quadriceps and shoulder girdle muscles to ensure safe mobilization with walking aids after immobilization (Pohlman et al 2010).

Spontaneously Breathing Patient with Traumatic Injury

After extubation, inspiratory lung volumes may be improved through the use of devices such as intermittent NIV in addition to the treatment interventions outlined in the previous paragraphs. However, the effectiveness of these techniques has not been demonstrated in trauma or in postoperative care, except for the use of non-invasive CPAP in amelioration of hypoxaemia. Non-invasive CPAP applied for patients after abdominal surgery is reported to significantly reduce the risk of development of atelectasis and pneumonia (Ferreyra et al 2008). There is a need for well-designed multi-centre trials to investigate the effectiveness of these adjuncts to physiotherapy in the management of patients who undergo surgery after traumatic injury. PEP devices such as bubble PEP or PEP mask may be used to improve lung capacity. If oscillating PEP (bubble PEP) is used, the physiotherapist should be aware that airway collapse may develop when the patient exhales beyond the level of functional residual capacity as intraluminal pressure is exceeded (Westerdahl et al 2005). A recent systematic review investigated the effectiveness of continuous PEP and oscillating PEP in patients after abdominal and thoracic surgery. PEP was not found to be any more effective than other techniques in the prevention of postoperative pulmonary complications. Furthermore, the authors stated that most of the trials included in their review were of low methodological quality (Orman & Westerdahl 2010).

Musculoskeletal and functional rehabilitation should be progressed daily using frequency and duration of activities as a guide (Figs 13-30 and 13-31). Progression of rehabilitation differs between individual patients and therefore frequent re-assessment of each patient's condition and response to treatment is of vital importance (NICE 2009).

Prior to hospital discharge, the patient should be provided with an individualized structured home rehabilitation programme and an appointment at the physiotherapy outpatient department for follow-up assessment 1 month after discharge. At the follow-up appointment the need for ongoing individual rehabilitation should be determined.

QUALITY OF LIFE AFTER TRAUMATIC INJURY

Long-term limitations in HRQoL related to physical function for survivors of critical illness have

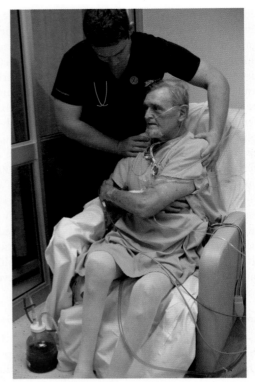

FIGURE 13-30 ■ Thoracic mobilization exercises in ICU following decortication surgery for empyema that developed secondary to haemothorax.

been widely reported in the critical care literature (Cuthbertson et al 2010, Herridge et al 2011). Trauma survivors suffer similar limitations in HRQoL after discharge. Musculoskeletal problems and pain secondary to the injury are common causes of limitations in physical functioning for long periods after discharge. Those who suffered penetrating injury to the abdomen and/or thorax and spent longer than 5 days on mechanical ventilation report significant limitations in muscle strength, exercise endurance and HRQoL related to physical functioning up to 6 months after discharge compared to those who spent less than 5 days on mechanical ventilation (Van Aswegen et al 2010, 2011). Limitations in most domains of HRQoL have been reported 5 years after the event for survivors of blunt or penetrating trauma in Sweden (Sluys et al 2005). Those who suffered pelvic and acetabular fractures report significant posttraumatic pelvic pain

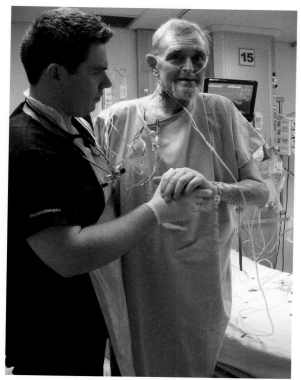

FIGURE 13-31 ■ Early mobilization in ICU following decortication surgery for empyema that developed secondary to haemothorax.

which negatively influences their HRQoL up to 4 years after the incident (Gerbershagen et al 2010).

The health benefits of regular exercise are well-known, yet there is a dearth of information available on the effect of exercise interventions after hospital discharge on the outcomes of survivors of critical illness. Only two groups have specifically investigated the effects of post-discharge exercise therapy on HRQoL of survivors of critical illness (Elliott et al 2011, Jones et al 2003). Unfortunately these groups reported conflicting results, as Jones et al (2003) reported significant improvement in HRQoL related to physical function for individuals in their experimental group who used a self-help rehabilitation manual compared to those who did not; however, Elliott et al (2011) reported that use of an 8-week home-based rehabilitation programme did not have significant effects on physical recovery or functional status of critical illness survivors in their multi-centre randomized controlled trial (RCT) (see the section on rehabilitation for survivors of intensive care in this chapter for more information on rehabilitation in critical care). No research evidence is currently available on the effectiveness of such interventions on the HRQoL outcomes of survivors of major trauma.

CONCLUSION

As the incidence of traumatic injury steadily increases throughout the world, physiotherapy becomes vitally important in the rehabilitation of survivors to ensure full functional ability, community integration and optimal HRQoL is regained after the injury. Little research evidence is currently available on the effectiveness of physiotherapy interventions utilized for this patient population in acute care and community settings. Such evidence is urgently needed to guide the clinical physiotherapy management of those who suffered traumatic injury.

Paediatrics

INTRODUCTION

Numerous adult-based studies have definitively established that physical activity and cardiorespiratory fitness are inversely correlated to morbidity and mortality. The evidence of the health benefits for physically active and fit adults is well-accepted (EU 2008, Morris et al 1953, WHO 2010). Over the last 60 years, a wealth of data has shown that physically active and fit adults can help attenuate the effects of hypertension, insulin resistance, hyperlipidaemia, obesity and cancer. Conversely, in adults there is also strong evidence that physical inactivity increases the risk of major non-communicable diseases such as breast and colon cancer, coronary heart disease and type 2 diabetes, and reduces life expectancy (Lee et al 2012).

However, the relationship between activity, fitness and the health benefits during childhood are less well established. It is intuitive to propose that an active child will become an active adult, but the research evidence is weak. Similarly, the extent to which children's fitness and activity must decrease to endanger their current or future health is also unknown. Nevertheless, there is increasing concern for the future health status of children due to the increased levels of overweight and obese children and the health consequences of leading a more sedentary lifestyle (Rowland 2007). For children with disease or disability there are substantial barriers to participating in physical activity (Rimmer 2005). As argued previously, being inactive is a serious health concern and for those children with disease or disability, there is greater risk of serious health consequences related to physical inactivity.

While the definitions for physical activity and fitness are well accepted, how much physical activity is required for children and adolescents and whether a minimum of fitness is required for optimal health is not known. Physical activity is a behaviour and therefore subject to a multitude of extraneous factors (Casperson et al 1985). Although physical activity is defined as any bodily movement produced by the skeletal muscles resulting in energy expenditure, knowing the situation for how and when young people move is important. Physical fitness defined as a trait or attribute and has usually been referenced in relation to physical work or exercise performance. Fitness is generally subdivided into endurance or cardiovascular fitness (often described as aerobic), strength, speed, power and flexibility.

There is general agreement worldwide that current recommendations for daily physical activity of healthy children and adolescents should be 60 minutes per day of moderate to vigorous activity. Physical activity should include a selection of aerobic activities, including some vigorous intensity activity and on at least 3 days per week, children should engage in activities that strengthen muscle and bone. For additional health benefits, children should engage in more activity – up to several hours per day (UK Department of Health Physical Activity Guidelines, British Heart Foundation, Centres for Disease Control and Prevention, and Australian Government guidelines).

There are, however, no informed recommendations with comparable evidence for children and adolescents with chronic conditions. There is a scarcity of data for children and adolescent with chronic diseases and all systematic reviews on physical activity and

fitness, e.g., asthma (Chandratilleke et al 2012), juvenile idiopathic arthritis (Takken et al 2008), cerebral palsy (Verschuren et al 2008), CF (Cox et al 2013, Bradley & Moran 2008) and congenital heart disease (CHD) (Klausen et al 2014), have highlighted the lack of well-controlled studies and called for more studies to be conducted.

Children with chronic diseases are likely to have their participation in activity reduced either by real or perceived limitations brought about by their specific condition. The consequence of this hypo-activity leads to a deconditioning effect which reduces functional capacity, e.g., reduced aerobic fitness, muscle mass and strength. This downward spiral is compounded by both the disease burden itself and the effect of physical inactivity. This situation is analogous to a healthy child who is hypoactive and at higher risk of associated sedentary lifestyle outcomes (cardiovascular disease, obesity and pre-diabetes). Therefore there has been considerable discussion by clinicians and their support teams on the efficacy of exercise and physical activity to reduce the combined effects of hypo-activity and the disease (Bar-Or & Rowland 2004, Painter 2008, Williams & Stevens 2013).

The utilization of exercise testing to determine the fitness levels of children with chronic disease is clinically important, not only due to its predictive capabilities of mortality and morbidity, but because it will assist in determining training intensity levels. Physical fitness training has been shown to be effective across a range of diseases and to be safe. But there is a need to focus on more individualized and specifically tailored training programmes, because not only is the exercise tolerance between individuals with the same disease large but between different diseases is also considerably wide. Therefore future research should focus on longitudinal data from childhood with chronic disease through adolescence and adulthood to elucidate the complexity of the physical fitness and activity relationships. In order to provide clinically relevant data, the most objective and accurate instruments must be utilized while minimizing the burden of the patient as a research participant. In addition, the factors associated with parental and patient fears about activity participation need addressing. In combination, clinicians and their support teams and researchers can advocate the words of Bar-Or and Rowland that by 'prescribing exercise we are signalling to the child that he or she can, and should, act like his or her healthy peers' (Bar-Or & Rowland 2004, p. 112).

REHABILITATION IN SPECIAL PAEDIATRIC POPULATIONS

It is well known that children with chronic disease have reduced levels of aerobic fitness and these reductions are caused by a combination of the condition-related pathophysiology itself, the treatment of the condition (such as certain medications), hypo-activity and de-conditioning (van Brussel et al 2011). It is therefore likely that children with chronic conditions will benefit from an increase in habitual activity and exercise training (van Brussel et al 2011). It is essential that clinicians can accurately identify if a child is actually de-conditioned. Once this has been objectively determined through exercise testing then it is essential to identify if the deconditioning is due to inactivity, medication, nutritional status or disease-related pathophysiology or due to a combination of these factors (van Brussel et al 2011).

The following sections outline some of the recommendations and evidence for incorporating exercise training into the management of children with CF, asthma, other respiratory disorders (interstitial lung disease, non-CF bronchiectasis), heart disease, transplantation (heart and lung) and in those with weight disorders.

CYSTIC FIBROSIS

The role of exercise in CF is well established and over the last 3 decades has become an important component in the management of all individuals including children with CF (Rand & Prasad 2012). The role of exercise as a prognostic indicator or as a therapeutic tool is also now an important area of research interest in CF care internationally. The safety of exercise in CF was first documented in the early 1980s (Cerny et al 1982). Exercise now plays an integral role in the physiotherapy treatment of individuals with CF, and one of the greatest developments in physiotherapy for CF is that exercise is now seen as 'medicine' (Wheatley et al 2011) and for some individuals is established as normal part of life rather than an increase in treatment burden.

Judgements of the benefits of exercise on long-term survival in CF to date can, however, only be extrapolated from relatively short-term (3 weeks–2

months) clinical trials (Dodd & Prasad 2005 Gruber et al 2011, Paranjape et al 2012, Selvadurai et al 2002). The current recommendations for exercise training in CF are based both on an understanding of the physiological mechanisms and clinical reasoning (Dwyer et al 2011).

The specific therapeutic effects of exercise in CF continue to be investigated. Both children and adults with CF have been shown to have the ability to increase exercise capacity with exercise training regardless of disease severity (Gruber et al 2008, Hebestreit et al 2010, Klijn et al 2004, Nixon et al 1992, Stevens et al 2009b and Stevens et al 2011). Regular exercise also has the potential both in the short- (Klijn et al 2004, Kulich et al 2003, Paranjape et al 2012) and long-term (Moorcroft et al 2004, Schneiderman-Walker 2000, Wilkes et al 2007) to slow down the annual rate of decline in lung function. It has also been shown that fitness can be maintained in the long term, despite deterioration in lung function (Moorcroft et al 2004). However, as more evidence emerges, it seems clear that the relationship between lung function and exercise may only become significantly stronger with severe disease, and that respiratory factors do not limit maximal symptom-limited exercise in individuals with mild-to-moderate CF lung disease (Stevens et al 2009a, b, Dodd et al 2006).

An association between aerobic capacity and survival in CF was first reported in 1992 with the demonstration of a significant positive correlation between aerobic fitness (VO_{2peak}) and 8-year survival (which remained intact after adjustment for other predictor variables such as age, sex, lung function, nutritional status and bacterial colonization) (Nixon et al 1992). An association between changes in exercise capacity measured by VO_{2peak} and survival has also been reported in a study of 28 children with CF aged 8–17 years (Pianosi et al 2005). It is therefore suggested that VO_{2peak} could be used as an independent predictor of survival, but as yet there is no longitudinal data to support this hypothesis. It is imperative that the works of Nixon (1992) and Pianosi (2005) be re-evaluated in light of the on-going increases in morbidity and mortality in CF.

Exercise ability may also be an important determinant of quality of life in CF (Orenstein et al 1989). A positive moderate association (r = 0.58, p < 0.01) between higher exercise capacity and better quality of life was reported in a study of a small group of children and adolescents with CF (Orenstein et al 1989). Improved body image following an exercise training programme may also improve the perception of quality of life (Sahlberg et al 2008). Exercise training in the out-patient setting has also been shown to result in benefits in quality of life for children, which was maintained at 2-year follow-up (Hebestreit et al 2010).

In mild to moderate CF lung disease, the current guidelines for physical activity for healthy children and adults are applicable in CF and have been recommended as the basis for exercise advice in CF. With increasing disease severity, a more considered approach to exercise programs is required, incorporating more interval-type training with frequent re-evaluation. Historically, exercise-training regimens for children have been extrapolated from the recommendations for adults (Selvadurai 2009). Recently published exercise training guidelines can now assist CF patients and health professionals to tailor exercise regimens in an appropriate and effective manner to ensure an exercise training effect for all individuals with CF (Williams et al 2010) (Table 13-16 and Figs 13-32 and 13-33).

ASTHMA

The prevalence of asthma in children and adolescents varies among countries and can be estimated to be somewhere between 5% and 20% (Hebestreit 2008). The UK has among the highest prevalence rates of asthma symptoms in children worldwide (Asthma UK, www.asthma.org.uk (accessed 13 Jan 2016)). There are 5.4 million people in the UK with a diagnosis of asthma, with one in 11 of these being children. This equates to approximately 2 asthmatic children in every classroom in the UK. Children with asthma may show less tolerance to exercise due to worsening symptoms during exercise or other reasons such as de-conditioning as a consequence of inactivity (Carson et al 2013). There remains, however, conflicting evidence to support or refute this hypothesis. But there is increasing evidence that a reduced level of physical activity in children with asthma is a more important predictor of low fitness than disease severity (Santuz et al 1997).

One of the main characteristics of asthma is that the airways are hyper-responsive to a variety of triggers, including airway infections, exposure to allergens or air pollutants, inhalation of dry or cold air and also exercise (Hebestreit 2008). This hyper-responsiveness

TABLE 13-16
General Exercise and Training Recommendations for Individuals with CF

	Patients with *Mild to Moderate* CF Lung Disease	Patients with *Severe* CF Lung Disease
Recommended activities	Walking, hiking, aerobics, cycling running, tennis, swimming strength training, trampolining, climbing, roller-skating,	Ergometric cycling, walking, strengthening and gym exercises everyday activities
Frequency and duration	3–5 times/week for 30–45 minutes	5 times/week for 20–30 minutes
Intensity and exercise prescription	70–85% HR_{max}; 60–80% VO_{2peak}; LT; GET intermittent and steady-state	60–80% HR_{max}; 50–70% VO_{2peak}; LT; GET intermittent
Supplemental oxygen	Indicated, if SaO_2 drops below 90% during exercise (resting hypoxia with severe CF)	
Activities to avoid	Bungee-jumping, high diving, scuba diving and hiking at altitude (severe CF)	
Potential risks	Dehydration, hypoxaemia, bronchoconstriction, pneumothorax, hypoglycaemia*	
	Haemoptysis, oesophageal bleedings, cardiac arrhythmias, rupture of liver and spleen, spontaneous fractures[†]	

Adapted from Williams et al 2010.

CF, Cystic fibrosis; *GET,* gas exchange threshold; HR_{max}, maximum heart rate; *LT,* lactate threshold; SaO_2, oxygen saturation; VO_{2peak}, peak oxygen consumption.

*Depending on the existence of an impaired glucose tolerance.

[†]Depending on the existence of untreated CF-related bone disease.

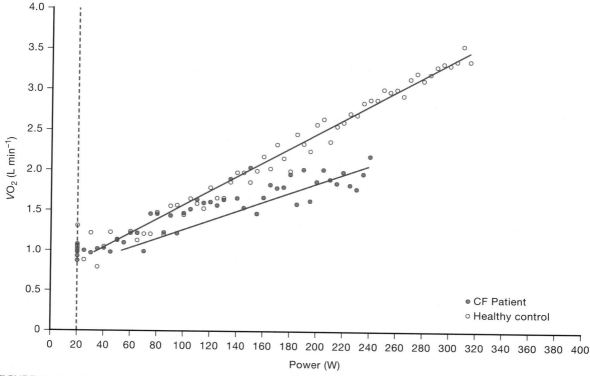

FIGURE 13-32 ■ The typical VO_2–WR relationship derived from a maximal ramp cycle ergometer test for one cystic fibrosis (CF) paediatric patient and one healthy control. Lines represent the slope of the VO_2–WR relationship. VO_2, Rate of oxygen consumption; *WR*, work rate.

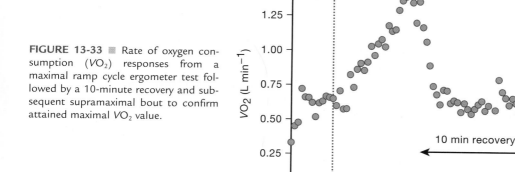

FIGURE 13-33 ■ Rate of oxygen consumption (VO_2) responses from a maximal ramp cycle ergometer test followed by a 10-minute recovery and subsequent supramaximal bout to confirm attained maximal VO_2 value.

leads to recurrent episodes of wheezing, breathlessness, chest tightness and coughing (Morton & Fitch 2011). Exercise induced bronchoconstriction (EIB) describes the acute airway narrowing that occurs as a results of exercise, usually after a period (≈6–8 minutes) of continuous aerobic exercise (Parsons et al 2013, Weiler et al 2007). It has been reported that most, if not all, of individuals with a diagnosis of asthma experience EIB (Weiler et al 2007). EIB has also been shown to occur in individuals with an overall prevalence of ≈20% (Weiler et al 2007) with no history of asthma (Parsons et al 2013). The diagnosis of EIB should always be based on changes in lung function (≥10% drop in $FEV_1\%$ predicted from baseline) provoked by exercise, not on the basis of symptoms (Parsons et al 2013).

The current exercise recommendations for individuals with EIB is the administration of an inhaled short acting β-agonist (SABA) usually taken 15 minutes before exercise (Parsons et al 2013). A controller agent is usually added whenever SABA therapy is used daily or more frequently. For those with continuing EIB symptoms despite the aforementioned approach, inhaled corticosteroids and other appropriate medications may be required (Parsons et al 2013) but this is outside of the scope of this document. It is well known that EIB after appropriate medical prophylaxis is extremely low (Orenstein 2002). In children, EIB symptoms (coughing, wheezing, and SOB shortly after exercise) usually resolves within 10–90 minutes of cessation of the exercise (Hebestreit 2008).

As breathlessness is a normal physiological response to exercise in all individuals, many asthmatic individuals and their families are unaware that they develop EIB with exercise (Morton & Fitch 2011). As a result these individuals often assume that their breathlessness is due to lack of fitness, fail to seek medical advice and exercise at a disadvantage due to lack of appropriate medication (Morton & Fitch 2011).

The primary medical management of asthma and EIB is pharmacological (Morton & Fitch 2011). Physiotherapy management includes medication-related education (e.g. inhaler technique) and airway clearance techniques as appropriate, with exercise playing a predominantly secondary role. The role of exercise training in asthma is to maintain cardiorespiratory fitness and to assist asthmatic individuals to lead as normal a physical lifestyle as possible, which should allow full participation in sports (Morton & Fitch 2011). Several studies have evaluated the benefits of increased physical activity in children and adolescents with asthma (Hebestreit 2008). The therapeutic effects of exercise are generally more pronounced in children with more severe disease compared to those categorized with moderate to severe asthma. Patients with mild asthma may not benefit from exercise training any more than healthy children (Hebestreit 2008).

The 2013 American College of Sports Medicine (ACSM) guidelines report that 'current evidence states that the standard principles of exercise prescription can be applied to patients with respiratory disease, including asthma'. Certain sports are considered more asthmagenic than others and physiotherapists should advise appropriately. Swimming has been reported to be less asthmagenic, as it has been demonstrated to provoke less EIB than running or cycling (Morton & Fitch 2011). However, it is now well known that breathing in air contaminated with chloramines in indoor pools may be problematic for some individuals.

Individuals with asthma and EIB should be encouraged to include an early warm-up session to produce a so-called 'refractory period' which has been shown to be useful as a preventative measure during which an individual has a reduced propensity to develop EIB (McKenzie et al 1994). However, it should be noted that not all individuals with EIB exhibit a refractory period and in those who do, the most effective preventative exercise protocol may vary (Hebestreit 2008). It is therefore essential that the exercise programmes are individualized to ensure the most effective routine. For exercise in the cold weather, the recommendations are that a device, e.g. a face mask, should be used to allow the air to be warmed and humidified on inhalation during exercise.

There is a lack of good quality intervention studies examining the effects of exercise training in asthma. A recent Cochrane review included 19 studies which examined the benefits of exercise training on individuals, a total of 695 children with asthma of all severities aged 8 years and older (Chandratilleke et al 2012). Twelve of the studies involved children and six of these 12 studies used swim training as the intervention. It was reported that physical training of any type (aerobic in nature but predominantly swim training in most of the studies and for greater than 20 minutes undertaken 2–3 times per week for a minimum of 4 weeks) was well tolerated with no adverse effects reported in any of the studies reviewed. It was also reported that none of the studies mentioned worsening of asthma symptoms following physical training. The authors concluded that physical training improved cardiopulmonary fitness as measured by a statistically and clinically significant increase in maximum oxygen uptake (VO_{2peak} (mean difference (MD) 5.57 mL.kg^{-1}.min^{-1}; 95% confidence interval (CI) 4.36 to 6.78; six studies on 149 participants) and maximum expiratory ventilation (VE 6.0 L/min, 95% CI 1.57 to 10.43; four studies on 111 participants) with no significant effect on resting lung function (performed in four studies). Although there were insufficient data to pool due to diverse reporting tools, there is some evidence available to suggest that physical training may have positive effects on HRQoL in asthma, with four of five studies producing a statistically and clinically significant benefit. This review demonstrated that physical training can improve cardiopulmonary fitness and was well tolerated among people with asthma in the included studies. As such, people with stable asthma should be encouraged to participate in regular exercise training without fear of symptom exacerbation.

Provided that the child with asthma and their parents/carers are well educated and trained in the management of asthma symptoms and EIB (if present), that the disease is treated adequately, and that the methods to prevent bronchial hyper-responsiveness with exercise are employed, exercise can be safe. Under these conditions nearly all patients with asthma can engage, and should engage, in all types of physical activities and exercise training. However, it must be recognized that it is a challenge for the three conditions to always be successfully achieved, so it is imperative that health professionals dealing with these children take these factors into account and make recommendations to the wider medical team if necessary.

OTHER RESPIRATORY CONDITIONS

Interstitial Lung Disease

The term 'childhood interstitial lung disease (chILD)' encompasses a broad group of pulmonary disorders that are associated with significant morbidity and sometime mortality (Kuo & Young, 2014). 'Interstitial lung disease (ILD)' is a term that refers to a heterogeneous collection of disorders characterized by abnormal gas exchange because of altered structure of the interstitial region of the lung, e.g. acinar dysplasia, chronic neonatal lung disease (bronchopulmonary dysplasia (BPD)), sarcoidosis (Kuo & Young 2014). ILD is rare in children with a prevalence of 3.6 cases per million in the UK and Ireland (Dinwiddie et al 2002). Physical training is well established in other chronic paediatric respiratory diseases such as CF but little is known regarding physical training in ILD (Holland & Hill 2008). A Cochrane review investigated the evidence for physical training in ILD (Holland & Hill 2008). Despite the fact that no age limit exclusions were applied, all of the data included were from adult studies which were either aerobic training or a combination of aerobic and resistance exercise training. The training programmes varied in duration (from 5 weeks to 6 months) and in terms of training frequency (2–5 sessions per week). The authors concluded that exercise training was safe for people with ILD and resulted in significantly improved functional exercise capacity, dyspnoea and HRQoL immediately following a period of exercise training (Holland & Hill 2008). However, there is currently little evidence of long-term benefit and there are no studies examining the effects of physical training in children with ILD.

Non-CF Bronchiectasis

Bronchiectasis unrelated to CF (non-CF bronchiectasis) is a chronic respiratory condition characterized by bronchial dilatation secondary to airway inflammation, infection and dysfunction of mucociliary clearance (Barker 2002). Current British Thoracic Society guidelines (Pasteur et al 2010) for the treatment of non-CF bronchiectasis recommend pulmonary rehabilitation with the aim of improving exercise tolerance and HRQoL. However, there is limited evidence of the effects of pulmonary rehabilitation in non-CF bronchiectasis (Mandal et al 2012, Newall et al 2005, Ong et al 2011, Zan Zellar et al 2012). Exercise training and education has been associated with a reduction in exacerbations and quality-adjusted life years in patients with non-CF bronchiectasis (Griffiths et al 2001). A recent randomized controlled, multi-site adult study in Australia investigated the short- and long-term effects of exercise training on exercise capacity, HRQoL and exacerbations over a 12-month follow-up period (Lee et al 2014a, b). The intervention group (n = 42) attended a twice weekly aerobic exercise training programme for 8 weeks, as well as a home exercise programme with the aim of achieving three to five unsupervised sessions per week. The results showed significant increases in exercise capacity and in the perception of dyspnoea and fatigue following the 8-week training period, but this was not sustained at 6 or 12 months after the training programme. Exercise training also reduced the number of exacerbations over the 12-month period, with a trend towards fewer exacerbations requiring antibiotics and a relative risk reduction of 0.69 (95% CI 0.49 to 0.98) in the intervention group compared to the control group. The evidence from these adult studies suggest that supervised exercise programmes for individuals with non-CF bronchiectasis may have benefits in the short term but there is a need to explore the effects of exercise training in children with non-CF bronchiectasis both in the short and long term. Despite the lack of evidence in the paediatric population, exercise training should be considered by health professionals as an important component in the management of children with non-CF bronchiectasis.

Lung Transplant

Lung transplantation has been shown to improve quality of life and survival in individuals with various end-stage lung diseases (Studer et al 2004). A 2010 systematic review of the effects of exercise training after lung transplantation in adults reported that there is some evidence to support a period of structured exercise training post lung transplantation to improve maximal and functional exercise capacity, skeletal muscle strength, and lumbar bone mineral density (Wickerson et al 2010).

There is limited evidence investigating the effects of exercise training in paediatric lung transplant recipients, however. Deliva et al (2012) investigated the effects of a 3-month hospital- or home-based exercise programme following paediatric heart and lung transplantation in children over the age of 6 years. The children were provided with ×3/week supervised sessions or ×3/week training programmes to be undertaken at home. A total of 39 participants were included in the

study, of which 12 were lung transplant recipients. Clinically and statistically significant improvements in 6-minute walk distance (6MWT) were observed over time (baseline 425.7 ± 109.4 m, 3 months 500.6 ± 93.6 m, at 1 year 528.6 ± 66.6 m). Further research is required to fully evaluate the effects of exercise training after paediatric lung transplantation.

OBESITY

The escalating epidemic of overweight and obesity has been termed 'globesity'. The United States is widely recognized as having the highest prevalence of childhood obesity and overweight, although the UK and Australia are now ranked fourth and eighth, respectively (Health Survey for England 2011). The UK has the highest rates of childhood obesity among European countries (OECD 2013). A position statement by the Royal College of Paediatrics and Child Health in 2012 reported that nearly one-third (31%) of children aged 2–15 years in the UK are overweight or obese (Health Survey for England 2011). The causes of obesity are complex but the problem is closely linked with obesogenic environments, which include, but are not confined to, a sedentary lifestyle and encouraging children to consume too much food. The management of children with weight problems needs to be sensitively addressed, as treatment may stigmatize them and put them at risk of bullying (NICE clinical guideline 47). Parental lifestyles can also have an impact on children's lifestyles, with a subsequent impact on body weight. The family environment and positive parental influences are invaluable in the management and treatment of childhood obesity. Parents should be encouraged to be active role models, encouraging children to be active (Hills et al 2008).

There is indisputable evidence that childhood obesity tracks into adulthood (Whitaker et al 1997) and is linked to adult obesity, cardiovascular disease, diabetes and the other obesity-related problems (Baird et al 2005). There is also evidence that adults whose obesity started in childhood are at greater risk than those who develop obesity later (Baird et al 2005). Appropriate management of childhood obesity is critical, since excess body weight (fat) in childhood is associated with a greater chance of high levels of adiposity in adulthood (Freedman et al 2005).

Children with chronic diseases are at risk of developing obesity either as a primary or secondary consequence to their disease. Health professionals, educators and parents have a responsibility to be vigilant and to ensure young people are protected from extraneous pressure to lose weight and to ensure that they have the knowledge that this can be achieved through a sensible approach to nutrition and exercise (Hills et al 2008).

The traditional 'treatment' for obesity is diet, exercise and behaviour modification. It is now well documented that the active involvement of parents and family members should be an additional element. Single interventions, for example diet alone, are limited. The treatment of obesity in children should aim to restore the balance between energy intake and energy expenditure (Speiser et al 2005) and this should be done by focussing on improving health rather than emphasizing weight loss (Golan & Crow 2004). Severe dietary restriction in children is contraindicated in children, as growth and development may be jeopardized. A Cochrane review in 2011 reported on the results from 55 international studies with a combined sample of 27 946 children, which were focused on interventions for preventing obesity in children. It was concluded that there was a wide heterogeneity in the study designs and variations in the approaches and interventions tested. The results demonstrated that short-term (<12 months) interventions predominantly conducted in educational settings and aimed at preventing obesity through strategies aimed at altering dietary or physical activity–related factors, or both combined, may be effective in reducing BMI. The magnitude of the change in BMI_z/BMI from pre to post intervention in the intervention group compared to the control was −0.15 units, which would equate to a reduction of 0.8% in BMI for a child aged 9.5 years with a BMI of 18.2 kg/m^2, which if sustained over several years would represent important reductions at a population level (Waters et al 2011). The authors also concluded that interventions focused on dietary or physical activity–related factors or both combined represent only some of the factors that are important in tackling childhood obesity and should be considered as part of a multi-modal approach.

The treatment and management of obesity in children and adolescents is challenging. Health professionals are in a key position to help to promote exercise as a means of achieving health and wellness, rather than helping to perpetuate the restrictive approach of using exercise merely as an avenue for weight control. The National UK physical activity guidelines should be used as a guide for physical activity levels for the different age groups; however, it should be noted that these guidelines are not specific for obese groups.

HEART DISEASE

Congenital Heart Disease

Many children with CHD have reduced exercise capacity and a reduced level of physical activity (Takken et al 2011). These children are often de-conditioned preoperatively and postoperatively, but most patients improve their functional ability and quality of life through exercise (Miller et al 2005). The reasons for this inactivity are multi-factorial: residual haemodynamic problems, chronotropic impairment, as well as psychosocial factors such as parental overprotection or restraints imposed by children's social surroundings and limited or inaccurate education, with resulting discouragement by healthcare professionals. Children may also have a lack of interest because they are deconditioned or they may fear to participate in activities (Miller et al 2005). Patients with CHD who participate in sports from an early age have a significantly lower chance of becoming sedentary adults (Moola et al 2009, Schickendantz et al 2007).

A relationship between exercise capacity, survival and morbidity has been shown in patients with CHD especially in those with repaired tetralogy of Fallot, transposition of the great arteries after atrial redirection and with Fontan circulation (Takken et al 2011). European consensus reports in 2006 and 2011 state that exercise should be performed and encouraged in children with CHD (Takken et al 2011). Children with CHD should be advised to comply with public health recommendations of daily participation in at least 60 minutes of moderate to vigorous physical activity that is developmentally appropriate and enjoyable and involves a variety of activities (Takken et al 2012), although these are evidence-informed rather than evidence-based recommendations. Those with specific lesions or complications may require counselling regarding precautions and recommendations (Takken et al 2012). However, healthcare professionals are often reluctant to recommend exercise for these children due to a lack of knowledge of cardiac effects and risks related to exercise. In addition 'over-protection' by parents, caregivers and educators by restricting physical activities for children with CHD may also be contributing to the observed reduction in exercise capacity and physical activity levels.

A recent systematic review (Duppen et al 2013) reviewed a total of 19 studies, of which 16 were paediatric, examining the effects of physical exercise training programmes in children and young adults with a wide variety of CHD. It was reported that for most studies participation in a physical exercise training programme was safe (Box 13-10). The reported duration of the training programmes varied between 6 and 52 weeks, with the majority using 12 weeks. The

---

BOX 13-10

THE FOLLOWING CONGENITAL HEART DEFECTS CAN PARTICIPATE IN ALL SPORTS WITHOUT RESTRICTIONS

- ASD (closed or small unoperated) and PFO (except scuba diving in PFO)
- VSD (closed or small unoperated)
- AVSD (only mild AV insufficiency; no significant sub-aortic stenosis or arrhythmia)
- Partial or complete anomalous pulmonary venous connection (no significant pulmonary or systemic venous obstruction, no pulmonary hypertension or exercise-induced arrhythmia)
- Persistent ductus arteriosus (operated) (6 months post closure and no residual pulmonary hypertension)
- Mild pulmonary stenosis (normal RV, normal ECG)
- Mild aortic stenosis (with the exception of high static, high dynamic) (mean gradient <21 mmHg; no history of arrhythmias, no dizziness, syncope, or angina pectoris)
- Transposition of the great arteries after arterial switch (with the exception of high static, high dynamic) (no or only mild neo-aortic insufficiency; no significant pulmonary stenosis; no signs of ischaemia or arrhythmia on exercise ECG)

Adapted from Ten Harkel and Takken 2010.
ASD, Atrioseptal defect; ASVD, atrioventricular septal defect; AV, atrioventricular; ECG, electrocardiogram; PFO, patent foramen ovale; RV, right ventricle; VSD, ventricular septal defect.

---

training regimens varied from 1 session per week up to daily sessions with an average of 3 sessions per week. Sessions varied in length of time from 5 to 60 minutes. Not all training programmes therefore complied with the Takken et al (2011) recommendations. Heart rate was used to set the training intensity, and steady state exercise protocols were used in all studies. Baseline mean VO_{2peak} was 32.2 mL.kg^{-1}.min^{-1} and the mean increase in fitness after the training period in VO_{2peak} was 2.6 mL/kg min^{-1} with 12 of 24 studies who used a maximal exercise test showing a statistically significant increase in exercise capacity (Duppen et al 2013).

Acquired Heart Disease

Children at risk of acquired heart disease include children with any chronic disease including cancer, renal disease, respiratory disease and HIV for example. Deconditioning can occur as a direct result of the disease process or as a secondary consequence of the disease due to the burden of treatment regime, medication-induced illness and secondary complications. Fear of participation and imposed restrictions on activity that is perceived to be 'safe' for that child can also play an important role in children with chronic disease levels of activity. The presence of cardiovascular risk factors (adiposity, decreased lean body mass, hyper-lipidaemia and insulin resistance) as a result of treatment or the disease process itself makes it essential to include exercise training as part of the management of children with chronic disease.

There is limited evidence, however, to demonstrate the effects of exercise in children at risk of acquired heart disease. Survivors of childhood cancer have been reported to have an eightfold increased risk of death from cardiovascular disease (Miller et al 2005), a lower aerobic capacity (van Brussel et al 2006) and lower physical activity levels (Winter et al 2009) than children who have not had cancer. A recent Cochrane review reviewed the physical exercise training interventions for children and young adults during and after treatment for cancer (Braam et al 2013). Five studies were included in the review with a combined sample of 131 participants. The authors reported that all interventions were implemented during chemotherapy treatment for acute lymphoblastic leukaemia (ALL). The duration of the training sessions ranged from 15 to 60 minutes per session. Both the type of intervention, as well as the intervention period, which ranged from 10 weeks to 2 years, varied in all the included studies. Exercise training resulted in positive changes in physical fitness, body composition and flexibility in some of the studies. Physical fitness was assessed using the 9-minute run-walk test, the timed up-and-down stairs test, and the 20-m shuttle run test. Only the up-and-down stairs test showed significant differences between the intervention and the control group, in favour of the intervention group (p value = 0.05). Bone mineral density was assessed in one study only and a statistically significant difference in favour of the exercise group was identified (SMD 1.07; 95% CI 0.48 to 1.66, p < 0.001). Flexibility was assessed in three studies. In one study the active ankle dorsiflexion method was used to assess flexibility and the second study used the passive ankle dorsiflexion test. No significant difference between the intervention and control group was identified with the active ankle dorsiflexion test, whereas with the passive test method a statistically significant difference in favour of the exercise group was found (MD 0.69; 95% CI 0.12 to 1.25; p = 0.02). A lack of methodological robustness and the fact that only the ALL population was included means the data should be interpreted with caution. The evidence of increased body weight and obesity in patients with and survivors of leukaemia is, however, overwhelming and obesity has also been described in survivors of paediatric brain tumours (Warner 2008).

There are few small studies that have investigated exercise in children with cancer. The available evidence suggests that supervised exercise training may increase the functional capacity of patients with childhood cancer and children who survive childhood cancer (van Brussel et al 2011). However, the practicalities and feasibility of participation in structured exercise therapy during remission may be challenging as children may wish to be 'free' of the disease at this stage (van Brussel et al 2011).

Abnormal cardiovascular risk factors as a result of highly active anti-retroviral therapy (HAART) or chronic viral infection may contribute to or be exacerbated by a sedentary lifestyle in children with HIV (Miller et al 2010). A recent US study of children (greater than 6 years of age) and young adults (median and range age of 15.5 years (6.0–22.6 years)) with HIV demonstrated that a 24-session supervised hospital and home-based exercise training programme was feasible and resulted in significant improvements in upper and lower extremity strength, flexibility and peak VO_2. The median increases in muscle endurance, relative VO_{2peak}, and lean body mass were 38.7% (95% CI 12.5–94.7; p < 0.006), 3.0 mL.kg^{-1}.min^{-1} (95% CI 1.5–6.0; p < 0.001), and 4.5% (95% CI 2.4–6.6; p < 0.001), respectively. Additional significant improvements in total lean mass measured using a dual-energy X-ray absorptiometry (DEXA) scan was also noted (Miller et al 2010).

The benefits of exercise for children without cardiovascular disease per se, but who are at risk for developing cardiovascular disease, are multidimensional. It is therefore essential that physical activity and exercise is incorporated into the management of these children with chronic disease.

Ventricular Assist Devices

A shortage of donor organs combined with the efficacy of mechanical circulatory support for adults and children has resulted in the increasing use of ventricular assist devices (VADs) worldwide. VADs are utilized in children with acute congestive heart failure associated with CHD, cardiomyopathy and myocarditis, both as a bridge to transplantation and to aid myocardial recovery (Gazit et al 2010). VADs are mainly used as a longer term option as opposed to ECMO, which is a technique of providing both cardiac and respiratory support oxygen to patients whose heart and lungs are so severely diseased or damaged that they can no longer serve their function and is used for short-term mechanical support (Gazit et al 2010). There are two main types of VAD used in children. The Berlin heart is a type of VAD, which is a simple air driven pump which takes over the work of one or both sides of the child's own heart. A single pump to support the left side of the heart, while the right side continues to work naturally, is known as an 'LVAD'. Some children need two pumps, one to support the left side of the heart and one to support the right. This is known as a bi-ventricular assist device or BiVAD.

There are currently no paediatric studies investigating the effect of VADs on exercise capacity. Adult studies have shown that the implantation of an LVAD is associated with improvements in exercise capacity (peak VO_2, cardiac output, heart rate, catecholamine levels and submaximal exercise performance) (Foray et al 1996, Jaski et al 1993, Kugler et al 2011, Morrone et al 1996). Most of these improvements are attributed to an increase in cardiac output which was directly measured from the LVAD device (Kennedy et al 2003). However, it is well known that despite these improvements, patients continue to have significant functional limitations, with exercise capacity below that reported for patients after heart transplantation and age-matched controls (Morrone et al 1996). A paucity of studies have examined the effects of exercise training on cardiovascular fitness in adult LVAD patients. These studies have reported that exercise is safe, feasible and may improve sub-maximal and maximal exercise performance. These training studies have used both supervised and unsupervised exercise programmes and have consisted of predominantly aerobic type exercise. A recent Australian randomized controlled study (n = 14) using an 8-week, gym-based, supervised exercise programme compared to a progressive mobilization control group (aiming to walk for 60 minutes at an intensity of 13 on the subjective Borg RPE scale). A significant improvement in VO_{2peak} and 6-minute walk distance (6MWT) was reported for both groups with no significant difference in the improvements between the groups (Hayes at al 2012). These results were in agreement with Laoutaris et al (2011), who also demonstrated that additional exercise training beyond a home walking programme did not significantly improve VO_{2peak}, 6MWD or quality of life. However, both of these studies had small sample sizes so the results should be interpreted with caution.

Despite the paucity of exercise training evidence, it is now well known that exercise training is safe and feasible in patients with VAD (Hayes et al 2012). Exercise training is therefore an important component of the physiotherapy management of these patients and should be included in the management of paediatric VAD patients. The basic principles of exercise prescription (frequency, intensity, time and type) are applicable to these patients (Kennedy et al 2003) and should be utilized as appropriate for each child individually.

Heart Transplant

Over the last 25 years with the introduction of the current immunosuppressant regimen, paediatric heart transplantation has increased dramatically (Takken et al 2011). Heart, lung and heart–lung transplantation has increased steadily since the 1980s. Long-term survival and recent reports of actuarial survival at 15 and 20 years have been reported as 80% and 53%, respectively, for paediatric heart transplants (Ross et al 2006).

There is very little data on exercise performance in children and adolescents following heart transplantation and even more limited data on the effects of exercise training in this population. There are also no recommendations for either recreational or competitive sports participation for children after transplant (Takken et al 2011). Data from adult studies is not extensive either; however, the adult studies can help to provide useful information on the nature of exercise limitations and the effects of training and rehabilitation programmes that have the potential to be extended to the paediatric population.

Exercise data from adult patients has reported either a progressive decrease in VO_2 with increasing time post transplant of about 5% per year or no change in maximum heart rate and VO_2 over time (Dipchand et al 2009). The few reports of exercise testing in paediatric heart transplants have reported VO_{2peak} of 50–60% of healthy age- and sex-matched controls (Davis et al 2006, Dipchand et al 2009, Patel et al 2008). The main reasons for these reductions are believed to be both central (e.g. reduced stroke volume, abnormalities in autonomic innervation, diastolic abnormalities) and peripheral (e.g. skeletal muscle mass and strength reduction) (Takken et al 2011).

There are a limited number of studies aimed at assessing the specific components of exercise training (mode, safety, physiological effects) for children after heart transplant. Studies of rehabilitation programmes in adults have shown that improvements in VO_{2peak}, muscle strength and endurance, as well as bone mineral density, can result from formal exercise training programmes both in the short and long term (Takken et al 2011). A study by Patel et al (2008) using a home exercise programme (endurance and strengthening) of 12 weeks' duration demonstrated a mean increase of 15% in VO_{2peak} in children (mean age at enrolment 14.7 ± 5.3 years (8–25 years) with an average of 5.26 years post-transplant).

Due to the combined effects of reduced exercise performance and the evidence from the adult literature, it is clear that exercise training is an important component in the management of children after heart transplantation. Please see Chapter 6 for more specific information on exercise testing: cardiopulmonary exercise test (CPET) field walking tests and other commonly used exercise outcomes in children. More studies are required to examine the relationship between sub-maximal and maximal exercise variables and clinical outcomes. Specific studies required include investigating the sensitivity of these exercise parameters to disease prognosis and evaluating therapeutic interventions. For a comprehensive review of the utility of CPET, readers are referred to Wasserman et al (2005).

EXERCISE PRESCRIPTION

An evaluation of exercise performance is important for the safe prescription of any training intervention (ACSM 2000). In relation to exercise prescription, the CPET has significant advantages over other available indirect tests, as it is possible to use the test data to set the intensity of exercise. A choice of submaximal data from the CPET can be usefully employed to set the exercise training intensity. e.g. RPE, heart rate, cycle power output (or treadmill speed) or oxygen consumption. If oxygen consumption is used, then identifying certain points can help demarcate the exercise intensity, i.e., below the gaseous exchange threshold (GET) is usually defined as easy to moderate exercise intensity. Above the GET but below the critical power (attainment of an elevated but stable blood lactate) is defined as 'heavy intensity domain exercise'. The latter example of using oxygen consumption to set the exercise intensity will require the expertise of an exercise physiologist and therefore most studies typically use heart rate or RPE.

However, the majority of clinical exercise training programmes have either poorly quantified training intensity or have failed to adequately describe it. It is therefore very difficult to prescribe anything other than very generic recommendations for training prescription within clinical groups. For example, in a Cochrane review in 2008 on physical training for CF

(Bradley & Moran 2008), of the 26 studies reviewed, only seven studies met the inclusion criteria. The authors found that there was some limited evidence for the beneficial effects of training on such variables as exercise capacity, strength and lung function, but there were inconsistent improvements between studies. It was concluded that more studies were needed to comprehensively examine training effects both in the short and long term and that both aerobic- and anaerobic-type training should be investigated. A more recent review of training for CF paediatric patients supported the findings of the Cochrane review but added that for training to be sustainable it must operate within an integrative support system involving both psychological and nutritional support (Williams & Stevens 2013).

Although the function of exercise as a therapy in children with chronic disease is becoming accepted, the clinical team are faced with a number of issues to resolve before the training can be implemented. These issues are likely to vary considerably not only between patients but between disease conditions. For these reasons, only general recommendations can be applied across disease conditions before individual circumstances are taken into account. However, as one key factor to any training programme is individualization, this should not be problematic. Once the contraindications for exercise training have been appropriately considered, specific aspects such as patient preferences for exercise, available facilities, and parental support should be factored into the programme. Next the training characteristics should be considered, including frequency, intensity, time and type (the FITT acronym, also used in Chapter 12, Cardiac Rehabilitation). In paediatric training studies of healthy children, *intensity* seems to be the key factor of FITT, but for children with chronic disease there is little evidence to support this proposal. In all likelihood, it would be better to focus on the frequency and time or duration of the training while maintaining intensity low until both the patient and clinical team become confident. Heart rate is the easiest indicator of training intensity, although the RPE is also a simple measure to teach patients. It should be borne in mind that patients with low fitness will perform the same activities as their healthy school-aged peers, but at a higher level of exertion (Bar-Or & Rowland 2004, Stevens et al 2011).

Exercise Training in Cancer Populations

INTRODUCTION

'Cancer' is a generic term for a large group of diseases that can affect any part of the body (World Health Organization 2015). The heterogeneous group of diseases occur as a result of 'abnormal cells not being destroyed by the normal metabolic processes but instead proliferate and spread (metastasize) out of control' (AIHW 2014). Overall lung cancer is the most frequent cancer diagnosed worldwide (Ferlay et al 2012). Breast cancer is the most common cancer diagnosed in females, followed by colorectal cancer, cancer of the cervix uteri and lung cancer (Ferlay et al 2012). Lung cancer is the most common cancer diagnosed in males, followed by prostate cancer, colorectal cancer and stomach cancer (Ferlay et al 2012). Lung cancer is the leading cause of cancer death, accounting for one in five cancer deaths (19% of total cancer-related deaths) (Ferlay et al 2012).

Over the past few decades there has been great progress made in terms of screening for cancer (allowing cancers to be detected earlier) and in the efficacy of cancer treatment, resulting in dramatically improved cancer survival rates. Commencing as an incurable disease with rising incidence and mortality rates, research and health care has now permitted cancer to be a curable disease for many, with mortality rates declining and a rise in the number of people living as cancer survivors. The 5-year survival rate for cancer in the 1960s was only 38% and projections suggest that beyond 2015 the cancer survival rate will rise above 80% (DeVita et al 2012). This means that there will continue to be a growth in the number of people living with cancer in the community. Despite promising improvements in the survival rate, cancer is still associated with significant morbidity to the individual and a huge burden to the healthcare system. With cancer transitioning into a 'chronic disease', there is now a push to implement strategies that address the morbidity associated with cancer. Physiotherapists, particularly through exercise intervention, play an important role in the prevention and treatment of cancer and cancer-related morbidity. Physical activity and exercise are now seen as vital components across three main areas of the cancer continuum:

1. cancer prevention
2. reducing cancer mortality (evidence only for some types of cancer)
3. reducing cancer morbidity: preventing deterioration, maximizing and restoring physical status of cancer survivors prior to, during and following cancer treatment.

PHYSICAL ACTIVITY FOR CANCER PREVENTION

Many people with cancer may have been inactive for a large proportion of their life. Physical inactivity, poor nutrition and obesity are some of the risk factors for the development of cancer. For the prevention of cancer, the American Cancer Society (2012) recommends that individuals maintain a physically active lifestyle, avoid smoking or exposure to second-hand smoke, maintain a healthy weight and consume a healthy diet. The specific physical activity guidelines are:

■ Adults should engage in at least 150 minutes of moderate intensity physical activity per week or 75 minutes of vigorous intensity physical activity per week and that the physical activity occasions should be spread throughout the week (American Cancer Society 2012, Rock et al 2013).
■ Children should engage in at least 60 minutes of moderate intensity or vigorous intensity physical activity per day and at least three occasions of vigorous activity per week (American Cancer Society 2012).

These recommendations are based on epidemiological evidence which shows that higher levels of physical activity may be protective against colon, breast, pancreatic, endometrial and prostate cancer (Courneya et al 2007). There is an approximate 40–50% risk reduction for the development of colorectal cancer and a 30–40% risk reduction for the development of breast cancer associated with increased levels of physical activity (Friedenreich 2001). Engagement in at least 3–4 hours of physical activity per week reduces females' risk of breast cancer development by 30–40% compared to sedentary individuals

(McTiernan 2008). Excessive sedentary time, independent to moderate and vigorous physical activity, is also associated with increased risk of cancer (Biswas et al 2015).

The postulated mechanisms linking higher levels of physical activity and the risk reduction associated with developing cancer varies slightly for each type of cancer. In general, physical activity reduces obesity and body fat content, enhances the body's immune function, lowers endogenous sex hormones and increases the activity levels of metabolic hormones and growth factors (Friedenreich 2001). The immune-related response to exercise includes a reduction in systemic inflammation. Lower body fat associated with exercise results in less inflammatory cytokines in adipose tissue and a reduction in the storage of carcinogens in visceral fat tissue (Friedenreich 2001, McTiernan 2008). Physical activity raises high-density lipoprotein cholesterol levels and reduces insulin resistance, hyperinsulinaemia, hyperglycaemia and triglyceride levels and the occurrence of type 2 diabetes, all of which are linked with cancer risk (Friedenreich 2001, McTiernan 2008). The strong association between physical activity and a reduced risk of colon cancer is hypothesized to be due to an increase in gut motility and a decrease in gastrointestinal transit time, and therefore a decrease in the exposure of gut mucosa to carcinogens (Friedenreich 2001). It is also thought to be due to an increase in prostaglandin F and decrease in circulating insulin and glucose resulting from exercise (Friedenreich 2001). The association between physical activity and breast cancer risk reduction is related to the effect of exercise on menstrual function and sex hormones, with an overall decreased lifetime exposure to oestrogen and progesterone and an increase in globulin levels associated with exercise (McTiernan 2008, Friedenreich 2001).

MEDICAL TREATMENT OF CANCER AND THE ASSOCIATED SIDE EFFECTS

There are many different forms of cancer treatment:

- surgery
- chemotherapy
- radiotherapy
- molecular targeted therapy.

The choice of treatment depends on the type of cancer, stage of cancer, tumour location and the individual's comorbid conditions and degree of frailty. Patients will often have a combination of treatments, for example, surgery followed by chemotherapy and or radiotherapy, or radiotherapy followed by surgery. Each cancer treatment is associated with side effects which add to the morbidity suffered by the individual (Table 13-17).

Surgical resection of the tumour normally offers the best curative potential for patients with cancer; however, in order for surgery to be an option the patient needs to be fit enough to withstand this insult.

TABLE 13-17	
Common Side Effects Resulting from Cancer Treatments	
Surgery	Exercise intolerance
	Pain
	Cough
	Fatigue
Chemotherapy	Fatigue
	Nausea and vomiting
	Diarrhoea or constipation
	Loss of appetite
	Hair loss
	Anaemia
	Infection (immunosuppression)
	Mouth ulcers or infection
	Weight gain or weight loss
Radiotherapy	Fatigue
	Skin erythema
	Oesophagitis
	Nausea and vomiting
	Diarrhoea
	Loss of appetite
	Hair loss
	Cough
	Rigors
	Flu-like symptoms
Molecular targeted therapies	Fatigue
	Skin and hair changes
	Nausea and vomiting
	Diarrhoea or constipation
	Loss of appetite

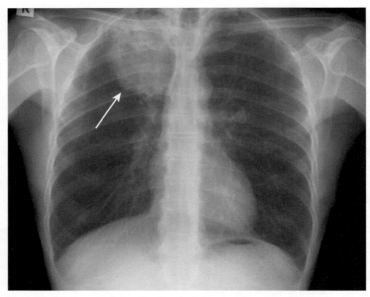

FIGURE 13-34 ■ Chest radiograph of an individual with a right upper lobe lung cancer.

For patients with lung cancer undergoing thoracic surgery, pulmonary resection directly impacts on their cardiorespiratory fitness (Fig. 13-34). By removing a section of the lung parenchyma, surgery alters the ventilation and diffusing capacity of the lungs. There is a known immediate reduction in peak oxygen consumption (VO_{2peak}) by approximately 12% and 18% post lobectomy and pneumonectomy, respectively (Brunelli et al 2009). Surgery is also associated with a risk of postoperative complications (see Chapter 11) and side effects (see Table 13-17).

Chemotherapy is the treatment of cancer using pharmacological medications. Chemotherapeutic therapeutic agents act by directly interfering with the process of mitosis and therefore kill rapidly dividing cells. Cytotoxic drugs inhibit cell division in both cancerous and non-cancerous cells and therefore result in many side effects from the damage caused to normal cells (see Table 13-17). Acutely, chemotherapy can cause bone marrow suppression with the production of white blood cells predominantly affected. Levels of white blood cells tend to fall about 5–7 days after a chemotherapy dose and are lowest about 2 weeks following treatment (Priestman 2008). At this time, patients are immunosuppressed and particularly susceptible to infections. Anaemia is another common side effect, with oxygen delivery affected by a reduction in haemoglobin. If severe enough, this can be treated with blood transfusions or erythropoietic agents (Priestman 2008). Some chemotherapeutic treatments are cardiotoxic and can also directly impact cardiac function during and following treatment resulting in acute and long-term cardiac impairments.

Radiotherapy is the treatment of cancer using ionizing radiation, which targets the cancerous cells. This can be delivered as either internal radiotherapy (brachytherapy) or external radiotherapy (which is more common). For internal radiotherapy, a radiation source is placed inside the body close to the tumour. For external radiotherapy, an external linear accelerator produces electron radiation which is specifically targeted at the tumorous cells. The radiation results in formation of free radicals, which in turn cause damage to cell DNA and subsequent apoptosis of cancer cells. However, the surrounding normal tissue can be damaged in this process. Normal rapidly dividing cells such as those in the oesophageal mucosa are particularly susceptible to damage from the radiotherapy (Hunt et al 2008). Radiotherapy results in a widespread inflammatory response and the release of cytokines, which cause systemic side effects for the patient. Acute side effects of radical radiotherapy include skin erythema, oesophagitis, cough, fatigue, rigors and flu-like symptoms and typically last for 4–6 weeks (Hunt et al 2008) (see Table 13-17). Patients receiving palliative radiotherapy typically only suffer from treatment-related side effects for a couple of days after treatment. This is because in palliative radiotherapy dosages are minimal and decided on the balance of symptom control versus treatment side effects.

Molecular targeted therapies are a more recent form of cancer treatment which are being increasingly understood and used for treatment. Tumours are driven by genomic mutations and the different genomes in cancer are becoming recognized and then targeted with these agents. Targeted agents are different to chemotherapy agents: chemotherapy agents act 'in the nucleus by inhibiting the division of any rapidly dividing cells', whereas molecular targeted agents act by 'inhibiting pathways outside of the nucleus that are required for malignant proliferation' (Heigener et al 2009).

Individuals with cancer often have more comorbidities than individuals who do not have cancer. Research suggests that people with lung cancer and renal cancer have the highest number of comorbidities and those with melanoma, non-Hodgkin lymphoma and prostate cancer have the lowest (Smith et al 2008). The presence of comorbidities can significantly impact the cancer treatment. Depending on coexisting medical conditions, patients may not be medically fit for surgery, chemotherapy or high-dose radical radiotherapy; may not be able to tolerate the full course of treatment (which is important for cure/survival) and may have worse postoperative outcomes (Hollaus et al 2003) and prognosis. The presence of coexisting medical conditions is also likely to influence the clinical profile of cancer by amplifying symptoms and functional limitations associated with each additional comorbid condition.

LACK OF PHYSICAL ACTIVITY AFTER A DIAGNOSIS OF CANCER

There are many reasons why people with cancer may be inactive; adverse physiological and psychological

TABLE 13-18	
Physical Activity in Different Patient Groups	
Patient Group	Mean Steps Per Day
Cardiac disease	4684
COPD	2237
Type 2 diabetes	6342
Breast cancer	7409
Neuromuscular diseases	5887
Arthritis	4086
Elderly with comorbidities	6078

From Tardon et al 2005.
COPD, Chronic obstructive pulmonary disease.

effects and complex symptom clusters arise from multiple causative factors including:

- the cancer itself
- the cancer treatment (see Table 13-17)
- pre-existing medical, physical and psychological comorbidities (Table 13-18)
- pre-existing risk-related health behaviours potentially involved in the aetiology of the cancer (such as lack of physical activity, smoking or obesity).

As a result people with cancer can experience a magnitude of symptoms and impairments (Fig. 13-35). Many of these are of particular importance to physiotherapists, including fatigue and loss of functional abilities through deconditioning, dyspnoea and physiological changes in muscles from the chemotherapy. The symptoms a patient experiences will vary on an individual basis but the most frequent symptom in cancer is cancer-related fatigue which affects between 40% and 100% of patients. Cancer-related fatigue is a type of fatigue that is unremitting and not alleviated by rest; however, this symptom is very problematic as it encourages patients to rest and reduce their level of physical activity.

Cancer cachexia is 'a multi-factorial syndrome defined by an ongoing loss of skeletal muscle mass (with or without loss of fat mass) that cannot be fully reversed by conventional nutritional support and leads to progressive functional impairment' (Blum

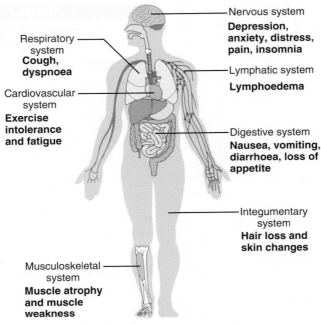

Respiratory
system
**Cough,
dyspnoea**

Cardiovascular
system
**Exercise
intolerance
and fatigue**

Musculoskeletal
system
**Muscle atrophy
and muscle
weakness**

Nervous system
**Depression,
anxiety, distress,
pain, insomnia**

Lymphatic system
Lymphoedema

Digestive system
**Nausea, vomiting,
diarrhoea, loss of
appetite**

Integumentary
system
**Hair loss and
skin changes**

FIGURE 13-35 ▪ Common symptoms in cancer.

et al 2011). Cancer cachexia occurs in approximately 50% of patients with cancer. Clinically cancer cachexia presents as a combination of anorexia, metabolic alterations, loss of fat mass, loss of skeletal muscle protein, loss of weight, impaired muscle strength and fatigue. There are many severe consequences of cancer cachexia, including a reduced ability to tolerate surgery, poor response to chemotherapy or radiotherapy, impaired resilience to treatment, worse HRQoL and ultimately increased mortality, highlighting the importance of strategies to attempt to prevent and also reverse the cachexia process and manifestation.

Cancer symptoms and cancer cachexia directly impact the individual's ability to maintain physical activity and their capacity to engage in exercise training programs. Symptoms can cause significant interference with daily activities, such as the ability of an individual to walk to the shops or to do the gardening. Avoidance of triggers for symptoms (i.e. physical activity) promotes a vicious cycle where individuals electively choose to decrease their level of physical activity. This leads to functional decline and deconditioning and ultimately impacts the ability to participate in ADLs and their HRQoL (Figs 13-36 and 13-37) (Granger

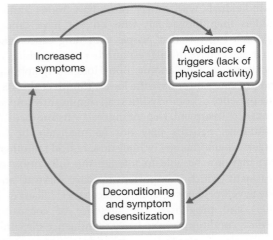

Increased
symptoms

Avoidance of
triggers (lack of
physical activity)

Deconditioning
and symptom
desensitization

FIGURE 13-36 ▪ Cycle of symptoms, inactivity and deconditioning in cancer.

et al 2014, Tanaka et al 2002, O'Driscoll et al 1999, Hewitt et al 2003). Physiotherapists play an important role in the prevention of functional decline through education regarding physical activity (to patients, carers and cancer healthcare professionals) and with

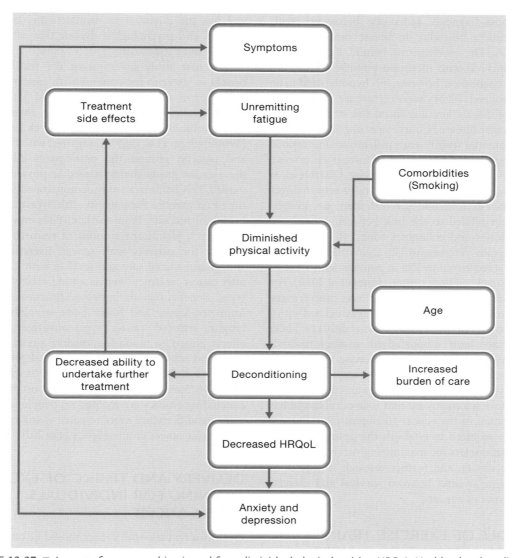

FIGURE 13-37 ■ Impact of cancer resulting in and from diminished physical activity. *HRQoL,* Health-related quality of life.

the delivery and prescription of exercise training to cancer survivors.

PHYSICAL ACTIVITY GUIDELINES FOR PEOPLE LIVING WITH CANCER

The World Health Organization recommends that older adults, aged 65 years and above, engage in 150 minutes of moderate intensity physical activity or 75 minutes of vigorous intensity physical activity throughout the week (WHO 2010). This is the same as the guidelines recommended by the American Cancer Society for individuals with cancer (Rock et al 2013). Consistent evidence links higher physical activity levels post diagnosis with reduced cancer-specific and all-cause mortality (breast, colon and prostate cancer) (Ballard-Barbash et al 2012, Lee et al 2014a, b). Additionally there is emerging evidence linking post-diagnosis sedentary behaviour with reduced cancer mortality in breast cancer (Biswas et al 2015). The mechanisms behind the improvement in survival with increased physical activity are still being established; however, it is hypothesized to be due to a reduced risk of cancer recurrence, slowed progression of disease and a reduced risk of non-cancer cardiovascular disease (Courneya et al 2007). Exercise has the potential to influence inflammation, tumour morphology, tumour growth and cancer recurrence (Antoni et al 2006, Davis et al 1998, Gleeson et al 2011). In lung cancer, while there is not a proven direct link between exercise and survival, there are promising findings related to the link between fitness and survival; Jones and colleagues found that for every 1.1 mL/kg min^{-1} increase in VO_{2peak} at time of diagnosis, survival improved by 7% in patients with stage I–IIIB non-small cell lung cancer (Jones et al 2010). For patients with inoperable metastatic lung cancer, every 50 m improvement in the 6MWD was associated with a 13% improvement in survival (Jones et al 2012). These findings have been supported by another research group (Kasymjanova et al 2009). Exercise, unlike other cancer treatments (surgery, chemotherapy and radiotherapy), is not associated with unwanted side effects and therefore is a treatment that is favourable and has great potential in the cancer treatment plan. Further research is required to establish the optimal exercise training parameters for maximizing survival in breast and colon cancer, and further research is require to establish similar links between survival and exercise in other types of cancers.

THE ROLE OF EXERCISE TRAINING IN THE MANAGEMENT OF CANCER

Exercise is a non-pharmacological intervention with great potential benefit for individuals with cancer. Exercise for the cancer population has been slower to develop than in other patient populations, such as COPD or cardiac disease. Physiotherapy and exercise rehabilitation are part of standard care for individuals with COPD and cardiac disease (via pulmonary rehabilitation or cardiac rehabilitation; see Chapter 12) in many places around the world; however, cancer exercise programs are much less frequent. Exercise in oncology is a growing area of physiotherapy practice

and has the potential to minimize the debilitating physical and psychological decline that often occurs with a cancer diagnosis.

The first study investigating the feasibility and benefit of exercise for patients with cancer was only published in 1988. This study exercised patients with breast cancer who were undergoing chemotherapy with aerobic exercise three times per week for 10 weeks (Winningham et al 1988). Compared with the control and placebo groups, the participants allocated to the exercise group demonstrated improved levels of nausea. This landmark study demonstrated for the first time that exercise for patients with breast cancer was beneficial and safe. From the late 1980s onwards there has been a significant amount of research targeting exercise for patients with cancer. Exercise training is now considered safe and feasible both during and after cancer treatment across a wide variety of cancer types. Benefits include improved functional capacity, improved upper and lower body strength, reduced fatigue, reduced cancer symptoms/treatment side effects, enhanced mood (depression, anxiety and distress) and enhanced HRQoL (Conn et al 2006, Cramp et al 2012, Knols et al 2005, Rock et al 2013, Schmitz K et al 2010, Speck et al 2010). However most of the RCTs concluding efficacy are focused on people with breast cancer and therefore more research is still required in non-breast cancer groups (Speck et al 2010).

DELIVERY AND TIMING OF EXERCISE TRAINING FOR INDIVIDUALS WITH CANCER

Ideally individuals with cancer should be offered exercise pre-treatment, during treatment and following treatment:

- Exercise pre-treatment occurs in the time between diagnosis and surgery, or in the time between diagnosis and the commencement of chemotherapy or radiotherapy. Exercise at this time point aims to maximize the patients' physical status, maximize cardiorespiratory fitness and enhance muscle strength prior to the insult of treatment.
- Exercise during chemotherapy or radiotherapy aims to enhance physical activity levels, reduce

symptoms, prevent functional decline and maximize HRQoL and psychological status.

■ Exercise following the conclusion of treatment aims to restore any loss in cardiorespiratory fitness and muscle strength that occurred during the period of treatment and maximize functional abilities, psychological status and HRQoL for the cancer survivor long term.

Exercise can be delivered in a group setting, similar to the pulmonary rehabilitation model, in which outpatients enrol and attend an exercise class which is run in a community-health or hospital-based gymnasium. Commonly such programs run two to three times per week, for 8–12 weeks. Ideally patients would attend an outpatient programme three times per week and then continue exercise in the home environment on the days they do not attend the programme. Alternatively, if patients live in a remote location or in an area without established outpatient programs (which is very common), the physiotherapist can design and teach a home-exercise programme for the patient to complete in their home environment. Ultimately the aim is to increase the patient's level of physical activity through a change in lifestyle behaviour so that following conclusion of the structured

exercise programme, the individual continues to exercise for the rest of their life.

EVALUATION OF EXERCISE TRAINING FOR INDIVIDUALS WITH CANCER

When designing an exercise programme the physiotherapist needs to take into consideration the type of cancer, type of treatment, baseline physical status and general medical condition of their patient. The ACSM has specific guidelines regarding exercise safety for people with cancer (Rock et al 2013, Schmitz K et al 2010). Prior to commencement of an exercise programme, the individual should have a comprehensive initial assessment by the physiotherapist. The purpose of this assessment includes screening for safety and obtaining a baseline level of physical and psychological status. This assessment should be repeated following conclusion of the exercise programme to evaluate success of the training programme. The initial assessment should cover an assessment of:

■ screening for contra-indications or precautions to exercise (Table 13-19)
■ baseline physical status: functional exercise capacity, function and muscle strength

TABLE 13-19		
Risk Factors to Screen during the Initial Pre-Exercise Assessment		
Cancer Type	**Assessment**	**Prior to Commencement of**
All	■ Comorbidities (and their associated risk with exercise) ■ Risk of fracture ■ Muscle atrophy or severe cancer cachexia (loss of >35% premorbid weight) ■ Peripheral neuropathy ■ Musculoskeletal injury ■ Known cardiac complication of treatment (patient needs a medical cardiac examination prior to commencement) ■ Wound healing (postoperative; may need clearance from surgeon for commencement)	Any exercise
Breast	■ Shoulder and upper limb range of motion, strength and function	Upper body exercise
Colon	■ Risk of infection (in patients postoperative with an ostomy) ■ Risk of hernia (in patients postoperative with an ostomy)	Any exercise Resistance exercise
Gynaecological	■ Lower limb lymphoedema ■ Swelling in abdomen or groin	Vigorous intensity exercise, resistance training or exercise of the lower limb Vigorous intensity exercise, resistance training or exercise of the lower limb

■ baseline psychological status: HRQoL and mood
■ cancer symptoms: type and severity (these may fluctuate on a daily basis)
■ current level of physical activity and engagement in exercise training
■ exercise history
■ the patient's goals
■ the patient's readiness for change in lifestyle behaviour
■ barriers and enablers to exercise and physical activity for the individual.

Potential outcome measures for these components are listed in Table 13-20. Refer to Chapter 6 for more details on many of these tests.

EXERCISE PRESCRIPTION FOR INDIVIDUALS WITH CANCER

Exercise prescription needs to be individualized and modified according to the individual patient. There have been a wide variety of exercise prescriptions used in the previous studies which include programs with only aerobic training, programs with only resistance training, programs with a combination of mixed aerobic–resistance training and other methods of exercise training such as yoga, Tai Chi, dance and NMES. There is currently not enough evidence to routinely recommend one type of exercise training over another. Therefore current recommendations state that people with cancer should follow the ACSM guidelines for healthy and older adults or the guidelines for adults with chronic diseases. Exercise programs should include a combination of aerobic and resistance training and stretches (Table 13-21):

■ Aerobic training should be undertaken 3–5 days per week, progressed up to target duration of 30 minutes. Intensity should initially commence at

TABLE 13-20
Suggested Outcome Measures for Use in the Initial Assessment Prior to Commencement of Exercise

Domain	Outcome Measure
Cardiorespiratory fitness	■ Cardiopulmonary exercise testing ■ Six-minute walk test ■ Incremental shuttle walk test ■ Endurance shuttle walk test
Function	■ Timed up-and-go test ■ Short physical performance battery
Muscle strength	■ Hand-held dynamometry ■ Hand-grip dynamometry ■ Cybex norm dynamometry ■ 1 repetition maximum
HRQoL	■ Functional Assessment of Cancer Therapy core questionnaire and supplementary tumour module (specific to cancer type) ■ European Organization for the Research and Treatment of Cancer core questionnaire and supplementary tumour module (specific to cancer type) ■ Short-Form 36
Mood	■ Hospital anxiety and depression scale

HRQoL, Health-related quality of life.

TABLE 13-21
General exercise prescription in cancer

Exercise Type	Frequency	Duration	Intensity	Example Exercises
Aerobic	■ 3–5 times per week OR	≥30 min per session	Moderate	Ground walking, treadmill walking, stationary bike cycling, stepping on machine, sit to stands, aerobics
	■ 3 times per week	≥20 min per session	Vigorous*	As above plus running
Resistance	■ 2–3 times per week			Exercises with the use of: gravity, Theraband, weight machines or free weights
Stretches	■ Days of exercise			

From Schmitz K et al 2010.
*Vigorous intensity exercise is generally not recommended for patients during active cancer treatment.

light intensity and be progressed during the pro-gramme to either a moderate or vigorous inten-sity depending on the individual patient. Patients with a previous exercise history may be able to commence at a moderate intensity – this can be determined during the initial pre-exercise assess-ment depending on the results of their functional exercise capacity tests. Vigorous intensity exercise is generally not recommended for patients during active cancer treatment, although following treatment some patients will be able to be pro-gressed up to vigorous intensity exercise, particu-larly younger patients such as those with breast cancer. Patients with cardiovascular limitations such as chemotherapy-induced left ventricular dysfunction or severe anaemia, patients with peripheral limitations such as severe cancer cachexia or muscle atrophy or patients post-haematologic stem cell transplant generally should only progress up to moderate intensity activity and not engage vigorous intensity aerobic exercise (Lakoski et al 2012). Such limitations should be identified during the initial pre-exercise assessment and this information can be used to individually tailor the exercise pro-gramme (commencement and progression) accordingly. Suggestions of methods to perform aerobic exercise are provided in Table 13-21.

■ Resistance training of large muscle groups and upper and lower limb muscles should be under-taken two to three times per week. The ACSM resistance training principles apply to individual with cancer and resistance exercises should be delivered using two to three sets of eight to 15 repetitions. There are many cancer groups in which resistance training should be prescribed with caution and close monitoring (or not at all). These patient groups are listed in Table 13-22.

MONITORING DURING EXERCISE FOR INDIVIDUALS WITH CANCER

Despite the fact that individuals will go through a detailed initial pre-exercise assessment prior to com-mencement of the exercise programme, patients should be briefly assessed on a daily basis before commencement of exercise on that particular day.

Physiotherapists should ask about any changes or events that have occurred since the prior exercise session. Cancer symptoms can fluctuate on a daily basis and need to be screened for both before, during and after exercise training. Patients with extreme fatigue should not exercise on those days. Patients during treatment or patients at risk of hypotension or hypertension should have their blood pressure taken before starting exercise and occasionally during exercise.

During exercise training the Borg scale can be used to assess and monitor the intensity of exercise (see Chapter 12). For moderate intensity aerobic exercise the patient should aim to be exercising at a Borg breathlessness level of three to five (moderate to hard) (Borg 1982). Patients should also be monitored with pulse oximetery measuring oxygen saturation (SpO_2) and heart rate. Exercise should be ceased if SpO_2 declines below 85%. A list of specific precautions and factors to monitor is provided in Table 13-22.

STRATEGIES FOR ADHERENCE TO INCREASED PHYSICAL ACTIVITY FOR INDIVIDUALS WITH CANCER

The evidence suggests that maintaining high levels of physical activity (i.e. meeting the physical activity guidelines) has a wealth of benefit for people with cancer with respect to reducing morbidity and poten-tially prolonging life. The time of cancer diagnosis is a 'window of opportunity' and a teachable moment that often will have the greatest success at behavioural change. From the time of diagnosis, physiotherapists and cancer healthcare professionals need to educate patients and their carers about the importance of maintaining physically active from that instance for-wards for the rest of their life. Exercise programs provide a structured environment for individuals with cancer to increase their level of physical activity; however, commonly after conclusion of such pro-grams people often revert back to their previous level of activity. Strategies should be put in place to maxi-mize sustainability of engagement in higher levels of physical activity for the longer term. Physiotherapists should discuss with their patient (both at commence-ment of the exercise programme and at conclusion of the programme) any barriers and enablers the patient

TABLE 13-22		
General Contraindications and Precautions to Exercise Training		
Exercise Type	**Patient Group**	**Details**

Any	■ Any type of cancer	■ Avoid exercise on days when:
		  ■ Haemoglobin level <80 g/L
		  ■ Neutrophil count ≤.5 × 10.9/μL
		  ■ Platelet count <50 × 109/μL
		  ■ Fever >38°C
		  ■ Extreme fatigue or severe nausea

	■ Upper or lower limb lymphoedema ■ Breast cancer	■ Wear compression garment during exercise ■ If there is an increase in upper limb swelling or lymphoedema with exercise, exercise should be temporarily ceased and medical opinion sought.
	■ Gynaecological cancer	■ If there is an increase in swelling in abdomen, groin or lower limb with exercise, exercise should be temporarily ceased and medical opinion sought.
Aerobic	■ Peripheral limitation, such as severe cancer cachexia or muscle atrophy	■ Commence with only resistance training and then progress to incorporate aerobic training after muscle bulk and strength is improved.
Resistance	■ Colon cancer post surgery with ostomy	■ Avoid activities which increase intra-thoracic pressure (such as sit-ups). ■ Progress slowly with resistance exercises to avoid hernia at the stoma (advise medical clearance before commencement after surgery).
	■ Known/high-risk bony metastases ■ High risk of osteoporosis (such as patients treated with hormonal therapy) ■ High risk of bone fracture ■ Cardiorespiratory limitation, such as chemotherapy-induced left ventricular dysfunction or severe anaemia	■ Prescribe with caution. ■ Prescribe with caution. ■ Prescribe with caution. ■ Generally contraindicated (advise medical clearance before commencement)
	■ Postoperative patients	■ Care with wound healing: often require 6–8 weeks postoperative for healing prior to commencement of resistance exercises (advise medical clearance before commencement postoperative)
Stretches	■ Postoperative patients	■ Care with wound healing: often require 6–8 weeks postoperative for healing prior to commencement of resistance exercises (advise medical clearance before commencement post-operative)

foresee that could impact on their ability to exercise. These barriers and enablers will be personal and different for each patient. Engaging the carers, friends and family is a common strategy to increase adherence and enjoyment of exercise. If possible, patients should be encouraged to walk with their carer or friends as the social interaction and engagement provides increased enjoyment. Another common barrier is lack of a suitable environment to exercise. For example, patients may identify that a barrier to them being able to walk outdoors is the fact that they live in a hilly neighbourhood. In this situation the physiotherapist should brainstorm with the patients for an alternative,

such as the option to drive to the local sports oval or park and then walk around that flatter area. Some general exercise recommendations and tips for individuals with cancer include:

■ Wear suitable footwear and clothing.
■ Keep hydrated with water.
■ Exercise with someone (a friend or family member).
■ Be aware of your symptoms and on 'very bad days' (often during treatment) modify your exercise programme by either reducing the duration and or intensity of exercise just for that day.

- Be aware of the intensity of exercise. One option to monitor intensity is the 'talk and walk test'; in this situation for moderate intensity exercise you should be 'puffed' but still able to talk in sentences. If you are not 'puffed' you are not working hard enough, alternatively if you cannot talk in sentences you may be working too hard.
- Keep a diary to record your daily exercise routine. This includes the duration, type and intensity of exercise. A diary will you help identify if you have decreased the amount of exercise you are doing over time. It will also help you progress and increase your exercise.
- Avoid exercise at times of extreme heat. On hot days do not exercise outdoors in the middle of the day (when temperatures are highest). Either exercise indoors (such as a shopping centre or gymnasium with air-conditioning) or exercise at the start or end of the day when temperatures are lower.
- Avoid exercise outdoors on days of extreme cold. In these situations either exercise indoors (such as a shopping centre or gymnasium) or in the middle of the day when temperatures are highest.
- Rest and getting adequate sleep is important to allow you to exercise sufficiently the next day.

Rehabilitation for Survivors of Intensive Care

Improved survival following critical illness in the last two decades has resulted in more patients admitted with critical illness living beyond hospital discharge. However, many of these survivors report ongoing muscle weakness and poor physical function as well as neurocognitive and psychiatric symptoms that impact their daily life. Referred to as 'post intensive care syndrome (PICS)' (Needham et al 2012) (Fig. 13-38), this constellation of symptoms can impact family roles and responsibilities, participation in social activities and the capacity for return to work (Davidson, Jones & Bienvenu 2011). Iwashyna and Netzer provide a conceptual model to guide choice of assessments and rehabilitation after critical illness, anchored in the International Classification of Functioning, Disease and Health (ICF) (Iwashyna & Netzer 2012). Within the ICF model, an assessment might focus on body function and structure (e.g. muscle atrophy or weakness on strength testing), on activity (e.g. performance on 6-minute walk testing), and on participation (e.g. ADLs) (Box 13-11). (See Chapter 6 for further information on outcome measures in ICU). This model is excellent, as it allows clinicians to focus on the limitations or disabilities that most affect individual

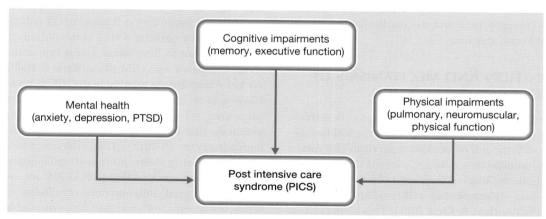

FIGURE 13-38 ■ Impairments that make up post intensive care syndrome (PICS). *PTSD,* Post-traumatic stress disorder. *(Needham et al.)*

patients and provides a basis for changing assessments to measure progress along the continuum of ICU recovery.

This section on ICU rehabilitation will review the underlying mechanisms responsible for PICS, the evidence base for the effectiveness of rehabilitation, describe the role of the physiotherapist in assessment and treatment, outline some of the treatment techniques currently used and discuss limitations to our current knowledge base.

DEFINITION AND MECHANISMS OF MUSCLE WEAKNESS IN ICU

Until recently medical care in ICU has concentrated almost exclusively on achieving physiological homoeostasis with the aim of improving survival. This model of care has necessitated 'taking over for the patient' by sedating them, keeping them immobile and manipulating fluid replacement as well renal and respiratory status (Schweickert & Kress 2011). This model of care has now been challenged, as the consequences of therapies administered in the ICU such as sedation and immobilization are shown to have detrimental short- and long-term effects on the body and the brain (Needham et al 2012). The most common complaint suffered by survivors of intensive care is muscle weakness (Herridge et al 2003). Referred to as 'ICU-AW', it has both short- and long-term consequences with prolonged muscle weakness being reported up to 5 years following hospital discharge (Herridge et al 2011).

ICU-AW is a clinical definition and is defined as weakness secondary to critical illness in the absence of any neurological or metabolic aetiology (Griffiths & Hall 2010). ICU-AW may be described as either a neuropathy – critical illness neuropathy (CIP), a myopathy – critical illness myopathy (CIM) or a combination of both, as there is significant overlap observed in critically ill patients with neuropathy and myopathy that may potentially be a continuum of the same disease process (Kress & Hall 2014). Both functional and structural abnormalities in muscle and nerve have been implicated (Bolton & Breuer 1999). CIP is characterized by a primary axonal degeneration that affects motor more than sensory nerves. Electrophysiological studies show reduced amplitude of compound motor and sensory nerves' action potentials with preservation of conduction velocity (Bolton et al 1986; Latronico & Bolton 2011). Specific diagnosis of CIP is difficult without electrophysiological testing. Distinguishing muscle and nerve injury from the effects of immobility in the diagnosis of ICU-AW is challenging, as it is impossible to know the impact of immobilization as distinct from critical illness highlighting the importance of activities to reduce immobility. However, the phenotype is important as it may impact patient outcomes whereby patients with a combination of CIP/CIM are shown to have worse 1-year functional outcomes compared with CIM alone (Kress & Hall 2014). We know that muscle wasting in the ICU is rapid with 15–30% of rectus femoris muscle cross-sectional area (measured using diagnostic ultrasound) being lost within the first 10 days of admission (Parry et al 2015, Puthucheary et al 2013). This evidence provides a rationale for early intervention with rehabilitation.

The mechanisms that lead to ICU-AW are complex and multifactorial. Inflammatory conditions such as sepsis, the systemic inflammatory response and bacteraemia, as well as the presence of septic encephalopathy and the use of vasopressors and aminoglycosides;

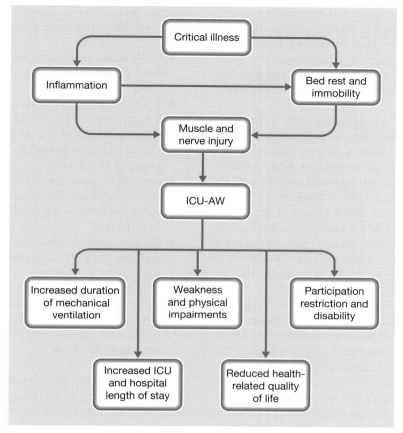

FIGURE 13-39 ▪ Possible mechanisms and sequelae for intensive care unit–acquired weakness (ICU-AW).

increasing severity of illness; hyperglycaemia and immobilization are all independent risk factors for the development of ICU-AW (Fig. 13-39) (Hermans et al 2015, Truong et al 2009).

Diagnosis of ICU-AW is clinical and involves strength testing using manual muscle testing of 12 muscle groups using the Medical Research Council (MRC) scale (Stevens et al 2009a, b). Each of six muscle groups (arm abduction, elbow flexion, wrist extension, hip flexion, knee extension and ankle dorsiflexion) bilaterally is tested and scored from 0 (no contraction) through 5 (normal strength). If the sum score is less than 48/60 (mean strength across all muscle groups less than 4/5), a positive diagnosis of ICU-AW is made. A limitation of manual muscle testing in the critical care setting is that it requires the active participation of the patient. This means that many patients cannot

be measured or have a delayed diagnosis that can often not be made until after ICU discharge (Connolly et al 2013). Despite limitations of reliability (Hough et al 2011), this method is currently accepted as the gold standard for diagnosis ICU-AW. More detail regarding testing of muscle strength is available in Chapter 6.

The impairments that result from an ICU stay, such as ICU-AW, may respond to early and intensive rehabilitation. The aim of the management of patients who are critically ill in ICU should be to minimize exposure to the severity and intensity of critical illness and to promote early rehabilitation (Hough 2013). The definition of what constitutes rehabilitation as opposed to (for example) physical therapy, early ambulation or early mobilization is unclear, with different definitions used by clinicians and researchers or indeed often no definition is provided (Gosselink et al 2012). Exercises along a continuum from passive movements to active movements and changes in position such as exercising over the edge of the bed or moving from sitting to standing are considered rehabilitation by some authors (Morris et al 2008), while others call this early mobilization and include bed, sitting and walking exercises.

Members of the rehabilitation team in the ICU (physicians, physiotherapists, occupational and respiratory therapists and nurses) need to understand the types of rehabilitation modalities, the safety parameters and monitoring around these in order to provide the best interdisciplinary care (Gosselink et al 2012). Physiotherapists are key to the success of the implementation of a rehabilitation strategy, as when they are a member of the multidisciplinary team, they provide over 80% of all mobilization activities (Berney et al 2012), achieving higher levels of mobilization for patients (Garzon-Serrano et al 2011).

The decision making process for working with patients who are critically ill requires the physiotherapist to collaborate with not only the patient and family but also the inter-professional team working in the unit. This team communication serves three important purposes by: (1) providing an overview of the patient's medical history and recovery potential, (2) establishing a dialogue regarding potential barriers to early rehabilitation, e.g. sedation, pain management and delirium and (3) further delineating the role each member of the team has regarding patient management. In addition to gathering data from the inter-professional team, physiotherapists are expected to synthesize data from the patient's electronic medical record regarding precautions, laboratory values and cardiopulmonary systems (see Box 13-11).

Currently, there are no universally accepted parameters for readiness for examination and intervention; however, recent clinical trials have integrated the factors listed to gauge safety and patient response to early intervention (Denehy et al 2013, Morris et al 2008, Schweickert et al 2009). Because patient acuity and therapist expertise varies greatly across ICUs, the physiotherapist must consult with the inter-professional team to determine appropriate safety parameters for the unit. Recently a traffic light system of safety criteria have been developed that may be useful for clinical settings. Readers are referred to Hodgson and colleagues (2014). As an exemplar, the respiratory parameters agreed upon included:

- *Endotracheal tube intubation is not in itself a contraindication to early mobilization (green light).*
- *A fraction of inspired oxygen (FiO$_2$) less than 0.6 is a safe criterion for in- and out-of-bed mobilization if there are no other contraindications (green). Caution or orange is needed if FiO$_2$ is >0.6.*
- *Caution (orange) should be taken with in bed exercises with arterial saturation <90%, while out of bed exercises are a red light and should not be performed.*
- *Caution should be taken if respiratory rate is >30 bpm, if PEEP is >10 cmH$_2$O and if also there is ventilator dysynchrony.*
- *If the patient is at the safety limits for several categories (e.g., low percutaneous oxygen saturation, high FiO$_2$ and high PEEP), an experienced medical team should be consulted prior to mobilization.*

Cardiovascular and neurological considerations are also described in the paper (Hodgson et al 2014).

To date, the safety profile of rehabilitation interventions for the critically ill has been satisfactory with randomized trials including more than 300 participants reporting only one serious adverse event and a large observational study of over 1000 patients receiving over 5000 physiotherapist interventions reporting only 34 safety events, of which only four (<0.001%) required treatment (Sricharoenchai et al 2014).

Once pertinent sources of information are collected from assessment, the physiotherapist must use clinical decision making skills to determine which interventions are indicated, how to implement the activities and how to determine intensity and frequency of the interventions. Because of the variability of patients' cognitive and physical status, three categories of patient abilities may be helpful to guide the therapists' thought processes: (1) patients who are unconscious, (2) patients who are conscious and medically stable and (3) patients who have experienced deconditioning due to extended inactivity and/or sedation (Table 13-23).

TABLE 13-23

Assessment Framework for a Critically Ill Patient

Patient is Conscious and Physiologically Stable	Patient is Unconscious
Interprofessional discussion, e.g. risk or benefit of early mobility	Interprofessional consultation, e.g. sedation, delirium, prevention of body system dysfunction
Assess precautions to early mobility	Assess cardiopulmonary reserve to determine safe intervention Use traffic light system (Hodgson et al 2014)
Assess cardiopulmonary reserve Use traffic light system (Hodgson et al 2014)	Primary interventions positioning, ROM, and patient family education
Intervention focus on functional goals and measuring responses to activity	Consider risk or benefit of supine cycling and/or NMES

NMES, Neuromuscular electrical stimulation; ROM, range of motion.

PATIENTS WHO ARE UNCONSCIOUS/SEDATED

Due to the high acuity of patients in critical care, sedation is often used to facilitate the establishment of physiological homoeostasis and medical management of multi-organ system failure. If patients are unable to actively follow commands, early interventions are important to consider due to the early detrimental effects on muscle previously discussed in this chapter. Expert opinion and recent trials have established the importance of inter-professional team discussions to optimize patient readiness for rehabilitation, e.g. reduce sedation, treatment of delirium or provision of pain management. During this early phase, management can include positioning, passive range of movement and patient/family education (Bailey et al 2007, Hanekom et al 2011, Morris et al 2008, Schweickert et al 2009). Positioning changes help to prevent pressure ulcers and to determine patients' response to more upright positions, which is critical to prepare for functional mobility.

In addition to positioning and ROM activities, several investigations have described protocols for NMES and cycling for patients who are unconscious.

There is a growing interest in the use of assistive technologies to enable patients to commence rehabilitation early in the ICU admission without the need for direct patient engagement (Needham et al 2009). Supine cycle ergometry can be utilized passively, actively (by patient effort), actively assisted using electrical muscle stimulation (EMS) or resisted. The safety (Kho et al 2015, Pires-Neto et al 2013), feasibility (Kho et al 2015) and efficacy of cycle ergometry (Burtin et al 2009) has been reported in several studies. Burtin and colleagues conducted an RCT in Belgium (Burtin et al 2009), examining 90 patients (mean Acute Physiology and Chronic Health Evaluation (APACHE) II score >25) in the ICU setting who underwent cycling five times a week for up to 30 minutes. Initially, cycling was passive and as the patient was able to engage in the therapy and actively cycle, resistance was added to increase the workload. The control comparison group received usual care physiotherapy, which involved standardized upper and lower limb exercises and mobilization once the patient was able to participate in therapy (Burtin et al 2009). The study found a significant difference in favour of the intervention cohort for 6MWD and improvement in isometric quadriceps strength at hospital discharge (Burtin et al 2009). Although this study demonstrated promising results for enhancing the recovery of muscle strength and functional outcomes, there was a delay of 14 days in the time to commencement of the intervention. Both Kho et al (n = 33; 2015) and Pires-Neto et al (n = 19; 2013) in two case series reported that cycling could be safely implemented early (within 4 days) of ICU admission. Pires-Neto and colleagues (2013) were able to provide cycle ergometry to six of the 19 patients within 24 hours with no adverse effect on haemodynamic, respiratory or metabolic parameters. Kho and colleagues (2015) reported a safety event rate of 2% for patients who commenced cycling (30 minutes/day) within 4 days following admission. Participants cycled for a mean distance of 11.2 ± 8.8 km, These investigators were also able to achieve a 92% consent rate in the study, demonstrating that cycling was acceptable to both patients and their families. These investigators are undertaking further cycling research in Canada, known as 'TryCYCLE' (www.clinicaltrials.gov/ct/show/ NCTT01885442 (accessed 14 Jan 2016)). The findings of this study will add to the knowledge around the use of assistive technology and the ability to provide rehabilitation earlier than traditional mobility.

EMS is another assistive modality which can be utilized without the need for volitional activation. It involves artificial stimulation of the skeletal muscles through the use of low-voltage electrical impulses delivered through the skin to the underlying muscle via surface electrodes (Maffiuletti 2010). It has been hypothesized that artificial stimulation may protect muscles from myopathic changes and thus could prevent the development of ICU-AW (Needham et al 2009). A systematic review has reported promising results in longer-stay ICU patients for the maintenance of muscle strength from seven studies using EMS in the ICU (Parry et al 2013). Functional electrical stimulation has also been reported in one case-matched study (Parry et al 2014) to maintain muscle strength and function. This involves the combined use of EMS with supine cycling in a functional pattern with stimulation of several muscle groups that are used in normal cycling (gluteals, calf, quadriceps and tibialis anterior). Further research is underway in a large international randomized trial in Australia and the USA examining this combined modality.

CONSCIOUS AND STABLE PATIENTS

Early Mobilization

The aim of the management of patients who are critically ill in ICU should be to minimize exposure to the severity and intensity of critical illness and to promote early rehabilitation (Hough 2013). The physiological demands are different depending on whether rehabilitation is provided in bed or out of bed and this needs to be taken into consideration, particularly as out-of-bed activities are more likely to present extra challenges in relation to cardiovascular stability.

Although early mobilization is shown to be safe and feasible in the ICU setting (Adler & Malone 2012, Bailey et al 2007, Morris et al 2008), two recent point prevalence studies demonstrated that the actual level of mobility of patients in ICU is low, particularly in patients who are mechanically ventilated (Berney et al 2013, Nydahl et al 2014). In both studies, physiotherapists were the main health provider instigating the mobilization of critically ill patients in the ICU setting.

At the time the main points raised by the point prevalence studies were the lack of a standardized consensus around safety parameters in terms of when to sit out of bed and to ambulate. There are now safety parameters published from a consensus but these are not validated in any trials to date.

Three RCTs have evaluated the efficacy of early mobilization in the ICU setting (Denehy et al 2013, Schweickert et al 2009). Schweickert and colleagues (2009) published a landmark and novel study examining the efficacy of early physical and occupational therapy compared to no therapy in mechanically ventilated individuals who were critically ill (Schweickert et al 2009). The study found a significantly higher percentage of individuals returned to independent functional status at hospital discharge in the intervention group (59%) compared to the control group (35%), and that there was a shorter duration of delirium in the intervention group (Schweickert et al 2009). Denehy and colleagues examined the efficacy of exercise rehabilitation commencing during the ICU admission and continuing across the continuum of recovery into the out-patient setting, compared to usual care practices (Denehy et al 2013). There was no significant difference found in 6-minute walk test (6MWT) results at 12 months; however, exploratory analyses demonstrated that the rate of change of the 6MWT distance and mean between group differences was higher in the intervention cohort. The key differences between these two RCTs are: (1) the standard care physiotherapy provided in the Australian trial and (2) timing of the intervention with the trial by Schweickert and colleagues commencing early (within 48 hours of admission) and that by Denehy commencing after day 5 (Parker et al 2013). These two factors may impact the outcomes between the two studies. A recent trial of 50 patients who were septic were randomized (Kayambu et al 2015) to receive standard care or early physical rehabilitation. Physical outcomes were measured. The authors found that implementation of early physical rehabilitation improved self-reported physical function measured using the SF-36 but not performance-based function, but it did induce systemic anti-inflammatory effects in the intervention group (Kayambu et al 2015).

There are also two RCTs that investigated interventions after ICU discharge (Elliott et al 2011, Walsh et al 2015). Walsh and colleagues (2015) investigated the effect of increasing physical and nutritional rehabilitation delivered during the post-ICU acute hospital stay in 240 patients. The authors did not find a difference in physical recovery or HRQoL in this study. Elliott and colleagues (2011) investigated the provision of home-based physical rehabilitation compared with usual care upon physical function measured using the 6MWT and HRQoL with the SF-36 at 3 and 6 months post discharge. They found no differences in either the 6MWT distance or HRQoL. No clinical assessments were undertaken at ICU discharge and so the sample may have included patients without identifiable muscle weakness, diminishing the optimal treatment effect (Elliott et al 2011). The evidence from these studies suggests that starting intensive rehabilitation earlier, while the patient is in ICU, to help to prevent muscle wasting and weakness may be a preferred management option rather than after discharge to the ward or home.

Although the evidence is supportive in favour of rehabilitation, there are still a number of limitations and gaps within the current knowledge base. To date there is no evidence that a particular type of intervention is more effective than another. Further research is required to elucidate the optimal type, intensity and dosage of exercise, as well as the timing and frequency. The challenge for the future will be in the ability to provide rehabilitation along the continuum of critical illness recovery, commencing on admission with the aid of assistive technology, then moving towards more functional tasks once the patient is able to actively engage and then utilizing strategies to maintain activity and keep patients active throughout the day and not just in their physical therapy sessions. There is particular interest in being able to examine interventions which can commence early to try to mitigate the rapid muscle wasting that occurs in individuals who are critically unwell.

Although it is known that patients can have ongoing significant impairments in strength and physical functioning years post the initial critical illness, it is currently unknown what the trajectory of the recovery pathway looks like. Critical care is a challenging setting to design rehabilitation interventions, as the patient cohort is heterogenous in terms of admission diagnosis and comorbidities (Deutschman et al 2012). Individualized assessment and treatment is important. It is also possible that there is heterogenity in the trajectory of recovery post critical illness (Iwashyna 2012). A thorough assessment of pre-morbid health state is essential in determining the likely trajectory of recovery for survivors of a critical illness (Puthucheary & Denehy 2015). Use of outcome measures by physiotherapist is very important in assessing treatment responses (Table 13-24). See also Chapter 6.

NEUROCOGNITIVE INTERVENTIONS

Long-term cognitive dysfunction is common after critical illness and may last up to 12 months (Pandharipande et al 2013). In a landmark study of 821 patients admitted to ICU, the incidence of delirium was 74%, occurred mainly in the first 10 days after admission and was associated with worse global cognition and executive function at 3 and 12 months

TABLE 13-24			
Potential Treatment Techniques Across the Continuum of ICU Survivorship			
Point on Recovery Trajectory	**Unable to Actively Participate**	**Actively Engaging**	**Progression to Ward and Discharge**
Possible techniques	Passive ROM	Active exercises	Nintendo Wii
	Supine cycling	Functional tasks	Exercises with family members
	NMES and FES	MOS, ambulation	Pedals
		Nintendo Wii	Weights
			Functional activity and ADLs
			Aerobic and resistance exercise

ADLs, Activities of daily living; *FES,* functional electrical stimulation; *ICU,* intensive care unit; *MOS,* marching on spot; *NMES,* neuromuscular electrical stimulation; *ROM,* range of motion.

(Pandharipande et al 2013). These findings were not related to age, sedatives or analgesics. It is not clear if specific interventions provide protection against later neurocognitive dysfunction; however, given the association between delirium and cognitive dysfunction, any treatment that may reduce the incidence of delirium may reduce brain injury. Early physical rehabilitation commenced in ICU was shown to reduced the incidence of delirium by 50% (Schweickert et al 2009) and may be a promising intervention, but more research is needed to further test this hypothesis.

RESOURCES

There are several online resources available now to assist ICU health teams to access the latest information about rehabilitation. The most recent and comprehensive of these is called ICU Recovery Network (IRN). It is a virtual community of clinicians and researchers interested in improving the recovery of critically ill patients, with a particular focus on early rehabilitation and related interventions. The provider of this network (MedConcert by CE City) is providing this service free of charge. If you have an iPhone, you can download the MedConcert app to view and access the network on your phone. The address is medconcert.com (accessed 14 Jan 2016).

SUMMARY

Rehabilitation in ICU is a field of growing importance, particularly for physiotherapists. There are many questions remaining to answer in this area, including identification of the most appropriate type, intensity, time of commencement and dose of exercise and mobilization; the most clinimetrically sound and clinically feasible outcome measures across the different stages of the rehabilitation continuum and the identification of prevention strategies for ICU-AW. There are currently studies being undertaken to address some of the remaining questions.

REFERENCES

Abel, R., Silke, R., Spahn, B., 2004. Cervical spinal cord injury and deglutition disorders. Dysphagia 19, 87–94.

Adler, J., Malone, D., 2012. Early mobilization in the intensive care unit: a systematic review. Cardiopulm. Phys. Ther. J. 23 (1), 5–13.

Aggarwal, S., Smailes, S., Dziewulski, P., 2009. Tracheostomy in burns patients revisited. Burns 35 (7), 962–966.

AIHW, 2014. Australian Institute of Health and Welfare & Australasian Association of Cancer Registries. Cancer in Australia: an Overview. Australian Institute of Health and Welfare, Canberra no. CAN 88.

Alderson, J.D., 1999. Spinal cord injuries. Care Crit. Ill 15 (2), 48–52.

Alvarez, S., Peterson, M., Lunsford, B., 1981. Respiratory treatment of the adult patient with spinal cord injury. Phys. Ther. 61 (12), 1737–1745.

American Burn Association Consensus Conference on Burn Sepsis and Infection Group, 2007. American Burn Association Consensus Conference to define sepsis and infection in burns. J. Burn Care Res. 28, 776–790.

American Cancer Society. Cancer prevention and early detection facts and figures 2012 [Online]. Atlanta. Available: <http://www.cancer.org/acs/groups/content/@epidemiologysurveilance/documents/document/acspc-033423.pdf>.

American College of Sports Medicine, 2000. ACSM's Guidelines for Exercise Testing and Prescription. Lippincott Williams & Wilkins, MD, USA.

Andreassen, A.K., 2008. Point: cardiac denervation does/does not play a major role in exercise limitation after heart transplantation. J. Appl. Physiol. 104, 559–560.

Antoni, M., Lutgendorf, S., Cole, S., et al., 2006. The influence of bio-behavioural factors on tumour biology: pathways and mechanisms. Nat. Rev. Cancer 6, 240–248.

Armstrong, A., 2009. Developing a breath-stacking system to achieve lung volume recruitment. British Journal of Nursing 18 (19), 1166–1169.

Arora, S., Flower, O., Murray, N.P., Lee, B.B., 2012. Respiratory care of patients with cervical spinal cord injury: a review. Crit. Care Resusc. 14 (1), 64–73.

Axen, K., Pineda, H., Shunfenthal, I., Haas, F., 1985. Diaphragmatic function following cervical cord injury: neurally mediated improvement. Arch. Phys. Med. Rehabil. 66, 219–222.

Bach, J.R., 1993. Mechanical insufflation-exsufflation: comparison of peak expiratory flows with manually assisted and unassisted coughing techniques. Chest 104, 1553–1562.

Bach, J.R., 2012. Noninvasive respiratory management of high level spinal cord injury. J. Spinal Cord Med. 35 (2), 72–80.

Bach, J.R., McDermott, I.G., 1990. Strapless oral-nasal interface for positive-pressure ventilation. Arch. Phys. Med. Rehabil. 71 (11), 910–913.

Bach, J.R., Smith, W.H., Michaels, J., et al., 1993. Airway secretion clearance by mechanical exsufflation for poliomyelitis ventilator-assisted individuals. Arch. Phys. Med. Rehabil. 74 (2), 170–177.

Bailey, P., Thomsen, G., Spuhler, V., et al., 2007. Early activity is feasible and safe in respiratory failure patients. Crit. Care Med. 35 (1), 139–146.

Baird, J., Fisher, D., Lucas, P., et al., 2005. Being big or growing fast: systematic review of size and growth in infancy and later obesity. BMJ 331 (7522), 929. [Epub 2005 Oct 14].

Ball, P.A., 2001. Critical care of spinal cord injury. Spine 26, S27–S30.

Ballard-Barbash, R., Friedenreich, C., Courneya, K., et al., 2012. Physical activity, biomarkers, and disease outcomes in cancer survivors: a systematic review. J. Nat. Cancer Inst. 104 (11), 815–840.

Bar-Or, O., Rowland, T.W., 2004. Children and exercise in a clinical context: an overview. In: Bar-Or, O., Rowland, T.W. (Eds.), Paediatric exercise medicine: from physiologic principles to health care application. Human Kinetics, Champaign, pp. 105–115.

Barker, A.F., 2002. Bronchiectasis. N. Engl. J. Med. 346 (18), 1383–1393.

Barratt, D.J., Harvey, L.A., Cistulli, P.A., et al., 2012. The use of bronchodilators in people with recently acquired tetraplegia: a randomized cross-over trial. Spinal Cord 50, 836–839.

Barthelemy, O., Toledano, D., Varnous, S., et al., 2012. Multislice computed tomography to rule out coronary allograft vasculopathy in heart transplant patients. J. Heart Lung Transplant. 31, 1262–1268.

Baydur, A., Adkins, R.H., Milic-Emili, J., 2001. Lung mechanics in individuals with spinal cord injury: effects of injury level and posture. J. Appl. Physiol. 90, 405–411.

Beauchamp, M.K., Nonoyama, M., Goldstein, R.S., et al., 2010. Interval versus continuous training in individuals with chronic obstructive pulmonary disease: a systematic review. Thorax 65, 157–164.

Benden, C., Edwards, L.B., Kucheryavaya, A.Y., et al., 2012. The registry of the International Society for Heart and Lung Transplantation: fifteenth paediatric lung and heart-lung transplantation report, 2012. J. Heart Lung Transplant. 31, 1087–1095.

Berlly, M., Shem, K., 2007. Respiratory management during the first five days after spinal cord injury. J. Spinal Cord Med. 30, 309–318.

Berlowitz, D.J., Brown, D.J., Campbell, D.A., Pierce, R.J., 2005. A longitudinal evaluation of sleep in the first year after cervical spinal cord injury. Arch. Phys. Med. Rehabil. 86 (6), 1193–1199.

Berney, S., Bragge, P., Granger, C., et al., 2011a. The acute respiratory management of cervical spinal cord injury in the first 6 weeks after injury: a systematic review. Spinal Cord 49 (1), 17–29.

Berney, S., Opdam, H., Bellomo, R., et al., 2008. An assessment of early tracheostomy after anterior cervical stabilization in patients with acute cervical spine trauma. J. Trauma 64, 749–753.

Berney, S., Stockton, K., Berlowitz, D., Denehy, L., 2002. Can early extubation and intensive physiotherapy decrease length of stay of acute quadriplegic patients in intensive care? A retrospective case control study. Physiother. Res. Int. 7 (1), 14–22.

Berney, S.C., Gordon, I.R., Opham, H.I., Denehy, L., 2011b. A classification and regression tree to assist clinical decision making in airway management for patients with cervical spinal cord injury. Spinal Cord 49 (2), 244–250.

Berney, S., Haines, K., Denehy, L., 2012. Physiotherapy in critical care in Australia. Cardiopulm. Phys. Ther. J. 23, 19–25.

Berney, S., Harrold, M., Webb, S., et al., 2013. Intensive care unit mobility practices in Australia and New Zealand: a point prevalence study. Crit. Care Resusc. 15 (4), 260–265.

Bhaskar, K.R., Brown, R., O'Sullivan, D.D., et al., 1991. Bronchial mucus hypersecretion in acute quadriplegia: macromolecular yields and glycoconjugate composition. Am. Rev. Respir. Dis. 143, 640–648.

Biswas, A., Oh, P., Faulkner, G., et al., 2015. Sedentary time and its association with risk for disease incidence, mortality, and hospitalization in adults: a systematic review and meta-analysis. Ann. Intern. Med. 162, 123–132.

Bittner, H.B., Lehmann, S., Binner, C., et al., 2011. Sternum sparing thoracotomy incisions in lung transplantation surgery: a superior technique to the clamshell approach. Innovations (Phila) 6, 116–121.

Blum, D., Omlin, A., Baracos, V., et al., 2011. Cancer cachexia: a systematic literature review of items and domains associated with involuntary weight loss in cancer. Crit. Rev. Oncol./Hematol. 80, 114–144.

Bolton, C., Breuer, A., 1999. Critical illness polyneuropathy. Muscle Nerve 22, 5.

Bolton, C., Laverty, D., Brown, J., et al., 1986. Critically ill polyneuropathy: electrophysiological studies and differentiation from Guillain-Barré syndrome. J. Neurol. Neurosurg. Psychiatry 49 (5), 563–573.

Boots, R.J., Dulhunty, J.M., Paratz, J.D., Lipman, J., 2009. Respiratory complications in burns. An evolving spectrum of injury. Clin. Pulm. Med. 16, 132–138.

Borel, J.F., 1980. Immunosuppressive properties of cyclosporin A (CY-A). Transplant. Proc. 12, 233.

Borg, G., 1982. Psychophysical bases for perceived exertion. Med. Sci. Sports Exerc. 14, 377–381.

Bott, J., Keilty, S.J., Noone, L., 1992. Intermittent positive pressure breathing: a dying art? Physiotherapy 78 (9), 656–660.

Braam, K.I., van der Torre, P., Takken, T., et al., 2013. Physical exercise training interventions for children and young adults during and after treatment for childhood cancer. Cochrane Database Syst. Rev. 4, CD008796, doi:10.1002/14651858.CD008796.pub2.

Bradley, J., Moran, F., 2008. Physical training for cystic fibrosis. Cochrane Database Syst. Rev. 1, CD002768.

Brady, J.E., Li, G., 2013. Prevalence of alcohol and drugs in fatally injured drivers. Addiction 108, 104–114.

Braith, R.W., 1998. Exercise training in patients with CHF and heart transplant recipients. Med. Sci. Sports Exerc. 30, S367–S378.

Braith, R.W., Beck, D.T., 2008. Resistance exercise: training adaptations and developing a safe exercise prescription. Heart Fail. Rev. 13, 69–79.

Braith, R.W., Conner, J.A., Fulton, M.N., et al., 2007. Comparison of alendronate vs alendronate plus mechanical loading as prophylaxis for osteoporosis in lung transplant recipients: a pilot study. J. Heart Lung Transplant. 26, 132–137.

Braith, R.W., Edwards, D.G., 2000. Exercise following heart transplantation. Sports Med. 30, 171–192.

Braith, R.W., Mills, R.M., Welsch, M.A., et al., 1996. Resistance exercise training restores bone mineral density in heart transplant recipients. J. Am. Coll. Cardiol. 28, 1471–1477.

Branch, K.R., Dembitsky, W.P., Peterson, K.L., et al., 1994. Physiology of the native heart and Thermo Cardiosystems left ventricular assist device complex at rest and during exercise: implications for chronic support. J. Heart Lung Transplant. 13, 641–650.

Bravo, G., Rojas-Martínez, R., Larios, F., et al., 2001. Mechanisms involved in the cardiovascular alterations immediately after spinal cord injury. Life Sci. 68 (13), 1527–1534.

British Thoracic Society, 2002. Non-invasive ventilation in acute respiratory failure. Thorax 57, 192–211.

Brooks, D., O'Brien, K., 2005. Is inspiratory muscle training effective for individuals with cervical spinal cord injury? A qualitative systematic review. Clin. Rehabil. 19, 237–246.

Brown, R., DiMarco, A.F., Hoit, J.D., Garshick, E., 2006. Respiratory dysfunction and managements in spinal cord injury. Respir. Care 51 (8), 853–870.

Brunelli, A., Belardinelli, R., Refai, M., et al., 2009. Peak oxygen consumption during cardiopulmonary exercise test improves risk stratification in candidates to major lung resection. Chest 135, 1260–1267.

Bull, F.C., Bellew, B., Schoeppe, S., Bauman, A.E., 2004. Developments in National Physical Activity Policy: an international review and recommendations towards better practice. J. Sci. Med. Sport 7 (1), 93–104.

Burns, S.P., Kapur, V., Yin, K.S., et al., 2001. Factors associated with sleep apnoea in men with spinal cord injury: a population based-case control-study. Spinal Cord 39, 15–22.

Burns, S.P., Little, J.W., Hussey, J.D., et al., 2000. Sleep apnea syndrome in chronic spinal cord injury: associated factors and treatment. Arch. Phys. Med. Rehabil. 81, 1334–1339.

Burns, S.P., Weaver, F.M., Parada, J.P., et al., 2004. Management of community-acquired pneumonia in persons with spinal cord injury. Spinal Cord 42, 450–458.

Burtin, C., Clerckx, B., Robbeets, C., et al., 2009. Early exercise in critically ill patients enhances short-term functional recovery. Crit. Care Med. 37 (9), 2499–2505.

Burton, J.H., Marshall, J.M., Munro, P., et al., 2009. Rehabilitation and transition after lung transplantation in children. Transplant. Proc. 41, 296–299.

Callahan, L.A., Supinski, G.S., 2009. Sepsis-induced myopathy. Crit. Care Med. 37, S354–S367.

Cameron, T., McKinstry, A., Burt, S., et al., 2009. Outcomes of patients with spinal cord injury before and after introduction of an interdisciplinary tracheostomy team. Crit. Care Resusc. 11, 14–19.

Cameron, G.S., Scott, J.W., Jousse, A.T., Botterell, E.H., 1955. Diaphragmatic respiration in quadriplegic patient and effect of position on his vital capacity. Ann. Surg. 141, 451–456.

Cancio, L.C., 2009. Airway management and smoke inhalation injury in the burn patient. Clin. Plast. Surg. 36 (4), 555–567.

Cantu, E. 3rd, Appel, J.Z. 3rd, Hartwig, M.G., et al., 2004. J. Maxwell Chamberlain Memorial Paper. Early fundoplication prevents chronic allograft dysfunction in patients with gastroesophageal reflux disease. Ann. Thorac. Surg. 78, 1142–1151.

Capoor, J., Stein, A.B., 2005. Aging with spinal cord injury. Phys. Med. Rehabil. Clin. N. Am. 16, 109–128.

Carrasco, C.E., Godinho, M., Barros, M.B., et al., 2012. Motor cycle crashes: a serious public health problem in Brazil. World J. Emerg. Surg. 7 (Suppl. 1), S5.

Carson, K.V., Chandratilleke, M.G., Picot, J., et al., 2013. Physical training for asthma. Cochrane Database Syst. Rev. 9, CD001116.

Carter, R.E., 1993. Experience with ventilator dependent patients. Paraplegia 31, 150–153.

Cartotto, R., 2009. Fluid resuscitation of the thermally injured patient. Clin. Plast. Surg. 36 (4), 569–581.

Casperson, C.J., Powell, K.E., Christenson, G.M., 1985. Physical activity, exercise, and physical fitness: definitions and distinctions for health-related research. Pub. Health Reports 100, 126–131.

Cassaburi, R., Oi, S., 1989. Effect of liver disease on the kinetics of lactate removal after heavy exercise. Eur. J. Appl. Physiol. Occup. Physiol. 59, 89–97.

Castriotta, R.J., Wilde, M.C., Sahay, S., 2012. Sleep disorders in spinal cord injury. Sleep Med. Clin. 7, 643–653.

Celis, M.M., Suman, O.E., Huang, T.T., 2003. Effect of a supervised exercise and physiotherapy program on surgical interventions in children with thermal injury. J. Burn Care Rehabil. 24, 57–61.

Centers for Disease Control and Prevention (CDC) and Centers for Disease Control and Prevention (CDC), 2008. How much physical activity do adults need. CDC, Atlanta, GA. Retrieved from: <http://www.cdc.gov/physicalactivity/everyone/guidelines/adults.html>.

Cerny, F.J., Pullano, T.P., Cropp, G.J., 1982. Cardiorespiratory adaptations to exercise in cystic fibrosis. Am. Rev. Respir. Dis. 126 (2), 217–220.

Chandratilleke, M.G., Carson, K.V., Picot, J., et al., 2012. Physical training for asthma. Cochrane Database Syst. Rev. 5, CD001116.

Chatwin, M., Ross, E., Hart, N., et al., 2003. Cough augmentation with mechanical insufflation-exsufflation in patients with neuromuscular weakness. Eur. Respir. J. 21, 502–508.

Chatwin, M., Simonds, A., 2002. Mechanical technique for assisted cough (Correspondence). Physiotherapy 88 (6), 381–382.

Chaw, E., Shem, K., Castillo, K., et al., 2012. Dysphagia and associated respiratory considerations in cervical spinal cord injury. Top. Spinal Cord Inj. Rehabil. 18 (4), 291–299.

Chen, C., Lien, I., Wu, M., 1990. Respiratory function in patients with spinal cord injuries: effects of posture. Paraplegia 28, 81–86.

Chevrolet, J., Deleamont, P., 1991. Repeated vital capacity measurements as predictive parameters for mechanical ventilation need and weaning success in Guillain-Barré syndrome. Am. Rev. Respir. Dis. 144, 814–818.

Chiodo, A.E., Scelza, W., Forchheimer, M., 2008. Predictors of ventilator weaning in individuals with high cervical spinal cord injury. J. Spinal Cord Med. 31, 72–77.

Choi, J.S., Jones, A.Y., 2005. Effects of manual hyperinflation and suctioning on respiratory mechanics in mechanically ventilated patients with ventilator-associated pneumonia. Aust. J. Physiother. 51, 25–30.

Christie, J.D., Edwards, L.B., Kucheryavaya, A.Y., et al., 2012. The Registry of the International Society for Heart and Lung Transplantation: 29th adult lung and heart-lung transplant report, 2012. J. Heart Lung Transplant. 31, 1073–1086.

Chughtai, T., Ali, S., Sharkey, P., et al., 2009. Update on managing diaphragmatic rupture in blunt trauma: a review of 208 consecutive cases. Can. J. Surg. 52 (3), 177–181.

Cirocchi, R., Montedori, A., Farinella, E., et al., 2013. Damage control surgery for abdominal trauma. Cochrane Database Syst. Rev. (3), Art. No.: CD007438, doi:10.1002/14651858.CD007438.pub3.

Clark, A.L., Poole-Wilson, P.A., Coats, A.J., 1996. Exercise limitation in chronic heart failure: central role of the periphery. J. Am. Coll. Cardiol. 28, 1092–1102.

Claxton, A.R., Wong, D.T., Chung, F., Fehlings, M.G., 1998. Predictors of hospital mortality and mechanical ventilation inpatients with cervical spinal cord injury. Can. J. Anaesth. 45 (2), 144–149.

Cohn, J.R., 1993. Pulmonary management of the patient with spinal cord injury. Trauma Q. 9 (2), 65–71.

Cohn, S.M., DuBose, J.J., 2010. Pulmonary contusion: an update on recent advances in clinical management. World J. Surg. 34, 1959–1970.

Colohan, S.M., 2010. Predicting prognosis in thermal burns with associated inhalational injury: a systematic review of prognostic factors in adult burn victims. J. Burn Care Res. 31 (4), 529–539.

Como, J.J., Sutton, E.R., McCunn, M., et al., 2005. Characterizing the need for mechanical ventilation following cervical spinal cord injury with neurological deficit. J. Trauma 59, 912–916.

Conn, V., Hafdahl, A., Porock, D., et al., 2006. A meta-analysis of exercise interventions among people treated for cancer. Support. Care Cancer 14, 699–712.

Connolly, B.A., Jones, G.D., Curtis, A.A., et al., 2013. Clinical predictive value of manual muscle strength testing during critical illness: an observational cohort study. Crit. Care 17 (5), R229. doi:10.1186/cc13052.

Cooper, J.D., Pearson, F.G., Patterson, G.A., et al., 1987. Technique of successful lung transplantation in humans. J. Thorac. Cardiovasc. Surg. 93, 173–181.

Cordova, F.C., Criner, G.J., 2002. Lung volume reduction surgery as a bridge to lung transplantation. Am. J. Respir. Med. 1, 313–324.

Couetil, J.P., Tolan, M.J., Loulmet, D.F., et al., 1997. Pulmonary bipartitioning and lobar transplantation: a new approach to donor organ shortage. J. Thorac. Cardiovasc. Surg. 113, 529–537.

Courneya, K., Friedenreich, C., 2007. Physical activity and cancer control. Semin. Oncol. Nurs. 23, 242–252.

Cox, N.S., Alison, J.A., Holland, A.E., 2013. Interventions for promoting physical activity in people with cystic fibrosis. Cochrane Database Syst. Rev. 12, CD009448.

Craig, R., Mindell, J. (Eds.), 2012. Health Survey for England 2011: Health, social care and lifestyles. The Information Centre, London.

Cramp, F., Daniel, J., 2012. Exercise for the management of cancer-related fatigue in adults. Cochrane Database Syst. Rev. 11, CD006145.

Cripps, R.A., Lee, B.B., Wing, P., et al., 2011. A global map for traumatic spinal cord injury epidemiology: towards a living data repository for injury prevention. Spinal Cord 49 (4), 493–501.

Cuthbertson, B., Roughton, S., Jenkinson, D., et al., 2010. Quality of life in the five years after intensive care: a cohort study. Crit. Care 14, R6.

Cypel, M., Yeung, J.C., Machuca, T., et al., 2012. Experience with the first 50 ex vivo lung perfusions in clinical transplantation. J. Thorac. Cardiovasc. Surg. 144, 1200–1206.

Date, H., 2011. Update on living-donor lobar lung transplantation. Curr. Opin. Organ. Transpl. 16, 453–457.

Davidson, J., Jones, C., Bienvenu, O., 2011. Family response to critical illness: postintensive care syndrome-family. Crit. Care Med. 40 (2), 618–624.

Davis, J., Kohut, M., Jackson, D., et al., 1998. Exercise effects on lung tumor metastases and in vitro alveolar macrophage antitumor cytotoxicity. Am. J. Physiol. 274 (5 Pt 2), R1454–R1459.

Davis, J.A., McBride, M.G., Chrisant, M.R., et al., 2006. Longitudinal assessment of cardiovascular exercise performance after pediatric heart transplantation. J. Heart Lung Transplant. 25 (6), 626–633. [Epub 2006 May 2].

Davies, R.R., Russo, M.J., Morgan, J.A., et al., 2010. Standard versus bicaval techniques for orthotopic heart transplantation: an analysis of the United Network for Organ Sharing database. J. Thorac. Cardiovasc. Surg. 140, 700–708.

de Lateur, B.J., Magyar-Russell, G., Bresnick, M., et al., 2007. Augmented exercise in treatment of deconditioning from major burn injury. Arch. Phys. Med. Rehabil. 88 (12 Suppl. 2), S18–S23.

De Man, F.S., Handoko, M.L., Groepenhoff, H., et al., 2009. Effects of exercise training in patients with idiopathic pulmonary arterial hypertension. Eur. Respir. J. 34, 669–675.

De Oliveira, N.C., Osaki, S., Maloney, J.D., et al., 2010. Lung transplantation with donation after cardiac death donors: long-term follow-up in a single center. J. Thorac. Cardiovasc. Surg. 139, 1306–1315.

De Troyer, A., Estenne, M., 1991. Review article: the expiratory muscles in tetraplegia. Paraplegia 29, 359–363.

De Troyer, A., Heilporn, A., 1980. Respiratory mechanics in quadriplegia: the respiratory function of the intercostal muscles. Am. Rev. Respir. Dis. 122, 591–600.

Del Rizzo, D.F., Menkis, A.H., Pflugfelder, P.W., et al., 1999. The role of donor age and ischemic time on survival following orthotopic heart transplantation. J. Heart Lung Transplant. 18, 310–319.

Deliva, R.D., Hassall, A., Manlhiot, C., et al., 2012. Effects of an acute, outpatient physiotherapy exercise program following pediatric heart or lung transplantation. Pediatr. Transplant. 16 (8), 879–886.

Demling, R.H., 1987. Fluid replacement in burned patients. Surg. Clin. North Am. 67 (1), 15–30.

Denehy, L., Elliott, D., 2012. Strategies for post ICU rehabilitation. Curr. Opin. Crit. Care 18 (5), 503–508.

Denehy, L., Skinner, H., Edbrooke, L., et al., 2013. Exercise rehabilitation for patients with critical illness: a randomized controlled trial with 12 months follow up. Critical Care 17 (4), R156.

Department of Health, Start Active, Stay Active: A Report on Physical Activity from the Four Home Countries' Chief Medical Officers (2011). <https://www.gov.uk/government/uploads/system/uploads/attachment_data/file/216370/dh_128210.pdf>.

Desai, M.H., Mlcak, R., Richardson, J., et al., 1998. Reduction in mortality in pediatric patients with inhalation injury with aerosolized heparin/N- acetylcystine therapy. J. Burn Care Rehabil. 19 (3), 210–212.

Deutschman, C., Ahrens, T., Cairns, C., et al., 2012. Multisociety task force for critical care research: key issues and recommendations. Chest 141 (1), 201–209.

DeVita, V., Rosenberg, S., 2012. Two hundred years of cancer research. NEJM 366, 2207–2214.

DeVivo, M.J., Krause, J.S., Lammertse, D.P., 1999. Recent trends in mortality and causes of death among persons with spinal cord injury. Arch. Phys. Med. Rehabil. 80, 1411–1419.

DiMarco, A.F., 1999. Diaphragm pacing in patients with spinal cord injury. Top. Spinal Cord Inj. Rehabil. 5 (1), 6–20.

DiMarco, A.F., 2005. Restoration of respiratory muscle function following spinal cord injury: review of electrical and magnetic stimulation techniques. Respir. Physiol. Neurobiol. 147, 273–287.

DiMarco, AF., et al., 2009. Lower thoracic spinal cord stimulation to restore cough in patients with spinal cord injury: results of a national institutes of health-sponsored clinical trial. Part I. Methodology and effectiveness of expiratory muscle activation. Arch. Phys. Med. Rehabil. 90 (5), 717–725.

Dinwiddie, R., Sharief, N., Crawford, O., 2002. Idiopathic interstitial pneumonitis in children: a national survey in the United Kingdom and Ireland. Pediatr. Pulmonol. 34 (1), 23–29.

Dipchand, A.I., Manlhiot, C., Russell, J.L., et al., 2009. Exercise capacity improves with time in pediatric heart transplant recipients. J. Heart Lung Transplant. 28 (6), 585–590. doi:10.1016/j.healun.2009.01.025.

Ditunno, J.F., Little, J.W., Tessler, A., Burns, A.S., 2004. Spinal shock revisited: a four-phase model. Spinal Cord 42, 383–395.

Do, J.G., Kim, D.H., Sung, D.H., 2013. Incidence of deep vein thrombosis after spinal cord injury in Korean patients at acute rehabilitation unit. J. Korean Med. Sci. 28 (9), 1382–1387.

Dodd, J.D., Barry, S.C., Barry, R.B., et al., 2006. Thin-section CT in patients with cystic fibrosis: correlation with peak exercise capacity and body mass index. Radiology 240, 236–245.

Dodd, M.E., Prasad, S.A., 2005. Physiotherapy management of cystic fibrosis. Chron. Respir. Dis. 2 (3), 139–149.

Dries, D.J., Endorf, F.W., 2013. Inhalation injury: epidemiology, pathology, treatment strategies. Scand. J. Trauma Resusc. Emerg. Med. 21, 31.

Dunn, J., Smith, M., 2008. Critical care management of head injury. Anaesth. Intensive Care Med. 9 (5), 197–201.

Duppen, N., Takken, T., Hopman, M.T., et al., 2013. Systematic review of the effects of physical exercise training programmes in children and young adults with congenital heart disease. Int. J. Cardiol. 168 (3), 1779–1787.

Dutton, R.P., McCunn, M., 2003. Traumatic brain injury. Curr. Opin. Crit. Care 9 (6), 503–509.

Dwyer, T.J., Elkins, M.R., Bye, P.T.P., 2011. The role of exercise in maintaining health in cystic fibrosis. Curr. Opin. Pulm. Med. 17, 455–460.

Dylewski, M.L., Baker, M., Prelack, K., et al., 2013. The safety and efficacy of parenteral nutrition among pediatric patients with burn injuries. Paediatr. Crit. Care Med. 14 (3), e120–e125.

El Masri, W., 2010. Management of traumatic spinal cord injuries: current standard of care revisited. Adv. Clin. Neurosci. Rehabil. 10 (1), 37–39.

El-Ansary, D., Waddington, G., Adams, R., 2007. Measurement of non-physiological movement in sternal instability by ultrasound. Ann. Thorac. Surg. 83, 1513–1516.

Elliott, D., McKinley, S., Alison, J., et al., 2011. Health-related quality of life and physical recovery after a critical illness: a multi-centre randomised controlled trial of a home-based physical rehabilitation program. Critical Care 15 (3), R142.

Endorf, F.W., Gamelli, R.L., 2007. Inhalation injury, pulmonary perturbations, and fluid resuscitation. J. Burn Care Res. 28 (1), 80–83.

Enkhbaatar, P., Murakami, K., Cox, R., et al., 2004. Aerosolized tissue plasminogen inhibitor improves pulmonary function in sheep with burn and smoke inhalation. Shock 22 (1), 70–75.

Epstein, S.K., 2004. Extubation failure: an outcome to be avoided. Critical Care 8 (5), 310–312.

Ersson, U., Carlson, H., Mellstrom, A., et al., 1990. Observations of intracranial dynamics during respiratory physiotherapy in unconscious neurosurgical patients. Acta Anaesthesiol. Scand. 34 (2), 99–103.

Estenne, M., Maurer, J.R., Boehler, A., et al., 2002. Bronchiolitis obliterans syndrome 2001: an update of the diagnostic criteria. J. Heart Lung Transplant. 21, 297–310.

European Union Sport and Health Working Group, 2008. European Union Physical Activity Guidelines. European Union, Brussels.

Fallon, M., Abrahams, G., 2000. Pulmonary dysfunction in chronic liver disease. Hepatology 32 (4), 859–865.

Faraklas, I., Cochran, A., Saffle, J., 2012. Review of a fluid resuscitation protocol: 'fluid creep' is not due to nursing error. J. Burn Care Res. 33 (1), 74–83.

Fehlings, M., Rabin, D., Sears, W., et al., 2010. Current practice in the timing of surgical intervention in spinal cord injury. Spine 35, 166–173.

Fehlings, M.G., Vaccaro, A., Wilson, J.R., et al., 2012. Early versus delayed decompression for traumatic cervical spinal cord injury: results of the surgical timing in acute spinal cord injury study (STASCIS). PLoS ONE 7 (2), E32037.

Feiereisen, P., Delagardelle, C., Vaillant, M., et al., 2007. Is strength training the more efficient training modality in chronic heart failure? Med. Sci. Sports Exerc. 39, 1910–1917.

Feldman, D., Pamboukian, S.V., Teuteberg, J.J., et al., 2013. The 2013 International Society for Heart and Lung Transplantation guidelines for mechanical circulatory support: executive summary. J. Heart Lung Transplant. 32, 157–187.

Ferlay, J., Soerjomataram, I., Ervik, M., et al. GLOBOCAN 2012 v1.0, Cancer Incidence and Mortality Worldwide: IARC CancerBase No. 11. Lyon, France: International Agency for Research on Cancer 2013. Available from: <http://globocan.iarc.fr> (accessed on 15.01.07.).

Ferreira, L., Valenti, V., Vanderlei, L., 2013. Chest physiotherapy on intracranial pressure of critically ill patients admitted to the intensive care unit: a systematic review. Rev. Bras. Ter. Intensiva 25 (4), 327–333.

Ferreyra, G., Baussano, I., Squadrone, V., et al., 2008. Continuous positive airway pressure for treatment of respiratory complications after abdominal surgery. Ann. Surg. 247, 617–626.

Fischer, S., Struber, M., Simon, A.R., et al., 2001. Video-assisted minimally invasive approach in clinical bilateral lung transplantation. J. Thorac. Cardiovasc. Surg. 122, 1196–1198.

Fishburn, M.J., Marino, R.J., Ditunno, J.F., 1990. Atelectasis and pneumonia in acute spinal cord injury. Arch. Phys. Med. Rehabil. 71, 197–200.

Fitzpatrick, D.C., Denard, P.J., Phelan, D., et al., 2010. Operative stabilization of flail chest injuries: review of literature and fixation options. Eur. J. Trauma Emerg. Surg. 36, 427–433.

Foray, A., Williams, D., Reemtsma, K., et al., 1996. Assessment of submaximal exercise capacity in patients with left ventricular assist devices. Circulation 94 (9 Suppl.), II222–II226.

Fox, B.D., Kassirer, M., Weiss, I., et al., 2011. Ambulatory rehabilitation improves exercise capacity in patients with pulmonary hypertension. J. Card. Fail. 17, 196–200.

Franciosa, J.A., Park, M., Levine, B., 1981. Lack of correlation between exercise capacity and indexes of resting left ventricular performance in heart failure. Am. J. Cardiol. 47, 33–39.

Freedman, D.S., Khan, L.K., Serdula, M.K., et al., 2005. The relation of childhood BMI to adult adiposity: the Bogalusa heart study. Pediatrics 115 (1), 22–27.

Friedenreich, C., 2001. Physical activity and cancer prevention: from observational to intervention research. Cancer Epidemiol. Biomarkers Prev. 10, 287–301.

Frisbie, J.H., Sharma, G.V., 2012. The prevalence of pulmonary embolism in chronically paralyzed subjects: a review of available evidence. Spinal Cord 50 (6), 400–403.

Frownfelter, D., Massery, M., 2006. Facilitating airway clearance with coughing techniques. In: Frownfelter, D., Dean, E. (Eds.), Cardiovascular and Pulmonary Physical Therapy Evidence and Practice, fourth ed. Mosby & Elsevier Health Sciences, St. Louis, MO, pp. 363–76. Chapter 22.

Fuehner, T., Kuehn, C., Hadem, J., et al., 2012. Extracorporeal membrane oxygenation in awake patients as bridge to lung transplantation. Am. J. Respir. Crit. Care Med. 185, 763–768.

Fujiwara, T., Hara, Y., Chino, N., 1999. Expiratory function in complete tetraplegics: study of spirometry, maximal expiratory pressure, and muscle activity of pectoralis major and latissimus dorsi muscles. Am. J. Phys. Med. Rehabil. 78, 464–469.

Fuller, L., El-Ansary, D., Nelson, E.M., Gooi, J., 2012. External chest brace for clam shell sternal instability following bilateral sequential lung transplant: a case series. Int. J. Ther. Rehabil. 19, 233–237.

Gabbay, E., Williams, T.J., Griffiths, A.P., et al., 1999. Maximizing the utilization of donor organs offered for lung transplantation. Am. J. Respir. Crit. Care Med. 160, 265–271.

Garrioch, M.A., 2004. The body's response to blood loss. Vox Sang. 87, S74–S76.

Garstang, S.V., Miller-Smith, S.A., 2007. Autonomic system dysfunction after spinal cord injury. Phys. Med. Rehabil. Clin. N. Am. 18, 275–292, vi-vii.

Garstang, S.V., Walker, H., 2011. Cardiovascular and autonomic dysfunctions after spinal cord injury. In: Kirshblum, S., Campagnolo, D.I. (Eds.), Spinal Cord Medicine, second ed. Lippincott Williams and Wilkins, Philadelphia.

Garvey, C., 2010. Interstitial lung disease and pulmonary rehabilitation. J. Cardiopulm. Rehabil. Prev. 30, 141–146.

Gary, R.A., Cress, M.E., Higgins, M.K., et al., 2011. Combined aerobic and resistance exercise program improves task performance in patients with heart failure. Arch. Phys. Med. Rehabil. 92, 1371–1381.

Garzon-Serrano, J., Ryan, C., Waak, K., et al., 2011. Early mobilization in critically ill patients: patients' mobilization level depends on health care provider's profession. PM R 3 (4), 307–313. doi:10.1016/j.pmrj.2010.12.022.

Gay, P.C., 2013. Counterpoint: should phrenic nerve stimulation be the treatment of choice for spinal cord injury? No. Chest 143 (5), 1203–1206.

Gazit, A.Z., Gandhi, S.K., Canter, C.C., 2010. Mechanical circulatory support of the critically ill child awaiting heart transplantation. Curr. Cardiol. Rev. 6 (1), 46–53. doi:10.2174/157340310790231617.

Gerbershagen, H.J., Dagtekin, O., Isenberg, J., 2010. Chronic pain and disability after pelvic and acetabular fractures-assessment with the Mainz pain staging system. J. Trauma 69, 128–136.

Gleeson, M., Bishop, N., Stensel, D., et al., 2011. The anti-inflammatory effects of exercise: mechanisms and implications for the prevention and treatment of disease. Nat. Rev. Immunol. 11 (9), 607–615.

Gloeckl, R., Halle, M., Kenn, K., 2012. Interval versus continuous training in lung transplant candidates: a randomized trial. J. Heart Lung Transplant. 31, 934–941.

Golan, M., Crow, S., 2004. Targeting parents exclusively in the treatment of childhood obesity: long-term results. Obes. Res. 12 (2), 357–361.

Goldbaum, L.R., Orellano, T., Dergal, E., 1976. Mechanism of the toxic action of carbon monoxide. Ann. Clin. Lab. Sci. 6 (4), 372–376.

Goldman, J., Rose, L., Williams, S., et al., 1986. Effect of abdominal binders on breathing in tetraplegic patients. Thorax 41, 940–945.

Gosselink, R., Bott, J., Johnson, M., 2008. Physiotherapy for adult patients with critical illness: recommendations of the European Respiratory Society and European Society of Intensive Care Medicine Task Force on physiotherapy for critically ill patients. Intensive Care Med. 34, 1188–1199.

Gosselink, R., Needham, D., Hermans, G., 2012. ICU-based rehabilitation and its appropriate metrics. Curr. Opin. Crit. Care 18 (5), 533–539.

Gotthardt, D., Riediger, C., Weiss, K., et al., 2007. Fulminant hepatic failure: etiology and indications for liver transplantation. Nephrol. Dial. Transplant. 22 (Suppl. 8), viii5–viii8.

Gouden, P., 1997. Static respiratory pressures in patients with post-traumatic tetraplegia. Spinal Cord 35, 43–47.

Granger, C., McDonald, C., Irving, L., et al., 2014. Low physical activity levels and functional decline in individuals with lung cancer. Lung Cancer 83, 292–299.

Greenhalgh, D., 2007. Wound healing. In: Herndon, D.N. (Ed.), Total Burn Care, third ed. Saunders, USA, pp. 578–595. Chapter 46.

Griffiths, R., Hall, J., 2010. Intensive care unit-acquired weakness. Crit. Care Med. 38 (3), 779–787.

Griffiths, T., Phillips, C., Davies, S., et al., 2001. Cost effectiveness of an outpatient multidisciplinary pulmonary rehabilitation program. Thorax 56, 779–784.

Grigioni, F., Carigi, S., Potena, L., et al., 2006. Long-term safety and effectiveness of statins for heart transplant recipients in routine clinical practice. Transplant. Proc. 38, 1507–1510.

Gruber, W., Orenstein, D.M., Braumann, K.M., Huls, G., 2008. Health-related fitness and trainability in children with cystic fibrosis. Pediatr. Pulmonol. 43 (10), 953–964.

Gruber, W., Orenstein, D.M., Braumann, K.M., et al., 2011. Effects of an exercise program in children with cystic fibrosis: are there differences between females and males? J. Pediatr. 158 (1), 58–63.

Guerrero, K., Wuyam, B., Mezin, P., et al., 2005. Functional coupling of adenine nucleotide translocase and mitochondrial creatine kinase is enhanced after exercise training in lung transplant skeletal muscle. Am. J. Physiol. Regul. Integr. Comp. Physiol. 289, R1144–R1154.

Guillemenault, C., Philip, P., Robinson, A., 1998. Sleep and neuromuscular disease: bilevel positive airway pressure by nasal mask as a treatment for sleep disordered breathing in patients with neuromuscular disease. J. Neurol. Neurosurg. Psychiatry 65, 225–232.

Gullestad, L., Haywood, G., Ross, H., et al., 1996. Exercise capacity of heart transplant recipients: the importance of chronotropic incompetence. J. Heart Lung Transplant. 15, 1075–1083.

Gunduz, M., Unlugenc, H., Ozalevli, M., et al., 2005. A comparative study of continuous positive airway pressure (CPAP) and intermittent positive pressure ventilation (IPPV) in patients with flail chest. Emerg. Med. J. 22, 325–329.

Gupta, S., Castel, H., Rao, R.V., et al., 2010. Improved survival after liver transplantation in patients with hepatopulmonary syndrome. Am. J. Transplant. 10, 354–363.

Gutierrez, C.J., Harrow, J., Haines, F., 2003. Using an evidence-based protocol to guide rehabilitation and weaning of ventilator-dependent cervical spinal cord injury patients. J. Rehabil. Res. Dev. 40 (5 Suppl. 2), 99–110.

Gutierrez, C.J., Steven, C., Merritt, J., et al., 2010. Trendelenburg chest optimization prolongs spontaneous breathing trials in ventilator-dependent patients with low cervical spinal cord injury. J. Rehabil. Res. Dev. 47, 261–272.

Haddad, S., Arabi, Y., 2012. Critical care management of severe traumatic brain injury in adults. Scand. J. Trauma Resusc. Emerg. Med. 20, 12.

Haines, K.J., Skinner, E.H., Berney, S., the Austin POST study investigators, 2013. Association of postoperative pulmonary complications with delayed mobilisation following major abdominal surgery: an observational cohort study. Physiotherapy 99 (2), 119–125.

Hanekom, S., Gosselink, R., Dean, E., et al., 2011. The development of a clinical management algorithm for early physical activity and mobilization of critically ill patients: synthesis of evidence and expert opinion and its translation into practice. Clin. Rehabil. 25 (9), 771–787.

Harrison, C.A., MacNeil, S., 2008. The mechanism of skin graft contraction: an update on current research and potential future therapies. Burns 34, 153–163.

Harrop, J.S., Sharan, A.D., Scheid, E.H., et al., 2004. Tracheostomy placement in patients with complete cervical spinal cord injuries: American Spinal Injury Association grade A. J. Neurosurg. 100 (Spine 1), 20–23.

Hassid, V.J., Schinco, M.A., Tepas, J.J., et al., 2008. Definitive establishment of airway control is critical for optimal outcome in lower cervical spinal cord injury. J. Trauma, Injury, Infect. Crit. Care 65, 1328–1332.

Hauer, T., Huschitt, N., Kulla, M., et al., 2011. [Bullet and shrapnel injuries in the face and neck regions: current aspects of wound ballistics]. HNO 59, 752–764.

Hayes, K., Leet, A.S., Bradley, S.J., Holland, A.E., 2012. Effects of exercise training on exercise capacity and quality of life in patients with a left ventricular assist device: a preliminary randomized controlled trial. J. Heart Lung Transplant. 31 (7), 729–734. doi:10.1016/j.healun.2012.02.021; [Epub 2012 Mar 14].

Health and Social Care Information Centre, The Health survey for England results <http://www.hscic.gov.uk/catalogue/PUB13218>.

Heary, F.H., Zuozias, A.D., Campagnolo, D.I., 2011. Acute medical and surgical management of spinal cord injury. In: Kirshblum, S., Campagnolo, D.I. (Eds.), Spinal Cord Medicine, second ed. Lippincott Williams and Wilkins, Philadelphia.

Hebestreit, H., 2008. Exercise, physical activity and asthma. In: Armstrong, N., van Mechelen, W. (Eds.), Paediatric Exercise Science and Medicine, second ed. Oxford University Press, UK.

Hebestreit, H., Kieser, S., Junge, S., et al., 2010. Long-term effects of a partially supervised conditioning programme in cystic fibrosis. Eur. Respir. J. 35 (3), 578–583.

Heigener, D., Reck, M., Gatzemeier, U., 2009. Targeted therapy in nonsmall cell lung cancer. Eur. Respir. Monogr. 44, 284–298.

Henderson, K., Marshall, G., Sambrook, P., et al., 1997. Two cases of hip pain in patients with heart transplantation. Aust. J. Physiother. 43, 131–133.

Hermans, G., Van den Berghe, G., 2015. Clinical review: intensive care unit acquired weakness. Critical Care 19, 274. doi:10.1186/s13054.

Herndon, D.N., Barrow, R.E., Rutan, R.L., et al., 1989. A comparison of conservative versus early excision: therapies in severely burned patients. Ann. Surg. 209 (5), 547–552.

Herndon, D.N., Traber, L.D., Linares, H., et al., 1986. Etiology of the pulmonary pathophysiology associated with inhalation injury. Resuscitation 14, 43–59.

Herridge, M., Cheung, A., Tansey, C., et al., 2003. One-year outcomes in survivors of the acute respiratory distress syndrome. N. Engl. J. Med. 348 (11), 683–693.

Herridge, M., Tansey, C., Matté, A., et al., 2011. Functional disability 5 years after acute respiratory distress syndrome. NEJM 364 (14), 1293–1304. doi:10.1056/NEJMoa1011802.

Hewitt, M., Rowland, J.H., Yancik, R., 2003. Cancer survivors in the United States: age, health, and disability. J. Gerontol. a-Biol. Sci. Med. Sci. 58, 82–91.

Hickman, I., Jonsson, J., Prins, J., et al., 2004. Modest weight loss and physical activity in overweight patients with chronic liver disease results in sustained improvements in alanine aminotransferase, fasting insulin and quality of life. Gut 53, 413–419.

Higenbottam, T., Jackson, M., Woolman, P., et al., 1989. The cough response to ultrasonically nebulized distilled water in heart-lung transplantation patients. Am. Rev. Respir. Dis. 140, 58–61.

Hills, A.P., Byrne, N.M., Wood, R.E., 2008. Exercise, physical activity and eating and weight disorders. In: Armstrong, N., van Mechelen, W. (Eds.), Paediatric Exercise Science and Medicine, second ed. Oxford University Press, UK.

Hodgson, C., Stiller, K., Needham, D., et al., 2014. Expert consensus and recommendations on safety criteria for active mobilization of mechanically ventilated critically ill adults. Critical Care 18 (5), 658.

Hogan, B.K., Wolf, S.E., Hospenthal, D.R., et al., 2012. Correlation of American Burn Association sepsis criteria with the presence of bacteraemia in burned patients admitted to the intensive care unit. J. Burn Care Res. 33 (3), 371–378.

Holland, A., Hill, C., 2008. Physical training for interstitial lung disease. Cochrane Database Syst. Rev. (4), CD006322.

Hollaus, P., Wilfing, G., Wurnig, P., et al., 2003. Risk factors for the development of postoperative complications after bronchial sleeve resection for malignancy: a univariate and multivariate analysis. Ann. Thorac. Surg. 75, 966–972.

Hoo, G.W., 2003. Nonpharmacologic adjuncts to training during pulmonary rehabilitation: the role of supplemental oxygen and noninvasive ventilation. J. Rehabil. Res. Dev. 40, 81–97.

Hosenpud, J.D., 1999. Coronary artery disease after heart transplantation and its relation to cytomegalovirus. Am. Heart J. 138, S469–S472.

Hough, C., 2013. Improving function during and after critical care. Curr. Opin. Crit. Care 19 (5), 488–495.

Hough, C., Lieu, B., Caldwell, E., 2011. Manual muscle strength testing of critically ill patients: feasibility and interobserver agreement. Critical Care 15 (1), R43.

Hsieh, P.L., Wu, Y.T., Chao, W.J., 2011. Effects of exercise training in heart transplant recipients: a meta-analysis. Cardiology 120, 27–35.

Hunt, I., Muers, M., Treasure, T., (Eds.), 2008. ABC of lung cancer [electronic resource]. Blackwell Pub, Malden, Mass.

Huzar, T.F., Cross, J.M., 2011. Ventilator associated pneumonia in burn patients: a cause or consequence of critical illness? Expert Rev. Respir. Med. 5 (5), 663–673.

Ipaktchi, K., Arbabi, S., 2006. Advances in burn critical care. Crit. Care Med. 34 (9 Suppl.), S239–S244.

Iwashyna, T., 2012. Trajectories of recovery and dysfunction after acute illness, with implications for clinical trial design. Am. J. Respir. Crit. Care Med. 186 (4), 302–304.

Iwashyna, T., Netzer, G., 2012. The burdens of survivorship: an approach to thinking about long-term outcomes after critical illness. Semin. Respir. Crit. Care Med. 33 (4), 327–338.

Jackson, A.B., Groomes, T.E., 1994. Incidence of respiratory complications following spinal cord injury. Arch. Phys. Med. Rehabil. 75, 270–275.

Jalan, R., Olde Damink, S.W., Hayes, P.C., et al., 2004. Pathogenesis of intracranial hypertension in acute liver failure: inflammation, ammonia and cerebral blood flow. J. Hepatol. 41, 613–620.

Jamieson, S.W., Stinson, E.B., Oyer, P.E., et al., 1984. Operative technique for heart-lung transplantation. J. Thorac. Cardiovasc. Surg. 87, 930–935.

Jarosz, R., Littlepage, M.M., Creasey, G., McKenna, S.L., 2012. Functional electrical stimulation in spinal cord injury respiratory care. Top. Spinal Cord Inj. Rehabil. 18 (4), 315–321.

Jaski, B.E., Branch, K.R., Adamson, R., et al., 1993. Exercise hemodynamics during long-term implantation of a left ventricular assist device in patients awaiting heart transplantation. J. Am. Coll. Cardiol. 22 (6), 1574–1580.

Jaski, B.E., Kim, J., Maly, R.S., et al., 1997. Effects of exercise during long-term support with a left ventricular assist device: results of the experience with left ventricular assist device with exercise (EVADE) pilot trial. Circulation 95, 2401–2406.

Jaski, B.E., Lingle, R.J., Kim, J., et al., 1999. Comparison of functional capacity in patients with end-stage heart failure following implantation of a left ventricular assist device versus heart transplantation: results of the experience with left ventricular assist device with exercise trial. J. Heart Lung Transplant. 18, 1031–1040.

Jawa, R.S., Anillo, S., Huntoon, K., et al., 2011. Interleukin-6 in surgery, trauma and critical care. Part II. Clinical implications. J. Intensive Care Med. 26, 73–87.

Jeschke, M.G., Gauglitz, G.G., Finnerty, C.C., et al., 2013. Survivors versus nonsurvivors postburn: differences in inflammatory and hypermetabolic trajectories. Ann. Surg. Apr 10. [epub ahead of print].

Jeschke, M.G., Gauglitz, G.G., Kulp, G.A., et al., 2011. Long term persistence of the pathophysiologic response to severe burn injury. PLoS ONE 6 (7), e21245.

Johnson, C., 1984. Physical therapists as scar modifiers. Phys. Ther. 64, 1381–1387.

Jonas, M., Fang, J.C., Wang, J.C., et al., 2006. In-stent restenosis and remote coronary lesion progression are coupled in cardiac transplant vasculopathy but not in native coronary artery disease. J. Am. Coll. Cardiol. 48, 453–461.

Jones, L., Hornsby, W., Goetzinger, A., et al., 2012. Prognostic significance of functional capacity and exercise behavior in patients with metastatic non-small cell lung cancer. Lung Cancer 76, 248–252.

Jones, C., Skirrow, P., Griffiths, R.D., et al., 2003. Rehabilitation after critical illness. Crit. Care Med. 31, 2456–2461.

Jones, L., Watson, D., Herndon, J. 2nd, et al., 2010. Peak oxygen consumption and long-term all-cause mortality in nonsmall cell lung cancer. Cancer 116, 4825–4832.

Karnak, D., Shah, S.S., Rozas, M.S., et al., 2006. Repair of sternal dehiscence after bilateral lung transplantation. J. Thorac. Cardiovasc. Surg. 132, 425–426.

Kasten, K.R., Makley, A.T., Kagan, R.J., 2011. Update on the critical care management of severe burns. J. Intensive Care Med. 26, 223–236.

Kasymjanova, G., Correa, J., Kreisman, H., et al., 2009. Prognostic value of the six-minute walk in advanced non-small cell lung cancer. J. Thorac. Oncol. 4, 602–607.

Kavanagh, T., 1996. Physical training in heart transplant recipients. J. Cardiovasc. Risk 3, 154–159.

Kayambu, G., Boots, R., Paratz, J., 2015. Early physical rehabilitation in intensive care patients with sepsis syndromes: a pilot randomised controlled trial. Intensive Care Med. 41 (5), 865–874. doi:10.1007/s00134-015-3763-8.

Kemp, B.J., Krause, J.S., 1999. Depression and life satisfaction among people aging with post-polio and spinal cord injury. Disabil. Rehabil. 21, 241–249.

Kennedy, M.D., Haykowsky, M., Humphrey, R., 2003. Function, eligibility, outcomes, and exercise capacity associated with left ventricular assist devices: exercise rehabilitation and training for patients with ventricular assist devices. J. Cardiopulm. Rehabil. 23 (3), 208–217.

Kho, M.E., Truong, A.D., Zanni, J.M., et al., 2015. Neuromuscular electrical stimulation in mechanically ventilated patients: a randomized, sham-controlled pilot trial with blinded outcome assessment. J. Crit. Care 30 (1), 32–39. doi:10.1016/j.jcrc.2014.09.014.

Kirk, R., Dipchand, A.I., Edwards, L.B., et al., 2012. The registry of the International Society for Heart and Lung Transplantation: fifteenth pediatric heart transplantation report, 2012. J. Heart Lung Transplant. 31, 1065–1072.

Kirkpatrick, A.W., Laupland, K.B., Karmali, S., et al., 2006. Spill your guts! Perceptions of trauma association of Canada member surgeons regarding the open abdomen and the abdominal compartment syndrome. J. Trauma 60 (2), 279–286.

Klausen, S.H., Buys, R., Andersen, L.L., et al., 2014. Interventions to increase physical activity for people with congenital heart disease (protocol). Cochrane Database Syst. Rev. CD0111030.

Klijn, P.H., Oudshoorn, A., van der Ent, C.K., et al., 2004. Effects of anaerobic training in children with cystic fibrosis: a randomized controlled study. Chest 125 (4), 1299–1305.

Knols, R., Aaronson, N., Uebelhart, D., et al., 2005. Physical exercise in cancer patients during and after medical treatment: a systematic review of randomized and controlled clinical trials. J. Clin. Oncol. 23, 3830–3842.

Kraft, R., Herndon, D.N., Branski, L.K., et al., 2013. Optimised fluid management improves outcomes of pediatric burn patients. J. Surg. Res. 181 (1), 121–128.

Kress, J., Hall, J., 2014. ICU-acquired weakness and recovery from critical illness. N. Engl. J. Med. 370 (17), 1626–1635.

Krishnan, P., Frew, Q., Green, A., et al., 2013. Cause of death and correlation with autopsy findings in burns patients. Burns 39 (4), 583–588.

Krowka, M.J., 2000. Hepatopulmonary syndromes. Gut 46, 1–4.

Kugler, C., Malehsa, D., Tegtbur, U., et al., 2011. Health-related quality of life and exercise tolerance in recipients of heart transplants and left ventricular assist devices: a prospective, comparative study. J. Heart Lung Transplant. 30 (2), 204–210. doi:10.1016/j.healun.2010.08.030; [Epub 2010 Oct 27].

Kulich, M., Rosenfeld, M., Goss, C.H., Wilmott, R., 2003. Improved survival among young patients with cystic fibrosis. J. Pediatr. 142 (6), 631–636.

Kumar, A., Parrillo, J.E., 2008. Shock: classification, pathophysiology and approach to management. In: Parrillo, J.E., Dellinger, R.P. (Eds.), Critical Care Medicine: Principles of Diagnosis and Management in the Adult, third ed. Mosby Elsevier, Philadelphia, pp. 379–422.

Kuo, C.S., Young, L.R., 2014. Interstitial lung disease in children. Curr. Opin. Pediatr. 26 (3), 320–327.

Lakoski, S., Eves, N., Douglas, P., et al., 2012. Exercise rehabilitation in patients with cancer. Nat. Rev. Clin. Oncol. 9, 288–296.

Lands, L.C., Smountas, A.A., Mesiano, G., et al., 1999. Maximal exercise capacity and peripheral skeletal muscle function following lung transplantation. J. Heart Lung Transplant. 18, 113–120.

Lang, P., Stoller, J., 1996. Hepatopulmonary syndrome: effects of liver transplantation. Clin. Chest Med. 17 (1), 115–123.

Langbein, W.E., Maloney, C., Kandare, F., et al., 2001. Pulmonary function testing in spinal cord injury: effects of abdominal muscle stimulation. J. Rehabil. Res. Dev. 38 (5), 591–598.

Lange, M., Hamahata, A., Traber, D.L., et al., 2011. Preclinical evaluation of epinephrine nebulization to reduce airway hyperemia and improve oxygenation after smoke inhalation injury. Crit. Care Med. 39 (4), 718–724.

Langer, D., Burtin, C., Schepers, L., et al., 2012a. Exercise training after lung transplantation improves participation in daily activity: a randomized controlled trial. Am. J. Transplant. 12, 1584–1592.

Langer, D., Cebria I Iranzo, M.A., Burtin, C., et al., 2012b. Determinants of physical activity in daily life in candidates for lung transplantation. Respir. Med. 106, 747–754.

Lanig, I.S., Peterson, W.P., 2000. The respiratory system in spinal cord injury. Phys. Med. Rehabil. Clin. N. Am. 11 (1), 29–43.

Laoutaris, I.D., Dritsas, A., Adamopoulos, S., et al., 2011. Benefits of physical training on exercise capacity, inspiratory muscle function, and quality of life in patients with ventricular assist devices long-term postimplantation. Eur. J. Cardiovasc. Prev. Rehabil. 18 (1), 33–40. doi:10.1097/HJR.0b013e32833c0320.

Larson, A., Curtis, J., 2006. Integrating palliative care for liver transplant candidates: 'too well for transplant, too sick for life'. J. Am. Med. Assoc. 295 (18), 2168–2176.

Latenser, B.A., 2009. Critical care of the burn patent: the first 48 hours. Crit. Care Med. 37, 2819–2826.

Latronico, N., Bolton, C.F., 2011. Critical illness polyneuropathy and myopathy: a major cause of muscle weakness and paralysis. Lancet Neurol. 10 (10), 931–941. doi:10.1016/S1474-4422(11)70178-8.

Le Guen, M.C., Cistulli, P.A., Berlowitz, D.J., 2012. Continuous positive pressure airway requirements in patients with tetraplegia and obstructive sleep apnoea. Spinal Cord 50, 682–685.

Ledsome, J., Sharp, J., 1981. Pulmonary function in acute cervical cord injury. Am. Rev. Respir. Dis. 124, 41–44.

Leduc, B.E., Dagher, J.H., Mayer, P., et al., 2007. Estimated prevalence of obstructive sleep apnoea–hypopnea syndrome after cervical cord injury. Arch. Phys. Med. Rehabil. 88, 333–337.

Lee, B.B., Cripps, R.A., Fitzharris, M., Wing, P.C., 2013. The global map for traumatic spinal cord injury epidemiology: update 2011, global incidence rate. Spinal Cord 52 (2), 110–116.

Lee, A.L., Hill, C.J., Cecins, N., et al., 2014a. The short and long term effects of exercise training in non-cystic fibrosis bronchiectasis: a randomised controlled trial. Respir. Res. 15, 44.

Lee, K., Rincon, F., 2012. Pulmonary complications in patients with severe brain injury. Crit. Care Res. Pract. 2012 (2012), 207247. doi:10.1155/2012/207247.

Lee, I.M., Shiroma, E.J., Lobelo, F., et al., 2012. Effect of physical inactivity on major non-communicable diseases worldwide: an analysis of burden of disease and life expectancy. Lancet 389 (9838), 219–229.

Lee, I., Wolin, K., Freeman, S., et al., 2014b. Physical activity and survival after cancer diagnosis in men. J. Phys. Act. Health 11, 85–90.

Lehmann, K., Lane, J., Piepmeier, J., et al., 1987. Cardiovascular abnormalities accompanying acute spinal cord injury in humans: incidence time course and severity. J. Am. Coll. Cardiol. 10, 46–52.

Levy, R.D., Ernst, P., Levine, S.M., et al., 1993. Exercise performance after lung transplantation. J. Heart Lung Transplant. 12, 27–33.

Lidofsky, S.D., Bass, N.M., Prager, N.M., et al., 1992. Intracranial pressure monitoring and liver transplantation for fulminant hepatic failure. Hepatology 16, 1–7.

Lin, V.W.H., Singh, H., Chitkara, R.K., Perkash, I., 1998. Functional magnetic stimulation for restoring cough in patients with tetraplegia. Arch. Phys. Med. Rehabil. 79, 517–522.

Linder, S.H., 1993. Functional electrical stimulation to enhance cough in quadriplegia. Chest 103, 166–169.

Linn, W.M., Adkins, R.H., Gong, H., Waters, R.L., 2000. Pulmonary function in chronic spinal cord injury: a cross-sectional survey of 222 Southern California adult outpatients. Arch. Phys. Med. Rehabil. 81, 757–763.

Livingstone, D.H., Hauser, C.J., 2004. Trauma to the chest wall and lungs. In: Moore, E.E., Feliciano, D.V., Mattox, K.L. (Eds.), Trauma, fifth ed. McGraw-Hill Professional, New York, pp. 507–538.

Lloyd-Williams, F., Mair, F.S., Leitner, M., 2002. Exercise training and heart failure: a systematic review of current evidence. Br. J. Gen. Pract. 52, 47–55.

Lucke, K.T., 1998. Pulmonary management following acute SCI. J. Neurosci. Nurs. 30 (2), 91–103.

MacBean, N., Ward, E., Murdoch, B., et al., 2009. Optimizing speech production in ventilator-assisted individual following cervical spinal cord injury: a preliminary investigation. Int. J. Lang. Comm. Dis. 44 (3), 382–393.

Macchiarini, P., Ladurie, F.L., Cerrina, J., et al., 1999. Clamshell or sternotomy for double lung or heart-lung transplantation? Eur. J. Cardiothorac Surg. 15, 333–339.

Madden, B.P., Kariyawasam, H., Siddiqi, A.J., et al., 2002. Noninvasive ventilation in cystic fibrosis patients with acute or chronic respiratory failure. Eur. Respir. J. 19, 310–313.

Maffiuletti, N., 2010. Physiological and methodological considerations for the use of neuromuscular electrical stimulation. Eur. J. Appl. Physiol. 110 (2), 223–234.

Mahanes, D., Lewis, R., 2004. Weaning of the neurologically impaired patient. Crit. Care Nurs. Clin. North Am. 16, 387–393.

Maiden, N., 2009. Ballistics reviews: mechanisms of bullet wound trauma. Forensic Sci. Med. Pathol. 5, 204–209.

Maiorana, A., O'driscoll, G., Cheetham, C., et al., 2000. Combined aerobic and resistance exercise training improves functional capacity and strength in CHF. J. Appl. Physiol. 88, 1565–1570.

Maltais, F., Leblanc, P., Simard, C., et al., 1996. Skeletal muscle adaptation to endurance training in patients with chronic obstructive pulmonary disease. Am. J. Respir. Crit. Care Med. 154, 442–447.

Mancini, D., Goldsmith, R., Levin, H., et al., 1998. Comparison of exercise performance in patients with chronic severe heart failure versus left ventricular assist devices. Circulation 98, 1178–1183.

Mandal, P., Sidhu, M.K., Kope, L., et al., 2012. A pilot study of pulmonary rehabilitation and chest physiotherapy versus chest physiotherapy alone in bronchiectasis. Respir. Med. 106 (12), 1647–1654.

Mandic, S., Tymchak, W., Kim, D., et al., 2009. Effects of aerobic or aerobic and resistance training on cardiorespiratory and skeletal muscle function in heart failure: a randomized controlled pilot trial. Clin. Rehabil. 23, 207–216.

Manito, N., Delgado, J.F., Crespo-Leiro, M.G., et al., 2010. Clinical recommendations for the use of everolimus in heart transplantation. Transplant. Rev. 24, 129–142.

Mansel, J., Norman, J., 1990. Respiratory complications and management of spinal cord injuries. Chest 97 (6), 1446–1452.

Marconi, C., Marzorati, M., 2003. Exercise after heart transplantation. Eur. J. Appl. Physiol. 90, 250–259.

Martinez, G.P., Barbera, J.A., Visa, J., et al., 2001. Hepatopulmonary syndrome in candidates for liver transplantation. J. Hepatol. 34, 651–657.

Martinu, T., Babyak, M.A., O'Connell, C.F., et al., 2008. Baseline 6-min walk distance predicts survival in lung transplant candidates. Am. J. Transplant. 8, 1498–1505.

Mateus, S.R., Beraldo, P.S., Horan, T.A., 2006. Cholinergic bronchomotor tone and airway caliber in tetraplegic patients. Spinal Cord 44, 269–274.

Mathur, S., Hornblower, E., Levy, R.D., 2009. Exercise training before and after lung transplantation. Phys. Sportsmed. 37, 78–87.

McCool, F.D., Pichurko, B.M., Slutsky, A.S., et al., 1986. Changes in lung volume and rib configuration with abdominal binding in quadriplegia. J. Appl. Physiol. 60 (4), 1198–1202.

McEvoy, D.R., Mykytyn, I., Sajkov, D., et al., 1995. Sleep apnoea in patients with quadriplegia. Thorax 50, 613–619.

McKenna, M.J., Fraser, S.F., Li, J.L., et al., 2003. Impaired muscle Ca^{2+} and K^+ regulation contribute to poor exercise performance post-lung transplantation. J. Appl. Physiol. 95, 1606–1616.

McKenzie, D.C., McLuckie, S.L., Stirling, D.R., 1994. The protective effects of continuous and interval exercise in athletes with exercise-induced asthma. Med. Sci. Sports Exerc. 26 (8), 951–956.

McKim, D., 2008. Keeping ventilated and 'at-risk' patients out of the intensive care unit. Can. Respir. J. 15 (Suppl. C), 9–10.

McTiernan, A., 2008. Mechanisms linking physical activity with cancer. Nat. Rev. Cancer 8, 205–211.

Mejaddam, A.Y., Velmahos, G.C., 2012. Randomized controlled trials affecting polytrauma care. Eur. J. Trauma Emerg. Surg. 38, 211–221.

Menter, R.R., Bach, J.R., Brown, D.J., et al., 1997. A review of the respiratory management of a patient with high level tetraplegia. Spinal Cord 35, 805–808.

Mereles, D., Ehlken, N., Kreuscher, S., et al., 2006. Exercise and respiratory training improve exercise capacity and quality of life in patients with severe chronic pulmonary hypertension. Circulation 114, 1482–1489.

Mettauer, B., Levy, F., Richard, R., et al., 2005. Exercising with a denervated heart after cardiac transplantation. Ann. Transplant. 10, 35–42.

Michael, D.B., Guyot, D.R., Darmody, W.R., 1989. Coincidence of head and cervical spine injury. J. Neurotrauma 6, 177–189.

Middleton, J.W., Dayton, A., Walsh, J., et al., 2012. Life expectancy after spinal cord injury: a 50-year study. Spinal Cord 50, 803–811.

Miller, T.L., Horgan, S., Lipshultz, S.E., 2005. Exercise rehabilitation of pediatric patients with cardiovascular disease. Prog. Pediatr. Cardiol. 20 (1), 27–37.

Miller, A.C., Rivero, A., Ziad, S., et al., 2009. Influence of nebulized unfractionated heparin and N- acetylcysteine in acute lung injury after smoke inhalation injury. J. Burn Care Res. 30 (2), 249–256.

Miller, T.L., Somarriba, G., Kinnamon, D.D., et al., 2010. The effect of a structured exercise program on nutrition and fitness outcomes in human immunodeficiency virus-infected children. AIDS Res. Hum. Retroviruses 26 (3), 313–319. doi:10.1089/aid.2009.0198.

Mitchell, M.J., Baz, M.A., Fulton, M.N., et al., 2003. Resistance training prevents vertebral osteoporosis in lung transplant recipients. Transplantation 76, 557–562.

Moller, S., Henriksen, J., 2006. Cardiopulmonary complications in chronic liver disease. World J. Gastroenterol. 12 (4), 526–538.

Moola, F., McCrindle, B.W., Longmuir, P.E., 2009. Physical activity participation in youth with surgically corrected congenital heart disease: devising guidelines so Johnny can participate. Paediatr. Child Health 14, 167–170.

Moorcroft, A.J., Dodd, M.E., Morris, J., Webb, A.K., 2004. Individualised unsupervised exercise training in adults with cystic fibrosis: a 1-year randomised controlled trial. Thorax 59 (12), 1074–1080.

Moore, K., Aithal, G., 2006. Guidelines on the management of ascites in cirrhosis. Gut 55 (Suppl. VI), vi1–vi12.

Morris, P., Goad, A., Thompson, C., et al., 2008. Early intensive care unit mobility therapy in the treatment of acute respiratory failure. Crit. Care Med. 36 (8), 2238–2243.

Morris, J.N., Heady, J.A., Raffle, P.A.B., et al., 1953. Coronary heart-disease and physical activity of work. Lancet 262 (6795), 1053–1057.

Morrone, T.M., Buck, L.A., Catanese, K.A., et al., 1996. Early progressive mobilization of patients with left ventricular assist devices is safe and optimizes recovery before heart transplantation. J. Heart Lung Transplant. 15 (4), 423–429.

Morton, A.R., Fitch, K.D., 2011. Australian association for exercise and sports science position statement on exercise and asthma. J. Sci. Med. Sport 14 (4), 312–316.

Mosier, M.J., Pham, T.N., 2009. American burn association practice guidelines for prevention, diagnosis and treatment of ventilator associated pneumonia (VAP) in burn patients. J. Burn Care Res. 30, 910–928.

Mosier, M.J., Pham, T.N., Park, D.R., et al., 2012. Predictive value of bronchoscopy in assessing the severity of inhalation injury. J. Burn Care Res. 33 (1), 65–73.

Mueller, G., de Groot, S., van der Woude, L., Hopman, M.T., 2008. Time-courses of lung function and respiratory muscles pressure generating capacity after spinal cord injury: a prospective cohort study. J. Rehabil. Med. 40, 269–276.

Mueller, G., Hopman, M.T., Perret, C., 2013. Comparison of respiratory muscle training methods in individuals with motor and sensory complete tetraplegia: a randomized controlled trial. J. Rehabil. Med. 45, 248–253.

Munro, P.E., Button, B.M., Bailey, M., et al., 2008. Should lung transplant recipients routinely perform airway clearance techniques? A randomized trial. Respirology 13, 1053–1060.

Munro, P.E., Holland, A.E., Bailey, M., et al., 2009. Pulmonary rehabilitation following lung transplantation. Transplant. Proc. 41, 292–295.

Myburgh, J.A., 2009. Chapter 67: severe head injury. In: Bersten, A.D., Soni, N. (Eds.), Oh's Intensive Care Manual, sixth ed. Butterworth-Heinemann, UK.

Myers, J., Gullestad, L., Vagelos, R., et al., 1998. Clinical, hemodynamic, and cardiopulmonary exercise test determinants of survival in patients referred for evaluation of heart failure. Ann. Intern. Med. 129, 286–293.

National Institute of Health and Care Excellence (NICE), 2009. Rehabilitation After Critical Illness. Mar, London (UK), p. 91. (Clinical guideline; no. 83).

Needham, D., Davidson, J., Cohen, H., et al., 2012. Improving long-term outcomes after discharge from intensive care unit: report from a stakeholders' conference. Crit. Care Med. 40, 502–509.

Needham, D., Truong, A., Fan, E., 2009. Technology to enhance physical rehabilitation of critically ill patients. Crit. Care Med. 37 (10 Suppl.), S436–S441.

New, P.W., Sundararajan, V., 2008. Incidence of non-traumatic spinal cord injury in Victoria, Australia: a population-based study and literature review. Spinal Cord 46 (6), 406–411.

Newall, C., Stockley, R.A., Hill, S.L., 2005. Exercise training and inspiratory muscle training in patients with bronchiectasis. Thorax 60 (11), 943–948.

Nguyen, H.B., Rivers, E.P., Abrahamian, F.M., et al., 2006. Severe sepsis and septic shock: review of the literature and emergency department management guidelines. Ann. Emerg. Med. 48, 28–54.

Nguyen, H.B., Smith, D., 2007. Sepsis in the 21st century: recent definitions and therapeutic advances. Am. J. Emerg. Med. 25, 564–571.

NICE public health guidance 47, 2013. Managing overweight and obesity among children and young people: lifestyle weight management serviceas. <http://guidance.nice.org.uk/ph47>.

Nici, L., Donner, C., Wouters, E., et al., 2006. American Thoracic Society/European Respiratory Society statement on pulmonary rehabilitation. Am. J. Respir. Crit. Care Med. 173, 1390–1413.

Nixon, P.A., Orenstein, D.M., Kelsey, S.F., Doershuk, C.F., 1992. The prognostic value of exercise testing in patients with cystic fibrosis. N. Engl. J. Med. 327 (25), 1785–1788.

NSCISC Report – National Spinal Cord Injury Statistical Center. Spinal cord injury: facts and figures at glance. Birmingham (AL): University of Alabama at Birmingham, National Spinal Cord Injury Statistical Center; 2013. Available at: <www.nscisc.uab.edu/PublicDocuments/> (accessed 14.02.)

Nydahl, P., Ruhl, A., Bartoszek, G., et al., 2014. Early mobilisation of mechanically ventilated patients: a one day point prevalence study in Germany. Crit. Care Med. 42 (5), 1178–1186.

O'Driscoll, M., Corner, J., Bailey, C., 1999. The experience of breathlessness in lung cancer. Eur. J. Cancer Care 8, 37–43.

O'Grady, J.G., Alexander, G.J., Hayllar, K.M., 1989. Early indicators of prognosis in fulminant hepatic failure. Gastroenterology 97 (2), 439–445.

OECD, 2013. Health at a Glance 2013: OECD Indicators. OECD Publishing. <http://dx.doi.org/10.1787/health_glance-2013-en>.

Oh, J.S., Chung, K.K., Allen, A., et al., 2012. Admission chest CT complements fiberoptic bronchoscopy in prediction of adverse outcomes in thermally injured patients. J. Burn Care Res. 33 (4), 532–538.

Olsson, J.K., Zamanian, R.T., Feinstein, J.A., Doyle, R.L., 2005. Surgical and interventional therapies for pulmonary arterial hypertension. Semin. Respir. Crit. Care Med. 26, 417–428.

Onders, R.P., Khansarinia, S., Weiser, T., et al., 2010. Multicenter analysis of diaphragm pacing in tetraplegics with cardiac pacemakers: positive implications for ventilator weaning in intensive care units. Surgery 148 (40), 893–898.

Ong, H.K., Lee, A.L., Hill, C.J., et al., 2011. Effects of pulmonary rehabilitation in bronchiectasis: a retrospective study. Chron. Respir. Dis. 8 (1), 21–30.

Oo, T., Watt, J.W., Soni, B.M., Sett, P.K., 1999. Delayed diaphragm recovery in 12 patients after high cervical spinal cord injury: a retrospective review of the diaphragm status of 107 patients ventilated after acute spinal cord injury. Spinal Cord 37 (2), 117–122.

Orenstein, D.M., 2002. Pulmonary problems and management concerns in youth sports. Pediatr. Clin. N. Am. 49 (4), 709–721.

Orenstein, D.M., Nixon, P.A., Ross, E.A., Kaplan, R.M., 1989. The quality of well-being in cystic fibrosis. Chest 95, 344–347.

Orman, J., Westerdahl, E., 2010. Chest physiotherapy with positive expiratory pressure breathing after abdominal and thoracic surgery: systematic review. Acta Anaesthesiol. Scand. 54, 261–267.

Painter, P., 2008. Exercise in chronic disease: Physiological research needed. Exerc. Sport Sci. Rev. 36 (2), 83–90.

Pandharipande, P., Girard, T., Jackson, J., et al., 2013. Long-term cognitive impairment after critical illness. NEJM 369 (14), 1306–1316.

Paranjape, S.M., Barnes, L.A., Carson, K.A., et al., 2012. Exercise improves lung function and habitual activity in children with cystic fibrosis. J. Cyst. Fibros. 11 (1), 18–23.

Paratz, J., Lipman, J., McAuliffe, M., 2002. Effect of manual hyperinflation on hemodynamics, gas exchange and respiratory mechanics in ventilated patients. J. Intensive Care Med. 17, 317–324.

Paratz, J.D., Stockton, K., Plaza, A., et al., 2012. Intensive exercise after thermal injury improves physical, functional and psychological outcomes. J. Trauma Acute Care Surg. 73, 186–194.

Parker, A., Tehranchi, K., Needham, D., 2013. Critical care rehabilitation trials: the importance of 'usual care'. Critical Care 17 (5), 183.

Parry, S., Berney, S., Granger, C., et al., 2013. Electrical muscle stimulation in the intensive care setting: a systematic review. Crit. Care Med. 41 (10), 2406–2418.

Parry, S., Berney, S., Warrillow, S., et al., 2014. Functional electrical stimulation with cycling in the critically ill: a pilot case-matched control study. J. Crit. Care 29 (4), 695.e691–695.e697.

Parry, S., El-Ansary, D., Cartwright, M., et al., 2015. Ultrasonography in the intensive care setting can be used to detect changes in the quality and quantity of muscle and is related to muscle strength and function. J. Crit. Care pii: S0883-9441(15)00332-9. [Epub Ahead of Print].

Parsons, J.P., Hallstrand, T.S., Mastronarde, J.G., et al., 2013. An official American Thoracic Society clinical practice guideline: exercise-induced bronchoconstriction. Am. J. Respir. Crit. Care Med. 187 (9), 1016–1027.

Pasteur, M.C., Bilton, D., Hill, A.T., 2010. British Thoracic Society guideline for non-CF bronchiectasis. Thorax 65 (Suppl. 1), i1–i58.

Patel, J.N., Kavey, R.E., Pophal, S.G., et al., 2008. Improved exercise performance in pediatric heart transplant recipients after home exercise training. Pediatr. Transplant. 12 (3), 336–340. doi:10.1111/j.1399-3046.2007.00806.x.

Patterson, G.A., Cooper, J.D., Goldman, B., et al., 1988. Technique of successful clinical double-lung transplantation. Ann. Thorac. Surg. 45, 626–633.

Peterson, P., Kirshblum, S., 2002. Pulmonary management of spinal cord injury. In: Kirshblum, S., Campagnolo, D., DeLisa, J. (Eds.), Spinal Cord Medicine. Lippincott, Williams & Wilkins Philadelphia, PA, pp. 136–155.

Pianosi, P., LeBlanc, J., Almudevar, A., 2005. Relationship between FEV_1 and peak oxygen uptake in children with cystic fibrosis. Pediatr. Pulmonol. 40 (4), 324–329.

Piepoli, M.F., Conraads, V., Corra, U., et al., 2011. Exercise training in heart failure: from theory to practice: a consensus document of the Heart Failure Association and the European Association for Cardiovascular Prevention and Rehabilitation. Eur. J. Heart Fail. 13, 347–357.

Pina, I.L., Apstein, C.S., Balady, G.J., et al., 2003. Exercise and heart failure: a statement from the American Heart Association Committee on Exercise, Rehabilitation, and Prevention. Circulation 107, 1210–1225.

Pires-Neto, R., Fogaca Kawaguchi, Y., Sayuri Hirota, A., et al., 2013. Very early passive cycling exercise in mechanically ventilated critically ill patients: physiological safety aspects, a case series. PLoS ONE 9 (8), e74182.

Pohlman, M.C., Schweikert, W.D., Pohlman, A.S., et al., 2010. Feasibility of physical and occupational therapy beginning from initiation of mechanical ventilation. Crit. Care Med. 38, 2089–2094.

Porot, V., Guerin, C., 2013. Bench assessment of a new insufflation-exsufflation device. Respir. Care 58 (9), 1536–1540.

Postma, K., Bussmann, J.B., Haisma, J.A., et al., 2009. Predicting respiratory infections one year after inpatient rehabilitation with pulmonary function measured at discharge in persons with spinal cord injury. J. Rehabil. Med. 41 (9), 729–733.

Priestman, T., 2008. Cancer Chemotherapy in Clinical Practice. Springer-Verlag, London.

Prigent, H., Lejaille, M., Terzi, N., et al., 2012. Effect of a tracheostomy speaking valve on breathing-swallowing interaction. Intensive Care Med. 38, 85–90.

Pruitt, B.A. Jr., Dowling, J.A., Moncrief, J.A., 1968. Escharotomy in early burn care. Arch. Surg. 96 (4), 502–507.

Pruitt, B.A. Jr., Erickson, D.R., Morris, A., 1975. Progressive pulmonary insufficiency and other pulmonary complications of thermal injury. J. Trauma 15, 369–379.

Pryor, J.A., 1999. Physiotherapy for airway clearance in adults. Eur. Respir. J. 14 (6), 1418–1424.

Punjabi, N.M., 2008. The epidemiology of adult obstructive sleep apnoea. Proc. Am. Thor. Soc. 5, 136–143.

Puthucheary, Z., Denehy, L., 2015. Exercise interventions in critical illness survivors: understanding inclusion and stratification criteria. Am. J. Respir. Crit. Care Med. 191 (12), 1464–1467.

Puthucheary, Z.A., Rawal, J., McPhail, M., et al., 2013. Acute skeletal muscle wasting in critical illness. JAMA 310 (15), 1591–1600.

Ragnarrson, K.T., 2012. Medical rehabilitation of people with spinal cord injury during 40 years of academic physiatric practice. Am. J. Phys. Med. Rehabil. 91, 231–242.

Rand, S., Prasad, S.A., 2012. Exercise as part of a cystic fibrosis therapeutic routine. Expert Rev. Respir. Med. 6 (3), 341–351, quiz 52.

Reedy, J.E., Swartz, M.T., Lohmann, D.P., et al., 1992. The importance of patient mobility with ventricular assist device support. ASAIO J. 38, M151–M153.

Reinsma, G.D., Ten Hacken, N.H., Grevink, R.G., et al., 2006. Limiting factors of exercise performance 1 year after lung transplantation. J. Heart Lung Transplant. 25, 1310–1316.

Reitz, B.A., Wallwork, J.L., Hunt, S.A., et al., 1982. Heart-lung transplantation: successful therapy for patients with pulmonary vascular disease. N. Engl. J. Med. 306, 557–564.

Rimmer, J.H., 2005. Exercise and physical activity in persons aging with a physical disability. Phys. Med. Rehabil. Clin. N. Am. 16 (1), 41–56.

Roberts, S., 2002. Respiratory management. In: Partridge, C. (Ed.), Neurological Physiotherapy. Bases of Evidence for Practice. Whurr Publishers Ltd, London.

Roberts, G., Lloyd, M., Parker, M., et al., 2012a. The Baux score is dead. Long live the Baux score: a 27-year retrospective cohort study of mortality at a regional burns service. J. Trauma Acute Care Surg. 72 (1), 251–256.

Roberts, D.J., Zygun, D.A., Grendar, J., et al., 2012b. Negative-pressure wound therapy for critically ill adults with open abdominal wounds: a systematic review. J. Trauma Acute Care Surg. 73, 629–639.

Rock, C., Doyle, C., Demark-Wahnefried, W., et al., 2013. Nutrition and physical activity guidelines for cancer survivors. CA Cancer J. Clin. 62, 215.

Rojas, Y., Finnerty, C.C., Radhakrishnan, R.S., et al., 2012. Burns: an update on current pharmacotherapy. Expert Opin. Pharmacother. 13 (17), 2485–2494.

Rosado, M., Banner, M., 1996. Ascites and its effects upon respiratory muscle loading and work of breathing. Crit. Care Med. 24 (3), 538–540.

Rosenberger, E.M., Dew, M.A., Dimartini, A.F., et al., 2012. Psychosocial issues facing lung transplant candidates, recipients and family caregivers. Thorac. Surg. Clin. 22, 517–529.

Rosenfeld, J., 2012. Practical Management of Head and Neck Injury, Churchill Livingstone. From Chapter 8: Operative Surgery. Churchill Livingstone Elsevier, UK.

Ross, M., Kouretas, P., Gamberg, P., et al., 2006. Ten- and 20-year survivors of pediatric orthotopic heart transplantation. J. Heart Lung Transplant. 25 (3), 261–270. [Epub 2006 Jan 6].

Ross, J., White, M., 2003. Removal of the tracheostomy tube in the aspirating spinal cord-injured patient. Spinal Cord 41 (11), 636–642.

Roth, E.J., Lu, A., Primack, S., et al., 1997. Ventilatory function in cervical and high thoracic spinal cord injury. Am. J. Phys. Med. Rehabil. 76 (4), 262–267.

Rowland, T.W., 2007. Promoting physical activity of children's health. Rationale and strategies. Sports Med. 37 (11), 929–936.

Sahlberg, M., Eriksson, B.O., Sixt, R., Strandvik, B., 2008. Cardiopulmonary data in response to 6 months of training in physically active adult patients with classic cystic fibrosis. Respiration 76 (4), 413–420.

Saffle, J.L., 2007. The phenomenon of "fluid creep" in acute burn resuscitation. J. Burn Care Res. 28 (3), 382–395.

Sagi, H.C., Beutler, W., Carroll, E., Connolly, P.J., 2002. Airway complications associated with surgery on the anterior cervical spine. Spine 27 (9), 949–953.

Saiman, L., Siegel, J., 2004. Infection control in cystic fibrosis. Clin. Microbiol. Rev. 17, 57–71.

Sajkov, D., Marshall, R., Walker, P., et al., 1998. Sleep apnoea related hypoxia is associated with cognitive disturbances in patients with tetraplegia. Spinal Cord 36, 231–239.

Sancho, J., Servera, E., Diaz, J., et al., 2004. Efficacy of mechanical insufflation-exsufflation in medically stable patients with amytrophic lateral sclerosis. Chest 125, 1400–1405.

Santuz, P., Baraldi, E., Filippone, M., Zacchello, F., 1997. Exercise performance in children with asthma: is it different from that of healthy controls? Eur. Respir. J. 10 (6), 1254–1260.

Sargent, S., 2006. The management and nursing care of cirrhotic ascites. Br. J. Nurs. 15 (4), 212–219.

Scanlon, P.D., Loring, S.H., Pichurko, B.M., et al., 1989. Respiratory mechanics in acute quadriplegia: lung and chest wall compliance and dimensional changes during respiratory maneuvers. Am. J. Respir. Crit. Care Med. 139 (3), 615–620.

Schickendantz, S., Sticker, E., Dordel, S., Bjarnason-Wehrens, B., 2007. Sport and physical activity in children with congenital heart disease. Dtsch Arztebl. 104, 6.

Schilero, G.J., Grimm, D.R., Bauman, W.A., et al., 2005. Assessment of airway caliber and bronchodilator responsiveness in subjects with spinal cord injury. Chest 127, 149–155.

Schmauss, D., Weis, M., 2008. Cardiac allograft vasculopathy: recent developments. Circulation 117, 2131–2141.

Schmitz, K., Courneya, K., Matthews, C., et al., 2010. ACSM roundtable on exercise guidelines for cancer survivors. Med. Sci. Sports Exerc. 42, 1409–1426.

Schneiderman-Walker, J., 2000. A randomized controlled trial of a 3-year home exercise program in cystic fibrosis. J. Pediatr. 136 (3), 304–310.

Schroeder, J.E., Weiss, Y.G., Mosheiff, R., 2009. The current state in the evaluation and treatment of ARDS and SIRS. Injury 40, S82–S89.

Schweickert, W.D., Kress, J.P., 2011. Implementing early mobilization interventions in mechanically ventilated patients in the ICU. Chest 140 (6), 1612–1617. doi:10.1378/chest.10–2829.

Schweickert, W., Pohlman, M., Pohlman, A., et al., 2009. Early physical and occupational therapy in mechanically ventilated, critically ill patients: a randomised controlled trial. Lancet 373 (9678), 1874–1882.

Scott, M.D., Frost, F., Supinski, G., 1993. The effect of body position and abdominal binders in chronic tetraplegic subjects more than 15 years post-injury. J. Am. Paraplegia Soc. 16 (2), 117.

Seidl, R.O., Nusser-Muller-Busch, R., Kurzweill, M., Niedeggen, A., 2010. Dysphagia in acute tetraplegics: a retrospective study. Spinal Cord 48, 197–201.

Selig, S.E., Levinger, I., Williams, A.D., et al., 2010. Exercise & Sports Science Australia Position Statement on exercise training and chronic heart failure. J. Sci. Med. Sport 13, 288–294.

Selvadurai, H., 2009. Exercise & exercise testing in health and in disease: what we know and what we need to know. Paediatr. Respir. Rev. 10, 81–82.

Selvadurai, H.C., Blimkie, C.J., Meyers, N., et al., 2002. Randomized controlled study of in-hospital exercise training programs in children with cystic fibrosis. Pediatr. Pulmonol. 33 (3), 194–200.

Servantes, D.M., Pelcerman, A., Salvetti, X.M., et al., 2012. Effects of home-based exercise training for patients with chronic heart failure and sleep apnoea: a randomized comparison of two different programmes. Clin. Rehabil. 26, 45–57.

Shamin, M., Syed, A., Syed, E., 2011. Non-operative management is superior to surgical stabilisation in spine injury patients with complete neurological deficits: a perspective study from a developing country, Pakistan. Surg. Neurol. Int. 2, 166.

Shane, E., Rivas, M.C., Silverberg, S.J., et al., 1993. Osteoporosis after cardiac transplantation. Am. J. Med. 94, 257–264.

Shirani, K.Z., Pruitt, B.A. Jr., Mason, A.D. Jr., 1987. The influence of inhalation injury and pneumonia on burn mortality. Ann. Surg. 205 (1), 82–87.

Slack, R.S., Shucart, W., 1994. Respiratory dysfunction associated with traumatic injury to the central nervous system. Clin. Chest Med. 15 (4), 739–749.

Sluys, K., Häggmark, T., Iselius, L., 2005. Outcome and quality of life 5 years after major trauma. J. Trauma 59, 223–232.

Smailes, S.T., Engelsman, K., Dziewulski, P., 2013a. Physical functional outcome assessment of patients with major burns admitted to a UK burn intensive care unit. Burns 39 (1), 37–43.

Smailes, S.T., Engelsman, K., Rodgers, L., Upson, C., 2016. Increasing the utility of the Functional Assessment for Burns Score: Not just for major burns. Burns 42, 163–168.

Smailes, S.T., Martin, R.V., McVicar, A.J., 2009a. Evaluation of the spontaneous breathing trial in burn intensive care patients. Burns 35, 665–671.

Smailes, S.T., Martin, R.V., McVicar, A.J., 2009b. The incidence and outcome of extubation failure in burn intensive care patients. J. Burn Care Res. 30 (3), 386–392.

Smailes, S.T., Martin, R.V., McVicar, A.J., 2013b. Cough strength, secretions and extubation outcome in burn patients who have passed a spontaneous breathing trial. Burns 39 (2), 236–242.

Smith, A., Reeve, B., Bellizzi, K., et al., 2008. Cancer, comorbidities, and health-related quality of life of older adults. Health Care Financ. Rev. 24, 41–56.

Solway, S., Brooks, D., Lau, L., Goldstein, R., 2002. The short-term effect of a rollator on functional exercise capacity among individuals with severe COPD. Chest 122, 56–65.

Speck, R., Courneya, K., Mâsse, L., et al., 2010. An update of controlled physical activity trials in cancer survivors: a systematic review and meta-analysis. J. Cancer Survivorship 4, 87–100.

Speiser, P.W., Rudolf, M.C., Anhalt, H., et al., 2005. Childhood obesity. J. Clin. Endocrinol. Metab. 90 (3), 1871–1887.

Sricharoenchai, T., Parker, A., Zanni, J., et al., 2014. Safety of physical therapy interventions in critically ill patients: a single-center prospective evaluation of 1110 intensive care unit admissions. J. Crit. Care 29 (3), 395–400.

Stanic, U., Kandare, F., Jaeger, R., Sorli, J., 2000. Functional electrical stimulation of abdominal muscles to augment tidal volume in spinal cord injury. IEEE Trans. Rehabil. Eng. 8 (1), 30–34.

Stark, R.P., McGinn, A.L., Wilson, R.F., 1991. Chest pain in cardiac-transplant recipients: evidence of sensory reinnervation after cardiac transplantation. N. Engl. J. Med. 324, 1791–1794.

Starnes, V.A., Woo, M.S., Maclaughlin, E.F., et al., 1999. Comparison of outcomes between living donor and cadaveric lung transplantation in children. Ann. Thorac. Surg. 68, 2279–2283.

Stehlik, J., Edwards, L.B., Kucheryavaya, A.Y., et al., 2012. The registry of the International Society for Heart and Lung Transplantation: 29th official adult heart transplant report-2012. J. Heart Lung Transplant. 31, 1052–1064.

Stepp, E.L., Brown, R., Tun, C.G., et al., 2008. Determinants of lung volumes in chronic spinal cord injury. Arch. Phys. Med. Rehabil. 89, 1499–1506.

Stevens, R.D., Bhardwaj, A., Kirsch, J.R., Mirski, M.A., 2003. Critical care and perioperative management in traumatic spinal cord injury. J. Neurosurg. Anesthesiol. 15 (3), 215–229.

Stevens, R., Marshall, S., Cornblath, D., et al., 2009a. A framework for diagnosing and classifying intensive care unit-acquired weakness. Crit. Care Med. 37 (10 Suppl.), S299–S308.

Stevens, D., Oades, P.J., Armstrong, N., Williams, C.A., 2009b. Early oxygen uptake recovery following exercise testing in children with chronic chest diseases. Pediatr. Pulmonol. 44 (5), 480–488.

Stevens, D., Oades, P., Armstrong, N., Williams, C.A., 2011. Intermittent exercise and CF patients. Appl. Physiol. Nutr. Metab. 36 (6), 920–927.

Stewart, S., Fishbein, M.C., Snell, G.I., et al., 2007. Revision of the 1996 working formulation for the standardization of nomenclature in the diagnosis of lung rejection. J. Heart Lung Transplant. 26, 1229–1242.

Stewart, S., Winters, G.L., Fishbein, M.C., et al., 2005. Revision of the 1990 working formulation for the standardization of nomenclature in the diagnosis of heart rejection. J. Heart Lung Transplant. 24, 1710–1720.

Stiebellehner, L., Quittan, M., End, A., et al., 1998. Aerobic endurance training program improves exercise performance in lung transplant recipients. Chest 113, 906–912.

Stiller, K., 2007. Safety issues that should be considered when mobilizing critically ill patients. Crit. Care Clin. 23, 35–53.

Stiller, K., Huff, N., 1999. Respiratory muscle training for tetraplegic patients: a literature review. Aust. J. Physiother. 45, 291–299.

Stockhammer, E., Tobon, A., Michel, F., et al., 2002. Characteristics of sleep apnea syndrome in tetraplegic patients. Spinal Cord 40, 286–294.

Stockton, K., 2001. Exercise training in patients with chronic liver disease. Physiother. Theory Pract. 17, 29–38.

Stockton, K.A., Davis, M.J., Brown, M.C., et al., 2012. Physiological responses to maximal exercise testing and modified incremental shuttle walk test in adults following thermal injury: a pilot study. J. Burn Care Res. 33 (2), 252–258.

Stravitz, R., Larsen, F., 2009. Therapeutic hypothermia for acute liver failure. Crit. Care Med. 37 (7 Suppl.), S258–S264.

Stravitz, T., Kramer, A.H., Davern, T., et al., 2007. Intensive care of patients with acute liver failure: recommendations of the US acute liver failure study group. Crit. Care Med. 35 (11), 2498–2508.

Studer, S.M., Levy, R.D., McNeil, K., Orens, J.B., 2004. Lung transplant outcomes: a review of survival, graft function, physiology, health related quality of life and cost-effectiveness. Eur. Respir. J. 24, 670–685.

Suiter, D., McCullough, G., Powell, P., 2003. Effects of cuff deflation and one-way tracheostomy speaking valve placement on swallow physiology. Dysphagia 18, 284–292.

Suman, O.E., Spies, R.J., Celis, M.M., et al., 2001. Effects of a 12-week resistance exercise program on skeletal muscle strength in children with burn injuries. J. Appl. Physiol. 91, 1168–1175.

Suman, O.E., Thomas, S.J., Wilkins, J.P., et al., 2003. Effect of exogenous growth hormone and exercise on lean mass and muscle function in children with burns. J. Appl. Physiol. 94, 2273–2281.

Takken, T., Christian Blank, A., Hulzebos, E., 2011. Respiratory gas exchange during exercise in children with congenital heart disease: methodology and clinical concepts. Curr. Respir. Med. Rev. 7 (2), 87–96.

Takken, T., Giardini, A., Reybrouck, T., et al., 2012. Recommendations for physical activity, recreation sport, and exercise training in paediatric patients with congenital heart disease: a report from the Exercise, Basic & Translational Research Section of the European Association of Cardiovascular Prevention and Rehabilitation, the European Congenital Heart and Lung Exercise Group, and the Association for European Paediatric Cardiology. Eur. J. Prev. Cardiol. 19 (5), 1034–1065.

Takken, T., van Brussel, M., Engelbert, R.H.H., et al., 2008. Exercise therapy in juvenile idiopathic arthritis. Cochrane Database Syst. Rev. 2, CD005954.

Tanaka, K., Akechi, T., Okuyama, T., et al., 2002. Impact of dyspnea, pain, and fatigue on daily life activities in ambulatory patients with advanced lung cancer. J. Pain Symptom Manage. 23, 417–423.

Tardon, A., Lee, W., Delgado-Rodriguez, M., et al., 2005. Leisure-time physical activity and lung cancer: a meta-analysis. Cancer Causes Control 16, 389–397.

Taylor, P.N., Tromans, A.M., Harris, K.R., Swain, I.D., 2002. Electrical stimulation of abdominal muscles for control of blood pressure and augmentation of cough in a C3/4 level tetraplegic. Spinal Cord 40, 34–36.

Ten Harkel, A.D., Takken, T., 2010. Exercise testing and prescription in patients with congenital heart disease. Int. J. Paediatr. 2010, pii: 791980. doi:10.1155/2010/791980.

Thabut, G., Mal, H., Cerrina, J., et al., 2005. Graft ischemic time and outcome of lung transplantation: a multicenter analysis. Am. J. Respir. Crit. Care Med. 171, 786–791.

The Acute Respiratory Distress Syndrome Network, 2000. Ventilation with lower tidal volumes as compared with traditional tidal volumes and for acute lung injury and the acute respiratory distress syndrome. N. Engl. J. Med. 342, 1301–1308.

The Brain Trauma Foundation, The American Association of Neurological Surgeons, The Joint Section on Neurotrauma and Critical Care, 2007. Intracranial pressure thresholds. J. Neurotrauma 24, S55–S58.

Thim, T., Krarup, N.H., Grove, E.L., et al., 2012. Initial assessment and treatment with the Airway, Breathing, Circulation, Disability, Exposure (ABCDE) approach. Int. J. Gen. Med. 5, 117–121.

Thomas, B., Aurora, P., Spencer, H., et al., 2012. Persistent disruption of ciliated epithelium following paediatric lung transplantation. Eur. Respir. J. 40, 1245–1252.

Thomas, E., Paulson, S.S., 1994. Protocol for weaning the SCI patient. SCI Nurs. 11 (2), 42–45.

Thorens, J.B., Junod, A.F., 1992. Hypoxaemia and liver cirrhosis: a new argument in favour of a 'diffusion-perfusion defect. Eur. Respir. J. 5, 754–756.

Tirdel, G.B., Girgis, R., Fishman, R.S., Theodore, J., 1998. Metabolic myopathy as a cause of the exercise limitation in lung transplant recipients. J. Heart Lung Transplant. 17, 1231–1237.

Torres-Castro, R., Vilaro, J., Vera-Uribe, R., et al., 2014. Use of air stacking and abdominal compression for cough assistance in people with complete tetraplegia. Spinal Cord 52 (5), 354–357.

Townsend, N., Wickramasinghe, K., Williams, J., et al., 2015. Physical Activity Statistics 2015. British Heart Foundation, London.

Tran, K., Hukins, C., Gerahty, T., et al., 2010. Sleep disordered breathing in spinal cord injured patients: a short-term longitudinal study. Respirology 15, 272–276.

Tromans, A.M., Mecci, M., Barrett, F.H., et al., 1998. The use of the BiPAP biphasic positive airway pressure system in acute spinal cord injury. Spinal Cord 36, 481–484.

Truong, A., Fan, E., Brower, R., Needham, D., 2009. Bench-to-bedside review: mobilizing patients in the intensive care unit – from pathophysiology to clinical trials. Critical Care 13 (4), 216.

Turner, D.A., Cheifetz, I.M., Rehder, K.J., et al., 2011. Active rehabilitation and physical therapy during extracorporeal membrane oxygenation while awaiting lung transplantation: a practical approach. Crit. Care Med. 39, 2593–2598.

Tzeng, A.C., Bach, J.R., 2000. Prevention of pulmonary morbidity for patients with neuromuscular disease. Chest 118 (5), 1390–1396.

Urdaneta, F., Layon, J., 2003. Respiratory complications in patients with traumatic cervical spine injuries: case report and review of the literature. J. Clin. Anaesth. 15, 398–405.

Van 'T Hul, A., Gosselink, R., Hollander, P., et al., 2006. Training with inspiratory pressure support in patients with severe COPD. Eur. Respir. J. 27, 65–72.

Van Aswegen, H., Eales, C., Richards, G.A., et al., 2010. The effect of penetrating trunk trauma and mechanical ventilation on the recovery of adult survivors after hospital discharge. S. Afr. J. Crit. Care 26, 25–32.

Van Aswegen, H., Myezwa, H., Mudzi, W., et al., 2011. Health-related quality of life of survivors of penetrating trunk trauma in Johannesburg, South Africa. Eur. J. Trauma Emerg. Surg. 37, 419–426.

Van Aswegen, H., Van Aswegen, A., Du Raan, H., et al., 2013. Airflow distribution with manual hyperinflation as assessed through gamma camera imaging: a crossover randomised trial. Physiotherapy 99, 107–112.

van Brussel, M., Takken, T., van der Net, J., et al., 2006. Physical function and fitness in long-term survivors of childhood leukaemia. Pediatr. Rehabil. 9 (3), 267–274.

van Brussel, M., van der Net, J., Hulzebos, E., et al., 2011. The Utrecht approach to exercise in chronic childhood conditions: the decade in review. Pediatr. Phys. Ther. 23 (1), 2–14.

Van der Vlies, C.H., Olthof, D.C., Gaakeer, M., et al., 2011. Changing patterns in diagnostic strategies and the treatment of blunt injury to solid abdominal organs. Int. J. Emerg. Med. 4, 47.

Van Houtte, S., Vanlandewijck, Y., Gosselink, R., 2006. Respiratory muscle training in persons with spinal cord injury: a systematic review. Respir. Med. 100 (11), 1886–1895.

Vazquez, R.G., Sedes, P.R., Farina, M.M., et al., 2013. Respiratory management in the patient with spinal cord injury. BioMed. Res. Int. 2013, Article ID 168757.

Venuta, F., Rendina, E.A., De Giacomo, T., et al., 2003. Bilateral sequential lung transplantation without sternal division. Eur. J. Cardiothorac Surg. 23, 894–897.

Verschuren, O., Ketelaar, M., Takken, T., et al., 2008. Exercise programs for children with cerebral palsy. Am. J. Phys. Med. Rehabil. 87, 404–417.

Vianello, A., Corrado, A., Arcaro, G., et al., 2005. Mechanical insufflation-exsufflation improves outcomes for neuromuscular disease patients with respiratory tract infections. Am. J. Phys. Med. Rehabil. 84 (2), 83–88.

Vintro, A., Krasnkoff, J., Painter, P., 2002. Roles of nutrition and physical activity in musculoskeletal complications before and after liver transplantation. Adv. Pract. Acute Crit. Care 13 (2), 333–347.

Vos, R., Vanaudenaerde, B.M., Ottevaere, A., et al., 2010. Long-term azithromycin therapy for bronchiolitis obliterans syndrome: divide and conquer? J. Heart Lung Transplant. 29, 1358–1368.

Wadsworth, B.M., Haines, T.P., Cornwell, P.L., Paratz, J.D., 2009. Abdominal binder use in people with spinal cord injuries: a systematic review and meta-analysis. Spinal Cord 47 (4), 274–285.

Wadsworth, B.M., Haines, T.P., Cornwell, P.L., et al., 2012. Abdominal binder improves lung volumes and voice in people with tetraplegic spinal cord injury. Arch. Phys. Med. Rehabil. 93 (12), 2189–2197.

Wagner, F.M., 2011. Donor heart preservation and perfusion. Appl. Cardiopulm. Pathophysiol. 15, 198–206.

Wallbom, A.S., Naran, B., Thomas, E., 2005. Acute ventilator management and weaning in individuals with high tetraplegia. Top. Spinal Cord Inj. Rehabil. 10, 1–7.

Walsh, T., Salisbury, L., Merriweather, J., et al., 2015. Increased hospital-based physical rehabilitation and information provision after intensive care unit discharge: the RECOVER randomised clinical trial. JAMA Int. Med. 175 (6), 901–910. doi:10.1001/jamainternmed.2015.0822.

Wang, A.Y., Jaeger, R.J., Yarkony, G.M., Turba, R.M., 1997. Cough in spinal cord injured patients: the relationship between motor level and peak expiratory flow. Spinal Cord 35, 299–302.

Wang, X.N., Williams, T.J., McKenna, M.J., et al., 1999. Skeletal muscle oxidative capacity, fiber type, and metabolites after lung transplantation. Am. J. Respir. Crit. Care Med. 160, 57–63.

Warden, G.D., 1992. Burn shock resuscitation. World J. Surg. 16 (1), 16–23.

Waring, W.P., Karunas, R.S., 1991. Acute spinal cord injuries and the incidence of clinically occurring thromboembolic disease. Paraplegia 29, 8–16.

Warner, J.T., 2008. Body composition, exercise and energy expenditure in survivors of acute lymphoblastic leukaemia. Pediatr. Blood Cancer 50 (2 Suppl.), 456–461.

Warrillow, S.J., Bellomo, R., 2014. Preventing cerebral oedema in acute liver failure: the case for quadruple-H therapy. Anaesth. Intensive Care. 42 (1), 78–88.

Wasenko, J.L., Hochhauser, L., 2009. Chapter 6: central nervous system trauma. In: Haaga, John R, Dogra, Vikram S, Forsting, Michael (Eds.), CT and MRI of the Whole Body, fifth ed. Mosby Elsevier, PA: Philadelphia.

Wasserman, K., Hansen, J.E., Sue, D.Y., et al., 2005. Principles of Exercise Testing and Interpretation: Pathophysiology and Clinical Applications. Lippincott Williams & Wilkins, MD, USA.

Waters, E., de Silva-Sanigorski, A., Hall, B.J., et al., 2011. Interventions for preventing obesity in children. Cochrane Database Syst. Rev. (12), CD001871, doi:10.1002/14651858.CD001871.pub3.

Weber, B., 1990. Cardiac surgery and heart transplantation. In: Hudak, C., Gallo, B., Benz, J. (Eds.), Critical Care Nursing: A Holistic Approach, fifth ed. JB Lippincott, Philadelphia, PA.

Weiler, J.M., Bonini, S., Coifman, R., et al., 2007. American Academy of Allergy, Asthma & Immunology work group report: exercise-induced asthma. J. Allergy Clin. Immunol. 119 (6), 1349–1358.

Westerdahl, E., Lindmark, B., Eriksson, T., et al., 2005. Deep breathing exercises reduce atelectasis and improve pulmonary function after coronary artery bypass surgery. Chest 128, 3482–3488.

Wheatley, C.M., Wilkins, B.W., Snyder, E.M., 2011. Exercise is medicine in cystic fibrosis. Exerc. Sport Sci. Rev. 39 (3), 155–160.

Whitaker, R.C., Wright, J.A., Pepe, M.S., et al., 1997. Predicting obesity in young adulthood from childhood and parental obesity. N. Engl. J. Med. 337 (13), 869–873.

White, H., Baker, A., 2002. Continuous jugular venous oximetry in the neurointensive care unit: a brief review. Neuroanesth. Intensive Care 49 (6), 623–629.

Whitney, J., Harden, B., Keilty, S., 2002. Assisted cough: a new technique. Physiotherapy 88 (4), 201–207.

Whittom, F., Jobin, J., Simard, P.M., et al., 1998. Histochemical and morphological characteristics of the vastus lateralis muscle in patients with chronic obstructive pulmonary disease. Med. Sci. Sports Exerc. 30, 1467–1474.

WHO, 2010. Global Recommendations on Physical Activity for Health. World Health Organization, Geneva.

Wickerson, L., Mathur, S., Brooks, D., 2010. Exercise training after lung transplantation: a systematic review. J. Heart Lung Transplant. 29, 497–503.

Wicks, A., Menter, R., 1986. Long-term outlook in quadriplegic patients with initial ventilator dependency. Chest 3, 406–410.

Wilkes, D., Schneiderman-Walker, J., Corey, M., 2007. Long-term effect of habitual physical activity on lung health in patients with cystic fibrosis. Pediatr. Pulmonol. 42 (S30), 358–359.

Williams, P., 1990. Use of intermittent stretch in the prevention of serial sarcomere loss in immobilised muscle. Ann. Rheum. Dis. 49, 316–317.

Williams, C.A., Benden, C., Stevens, D., Radtke, T., 2010. Exercise training in children and adolescents with cystic fibrosis: theory into practice. Int. J. Pediatr. 2010, 1–7.

Williams, T.J., Patterson, G.A., McClean, P.A., et al., 1992. Maximal exercise testing in single and double lung transplant recipients. Am. Rev. Respir. Dis. 145, 101–105.

Williams, C.A., Stevens, D., 2013. Physical activity and exercise training in young people with cystic fibrosis: current recommendations and evidence. J. Sport Health Sci. 2, 39–46.

Winck, J.C., Goncalves, M.R., Lourenco, C., et al., 2004. Effects of mechanical insufflation-exsufflation on respiratory parameters for patients with chronic airway secretion encumbrance. Chest 126, 774–780.

Winkelman, C., 2004. Inactivity and inflammation: selected cytokines as biologic mediators in muscle dysfunction during critical illness. AACN Clin. Issues 15, 74–82.

Winkelman, C., Higgins, P.A., Chen, Y.J., et al., 2007. Cytokines in chronically critically ill patients after activity and rest. Biol. Res. Nurs. 8, 261–271.

Winninghan, M.L., MacVicar, M.G., 1988. The effect of aerobic exercise on patient reports of nausea. Oncol. Nurs. Forum 15, 447–450.

Winslow, C., Bode, R.K., Felton, D., et al., 2002. Impact of respiratory complications on length of stay and hospital costs in acute cervical spine injury. Chest 121, 1548–1554.

Winter, C., Müller, C., Brandes, M., et al., 2009. Level of activity in children undergoing cancer treatment. Pediatr. Blood Cancer 53 (3), 438–443.

Wolfe, L.F., 2013. Point: should phrenic nerve stimulation be the treatment of choice for spinal cord injury? Yes. Chest 143 (5), 1201–1203.

Wong, S.L., Shem, K., Crew, J., 2012. Specialized respiratory management of acute cervical spinal cord injury: a retrospective analysis. Top. Spinal Cord Inj. Rehabil. 18 (4), 283–290.

World Health Organisation, 2011. Global Burden of Disease Report <http://www.who.int/healthinfo/global_burden_disease/en>.

World Health Organization, 2015. Cancer, Fact sheet N°297 [Online]. Available: <http://www.who.int/mediacentre/factsheets/fs297/en/index.html>.

Wright, P., 1984. Fundamentals of acute burn care and physical therapy management. Phys. Ther. 64, 1217–1231.

Wright, C.D., 2003. Minitracheostomy. Clin. Chest Med. 24, 431–435.

Wu, L.J., Wu, M.S., Lien, G.S., et al., 2011. Fatigue and physical activity levels in patients with liver cirrhosis. J. Clin. Nurs. 21, 129–138.

Wyndaele, M., Wyndaele, J.J., 2006. Incidence, prevalence and epidemiology of spinal cord injury: what learns a worldwide literature survey? Spinal Cord 44, 523–529.

Yamamoto, Y., Enkhbaatar, P., Sousse, L.E., et al., 2012. Nebulization with gamma-tocopherol ameliorates acute lung injury after burn and smoke inhalation in the ovine model. Shock 37 (4), 408–414.

Yardley, C.P., Fitzsimons, C.L., Weaver, L.C., 1989. Cardiac and peripheral vascular contributions to hypotension in spinal cats. Am. J. Physiol. 257, H1347–H1353.

Yeo, J.D., Walsh, J., Rutkowski, S., et al., 1998. Mortality following spinal cord injury. Spinal Cord 36, 329–336.

Yugue, I., Okada, S., Ueta, T., et al., 2012. Analysis of the risk factor for tracheostomy in traumatic cervical spinal cord injury. Spine 37, E1633–E1638.

Yung, G.L., Kriett, J.M., Jamieson, S.W., et al., 2001. Outpatient inhaled nitric oxide in a patient with idiopathic pulmonary fibrosis: a bridge to lung transplantation. J. Heart Lung Transplant. 20, 1224–1227.

Zan Zellar, M., Caetano, P., Amorim, A., et al., 2012. Pulmonary rehabilitation in patients with bronchiectasis: pulmonary function, arterial blood gases and the 6-minute walk test. J. Cardiopulm. Rehabil. 32, 278–283.

Zupan, A., Savrin, R., Erjavec, T., et al., 1997. Effects of respiratory muscle training and electrical stimulation of abdominal muscles on respiratory capabilities in tetraplegic patients. Spinal Cord 35, 540–545.

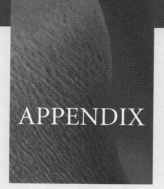

APPENDIX

NORMAL VALUES, CONVERSION TABLE AND ABBREVIATIONS

NORMAL VALUES

Age Group	Heart Rate Mean (range) (beats/min)	Respiratory Rate (range) (breaths/min)	Blood Pressure Systolic/Diastolic (mmHg)
Preterm	150 (100–200)	40–60	39–59/16–36
New-born	140 (80–200)	30–50	50–70/25–45
<2 years	130 (100–190)	20–40	87–105/53–66
>2 years	80 (60–140)	20–40	95–105/53–66
>6 years	75 (60–90)	15–30	97–112/57–71
Adults	70 (50–100)	12–16	95–140/60–90

Arterial Blood

pH	7.35–7.45 [H^+] 45–35 nmol/L
PaO_2	10.7–13.3 kPa (80–100 mmHg)
$PaCO_2$	4.7–6.0 kPa (35–45 mmHg)
HCO_3^-	22–26 mmol/L
Base excess	−2 to +2

Venous Blood

pH	7.31–7.41 [H^+] 46–38 nmol/L
PO_2	5.0–5.6 kPa (37–42 mmHg)
PCO_2	5.6–6.7 kPa (42–50 mmHg)

Ventilation/Perfusion

Alveolar–Arterial Oxygen Gradient (A–aPO$_2$):

Breathing air	0.7–2.7 kPa (5–20 mmHg)
Breathing 100% oxygen	3.3–8.6 kPa (25–65 mmHg)

757

Pressures

		mmHg	kPa
Right atrial (RA) pressure	Mean	−1–+7	−0.13 to 0.93
Right ventricular (RV) pressure	Systolic	15–25	2.0–3.3
	Diastolic	0–8	0–1.0
Pulmonary artery (PA) pressure	Systolic	15–25	2.0–3.3
	Diastolic	8–15	1.0–2.0
	Mean	10–20	1.3–2.7
Pulmonary capillary wedge pressure (PCWP)	Mean	6–15	0.8–2.0
Central venous pressure (CVP)		3–8	
Intracranial pressure (ICP)		<10	<1.3
Peak inspiratory mouth pressure (Pi_{max})	Male	103–124 cmH$_2$O (age dependent)	
	Female	65–87 cmH$_2$O (age dependent)	
Peak expiratory mouth pressure (Pe_{max})	Male	185–233 cmH$_2$O (age dependent)	
	Female	128–152 cmH$_2$O (age dependent)	

Blood Chemistry

Albumin	37–53 g/L
Calcium (Ca^{2+})	2.25–2.65 mmol/L
Creatinine	60–120 μmol/L
Glucose	4–6 mmol/L
Potassium (K$^+$)	3.4–5.0 mmol/L
Sodium (Na$^+$)	134–140 mmol/L
Urea	2.5–6.5 mmol/L
Haemoglobin (Hb)	14.0–18.0 g/100 mL (men), 11.5–15.5 g/100 mL (women)
Platelets	150–400 × 10^9/L
White blood cell count (WBC)	4–11 × 10^9/L
Urine output	1 mL/kg h^{-1}

CONVERSION TABLE

0.133 kPa = 1.0 mmHg

pH = 9 − log [H$^+$], where [H$^+$] is in nmol/L

kPa	mmHg	pH	[H$^+$]
1	7.5	7.52	30
2	15.0	7.45	35
4	30.0	7.40	40
6	45.0	7.35	45
8	60.0	7.30	50
10	75.0	7.26	55
12	90.0	7.22	60
14	105.0	7.19	65

ABBREVIATIONS

1RM	one repetition maximum
6MWD	6-minute walk distance
6MWT	6-minute walk test
A–a gradient	alveolar–arterial oxygen gradient
AACVPR	American Association of Cardiovascular and Pulmonary Rehabilitation
AAD	assisted autogenic drainage
AARC	American Association for Respiratory Care
ABCDE	airway, breathing, circulation, disability and exposure
ABG	arterial blood gas
ABI	ankle–brachial index
ABPA	allergic bronchopulmonary aspergillosis

ACBT	active cycle of breathing techniques	ASA	American Society of Anesthesiologists
ACC	American College of Cardiology	ASD	atrial septal defect
ACCP	American College of Clinical Pharmacy	ASIA	American Spinal Injury Association
ACE	angiotensin-converting enzyme	ASL	airway surface liquid
ACPICR	Association of Chartered Physiotherapists in Cardiac Rehabilitation	ATP	adenosine triphosphate
		ATS	American Thoracic Society
		AV	atrioventricular
ACSM	American College of Sports Medicine	AVAS	absolute visual analog scale
		a-vO$_{2diff}$	arteriovenous oxygen difference
ACT	airway clearance technique	AVR	aortic valve replacement
AD	autogenic drainage	AVSD	atrioventricular septal defect
ADH	anti-diuretic hormone	BAL	bronchoalveolar lavage
ADL	activity of daily living	BBB	blood–brain barrier
AECOPD	acute exacerbation chronic obstructive pulmonary disease	BC	breathing control
		BE	base excess
AED	automated external defibrillator	BiPAP	bi-level positive airway pressure
AF	atrial fibrillation	BiVAD	bi-ventricular assist device
AHA	American Heart Association	BLS	Basic Life Support
AHC	anterior horn cell	BMI	body mass index
AHRF	acute hypoxaemic respiratory failure	BNP	brain natriuretic peptide
		BOS	bronchiolitis obliterans syndrome
AIS	ASIA Impairment Scale	BP	blood pressure
ALI	acute limb ischaemia, acute lung injury	BPD	bronchopulmonary dysplasia
		bpm	beats per minute
ALL	acute lymphoblastic leukaemia	BSLTx	bilateral sequential lung transplantation
AMI	acute myocardial infarction		
AMP	adenosine monophosphate	Ca+	calcium ion
AMR	antibody-mediated humoral rejection	CABG	coronary artery bypass graft
		CAL	chronic airflow limitation
ANS	autonomic nervous system	CAM-ICU	Confusion Assessment Method for the ICU
AP	antero-posterior		
APACHE	Acute Physiology and Chronic Health Evaluation	CAV	cardiac allograft vasculopathy
		CBF	cerebral blood flow
APO	acute pulmonary oedema	CC	closing capacity
APRV	airway pressure release ventilation	CCS	Canadian Cardiovascular Society
AQoL, AQoL-8D	Assessment of Quality of Life	CDH	congenital diaphragmatic hernia
AR	aortic regurgitation	CF	cystic fibrosis
ARDS	acute respiratory distress syndrome	CFI	cardiac function index
		CFTR	cystic fibrosis transmembrane conductance regulator
ARVC	arrhythmogenic right ventricular dysplasia/ cardiomyopathy	CHD	congenital heart disease, coronary heart disease
AS	aortic stenosis	CHF	chronic heart failure

chILD	childhood interstitial lung disease	DC	direct current
CI	confidence interval	DCD	donation after cardiac death
CICR	calcium-induced calcium release	DCM	dilated cardiomyopathy
CIM	critical illness myopathy	DEMMI	de Morton mobility index
CIP	critical illness polyneuropathy	DEXA	dual-energy X-ray absorptiometry
CLD	chronic liver disease, chronic lung disease	DH	drug history
CLI	critical limb ischaemia	DKA	diabetic ketoacidosis
CMR	cardiac magnetic resonance	DMD	Duchenne muscular dystrophy
CMV	cytomegalovirus	dP	driving pressure
CO	cardiac output	DPG	diphosphoglycerate
CO_2	carbon dioxide	DRG	dorsal respiratory group
COAD	chronic obstructive airways disease	DVT	deep vein thrombosis
COLD	chronic obstructive lung disease	EBV	Epstein-Barr virus
COPD	chronic obstructive pulmonary disease	$ECCO_2R$	extracorporeal carbon dioxide removal
COSMIN	COnsensus-based Standards for the selection of health Measurement INstruments	ECG	electrocardiogram, electrocardiography
		ECMO	extracorporeal membrane oxygenation
COT	continuous oxygen therapy	EGDT	early goal-directed therapy
CPAP	continuous positive airway pressure	EIA	exercise-induced asthma
		EIB	exercise-induced bronchoconstriction
CPAx	Chelsea Critical Care Physical Assessment Tool	EMG	electromyography
		EMS	electrical muscle stimulation
CPB	cardiopulmonary bypass	EORTC QLQ-C30	European Organization for Research and Treatment of Cancer Quality of Life Questionnaire
CPET, CPEX	cardiopulmonary exercise test		
CPF	cough peak flow		
CPG	central pattern generator		
CPP	cerebral perfusion pressure	EPAP	expiratory positive airway pressure
CR	cardiac rehabilitation		
CRQ	Chronic Respiratory Disease Questionnaire	EPP	equal pressure point
		EPS	electrophysiological study
CRT	capillary refill time, cardiac resynchronization therapy	EQ-5D	EuroQol five dimensions questionnaire
CSF	cerebrospinal fluid	ERAS	enhanced recovery after surgery
CT	computed tomography	ERCP	endoscopic retrograde cholangiopancreatography
CTPA	computed tomographic pulmonary angiography		
		ERS	European Respiratory Society
CVD	cardiovascular disease	ERV	expiratory reserve volume
CVP	central venous pressure	ESWT	endurance shuttle walk test
$\dot{D}O_2$	oxygen delivery	ET	endotracheal
DB/HVS	dysfunctional breathing/ hyperventilation syndrome	ETT	endotracheal tube, exercise tolerance test
DB	dysfunctional breathing	EVAR	endovascular aneurysm repair
DBE	deep breathing exercise	EVLWI	extravascular lung water index

EWS	Early Warning Scores	HFCFC	high-frequency chest wall compression
FAB	Functional Assessment for Burns	HFCWO	high frequency chest wall oscillation
FBC	fluid balance chart	HFNC	high-flow nasal cannula
FDG	$[^{18}F]$fluorodeoxyglucose		
FEF_{25-75}	forced expiratory flow at 25–75% of forced vital capacity	HFnlEF	heart failure with normal ejection fraction
FET	forced expiration technique	HFNP	high flow nasal prong
FEV_1	forced expiratory volume in 1 second	HFOO	high-frequency oral oscillation
		HFOV	high-frequency oscillatory ventilation
FG	French gauge		
FH	family history	HFpEF	heart failure with preserved ejection fraction
FHF	fulminant hepatic failure		
FIM	Functional Independence Measure	HFrEF	heart failure with reduced ejection fraction
FiO_2	fraction of inspired oxygen, inspired oxygen concentration	HiPEP	high-pressure positive expiratory pressure
FITT	frequency, intensity, time and type	HIV	human immunodeficiency virus
		HME	heat and moisture exchanger
FOB	fibre-optic bronchoscopy	HPC	history of presenting condition
FRC	functional residual capacity	HPS	hepatopulmonary syndrome
FSS-ICU	Functional Status Score for the Intensive Care Unit	HPV	hypoxic pulmonary vasoconstriction
FVC	forced vital capacity	HR	heart rate
GA	general anaesthesia, gestational age	HRCT	high-resolution computed tomography
GAP	gravity-assisted positioning	HR_{max}	maximal heart rate
GCS	Glasgow Coma Scale	HRQoL	health related quality of life
GET	gas exchange threshold	HRR	heart rate reserve
GIQoL	Gastrointestinal Quality of Life Index	HRS	hepatorenal syndrome
		I : E ratio	ratio of inspiratory to expiratory time
GOR	gastro-oesophageal reflux		
GPB	glossopharyngeal breathing	IABP	intra-aortic balloon pump
GUCH	grown-up congenital heart disease	IASP	International Association for the Study of Pain
H+	hydrogen ion	ICC	intercostal catheter
H_2O	water	ICD	implantable cardioverter–defibrillator, intercostal drain
HAART	highly active anti-retroviral therapy	ICF	International Classification of Functioning, Disability and Health
Hb	haemoglobin		
$HbCO_2$	carbaminohaemoglobin		
HCM	hypertrophic cardiomyopathy	ICP	intracranial pressure
HCO_3^-	bicarbonate concentration	ICU	intensive care unit
HCP	healthcare professional	ICU-AW	intensive care unit–acquired weakness
HDL	high-density lipoprotein		
HFCC	high-frequency chest compression	IgE	immunoglobulin E
		IHD	ischaemic heart disease

IL	interleukin (IL-1, -6, etc)
ILD	interstitial lung disease
IMA	internal mammary artery
IMT	inspiratory muscle training
INR	International Normalized Ratio
IPAP	inspiratory positive airway pressure
IPAQ	International Physical Activity Questionnaire
IPF	idiopathic pulmonary fibrosis
IPPB	intermittent positive pressure breathing
IPPV	intermittent positive pressure ventilation
IPV	intrapulmonary percussive ventilation
IRDS	infant respiratory distress syndrome
IRN	ICU Recovery Network
IR-PEP	inspiratory resistance-positive expiratory pressure
IRV	inspiratory reserve volume
IS	incentive spirometry
ISWT	incremental shuttle walk test
ITBVI	intrathoracic blood volume index
IUGR	intrauterine growth restriction
IV	intravenous
IVH	intraventricular haemorrhage
IWQoL-Lite	Impact of Weight on Quality of Life-Lite
JVP	jugular venous pressure
K+	potassium ion
KDQoL	Kidney Disease Quality of Life
LAD	left anterior descending
LIP	lower inflection point
LLQ	left lower quadrant
LMWH	low–molecular-weight heparin
LOS	length of stay
LTOT	long-term oxygen therapy
LUQ	left upper quadrant
LVAD	left ventricular assist device
LVEF	left ventricular ejection fraction
LVH	left ventricular hypertrophy
LVRS	lung volume reduction surgery
MAP	mean arterial pressure

MAPCA	major aortopulmonary collateral artery
MAS	meconium aspiration syndrome
MBTS	modified Blalock–Taussig shunt
MCC	mucociliary clearance
MCT	mucociliary transport
MD	mean difference
MDCT	multi-detector computed tomography
MDT	multidisciplinary team
MEP	maximal expiratory pressure
MET	metabolic equivalent of task
MGS	Melbourne Group Scale
MHI	manual hyperinflation
MI	myocardial infarction
MID	minimal important difference
Mini-AQLQ	Mini-Asthma Quality of Life Questionnaire
MIP	maximal inspiratory pressure
MIP$_{uni}$	maximal inspiratory pressure measured with a univalve
MoCA	Montreal Cognitive Assessment
mPD&P	modified postural drainage and percussion
mPD	modified postural drainage
MR	mitral regurgitation
MRA	magnetic resonance angiography
MRC	Medical Research Council
MRC-SS	Medical Research Council Sum-score
MRI	magnetic resonance imaging
MRSA	methicillin-resistant *Staphylococcus aureus*
MS	mitral stenosis
MSE	muscle strength endurance
MVO_2	myocardial oxygen consumption
MVV	maximum voluntary ventilation
MWST	modified shuttle walk test
Na$^+$	sodium ion
NG	nasogastric
NHP	Nottingham Health Profile
NIBP	non-invasive blood pressure
NICE	National Institute of Health and Care Excellence
NICU	neonatal intensive care unit
NIPPV	non-invasive positive pressure ventilation

NIV	non-invasive ventilation
NJ	nasojejunostomy
NMES	neuromuscular electrical stimulation
NNU	neonatal unit
NO	nitric oxide
NPPV	non-invasive positive pressure ventilation
NRS	numerical rating scale
NSAID	non-steroidal anti-inflammatory drug
NSCLC	non–small cell lung cancer
NSTEMI	non–ST-segment elevation myocardial infarction
NYHA	New York Heart Association
O_2	oxygen
OHS	open heart surgery
OI	oxygenation index
OP	off-pump
OPCAB	off-pump coronary artery bypass
OPCPB	off-pump cardiopulmonary bypass
OPEP	oscillating positive expiratory pressure
OR	odds ratio
OSA	obstructive sleep apnoea
PA	postero-anterior
$PaCO_2$	alveolar partial pressure of carbon dioxide
$PaCO_2$	partial pressure of carbon dioxide in arterial blood
PACS	picture archiving and communication systems
PAD	peripheral artery disease
PAF	paroxysmal atrial fibrillation
PAH	pulmonary arterial hypertension
PAL	persistent air leak
PALISI	Pediatric Acute Lung Injury and Sepsis Investigators
PaO_2	partial pressure of oxygen in arterial blood
PAOP	pulmonary artery occlusion pressure
PAPVC	partial anomalous pulmonary venous connection

PASE	Physical Activity Scale for the Elderly
PCA	patient-controlled analgesia
PCD	primary ciliary dyskinesia
PCF	peak cough flow
PCI	percutaneous coronary intervention
PC–IRV	pressure control–inverse ratio ventilation
PCO_2	partial pressure of carbon dioxide
pCPAP	periodic continuous positive airway pressure
PCV	pressure control ventilation
PD&P	postural drainage and percussion
PD	postural drainage
PDA	patent ductus arteriosus
Pdi	trans-diaphragmatic pressure
PE	pulmonary embolism
PEDI	Paediatric Evaluation of Disability Inventory
PEDro	physiotherapy evidence database
PEEP	positive end-expiratory pressure
PEF	peak expiratory flow
PEG	percutaneous endoscopic gastrostomy
PEmax or MEP	maximum expiratory pressure
PEP	positive expiratory pressure
PERL	pupils equal and reactive to light
PET	positron emission tomography
PFIT-s	Physical Function in Intensive Care Test-scored
PFO	patent foramen ovale
Pi	pulmonary interstitial pressure
PICC	peripherally inserted central catheter
PICS	post intensive care syndrome
PICU	paediatric intensive care unit
PIE	pulmonary interstitial emphysema
PIF	peak inspiratory flow rate
Pi_{max}	maximal inspiratory pressure
Pip	intrapleural pressure
PIP	positive inspiratory pressure
PLT	postero-lateral thoracotomy

PMH	previous medical history	SBOT	short burst oxygen therapy
PND	paroxysmal nocturnal dyspnoea	SBP	systolic blood pressure
PNS	parasympathetic nervous system	SCD	sudden cardiac death
PO_2	partial pressure of oxygen	SCI	spinal cord injury
PPC	postoperative pulmonary complication	SF-12	Short-Form 12
		SF-36	Short-Form 36
PPM	permanent pacemaker	SGA	small for gestational age
Ppul – Pip	transpulmonary pressure	SH	social history
Ppul	intrapulmonary pressure	SIMV	synchronized intermittent mandatory ventilation
PR	pulmonary regurgitation; pulmonary rehabilitation	SIP	sickness impact profile
PRVC	pressure-regulated volume control	SIRS	systemic inflammatory response syndrome
PT	physiotherapist	SIS	Sternal Instability Scale
$PvCO_2$	partial pressure of venous carbon dioxide	$SjvO_2$	jugular venous saturation of oxygen
PVH	periventricular haemorrhage	SLTx	single lung transplantation
PVL	periventricular leucomalacia	SMA	spinal muscular atrophy
PVO_2	partial pressure of venous oxygen	SMART	specific, measurable, attainable, realistic and time based
$\dot{Q}$	perfusion	SNS	sympathetic nervous system
QOL	quality of life	SOB	shortness of breath
RASS	Richmond Agitation Sedation Scale	SpO_2	oxyhaemoglobin saturation by pulse oximeter
RBC	red blood cell	SRT	steep ramp test
RCC	respiratory control centre	STEMI	ST-segment elevation myocardial infarction
RCT	randomized controlled trial		
RDS	respiratory distress syndrome	STOT	short-term oxygen therapy
REM	rapid eye movement	SV	stroke volume
RER	respiratory exchange ratio	SVC	superior vena cava
RFA	radiofrequency ablation	SVRI	systemic vascular resistance index
rhDNase	recombinant human deoxyribonuclease	TAPVC	total anomalous pulmonary venous connection
RLQ	right lower quadrant		
RM	repetition maximum	TASC	Trans-Atlantic Inter-Society Consensus
ROM	range of motion		
RPE	rating of perceived exertion	TAVI	transcatheter aortic valve implantation
RPP	rate pressure product		
RR	respiratory rate	TB	tuberculosis
RSV	respiratory syncytial virus	TBB	transbronchial biopsy
RUQ	right upper quadrant	TBI	traumatic brain injury
RV	residual volume	TBSA	total body surface area
SA	sino-atrial	TEE	thoracic expansion exercise
SABA	short-acting β-agonist	TENS	transcutaneous electrical nerve stimulation
SaO_2	oxyhaemoglobin saturation by arterial blood gas		
SAQ	Seattle Angina Questionnaire	TGA	transposition of the great arteries

TIPS	transjugular intrahepatic portosystemic shunt	VCV	volume control/cycled ventilation
TLC	total lung capacity	V_D	dead space volume
TL_{CO}	transfer factor for carbon monoxide	$V_D{:}V_T$	dead space to tidal volume ratio
TOE	transoesophageal echocardiogram	VDS	verbal descriptor scale
		V_E	expiratory volume
TPN	total parenteral nutrition	VF	ventricular fibrillation
TR	tricuspid regurgitation	VHI	ventilator hyperinflation
TTE	transthoracic echocardiogram	VILI	ventilator induced lung injury
UAP	unstable angina pectoris	VO_2	rate of oxygen consumption
UAS	upper abdominal surgery	VO_{2max}	maximal oxygen consumption
UWSD	underwater sealed drainage	VO_{2peak}	peak oxygen consumption
$\dot{V}$	ventilation	VO_2R	oxygen consumption reserve
$\dot{V}_A$	alveolar ventilation	VR	venous return
$\dot{V}_E$	minute ventilation	VRG	ventral respiratory group
$\dot{V}/\dot{Q}$	ventilation–perfusion	VSD	ventricular septal defect
VAD	ventricular assist device	V_T	tidal volume
VAE	ventilator-associated event	VT	ventricular tachycardia
VAP	ventilator-associated pneumonia	VTE	venous thromboembolism
		W	watt
VAS	visual analogue scale	WBC	white blood cell
VATS	video-assisted thoracic surgery	WBV	whole body vibration
		WeeFIM	Functional Independence Measure for Children
VC	vital capacity	WHO	World Health Organization
VCO_2	volume of carbon dioxide	WHOQoL-BREF	WHO Quality of Life-BREF

INDEX

Page numbers followed by '*f*' indicate figures, '*b*' indicate boxes, and '*t*' indicate tables.

A

AAD. *see* Assisted autogenic drainage (AAD)
AARC. *see* American Association for Respiratory Care (AARC)
Abdomen
 assessment, 70
 co-contraction of, 374*f*, 376–377
Abdominal aortic aneurysm surgery, 555*t*–557*t*
Abdominal binders, 678–679, 679*f*
Abdominal distension, 56
Abdominal injury, 702–703, 703*f*–704*f*
 management of, precautions and contraindications to, 705*b*
Abdominal movement, 56–57
Abdominal muscles, 371–372
Abdominal palpation, 70
Abdominal surgery, 526–527, 528*b*–531*b*, 555*t*–557*t*
 physiotherapy evidence in, 532
Abdomino-perineal resection, 528*t*–531*t*
Absent breath sounds, 62*t*
Absolute visual analogue scale (AVAS), 358
Acapella
 clinical application of, 282
 for oscillating PEP, 279, 282, 283*f*–284*f*
ACBT. *see* Active cycle of breathing techniques (ACBT)
Accelerometers, 226
Acceptance, end stage of life, 410
Accessory inspiratory muscle, 57
Accessory muscles, 9
 of inspiration, 13
ACCP. *see* American College of Clinical Pharmacy (ACCP)
ACE inhibitors. *see* Angiotensin-converting enzyme (ACE) inhibitors
Acquired heart disease, 718–719

Active cycle of breathing techniques (ACBT), 266–270, 267*f*
 breathing control, 266
 clinical application and evidence for, 269–270
 forced expiration technique, 268–269, 268*f*, 270*f*
 thoracic expansion exercises, 266–268
 see also individual techniques
Active recovery (AR) stations, 612
Activities of daily living (ADLs), in acute care, 217–218
Activity limitations, measurement of, 211–226
 exercise testing, 218–221
 field walking test, 221–223, 224*t*
 mobility and activities of daily living, 212*t*–216*t*, 217–218
 physical activity, 223–226
 physical function and mobility, 211–217, 212*t*–216*t*
 summary of, 226*b*
ACTs. *see* Airway clearance techniques (ACTs)
Acute aortic dissection, 152
Acute bronchiolitis, paediatrics, ventilation strategies for, 467–469, 468*b*
Acute cardiopulmonary dysfunction, improving oxygen transport in, 320–324, 321*t*
 mobilization, 322–324
 physiological and scientific rationale, 322–324
 positioning, 321–322
Acute coronary syndromes, 52*t*–54*t*, 128
Acute hypoxaemic respiratory failure, 458
 ventilation strategies for, 469
Acute laryngotracheobronchitis (croup), 494
Acute pain, definition of, 516

Acute rejection, 688–689, 689*f*, 689*t*
Acute respiratory distress syndrome (ARDS), 430–431
 in burn patients, 650
 diagnostic criteria for, 458
 pathogenesis of, 431
 radiographic appearance, 104, 105*f*
Acute respiratory failure
 in children, epidemiology of, 456–458
 non-invasive ventilation for, 299
 pattern and time course of, 457–458, 457*t*
Acutely Ill/deteriorating patient, 77–80
 action and communication in, 80
 assessment technique for, 77–80
 airway, 78
 breathing, 78–79
 circulation, 79
 disability, 79–80
 exposure, 80
AD. *see* Autogenic drainage (AD)
Adjunctive techniques, for incontinence management, 292
ADLs. *see* Activities of daily living (ADLs)
Adolescent(s), engagement with medical teams, 410–411
β_2-Adrenergic agonists, for asthma, 182–184
'Adult hyaline membrane disease.' *see* Acute respiratory distress syndrome (ARDS)
Aegophony, 61
Aerobic conditioning, 610–613, 611*b*, 612*t*
Aerobic exercise, for burn patients, 656*b*
Aerobika, 279
Air bronchogram, 95
Air entrainment mask, 329–330
Air entrainment nebulizer, 330
'Air hunger', 186
Air pollution, height and exposure to, child *vs.* adult, 38

Airflow limitation
  chronic, 106–108
  clinical signs of, 17
  in COPD, 165–167, 166f–167f, 168t
  problems associated with, 17
  reversal of, 17–18
Airway(s)
  assessment, 54–55
  diameter, child *vs*. adult, 36
  innervation, 16
  moisture to, increased, in critically ill
    patients, 426–429
Airway clearance, impaired, 198–199, 199b
Airway clearance techniques (ACTs),
    250–292
  for babies and children, 253–254,
    254f–255f
  in complex patients, 175–176
  for COPD, 169
  for cystic fibrosis, 175–177
    infants and young children, 175
  device-dependent, 274–284
  independently performed, 266–291
  machine-dependent, 284–291
  manual, 252–254, 258–265
    chest percussion/clapping, 259–261,
      260f, 261b
    clinical application and evidence for,
      264–265
    contraindications and precautions
      for, 265b
    for musculoskeletal dysfunction,
      355–366, 357f–358f
    shaking, chest compression and rib
      springing, 263–265
    suction, 265–266
    vibrations/chest shaking and
      compression, 261–263, 262f–263f,
      263b
  modified postural drainage, 255–258,
    255f–257f, 258t
  mucociliary clearance and, 250
  postural drainage, 255–258, 255f–257f,
    258t
  traditional, 252–254
  see also individual technique
Airway disease, 115–123
Airway management, for spinal cord
    injury, 679–680
  extubation, 679
  speech options with tracheostomy, 680
  tracheostomy, 679–680
  tracheostomy decannulation, 680
  from ventilation, 679–680
Airway pressure release ventilation
    (APRV), 416

Airway resistance, 16–18
  highest, site of, 16
  increased, consequences of, 17
Airway suction. *see* Suction, airway
Aldosterone, 45
Allografts, for burn, 647t–648t
Alveolar dead space, 25
Alveolar interdependence, 267f
Alveolar membrane
  surface area of, 28
  thickness of, 28
Alveolar ventilation, 25–26
Alveoli, child *vs*. adult, 36–37
Ambulatory oxygen
  in conjunction with COT, 333
  domiciliary, 326t, 333
American Association for Respiratory
    Care (AARC), on nasopharyngeal
    suctioning, 266
American College of Clinical Pharmacy
    (ACCP), 220–221
American Spinal Injury Association (ASIA)
    Impairment Scale (AIS), 669, 670f–671f
    International Standards Worksheet,
      670f–671f
Anaesthesia
  epidural, 521f
  general, 515–516
  induction of, 515–516
  spinal, 521f
Analgesia
  epidural, 519
  multimodal, 519
  patient-controlled, 517t, 519
  physiotherapy keypoints with regard to,
    522b
  pre-emptive, 515
Anatomical dead space, 25
Anger, end stage of life, 410
Angina, 52t–54t
Angiography, in paediatrics, 110
Angiotensin I, 45
Angiotensin II, 45
Angiotensin II receptor blockers, for
    ischaemic heart disease, 131t
Angiotensin-converting enzyme (ACE)
    inhibitors, for ischaemic heart
    disease, 131t
Anterior resection, 528f
Anterior-stretch basal lift, 374f, 375
Anthropometry, in muscle measurement,
    201–202
Antiarrhythmic medications, 149t
Antibiotics
  for bronchiectasis, 171
  for cystic fibrosis, 174–175

Anticoagulants, for ischaemic heart
    disease, 131t
Anti-contracture positions, 656, 657t
Antiplatelet agents, for ischaemic heart
    disease, 131t
Anxiety, 409, 409f
Aorta, coarctation of, 499
Aortic aneurysm, 52t–54t
  abdominal, surgery for, 555t–557t
  thoracoabdominal, repair of, 555t–557t
Aortic arch, interrupted, 502
Aortic disease, 152–154
  aetiology and pathophysiology of, 152
  classification of, 153
  diagnosis of, 153
  medical management of, 153–154
  physiotherapy-specific management of,
    154
  symptoms and signs of, 152–153
Aortic dissection, acute, 152
Aortic opening, diaphragm and, 11
Aortic regurgitation, 133
  medical management of, 136
  symptoms and signs of, 134
Aortic stenosis, 133, 502
  medical management of, 136
  symptoms and signs of, 134
Aortic valve surgery, 547
Apneustic breathing, 58t–59t, 59f
Apnoea, 58f, 58t–59t
APRV. *see* Airway pressure release
    ventilation (APRV)
Aqueous (sol) layer, of mucociliary
    transport system, 15
ARDS. *see* Acute respiratory distress
    syndrome (ARDS)
Arrhythmias, cardiac, 147–150, 147b
  aetiology and pathophysiology of,
    147–148, 147t
  classification of, 148
  diagnosis of, 148, 148b, 149f
  medical management of, 148–149, 148b,
    149t
  physiotherapy-specific management of,
    149–150
  symptoms and signs of, 148
Arrhythmogenic right ventricular
    dysplasia/cardiomyopathy (ARVC),
    138
Arterial blood, reference ranges for, 326t
Arterial blood gases
  assessment of, 63, 63t
  in critically ill patient, 419
Arterial blood pressure, critically ill
    patient, 419–420
Arterial oxygen tension, 322

Arteries, 40
ARVC. *see* Arrhythmogenic right ventricular dysplasia/cardiomyopathy (ARVC)
Ascites, in liver disease, 661
ASD. *see* Atrial septal defect (ASD)
ASIA. *see* American Spinal Injury Association (ASIA)
Aspiration pneumonia, radiographic appearance, 104
Assessment, patient, 47–82
    cardiac rehabilitation, 615–616, 617t–622t
    documentation in, 71–73, 73f
    functional ability, 51, 68–69
    information gathering, 48
    information used in, 71
    objective, 51–71, 73f
        airway, 54–55
        breathing, 55–64, 55f
        circulation, 64–65
        disability, 67–69
        exposure, 69–71
    outcome evaluation in, 73
    quality of life, 69, 228t–232t
    subjective, 48–51, 52t–54t, 73f
    thoracic organ transplantation, 684–685, 685b
Assisted autogenic drainage (AAD), 271–274
Asthma, 182–185, 491
    aetiology of, 182
    in children, 712–715
    clinical features of, 182
    diagnosis/investigations of, 182
    exercise training and, 593
    medical management of, 182–184, 183t
    pathophysiology of, 182
        pathological changes consequences, 182
    physiotherapy management of, 184–185
        breathing techniques, 185
        education, 184, 184f
        exercise, 184–185
    radiographic appearance, 113f, 120
'Asthma Management Plans', 182–184
Asymmetry, of chest, 56
Ataxic breathing, 58t–59t, 59f
Atelectasis, radiographic appearance, 95–97, 97b
    fissure shift, 97
    individual lobes, 97–99
    in paediatrics, 112, 113f
    postoperative, 104
Atherosclerosis, 127
'Atmospheric pressure', 13

Atrial septal defect (ASD), 499
Atrioventricular septal defect (AVSD), 500
Attention Screening Examination, 202–204
Auscultation, 60–61, 198–199
    of infant and child, 76
    in major burn/smoke inhalation patients, 653–654
Autogenic drainage (AD), 271–274, 271f, 272t, 273f
Autonomic nervous system, spinal cord injury and, impact on respiration, 670–671
AVAS. *see* Absolute visual analogue scale (AVAS)
AVSD. *see* Atrioventricular septal defect (AVSD)

B
Bacterial infection, in children, radiographic appearance, 111f, 118
Balance training, 590
Bargaining, end stage of life, 410
Bariatric surgery, 527–532
Barium studies, children, 110–111
Barrel chest, in patients with COPD, 167
Beating heart bypass surgery, 548
Berg balance scale, 217
Bicarbonate, carbon dioxide as, 33
Bi-level positive airway pressure (BiPAP), 416, 417f
    in children, 472
    hypoxia, 459
Bi-level ventilation, 416
Bilobectomy, 535t–536t
Biobrane, 647t–648t
Biots breathing, 58f, 58t–59t
BiPAP. *see* Bi-level positive airway pressure (BiPAP)
Biphasic positive airway pressure, 416, 417f
Bird Mark 7 ventilator, 293f, 294
β-Blockers, for ischaemic heart disease, 131t
Blood glucose, assessment, 68
Blood pressure (BP), 44
    assessment, 66
    auto regulation of, 45–46
'Blue dye' test, 447
Body composition analysis, in muscle measurement, 200–201
Body structure/functions level, measurement of impairment at, 198–211

Body systems, monitoring of, critically ill patient, 419–423
    cardiovascular system, 419–420
    neurological system, 420–423
    respiratory system, 419
Body temperature, assessment, 65–66
Body weight, assessment, 70–71
BOS. *see* Bronchiolitis obliterans syndrome (BOS)
'Bovine', 50
Bowel sounds, assessment, 70
BP. *see* Blood pressure (BP)
Bradypnoea, 58f, 58t–59t
Brain centres, higher, 20
Brain death, 686–687
Brain injury, 433–435
Breath sounds
    absent, 62t
    assessment of, 60, 62t
    bronchial, 62t
    normal, 62t
    reduced, 62t
Breath stacking, 678
    abdominal binders, 678–679, 679f
    glossopharyngeal breathing, 678
Breathing
    assessment, 55–64, 55f
    control of, 19–23
    origin of, 19
    see also Respiration
Breathing control (BC), 266
    for dyspnoea, 350–354, 351f–352f
    while stair climbing, 354, 354f
Breathing patterns, 58t–59t
    child *vs.* adult, 39
Breathing techniques, 266–274
    active cycle of, 266–270
    assisted autogenic drainage, 271–274
    for asthma, 185
    autogenic drainage, 271–274, 271f, 272t, 273f
        clinical application and evidence for, 273–274
    postural drainage and, 250
    pulmonary rehabilitation, 596
Breathlessness
    assessment, 49, 64
    see also Dyspnoea
Bronchial arteriography, 90
Bronchial breath sounds, 62t
Bronchial fremitus, 60
Bronchial mucosa, in chronic bronchitis, 165f
Bronchial tree, 4–5
Bronchial walls, child *vs.* adult, 36

Bronchiectasis, 170–172
  aetiology of, 170
  clinical features of, 170–171
  diagnosis/investigations of, 171
  medical management of, 171–172
  non-CF, in children, 715–716
  pathophysiology of, 170, 170f
  physiotherapy management of, 172
    excess bronchial secretions, 172
    exercise training, 172
  radiographic appearance, 106, 107f, 121,
    123f
  rehabilitation for, 592–593
  vicious cycle of, 170f
Bronchiole response, 30–31
Bronchiolitis, 493
  acute, paediatrics, ventilation strategies
    for, 467–469, 468b
Bronchiolitis obliterans syndrome (BOS),
  121, 689–690
Bronchoconstriction, exercise induced,
  712–714
Bronchodilators, 340–341
  for asthma, 182–184
  for bronchiectasis, 171
Bronchophony, 61
Bronchopulmonary dysplasia, 484–485,
  494–495
  physiotherapy for, 495
Bronchopulmonary segments, 6–7
Bubble/bottle positive expiratory pressure,
  279–284, 285f
'Bucket handle movement', 9, 11f
Bupivacaine, 518t–519t
Burkholderia cepacia, 173
Burn
  acute management of, 641–658, 642t
  cardiorespiratory physiotherapy
    assessment, 653–654
    auscultation, 653–654
    cardiovascular system, 653
    core and peripheral temperature,
      653
    fluid balance, 653
    respiratory system, 653
  cardiorespiratory physiotherapy
    treatment of
    autografts to the chest wall, 654
    extubation, readiness for, 655
    pain control, 654
    self ventilating patients, 654–655
  classification of, 642–645, 643t
    full thickness burns, 643t, 644–645,
      644f–645f
    spontaneously healing wound,
      643–644, 644f

exercise prescription, 656–658, 656b,
  657t
pathophysiological response to major,
  645–650
  fluid shifts, 646–649
  hypermetabolism, 649
  systemic inflammatory response
    syndrome (SIRS), 649–650, 650f,
    651b
physical rehabilitation for, 655–658
smoke inhalation injury, 650–652
  chemical injury, 651
  management of, 652
  systemic intoxication, 651–652
surgery for, 645, 646f, 647t–648t
Burn shock, 646–649

C

CABG. see Coronary artery bypass
  grafting (CABG)
CABG surgery. see Coronary artery bypass
  grafting (CABG) surgery
Caffeine, 486
Calcium channel blockers, for ischaemic
  heart disease, 131t
CAM-ICU. see Confusion Assessment
  Method for the ICU (CAM-ICU)
Canadian Health Utilities Index (HUI),
  228t–232t
Canalicular period, lung, 34
Cancer
  definition of, 722
  diagnosis of, lack of physical activity
    after, 725–727, 725t, 726f–727f
  exercise prescription for, 730–731, 730t,
    732t
  exercise training for, 722–733
    delivery and timing of, 728–729
    evaluation of, 729–730, 729t–730t
    medical treatment of, and associated
      side effects, 723–725, 723t, 724f
  monitoring during exercise, 731
  physical activity, 722–723
    guidelines for, 727–728
  radiotherapy for, 724–725
  strategies for adherence to increased
    physical activity for individuals
    with, 731–733
Cancer cachexia, 725–726
Cannula(e)
  nasal, 328
    high-flow, 487
  reservoir, 328
Capillary refill time (CRT), assessment,
  64–65

Carbon dioxide (CO$_2$)
  as bicarbonate, 33
  haemoglobin and, 33
  partial pressure of, 659
  transport of, 33
Carbon dioxide pathway, 319
Carbon dioxide retention, 319
Carbon dioxide theory, 185, 185f
Carboxyhaemoglobin, 651
Cardiac allograft vasculopathy (CAV), 690
Cardiac arrhythmias, 147–150, 147b
  aetiology and pathophysiology of,
    147–148, 147t
  classification of, 148
  diagnosis of, 148, 148b, 149f
  medical management of, 148–149, 148b,
    149t
  physiotherapy-specific management of,
    149–150
  symptoms and signs of, 148
Cardiac catheterization, 129, 129b, 130f
  in paediatrics, 110
Cardiac cycle, 41–42
Cardiac denervation, 690–691
Cardiac failure. see Heart failure
Cardiac magnetic resonance imaging
  (CMR), 151b
Cardiac manifestations, of respiratory
  distress, in infant, 76
Cardiac output, child vs. adult, 39
Cardiac pacemaker, 150b
Cardiac pacemaker wire, 103
Cardiac rehabilitation, 597–638
  contemporary models to broaden
    delivery, emergence of, 603–604
  exercise prescription, 607–614
    cool-down, 613
    frequency of, 607–608
    heart rate, use of, 609
    intensity of, 608–610
    metabolic equivalent values (METs),
      use of, 609–610
    mode of, 608
    perceived exertion, rating of, 608–609
    principles of, 607, 608t
    progression of, 613–614
    resistance training, 608t, 613
    type of, 608, 610
    typical exercise session warm-up,
      format of, 610–613
  exercise training
    benefits of, 605–606
    in secondary prevention
      programmes, 604–605
    long-term community-based exercise
      provision, 626–627

past, present and future directions, 598–605, 599f
programme implementation, 614–627
  assessment and risk stratification, 615–616, 617t–622t
  exercise considerations, for special cardiac groups, 623–626, 624t–625t
  first 3 months, 615
  health and safety protocols, 623
  immediate post-discharge phase, 614–615
  in-hospital activity component, 614
  long-term community-based exercise provision, transition of, 626–627
  outcome measures, 623
  patient induction, 616–623
  patient supervision and staffing, for group exercise sessions, 616
  safe delivery and programme management, 616–623
  secondary prevention delivery, 599f, 601–603
  secondary prevention programmes availability, 601
  secondary prevention-evidence of effectiveness and, 600–601
Cardiac surgery, 540t–541t, 545–553, 560t–570t
  in children, 498
    closed procedures, 498–499
    open procedure, 499–502
    palliative procedures, 498
  definition of, 545–546
  haemodynamic management, 548–549
  physiotherapy evidence in, 550–553
    considerations for women undergoing cardiac surgery, 553, 553b
    postoperative exercise training, 550–551
    postoperative pulmonary complications, prevention of, 550, 551b
    sternal instability, 552–553, 552t, 553f
    sternal precautions, 551–552
  postoperative management in, 549
  post-sternotomy pain, 549–550
  sternal management, 550
  types of, 546
    minimally invasive heart surgery, 546
    open heart surgery, 546–549
  see also individual procedures
Cardiac valve abnormalities, 502–503
Cardiac valve disease, 132–137, 132b
  classification of, 136
  diagnosis of, 134–136, 134b, 135f

medical management of, 136–137, 136b
  physiotherapy-specific management of, 137
  right-sided, 133–134
    medical management of, 137
    symptoms and signs of, 134
  symptoms and signs of, 134
Cardiac valve prostheses, 547
Cardiogenic pulmonary oedema, non-invasive ventilation for, 300–301
Cardiomyopathy, 137–140, 137b
  aetiology and pathophysiology of, 137–138
  diagnosis of, 138–139
  dilated, 137–138
  hypertrophic, 138
  medical management of, 139–140, 139f
  physiotherapy-specific management of, 140
  restrictive, 138
  symptoms and signs of, 138
Cardiopulmonary bypass, 547–548
Cardiopulmonary dysfunction
  factors contributing to, 319b
  improving oxygen transport in acute, 320–324, 321t
    mobilization, 322–324
    positioning, 321–322
    post-acute, 324–325
    post-chronic, 324–325
Cardiopulmonary exercise test (CPET/CPEX), 218
  physiological measurements during, 220t
Cardiorespiratory fitness, 581
Cardio-respiratory illness, living with, 405–410
  emotional impact of, 407–410
    anxiety, 409, 409f
    depression, 409–410
    end stage of life, 410
  managing treatment regimens, 405–407
    collaborative care, 406
    role of parenting in, 406–407
    self-management, 406
  peer relationships, 407
  social relationships, 407
Cardiorespiratory physiotherapy practice, outcome measurement in, 195–247
Cardiovascular disease (CVD), field walking tests for, 224t
Cardiovascular system
  assessment of, in major burn/smoke inhalation patients, 653

monitoring of, in ICU patients, 419–420
  spinal cord injury and, impact on respiration, 670–671
Cardioverter defibrillator, implantation of, 625–626
'Carina', 4
Carpentier's pathophysiological triad, 133
Cause, illness representation, 404
CAV. see Cardiac allograft vasculopathy (CAV)
CEAs. see Cultured epithelial autografts (CEAs)
Central changes, in exercise training, 606
Central pattern generator (CPG), 366–367
Central venous pressure (CVP)
  assessment, 66
  critically ill patients, ICU, 420
Cerebral contusions, 658
Cerebral perfusion pressure (CPP), calculation of, 423b
CF. see Cystic fibrosis (CF)
CFTR. see Cystic fibrosis transmembrane conductance regulator (CFTR)
Chelsea Critical Care Physiotherapy Assessment Tool, 211
Chemical injury, 651
Chemoreceptors, 21
  central, 22
    COPD and, 22
    stimulation of, 22
  peripheral, 22
Chemotherapy, 724
  side effects of, 723t
Chest
  auscultation. see Auscultation
  congenital abnormalities of, 115–123
  expansion, 59, 59f
  flail, 57
  movement, 56–57
  neurophysiological facilitation for, 373t
  normal, 91–95, 91f
Chest clapping. see Chest percussion/clapping
Chest compression, 261–265, 262f–263f, 263b
Chest infection, readmission to hospital with, spinal cord injury and, 681
Chest pain
  assessment, 51
  differential diagnosis of, 52t–54t
  musculoskeletal, 174, 356
Chest percussion/clapping, 259–261, 260f, 261b
  in children, 477–479, 478f
  cystic fibrosis, 260, 264

Chest percussion/clapping *(Continued)*
  self, 259–260
  single-handed, 259–260, 260*f*
Chest radiograph, 84–90
  basic signs on plain, 111–114
  for bronchiectasis evaluation, 171
  children, 109
    signs, 95–103
  for emphysema, 166*f*
  factors influencing the quality of,
    84–85, 85*f*
  lateral decubitus view, 84
  lateral view of, 93–94, 93*f*
  lordotic view, 84
  types of, 84
  useful points in interpretation of, 94–95
    documentary information, 94
    inspiration/expiration, state of, 95
    patient rotation, 94–95
    radiograph projection, 94
    supine *vs.* prone position, 94
Chest shaking, 261–265, 262*f*–263*f*, 263*b*
Chest shape, child *vs.* adult, 35
Chest trauma, 536–537, 538*b*
  in ICU patients, 432, 434*f*
'Chest wall', 9
Chest wall vibrations, 261–263, 262*f*–263*f*,
  263*b*, 426
  in children, 477–479
Cheyne-Stokes breathing, 58*f*, 58*t*–59*t*
CHFQ. *see* Chronic heart failure
  questionnaire (CHFQ)
Children. *see* Paediatrics
Chronic graft dysfunction, 689–690
Chronic Heart Failure Questionnaire
  (CHFQ), 233*t*–236*t*
Chronic hyperventilation, 185
Chronic liver disease, 662–663
  physiotherapists, considerations for, 663
'Chronic lung disease (CLD)'. *see*
  Bronchopulmonary dysplasia
Chronic obstructive pulmonary disease
  (COPD), 164–170
  acute exacerbation of, 251, 264
  aetiology of, 164
  aims of rehabilitation in, 586–587
  airflow limitation in, 165–167,
    166*f*–167*f*, 168*t*
  central chemoreceptors and, 22
  clinical features of, 167–168
  co-morbid conditions in, 168
  diagnosis/investigations of, 166*f*, 168,
    168*t*
  dyspnoea in, 166
  field walking tests for, 224*t*
  gas exchange abnormalities in, 165–166

hypercapnic, clinical relevance of, 23
lung hyperinflation in, 165–167,
  166*f*–167*f*
medical management of, 168–169
  medications, 169, 183*t*
  oxygen therapy, 169
  smoking cessation, 168
  surgical interventions, 169
  vaccinations, 169
  ventilatory support, 169
non-invasive ventilation for, 300
pathophysiology of, 164–167, 165*f*
  pathological changes consequences,
    165–167
physiotherapy management of, 169–170
  airway clearance, 169
  breathing exercises, 169
  during exacerbation, 169–170
  pulmonary rehabilitation, 169
predisposing factors for, 164*f*
reduced cardiac output in, 167
reduced exercise tolerance in, 166–167
skeletal muscle dysfunction in, 167
Chronic organ failure, 583–584
Chronic respiratory failure, non-invasive
  ventilation for, 297, 298*b*, 298*f*
Chronic Respiratory Questionnaire
  (CRQ), 233*t*–236*t*
CICU, clinical problem encountered in,
  504
Cilia
  child *vs.* adult, 36
  description of, 3
  in mucociliary transport system, 15
Circulation, assessment, 64–67
Circulatory deficits, trauma and, 701
Closing capacity, effects of surgical process
  on, 522–523
Closing volume, 18
  child *vs.* adult, 38
CMR. *see* Cardiac magnetic resonance
  imaging (CMR)
Coagulopathy, in liver disease, 662
Codeine, 518*t*–519*t*
Cognitive behavioural interventions,
  self-management, 406
Cold response, child *vs.* adult, 39–40
Collaborative care, improving, 406
Collapse. *see* Atelectasis
Collateral ventilation, 15–16, 16*f*
  child *vs.* adult, 37
Colostomy, 529*f*
  double-barrelled, 529*f*
  loop, 530*f*
  sigmoid, 528*t*–531*t*
  single-barelled, 529*f*

Combustion, of oxygen therapy, 334
Comfort scale, 420
Community-based cardiac rehabilitation
  programmes, 603–604
Compliance, altered chest wall, 19
Compressed gas cylinders, 332
Computed tomographic pulmonary
  angiography (CTPA), 157, 158*b*
Computed tomography (CT), 86–87,
  87*f*–88*f*
  cranial, in ICU patients, 422
  indications for, 87–88
  interventional procedures for, 90
  in paediatrics, 110
  see also High-resolution computed
    tomography (HRCT)
Concentration gradient, 27–28
Conducting zone, 5, 5*f*
Confusion Assessment Method for the
  ICU (CAM-ICU), 202–204
Congenital abnormalities, 483
Congenital cardiac anomalies,
  radiographic appearance, 116
Congenital cystic adenomatoid
  malformation, radiographic
  appearance, 115
Congenital diaphragmatic hernia, 483
  radiographic appearance, 115, 117*f*
Congenital heart disease, 717–718, 718*b*
Congenital lobar emphysema,
  radiographic appearance, 115–116,
  117*f*
Congenital pulmonary airways
  malformation, radiographic
  appearance, 115
Consciousness level
  alteration in, in infant, 76
  in ICU patients, 420
Consequences, illness representation, 404
Conservation devices, 332
Consolidation, radiographic appearance,
  95, 96*f*, 111*f*
  in paediatrics, 111–112, 112*f*, 112*t*
  silhouette sign, 95
  widespread, in adults, 95*t*
'Conspiracy of silence', 403
Constrictive obliterative bronchiolitis. *see*
  Bronchiolitis obliterans syndrome
  (BOS)
Continuous exercise training. *see*
  Endurance exercise training
Continuous lateral rotation therapy, 430
Continuous oxygen therapy (COT), 328,
  332
  ambulatory oxygen in conjunction with,
    333

Continuous positive airway pressure (CPAP), 416, 707–708
  acute bronchiolitis, 468
  hypoxia, in children, 459
  in neonate, 487
  pulmonary oedema, 300
Contractures, 656
Control, illness representation, 404
Cool pale limbs, 65
Cool-down, cardiac rehabilitation, 613
COOP-WONCA charts, 228t–232t
COPD. see Chronic obstructive pulmonary disease (COPD)
Coping, 408
Core temperature, assessment of, in burn/smoke inhalation patients, 653
Coronary angiography, 128
Coronary artery, 127
Coronary artery bypass grafting (CABG) surgery, 131–132, 540t–541t, 546–547, 560t–570t
Coronary atherosclerosis, 127–128
Coronary circulation, 41, 42f
Coronary revascularization, 130–132
Corticosteroids
  for asthma, 182–184
  for respiratory conditions, 486
Costal fibres, 11
Costochondritis, 52t–54t
Costotransverse joint, 9
Costovertebral joints, 9
COT. see Continuous oxygen therapy (COT)
Cough, 252
  assessment, 49–50
  quality of, 60
  spinal cord injury and, 673
Cough assistance devices, 675–678, 677f
CoughAssist, 285, 287, 287f
Coughing, assisted, 675, 676f–677f
  mechanical aids for, 675–678, 677f
CPAP. see Continuous positive airway pressure (CPAP)
CPET. see Cardiopulmonary exercise test (CPET/CPEX)
CPEX. see Cardiopulmonary exercise test (CPET/CPEX)
CPG. see Central pattern generator (CPG)
CPP. see Cerebral perfusion pressure (CPP)
Critically ill patients, ICU, 424–426
  decreased mucociliary clearance, 424–425
  gas exchange, 424
  increased work of breathing, 425–426, 425t

lung compliance, 424
lung volumes, 424
peripheral muscle weakness, 425
respiratory weakness, 425
secretion clearance, 424–425
see also Intensive care unit (ICU) patients
Croup, 494
CRQ. see Chronic Respiratory Questionnaire (CRQ)
CRT. see Capillary refill time (CRT)
CT. see Computed tomography (CT)
CTPA. see Computed tomographic pulmonary angiography (CTPA)
Cultured epithelial autografts (CEAs), 647t–648t
CVD. see Cardiovascular disease (CVD)
CVP. see Central venous pressure (CVP)
Cyanosis, 76
Cystic fibrosis (CF), 172–177
  acute exacerbation of, definition of, 173b
  aetiology of, 172–173
  in children, 711–712, 712t, 713f
  clinical features of, 173–174
  diagnosis and investigations of, 174
  field walking tests for, 224t
  inhalation therapy for, 176
  medical management of, 174–175
    end stage disease, 175
  musculoskeletal dysfunction in, 174
  new-born screening and, 174
  pathophysiology of, 173
  physiotherapy management of, 175–177
    airway clearance techniques, 175–177
    in end stage disease, 177
    infection control, 177
    musculoskeletal complications, 176
    pregnancy and continence, 176–177
  radiographic appearance, 107f, 121, 123f
Cystic fibrosis transmembrane conductance regulator (CFTR), 172–173

D

DCD. see Donation after cardiac death (DCD)
De Morton Mobility Index (DEMMI), 217
Death/dying
  bereavement, 410
  family member request, 410
Decannulation, suggested guidelines for, 448t
Decortication, 535t–536t
Deep partial thickness burns, 643t

Deep vein thrombosis, 156, 156t
  symptoms and signs of, 157
DEMMI. see De Morton Mobility Index (DEMMI)
Denervation, 690–691
  heart transplantation, 690–691
  lung transplantation, 691
Denial, end stage of life, 410
Departmental radiograph, 84
Depression, 409–410
  end stage of life, 410
Dermal wounds, deep, 643
Developmental care, 489
Diagnosis
  following, 404–405
  impact of, 402–405
    in adulthood, 403–404
    in childhood, 402–403
Diagphragmatic breathing. see Breathing control (BC)
Diaphragm, 11, 368–369
  child vs. adult, 35
  radiographic appearance, 92
    elevation, 100–101
Diaphragmatic hernia, congenital. see Congenital diaphragmatic hernia
Diastole, 41
Diffuse axonal injury, 658, 658f
Digitalis preparations, for ischaemic heart disease, 131t
Dilated cardiomyopathies, 137–138
Dipalmitoylphosphatidylcholine, 18
Diphosphoglycerate (DPG), 32–33
Disability, assessment, 67–69
Disease awareness, patient, 51
Diuretics, for ischaemic heart disease, 131t
DMD. see Duchenne muscular dystrophy (DMD)
Documentation, assessment, 71–73
Domiciliary ambulatory oxygen, 326t, 333
Domiciliary oxygen therapy, 330–333
  prescription, 331t, 332
Donation after cardiac death (DCD), 687
Dornase alpha
  evidence about efficacy, 339–340
  physiotherapy interaction with, 340
Double lung/bilateral sequential lung transplantation, 686
Double-barrelled colostomy, 529f
DPG. see Diphosphoglycerate (DPG)
Drug history, patient, 48
Duchenne muscular dystrophy (DMD), with intrapulmonary percussive ventilation, 288
Duplex compression ultrasonography, 157, 158b

Dying. *see* Death/dying
Dynamometry, of peripheral muscle strength measurement, 209
Dysfunctional breathing, 185–188
 aetiology of, 186
 compensatory breath holds for, 187–188
 diagnosis of, 186
 exercise and, 188
 management of, 186–187
 rescue techniques for, 188
 speech and, 188
 techniques for improving, 355–377
  manual therapy techniques for, 355–366
Dyspnoea, 49
 assessment of, 345–346, 345*f*
 breathing control for, 350–354, 351*f*–352*f*
 in COPD, 166
 definition of, 199, 342
 inspiratory muscle training for, 348–350
 management strategies for, 346–348, 347*t*
 mechanisms underpinning, 343–345, 344*f*
 versus shortness of breath, 342–343, 342*f*
 short-term relief of, 346
 techniques for improving, 342–354
Dyspnoea-12, 345

E
'Ebb' phase, 649
Echocardiography, 134–136, 135*b*, 144
 for cardiac valve disease, 134–136
 for GUCH, 150–151
 use of, for pulmonary arterial hypertension, 180–181
ECMO. *see* Extracorporeal membrane oxygenation (ECMO)
Education and self-efficacy, 589–591
 balance training, 590
 neuromuscular electrical stimulation, 590
 whole body vibration (WBV), 590–591
Effectors, clinical failure of, 20
EIB. *see* Exercise induced bronchoconstriction (EIB)
Elderly Mobility Scale, 217
Electrical conductivity
 electrocardiogram and, 43–44, 43*f*
 of heart, 42–43, 43*f*
Electrical stimulation, of breathing, for spinal cord injury, 682

Electrocardiogram (ECG)
 assessment, 66
 critically ill patient, 420, 421*t*–422*t*, 423*f*
 electrical conductivity and, 43–44, 43*f*
 12-lead, 128, 129*b*, 129*f*
Electroimpedance tomography, 471
Electromyography (EMG), 370
Electrophysiological studies, 148, 148*b*
Embryonic period, lung, 34
EMG. *see* Electromyography (EMG)
Emotional impact, of medical illness, 407–410
Emphysema, radiographic appearance, 106–108, 107*f*
 lung overinflation, 106–108, 107*f*
 pruning of the vessels, 106–108
Emphysematous lung tissue, 165*f*
Empyema, drainage of, 535*t*–536*t*
Encephalopathy
 grades of, 661*t*
 in liver disease, 661
Enclosure systems, of oxygen therapy, 330
End stage of life, 410
Endoscopy, 527
Endotracheal airway suction, in children, 480, 480*f*
Endotracheal intubation, 460–461, 461*t*, 462*f*
Endurance exercise training, 588
Endurance Shuttle Walk Test (ESWT), 222–223, 595
Epidural anaesthesia, 521*f*
Epidural analgesia, 519
Epidural route, for postoperative analgesia administration, 517*t*
Epiglottitis, acute, 494
ERS. *see* European Respiratory Society (ERS)
Erythema, 643
Eschar, 644
Escharotomy, for circumferential full thickness wound, 644–645, 645*f*
ESWT. *see* Endurance Shuttle Walk Test (ESWT)
Eupnoea, 58*f*, 58*t*–59*t*
European Respiratory Society (ERS), 220–221
EuroQoL 5D, 228*t*–232*t*
Excess bronchial secretions, in bronchiectasis, 172
Exercise
 for airway clearance, 291–292
 for asthma, 184–185
 for cystic fibrosis, 711
  airway clearance, 176–177
 dysfunctional breathing and, 188

levels of, 606–607
 limitation, thoracic organ transplantation, 697–699
 non-invasive ventilation as an adjunct to, 307, 308*f*
 for oxygen transport improvement programme planning, 324–325
  progression, 325
 as physiotherapy intervention, 341
 see also Exercise training
Exercise capacity
 in cystic fibrosis, 711
 in heart failure, 692
 improvement, 605–606
  central changes, 606
  maximal oxygen uptake, consequences of, 606
  peripheral changes, 606
  risk factor modification, benefits of exercise in, 606
 maximizing, for cystic fibrosis, 176
Exercise induced bronchoconstriction (EIB), 712–714
Exercise prescription
 for burn patients, 656–658, 656*b*, 657*t*
 for cancer patients, 730–731, 730*t*, 732*t*
 in cardiac rehabilitation, 607–614
  cool-down, 613
  frequency of, 607–608
  heart rate, use of, 609
  intensity of, 608–610
  metabolic equivalent values (METs), use of, 609–610
  mode of, 608
  perceived exertion, rating of, 608–609
  principles of, 607, 608*t*
  progression of, 613–614
  resistance training, 608*t*, 613
  training, type of, 610
  type of, 608
  typical exercise session warm-up, format of, 610–613
 paediatrics, 721
 in pulmonary rehabilitation, 587
Exercise testing, 218–221
 activity limitations, measurement of, 218–221
 cardiopulmonary, 218
  physiological measurements during, 220*t*
 criteria to determine maximal, 219–220
 maximal. *see* Maximal exercise testing
 reasons to terminate, 220–221, 221*t*
Exercise training
 benefits of, 605–606, 605*f*
 for bronchiectasis, 172

for cancer management, 722–733
  delivery and timing of, 728–729
  evaluation of, 729–730, 729t–730t
  endurance. *see* Endurance exercise
    training
  exercise capacity, 605–606
    central changes, 606
    maximal oxygen uptake,
      consequences of, 606
    peripheral changes, 606
    risk factor modification, benefits of
      exercise in, 606
  individuality, 607
  progression of, 613–614
  progressive overload, 607
  regression or reversibility, 607
  specificity, 607
  thoracic organ transplantation, 691–692
Exomphalos, 483–484
Expiration
  active, 57
  prolonged, 57
'Expiratory flow increase techniques.' *see*
  Chest wall vibrations
Exposure, assessment, 69–71
External intercostals, 13
External respiration, definition of, 2–3
Extracorporeal carbon dioxide removal,
  418
Extracorporeal membrane oxygenation
  (ECMO), 418, 466–467, 467f,
  503–504
Extradural haematoma, 658–659, 659f
Extrapleural pneumonectomy, 535t–536t
Extrapulmonary air, radiographic
  appearance, 105
Extubation, 679
  readiness for, in burn patients, 655
Eyes, assessment, 69

F

Facemask
  for intermittent positive pressure
    breathing, 295
  for non-invasive ventilation, 473f
  percussion with, 260f
FACT. *see* Functional assessment of cancer
  therapy (FACT)
False ribs, 9
Family history, 48
Fast-track, 549
Fatigue, in liver disease, 662
Fentanyl, 518t–519t
FET. *see* Forced expiration technique
  (FET)

FEV$_1$. *see* Forced expiratory volume in 1
  second (FEV$_1$)
Fever, 51
FHF. *see* Fulminant hepatic failure (FHF)
Fibre-optic bronchoscopy (FOB), 652
Fick's law, 27
  gas exchange and, 27, 27f
Field walking tests, 217, 221–223, 224t
FiO$_2$/PaO$_2$ ratio, assessment, 63
Fissures
  of lungs, 6, 6f–7f
  radiographic appearance, 92
Five Times Sit to Stand Test, 217
Fixed performance systems, of oxygen
  therapy, 329–330
  interface devices for, 330
Flail chest, 57
Flange mouthpiece, for intermittent
  positive pressure breathing, 294,
  294f
Floating ribs, 9
Fluid balance, assessment of, 66–67
  in major burn/smoke inhalation
    patients, 653
Fluid creep, 646–649
Fluoroscopy, 85
  in paediatrics, 109
Flutter
  clinical application and evidence for,
    280–281
  key points when using, 280b
  for oscillating PEP, 279–280, 280f
FOB. *see* Fibre-optic bronchoscopy (FOB)
Forced expiration, muscles of, 13
Forced expiration technique (FET), 266,
  267f–268f, 268–269
Forced expiratory volume in 1 second
  (FEV$_1$), 63, 689–690
  cystic fibrosis, 260–261
  in spinal cord injury, 674
Forced vital capacity (FVC), 63
  in spinal cord injury, 674
  in tetraplegic patients, 673
Foreign body
  inhaled, in children, 496
    management of, 496
    physiotherapy of, 496
  obstruction, radiographic appearance,
    120, 122f
Forwards lean standing, 352, 352f
Four-wheeled rollator, diagrammatic
  representation of, 355f
Fraction of inspired oxygen (FiO$_2$)
  assessment, 63
  hypoxia, in children, 459
Frank haemoptysis, 50

FRC. *see* Functional residual capacity
  (FRC)
Fremitus, 60, 60f
'Frog breathing.' *see* Glossopharyngeal
  breathing (GPB)
FSS-ICU. *see* Functional status score for
  intensive care unit (FSS-ICU)
FTGs. *see* Full thickness skin grafts (FTGs)
Full thickness burns, 643t, 644–645,
  644f–645f
Full thickness skin grafts (FTGs),
  647t–648t
Fulminant hepatic failure (FHF), 664–667
  intracranial dynamics, 664–665, 665f
  management of, 665–666, 665t, 666f
  physiotherapists, considerations for,
    666–667
Functional ability, assessment, 51, 68–69
Functional ambulation classification, 217
Functional Assessment of Cancer Therapy
  (FACT), 233t–236t
Functional disability scale, 358
'Functional Independence Measure for
  Children', 217–218
Functional residual capacity (FRC), 18, 253
  effects of surgical process on, 522, 523f
Functional Status Score for Intensive Care
  Unit (FSS-ICU), 211
Functional strength testing, for peripheral
  muscle strength measurement, 210
FVC. *see* Forced vital capacity (FVC)

G

Gas cylinders, compressed, 332
Gas exchange, 26–34
  alveolar, 27, 27f
  critically ill patient, ICU, 424
  Fick's law and, 27, 27f
  impaired. *see* Impaired gas exchange
  techniques for improving, 317–334
    positioning and mobilization,
      317–325, 318f
Gas solubility, 27–28
Gas transport, definition of, 3
Gastrectomy, 531f
  partial
    Bill Roth I, 531f
    Bill Roth II, 531f
Gastrointestinal Quality of Life Index
  (GIQLI), 227–239
Gastroschisis, 483–484
GCS. *see* Glasgow Coma Scale (GCS)
Gel (mucus) layer, of mucociliary
  transport system, 15
General anaesthesia, 515–516

GIQLI. *see* Gastrointestinal Quality of Life Index (GIQLI)

Glasgow Coma Scale (GCS), 67–68, 67*t*, 202–204, 420
head injury in children, 490

Glenohumeral rotation, range of, 360

Glossopharyngeal breathing (GPB), 313–317, 678
nasal, stages with, 316*b*
stage 1 of, 314*b*, 314*f*
stage 2 of, 314*f*, 315, 315*b*
stage 3 of, 314*f*, 315, 315*b*
three stages for each gulp in, 314–315, 314*b*
uses of, 313*b*

Goblet cells, 3

Godin Exercise Leisure Time Questionnaire, 223

GPB. *see* Glossopharyngeal breathing (GPB)

Gravity-assisted positioning (GAP), 6–7, 255–256, 258*t*
ICU patients, 429

Great artery, transposition of, 501–502, 501*f*

Grown up congenital heart disease (GUCH), 150–152
aetiology and pathophysiology of, 150
classification of, 151
diagnosis of, 150–151, 151*b*
medical management of, 151
physiotherapy-specific management of, 151–152
signs and symptoms of, 150

Grunting, 76

GUCH. *see* Grown up congenital heart disease (GUCH)

H

Haematoma
extradural, 658–659, 659*f*
subdural, 659, 659*f*

Haemodynamic management, in cardiac surgery, 548–549

Haemodynamic stability, cardiac surgery and, 548

Haemoglobin (Hb)
carbon dioxide and, 33
oxygen and, 31

Haemoptysis, 50, 50*t*

Haldane effect, 23

Hamberger theory, 370

Handgrip dynamometry, for peripheral muscle strength measurement, 209–210, 210*f*

Hands, assessment, 69, 70*f*

Hartmann procedure, 526

Head bobbing, in infant, 76

Head injury
intracranial hypertension management in, 659–660
management of, 658–660
physiotherapy management in, 660
severe acquired, respiratory consequences in, 660
types of, 658–659
cerebral contusions, 658
diffuse axonal injury, 658, 658*f*
extradural haematoma, 659*f*
subdural haematoma, 659, 659*f*

Headache, 51

Health and disease, long-term activity behaviour in, 584–585, 585*f*

Health and safety protocols, in cardiac rehabilitation, 623

Health-related quality of life (HR-QoL), 227–239
outcome measures, 227
dimension-specific, 227
disease-specific, 227–239, 233*t*–236*t*
generic, 227, 228*t*–232*t*
method of administration and, 239
paediatric, 239
psychometric properties of instruments, 227, 238*t*

Heart
anatomy of, 40–46, 40*f*
electrical conductivity of, 42–43, 43*f*
radiographic appearance, 91–92
see also entries beginning cardiac

Heart block, 147*t*

Heart disease
acquired, 718–719
congenital, 717–718, 718*b*
ventricular assist devices, 719–720

Heart failure, 142–146, 142*b*
aetiology and pathophysiology of, 142–143, 142*t*
cardiac rehabilitation for, 623–625
classification of, 144–145, 145*t*
depression and, 409
diagnosis of, 144, 144*b*, 144*f*
exercise intensity, 625
hospitalization for, 146
medical management of, 145–146, 145*b*, 146*f*
physiotherapy-specific management of, 146
radiographic appearance, 105
symptoms and signs of, 143, 143*t*

Heart rate
autonomic regulation of, 44
use of, 609

Heart sounds, 42

Heart transplantation
acute cellular rejection grading in, 689*t*
in children, 720–721
considerations for, 700*t*

Heart valves, 41

Heart wall, layers of, 41

Heart-lung transplantation, 686

Heat and moisture exchanger (HME), 429

Heated humidifier systems, 330

Hemicolectomy, right, 528*f*

Hemithorax
decreased, density of, 100
opaque, radiographic appearance, 99–100

Hepatic hydrothorax, in liver disease, 661–662

Hepatopulmonary syndrome (HPS), 663–664
physiotherapists, considerations for, 664

Hepatorenal syndrome (HRS), in liver disease, 662

Hernia, congenital diaphragmatic, 483
radiographic appearance, 115, 117*f*

HFCC. *see* High-frequency chest compression (HFCC)

HFCWO. *see* High-frequency chest wall oscillation (HFCWO)

HFOV. *see* High-frequency oscillatory ventilation (HFOV)

High peak airway pressure, cause of, 436

High side lying, 352, 352*f*

High-frequency chest compression (HFCC), 289
see also High-frequency chest wall oscillation (HFCWO)

High-frequency chest wall oscillation (HFCWO), 289–291, 290*f*

High-frequency oscillatory ventilation (HFOV), 418
for children, 466, 466*f*
indication for, 466

High-frequency ventilation, 418

High-pressure positive expiratory pressure (HiPEP), 277*b*, 278–279, 279*f*

High-resolution computed tomography (HRCT), 110
in diagnosing bronchiectasis, 171

Hila
radiographic appearance, 92
shadow abnormalities, 92

HiPEP. *see* High-pressure positive expiratory pressure (HiPEP)
History of presenting condition (HPC), 48
HME. *see* Heat and moisture exchanger (HME)
Hoover sign, 57
Horizontal fissure, lung, 8
Hospitalization, heart failure requiring, 146
HPC. *see* History of presenting condition (HPC)
HPS. *see* Hepatopulmonary syndrome (HPS)
HPV. *see* Hypoxic pulmonary vasoconstriction (HPV)
HRCT. *see* High-resolution computed tomography (HRCT)
HR-QoL. *see* Health-related quality of life (HR-QoL)
HRS. *see* Hepatorenal syndrome (HRS)
HUI. *see* Canadian Health Utilities Index (HUI)
Human cadaver allograft, 647t–648t
Human recombinant dornase alfa, for cystic fibrosis, 175
Humidification
    critically ill patient, ICU, 426–429
    in mechanical ventilation, 470
    in non-invasive ventilation, 305b
HVS. *see* Hyperventilation syndrome (HVS)
Hydrogen cyanide, 651
Hyperacute rejection, 688
Hypercapnia, 325
Hypercarbia, in children, 459–460
Hyperglycaemia, 68
Hyperinflation, 56, 311
    in children, 479
    in COPD, 165–167, 166f–167f
    manual, 310–313, 311b, 426
        procedure of, 311–313, 311f
        precautions and contraindications for, 311b
    techniques, for critically ill patient, ICU, 426
    ventilator, 310–313, 426
Hypermetabolism, 649
Hyperoxygenation, in children, 479
Hyperpnoea, 58f, 58t–59t
Hypertension, 66
Hypertonic saline, 335–337, 665
    for bronchiectasis, 171
    evidence about efficacy, 336–337
    mechanism of action, 336
    physiotherapy interaction with, 337
Hypertrophic cardiomyopathy, 138

Hyperventilation, 58f, 58t–59t
    in children, 479–480
    chronic. *see* Chronic hyperventilation
    vicious cycle of, 185f
    see also Dysfunctional breathing
Hyperventilation syndrome (HVS), 185
Hypocapnia, effects of, 185–186
Hypoglycaemia, 68
Hypoplastic left heart syndrome, 503
Hypotension, 66
Hypothermia, in neonates, 39–40
Hypoventilation, 58f, 58t–59t
    alveolar, definition of, 26
Hypoxaemia, 325
    refractory, 466
    severe, 322
Hypoxia
    in children
        initial treatment of, 460b
        oxygen administration, 459, 459t
        supportive respiratory therapy for, 458–459, 459t, 460b
    response to, child *vs.* adults, 39
Hypoxic drive, loss of, 23
Hypoxic pulmonary vasoconstriction (HPV), 30

I

IABP. *see* Intra-aortic balloon pump (IABP)
ICCs. *see* Intercostal catheters (ICCs)
ICDs. *see* Implantable cardioverter-defibrillators (ICDs)
ICF framework. *see* International Classification of Functioning (ICF) framework
ICP. *see* Intracranial pressure (ICP)
ICU. *see* Intensive care unit (ICU)
ICU Mobility Scale, 211
ICU-AW, 734
    diagnosis of, 735
Identity, illness representation, 404
IHD. *see* Ischaemic heart disease (IHD)
ILD. *see* Interstitial lung disease (ILD)
Ileostomy, 529f
Illness
    emotional impact of, 407–410
    representation, 404
IMA. *see* Internal mammary artery (IMA)
Immunosuppression, 687–690, 688t
Impact of Weight on Quality of Life-Lite (IWQOL-Lite), 227–239
Impaired airway clearance, impaired, se Airway clearance
Impaired gas exchange, 156–157

Implantable cardioverter-defibrillators (ICDs), 149, 150b
Incentive spirometry, 308–310, 309f
Incontinence, assessment, 51
Incremental Shuttle Walk Test (ISWT), 222, 222f
Infant(s), 74–77
    airway clearance strategies for, 253–254, 254f–255f
    alteration in level of consciousness, 76
    carers, discussion with, 75
    communication in, 74–75
    cystic fibrosis in, airway clearance techniques for, 175
    medical notes for, 74
    physical examination for, 75
    positive expiratory pressure therapy for, 274–279, 276f
    respiratory distress in, clinical signs of, 75–76, 76b
    see also Paediatrics
Infections
    bacterial, in children, radiographic appearance, 111f, 118
    chest, readmission to hospital with, spinal cord injury and, 681
    control, in cystic fibrosis, 177
    Mycoplasma, radiographic appearance, 111f, 118
    pleural, 494
    respiratory tract, radiographic appearance, 118–119
    in transplant recipients, 690, 690b
    viral, radiographic appearance, 118, 120f
Inhalation therapy, 334–341, 335t
    bronchodilators, 340–341
    dornase alpha, 339–340
        evidence about efficacy, 339–340
        physiotherapy interaction with, 340
    hypertonic saline, 335–337
        evidence about efficacy, 336–337
        mechanisms of action, 336
        physiotherapy interaction with, 337
    mannitol, 337–339
        evidence about efficacy, 338–339
        mechanisms of action, 338
        physiotherapy interaction with, 339
    structuring airway clearance session, 341
        combining interventions, 341
        order of interventions, 341
Innermost intercostals, 13
Inspiration, accessory muscles of, 13, 371
Inspiratory flow rate, inadequate, troubleshooting for, 437, 438t

Inspiratory muscle training, 348–350
Inspiratory resistance-positive expiratory
    pressure (IR-PEP), 279
Insufflation/exsufflation, mechanical
    and assisted cough, 285–287
    devices for, 287, 287f
        for assisted coughing, 675
Integra, 647t–648t
Intensive care unit (ICU) patients
    abdominal injury, 702–703, 703f–704f
    burn, 645–646
    conscious and stable, 738–739
        early mobilization in, 738–739, 739t
    critically ill patient, 415–454
        acute respiratory distress syndrome,
            430–431
        brain injury, 433–435
        chest trauma, 432, 434f
        haematological problems, 433
        high flow oxygen, 430
        hyperinflation techniques, 426
        increased moisture to airways,
            426–429
        manual techniques, 426
        mechanical support for, 416–423
        mobilization in, 430
        monitoring of, 416–423
        non-invasive ventilation, 430
        physiotherapy interventions in,
            426–430, 427f–428f
        positioning, 429–430
        problem identification of, 423–435
        secretion removal techniques, 426
        sepsis, 432
        severe neuromuscular disease, 435
        specific conditions in, 430–435
        systemic inflammatory response
            syndrome, 432
        ventilator-associated events, 431
        ventilator-associated pneumonia,
            431
    field walking tests on, 224t
    muscle weakness in, definition and
        mechanisms of, 734–736, 734b,
        735f, 737t
    neurocognitive interventions in,
        739–740
    pelvic injury, 705
    physical function and mobility
        measurement in, 211–217,
        212t–216t
    rehabilitation for survivors in, 733–740,
        733f, 734b
    thoracic injury, 703–705, 704f
    thoracic organ transplantation, 695,
        695f

trauma and, 702–705
unconscious/sedated, 737–738
Intercostal catheters (ICCs), 542–543,
    543b
Intercostal drains, 56
Intercostal indrawing, 57
Intercostal muscles, 13, 370
    external, 13
    innermost, 13
    internal, 13
Intercostal stretch, 372, 374f
Interface devices, for fixed performance
    systems, 330
Intermittent oxygen therapy, 333
Intermittent positive pressure breathing
    (IPPB), 257–258, 292–296, 293f
    apparatus, preparation of, 294–295
    contraindications for, 296
    facemask for, 295
    patient treatment of, 295–296
    preparation of, 294–295
    use of, 274
Intermittent positive pressure ventilation,
    487
Internal intercostals, 13
Internal mammary artery (IMA), 547f
Internal organs, child vs. adult, 37, 37f
Internal respiration, definition of, 3
International Classification of Functioning
    (ICF) framework, 196
International Physical Activity
    Questionnaire (IPAQ), 223
Interrupted aortic arch, 502
Interstitial lung disease (ILD), 177–179
    in children, 715
    classification of, 177b
    clinical features of, 178
    diagnosis and investigations of, 178
    field walking tests for, 224t
    medical management of, 178–179
    pathophysiology of, 178
    physiotherapy management of, 179
    rehabilitation of, 592
Interstitial pulmonary oedema,
    radiographic appearance, 105,
    105f
Interval training
    cardiac rehabilitation, 610
    pulmonary rehabilitation, 588
Intra-aortic balloon pump (IABP), 85f,
    103, 548–549
Intracranial hypertension, management of,
    659–660
Intracranial pressure (ICP)
    assessment, 68
    in children, 490

definition of, 659
in ICU patients, 422–423
measurement of, 664–665
Intramuscular route, for postoperative
    analgesia administration, 517t
Intrapleural pressure (P_{ip}), 13–14
Intrapulmonary percussive ventilation
    (IPV), 287–289, 290f
Intrapulmonary pressure (P_{pul}), 13, 14f
Intravenous route, for postoperative
    analgesia administration, 517t
IPAQ. see International Physical Activity
    Questionnaire (IPAQ)
IPPB. see Intermittent positive pressure
    breathing (IPPB)
IPV. see Intrapulmonary percussive
    ventilation (IPV)
IR-PEP. see Inspiratory resistance-positive
    expiratory pressure (IR-PEP)
Irritant receptors, 21
Ischaemic heart disease (IHD), 127–132,
    127b–128b
    aetiology and pathophysiology of,
        127–128, 133–134
    classification of, 129–130
    diagnosis of, 128–129
    medical management of, 130–132, 130b,
        131t
    physiotherapy-specific management of,
        132
    risk factors for, 127t
    signs and symptoms of, 128
ISWT. see Incremental Shuttle Walk Test
    (ISWT)
IWQOL-Lite. see Impact of Weight on
    Quality of Life-Lite (IWQOL-Lite)

J
Jaundice
    in liver disease, 661
    physiological, 486
Jugular venous pressure (JVP), assessment,
    65
Jugular venous saturation of oxygen
    (SjvO$_2$), 665
Juxta-capillary receptors, 21
JVP. see Jugular venous pressure (JVP)

K
KDQOL. see Kidney Disease Quality of
    Life (KDQOL)
Ketamine, 518t–519t
Kidney Disease Quality of Life (KDQOL),
    227–239

Kinetic therapy, for ICU patients, 430
'The Knack', 292
Kneeling position, 352, 353f
Kussmaul breathing, 58f, 58t–59t
Kyphoscoliosis, 56
    radiographic appearance, 106
Kyphosis, 56

L

Laboratory investigations, assessment, 71,
    72t
Laparoscopy, 527
Larynx, 4
    position of, child vs. adult, 35–36
Lateral positioning, in ICU patients,
    429–430
12-lead electrocardiogram (ECG), 128,
    129b, 129f
Left lower lobe collapse, radiographic
    appearance, 98f, 99
Left lung, 8
Left upper lobe collapse, radiographic
    appearance, 98–99, 99f
Level of consciousness
    alteration in, in infant, 76
    in ICU patients, 420
Limb exposure, assessment, 69
'Lip phenomenon', 376
Lipomas, 70
Liquid oxygen systems, 332
Liver, 661
Liver disease, 661–667
    chronic, 662–663
    hepatopulmonary syndrome (HPS) in,
        663–664
    signs and symptoms of, 661–662
Liver transplantation, pulmonary problem
    following, in children, 497–498
Living donor lobar lung transplantation,
    687
Lobar emphysema, congenital,
    radiographic appearance, 115–116,
    117f
Lobectomy, 535t–536t
Lobes, of lungs, 6, 6f–7f
    collapse of, radiographic appearance,
        97–99, 97f
Long-term oxygen therapy (LTOT), 332,
    595
Loop colostomy, 530f
Low birth weight, 482–483
Low tidal volume ventilation, 465
LTOT. see Long-term oxygen therapy
    (LTOT)
Lumbar fibres, 11

Lung(s)
    capacities of, 23, 24t
        clinical relevance of, 24–25
        measuring, 25
    carriage from tissue to, 33–34
    chronic graft dysfunction, 689
    compliance, 18
        altered, 18
        critically ill patient, ICU, 424
        factors affecting, 18
        reduced total, consequences of, 19
    distribution of
        perfusion in, 29, 29f
        ventilation in, 28–29, 29f
    left, 8
    mechanics of, in ICU patients, 419
    pathology, CT, 110
    pleurae and, 5–8
    right, 8
    surface markings of, 8–9
Lung cancer, field walking tests for,
    224t
Lung contusion, 541
Lung denervation, 691
The Lung Flute, 279, 283–284, 285f
Lung function test, assessment, 63
Lung hyperinflation
    in COPD, 165–167, 166f–167f
    precautions and contraindications for,
        311b
Lung resection, 558t–559t
Lung transplantation, 686
    in children, 716
        considerations for, 700t
    double lung/bilateral sequential, 686
    heart-lung transplantation, 686
    single, 686
    techniques for, 686
Lung volume(s), 23, 24t
    clinical relevance of, 24–25
    critically ill patient, ICU, 424
    effects of surgical process on, 522
    factors affecting, 23–24
    glossopharyngeal breathing, 313–317
        nasal, stages with, 316b
        stage 1 of, 314b, 314f
        stage 2 of, 314f, 315, 315b
        stage 3 of, 314f, 315, 315b
        three stages for each gulp in,
            314–315, 314b
        uses of, 313b
    improvement of, techniques for,
        292–317
    incentive spirometry, 308–310, 309f
    intermittent positive pressure breathing,
        292–296, 293f

    manual hyperinflation, 310–313, 311b
        procedure of, 311–313, 311f
    measurement of, 25
    non-invasive ventilation, 296–307
        definition of, 296–297
        description of, 296
        indications for, 297–302
        in spinal cord injury, 672–673
        maximizing, 678
        ventilator hyperinflation, 310–313
Lung volume reduction surgery (LVRS),
    535t–536t
LVRS. see Lung volume reduction surgery
    (LVRS)
Lymphatic tissue, child vs. adult, 37, 37f

M

Magnetic resonance imaging (MRI), 88,
    89f, 422
    contraindications to, 88
    gadolinium for, 110
    in paediatrics, 110
    principles of, 88
Magnetic stimulation, of breathing, for
    spinal cord injury, 682
Maintained manual pressure, 375
Mannitol, 337–339
    for bronchiectasis, 171–172
    evidence about efficacy, 338–339
    mechanisms of action, 338
    physiotherapy interaction with, 339
Manual hyperinflation (MHI), 310–313,
    311b, 426
    procedure of, 311–313, 311f
Manual lung inflation, 476f, 479–480
Manual muscle strength testing, for
    peripheral muscle strength
    measurement, 205–209, 205t–208t
Manual resuscitation bag, 312, 312f
Manual techniques, of airway clearance,
    258–265
    chest percussion/clapping, 259–261,
        260f
        key points for, 261b
    clinical application and evidence for,
        264–265
    contraindications and precautions for,
        265b
    for musculoskeletal dysfunction,
        355–366, 357f–358f
        mobilization techniques, 361–362,
            361f–363f
        motor control training for, 361
        muscle retraining, 364–365,
            365f–366f, 365t

Manual techniques, of airway clearance
    (Continued)
    muscle-lengthening techniques, 362,
        364t
    neural tissue techniques, 365
    physiotherapy management of, 360
    postural correction for, 361
    posture, 358f, 359
    range of motion, 359–360, 360f
    subjective assessment of, 358–359
    summary of, 365–366
    taping, 362–364
    shaking, chest compression and rib
        springing, 263–265
    suction, 265–266
    vibrations/chest shaking and
        compression, 261–263, 262f–263f
    key points for, 263b
MAP. see Mean arterial pressure (MAP)
Maximal exercise testing, 581
    determination of, criteria for, 219–220
Maximal expiratory pressure (MEP), 447
Maximal heart rate, 582
Maximal inspiratory pressure testing, for
    respiratory muscle strength
    measurement, 204
Maximal oxygen uptake
    in exercise, 218, 606
    measurement of, 67
Maximum expiratory pressure (P$_e$max), 64
MBTS. see Modified Blalock-Taussig
    shunt; Modified Blalock-Taussig
    shunt (MBTS)
MCC. see Mucociliary clearance (MCC)
McGill pain questionnaire, 520–521
Mcleod syndrome, 123
Mean arterial pressure (MAP), 419–420
Mechanical insufflation/exsufflation. see
    Insufflation/exsufflation,
    mechanical
Mechanical support, in children,
    456–473
    for respiratory conditions, 487
        continuous positive airway pressure,
            487
        high-flow nasal cannulae, 487
        intermittent positive pressure
            ventilation, 487
        non-invasive ventilation, 487
    supportive respiratory therapy,
        indications for, 458–461
Mechanical ventilation, 416–419,
    417f–418f
    adjuncts to, 418
    airway pressure release ventilation, 416
    airway secretions in, 437, 439t

in children, 461–466
    acute deterioration, 461t, 464, 475t
    considerations during, 470
    general ventilation care, 461–464,
        463b, 463f
    humidification, 470
    modes of, 464–466
    monitoring during, 470–471
    non-invasive support, 472–473,
        472f–473f
    physiotherapy, 470
    positioning in, 470, 489
    suctioning, 470
    'troubleshooting', 461t, 464, 475t
    weaning from, 471, 471b
high-frequency ventilation, 418
monitoring of patients on, 418–419
    lung mechanics, 419
    respiratory muscle function, 419
other forms of, 418
pressure control-inverse ratio
    ventilation, 416
waveform analysis, 436–437, 438t–439t
weaning from, 441–447, 441b–442b
    concepts of, 435–447
    physiotherapist's role in, 441–442
    strategies, 441
    see also individual types
Mechanoreceptors, 21
Meconium aspiration, 485
Meconium aspiration syndrome,
    radiographic appearance, 118, 120f
Median sternotomy, exercise following,
    626
Mediastinum, radiographic appearance, 91
Medical teams
    engagement with, 410–412
    team work of, 411–412
    technology and, 411–412
Medullary control centres, 19–20
Melbourne Group Scale, 525, 525b
MEP. see Maximal expiratory pressure
    (MEP)
Metabolic equivalent values (METs),
    609–610
Methylxanthines, for respiratory
    conditions, 486
METs. see Metabolic equivalent values
    (METs)
MHI. see Manual hyperinflation (MHI)
Microchip technology, 412
Microprocessor pump, 520f
Mini-AQLQ. see Mini-Asthma Quality of
    Life Questionnaire (mini-AQLQ)
Mini-Asthma Quality of Life Questionnaire
    (mini-AQLQ), 227–239

Minimal access surgery, 527
Minitracheotomy, in ICU patient, 426
Minnesota Living with Heart Failure
    Questionnaire (MLHFQ),
    233t–236t
6-minute walk test (6MWT), 221–222,
    551
Mitral regurgitation, 133
    medical management of, 137
    symptoms and signs of, 134
Mitral stenosis, 133
    medical management of, 136–137
    symptoms and signs of, 134
Mitral valve, 503
    surgery for, 547
MLHFQ. see Minnesota Living with
    Heart Failure Questionnaire
    (MLHFQ)
Mobilization
    in ICU patients, 430, 738–739, 739t
    for improving gas exchange, 317–325,
        318f
    monitoring, 323
    oxygen transport effects, 321t,
        322–324
    physiological rationale, 322–324
    scientific rationale, 322–324
    techniques, for musculoskeletal
        dysfunction, 361–362, 361f–363f
    see also Positioning
Moderate intense exercise, 582
Modified 6-minute walk assessment
    (6MWA), 551
Modified Blalock-Taussig shunt (MBTS),
    498
Modified Shuttle Walk Test (MSWT),
    223
Monro-Kellie doctrine, 664
Morphine, 518t–519t
Motion sensors, 226
Motivational interviewing, 406
Motor control training, for
    musculoskeletal dysfunction, 361
Motor Neurone Disease Dyspnoea Rating
    Scale, 345
'Mouth phenomenon', 376
MRI. see Magnetic resonance imaging
    (MRI)
MSWT. see Modified Shuttle Walk Test
    (MSWT)
Mucociliary clearance (MCC)
    airway clearance techniques and, 250
    decreased, critically ill patient, ICU,
        424–425
    effects of surgical process on, 523,
        524b

Mucociliary transport system, 15, 15f
Multidimensional Dyspnoea scale, 345
Multidisciplinary transplant team, 685b
Multimodal analgesia, 519
Multi-organ dysfunction, after burn injury, 642t
Muscles
 of forced expiration, 13
 measurement of, 199
Muscle fatigue, child vs. adult, 39
Muscle mass, 199–202
 anthropometry in, 201–202
 body composition analysis in, 200–201
 definition of, 199–200
 impairment
  assessment of, 202b
  measurement of, 201t
 neuromuscular ultrasound imaging in, 200, 200f
Muscle retraining, for musculoskeletal dysfunction, 364–365, 365f–366f, 365t
Muscle strength, 202–211
 definitions of, 202
 evaluation of impairment, 211b
 increase, for spinal cord injury, 679
  respiratory muscle training, 679
 peripheral, 205–211
  dynamometry, 209
  functional strength testing, 210
  handgrip dynamometry, 209–210, 210f
  manual muscle strength testing, 205–209, 205t–208t
  peripheral nerve stimulation, 210–211
 respiratory, 204–205
  maximal inspiratory pressure testing, 204
  phrenic nerve stimulation, 204–205
 volitional and non-volitional assessment of, 202–204, 203f, 206t–208t
Muscle wasting, in liver disease, 662
Muscle weakness
 ICU patients, definition and mechanisms of, 734–736, 734b, 735f, 737t
 trauma and, 701–702
Muscle-lengthening techniques, for musculoskeletal dysfunction, 362, 364t
Musculoskeletal dysfunction
 assessment of
  posture, 359
  range of motion, 359–360, 360f
  subjective, 358–359

 in cystic fibrosis, 174
 manual therapy techniques for, 355–366, 357f–358f
  mobilization techniques, 361–362, 361f–363f
  muscle retraining, 364–365, 365f–366f, 365t
  muscle-lengthening techniques, 362, 364t
  neural tissue techniques, 365
  summary of, 365–366
  taping, 362–364
 motor control training for, 361
 physiotherapy management of, 360
 postural correction for, 361
Mycoplasma infection, radiographic appearance, 111f, 118
Myocardial infarction, 52t–54t
 diagnosis of, 128–129

N
Nasal cannula(e), 328
 high-flow, 487
Nasal catheter, 328
Nasal flaring, 57, 76
Nasal turbinates, 3–4
Nasal vestibule, 3–4
Nasal vibrissae, 3–4
Nasopharyngeal suction
 in children, 480, 480f
 in ICU patients, 426
Naso-pulmonary reflexes, 21
Nasotracheal suction, 265
Nebulizer/nebulization
 air entrainment, 330
 airway clearance session, 341
 antibiotics and, 171
 cystic fibrosis, 340
 intermittent positive pressure breathing, 293
Neck Disability Index, 358
Nedocromil sodium, for asthma, 182–184
Neonatal intensive care unit (NICU), 482–484
 admission reasons, 482–483, 490–491
 clustering of care, 489
 considerations in, 489–490
 general paediatric intensive care, 490
 level of perinatal care, 482
 parent-infant bonding in, 490
 physiotherapy intervention in, 488
 sepsis in, 489
 temperature control, 489–490
 see also Special care nurseries

Neonate(s)
 chest percussion/clapping, 259–260, 260f, 477
 chest problem, 116–118
 continuous positive airway pressure (CPAP), 487
 hypothermia, 39–40
 non-invasive positive pressure ventilation for, 472
 respiratory compliance, 38
 see also Paediatrics
Neural control, 367–368, 367f
Neural tissue techniques, for musculoskeletal dysfunction, 365
Neuralgia, 52t–54t
Neurocognitive interventions, in ICU patients, 739–740
Neurological and neuromuscular impairment, children with, 496
Neurological level and completeness, for spinal cord injury, 669, 670f–671f, 672t
Neurological system, monitoring of, in ICU patients, 420–423
Neuro-motor exercise, 583
Neuromuscular electrical stimulation, 590
Neuromuscular ultrasound imaging, in muscle measurement, 200, 200f
Neurophysiological facilitation, of respiration, 366–377
 clinical application of, 377
 neural control, 367–368, 367f
 respiratory muscles, 368–372
  abdominal muscles, 371–372
  accessory muscles of inspiration, 371
  diaphragm, 368–369
  intercostal muscles, 370
 stimuli, 372–377, 373t
  anterior-stretch basal lift, 374f, 375
  co-contraction of abdomen, 374f, 376–377
  intercostal stretch, 372, 374f
  maintained manual pressure, 375
  perioral pressure, 374f, 375–376
  vertebral pressure, 372–375, 374f
NHP. see Nottingham Health Profile (NHP)
NICU. see Neonatal intensive care unit (NICU)
Nijmegen questionnaire, 186, 187f
NIPPY Clearway, 285, 287, 287f
Nitric oxide
 for ARDS, 469–470
 inhaled, ventilation and, 418
NIV. see Non-invasive ventilation (NIV)
Nociception, 516

Nocturnal hypercapnic respiratory failure, 298b
Nocturnal oxygen, 333
Non-invasive positive pressure ventilation, 296–297, 652
Non-invasive ventilation (NIV), 595–596
  adverse effects of, 306
  for airway clearance, 284–285, 306–307
  as an adjunct to exercise, 307, 308f
  assessing the need for, 299–302
  for children, 472–473, 472f–473f, 487
  contraindications for, in acute setting, 300b
  definition of, 296–297
  description of, 296–307
  humidification in, 305
  in ICU patients, 430
  indications for, 297–302
    acute respiratory failure, 299
    in acute setting, 300b
    assessing 'at-risk' patients, 297–299
    cardiogenic pulmonary oedema, 300–301
    chronic obstructive pulmonary disease, 300
    chronic respiratory failure, 297, 298b, 298f
    evidence for other, 301–302
    immunocompromised patients, 301
    weaning and post extubation respiratory failure, 301
  initiating and monitoring therapy for, 302–306, 304f, 305b
  interfaces for, 302, 303f
  oxygen therapy in, 306
  physiotherapy in management of, 305b
  practical issues in application of, 302–307
  steps in, for home ventilatory support, 305b
Non-pulsatile open heart surgery, 547–548
Non-rebreathing mask, of reservoir masks, 329
Nose, 3
Nottingham Health Profile (NHP), 227–239, 228t–232t
NSAIDs, 518t–519t
Numeric rating scales, for intensity or unpleasantness, 345
Nutrition, assessment, 69–70

O
Obesity, in children, 716–717
Objective assessment. see Assessment, patient

Oblique fissure, 8
Obstructive sleep apnoea, in spinal cord injury, treatment of, 681–682, 681f
Oedema
  in liver disease, 662
  peripheral, 65
  pulmonary, 671–672
    cardiogenic, non-invasive ventilation for, 300–301
    continuous positive airway pressure, 300
    interstitial, radiographic appearance, 105, 105f
Oesophageal atresia, congenital, 483
Oesophageal opening, 11
Oesophageal surgery, 534–536, 537b
  evidence in, 538–539
Oesophageal varices, in liver disease, 662
Oesophagectomy, 515, 535t–536t
Oesophagogastrectomy, 535t–536t
Off-pump coronary artery bypass surgery (OPCAB), 548
Older people
  chest trauma, 432
  decreased exercise tolerance, 583–584
  pulmonary rehabilitation safety issues, 596
Omphalocoele, 483–484
Ondine curse, 20
Opaque hemithorax, radiographic appearance, 99–100
OPCAB. see Off-pump coronary artery bypass surgery (OPCAB)
Open abdominal surgery, 555t–557t
'Open lung/protective ventilation', 416
Opioids, 516
Oral route, for postoperative analgesia administration, 517t
Organ donation, for transplantation, 686–687
Oropharyngeal suction, 266
  in ICU patients, 426
Orthodeoxia, 663
Orthopaedic management, for spinal cord injury, 669–670
Orthotopic heart transplantation, 685–686
Oscillation of airflow, 253, 253f
  physiological effects of, 253
Osteoporosis, in liver disease, 662
Outcome measurement
  activity limitations, 211–226
    exercise testing, 218–221
    field walking tests, 221–223, 224t
    mobility and activities of daily living, 212t–216t, 217–218

physical activity, 223–226
physical function and mobility, 211–217, 212t–216t
body structure/functions level impairment, 198–211
in cardiorespiratory physiotherapy practice, 195–247
choice of, 196–198
considerations in choosing, 198b
definition of, 196
health-related quality of life, 227
  dimension-specific measures, 227
  disease-specific measures, 227–239, 233t–236t
  generic measures, 227, 228t–232t
  paediatric, 239
  psychometric properties of instruments, 227, 238t
International Classification of Functioning (ICF) framework, 196
measurement properties of, 197t
muscle, 199
  mass, 199–202
  strength, 202–211
participation restriction, 226–239, 240b
respiratory, 198–199
  assessment of impairment, 199b
  breathlessness, 198–199
  dyspnoea, 199–202
  impaired airway clearance, 198–199
  low lung volumes, 198–199
selection of, 196–198
Outpatient rehabilitation, thoracic organ transplantation, 696–697, 696f–697f, 698b
Oximetry, 326
Oxycodone, 518t–519t
Oxygen, 31
  dissociating, 32
  haemoglobin's affinity for, 32
    factors affecting, 32
  high flow, 430
  nocturnal, 333
  training, 333
  transport of, 31
Oxygen concentrators, 331
Oxygen consumption, child vs. adult, 39
Oxygen delivery systems, 327–330, 327t
  devices for, 331–332
Oxygen dissociation curve, 32, 32f
Oxygen saturation
  assessment, 63
  range of, 326–327

Oxygen therapy
in acute setting, 326–334
delivery systems, 327–330, 327*t*
enclosure systems, 330
fixed performance systems, 329–330
general principles of, 326–327
variable performance systems, 327–329
combustion, 334
continuous, 328, 332
for COPD, 169
description of, 325–326
domiciliary, 330–333, 331*t*
hazards of, 334
physiological, 334
intermittent, 333
other uses of, 333
long-term, 332
in non-invasive ventilation, 306, 326–334
short-term, 332–333
Oxygen transport
in acute cardiopulmonary dysfunction, 320–324, 321*t*
mobilization, 322–324
physiological and scientific rationale, 322–324
positioning, 321–322
in post-acute and chronic cardiopulmonary dysfunction, 324–325
physiological and scientific rationale, 324, 324*t*
Oxygenation
deficits in, trauma and, 701
monitoring of, in ICU patients, 419

P
PaCO₂
hypercapnia, 325
hypocapnia, 185, 185*f*
normal values, 63*t*
Paediatric Evaluation of Disability Inventory (PEDI), 217–218
Paediatric intensive care unit (PICU)
admission reasons, 490–498
cardiac problems, 498–505
equipment, 474, 475*f*
Paediatrics, 74–77, 709–721
acquired heart disease in, 718–719
airway clearance strategies for, 253–254, 254*f*–255*f*
asthma in, 712–715
carers, discussion with, 75
communication in, 74–75

congenital heart disease, 717–718, 718*b*
considerations for, 699
cystic fibrosis in, 711–712, 712*t*, 713*f*
airway clearance techniques, 175
diagnosis in, 402–403
exercise prescription for, 721
health-related quality of life outcome measures for, 239
heart transplantation in, 720–721
medical notes for, 74
obesity in, 716–717
peer relationships, 407
physical examination for, 75
rehabilitation in, 711
respiratory conditions in, 715–716
interstitial lung disease, 715
lung transplant, 716
non-CF bronchiectasis, 715–716
respiratory distress in, clinical signs of, 75–76, 76*b*
thoracic imaging, 108–123
issues in, 108–109
understanding of illness, 403
ventricular assist devices for, 719–720
PAH. *see* Pulmonary arterial hypertension (PAH)
Pain
acute, definition of, 516
measurement of, 520–521, 522*b*
instruments, 520
postoperative. *see* Postoperative pain
post-sternotomy, in cardiac surgery, 547*f*, 549–550
Pallor, in infant, 76
Pancreatic enzyme supplementation, for cystic fibrosis, 175
PaO₂
normal values, 63*t*
Paracetamol, 518*t*–519*t*
Paradoxical breathing, 57
in supine, 668, 669*f*
Parent management training, 406–407
Parietal pleura, 7–8
Partial pressure of carbon dioxied in arterial blood. *see* PaCO₂
Partial rebreathing mask, 329
Partial/total anomalous pulmonary venous connection (PAPVC or TAPVC), 502
Participation restriction
definition of, by World Health Organization, 226
measurement of, 226–239, 240*b*
PASE. *see* Physical Activity Scale for the Elderly (PASE)
Passy-Muir valve, 316–317

Patent ductus arteriosus, 485–486, 498–499
Patent foramen ovale, 151
Patient examination, 48
Patient-centred approach, 404–405
Patient-controlled analgesia, 517*t*, 519
Patient-ventilator synchrony, assessment of, 436–437
PC-IRV. *see* Pressure control-inverse ratio ventilation (PC-IRV)
Peak cough flow (PCF), assessment, 63
Peak expiratory flow, 63
Pectus carinatum, 56
Pectus excavatum, 56
PEDI. *see* Paediatric Evaluation of Disability Inventory (PEDI)
Pedometer, 584
PEEP. *see* Positive end-expiratory pressure (PEEP)
Peer relationships, 407
Pelvic injury
ICU patients, 705
management of, precautions and contraindications to, 706*t*
Pendelluft flow, 267
Perceived exertion, rate of, 608–609
Percussion, 60, 60*f*–61*f*
in ICU patient, 426
Percutaneous coronary intervention, 130*f*, 131
Percutaneous needle biopsy, 90
Perfusion
child *vs.* adult, 38–39
distribution of, in healthy lung, 29, 29*f*
Perfusion matching, ventilation and, 28
Pericardial disease, 140–142
aetiology and pathophysiology of, 140
classification of, 141
diagnosis of, 141
medical management of, 141–142
physiotherapy-specific management of, 142
symptoms and signs of, 140–141
Pericardial effusion, 141
Pericardial fluid, 140
Pericardium, 52*t*–54*t*, 140
Peri-exacerbation, 591–592
Perinatal care, level of, 482
Perioral pressure, 374*f*, 375–376
Peripheral artery disease, 154–155
aetiology and pathophysiology of, 154
diagnosis of, 155
medical management of, 155
physiotherapy-specific management of, 155
symptoms and signs of, 154

Peripheral blocks, 517t
Peripheral changes, in exercise training, 606
Peripheral muscle strength measurement, 205–211
Peripheral muscle weakness, critically ill patient, ICU, 425
Peripheral nerve stimulation, of peripheral muscle strength measurement, 210–211
Peripheral oedema, 65
Peripheral pulses, assessment, 65
Peripheral temperature, assessment of, in burn/smoke inhalation patients, 653
Periventricular haemorrhage, 485
Periventricular leucomalacia, 485
Persistent air leak (PAL), in UWSD, 544–545
Pertussis, 493
Pethidine, 518t–519t
PFIT-s. see Physical Function in Intensive Care Test-scored (PFIT-s)
Pharynx, 4
Phrenic nerve damage, 505
Phrenic nerve stimulation, in respiratory muscle strength measurement, 204–205
Physical activity, 223–226, 580–582
    definition of, 580
    levels of, 606–607
    and rehabilitation, 579–638
    vs. physical fitness, 580–581
Physical Activity Scale for the Elderly (PASE), 223
Physical fitness, 581–582
    physical activity vs., 580–581
    strategies for improving and maintaining, 582–585
        chronic organ failure, 583–584
        general principles, 582–583, 583t
        for long-term activity behaviour in health and disease, 584–585, 585f
Physical Function in Intensive Care Test-scored (PFIT-s), 211
Physiological dead space, 25
Physiological jaundice, 486
Physiotherapists, cardiorespiratory, 196
Physiotherapy
    management, of ventilated infants and children, 462f, 473–481, 475f–477f
    in mechanical ventilation, 470
    preoperative, and prehabilitation, 514–515

Physiotherapy interventions, 248–401
    airway clearance techniques, 250–292
        for babies and children, 253–254, 254f–255f
        breathing techniques, 266–274
        independently performed, 266–291
        manual, 252–254, 258–265
        modified postural drainage, 255–258, 255f–257f, 258t
        postural drainage, 255–258, 255f–257f, 258t
        secretion clearance interventions rationale, 252–253
        traditional, 252–254
    dysfunctional breathing, techniques for improving, 355–377
        manual therapy techniques for, 355–366
        mobilization techniques for, 361–362, 361f–363f
        muscle retraining for, 364–365, 365f–366f, 365t
        muscle-lengthening techniques for, 362, 364t
        neural tissue techniques for, 365
        summary of, 365–366
        taping for, 362–364
    dyspnoea, techniques for improving, 342–354
    gas exchange, techniques for improving, 317–334
        positioning and mobilization, 317–325, 318f
    inhalation therapy, 334–341, 335t
        bronchodilators, 340–341
        dornase alpha, 339–340
        hypertonic saline, 335–337
        mannitol, 337–339
        structuring airway clearance session, 341
    intrapulmonary percussive ventilation, 287–289, 290f
    lung volumes, techniques for improving, 292–317
        glossopharyngeal breathing, 313–317, 313b
        incentive spirometry, 308–310, 309f
        intermittent positive pressure breathing, 292–296, 293f
        manual hyperinflation, 310–313, 311b
        non-invasive ventilation, 296–307
        ventilator hyperinflation, 310–313
    mechanical insufflation/exsufflation and assisted cough, 285–287

oxygen therapy
    in acute setting, 326–334
    description of, 325–326
Physiotherapy interventions, in ICU patient, 426–430, 427f–428f
PiCCO device, 423f
PICS. see Post intensive care syndrome (PICS)
PICU. see Paediatric intensive care unit (PICU)
PIE. see Pulmonary interstitial emphysema (PIE)
P_{ip}. see Intrapleural pressure (P_{ip})
Plain chest radiograph, in children, 109
Platypnoea, 663
Pleura(e), 9, 52t–54t
    lungs and, 5–8
Pleural disease, radiographic appearance, 101, 101f
Pleural effusion, 101f
Pleural fluid, 7–8
    in paediatrics, 112–114, 114f
Pleural fremitus, 60
Pleural infection, 494
Pleural layers, 8f
'Pleural membrane', 7–8
Pleural rub, 62t
Pleural surgery, 534
Pleurectomy, 535t–536t
Pleurodesis, 535t–536t
PMH. see Previous medical history (PMH)
Pneumonectomy, 535t–536t
Pneumonia, 493–494
    aspiration, radiographic appearance, 104
    radiographic appearance, 104–105
    ventilator-associated, 429, 431
        in burn patients, 650
        specific criteria for diagnosis of, 431–432
        treatment of, 431–432
'Pneumotaxic centre', 368
Pneumothorax, 52t–54t, 539–543
    primary spontaneous, 539–541
    radiographic appearance, 99, 100f
        in paediatrics, 114, 115f–116f
    risk from mechanical insufflation/exsufflation, 286
    secondary, 541
    tension, 541, 542f
        radiographic appearance, 100f, 114
    traumatic, 541
Poiseuille's law, 16
    clinical relevance of, 16–17
Polycythaemia, secondary, 332

Pontine control centres, 20
Positioning
    for critically ill patient, ICU, 429–430
    gravity-assisted, 6–7, 255–256, 258t
        ICU patients, 429
    for improving gas exchange, 317–325,
        318f
    mechanical ventilation and
        case study, 440b
        in children, 470, 489
    oxygen transport effects, 321–322, 321t
    recumbency, 322–323
    for spinal cord injury, 673, 673f
    work of breathing and, 322
    see also Mobilization; individual
        positions
Positive end-expiratory pressure (PEEP)
    hypoxia, children, 460b
    intrinsic, 437, 438t–439t
Positive expiratory pressure therapy,
        274–279, 275f–276f, 277b
    bubble/bottle, 279–284, 285f
    clinical application and evidence for,
        277–278
    clinical precautions for, 277b
    high-pressure, 278–279, 278b, 279f
        clinical application and evidence for,
            279
    infant, 274–279, 276f
    inspiratory resistance, 279
    key points when using, 276b
    oscillating, 279–284
Positive pressure treatment, for spinal
        cord injury, 678
Positron emission tomography, 89–90, 90f
    in paediatrics, 111
Post extubation respiratory failure,
        non-invasive ventilation for, 301
Post intensive care syndrome (PICS),
        733–734, 733f
Post-exacerbation, 591
Postoperative pain
    acute, management of, 516
    pharmacological management of,
        516–520, 517t–519t, 520f–521f
Postoperative pulmonary complications,
        524–526, 525b
    risk factors for, 525–526
Post-sternotomy pain, in cardiac surgery,
        547f, 549–550
Postural correction, for musculoskeletal
        dysfunction, 361
Postural drainage
    in airway clearance techniques,
        255–258, 255f–257f, 258t
    breathing techniques and, 250

modified, in infant, 481f
    see also Gravity-assisted positioning
        (GAP)
Postural hypotension, 66
Posture, physical assessment, 359
P_{pul}. see Intrapulmonary pressure (P_{pul})
Pre-emptive analgesia, 515
Preferential nasal breathing, child vs.
        adult, 35
Prehabilitation, preoperative
        physiotherapy and, 514–515
Pressure control ventilation, 416
    versus volume control ventilation,
        464–465, 465t
Pressure control-inverse ratio ventilation
        (PC-IRV), 416
Pressure gradient, creation of, 543
Pressure-regulated volume control (PRVC)
        ventilation, 465–466
Pressure-supported ventilation, 416
Preterm birth, 482
Pre-transplant education, 693
Previous medical history (PMH), 48
Primary spontaneous pneumothorax,
        539–541
Prone positioning
    for acute hypoxaemic respiratory
        failure, 469
    for ICU patients, 429
Proprioceptors, 21
'Protective ventilation', 416, 431
Proxy respondents, 239
Pruritus, in liver disease, 662
PRVC ventilation. see Pressure-regulated
        volume control (PRVC) ventilation
Pseudoaneurysms, 152
Pseudoglandular period, lung, 34
Pseudomonas aeruginosa, 336
    eradication therapy for, 174–175
Pulmonary arterial hypertension (PAH),
        179–182, 180b
    aetiology of, 179–180
    clinical features of, 180
    diagnosis and investigations of, 180–181
    field walking tests for, 224t
    medical management of, 181
    pathophysiology of, 180
    physiotherapy management of, 181–182
Pulmonary arteriography, 90
Pulmonary artery band, 498
Pulmonary atresia, 501
Pulmonary capillary recruitment, 30
Pulmonary embolism, 156–157, 671–672
    radiographic appearance, 88f, 105–106
    symptoms and signs of, 157
Pulmonary embolus, 52t–54t

Pulmonary gas exchange, 2–3
Pulmonary graft rejection, 689t
Pulmonary haemorrhage, NICU, 485
Pulmonary hypertensive crisis, 504–505
Pulmonary interstitial emphysema (PIE),
        radiographic appearance, 117, 118f
Pulmonary lesion, radiographic
        appearance, 102–103, 102f
Pulmonary mass, radiographic
        appearance, 87f, 101
Pulmonary nodule, radiographic
        appearance, 101, 102f
Pulmonary oedema, 671–672
    cardiogenic, non-invasive ventilation
        for, 300–301
    continuous positive airway pressure, 300
    interstitial, radiographic appearance,
        105, 105f
Pulmonary rehabilitation, 586–597
    aims of, in chronic obstructive
        pulmonary disease, 586–587
    for airway clearance, 291–292
    definition of, 586
    education and self-efficacy in, 589–591
        balance training, 590
        neuromuscular electrical stimulation,
            590
        whole body vibration (WBV),
            590–591, 591b
    exercise prescription in, 587
    long-term effects of, 596–597
    non-COPD population, 592–593
        asthma, 593
        bronchiectasis, rehabilitation for,
            592–593
        interstitial lung disease, rehabilitation
            for, 592
    practical aspects of, 593–596
        breathing techniques for, 596
        equipment in, 593, 594f
        location of, 593, 594f
        non-invasive ventilation, 595–596
        nutrition, 596
        safety issues, 596
        supplemental oxygen, 593–595
    timing of, 591–592
        disease stability, 591
        peri-exacerbation, 591–592
        post-exacerbation, 591
    training programme in, 587–589
        duration of, 587
        frequency of, 587
        intensity of, 587–588
        respiratory muscle training, 589
        training modality, 588–589
        water-based training, 589

Pulmonary sepsis, in burn patients, 650
Pulmonary stenosis, 502–503
Pulmonary surfactant, 18–19
Pulmonary vessel dilatation, mechanism of, 663
Pulse rate, assessment, 65
Pulse rhythm and quality, assessment, 65
Pulsus paradoxus, 65
'Pump handle movement', 9
Pupillary response, assessment, 68
Pupils equal and reactive to light (PERL), 420
Pursed-lip breathing, 57

Q
The Quake, 279, 283, 285f
Quality of life, 226–227
    after trauma, 708–709
    assessment of, 69, 228t–232t
    definition of, by World Health Organization, 226
    health-related, 227–239
        psychometric properties of instruments, 227, 238t
QWB, 228t–232t

R
Radiation dose, in children, 108
Radiograph, chest. see Chest radiograph
Radionuclide imaging, 88–89
Radionuclide studies, in paediatrics, 111
Radiotherapy, 724–725
Range of motion, assessment of, 359–360, 360f
Rapid eye movement sleep, child vs. adults, 39
RASS. see Richmond Agitation Sedation Scale (RASS)
RBC. see Red blood cell (RBC)
RC-Cornet
    evidence for, 282
    key points when using, 282b
    for oscillating PEP, 279, 281–282, 281f
RCCs. see Respiratory control centres (RCCs)
Recession, 75–76
Recruitment manoeuvres, paediatrics, 469–470
Red blood cell (RBC), transit time of, 28
Refractory hypoxaemia, 466
Rehabilitation
    cardiac. see Cardiac rehabilitation
    pulmonary. see Pulmonary rehabilitation

Rejection, 687–690
    acute, 688–689, 689f, 689t
    chronic graft dysfunction, 689–690
    hyperacute, 688
Relaxed sitting, 351f, 352
Relaxed standing, 352, 353f
Reluctance to feed, in infant, 76
Renal system, 45
Renin, 45
Rescue techniques, for dysfunctional breathing, 188
Resection
    abdomino-perineal, 528t–531t
    anterior, 528f
    for bronchiectasis, 172
    lung, 558t–559t
    segmental, 535t–536t
    sleeve, 535t–536t
    thoracoabdominal, 558t–559t
    wedge, 535t–536t
Reservoir cannulae, 328
Reservoir masks, 329
Resistance training
    for burn patients, 656b
    for cancer patients, 731
    cardiac rehabilitation, 608t, 613
    heart transplant recipients, 697–698
Respiration, 2–3
    growth and ageing effect of, 34–35
    muscles of, 11–13, 12f
    neurophysiological facilitation of, 366–377
        abdominal muscles, 371–372
        accessory muscles of inspiration, 371
        anterior-stretch basal lift, 374f, 375
        clinical application of, 377
        co-contraction of abdomen, 374f, 376–377
        diaphragm, 368–369
        intercostal muscles, 370
        intercostal stretch, 372, 374f
        maintained manual pressure, 375
        neural control, 367–368, 367f
        perioral pressure, 374f, 375–376
        respiratory muscles, 368–372
        stimuli, 372–377, 373t
    spinal cord injury and, 668–674
        cardiovascular and autonomic impact on, 670–671
    spinal innervation, 668, 668f
Respiratory assessment
    in burn/smoke inhalation patients, 653
    in spinal cord injury, 674
Respiratory compliance, 18–19
    child vs. adults, 38
    reduced, 18

Respiratory conditions, in NICU
    manual techniques in, 488–489
    pharmaceutical intervention for, 486–487
    physiotherapy in, 491, 492f
    treatment available for, 486–490
Respiratory control centres (RCCs), 19
    clinical failure of, 20
    sensors and, 21f
Respiratory control feedback mechanism, 20, 21f
Respiratory diseases, 163–194
Respiratory distress, in infant and child, clinical signs of, 76b
Respiratory distress syndrome, 484
    radiographic appearance, 115f, 116–118, 118f–120f
Respiratory failure
    acute
        epidemiology of, in children, 456–458
        non-invasive ventilation for, 299
        pattern and time course of, 457–458, 457t
    chronic, non-invasive ventilation for, 297, 298b, 298f
    nocturnal hypercapnic, 298b
    post extubation, non-invasive ventilation for, 301
Respiratory gating model, 344f
Respiratory management, in cardiac surgery, 549
Respiratory mechanics, 13–14
Respiratory muscle function, effects of surgical process on, 523–524, 524b
Respiratory muscle strength
    assessment of, 64
    measurement of, 204–205
    and weaning, in ICU patients, 440–441
Respiratory muscle training, 589
    for spinal cord injury, 679
Respiratory muscles, 368–372
Respiratory rate, assessment, 62
Respiratory system
    adult vs. child
        anatomical differences, 35–40
        physiological differences, 35–40
    anatomy and physiology of, 1–46
        bronchial tree, 4–5, 4f
        lungs and pleurae, 5–8
        muscles of respiration, 11–13, 12f
        surface markings of lungs, 8–9
        thoracic cage, 9–11, 10f
        upper respiratory tract, 3–4, 3f
    collateral ventilation, 15–16, 16f
    control of breathing, 19–23

gas exchange, 26–34
  Fick's law and, 27, 27f
lung volumes and ventilation, 23–26, 24f
monitoring of, in ICU patients, 419
mucociliary transport system, 15
oxygen and carbon dioxide transport, 31
primary function of, 2
respiratory mechanics, 13–14
Respiratory system sensors, 21
Respiratory tract infection, radiographic appearance, 118–119
Respiratory walking frame, 354, 355f
Respiratory weakness, critically ill patient, ICU, 425
Respiratory zone, 5, 5f
Restrictive cardiomyopathies, 138
Resuscitation, of vital functions, for trauma, 702
Retrosternal line, 94
Rhonchal fremitus, 60
Rib(s)
  false, 9
  floating, 9
  head of, 9
  movements of, 9–11, 11f
  neck of, 9
  shaft of, 9
  true, 9
Rib angle, 9
Rib cage, child vs. adult, 35
Rib fracture, 52t–54t
Rib springing, 263–265
Richmond Agitation Sedation Scale (RASS), 202–204, 420
Right hemicolectomy, 528f
Right lower lobe collapse, radiographic appearance, 97, 98f
Right lung, 8
Right middle lobe collapse, radiographic appearance, 97, 98f
Right upper lobe collapse, radiographic appearance, 97, 97f
Right-sided cardiac valve disease, 133–134
  medical management of, 137
  symptoms and signs of, 134
Riker scale, 420
Rollator, 593

S

SABA. see Short acting β-agonist (SABA)
Saline instillation, 429, 481
  see also Hypertonic saline

SAQ. see Seattle Angina Questionnaire (SAQ)
SBOT. see Short burst oxygen therapy (SBOT)
Scalenes, 13
Scapulae
  radiographic appearance, 94
  secondary malalignment of, 356
SCI. see Spinal cord injury (SCI)
Scoliosis, 56
Seattle Angina Questionnaire (SAQ), 227–239
Secondary polycythaemia, 332
Secretion clearance
  for assisted cough, 675
  critically ill patient, ICU, 424–425
  see also Airway clearance techniques (ACTs)
Secretion removal techniques, for ICU patients, 426
'Sedation breaks', 416
Segmental bronchi, radiographic appearance, 92
Segmental resection, 535t–536t
Self-efficacy, education and, in pulmonary rehabilitation, 589–591
Self-management
  concerns about medication, 406
  improvement, 406
  necessity of medication, 406
Self-report, 411
Sepsis
  in ICU patients, 432
  in NICU patients, 489
  trauma and, 701–702
'Sepsis care bundle', 432
Septic shock, 432
  case study, 433b
Septostomy, 498
Severe acquired brain injury, respiratory consequences in, 660
Severe neuromuscular disease, in ICU patients, 435
SF-36. see Short-Form 36 (SF-36)
SGRQ. see St. George's Respiratory Questionnaire (SGRQ)
Shaker classic/shaker deluxe, 283
Shaking. see Chest wall vibrations
'Shock lung.' see Acute respiratory distress syndrome (ARDS)
Short acting β-agonist (SABA), 714
Short burst oxygen therapy (SBOT), 333
Short-Form 6D, 228t–232t
Short-Form 36 (SF-36), 227, 228t–232t
Short-term oxygen therapy (STOT), 332–333

Sickness Impact Profile (SIP), 227–239
Sigmoid colostomy, 528t–531t
Simple oxygen mask, 328–329
Single lung transplantation, 686
Single-barelled colostomy, 529f
Single-handed percussion, 259–260, 260f
SIP. see Sickness Impact Profile (SIP)
SIRS. see Systemic inflammatory response syndrome (SIRS)
SIS. see Sternal Instability Scale (SIS)
SjvO$_2$. see Jugular venous saturation of oxygen (SjvO$_2$)
Skin colour and condition, assessment, 69
Skin turgor, assessment, 64
Sleep apnoea syndrome, spinal cord injury and, 673–674
Sleep-disordered breathing, spinal cord injury and, 673–674
Sleeve resection, 535t–536t
Slide tracheoplasty, 504
SMA. see Spinal muscular atrophy (SMA)
Small airway disease, radiographic appearance, 121–123, 123f
Smoke inhalation injury, 650–652
  cardiorespiratory physiotherapy treatment of, 654–655
  indicators of, 653t
  management of, 652
  thermal injury, 650–651
Smoking cessation, for COPD, 168
'Sniff' manoeuvre, 267–268
'Snout phenomenon', 376
Social history, 48
Social relationships, 407
Sodium cromglycate, for asthma, 182–184
Special care nurseries, 482–484
Speech, dysfunctional breathing and, 188
Spinal anaesthesia, 521f
Spinal cord injury (SCI), 667–682
  cough and, 673
  effects of, 668–669, 668f–669f
  long-term ventilation for, 680, 681f
  lung volumes and, 672–673
  neurological level and completeness, 669, 670f–671f, 672t
  orthopaedic management in, 669–670
  physiotherapy treatment of, 674–680
  positioning for, 673, 673f
  respiration and, 668–674
    cardiovascular and autonomic impact on, 670–671, 672t
  respiratory assessment in, 674
  respiratory management, long-term, 680–682
  sleep apnoea syndrome, 673–674
  sleep-disordered breathing, 673–674

Spinal cord reflexes, 21
Spinal muscular atrophy (SMA), 316
Spirometry, 25
    incentive, 308–310, 309f
Split thickness skin grafts, 647t–648t
Spontaneous pneumothorax, 100f
Spontaneously healing wounds, 643–644,
    644f
Sputum, assessment, 50, 50t
SRT. see Steep Ramp Test (SRT)
St. George's Respiratory Questionnaire
    (SGRQ), 233t–236t
Stair climbing, breathing control, 354,
    354f
Statins, for ischaemic heart disease, 131t
Steep Ramp Test (SRT), 219
Stenosis
    aortic, 133, 502
        medical management of, 136
        symptoms and signs of, 134
    mitral, 133
        medical management of, 136–137
        symptoms and signs of, 134
    pulmonary, 502–503
    tracheal, 504
Step test, 223
Sternal fibres, 11
Sternal Instability Scale (SIS), 552, 552t
Sternocleidomastoid, 13
Sternotomy procedure, 546–547, 547f
Sternum, delayed closure of, 505
'Stiff lung syndrome.' see Acute respiratory
    distress syndrome (ARDS)
STOT. see Short-term oxygen therapy
    (STOT)
Strength (resistance) training, 588
Stress, 408
Stress incontinence, management of, 292
Stridor, 76
Stroke volume (SV), 44–45
Subcutaneous air, 59
Subcutaneous route, for postoperative
    analgesia administration, 517t
Subdural haematoma, 659, 659f
Substantial fluid resuscitation, 646–649
Suction, airway
    in children, 480
        adverse effects, 480
        complications, 480
    effects of, 265–266
    in ICU patient
        nasopharyngeal/oropharyngeal, 426
        open/closed, 426
    in mechanical ventilation, 470
    for non-intubated adult, 265–266
Superficial burns, 643t

Superficial partial thickness burns, 643t,
    644f
Superior vena cavography, 90
Supplemental oxygen, 593–595
    for respiratory conditions, 487
    see also Oxygen therapy
Support and monitoring apparatus, 85f,
    103–104
Supportive respiratory therapy, indications
    for, 458–461
Supraclavicular indrawing, 57
Supramaximal transient expiratory flow,
    rates of, 252
Supraventricular arrhythmias, 147t
Surfactant, 36–37, 470
    therapy , for respiratory conditions,
    486–487
Surfactant-deficient disease, radiographic
    appearance, 116–118
Surgery
    abdominal, 526–527, 528b–531b
        physiotherapy evidence in, 532
    bariatric, 527–532
    special considerations in, 553–554, 554b
    thoracic, 532–539, 535t–536t, 540t–541t
        physiotherapy in, 537b
        postoperative exercise training in,
        539, 540t–541t
        risk assessment for patients
        undergoing, 532–533
        surgical approach for, 533–534, 533f
        types of, 534–538
    types of, 526–553, 527t
Surgical ICU Optimal Mobilization Score,
    211
Surgical patients
    postoperative management of, 497
    preoperative management of, 497
Surgical process, 515–526
    acute postoperative pain, management
    of, 516
    anaesthesia, induction of, 515–516
    effects, on respiratory function,
    521–526
        functional residual capacity and
        closing capacity, 522–523, 523f
        lung volume, 522
        mucociliary clearance, 523, 524b
        postoperative pulmonary
        complications, 524–526, 525b
        respiratory muscle function, 523–524,
        524b
    general anaesthesia, 515–516
    pain, measurement of, 520–521, 522b
Surgical resection, for bronchiectasis, 172
Surgical terminology, 527t

'Surviving Sepsis Campaign', 432
SV. see Stroke volume (SV)
'Swallow breath', 376
Swallowing, 376
Swyer-James syndrome, 123
Systemic inflammatory response
    syndrome (SIRS)
    in burn patients, 649–650, 650f, 651b
    case study, 433b
    in ICU patients, 432
    trauma and, 701–702
Systemic intoxication, smoke inhalation
    injury and, 651–652
Systole, 41

T
Tachypnoea, 57, 58f, 58t–59t, 76
Taping, for musculoskeletal dysfunction,
    362–364
TEEs. see Thoracic expansion exercises
    (TEEs)
TENS. see Transcutaneous electrical
    stimulation (TENS)
Tension pneumothorax, 541, 542f
    radiographic appearance, 100f, 114
Terminal sac period, lung, 34–35
Tetralogy of Fallot, 500–501, 501f
Tetraplegia. see Spinal cord injury (SCI)
'The Knack', 292
The Lung Flute, 279, 283–284, 285f
The Quake, 279, 283, 285f
Thermal injury, 650–651
Thoracic cage, 9–11, 10f
    radiographic appearance, 92
Thoracic expansion exercises (TEEs),
    266–268, 267f–268f
Thoracic imaging, 83–124
    adults, 84–108
    for assessment, 64
    critically ill patient, 103–106
    paediatrics, 108–123
        issues particular to, 108–109
    see also individual techniques
Thoracic injury
    ICU patients, 703–705, 704f
    management of, precautions and
    contraindications to, 706b
Thoracic organ transplantation, 682–699
    assessment in, 684–685, 685b
    physiotherapy, 685
    candidates, selection of, 683
    contraindications to, 684
    denervation, 690–691
    exercise limitation and function,
    697–699

history of, 682–683, 683f–684f
ICU management, 695, 695f
immunosuppression and rejection, 687–690, 688t
indications for, 683, 684t
infections in, 690, 690b
long-term management in, 699
organ donation, 686–687
outpatient rehabilitation, 696–697, 696f–697f, 698b
paediatrics, considerations for, 699, 700t
postoperative management in, 694–696, 694b
ward management, 695–696
preoperative rehabilitation, 691–694
bridge to transplant, 693–694
exercise training, 691–692
pre-transplant education, 693
pre-transplant exercise guidelines, 693
rejection. see Rejection
surgical procedures, 685–686
lung transplantation, 686
orthotopic heart transplantation, 685–686
Thoracic surgery, 532–539, 535t–536t, 540t–541t, 558t–559t
physiotherapy in, 537b, 538–539
evidence in, 538–539
postoperative exercise training in, 539, 540t–541t
risk assessment for patients undergoing, 532–533
surgical approach for, 533–534, 533f
types of, 534–538
chest trauma, 536–537, 538b
oesophageal surgery, 534–536, 537b
pleural surgery, 534
Thoracoabdominal aortic aneurysm repair, 555t–557t
Thoracoabdominal resection, 558t–559t
Three-wheeled walker, 355f
Throat, 4
Tidal volume, 465
Tietze syndrome, 52t–54t
Timed Up and Go test, 217
Time-line, illness representation, 404
TOE. see Transoesophageal echocardiography (TOE)
Total peripheral resistance (TPR), 45
TPR. see Total peripheral resistance (TPR)
Trachea, 4
position of, assessment, 59, 59f
radiographic appearance, 92
Tracheal stenosis, 504
Tracheitis, 52t–54t

Tracheo-oesophageal fistula, congenital, 483
Tracheostomy, 442–447
decannulation, 680
for long-term support, 103–104
for smoke inhalation injury, 652
speech option with, 680
for spinal cord injury, 679–680
Training oxygen, 333
Tramadol, 518t–519t
Transcutaneous electrical stimulation (TENS), 432
Transoesophageal echocardiography (TOE), 135
Transplant rejection. see Rejection
Transplantation surgery
in children, 503
see also Heart transplantation; Thoracic organ transplantation
Transpulmonary pressure (P_{pul}-P_{ip}), 14
Transtracheal catheter, 328
Trauma, 700–709
cause of, 700–701
chest, 536–537, 538b
complications related to, 701–702
circulatory deficits, 701
oxygenation deficits, 701
systemic inflammatory response syndrome, sepsis and muscle weakness, 701–702
immobility, complications develop due to, 706–708
responsive intubated patients, 705b–706b, 706t, 707
responsive patients with, and prolonged ICU stay, 707
spontaneously breathing patient with, 707–708, 708f–709f
unresponsive patient, 706–707
mechanism of, 700–701
medical and surgical management of, 702–705
definitive care, 702–705
primary survey and resuscitation of vital functions, 702
secondary survey, 702
physiotherapy intervention for, 705–708, 705b–706b, 706t
quality of life after, 708–709
Traumatic pneumothorax, 541
Tricuspid valve, 503
True ribs, 9
Truncus arteriosus, 502
Tubercle, 9
Tuberculosis, radiographic appearance, 118–119, 121f

Tumours, pulmonary, 52t–54t
Tussive fremitus, 60
'Two-way gas-liquid flow', 312

U
Ultrasonography, 85–86, 86f
in paediatrics, 109–110, 109f
Ultrasound. see Ultrasonography
Underwater seal, 543
Underwater seal drainage (UWSD) units, 543–545, 543b, 545b
implications for physiotherapists, 543–545
bubbling, 544
drainage, 544
persistent air leak, 544–545
suction, 544
swing, 544
types of, 543, 544f
Unobstructed gravity assisted drainage, 543
Upper limb training, 588–589
Upper respiratory tract, 3–4, 3f
Upright positioning, mobilization and, in oxygen transport, 321t
Urine colour and quality, assessment, 65
Urine incontinence, 292
Urine output, in ICU patients, 420
UWSD units. see Underwater seal drainage (UWSD) units

V
Vaccinations
for bronchiectasis, 172
for COPD, 169
VAEs. see Ventilator-associated events (VAEs)
Valve surgery, 547
aortic valve surgery, 547
cardiac valve prostheses, 547
mitral valve surgery, 547
Valvular heart disease, 546
VAP. see Ventilator-associated pneumonia (VAP)
Variable performance systems, of oxygen therapy, 327–329
Vascular ring, 499
Vasodilators, for ischaemic heart disease, 131t
Veins, 40
Vena caval opening, 11
Venous thromboembolism, 156–159
aetiology and pathophysiology of, 156–157
classification of, 157–158

Venous thromboembolism *(Continued)*
  diagnosis of, 157, 158*b*
  medical management of, 158
  physiotherapy-specific management of, 158–159
  risk factors for, 156*t*
  symptoms and signs of, 157
Ventilation, 14
  alveolar, 25–26
    alteration of, 26
    clinical relevance, 26
  child *vs.* adult, 38–39
  collateral, 15–16, 16*f*
  definition of, 2–3
  distribution of, in healthy lung, 28–29, 29*f*
  lung volumes and, 23–26
  strategy, for specific disease, 467–470
  terminology, 25
Ventilation-perfusion matching, 28
  maintaining, 30
  in self-ventilating adult, 29–30, 30*f*
Ventilation-perfusion mismatching, 88–89, 89*f*
  arterial hypoxaemia, 157
  decreased lung volumes and, 424
  diagnosis of, 30, 31*f*
  increased, 23
Ventilation-perfusion scanning, 88–89, 89*f*
Ventilator hyperinflation (VHI), 310–313, 426
Ventilator therapy, complications of, 462–464
Ventilator triggering, troubleshooting for, 437, 438*t*
Ventilator waveforms
  gas trapping, 437, 439*t*
  inadequate inspiratory flow rate, 437, 438*t*

inspiration-expiration cycling, 437, 438*t*
  intrinsic PEEP, 437, 439*t*
  ventilator triggering, 437, 438*t*
Ventilator-associated events (VAEs), 431
Ventilator-associated pneumonia (VAP), 429, 431
  in burn patients, 650
  specific criteria for diagnosis of, 431–432
  treatment of, 431–432
Ventilator-induced lung injury (VILI), 464
Ventilators
  familiarization, 436–437
  see also individual types
Ventilatory support techniques, 466–467, 466*f*
Ventricular arrhythmias, 147*t*
Ventricular assist devices, 719–720
Ventricular septal defect (VSD), 499–500, 500*f*
Venturi mask, 329–330
Vertebral pressure, 372–375, 374*f*
Vessels, radiographic appearance, 92
VHI. *see* Ventilator hyperinflation (VHI)
Video-assisted thoracoscopic surgery (VATS), 534
Vigorous intense exercise, 582
VILI. *see* Ventilator-induced lung injury (VILI)
Viral infection, radiographic appearance, 118, 120*f*
Visceral pleura, 7–8, 8*f*
Visual analogue scales, 345
Vocal resonance, 61, 61*f*
Volume control ventilation, 416
  pressure control ventilation *versus*, 464–465, 465*t*
VSD. *see* Ventricular septal defect (VSD)

W
Ward management, thoracic organ transplantation, 695–696
Warm-up, cardiac rehabilitation, 610–613, 611*b*, 612*t*
Water-based training, 589
WBV. *see* Whole body vibration (WBV)
Weaning, mechanical ventilation, 441–447, 441*b*–442*b*
  in children, 471, 471*b*
  concepts of, 435–447
  non-invasive ventilation for, 301
  physiotherapist's role in, 441–442
  for spinal cord injury, 679–680
  strategies, 441
Wedge resection, 535*t*–536*t*
'WeeFIM', 217–218
Welfare benefits, 408
Wells score, 157
'Wet' or 'dry' system, 543
Wheeze, assessment, 50–51, 62*t*
Whipple procedure, 530*f*
Whispered pectoriloquy, 61
WHO Quality of Life-BREF (WHOQOL-BREF), 227, 228*t*–232*t*
Whole body vibration (WBV), 590–591, 591*b*
WHOQOL-BREF. *see* WHO Quality of Life-BREF (WHOQOL-BREF)
Windpipe, 4
Work of breathing, 436
  increased, ICU patients, 425–426, 425*t*
  measures, 425*t*
  mechanical ventilation, 425
    airway resistance, 440, 440*b*
    lung/thoracoabdominal compliance, 440, 440*b*
  patient positioning and, 322
  physiotherapy management of, 435–447